Handbook of Home Health Care Administration

Second Edition

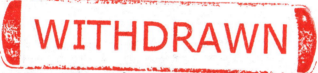

Marilyn D. Harris, RN, MSN, CNAA, FAAN

Executive Director
Abington Memorial Hospital Home Care
Willow Grove, Pennsylvania

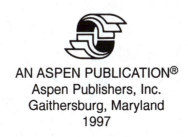

AN ASPEN PUBLICATION®
Aspen Publishers, Inc.
Gaithersburg, Maryland
1997

Library of Congress Cataloging-in-Publication Data

Handbook of home health care administration / edited by Marilyn D.
Harris.—2nd ed.
p. cm.
Includes bibliographical references and index.
ISBN 0-8342-0918-7
1. Home care services—Administration. 2. Home care services—
United States—Administration. I. Harris, Marilyn D.
[DNLM: 1. Home Care Services—organization & administration. WY
115 H236 1997]
RA645.3.H355 1997
3621'4'068—dc21
DNLM/DLC
for Library of Congress 97-6069
CIP

Orders: (800) 638-8437
Customer Service: (800) 234-1660

About Aspen Publishers • For more than 35 years, Aspen has been a leading professional
publisher in a variety of disciplines. Aspen's vast information resources are available in both
print and electronic formats. We are committed to providing the highest quality information
available in the most appropriate format for our customers. Visit Aspen's Internet site for
more information resources, directories, articles, and a searchable version of Aspen's full
catalog, including the most recent publications: **http://www.aspenpub.com**
Aspen Publishers, Inc. • The hallmark of quality in publishing
Member of the worldwide Wolters Kluwer group

The authors have made every effort to ensure the accuracy of the information herein. However,
appropriate information sources should be consulted, especially for new or unfamiliar procedures. It is
the responsibility of every practitioner to evaluate the appropriateness of a particular opinion in the
context of actual clinical situations and with due considerations to new developments. Authors, editors,
and the publisher cannot be held responsible for any typographical or other errors found in this book.

Editorial Resources: Ruth Bloom
Library of Congress Catalog Card Number: 97-6069
ISBN: 0-8342-0918-7

Printed in the United States of America

1   2   3   4   5

The book is dedicated to
my husband Charles, my colleagues, and hospital administration
for their support and encouragement;
also to the staff of Abington Memorial Hospital Home Care
who work with me as a team
to provide high-quality, compassionate home health and hospice care
to thousands of patients each year.

Table of Contents

Contributors xxiv

Foreword xxxi

Introduction xxxiii

Part I—Home Health Administration 1

Chapter 1—Home Health Administration: An Overview 3
    Janna Dieckmann
    Definition of Home Health Care 3
    Description of Home Health Care 4
    Initiation of Home Health Care Services 5
    Early Sources for Home Health Care 6
    Reasons for the Growth of Home Health Care 11
    Conclusion 13

Chapter 2—The Home Health Agency 15
    Judith A. Baigis and Kathleen E. Williams
    Historical Overview 15
    Recent History 15
    Financial Concerns 16
    Scope of Home Care 17
    Range of Home Health Agencies 17
    Conclusion 22

PART II—STANDARDS FOR HOME HEALTH AGENCIES 23

Chapter 3—Medicare Conditions of Participation 25
    Peggie Reid Webb
    Subpart B: Administration 25
    Subpart C: Furnishing of Services 43
    Conclusion 55

Chapter 4—The Joint Commission's Home Care Accreditation Program **57**
Maryanne L. Popovich and Richele C. Armstrong Schaffer
The Joint Commission's Home Care Accreditation Program 57
The Home Care Standards 58
The Survey Process 60
Unscheduled, Unannounced, and Random Unannounced Surveys 62
The Accreditation Decision Process 62
The Accreditation Decision Grid 63
Early Survey Policy 63
Deemed Status Option for Medicare Certification 65
Benefits of Accreditation 65
Conclusion 66

Chapter 5—CHAP Accreditation: Standards of Excellence for Home Care
        and Community Health Organizations **67**
Theresa Sekan Ayer
Purpose of Accreditation 68
Benefits of Accreditation 68
The CHAP Philosophy and Vision 69
The CHAP Mission and Purpose 69
The Objectives of CHAP... 70
The Governance of CHAP 70
Public Disclosure under CHAP..................................... 71
Expert Site Visitors 71
CHAP's Consumer Focus for Quality Improvement 71
Key Concepts in CHAP Accreditation: Standards of Excellence 71
Example of CHAP Standards: Outcome Measures 73
Benchmarking.. 73
The Advantages of CHAP Accreditation 73
Overview of the Accreditation Process 74
Types of Organizations Eligible for CHAP Accreditation 75
Conclusion... 75
Postscript 76

Chapter 6—Accreditation by the Foundation for Hospice and Home Care,
        National HomeCaring Council **77**
Ken Wessel
History 77
Structure.. 77
Standards 77
Process 78
Recent Developments 79
Conclusion... 79

Chapter 7—Certificate of Need and Licensure **81**
E. Michael Flanagan
HHA CON Requirements 81

HHA Licensure   85
Conclusion   87

Chapter 8—Professional Credentialing for Home Care/Hospice Personnel   90
Ann H. Cary
Current Guidelines for Nonadministrators   92
Credential Options Utilized by Home Care Administrators   94
Conclusion   96

**Chapter 9—The Relationship of the Home Health Agency to the State
    Trade Association 99**
Mary Kay Pera
Association Structure   99
What Associations Do   100
Getting the Most Out of Membership   101
Conclusion   102

Chapter 10—The National Association for Home Care   103
Val J. Halamandaris
How NAHC Works   103
Code of Ethics   104
NAHC's Mission   104
NAHC's Values   104
NAHC's Goals   105
Governance   107
Committees   108
Communications and Information Dissemination   109
Departments   109
Affiliate Organizations   111

PART III—CLINICAL ISSUES   113

Chapter 11—Self-Care Systems in Home Health Care Nursing   115
Joan Reynolds Yuan
Conclusion   118

Chapter 12—Home Health Care Documentation and Recordkeeping   119
Elissa DellaMonica
The Changing Health Care Environment   119
Regulations Governing Home Health Care Documentation   120
Clinical Record Policy   121
Reasons for Documentation   121
The Key to Successful Documentation   124
Documentation of Skilled Care   125
Current Trends in Documentation   127
Critical Pathways   128
Computerized Documentation   128

Medical Record Department 129
Conclusion 129
Appendix 12-A—COP Standards Pertaining to HHA Clinical Record Policy . . 131
Appendix 12-B—Abington Memorial Hospital Home Care Policy for Clinical
    Records 134

Chapter 13—Computerized Clinical Documentation. 144
    Donna R. Baldwin
Documentation Process 144
Defining Computerized Clinical Documentation 145
Impact of Health Care Trends on Documentation 145
Framework for Computerizing Documentation 147
Example of a Successful Computer Implementation 151
Conclusion 159

Chapter 14—Implementing a Competency System in Home Care 160
    Carol Clarke, Charlotte Banacki, and Margaret Golden
Organizational Assessment 160
Job Descriptions 161
Supervisor Competencies 162
Application Phase 163
Interview Phase 165
Orientation 169
Competency Assessment 170
Sign-Off. 175
On-Going Assessment of Competency 175
Quality Improvement Program 178
Occurrence Monitoring 178
Continuing Education 178
Methods 178
Policies And Procedures 179
Performance Evaluations. 179
Conclusion 181

Chapter 15—A Patient Classification Outcome Criteria System 182
    Elizabeth A. Daubert
The Patient Classification Outcome System 183
Patient Groups and Objectives 183
Patient Admission 186
Advantages 188
Validating Reliability 190
Conclusion. 191

Chapter 16—Classification: A Tool for Managed Care. 192
    Donna Ambler Peters
Classification Theory 192
Patient Classification Systems. 193

Nursing Diagnosis Taxonomy 193
Clinical Management 194
Administrative Management 197
Conclusion.. 201

**Chapter 17—Analysis and Management of Home Health Nursing Caseloads and
    Workloads 204**
Judith Lloyd Storfjell, Carol Easley Allen, Cheryl E. Easley
Background 204
Purpose of the Easley-Storfjell Caseload/Workload Analysis Instruments 204
Description of the CL/WLA Process 205
Instructions for Use of CL/WLA Instruments 206
Implications 210
Conclusion 214

**Chapter 18—The Home Health Care Classification of Nursing: Diagnoses and
    Interventions 215**
Virginia K. Saba
Home Health Care Components 215
Developmental Strategy 215
Nursing Diagnoses... 216
Nursing Interventions 216
Coding Framework 217
Analysis 217
Implications 219

Chapter 19—Nursing Diagnoses in Community Health Nursing 225
Carol Ann Parente
The Concept 225
The Process 228
The Effects 234

Chapter 20—Maternal–Child Health Program 242
Louise A. Harmer
Goals of Pediatric Home Care 244
Prenatal and Postpartal Home Care Program 247
Conclusion 248

Chapter 21—High-Technology Home Care Services 250
Vincent C. DiTrapano and James J. Williams
The Planning Process 251
Delivering High-Technology Services 253
Conclusion 270

Chapter 22—Discharge of a Ventilator-Dependent Child from the Hospital to Home .. 271
Andrea Gendelman and Zoe Ann Kinney
Funding for Home Care 272

Teaching Plan 272
Selection of a DME Vendor 273
Home Nursing Care 273
Home Assessment 274
Developmental Needs 274
Emergency Resources 274
The Home Nursing Care Plan 275
Conclusion 277

PART IV—QUALITY ASSESSMENT AND IMPROVEMENT **279**

Chapter 23—Performance Improvement **281**
Nancy L. Bohnet
Initiation and Implementation 282
Variation and Benchmarking. 288
Acceleration. 288
Process Measurement and Improvement. 288
Conclusion 289

Chapter 24—Quality Assessment/Performance Improvement: An Administrator's
      Viewpoint **290**
Marilyn D. Harris
Needs And Expectations For Survival And Growth 291
Evaluating Clinical and Financial Data To Improve Quality of Care 295
Analyzing Resources 297
Conclusion 301
Appendix 24–A: Policies and Forms for Evaluation of Clinical
    and Financial Data 304
Appendix 24–B: Field Agency Agreement 317

Chapter 25—Quality Planning for Quality Patient Care **319**
Marilyn D. Harris and Joan Reynolds Yuan

Chapter 26—Program Evaluation **324**
Nancy DiPasquale Ruane and Joseph W. Ruane
Definitions and Characteristics 324
Issues 325
Influences on Program Evaluation 326
Development of a Program Evaluation System. 329
Evaluation Models 332
Program Evaluation Tools. 333
Collection of Information 334
Program Evaluation Report 335
Systematic Approach to Program Evaluation 335
Operational Considerations in Program Evaluation 340
Appendix 26–A: Formats for Presenting Program Evaluation Tools 340

Chapter 27—Clinical and Financial Evaluations of Patient Care **345**
    Marilyn D. Harris
    Patient Classification System: Background and Significance 345
    ND Data Collection 346
    Development of Standardized Flow Sheets 347
    Staff Education 348
    QA/PI 348
    Data Analysis 349
    Conclusion 352
    Appendix 27–A: Data Collection Forms and Flow Sheets 353

Chapter 28—Critical Pathways **365**
    M. Kelly Cooke and Theresa M. Brodrick
    Pathway Development 365
    Variance Analysis 367
    Guidelines for Pathway Utilization 368
    Sample Pathway 369
    Benefits of Pathway Use 369
    Cost versus Quality 375
    Conclusion 375

Chapter 29—Outcome-Based Quality Improvement **377**
    Peter W. Shaughnessy and Kathryn S. Crisler
    Types of Outcomes 378
    Data Item Set 379
    Two-Stage Continuous Quality Improvement Screen 380
    Sample Outcome Report 382
    Current OBQI Demonstration Programs 383
    Conclusion 384

Chapter 30—Evaluating the Quality of Home Care Services Using
        Patient Outcome Data **387**
    Marilyn D. Harris and Michael Dugan
    Procedure 388
    Findings 389
    Implication for Home Health Care Nurses 392

Chapter 31—Implementing the Agency for Health Care Policy and Research Urinary
        Incontinence Guideline in a Home Health Agency **394**
    Diane K. Newman, Carol Ann Parente, and Joan Reynolds Yuan
    Managing UI in the Homebound 394
    Catheter Use in the Home 395
    Current Nursing Research on UI in the Homebound 395
    One Agency's UI Dilemma 396
    Identification of Catheter-Related Problems 396
    Conclusion.. 401
    Appendix 31–A: Tools for UI Assessment and Intervention 403

Chapter 32—Home Health Care Benchmarking **409**
Michael F. Kaufman
Background 410
The Benchmarking Process 411
Benchmarking Keys to Success 419
Conclusion 420

PART V—MANAGEMENT ISSUES IN HOME HEALTH ADMINISTRATION **421**

Chapter 33—Administrative Policy and Procedure Manual **423**
Marilyn D. Harris
Policy Development 423
Role of the Professional Advisory Committee in Policy Development
    and Review 424
Policy Review Procedure 425
Approval Process 425
Conclusion 425

Chapter 34—Discharge Planning **427**
Joann K. Erb
Historical Development... 427
Conceptual Framework for Discharge Planning 429
Goals and Objectives of Discharge Planning 429
Components of the Discharge Plan 430
Multidisciplinary Collaboration 431
Resources 432
Regulations 433
Integration of Discharge Planning Activities 434
Research Results 434
Steps in the Discharge Planning Process 435
Planning... 436
High-Technology Therapy 436
Implementation Evalution 437
Discharge Planning Models.. 438
Quality Assurance in Discharge Planning........................... 443
Ethical Issues in Discharge Planning............................... 443
Interface with the Home Health Agency 444
Conclusion 444

Chapter 35—Referral Sources in Home Health Care.......................... **447**
Domenica M. Chromiak
Referral Sources 447
Referral Information 448
Criteria for Service 449
Rejection of Referrals 449
Intake Person 450
Liaison 451

Seasonal Trends 452
Marketing 452
Legal Issues 453
Antitrust Issues 454
Conclusion 454

Chapter 36—Administrative Priorities: Decisions and Strategies That Attract
    and Retain Quality Staff **455**
    Elissa DellaMonica, Marilyn D. Harris, and Joan Reynolds Yuan
    Part I 455
        External Forces That Have an Impact on Home Care Staff 455
        Job and Personnel Characteristics in Home Care 456
        Hiring in an Era of Personnel Shortage 457
        Interviewing Prospective Team Members 457
        Retention and Quality Care 458
    Part II 459
        Structural Components Necessary To Attract and Retain Quality Staff 459
        Retention Issues within Administrative Control 460
        Characteristics of Participation and Collaboration 460
        Conclusion 461

Chapter 37—Flextime Scheduling **462**
    Diane T. Cass and Sharon D. Martin
    Background 462
    Task Force on Flextime 463
    The Pilot Project 464
    Results of the Pilot Project 466
    Limitations of the Study 466
    Experience Over Time 467
    Conclusion 468

Chapter 38—Evaluating Productivity **469**
    Lazelle E. Benefield
    What Is Productivity? 469
    What We Know about Productivity 471
    Analyze Service Delivery: Efficiency, Effectiveness, and Equity 472
    Evaluate Current Productivity 473
    The Next Step 478
    Conclusion 479

Chapter 39—Labor–Management Relations **481**
    Jessie F. Rohner
    Conceptual Framework 481
    Factors Influencing the Labor Relations Climate 481
    Communication and Interpersonal Skills 483
    Problem Solving 485
    General Recommendations 487

Collective Bargaining 489
Conclusion 490

Chapter 40—Human Resource Management **492**
Robert J. Tortorici
The Human Resource Defined 492
The Personnel Department and Its Role, Goal, and Structure 493
The Personnel Department Staff 496
Finding the Right Candidate for Employment 498
Selection and the Hidden Agenda 500
Making a Meaningful Employment Offer 503
Benefits 504
Employee Relations for Retention 504

Chapter 41—Staff Development in a Home Health Agency **507**
Joan Reynolds Yuan
Role And Responsibilities of the Educator 508
Orientation 508
Inservice Education 509
Continuing Education 515
Academic Education 515

Chapter 42—Transitioning Hospital Nurses to Home Care **517**
Carolyn J. Humphrey and Paula Milone-Nuzzo
Definition of Home Care Nursing 517
Differences between Hospital and Home Care Nursing 518
Key Content Areas Found in Orientation 521
Teaching Strategies 525
Conclusion 525

Chapter 43—Case Management **526**
Linda A. Billows
Case Management Defined 526
Components of Case Management 527
Quality Assurance 528
Research on Case Management 528
Training of Home Health Agency Staff 529
Conclusion 529

Chapter 44—Managed Care **531**
Nina M. Smith
History of Managed Care 532
Growth and Development of Managed Care 532
Structure of Managed Care 533
Stages of Managed Care Development 535
Payment Mechanisms and Pricing Strategies in Managed Care 535
Implications of Managed Care in Home Care 536
Networks 536

Contracting with Managed Care Companies   537
Dilemmas in Managed Care   538
The Future of Managed Care   541

Chapter 45—Working with Managed Care Networks: Strategies for Success   543
Marilyn D. Harris and Sharon A. Lynch
Managed Care versus Case Management   545
Advantages and Disadvantages of Contracting with Managed Care Companies .   545
Role of the Home Care Clinical Care Manager versus Payer Case Manager . . .   545
Strategies for Cultivating a Successful Relationship   546
Quality Assessment/Performance Improvement Issues   547
Conclusion   552
Postscript   552

Chapter 46—Community-Based Long-Term Care: Preparing for a New Role   555
Emily Amerman and David M. Eisenberg
Long-Term Care Defined   555
Current Policy and Program Trends   556
The Area Agency on Aging: A Partner in Service Delivery   557
The Philadelphia Model   558
Becoming a Long-Term Care Provider: Observations and Recommendations . .   560

PART VI—FINANCIAL ISSUES   563

Chapter 47—Understanding the Exposures of Home Health Care:
   An Insurance Primer   565
Brian M. Block
Types of Insurance   565
Risk Management   570
Purchasing Insurance   570
Conclusion   571

Chapter 48—Budgeting for Home Health Services   572
Gregory J. Brown
Program Planning and Evaluation   572
Statistical and Operational Budget Development   573
Analytical Budget Controls   583

Chapter 49—Reimbursement   585
Charlotte L. Kohler
Current Medicare Reimbursement Trends   586
Basic Tenets of Medicare Reimbursement   588
General Discussion of Increasing Reimbursement   602
Some Thoughts about the Future.   605

Chapter 50—How To Read, Interpret, and Understand Financial Statements   607
D. Scott Detar
Cash Basis or Accrual Basis   607

Schedule of Statistics 608
Income Statement 608
Balance Sheet 610
Functional Expenses 612
Cash Flows 614
Conclusion 615

Chapter 51—Management Information Systems **616**
Charlotte L. Kohler
The Expansiveness of a Management Information System 616
Why Computerize with a System That Allows Data Analysis? 617
Current Computer Technology 617
Approach to Selecting Automation and MIS 618
Types of Systems and Features 620
Why Should an HHA Computerize? 622
When Should an HHA Computerize? The Answer Is: "Yesterday." 623
Developing Your Own Software 624
Are There Any Guarantees? 625
Acceptance Testing for Software 625
Final Thoughts about Customized and Purchased Software 626
Appendix 51–A—Glossary 628

**Chapter 52—An Overview of One Home Health Agency Management
      Information System** **634**
Charles G. Farber
Generalized System Architectures 634
Data Collection 635
Master File Maintenance 636
Patient Master Update Forms 636
Daily Report Form 638
Year-to-Date Visits 640
Accounts Receivable File 640
Ad Hoc Reporting 640
Financial Management Reports...................................... 643
Activity Reports.. 643
Statistical Reports 643
Quality Assurance Reports 644
Clinical-Link Field Automation 644
Other Modules 649
Conclusion 650

PART VII—Legal/Ethical/Political Issues **651**

Chapter 53—Legal Issues of Concern to Home Care Providers **653**
Ann P. Sherwin
Introduction 653
Antitrust 653

Corporate Liability of Providers 654
Torts and Civil Liability 655
Fraud and Abuse 656
Decision Making, Privacy, and Informed Consent 658
Advance Directives 659
Labor and Employment Issues 661
Americans with Disabilities Act 662
Tax Matters 667
Environmental Issues 667
What To Consider in Selecting an Attorney 669

Chapter 54—Ethical Issues 671
Charmaine M. Fitzig
Ancient Beginnings 673
Selected Ethical Theories 673
Characteristics of Ethical Issues 674
Ethical Issues in the Administrative and Clinical Areas of
    Home Health Care 675
Strategies 680
Conclusion 681

Chapter 55—Understanding the Political Process 683
Kathleen Carlson Mebus and Elizabeth Z. Cathcart
Building Relationships 683
Local Government 684
Legislative Process 685
Regulatory Process 686
Political Action 687
Conclusion 688

PART VIII—STRATEGIC PLANNING/MARKETING/SURVIVAL ISSUES 691

Chapter 56—Strategic Planning 693
Edward R. Balotsky and David B. Smith
Introduction 693
How Organizations Change 694
How Strategic Planning Shapes Change in Organizations 701
Steps in Developing Strategic Planning Capacity 702
Pitfalls To Avoid in the Strategic Planning Process 704
Conclusion 705

Chapter 57—Marketing: An Overview 708
Karen L. Carney
What Marketing Is and Isn't 708
The Role of Marketing in Home Care 709
The Market Analysis 711
Market Trends and Forces 714

Market Preparation and Planning 715
The Marketing Mix 717
Implementation 720
Measurement and Adaptation 720
Conclusion 721

Chapter 58—Corporate Reorganization **723**
Bernard R. Lorenz
Single Corporate Organizations 726
Multicorporate Organizations 726
Conclusion 727

Chapter 59—An Experience in Diversification **728**
Mary Ann Keirans
Introduction 728
Why We Decided To Diversify 728
Choosing a Model 730
Funding Considerations 731
The Legal Aspects 732
Conclusion 733

**Chapter 60—The Process of Visiting Nurse Association Affiliation
    with a Major Teaching Hospital** **736**
Marilyn D. Harris
The Negotiation Process 736
The Decision-Making Process 737
The Transition Process 738
"Feelings": The Impact on Board and Staff 744
Adjustments for Staff 745
Change in Professional Relationship with Peers 745
Conclusion 746

Chapter 61—Integrated Delivery Systems. **748**
Warren Lyons
Introduction 748
Integrated Delivery Systems—Definition and Assessment 749
Description of "At-Risk" IDS Contracts 749
Disease State Management Issues 750
Integrated Delivery Systems Strategies 750
Implications for Home Health Care Agencies............................. 751
Recommendations for Home Health Agency Survival and Success 751

PART IX—OTHER TYPES OF RELATIONSHIPS **753**

Chapter 62—Resource Development for Home Health Care Providers **755**
Barbara Klaczynska
Introduction 755

Preliminary Preparation for Successful Fund-Raising 755
Improving the Probability of Receiving Funds 756
Fundraising Sources 756
Researching Foundations and Corporations As Potential Funding Sources 756
Researching Government Sources 757
Types of Fund-Raising Projects 757
Elements of a Successful Proposal 758
Submitting Proposals/Follow-Up 760
Stewardship of Funds 760
Conclusion 761

Chapter 63—Home Care Volunteer Program 762
Carol-Rae Green Sodano
The Notion of Volunteerism 762
Health Care Volunteerism 763
Home Care Volunteerism 764
The Philosophical Basis for a Successful Volunteer Program 765
Program Design 768
Program Structure 770
Conclusion 779

Chapter 64—The Peer Review Organization 781
Marilyn D. Harris and Maryanne McDonald
Overview of Process 781
Agency-Specific Findings 782
National Findings 783
Conclusion 783
Postscript 784
Appendix 64–A—Keystone Peer Review Organization HCFA Generic Quality
     Screens for Home Health Agency Review 786

Chapter 65—The Manager As Published Author: Tips on Writing for Publication 795
Suzanne Smith Blancett
Blocks to Writing 795
Rejection 797
Manuscript Critique 797
Getting Started 798
Selecting the Appropriate Journal 799
Writing the Paper 801
Submission Checklist 802
Research 803
The Publishing Process 805
Ethics 805
The Benefits of Publishing 806
Conclusion 806

**Chapter 66—Student Placements in Home Health Care Agencies: Boost or Barrier
to Quality Patient Care?** **808**
Ida M. Androwich and Pamela A. Andresen
Boosts 808
Barriers 810
Graduate Students 811
Recommendations 812
Cost-Benefit Considerations 814

Chapter 67—A Student Program in One Home Health Agency **816**
Marilyn D. Harris

Chapter 68—The Role of the Physician in Home Care **823**
Kenneth W. Hepburn and Joseph M. Keenan
Physician Involvement 824
The Home Care Administrator's Role 825

Chapter 69—The Physician Connection **831**
Marilyn D. Harris
Legislative or Regulatory and Clinical Issues 831
Administrative Issues 832
Conclusion 833

**Chapter 70—The Role of the Medicare Fiscal Intermediary and the Regional
Home Health Intermediary.** **836**
Deborah A. Randall
Part I 836
Functions of the Fiscal Intermediary 837
Part II 843
Provider Audit 843
Resolution of Cost Report Disputes and Reimbursement Appeals 846
Conclusion 849

**Chapter 71—The Appeal Process: Reopening, Reconsiderations, Administrative
Law Judge Hearings and Appeal Council** **851**
Louisa M. Jordan
Introduction 851
Background 851
Climate for Action 852
Types of Denials 853
Impacts of Denials 853
Examples of Denials 854
Actions 855
Steps in the Appeal Process 856
Opinions of Expert Nurse Presenters at the ALJ Level 863
Why Should Denials Be Appealed? 864
Conclusion 864

Chapter 72—Nursing Research in Home Health Agencies **867**
    Marilyn D. Harris
    Types of Research Projects 867
    Project Essentials 868
    The Cost in Time 869
    Conclusion 870

Chapter 73—Hospice Care **872**
    Rosemary Johnson Hurzeler, Evelyn A. Barnum, Sandra J. Klimas,
    and Eugene G. Michael
    Introduction 872
    Hospice Defined 872
    Regulation Issues... 874
    Financing 875
    Trends in Hospice Care 878

PART X—THE FUTURE OF HOME CARE **883**

Chapter 74—Electronic Home Visits To Improve Care and Decrease Costs **885**
    Ilene Warner and Alexander S. Beller
    The History of Telemedicine 885
    The Design of Telehealth Systems 886
    Scope of Telehealth Activities... 886
    The Delivery of Nursing Care 887
    The Delivery of Ancillary Services 887
    Agency Configuration 888
    Utilization by Diagnosis 888
    Patient Selection Process... 888
    Quality of Care Issues 889
    Legal Implications 889
    Reimbursement and Cost Issues 890
    The Future of Telehealth for Home Care 891

Chapter 75—Using the Internet for Home Health and Hospice Care **892**
    Susan M. Sparks
    Just What Is the Internet? 893
    Some Issues 895
    Search Tools for Finding the Information You Want 896
    Other Interesting Sites 897

Chapter 76—Developing a Home Page for the World Wide Web..................... **898**
    Virginia K. Saba
    World Wide Web 898
    Browsers 898
    The Home Page 898
    Appendix 76–A—Glossary 902

Chapter 77—Planning, Implementing, and Managing a Community-Based Nursing Center: Current Challenges and Future Opportunities **903**
Katherine K. Kinsey and Patricia Gerrity
Introduction 903
Overview 904
Evolution of One Urban Academic Nursing Center Model 904
Assessment 907
Strategic Planning 908
Program Development and Information Systems 909
Human Resource and Fiscal Management 910
The Future of Advocacy and Nursing Centers 911

Chapter 78—Adult Day Services—The Next Frontier **913**
Joanne Handy, Judith A. Bellome, and Nancy Moldenhauer
History of Adult Day Services 913
The Adult Day Care Service Market 914
Financing Adult Day Care 916
Operational Issues in Adult Day Care 916
Consumer Demand 917
The Home Care-Day Service Connection 918
Adult Day Care in a New Health Care Market 918
Conclusion 920

Chapter 79—Basics for Beginning a Parish Nurse Program **921**
Janice M. Striepe and Jean M. King
Jan's Story: Congregational-Based Model 921
Jean's Story: Director of Religious Education Model 922
Sally's Story: Co–Parish Nurse Model 922
Evelyn's Story: Team Model.. 922
Community Models 923
Non–Parish Nurse Model 923
Mary's Story: Barriers... 923
Issues: Funding 924
Be a Parish Nurse Pioneer 926

Chapter 80—Surviving the Present Challenges and Thriving in the Future: A Personal Viewpoint **927**
Marilyn D. Harris
Today's Health Care Climate 927
Strategies for Survival 929
Conclusion... 931

Appendix A—Abbreviations **932**

Appendix B—"Managed Competition 101" Syllabus **935**
Mary M. Nearpass

Appendix C—Home Health Agency Reorganization Checklist **940**
   William J. Simione, Jr.

Appendix D—Glossary of Insurance Terms **942**
   William W. Fonner
Index **945**

Contributors

Carol Easley Allen, PhD, RN
Vice President
Planning and Development
Academic Paradigms Online
Silver Spring, Maryland

Emily Amerman, MSW, ACSW
Director
Community Care Management
Managed Care Division
Genesis Health Ventures
Kennett Square, Pennsylvania

Pamela A. Andresen, PhD
Associate Professor
Community Health Nursing
Director, Loyola University Nursing Center
Loyola University Chicago
Chicago, Illinois

Ida M. Androwich, PhD, RN, FAAN
Associate Professor
Community and Administrative Nursing
Niehoff School of Nursing
Loyola University Chicago
Chicago, Illinois

Theresa Sekan Ayer, MS, RN, CNAA
President and Chief Operating Officer
CHAP—Community Health Accreditation
    Program, Inc.
New York, New York

Judith A. Baigis, PhD, RN, FAAN
Professor and Associate Dean for Research and
    Scholarship
Georgetown University School of Nursing
Washington, DC

Donna R. Baldwin, MSN, RN
Assistant Executive Director
Home Health Agency
Trinity Health Care Services
Memphis, Tennessee

Edward R. Balotsky, AbD
Assistant Professor, Health Administration
College of Business Administration
Department of Management and Marketing
Winthrop University
Rock Hill, South Carolina

Charlotte Banacki, BA, RN
Director
Client Services
Gotham Per Diem, Inc., Home Care
New York, New York

Evelyn A. Barnum, JD
Corporate Counsel
The Connecticut Hospice, Inc.
Branford, Connecticut

Alexander S. Beller, BA
President and Chief Executive Officer
Tevital Inc.
Berwyn, Pennsylvania

Judith A. Bellome, MS, RN
Vice President of Northern Operations
GranCare Home Health Care
Atlanta, Georgia

Lazelle E. Benefield, PhD, RN
Associate Professor
Texas Christian University
Harris College of Nursing
Fort Worth, Texas

Linda A. Billows, MS, RN
President
Linda A. Billows, Inc.
Marblehead, Massachusetts

Suzanne Smith Blancett, EdD, RN, FAAN
Editor-in-Chief
Journal of Nursing Administration
Philadelphia, Pennsylvania

Brian M. Block, MA
Director of Risk Management
Henry S. Lehr, Inc.
Bethlehem, Pennsylvania

Nancy L. Bohnet, MN, RN, FAAN, FACHE
President and Chief Operating Officer
VNA Services and Foundation, Western
    Pennsylvania
Butler, Pennsylvania
Adjunct Faculty
University of Pittsburgh Graduate School of
    Nursing
Pittsburgh, Pennsylvania

Theresa M. Brodrick, MSN
Director of Medical/Surgical and Outpatient
    Nursing
University of Pennsylvania Health System
Presbyterian Medical Center
Philadelphia, Pennsylvania

Gregory J. Brown, BBA
Director of Finance
Abington Memorial Hospital Home Care
Willow Grove, Pennsylvania

Karen L. Carney
President
Carney Communications
Editor and Publisher
The Home Advantage Newsletter
Andover, Massachusetts

Ann H. Cary, PhD, MPH, RN, A-CCC
Professor and Doctoral Program Coordinator
George Mason University, CNHS
Fairfax, Virginia

Diane T. Cass, RN, MS
Supervisor
Androscoggin Home Health Services
Lewiston, Maine

**Elizabeth Z. Cathcart, MPH, BSN, RN,
    CNAA**
Executive Director
Family Health Services of South Central
    Pennsylvania
Dry Run, Pennsylvania

Domenica M. Chromiak, BS, RN, CNAA
Director
Jeanes Home Health
Department of Jeanes Hospital
Philadelphia, Pennsylvania

Carol Clarke, MA, RN
President/Owner
Clarke Health Care Consultants
Seminole, Florida

M. Kelly Cooke, MSN, RN
Regional Manager for Home Care Coordination
Home Health Care Department
Allegheny University Hospitals
Philadelphia, Pennsylvania

Kathryn S. Crisler, RN, MS
Senior Research Associate
Center for Health Services Research
University of Colorado Health Sciences Center
School of Nursing
Denver, Colorado

Kaye Daniels
President
Hospital Home Health Care Agency of
    California
Torrance, California

Elizabeth A. Daubert, RN, MPH
Special Assistant to the President
Visiting Nurse Services of Connecticut, Inc.
Bridgeport, Connecticut

Elissa DellaMonica, MSN, RN, CNA
Director of Professional Services
Abington Memorial Hospital Home Care
Willow Grove, Pennsylvania

D. Scott Detar, CPA
Partner
Maillie, Falconiero & Company, LLP
Oaks, Pennsylvania

Janna Dieckmann, MSN, RN
Assistant Professor
School of Nursing
La Salle University
Philadelphia, Pennsylvania

Vincent C. DiTrapano, RPh
Senior Vice President, Operations
Vitalink Pharmacy Services
Naperville, Illinois

Michael Dugan, MBA
Regional Practice Manager
Abington Memorial Hospital
Physician Practice Network
Abington, Pennsylvania

Cheryl E. Easley, PhD, RN
Dean and Professor
College of Nursing and Allied Health Sciences
Saginaw Valley State University
University Center, Michigan

David M. Eisenberg, PhD
Partner
Eisenberg & Carrilio
Chula Vista, California

Joann K. Erb, RN, MSN
Level Coordinator
Abington Memorial Hospital
School of Nursing
Willow Grove, Pennsylvania

Charles G. Farber
Director of Systems and Architectures
Delta Health Systems
Altoona, Pennsylvania

Charmaine M. Fitzig, RN, DrPH
Senior Management Consultant
Health and Hospitals Corporation
Clinical Affairs
New York, New York

E. Michael Flanagan, JD
Partner, Health Law Group
Gardner, Carton & Douglas
Washington, DC

William W. Fonner
President
Knowles, Fonner & Associates, Inc.
Abington, Pennsylvania

Andrea Gendelman, RN
Home Care Nurse
Blue Bell, Pennsylvania

Patricia Gerrity, RN, PhD, FAAN
Associate Dean for Community Programs
Allegheny University
School of Nursing
Philadelphia, Pennsylvania

Margaret Golden, MBA, RN
Executive Director
Gotham Per Diem, Inc.
New York, New York
Midpoint Healthcare Services, Inc.
East Orange, New Jersey

Val J. Halamandaris, JD
President
National Association for Home Care
Washington, DC

Joanne Handy, MS, RN
President
Goldman Institute on Aging
Administrative Director
UCSF/Mount Zion Center on Aging
San Francisco, California

Louise A. Harmer, MSN, RN, CRNP
Pediatric Nurse Practitioner
Maternal Child Health Home Care Department
Abington Memorial Hospital Home Care
Willow Grove, Pennsylvania

Marilyn D. Harris, RN, MSN, CNAA, FAAN
Executive Director
Abington Memorial Hospital Home Care
Willow Grove, Pennsylvania

Kenneth W. Hepburn, PhD
Assistant Professor
Department of Family Practice and Community
   Health
University of Minnesota Medical School
Minneapolis, Minnesota

Carolyn J. Humphrey, MS, RN
Home Care Consultant
Editor
Home Healthcare Nurse
Louisville, Kentucky

Rosemary Johnson Hurzeler, MPH, RN, HA
President and Chief Executive Officer
The Connecticut Hospice, Inc.
Branford, Connecticut

Louisa M. Jordan, MSN, RN, CNAA, CHCE
Executive Director
Red Lion Visiting Nurse Association
Red Lion, Pennsylvania

Michael F. Kaufman, MHA, MBA
Consultant
Cincinnati, Ohio

Joseph M. Keenan, MD
Professor
Residency Program Director
University of Minnesota Medical School
Department of Family Practice and Community
   Health
Minneapolis, Minnesota

Mary Ann Keirans, BSN, MA, MBA, CNAA
Administrator
Visiting Nurse Association/Management
   Services of Luzerne County
Wilkes-Barre, Pennsylvania

Jean M. King, MSN, RN
Faculty Facilitator
RN-BSN Satellite Center
The University of Iowa
College of Nursing
Iowa City, Iowa

Zoe Ann Kinney, RN
Pennsylvania Ventilator Assisted Children
   Home Program
Children's Hospital of Philadelphia
Philadelphia, Pennsylvania

Katherine K. Kinsey, PhD, RN, FAAN
Associate Professor of Nursing
Director
La Salle University Neighborhood Nursing
　Center
La Salle University
Philadelphia, Pennsylvania

Barbara Klaczynska, PhD
Development Consultant
Health Care, Education, and Human Service
　Programs
Melrose Park, Pennsylvania

Sandra J. Klimas, MPH, RN
Director of Home Care
The Connecticut Hospice, Inc.
Branford, Connecticut

Charlotte L. Kohler, RN, CPA, CVA, CPAM
Vice President, Finance
Helix Health, Inc.
Lutherville, Maryland

Bernard R. Lorenz, CPA
Bernard R. Lorenz & Associates
Baltimore, Maryland

Sharon A. Lynch, MSN, RN
Clinical Supervisor
Abington Memorial Hospital Home Care
Willow Grove, Pennsylvania

Warren Lyons, MBA, MPH, FACHE
Executive Director, Chief Executive Officer
Abington Health Services
Abington Memorial Hospital Home Care
Abington, Pennsylvania

Sharon D. Martin, MSN, RN, CS
Assistant Professor
Department of Nursing
St. Joseph's College
Standish, Maine

Maryanne McDonald, MSN
Instructor
Department of Nursing
College of Allied Health Sciences
Thomas Jefferson University
Philadelphia, Pennsylvania

Kathleen Carlson Mebus, MSN, RN, CAE
Director, State Legislation
Legislative Services
The Hospital Association of Pennsylvania
Harrisburg, Pennsylvania

Eugene G. Michael, MSW
Senior Planning Advisor
Director of Managed Care
The Connecticut Hospice, Inc.
Branford, Connecticut

Paula Milone-Nuzzo, PhD, RN
Associate Professor and Chair
Specialty Care and Management Division
Yale School of Nursing
New Haven, Connecticut

Nancy Moldenhauer, MSW, ACSW
Former Director
The National Council on the Aging
National Adult Day Services Association
Washington, DC

Mary M. Nearpass, MA, MS
Community and Program Development
　Coordinator
The Becoming Center
Ambler, Pennsylvania

**Diane K. Newman, MSN, RNC, CRNP,
　FAAN**
Adult Nurse Practitioner
Access to Continence Care and Treatment
Philadelphia, Pennsylvania

Carol Ann Parente, MSN, RN, CRNP
Adult Nurse Practitioner
Abington Memorial Hospital Home Care
Willow Grove, Pennsylvania

Mary Kay Pera, BSN, RN
Program Manager, Home Health and Hospice
Medical Assistance Division
State of New Mexico
Santa Fe, New Mexico

Donna Ambler Peters, PhD, RN, FAAN
Senior Product Consultant
Delta Health Systems
Forked River, New Jersey

Maryanne L. Popovich, MPH, RN
Director
Home Care Accreditation Services
Joint Commission on Accreditation of
   Healthcare Organizations
Oakbrook Terrace, Illinois

Deborah A. Randall, Esq.
Partner
Health Practice
Arent Fox Kintner Plotkin & Kahn
Washington, DC

Jessie F. Rohner, DrPH, RN
Executive Administrator
Pennsylvania Nurses Association
Harrisburg, Pennsylvania

Joseph W. Ruane, PhD
Associate Professor of Sociology
Department of Social Sciences
Philadelphia College of Pharmacy and Science
Philadelphia, Pennsylvania

Nancy DiPasquale Ruane, MA, RN
Community Health Specialist
Keystone Hospice
Fort Washington, Pennsylvania

Virginia K. Saba, EdD, RN, FAAN, FACMI
Clinical Associate Professor
Georgetown University
School of Nursing
Washington, DC

Richele C. Armstrong Schaffer, MA
Manager of Home Care Accreditation Services
Joint Commission on Accreditation of
   Healthcare Organizations
Oakbrook Terrace, Illinois

Peter W. Shaughnessy, PhD
Professor and Director of Center for Health
   Services Research
University of Colorado Health Sciences Center
Department of Medicine
Denver, Colorado

Ann P. Sherwin, MSN, JD
Principal
Ann P. Sherwin, P.C.
Wilmette, Illinois

William J. Simione, Jr., CPA
Vice Chairman and Executive Vice President
Simione Central
Atlanta, Georgia

David B. Smith, PhD
Professor
Department of Health Administration
Temple University
Philadelphia, Pennsylvania

Nina M. Smith, MEd, RNC
President
Integrated Behavioral Health Consultants
Consultant, National Behavioral Health
   Programs
Western Medical Services
Fort Collins, Colorado

Carol-Rae Green Sodano, PhD
Dean
West Campus
Montgomery County Community College
Pottstown, Pennsylvania

Susan M. Sparks, PhD, RN, FAAN
Senior Education Specialist
Extramural Programs
National Library of Medicine
Bethesda, Maryland

Judith Lloyd Storfjell, PhD, RN
President
Storfjell Associates
Berrien Springs, Michigan
Assistant Professor
Department of Public Health, Mental Health
   and Administrative Studies
University of Illinois at Chicago
College of Nursing
Chicago, Illinois

Janice M. Striepe, MS, RN
Parish Nurse Coordinator
Northwest Aging Association
Spencer, Iowa

Robert J. Tortorici, BA
President
The HR Forum
Formerly, Senior Vice President, Human
   Resources
Visiting Nurse Service of Rochester and
   Monroe County, Inc.
Rochester, New York

Ilene Warner, MA, RN, MLSP
Vice President, Clinical Applications
Tevital, Inc.
Berwyn, Pennsylvania

Peggie Reid Webb, MS, RN
President
Home Health Development Corporation, Inc.
Blue Bell, Pennsylvania

Ken Wessel, MSW, ACSW
Executive Director
Visiting Homemaker Service of Passaic County
Paterson, New Jersey

Kathleen E. Williams, MSN, RN
Program Nurse Specialist
Medical University of South Carolina Medical
   Center
Charleston, South Carolina

James J. Williams, RN, NHA
Pharmacy Manager
Vitalink Pharmacy Services, Inc.
Allentown, Pennsylvania

Joan Reynolds Yuan, MSN, RNC
Director of Education/Quality Assessment
   Improvement
Abington Memorial Hospital Home Care
Willow Grove, Pennsylvania

Foreword

Home health care and hospice have found themselves doing a paradigm leap rather than the paradigm shift that many industries have experienced during the first part of the 1990s. Administrators have become chief executive officers or presidents. Nursing directors have become vice presidents of patient/client services, and controllers are now vice presidents of finance. Computers have become essential in managing the day-to-day business operations of an agency as well as the clinical care of the patient/client. Benchmarking, outcome-based care, and critical pathways are part of patient care planning. Managed care has spread like wildfire throughout the industry, and a prospective payment system for Medicare reimbursement looms on the horizon. Downsizing, rightsizing, mergers, acquisitions, and partnering among previously unlikely organizations have affected large and small agencies. New regulations imposed by federal and state legislation abound. Some form of outside evaluation or accreditation, such as offered by the Joint Commission on Accreditation of Healthcare Organizations and Community Health Accreditation Program, is becoming essential for contracts with third party payers. Evidence of quality assurance plans is often requested by referral sources.

Competition from large national providers, heavily financed regional providers, and investors from Wall Street has presented challenges. Telemedicine, more high-tech skills for field staff, expansion of the role of family caregivers, and utilization of volunteers trained in disease-specific interaction have become other areas that managers must explore to prepare for the future. In the midst of all these challenges to people working in the industry as well as new players, there has been a constant request for written information to help home care and hospice managers keep abreast.

The updating of the *Handbook of Home Health Care Administration* has brought together some of the finest minds in home health care and hospice, who share their experience in helping guide agency operations for today and the future. Marilyn Harris has sought out authors who work day to day in home health care. The equivalent of many thousands of years of practical home care and hospice experience can be found in this compendium. Answers to basic day-to-day operational issues blended with frameworks for the future will give readers references to guide them on a daily basis and plan for tomorrow.

Marilyn Harris herself has devoted her career to effective, caring home care administration. She has influenced home health in the United States and Europe. She is a personal role model who stands out in the industry for her integrity, good management, and forward thinking. Many of us who have had the good fortune to work with Marilyn Harris truly appreciate her ability to bring together this incredible reference book to help us participate in today's home health paradigm leap.

Kaye Daniels
President
Hospital Home Health Care Agency of California
Torrance, California

Introduction

It has been three short years since the *Handbook of Home Health Care Administration* was published. The number of changes that are taking place in home health care and the pace at which they are occurring are mind boggling. Every day there are reports of more mergers, affiliations, acquisitions, and integrated health care networks. The enrollment of individuals, both younger and older than 65 years, in managed care plans continues to increase. About 10 percent of the Medicare market is now in managed care. That number is expected to climb to 25 percent by 2002. The impact of Medicare managed care will extend far beyond the borders of the Medicare program ("Increasing Medicare Managed Care Enrollment," 1996). Administrators, supervisors, staff, and students of home health and hospice care need current information about a wide array of topics to meet the challenges that are encountered each day.

The strategic consensus report of the National Consensus Conference on the Educational Preparation of Home Care Administrators (Cary, 1989) contains 12 cluster areas of knowledge and skills recommended for home care administrators. Primary areas reflect the essential knowledge and skills that a home health administrator needs to achieve a beginning competency level. Secondary areas reflect knowledge needed to identify priorities and resources. This book incorporates information related to many of these cluster areas (Exhibit 1 and Table 1).

Scalzi and Wilson (1990,1991) completed a study to identify the relative amount of time spent and the relative importance attributed to specific job activities of nurse executives. The 184 nurse executives who participated in the study identified 11 curriculum areas by time spent and by practice settings, including home care, long-term care, occupational health, and acute care. The nurse executives in home care identified a stronger need for legal, health care policy, financial, and marketing acumen. Also, they indicated that they spent more time on clinical activities (Table 2). The chapters in this book address the areas of need that home care administrators identified as being important and as requiring the most time.

The original idea for this book started with an identified need for an in-house manual to be used by the students who come to the Visiting Nurse Association of Eastern Montgomery County/A Department of Abington Memorial Hospital (VNA) for a practicum in home health administration. Many times, administrators, the clinical educator, supervisors, and other staff spend much time explaining to students the programs and services of the agency and describing the services that are offered, types of funding, and other important issues. The purpose of this book is to present an overview of the administration of home health and hospice services. Each chapter could be expanded into a book-length publication. Not all topics are addressed in detail, but principles that apply to one discipline can be applied to others. For example,

Exhibit 1 Cluster Areas of Knowledge and Skill Recommended for Home Care Administration

- Finance/fiscal
- Human resource development
- Legal/ethical
- Management information systems
- Marketing
- Nursing science
- Operations
- Organization/management
- Policy
- Public health science
- Quality management
- Research

In an attempt to refine the clusters, the panel generated primary and secondary areas within each where appropriate.

1. *Primary areas* were defined as reflecting the essential knowledge and skill areas for a home health administrator to achieve a beginning competency level. As illustrated in the previous section, educational institutions are to assume the major responsibility for this content, with service organizations playing a minor role.
2. *Secondary areas* were defined as those for which a home care administrator needs some knowledge to identify priorities and resources as the basis for developing further competencies. As illustrated in the secondary areas, education and service organizations have equal responsibility for reinforcing this content.

Table 1 reflects the primary and secondary areas within the clusters generated by the consensus panel.

Source: Copyright © Ann H. Cary, PhD, RN.

accreditation standards and documentation principles apply to therapy and paraprofessional services as well as to nursing. Chapter authors have included a bibliography in addition to the reference list so that interested readers can pursue a particular topic in more detail.

All the contributors to this book are involved in some aspect of home health or hospice care. They include staff members, board members, nurse practitioners, consultants, accountants, lawyers, teachers, supervisors, administrators, and representatives from national and state organizations. Contributors represent various auspices and sizes of home health care agencies and geographical areas.

Part I provides an overview of home health administration. It includes a brief history and a description of the types of agencies. Part II addresses standards for home health agencies. Agency standards, including certification, accreditation, certificate of need, and licensure, are described. Professional standards such as credentialing of staff and administrators are included. The benefits of membership in national and state organizations are described by the staff of these organizations. The Joint Commission on Accreditation of Healthcare Organizations' *1997–98 Comprehensive Accreditation Manual for Home Care* was published in 1996. The revised standards are reviewed by

Table 1 Primary and Secondary Areas of Knowledge and Skill within 12 Individual Clusters

Cluster	Primary Areas	Secondary Areas
1. Finance/fiscal	p1 Read and interpret financial statements p2 Prepare a basic budget p3 Develop a basic budget p4 Develop financial controls	s1 Basic principles of economics (costing) s2 Basic principles of accounting s3 Principles of finance (resource) utilization, capital acquisition, cash flow management s4 Reimbursement systems s5 Ratio analysis s6 Small business administration (examples: payroll, taxes, banking, prudent buyer concept)
2. Human resource development	p1 Personnel practices (recruitment, retention, evaluation, termination, compensation) p2 Job analysis/staffing p3 Efficiency/effectiveness (productivity) p4 Supervision (orientation, evaluation, coaching, mentoring, maintenance, development)	s1 Staff development (orientation, continuing education, on-the-job/inservice training) s2 Personnel/legal aspects s3 Team building s4 Leadership
3. Legal/ethical		s1 Business law (introduction to corporate law, tort, labor relations, regulatory, legal reporting requirements) s2 Issues/ethical decision making, including confidentiality s3 Legal aspects of personnel administration
4. Management information systems	p1 Basic systems analysis/manual and automated information p2 Efficient use of management information systems, including system confidentiality p3 Computer literacy	s1 Appreciate technological state of the art
5. Marketing		s1 Marketing theory (basic)
6. Nursing science	p1 Apply appropriate models/theories to target populations	s1 Nursing theories s2 Family developmental theories s3 Communication and teaching/learning theories s4 Social/psychological theories

continues

Table 1 continued

Cluster	Primary Areas	Secondary Areas
7. Operations	p1 Program/product line design theory p2 Competencies in aggregate-based clinical care p3 Identify researchable problems p4 Problem-solving process p5 Behavioral objectives p6 Standards of practice p7 Community assessment/needs assessment p8 Program planning process—assessment/planning/implementation/evaluation p9 Community interactions/networking	s1 Patient delivery systems s2 Reimbursement/regulatory activities s3 Grantsmanship, applied s4 Case management/continuity of care s5 Policy and procedure development s6 Planning processes—types, models
8. Organization/management	p1 Principles and functions of management (controls, policy and procedure) p2 Organizational behavior (board/stockholder consultation, negotiation, collaboration, leadership, motivation, conflict management, implementing change) p3 Organizational structure	s1 Contract management
9. Policy	p1 Knowledge of health care delivery systems p2 Knowledge of public policy and implications p3 Legal/ethical implications of public policy p4 Case management/continuity of care p5 Political involvement	s1 Community standards s2 Regulations and regulatory bodies (Occupational Safety and Health Administration, Health Care Financing Administration), state licensure, etc. s3 Legislation/reimbursement s4 Entitlement programs s5 Standards of practice s6 Local/state/national advocacy programs and organizations

10. Public health science	p1 Epidemiology, population and demography p2 Health behaviors—culture, risk factors/ reductions, wellness concepts p3 Community theory	s1 Major health problems
11. Quality management	p1 Risk-management problems (prevention strategies/identification of risk, legal parameters, laws affecting home care) p2 QM theory—structure, process, outcome, design of QM program p3 Implement, evaluate QM program p4 Standards of practice p5 Infection control p6 Developing standards	s1 Community standards s2 Applicable regulations s3 Credentialing/licensure/certification/accreditation
12. Research	p1 Basic statistics (prerequisite) p2 Research designs p3 Analyze research reports p4 Interpret and apply findings p5 Knowledge of research process (prerequisite) p6 Basic research skills p7 Biostatistics p8 Support research/collaborate with researchers	

Table 2 Rank of Curriculum Areas by Time Spent (1, Low; 4, High)

Area of Need	Home Care	Overall Average
Law and health care policy	3.07	2.95
Finance	2.79	2.56
Marketing	2.67	2.51
QA	2.53	2.55
Organizational behavior	2.52	2.67
Organizational strategy	2.51	2.61
Risk management	2.31	2.39
Clinical nursing	2.26	2.14
Resource management	2.25	2.22
Management information systems	2.23	2.18
Ethics	2.11	2.11

Courtesy of Cynthia C. Scalzi, PhD, RN, University of Pennsylvania, Philadelphia, Pennsylvania with permission.

Joint Commission staff. The 1996 revisions to the Medicare conditions of participation (COPs) are presented. The anticipated total revision of the COPs was not available when this book went to press.

Part III explores a limited number of clinical issues that affect service delivery or cost identification. Documentation, patient classification systems, patient outcome systems, nursing diagnoses, maternal and child health programs, high-technology issues, and others are presented from the administrator's viewpoint. New chapters include a description of one computerized clinical documentation system. There is increased emphasis on determining and documenting the competency of personnel, including staff, contractors, and volunteers. The authors of a new chapter share their strategies and methods for meeting the challenge of competency evaluation of personnel.

Part IV describes the components of a quality assessment/performance improvement program, program and service evaluation, critical pathways, and performance improvement in home health agencies. Four new chapters are included in this section that address emerging issues. The authors describe outcome-based quality improve-

ment, implementation of the Agency for Health Care Policy and Research guidelines, and benchmarking as a performance improvement process.

Part V lists selected management issues that are important to home care administrators. Such issues as referral sources, staffing, productivity, labor relations, human resources, case management, staff education, and long-term care are addressed. Three new chapters appear in this part of the book that address two challenges to administrators and managers: managed care and transitioning of staff from acute care to home care. The authors describe the managed care concept and strategies for success in dealing with managed care organizations. The challenges and opportunities related to transitioning nurses from hospital to home care are shared by two experts in this process.

Part VI deals with financial issues. The current insurance/litigation climate, budgets, reimbursement, management information systems, and how to read and interpret financial audits are explored in detail. Part VII addresses legal, ethical, and political issues. Contracts, informed consent, and liability are discussed. Administrators must be aware of the many legislative and regulatory issues that affect home care at both state and national levels. The authors provide information about the political process and how personnel in home health agencies can become involved in the process. Ethical concerns surface at the clinical and administrative levels. A myriad of concerns are explored from theoretical and practical viewpoints.

Part VIII includes strategic planning, marketing, and survival issues. Topics such as diversification, corporate restructuring, mergers, acquisitions, and marketing are included. A new chapter explains the integrated health care networks that are being developed and the opportunities and challenges for home health agency administrators who are involved with such networks or may be in the future.

Part IX addresses areas of opportunity for administrative staff to serve as resource personnel and innovators. Student and volunteer programs are two areas of administration that may not be present in all agencies, but these programs present multiple opportunities for collaborative relationships with other agencies or educational institutions. The physician's role in home care is addressed by a physician. The role of the fiscal intermediary is also reviewed. Other topics include research, publishing, applying for grants, and administrative law judge (ALJ) hearings.

Part X includes new chapters that will help administrators meet the challenges that home health care and hospice leaders are facing in 1997. Telemedicine in home care will become more important as administrators seek to maintain high-quality care with decreased financial resources. Experienced authors describe how electronic visits can benefit home care patients and staff. Advice on how to use the Internet and how to develop one's own home care site on the World Wide Web are shared by experts on these issues.

Home care administrators are assuming responsibility for an ever-widening array of health care services in the community. Day care, community nursing centers, and community/interfaith parish nurse programs are logical extensions of the administrator's range of expertise as more and more services move into the community. Several authors share their expertise and experiences with these new responsibilities. Others attempt to put the administration of home health, hospice, and expanded programs into perspective and share their viewpoints on administration in today's economic, political, and health care climate.

Although issues are addressed on a chapter-by-chapter basis, many of the topics overlap one another. For example, ethical issues are mentioned in the chapters on discharge planning and high-technology procedures. Financial issues surface in reference to budgeting, reimbursement, and documentation. Productivity is common to staffing, budgeting, and ethical issues.

Today's home health care climate is ever changing. Information included in this book was current as of December 1996. Readers are encouraged to review current guidelines and regulations, specifically in such areas as reimbursement, certification and accreditation standards, documentation requirements, and Medicare forms, to keep informed of important changes that may have occurred since this book went to press.

As an administrator, I have had many new experiences during the past 3 years in my role as director of home health and hospice care. For example, I have had the opportunity to talk with colleagues throughout the United States through the sharing of benchmarking reports. The staff have planned for and implemented a computerized clinical documentation system. My responsibilities have also expanded to include planning and implementing health care services that are taken into the community. I have worked with community organizations and other hospital department directors and staff to plan for, establish, and open a community health center where direct care is provided by nurse practitioners and educational and health promotion programs are offered in response to requests for health information. I am part of a planning committee for implementing a community/interfaith parish nurse resource center.

The opportunities to meet the health care needs of the community we serve by providing high-quality health care services to individuals in a compassionate, caring, and cost-effective manner are endless.

It is my hope that each reader will find this publication to be a ready reference for the multifaceted aspects of home health care administration. I welcome your comments and look forward to hearing from many of you.

REFERENCES

Cary, A. 1989. *Strategies for a collaborative future: The consensus report for the National Consensus Conference on the Educational Preparation of Home Care Administrators.* Washington, DC: Catholic University of America School of Nursing.

Increasing Medicare managed care enrollment will have wide-ranging impact on health care. 1996. *State Health Watch* 3(9):5.

Joint Commission on Accreditation of Healthcare Organizations. 1996. *1997–98 Comprehensive accreditation manual for home care.* Oakbrook Terrace, IL: Joint Commission.

Scalzi, C., and D. Wilson. 1990. Empirically based recommendations for content of graduate nursing administration programs. *Nursing & Health Care* 11(10):522–525.

Scalzi, C., and D. Wilson. 1991. Future preparation of home health nurse executives. *Home Health Care Services Quarterly* 12(1):13,21.

Marilyn D. Harris

PART I

Home Health Administration

CHAPTER 1

Home Health Administration: An Overview

Janna Dieckmann

DEFINITION OF HOME HEALTH CARE

Home health care is the provision of health care services to people of any age at home or in other noninstitutional settings. Contemporary home health care is based on nursing service models developed within the visiting nurse association movement beginning in the late 19th century. Home health care has continued to evolve and change in response to social, economic, political, and scientific innovation during the 20th century. As health care professionalism has grown and differentiated, many health care occupations have become linked to home health care, including occupational therapy, home economics, social work, nutrition services, and, during World War II, physical therapy. Auxiliary workers, today called home health aides and homemakers, have frequently been part of home health care services. Physicians have a complex history in home care. Although medical practitioners have always made home visits and have always certified orders for home nursing care for their patients, direct physician participation within the home health multidisciplinary team has varied. During the last few decades, medicine has usually been more detached from proliferating home care agencies, although some physicians continue to participate fully in home health care. Other services, including transportation, laboratory services, home Meals-on-Wheels programs, and more, have usually been secured from outside agencies, although these have occasionally been directly incorporated into home health care agencies.

Two key goals of home health care have remained constant during more than 100 years of change: direct provision of health care services to those at home and education of both client and family toward the goals of health and independence from formal care systems. Contemporary home health care reflects most strongly the impact of the government-funded medical programs that began in the 1960s, Medicare and Medicaid. Nevertheless, public health initiatives, private insurance benefit regulation, and newly emerging health problems contribute to a constantly changing picture. Home health care services secured in a particular case ultimately depend on the complex interaction among client, family, and community needs as well as client–professional goals and the payment sources available to fund service organizations such as home health care agencies.

Four prominent national organizations involved in home health care provision—the Council of Home Health Agencies and Community Health Services, National League for Nursing; the National Home Caring Council (formerly the National Home Care Council); the National Association of Home Health Agencies; and the Assembly of Outpatient and Home Care Institutions of the American Hospital Association—provide a formal definition of home health care:

Home health service is that component of comprehensive health care whereby services are provided to individuals and families in their places of residence for the purpose of promoting, maintaining, or restoring health or minimizing the effects of illness and disability. Services appropriate to the needs of the individual patient and family are planned, coordinated, and made available by an agency or institution, organized for the delivery of health care through the use of employed staff, contractual arrangements, or a combination of administrative patterns. (McNamara, 1982, 61)

DESCRIPTION OF HOME HEALTH CARE

Home health care begins with the client, the individual identified as requiring home nursing or therapy services. Although this identified individual is the focus of the home health care services, professional goals for client development are implemented in the context of family and community. The family, neighbors, and other members of the client's informal support system generally provide the 24-hour care and support necessary during the client's period of illness or dependency. Formal services from home health agencies or the community's social service network can only supplement what family and friends provide. The more dependent the client, the greater the skill and commitment demanded from the informal caregiving system. If family and friends are unable to provide adequate care, and clients require more intensive services than available from the home health agency, consideration of nursing home, sheltered care, or other institutional placement becomes critical.

Because of this interactive reliance on informal supports in home health care, it is most practical to define a family in a flexible manner. Traditional definitions of family that include only close biological relatives are inadequate and can limit caregiving resources. In practice, the term *family* must include anyone the client so identifies. In addition to the nuclear family, persons included may be a significant other, distant relatives, a boarder who has lived in the home for years, close friends, or neighbors who perceive a mutual obligation with the client. This flexible definition of family increases the pool of available helpers for the dependent client, but it also requires that nursing and other home health care workers incorporate the needs of this extended family system into plans of care. In providing care, nursing considers both the learning needs of support system members and the psychosocial supports required to maintain their caregiving roles. It is not enough to provide instruction; meeting the needs of the informal support system requires complex coordination and problem solving as well.

The client's community may facilitate or detract from the provision of professional care and fulfillment of home health care service objectives. Communities vary from densely concentrated urban neighborhoods, to sprawling suburban towns, to lonesome rural back roads. Although a client may be isolated from supports in any environment, the concentration of people and services, the availability of transportation, and the proximity and diversity of pharmacy and grocery services constitute quantitative differences in the challenges faced by home health care clients and families.

The community, and the membership of the client and the family within it, have further effects on the client and family system and their presenting needs for home health care. The client's and family's socioeconomic background and class status frequently influence their access to care. The family's cultural and ethnic background may influence its expectations for health and health care services and its ability to meet those needs within the American health care system. Individuals, families, and communities have particular ways of defining health, illness, and dying that home health care professionals must recognize and address. For example, many religious groups have prohibitions of which formal caregivers should be aware. Home care professionals must acquire the ability to practice within diverse cultural parameters.

Health professionals, usually trained to hospital goals and values, find differences at every step toward home care. The most obvious difference cannot be minimized: The home, in all its many variations, has replaced the hospital. Rather than clients adapting to the foreign environment of the hospital, it is home health care providers themselves who must adapt to the family and community. Home care nurses are liaisons, expert consultants who adapt complex treatment plans to homes. This may involve, for example, obtaining equipment, making referrals to other services, or negotiating with physicians to alter medication programs.

INITIATION OF HOME HEALTH CARE SERVICES

Home health clients are visited by home care agencies after referrals are made for the clients' care. Referrals may originate from the client, the family, a community social service agency, a local physician, or almost anyone else. Many home care referrals are initiated by a nurse or discharge planner attached to a hospital. These referrals are made to home health agencies from hospitals when client needs for continuing care are identified during the hospitalization or while the client is under care at an ambulatory clinic or emergency department. Other referrals are received from nursing homes, community clinics and physicians' offices, area agencies on aging, and social work agencies.

A referral to home health care services usually includes client demographic information, family contacts, diagnoses, medications, and proposed treatment measures ordered by the physician. Professional disciplines to be provided to the client are specified. This referral is often not overly complex, generally focusing on the basic, immediate needs of the client. Nevertheless, it is most helpful for the referral to include a brief medical and surgical history for the client, recent laboratory findings, baseline vital sign readings, and history and course of the present illness. Because the client's social context suggests both needs for and limitations of care, knowledge of client and family strengths and weaknesses pertaining to the illness and home management will provide a head start for home health agency professionals. Thus comments and recommendations from members of the multidisciplinary team will contribute to accurate and relevant home care service decisions.

One consideration for Medicare home care referrals is clients' functional abilities: Are they substantially confined to the home? Several contemporary payment sources for home care require that clients receiving services be homebound. Although the definition of homebound status has varied, it has generally been interpreted to mean that the client's health and functional impairment is so great that he or she is unable to seek health services outside the home. Additional variables, such as the presence or absence of a safe environment and a reliable caregiver, may influence whether services can be provided in the home.

The organizations that provide home health care may be voluntary agencies including visiting nurse associations, proprietary agencies, official health departments, social service agencies, or hospital-based home care departments. Whatever the organizational structure, most agencies visit postacute home health care clients within 24 hours of the initial referral. This first visit will probably be the most complex of the entire service period. During this admission visit, the nurse conducts an assessment and evaluation of the client and family, assesses the environmental milieu, analyzes the impact of disease(s) on the client, identifies functional impairments of the client, determines the client's knowledge of and adherence to prescribed treatment for the disease, and identifies client/ family desires for care and eventual goals. Nurses establish the groundwork for needed services, ensuring the safety of clients until the next home care visit. Physical therapists or speech therapists may also take primary responsibility for a home health care case. Active participation of clients and families in establishing the goals of treatment and plan of care is sought and utilized to the fullest extent.

Clients receive services for variable periods of times, from a single visit to service durations of several weeks or months or even years. Visit patterns are usually directed by reimbursement regulations, resulting in varying patterns of care controlled from outside the client–provider nexus. Under Medicare, visits continue until the client's skilled care needs are met. This period is usually short, most often less than 2 months. Clients requiring technical interventions, such as dressing changes or indwelling urinary catheter management, may receive intermittent services over several years. Case management systems within health maintenance organizations or managed care health plans are often the most restrictive, sometimes allowing only two or three visits to complete all instruction and services, even for cases such as new insulin-dependent diabetics. Other reimbursement sources demand specialized requirements, resulting in varying patterns of care. An example is maternal–child programs with state or federal public health initiatives. In these programs, at-risk infants and their families may be visited monthly during the first year of life. In long-term home care programs for the aged, where available, nursing visits may be spaced at long intervals to provide skilled management of chronic conditions. Home-based hospice program visits may be frequent (sometimes daily), particularly for clients in late stages of a terminal disease.

Home care professionals work with clients and families to establish plans of care that address the long-term goals of the case, working toward incremental change during each visit. The home health care nurse utilizes many resources to facilitate client and family progress. Services of additional multidisciplinary team members, such as the physical therapist, occupational therapist, social worker,

speech therapist, and home health aide, may be utilized for the client's benefit. If rehabilitation goals predominate in the case, physical therapy or speech therapy may be the only discipline providing services. Home health care professionals communicate with the client's physician to coordinate the treatment plan to reflect client status changes (e.g., progress in rehabilitation, difficulty in wound healing, or persistent challenges of the terminal phase of illness).

The home health care team relies heavily on ongoing services provided by the community's formal support network as well as the family's own informal support system. Ongoing support systems are essential to prepare the client for discharge from home health care and to provide needed services when skilled care through the home health agency is terminated. The nurse or other professional will make, or suggest that the client or family make, appropriate referrals to formal care networks. The nurse will also seek to develop and support informal systems based in the family, neighborhood, or social groups.

Although actual home health care service outcomes vary significantly among clients and families, case discharge usually occurs when the client has met the goals of care. Some clients progress easily and completely to meet mutually set goals for care, whereas others may achieve only partial outcomes. The client is prepared for discharge during the entire period of home health care provision by being taught the skills required to resume independent management of health care needs. At discharge, the nurse or other home health care provider usually notifies the physician and other involved services that the case is closed. Discharged cases are reopened when clients are referred for new problems or exacerbations of health problems that were previously addressed.

EARLY SOURCES FOR HOME HEALTH CARE

An appreciation of the history of home health care accomplishments is important to understand its current status, including both the strengths and the limitations of the field (Exhibit 1–1). The history of home health care is also an ongoing case study in organizational styles and reimbursement patterns resulting from past patterns of social and economic change. For example, in the early 1900s home health care was part of the public health campaign that improved the health of all Americans. Home health care has frequently changed direction, often suddenly and sharply, as the direct result of changing reimbursement practices, which mirror the contemporary experience. Analysis and review of the history of home health care have implications for home health care services in the 1990s and beyond. An opportunity to avoid the pitfalls of the past emerges when similar patterns in the present are identified. The following brief sketch is but a beginning.

Until the 20th century, care of the sick was usually informal, provided by household members, almost always women. Historians today are aware of early experiments in home health nursing that developed during the early 19th century in the United States. Reflecting then contemporary ideas, these programs focused on moral elevation as well as illness intervention. The Ladies' Benevolent Society of Charleston, South Carolina provided charitable works to the poor and ill beginning in 1813. In Philadelphia, lay nurses who attended a short training program were sent to care for the newborns and postpartum mothers of all social strata. Significant in time and place, these early programs do not seem to have spread, and their influence on the development of visiting nurse associations and organized home health care in the late 19th century is unclear.

Florence Nightingale's innovations in training English nurses to replace untrained lay nurses influenced the late 19th century pattern of nursing education and service provision in the United States. William Rathbone established the first District Nursing Association in 1859 in Liverpool, England. It was not until 1877, however, that district nursing utilizing

graduates of the new nurse training schools was introduced into the United States.

Before 1900, nurses who had graduated from the early training programs usually worked in private duty nursing or held the few positions as hospital administrators and instructors. The new field of public health nursing began to employ a few nurses, often adopting the model of service provision used by the private duty nurse in middle- and upper-class homes. Whereas private duty nurses lived in with the clients and their families, the public health nurses visited several families in one day, providing personal care to the sick and health teaching to families. Many agencies hired only one nurse. Agency administration and direct supervision of the nurses were the responsibility of the agency board, usually comprised of wealthy or socially prominent women of the community. Their charitable community service was to direct both health care and good works by the nurse.

At the turn of the century, public health nursing was defined as "primarily family health work of an educational and preventive character but including restorative work" (Dock and Stewart, 1925, 213), which utilized a large and comprehensive plan for uplifting the general health level through outreach to the community. Although services were offered to individuals and families, the public health nurse sought to ensure the community's health. The focus of the public health nurse's work was the poor and immigrants.

Visiting nursing proved successful in the United States at meeting the public health challenges of that era. High incidence and mortality rates of communicable diseases such as tuberculosis, diphtheria, and typhoid fever affected the entire population. Increased urbanization and industrialization also increased human diseases. The late 19th century benefited from the new scientific explanations of disease, and the public health nurse became the agent for preventive education to the lay public. Nursing interventions, improved urban sanitation, economic improvements, and better nutrition were

Exhibit 1–1 Chronology of Home Health Care in the United States

1813	Ladies' Benevolent Society of Charleston, South Carolina is founded to provide relief of distress and aid to the sick poor.
1832	The Nurse Society of Philadelphia provides care for sick poor in their homes.
1859	First District Nursing Association established in Liverpool, England, by William Rathbone.
1875	First United States nurse training schools using the Nightingale model.
1877	New York City Mission sends trained nurses into homes of the sick poor.
1886	Visiting Nurse Society of Philadelphia and the Boston Instructive District Nursing Association are established.
1893	Henry Street Nurses' Settlement founded on the lower East Side of New York City by Lillian Wald and Mary Brewster.
1898	First municipal home care nurse employed in the United States at Los Angeles to visit the sick poor.
1901	58 organizations provide public health nursing, employing 130 nurses.
1907	Alabama legally approves employment of public health nurses by local boards of health.
1909	*Visiting Nurse Quarterly*, first ongoing specialty journal in the field, begins publication.
1909	Metropolitan Life Insurance Company offers home nursing to its industrial policyholders.
1912	National Organization for Public Health Nursing (NOPHN) is founded.
1912	Rural Nursing Service of the American Red Cross is established, later renamed the Town and Country Nursing Service.
1916	1,922 public health nursing organizations employ 5,150 nurses, a 30-fold increase over 1901 figures.
1921	Sheppard-Towner Act provides federal matching funds for prenatal and infant care programs supporting home care by nurses.
1922	4,040 public health nursing organizations employ 11,550 nurses, double the 1916 total.
1925	Kentucky Committee for Mothers and Babies, later the Frontier Nursing Service, is founded by Mary Breckenridge.
1925	First NOPHN statement of qualifications for public health nurses is published.
1931	4,250 public health nursing agencies employ 15,850 nurses, demonstrating only slight growth since 1922.
1935	Government funding of public health nursing emphasizes health departments over nonofficial agencies.
1935	Joint Committee of the American Nurses Association and NOPHN To Study Health Insurance and Its Implications for Nursing forms to seek health insurance funding for nursing care.
1935	The Association of State and Territorial Directors of Nursing forms.
1944	First basic nursing program is accredited as including sufficient public health nursing content.
1947	First "coordinated" home medical care program is established at Montefiore Hospital, Bronx, New York.
1950	25,100 public health nurses are employed.
1950	Red Cross Rural Nursing Service is discontinued.
1953	NOPHN merges with other organizations to form the National League for Nursing (NLN).
1953	Publication of *Public Health Nursing* ends.
1953	Life insurance companies cease supporting home nursing service.
1955	27,100 public health nurses are employed.
1956	Feasibility study is conducted for Blue Cross reimbursement for home nursing care in New York City.
1960	Kerr-Mills legislation provides Medical Aid for the Aged, including a home care benefit in selected states.

continues

Exhibit 1–1 Chronology of Home Health Care in the United States continued

1966	Home health services under Medicare and Medicaid begin providing support for official and nonofficial agencies in caring for the sick.
1982	National Association for Home Care forms from the combination of the National Association of Home Health Agencies and the NLN Council of Home Health Agencies/Community Health Services.
1983	Health Care Financing Administration implements medical prospective payment, restricting hospital admissions and length of stay and ultimately increasing the acuity of home care clients.
1983	Medicare hospice care benefit is implemented.
1988	*Duggan et al. v. Bowen et al.*, 691 F. Supp. 1487 (D.C. 1988) is decided (the Staggers lawsuit).
1993	World Organization for Care in the Home and Hospice is organized.

the bases for significant reductions in the incidence of deadly communicable disease by 1910.

Early visiting nurse agencies also sought to develop innovative services, whose ongoing maintenance and income support they expected to shift to government auspices. In New York City, Lillian Wald and her coworkers at the Henry Street Nurses' Settlement (later the Visiting Nurse Service) initiated several new services. From public health nursing practice emerged other nursing specialties, such as school nursing and occupational health nursing. In this period, these specialties were truly branches of home health care. Clients identified within the institutional setting were visited in the home, where health promotion and family education were the focus of the nurses' efforts.

Both nurses and lay supporters of the new visiting nurse agencies sought means to expand the visiting nurse movement through exchange of information and development of a professional identity. Publication of the *Visiting Nurse Quarterly* in 1909 established a professional medium of communication for clinical and organization concerns. Establishment of the National Organization for Public Health Nursing (NOPHN) in 1912, whose membership included both nurses and lay supporters, provided an accessible network for the developing leadership in the field. The organizational focus of the NOPHN was "improving the educational and service standards of the public health nurse,

and promoting public understanding of and respect for her work" (Rosen, 1958, 381). The NOPHN was soon a dominant force in public health nursing and endured until 1953, when it merged with other nursing organizations to form the National League for Nursing. The loss of this distinct community health nursing organization, which had joined public health and visiting nurses, remains an obstacle to unifying the specialty of public health/community health nursing.

Rapid growth of the practice field highlighted the need to provide effective educational preparation for current and future public health nurses. Education for public health nursing was initiated separately; graduates of the established nurse training schools were accepted after about 1906. These certificate programs offered lectures in public health nursing theory and practice in a program that might be familiar to contemporary nurses. Public health nursing did not become a regular part of most baccalaureate nursing education programs until much later.

Mechanisms for payment for home health care services were initially much simpler than today. Often through its social networks, the visiting nurse agency board of trustees raised funds to support the work with the poor and needy. Yet clients were encouraged to pay a small fee for nursing services, even as little as a nickel, reflecting social welfare concerns against promoting economic dependency by providing charity. An innovation at the time of its creation in 1909, the special nursing service provided by the Metropolitan Life Insurance Company for its policyholders served as a model for life insurance company sponsorship of nursing care. Nurses in existing agencies, or in agencies developed specifically by the life insurance companies, provided home care services in a significant amount until the early 1950s.

Agencies such as the American Red Cross also provided home care in areas outside the larger cities. Through the Rural Nursing Service, later the Town and Country Nursing Service, the Red Cross developed and passed to local voluntary or public administration almost 3,000 generalized programs of public health nursing services.

Beginning in Los Angeles in 1898, municipalities, and eventually the federal government, took on the task of providing financial support for home health care. Government funding emphasis gradually began to shift to official health departments. Although the economic impact of the 1930s Depression reduced both charitable and public funding for home health care, resulting in cutbacks in personnel and traditional services, New Deal legislation created new employment opportunities for nurses in official health programs. As had the Sheppard-Towner Act of 1921, which targeted improvements in maternal and child health care, Public Health Title VI of the 1935 Social Security Act focused available financial resources toward the nonofficial voluntary agencies.

Mobilization for World War II brought significant changes in nursing education. An increasing emphasis on baccalaureate nursing programs saw the first inclusion of public health nursing in the required coursework. By the mid-1950s, the National League for Nursing required public health nursing courses, but only in baccalaureate-level programs. Clinical practice in home health care remains absent from many diploma and associate degree programs and from the nursing licensure examinations.

The influence of the NOPHN in connecting different agencies and in increasing the spread of knowledge and information relating to practice had gradually decreased by the late 1940s. The challenges of securing financial support for the NOPHN and the popular trend toward centralization of professional nursing organizations laid the groundwork for the end of the NOPHN. In 1953, the NOPHN merged with other specialty nursing organizations to constitute the National League for Nursing. The journal *Public Health Nursing* (first called *Visiting Nurse Quarterly*) ceased publication.

The early 1950s saw other significant changes in visiting nurse sponsorship and organization. Insurance companies, including Metropolitan Life and John Hancock, and the American Red Cross discontinued their support of home health care and the voluntary agencies that had provided the nursing services. With the decrease in the incidence rate of acute, communicable diseases and distinct and progressive increases in chronic illness prevalence, the sponsoring life insurance companies doubted their financial ability to continue to support home nursing care.

During the 1950s, the organizational form of home health care service delivery was also reconsidered. Concern over duplication and a desire for excellent, comprehensive service provision fueled a movement toward combination agencies, defined as a merger of official and voluntary nursing services in a geographical area to provide joint public health and home health care nursing service. Although this was a long-sought and innovative format, declining municipal income and services severely threatened some combination agencies during the 1970s. Some previously combined services were separated into their components for reasons of economic survival. A second organization form emerged in hospital-based home care, particularly influenced by the home medical care program of Montefiore Hospital, Bronx, New York.

Initiation of Medicare and Medicaid health insurance benefits for the elderly and the poor in July 1966 formed an essential basis for the current home health care structure. Adequate funding for home health care was an infusion to voluntary organizations, resulting in increased breadth and amount of services provided. Where a few hospital-based programs had developed in the late 1940s, many more now operated and were joined by growing numbers of entrepreneurial groups drawn by profit-making opportunities, which recognized that a predictable source of home health care funding was now available. Although in 1960 only 250 official health agencies provided nursing care for the sick on a regular basis, by 1968 1,328 public health nursing agencies—50 percent of all official agencies—provided this service. Further refinement of Medicare through congressional amendment and administrative control during the 1970s and 1980s progressively refocused the home care benefit on postacute services. This change from 1960s Medicare home care practices constricted medium-term and long-term home health services as well as care of the chronic client.

REASONS FOR THE GROWTH OF HOME HEALTH CARE

Not only has home health care expanded in the last century, but it may continue to grow in response to the expected changes in the contemporary sociopolitical and economic forces influencing the home health care environment. Changing patterns of disease and population aging, emerging economic reimbursement mechanisms, and changing social values draw together to construct the contemporary home health care delivery system.

The change in the distribution of disease since the turn of the century represents the first factor in the growth of home health care. Improved scientific knowledge of disease agents, regular immunizations, availability of antibiotics, provision of basic nutrition to most people, pasteurization of milk, and other factors have decreased the risk of developing and dying of 19th century disease threats such as communicable diseases, tuberculosis, severe diarrheal illnesses, cholera, and many others. In place of the acute illnesses, chronic illnesses are now the primary causes of death in the United States. These illnesses, such as hypertension, cardiac disease, pulmonary disease, and diabetes, have a long period of development leading to irreversible changes in the body and frequently permanent impairment of the individual's functional abilities. Although early intervention may limit the effect of chronic disease exacerbations, affected individuals generally experience long periods of debility necessitating rehabilitation, during which they may fail to regain their previous abilities. The health care delivery system is faced with making policy decisions about people for whom illness and disease is irreversible, degenerative, and functionally impairing. Chronic illness reduces individual and family resources and decreases the ability to pay privately for needed services. It will be a challenge to society to develop systems that are efficient in meeting client needs and effective in controlling overall costs. Home care has shown promise in being the alternative of choice to meet this large and growing need.

A second and related set of changes affecting the growth of home health care is the changes in the distribution of the population of the United States. This nation is growing older as a whole. Although in 1900 only 4.1 percent of Americans were older than 65 years, by 1994 this number had more than tripled, to 12.7 percent of the U.S. population, a change in real numbers from 3.1 million to 33.2 million (American Association of Retired Persons, 1995). This change in the population older than 65 years is related to the changes in the distribution of disease toward increased prevalence of chronic illnesses. With decreased mortality due to acute illnesses in the younger population, more individuals are living into their later years, the period in which chronic illness is most likely to appear. Additionally, better treatment of complications of older age and chronic illness mean that, even with serious diseases, people tend to live longer than previously.

Complicating this population trend toward longer life have been changes in the social behavior of families. Changing distribution of employment, economic recession, and improved transportation have dispersed families across the country more than ever before. Fewer relatives live in proximity to elderly individuals, reducing available assistance during illness. Changing patterns of female employment, which have increased the percentage of women in the workforce, have simultaneously reduced the number of female family members available for full-time care of the chronically ill. As a result of all these functional changes in the family, care of the impaired elderly has required an increased social and governmental responsibility.

A third factor in the growth of home health care, and an indirect effect of the increase in chronic illness prevalence, has been the expansion of rehabilitative services for those at home with chronic illnesses. Rehabilitation is a long-term process requiring adaptation of the impaired individual to the home environment. This adaptation may require diverse professional services. Home health care has expanded its utilization of the therapies—physical therapy, occupational therapy, and speech therapy—in home rehabilitation efforts. Social work also has a place in the care of the homebound individual. When individuals require a diversity of services, overall utilization of home health care increases.

Changing reimbursement patterns have had such a profound effect on the outline of services provided under home health care that reimbursement is said to set the direction for home health care. Although analysis of home health care development substantiates this position, this fourth reason for the rise in home health care has had an especially strong impact since the passage of Medicare and Medicaid home care coverage with the 1965 Social Security Amendments. The Medicare focus on short-term, intermittent interventions has limited funding to develop new concepts for long-term home care management. Furthermore, Medicare reimbursement has made home health care a

profitable venture for proprietary agencies and hospitals. This has multiplied the number of agencies in a given area both with and without certificates of need. Competition has thus far led to home health care growth, but it has also opened the question of quality assurance and the adequacy of specific training of staff in home health care skills in the new agencies.

The search for health care cost containment has sometimes encouraged the growth of home health care, a fifth reason for its expansion. Changes in Medicare reimbursement for hospitalization toward prospective payment in the early 1980s, popularly known as the diagnosis-related group system, have given fiscal encouragement to limit the length of acute hospitalizations. A result has been the discharge to nursing home or private home of individuals who, in earlier years, may have remained in the acute care institution. The phrase *sicker and quicker* has been used to describe the situation of those released to home care under this policy. Increased acuity of home care clients implies more frequent skilled visits, more time-consuming visits as a result of increased complexity, and clients at greater risk for decompensation and rehospitalization. A shift of care from acute institutions to home care provides only a beginning for still further changes in home health care.

The optimistic belief that cost containment motives will increase home health care utilization is tempered by at least two different problems. On the one hand, the desire for overall cost containment in health services, instead of increasing reimbursement to encourage hospital discharge, is paradoxically curtailing home care services. Medicare intermediaries and managed care programs in particular have attempted to limit strictly the client categories reimbursed under regulations of skilled care, intermittent services, and homebound status. Managed care also emphasizes linkages between achievement of specific client care outcomes and reimbursement. On the other hand, some experts have questioned whether the real total cost of care for the client has been identified to compare with costs of acute hospital care. Lost income to the family caregiver, cost of physical maintenance of the home, and other informal costs have not usually been part of the comparison equation.

Earlier acute care discharge combined with increased home care availability of sophisticated biomedical equipment leads to the sixth factor increasing home health care. Complex services once rarely seen in the home, such as renal hemodialysis, ventilators, and infusion therapy, are more frequently an option for clients who prefer to be at home rather than endure long hospital stays. Simplified technology, effective teaching of clients' caregivers, and efficient supplier networks providing diverse equipment have assured complex care a place in the home environment.

A seventh and last area affecting the growth in home health care is the question of quality of life. The elderly and the chronically ill often prefer to remain in their independent living situations than be institutionalized in, for instance, a nursing home. Many families negatively value institutionalization and separation of the family members. Some cultural and ethnic groups are especially reluctant to treat the chronically ill and elderly in this manner. A desire for self-care as part of significant long-term changes in popular philosophy has also supported increases in home health care. Despite these significant trends in societal values, needed social and economic supports for clients and family caregivers involved in long-term home care are rarely provided.

CONCLUSION

Home health care has become an essential aspect of health care. The challenge will be to draw from home health care's past, to anticipate its future potential, and to provide effective services to contemporary clients and families.

SUGGESTED READING

American Association of Retired Persons (AARP). 1995. *Profile of older Americans.* Washington, DC: AARP.

Anderson, E.T. 1983. Community focus in public health nursing: Whose responsibility? *Nursing Outlook* 31: 44–48.

Brickner, P.W. 1978. *Home health care for the aged: How to help older people stay in their own homes and out of institutions.* New York: Appleton-Century-Crofts.

Buhler-Wilkerson, K. 1983. False dawn: The rise and decline of public health nursing in America, 1900–1930. In *Nursing history: New perspectives, new possibilities,* edited by E.G. Lagemann, 89–106. New York: Teachers College Press.

Buhler-Wilkerson, K. 1985. Public health nursing: In sickness or in health? *American Journal of Public Health* 75:1155–1161.

Buhler-Wilkerson, K. 1991. Home care the American way: An historical analysis. *Home Health Care Services Quarterly* 12:5–17.

Clemen-Stone, S., et al. 1995. *Comprehensive family and community health nursing: Family, aggregate, and community practice.* 4th ed. St. Louis: Mosby.

Division of Nursing, Bureau of Health Professions, Health Resources and Services Administration, Public Health Service. 1985. *Consensus conference on the essentials of public health nursing practice and education.* Washington, DC: U.S. Department of Health and Human Services.

Dock, L.L., and A.M. Stewart. 1925. *A short history of nursing: From the earliest times to the present day.* 2d ed. New York: G.P. Putnam's Sons.

Fitzpatrick, M.L. 1975. *The National Organization for Public Health Nursing, 1912–1952: Development of a practice field.* New York: National League for Nursing.

Fry, S.T. 1983. Dilemma in community health ethics. *Nursing Outlook* 31:176–179.

Gardner, M.S. 1932. *Public health nursing.* New York: Macmillan.

Heinrich, J. 1983. Historical perspectives on public health nursing. *Nursing Outlook* 31:317–320.

Hogstel, M.O. 1985. *Home nursing care for the elderly.* Bowie, MD: Brady Communications.

McNamara, E. 1982. Home care: Hospitals discover comprehensive home care. *Hospitals* 56(21):60–66.

Melosh, B. 1982. *"The physician's hand": Work culture and conflict in American nursing.* Philadelphia: Temple University Press.

Milio, N. 1981. *Promoting health through public policy.* Philadelphia: Davis.

Monteiro, L.A. 1985. Florence Nightingale on public health nursing. *American Journal of Public Health* 75:181–186.

Mundinger, M.O. 1983. *Home care controversy: Too little, too late, too costly.* Rockville, MD: Aspen.

National League for Nursing (NLN). 1979. *Community health: Today and tomorrow.* New York: NLN.

Roberts, D.E., and J. Heinrich. 1985. Public health nursing comes of age. *American Journal of Public Health* 75:1162–1172.

Rosen, G. 1958. *A history of public health.* New York: MD Publications.

Stanhope, M., and L. Lancaster. 1992. *Community health nursing: Promoting health of aggregates, families, and individuals.* 4th ed. St. Louis: Mosby.

Stewart, J.E. 1979. *Home health care.* St. Louis: Mosby.

Wald, L.D. 1915. *The house on Henry Street.* New York: Holt.

White, M.S. 1982. Construct for public health nursing. *Nursing Outlook* 30:527–530.

Williams, C.A. 1977. Community health nursing—What is it? *Nursing Outlook* 25:250–254.

CHAPTER 2

The Home Health Agency

Judith A. Baigis and Kathleen E. Williams

HISTORICAL OVERVIEW

The informal, sympathetic care of the sick in their homes by relatives and friends has a long history indeed. The delivery of systematic nursing care in the home, based on the best available knowledge of the natural history of disease, is a much more recent undertaking and is a result of Florence Nightingale's program of secular scientific education for nurses (Smith, 1983). Admiring the skills of the Nightingale nurses, William Rathbone supported philanthropic projects aimed at the sick poor in Liverpool. The Nightingale nurses ran and staffed some of the projects (Woodham-Smith, 1970).

This notion of delivering skilled nursing services to the sick poor was also developing in the United States. Philanthropists in this country provided funds for the start-up of voluntary organizations, forerunners of our visiting nurse associations (VNAs), with trained nurses hired to deliver home nursing services similar to those of their English counterparts. As local health departments developed and expanded in the early years of the 20th century, health officers in charge of these so-called official agencies also added nurses to their staffs. One of the nursing responsibilities was the delivery of services in the home. By the middle part of this century, a number of these voluntary and official agencies had combined their resources to various degrees to streamline their operations and thus decrease overhead, costs, and service

duplication. Such organizations became known, not surprisingly, as combination agencies.

In 1947, another innovative service model was instituted. E.M. Bluestone, a physician at Montefiore Hospital in Bronx, New York, introduced the notion of hospital-based home care. Patients discharged from that hospital were entitled to a wide range of nursing, social, and other related services, all delivered in their own homes (Cherkasky, 1949). Such an arrangement—a health care institution operating a department of home care—is not limited to hospitals any longer. Rehabilitation centers and skilled nursing facilities also offer home health services. These departments of home care are referred to as institution-based agencies. In contrast, those agencies that are not part of an institution are referred to as freestanding agencies.

RECENT HISTORY

By the mid-1960s, there were approximately 1,200 of the aforementioned agencies delivering home health services (Mundinger, 1983), most of which were paid for by donations through organizations such as local community chests or by the recipients of the care. The passage of Medicare, and to a lesser extent Medicaid, in the mid-1960s spurred the growth of the home health industry because these federal insurance programs ensure a stable source of income for the agencies that are eligible to participate in them. The growth of the private agency, another type of agency for the delivery of home health services, was further stimulated in 1982 when Congress and the Health Care Financing Administration (HCFA) opened up home health care to the for-profit sector for Medicare reimbursement. Table 2–1 shows the effect of the Medicare program on the growth in numbers of Medicare-certified home health agencies over the past 28 years.

Since 1982, the growth in numbers of both hospital-based and proprietary agencies has been pronounced. The growth spurt between 1984 and 1995 was due to the passage of the prospective payment system by Congress and, more recently, to the clarification of Medicare coverage by HCFA. Increasing numbers of acute care hospitals were diversifying to broaden their revenue base, and home health care was one of the areas targeted for this diversification (Ginzberg et al., 1984). There are currently about 7,019 noncertified agencies (National Association for Home Care, 1995). These noncertified agencies, such as homemaker–home health aide agencies, do not provide the kinds of services necessary to be certified by Medicare.

This chapter provides an outline of the similarities and differences among the various types of home health agencies (voluntary, official, and private). They are similar in administrative structure and sources of funding. The major differences among the aforementioned types of agencies are positioning for tax purposes and financial control or ownership.

FINANCIAL CONCERNS

The term *not for profit* is a designation that exempts organizations from taxation on profits or excess income under Section 501 of the Internal Revenue Code of 1954. This excess is put back into the organization, and no part of the net earnings can be used for the private benefit of owners, partners, or shareholders. Thus a voluntary organization such as a VNA or a community-owned hospital would usually be not for profit. If a not-for-profit organization wants to engage in activities intended to make a profit or surplus that is shared or distributed, it would have to form holding companies or separate corporate entities to deal with those profit-making actions. Many VNAs and hospitals are doing this in today's competitive market. The term *for profit* or *profit making* is also a designation for tax purposes. Agencies with this designation are called proprietary agencies, and they are not eligible for tax exemption under Section 501 of the Internal Revenue Code.

Such designations for tax purposes, however, are not true differentiations of financial status. For example, all business organizations (voluntary and private) must make profits or at least have income equal to expenses to continue to

---

Table 2–1 Medicare-Certified Home Care Agencies, 1967–1995

Year	Total	VNA	Public/ Official	Hospital	Private Proprietary	Private Nonprofit	Other
1967	1,753	549	939	133	0	0	39
1977	2,496	546	1,242	281	81	309	37
1987	5,923	500	1,172	1,382	1,882	803	1
1995	8,747	579	1,161	2,357	3,730	667	59
Change in Number from 1967 through 1995	+6,994	+30	+222	+2,224	+3,730	+667	+20

Source: Reprinted from National Association for Home Care, *NAHC Report No. 511* (7 May 1993) and *NAHC Basic Statistics* (September 1995).

exist. Terms such as *government agency, non-governmental, private, church affiliated,* and the like all refer to control or ownership, not to positioning for tax purposes. A health department is an example of an official government agency created to perform specified public functions, such as drinking water purification, and services, such as public health nursing. It is maintained from revenues such as taxes and fees collected from the people who are benefitting from its services or functions. Within this context, then, a community-owned agency would usually be not for profit, but a privately owned organization such as a home health agency could be either for profit or not for profit.

SCOPE OF HOME CARE

Home care is one of many service components in the arena of long-term care, although it is not limited to long-term care. Other service components of long-term care include, for example, nursing homes and programs for substance abusers, the mentally retarded, the occupationally disabled, and the handicapped. In other words, many different age and population groups require continuing care. Within this long-term care context, however, the phrase *home health care* is used in two ways. On the one hand, it is used to refer to the range of in-home services provided to chronically ill people over a long period of time. On the other hand, it is also used to refer to the Medicare-reimbursed home-based services that are primarily for the acutely ill elderly and are skilled, short term, and intermittent (Moyer, 1986). Regardless of how home health is defined, however, nursing care is the foundation of the entire system.

RANGE OF HOME HEALTH AGENCIES

The Medicare conditions of participation for home health agencies define a home health agency as a public agency or private organization primarily engaged in providing skilled nursing services and other therapeutic services

("Conditions of Participation," 1968; HCFA, 1996). Common to certified home health agencies, because it is required for participation in the Medicare program, is the professional advisory committee. This group of professional persons establishes policies and governs the services provided by the home health agency. Appropriate professional discipline representation is required in addition to a minimum of one physician and one registered nurse. In recent years, consumer representation has been strongly encouraged by the Medicare auditing agencies. This committee must review the agency's policies on an annual basis and fulfill an advisory function on a timely, regular, and planned basis.

Government Agencies

Government (official) home health agencies are "created and given their power through statutes enacted by legislators" (Stewart, 1979, p. 25). Home health services are frequently provided by the nursing division of state or local health departments. The organizational structure within the nursing divisions varies among agencies, with some agencies opting to have their public health nurses include their home health clients within their overall public health caseload. Other government agencies choose to form home health teams within their nursing departments. These teams' primary function is to provide home health services. Local health departments may have a combination of public health nurses and home health team nurses providing home health services. In addition to home health services, government agencies usually provide services such as disease prevention, health promotion, communicable disease investigation, environmental health, maternal–child health, and family planning.

Fiscal responsibility for the government home health agency rests with the city, county, or state government units or a combination of such organizations. The overall county/city/state budget restrictions can directly influence the provision of health services in a particular area. Home health caseloads of government agencies frequently include a disproportionate number of indigent patients because the agency cannot refuse services based on the client's ability to pay.

Voluntary Agencies

Home health agencies that do not depend on state and local tax revenues but are financed primarily with nontax funds, such as donations, endowments, United Way contributions, and third party insurance providers (Medicare, Medicaid, and Blue Cross), are referred to as voluntary agencies; an example is a VNA. Voluntary agencies are governed by a board of directors of interested individuals, frequently respected members of the surrounding community or service area.

These agencies are considered community-based agencies because they provide services within a fairly well-defined geographical location or community. In recent years, however, traditional VNA boundaries have become less distinct as a result of increased competition for clients. In the past, voluntary agencies could depend on virtually all the home health clients within their own catchment areas, but the growth of proprietary and institution-based home health agencies has now eroded their traditional referral base. The relationship between neighboring VNAs has turned in many instances from cooperation to competition.

Private Agencies

Private home health agencies can be for-profit or not-for-profit organizations. Some proprietary (for-profit) agencies participate in the Medicare home health program as part of national chains and are administered through a corporate headquarters. Recently, there has been a merger of several proprietary chain providers that may forecast a consolidation of the proprietary home health industry into larger, national firms. These larger companies are able to generate sufficient revenues to cover overhead costs (Anderson, 1986).

Although revenues are generated by some proprietary agencies through third party payers such as Medicare and Blue Cross, other proprietaries rely on private pay clients. These private pay agencies offer services such as private duty nursing to both acutely and chronically ill patients; this is a difference from most Medicare-certified providers, which provide most of their services to clients who have had a recent acute change in their medical condition. These private services are often on an extended hours basis (2 to 24 hours) rather than on a per visit basis (O'Malley, 1986). Many agencies also provide hospital staffing services.

Institution-Based Agencies

Home health agencies operating as departments in sponsoring health care organizations are certified under Medicare and hold a separate provider number, but they are governed by the sponsoring organization's board of trustees or directors. In the past, home health services provided by institution-based providers consisted of intensive-level services intended for those clients requiring multiple-discipline services and supplies. The client case mix of today's institution-based agencies reflects the change to a more balanced caseload, with clients requiring differing degrees of services. The principal source of referrals for these agencies is the inpatient population of the facility, with discharge planning/social services being the case finder of potential home health clients.

The philosophy of the institution-based agency usually coincides with that of the sponsoring organization. Good continuity of care is frequently cited by these agencies as their primary advantage over other types of home health agencies (Stewart, 1979). This continuity can be sold to the medical staff of the institution by promotion of the fact that the home care of the physicians' clients is being coordinated by persons familiar with the physicians and the institution. Until recently, a fiscal advantage of institution-based home health providers was the allowance by Medicare of the inclusion of a percentage of administrative and general overhead in the calculation of the visit costs. The Medicare home health reimbursement system also recognized the higher costs of office space in hospitals and permitted an add-on amount in the calculation of the visit costs. This add-on was eliminated as a result of tax reform legislation of 1993 (National Association for Home Care, 1993). Another advantage enjoyed by the institution-based home health agency is the ability to draw from the resources of the other departments of the facility for service provision as well as for formal and informal consultation services.

Hospice

An agency in which services are provided by a medically supervised interdisciplinary team of professionals and volunteers for terminally ill clients is defined as a hospice by the National Hospice Organization (1984). There are variations among home care hospice programs in their structure and staffing, but all profess to foster the provision of palliative and supportive services to the patient as well as to the family after the patient's demise (Morris and Christie, 1995). This service is unique to hospice agencies because other home health agencies cease services upon the death of the client. The hospice concept was imported from Britain into the United States at New Haven, Connecticut in the mid-1970s and has grown to more than 2,500 programs. In the 1990s, new hospices have experienced an annual growth of 8 percent, and the number of hospice patients has grown at an annual rate of 13 percent, to an estimated 340,000 patients served in 1994 (National Hospice Organization, 1995).

Hospice services are reimbursed by many health insurance plans, such as Blue Cross/Blue Shield, as well as by the home hospice service Medicare benefit provided in the Tax Equity and Fiscal Responsibility Act of 1982 (Cunningham, 1985). Many hospice agencies have chosen to obtain Medicare certification because of the improved reimbursement schedule outlined by recent regulations. Approximately 75 percent of hospices are Medicare certified or have certification pending. The hospice benefit is also covered by Medicaid in 36 states and the District of Columbia and has been authorized under the Civilian and Medical Program of the Uniformed Services (National Hospice Organization, 1995). Structurally, hospices can be institution based, owned by or affiliated with a certified home health agency, or independent agencies.

Homemaker–Home Health Aide Agencies

Agencies providing homemaker–home health aide services are frequently private agencies in which clients pay for the home care services or in which the care is financed by private insurance policies (Stewart, 1979). These agencies can provide home health aides who are Medicare certified; that is, they have completed a Medicare-approved home health aide course of study (75 hours in length) and/or have passed competency evaluation procedures. With these certified aides, homemaker–health aide agencies are able to contract with Medicare-certified home health agencies, which in turn are reimbursed by Medicare for the home health aide services. The Medicare-certified agency pays the homemaker–home health aide agency directly on an hourly basis. Such contracts are lucrative because they are guaranteed income for the homemaker–home health aide agency.

The distinction between homemakers and home health aides can at times be difficult to ascertain because both functions are often provided by a single employee. Homemakers function primarily as house cleaners, whereas the principal duties of home health aides are in the area of personal care, such as bathing. Other, more complex services, such as range-of-motion exercises, can be performed by the home health aide after proper instruction by a registered nurse. Homemaker–home health aide agencies are required to ensure that their per-

Table 2–2 Types of Agencies

Point of Comparison	Government	Voluntary	Proprietary	Institution Based	Hospice	Homemaker–Home Health Aide
Governing body	Local government units (boards of supervisors, local board of health) by way of local health officer	Board of directors comprising members of service area and local community	Individual owner(s) or corporate headquarters (chain)	Sponsoring health organization's board of trustees	Board of directors comprising members of local community and services area (independent) or board of trustees of sponsoring health organization (institution based)	Individual owner(s) or corporate headquarters (chain)
Role of professional advisory committee	Functions in advisory capacity as defined in Medicare regulations	Functions in advisory capacity as defined in Medicare regulations	Functions in advisory capacity as defined in Medicare regulations	Functions in advisory capacity as defined in Medicare regulations	Closely knit team of professionals and volunteers provide services as well as consultation	Usually no professional advisory committee; complies with appropriate Medicare personnel standards if contracted by a Medicare-certified agency

Client case/mix of services provided	Skilled home health clients; may have higher percentage of indigent; also provides public health services such as maternal–child health, family planning, environmental health	Skilled home health clients of all ages; some screening activities such as health maintenance; other community health activities in senior centers, etc.; services becoming more diverse	Skilled home health clients of all ages; private duty services, hospital-staffing services	Skilled home health clients of all ages; some custodial or private duty care	Terminally ill clients (usually with less than 6-month life span prognosis); much involvement with significant others; bereavement services also provided; volunteers used for services provided	Skilled and unskilled (custodial) home health clients of all ages; personal care and housekeeping services provided
Revenue sources	Primarily from tax revenues, third party insurance payers (Medicare, Medical Assistance, Blue Cross/Blue Shield, etc.)	Donations (e.g., United Way), endowments, fund raising, third party insurance payers, private pay (usually on sliding fee basis)	Third party insurance payers, private pay	Third party insurance payers, private pay, donations, endowments, fund raising (usually in conjunction with sponsoring institution)	Third party insurance payers (including Medicare hospice benefit), self-pay, donations, grants	Contract revenues from Medicare, certified home health agencies, private pay

Source: Data from J. Stewart, *Home Health Care.* Copyright © 1979 Mosby-YearBook, Inc.

sonnel complete 12 hours of inservice programs per year to meet Medicare standards. In addition, on-site performance evaluations are conducted by professionals, such as registered nurses.

Other Home Health Care Providers

In addition to the types of home health agencies discussed in this chapter, there are home health services provided by durable medical equipment companies, high-technology service companies (ventilators, total parenteral nutrition, etc.), home telephone reassurance programs, and companion services, to name a few. Many of these organizations refer to themselves, even in their titles, as home care. With the increase in consumer awareness of and demand for home care services, and as a result of the aging of the American population, all types of health care services provided in the home may blend with each other, thus creating

even more confusion among consumers and professionals alike about types of home health agencies.

CONCLUSION

The categorization of types of home health agencies has changed in the past decades, and the future may bring new organizational structures that are now beginning to evolve. These new alliances, formed mostly out of economic necessity and the growth of managed care, may continue to blur the distinctions among types of home health agencies, thus creating even more complexities with which a home health administrator must cope. Table 2–2 summarizes the preceding discussion of types of agencies, comparing each type of agency according to governing body, role of the professional advisory committee, client case mix/services provided, and revenue sources.

REFERENCES

Anderson, H.J. 1986. Two recent home healthcare mergers may signal consolidation. *Modern Healthcare* 16:118–119.

Cherkasky, M. 1949. The Montefiore Hospital home care program. *American Journal of Public Health* 39:163–166.

Conditions of participation. Home health agencies. 1968. *Federal Register* 33:12090–12098.

Cunningham, R.M. Jr. 1985. The evolution of hospice. Part 1. *Hospitals* 59:124–126.

Ginzberg, E., et al. 1984. *Home health care.* Totowa, NJ: Rowman & Allanheld.

Health Care Financing Administration (HCFA). 1996. *Medicare Home Health Agency Manual.* HCFA Pub. 11, Transmittal 277 (rev). Washington, DC:U.S. Department of Health and Human Services.

Morris, R., and K. Christie. 1995. Initiating hospice care. *Home Healthcare Nurse* 13:21–26.

Moyer, N. 1986. Public policy, politics, and home health care. *Home Healthcare Nurse* 4:7–12.

Mundinger, M.O. 1983. *Home care controversy.* Gaithersburg, MD: Aspen.

National Association for Home Care (NAHC). 1993. *NAHC Report.* Report no. 528. Washington, DC: NAHC.

National Association for Home Care (NAHC). 1995. *Basic statistics about home care.* Washington, DC: NAHC.

National Hospice Organization (NHO). 1984. *The Basics of Hospice* (pamphlet). Arlington, VA.

National Hospice Organization (NHO). 1995. *Hospice fact sheet.* Arlington, VA.

O'Malley, S.T. 1986. Reimbursement issues. In *Home health care nursing: Administrative and clinical perspectives,* edited by S. Stuart-Siddal, 23–82. Gaithersburg, MD: Aspen.

Smith, J.A. 1983. *The idea of health.* New York: Teachers College Press.

Stewart, J.E. 1979. *Home health care.* St. Louis: Mosby.

Woodham-Smith, C. 1970. *Florence Nightingale: 1820–1910.* London: Fontana.

PART II

Standards for Home Health Agencies

CHAPTER 3

Medicare Conditions of Participation

Peggie Reid Webb

This chapter presents a discussion of the major regulatory requirement that affects the operation of the Medicare-certified home health agency (HHA): the Medicare conditions of participation (Department of Health and Human Services, August 1989, July 1991, September 1991). The conditions of participation are given in a document by the same name that sets forth the requirements that must be met by an organization to achieve and maintain designation as a Medicare-certified provider of home health services. As home health care agencies struggle to design service delivery systems that can successfully accommodate the demands imposed by an ever-changing health care environment, a basic understanding of the conditions of participation remains essential. The following discussion is intended to enhance the reader's understanding of the conditions and how they may be operationalized by the HHA to demonstrate the compliance necessary to remain a Medicare-certified home health agency.

Each of the conditions in Subpart B, Administration, and Subpart C, Furnishing of Services, is presented below as written in Part 484, Conditions of Participation: Home Health Agencies (authority: §§1102, 1861, 1871, and 1891 of the Social Security Act [42 U.S.C. 1302, 1395x, 1395hh, and 1395bbb]). With one exception, this is followed by a discussion of the conditions and related policies, procedures, and practices that reflect the intent of the conditions. A full discussion of §484.38, Condition of Participation: Qualifying To Furnish Outpatient Physi-

cal Therapy or Speech Pathology Services, is beyond the scope of this chapter. For detailed information, the reader is referred to the sources (conditions) cited therein.

Although the content of each condition has been extrapolated, the reader should have Part 484, Conditions of Participation: Home Health Agencies, available in its entirety because Subpart A, General Provisions, which defines the basis and scope of the home health agency program, definitions relative to the operation of the home health agency and personnel qualifications, is not reported in detail here. Furthermore, the appendix, which includes the addenda for states incorporating requirements higher than those imposed by the conditions, is not included in this chapter.

SUBPART B: ADMINISTRATION

§486.10—Condition of Participation: Patient Rights

The patient has a right to be informed of his or her rights. The HHA must promote and protect the exercise of these rights.

(a) Standard: Notice of rights.

    (1) The HHA must provide the patient with a written notice of the patient's rights in advance of furnishing care to the patient or during the initial evaluation visit before the initiation of treatment.

(2) The HHA must maintain documentation showing that it has complied with the requirements of this section.

(b) Standard: Exercise of rights and respect for property and person.

(1) The patient has the right to exercise his or her rights as a patient of the HHA.

(2) The patient's family or guardian may exercise the patient's rights when the patient has been judged incompetent.

(3) The patient has the right to have his or her property treated with respect.

(4) The patient has the right to voice grievances regarding treatment or care that is (or fails to be) furnished or regarding the lack of respect for property by anyone who is furnishing services on behalf of the HHA and must not be subjected to discrimination or reprisal for doing so.

(5) The HHA must investigate complaints made by a patient or the patient's family or guardian regarding treatment or care that is (or fails to be) furnished or regarding the lack of respect for the patient's property by anyone furnishing services on behalf of the HHA and must document both the existence of the complaint and the resolution of the complaint.

(c) Standard: Right to be informed and to participate in planning care and treatment.

(1) The patient has the right to be informed, in advance, about the care to be furnished and the frequency of visits proposed to be furnished.

(i) The HHA must advise the patient in advance of the disciplines that will furnish care and the frequency of visits proposed to be furnished.

(ii) The HHA must advise the patient in advance of any changes in the plan of care before the change is made.

(2) The patient has the right to participate in the planning of the care.

(i) The HHA must advise the patient in advance of the right to participate in planning the care or treatment and in planning changes in the care or treatment.

(ii) The HHA complies with the requirements of Subpart I of part 489 of this chapter relating to maintaining written policies and procedures regarding advance directives. The HHA must inform and distribute written information to the patient, in advance, concerning its policies on advance directives, including a description of applicable State law.

(d) Standard: Confidentiality of medical records.

The patient has the right to confidentiality of the clinical records maintained by the HHA. The HHA must advise the patient of the agency's policies and procedures regarding disclosure of clinical records.

(e) Standard: Patient liability for payment.

(1) The patient has a right to be advised, before care is initiated, of the extent to which payment for the HHA services may be expected from Medicare or other sources and the extent to which payment may be required from the patient. Before the care is initiated, the HHA must inform the patient, orally and in writing, of—

(i) The extent to which payment may be expected from Medicare, Medicaid, or any other Federally funded or aided programs known to the HHA;

(ii) The charges for services that will not be covered by Medicare; and

(iii) The charges that the individual may have to pay.

(2) The patient has the right to be advised orally and in writing of any changes in the information provided in accordance with paragraph (e)(1) of this section when they occur. The HHA must advise the patient of these changes orally and in writing as soon as possible, but no later than 30 calendar days from the date that the HHA becomes aware of the change.

(f)   Standard: Home health hotline.

The patient has the right to be advised of the availability of the toll-free HHA hotline in the State. When the agency accepts the patient for treatment or care, the HHA must advise the patient in writing of the telephone number of the home health hotline established by the State, the hours of its operation, and that the purpose of the hotline is to receive complaints or questions about the local HHAs.

Clearly, these standards require the HHA to have available for each patient accepted for care written material that delineates the patient's rights while he or she is a recipient of the HHA's care and services. These rights are applicable for all patients accepted for care by the HHA, not just those accepted for care under the Medicare benefit. These rights are specified in a document, usually titled "Bill of Rights" or "Patient Bill of Rights." The document must be written with clarity in language that the patient can reasonably be expected to understand to enable the patient to identify his or her rights while receiving HHA care and services and the recourse available in the event that a patient believes these rights are not being honored. There should be guidelines for review of the document when the patient has limited facility with English and/or limited vision. If the HHA has a significant population, generally 25 percent or more of the HHA's total patient population, for whom English is a secondary language, it is recommended that the HHA have patient rights materials developed in that population's primary language.

At minimum, the document must address the areas cited in standards (a) through (f). In addition to stating the patient's rights, this document may also be used to inform the patient of his or her responsibilities while receiving care. These responsibilities include, but may not be limited to, notifying the HHA when he or she will not be home for a scheduled visit, providing essential medical/psychosocial information to assist in the development of the plan of care, and providing such other information as necessary to enable the HHA to obtain payment for the service(s) rendered. The bill of rights or some other document, signed and dated by the patient, should be incorporated into the clinical record as evidence that a review of patient rights was completed. Other materials may also be reviewed and, where appropriate, signed by the patient before the initiation of care as part of the presentation of patient rights and/or to demonstrate compliance with applicable state requirements, such as advance directives.

Standard (b)(2) states that the patient's family or guardian may exercise the patient's rights when the patient has been judged incompetent. Competence is a legal concept determined by the court. There are often instances, however, in which there are questions regarding the individual's competence in the absence of a legal judgment. In these instances, the question of competence should focus on the patient's decision-making capacity. Suggested criteria for assessing the patient's capacity to make a decision regarding care include the following: the ability to understand relevant facts and values, the ability to weigh a decision within a framework of values and goals, the ability to reason and deliberate about the information received, and the ability to give reasons for the decision considering known facts, the alternatives, and the consequence of the decision to the patient. Whereas competence is a legal absolute, decision-making capacity is relative, dependent on the type of decision that needs to be made vis-à-vis the patient's shifting abilities. To ensure uniformity in determinations about the patient's decision-making capacity, guidelines should be developed for staff. If the patient's condition necessitates the review of patient rights and planning for care with an individual acting on the patient's behalf, this should be thoroughly documented in the admission note.

Although the bill of rights may be considered a "stand alone" document, the HHA must demonstrate congruence between its operational practices and the assurances made in the document. The orientation for staff, including contracted providers, should include a thorough review of patients' rights and staff members' responsibilities relative to these rights. The review of policies, procedures, rules of conduct, standards of care, other related materials, and clinical records should provide evidence of the HHA's awareness of and commitment to patient rights. For example, written policy statements and/or procedures should specify how the HHA accepts, registers, and investigates patient grievances and the person(s) responsible for investigating patient grievances. This responsibility should also be identified in the appropriate position description. Reports of grievances and subsequent follow-up actions should be maintained apart from the clinical records. The report should document the specific redress offered the complainant. A periodic review of these reports, as part of the HHA's performance improvement program, should be conducted to determine whether further study is warranted and to ascertain whether practices in specific operational areas—human resources, administrative, financial, or patient services—contribute to a pattern of recurring grievances.

Another example is the existence of policies/procedures/protocols statements and attendant mechanisms to ensure that the right to be informed and to participate in planning care and treatment is demonstrated as specified in standard (c). Clinical record documentation should consistently reveal recording practices that demonstrate patient–provider interaction in planning for care and evidence that visiting personnel are cognizant of the patient's rights while they are providing care. At minimum, the clinical record should document that the patient was given the opportunity to participate in planning care through mutual determination of the goals or outcomes for care and in the attendant discussion of the disciplines involved in furnishing the care, the treatments/interventions to be provided, the frequency of visits, and the anticipated duration of services. Subsequently, the clinical notes should establish that any modifications to the plan of care, such as a change in a treatment, medication, or visit pattern, and/or

the termination or addition of therapeutic service was discussed with the patient.

Standard (c)(2)(i) requires the agency to ensure that its policies regarding advance directives are made known to the patient before furnishing care and services. Detailed written materials concerning the agency's policies regarding advance directives as well as materials describing applicable state laws must be given to and reviewed with the patient. Evidence that this review has been completed should be documented in the record, whether on a designated form completed as part of the initial evaluation visit or by having the patient or his or her representative sign copies of the advance directive materials for incorporation into the clinical record. Questioning during the interview process should determine whether the patient has an advance directive. The existence of an advance directive, or lack thereof, should be documented in the clinical record. The agency should make known, in writing, community resources that are available to assist the patient who wishes to make an advance directive. The patient must be informed of his or her right to contact the State Agency Hotline with complaints regarding implementation of the advance directive requirement.

Standard (d) requires the HHA to ensure the confidentiality of the patient's clinical record. If the HHA allow portions of the record to remain in the patient's home, HHA staff must instruct the patient and/or primary caregiver(s) regarding their responsibility to maintain the confidentiality of the clinical record and its contents. There should be documentation in the clinical record to substantiate that, when applicable, such instruction has been furnished by HHA staff.

Standard (e) requires the HHA to notify the patient of those services that will be reimbursed by Medicare or other sources and those services that are not covered. Specifically, the patient must be informed orally and in writing of the information stated in standard (e)(1)(i), (ii), and (iii). Documentation in the clinical record must establish that this requirement has been satisfied. Additionally, in the event that there is a change in the payment information initially discussed with the patient, the HHA must have in place a process to ensure that the patient is notified of the change orally and in writing no later than 30 calendar days from the date the HHA becomes aware of the change.

To demonstrate compliance with standard (f), the HHA must provide written information to the patient about the State Hotline number, its purpose, and hours of operation. The HHA must be able to document that this information was given to and reviewed with the patient as part of the admission process.

§484.12—Condition of Participation: Compliance with Federal, State, and Local Laws; Disclosure and Ownership Information; and Accepted Professional Standards and Principles

(a) Standard: Compliance with Federal, State, and local laws and regulations.

The HHA and its staff must operate and furnish services in compliance with all applicable Federal, State, and local laws and regulations. If State or applicable local law provides for the licensure of HHAs, an agency not subject to licensure is approved by the licensing authority as meeting the standards established for licensure.

(b) Standard: Disclosure of ownership and management information.

The HHA must comply with the requirements of Part 420, Subpart C of this chapter. The HHA also must disclose the following information to the State survey agency at the time of the HHA's initial request for certification, for each subsequent survey, and at the time of any change in ownership or management:

(1) The name and address of all persons with an ownership or control interest in the HHA as defined in §§420.201, 420.202, and 420.206 of this chapter.

(2) The name and address of each person who is an officer, a director, an agent, or a managing employee of the HHA as defined in §§420.201, 402.202, and 420.206 of this chapter.

(3) The name and address of the corporation, association, or other company that is responsible for the management of the HHA and the name and address of the chief executive officer and the chairman of the board of directors of that corporation, association, or other company responsible for the management of the HHA.

(c) Standard: Compliance with accepted professional standards and principles.

The HHA and its staff must comply with accepted professional standards and principles that apply to professionals furnishing services in an HHA.

Standard (a) requires that the HHA comply with all applicable federal, state, and local laws and regulations. It is not sufficient to attempt to meet this standard with a single policy that states "The agency will comply with all applicable federal, state, and local laws and regulations." State practice acts, professional standards of practice, codes, and ethics should be available within the agency, as should any applicable local or state communicable disease reporting requirements, Occupational Safety and Health Administration regulations, employment statutes, and other applicable laws, codes, statutes, and regulations. These materials should serve as additional guidelines for the written materials that direct the HHA's operational practices and performance expectations. Evidence of current licensure must be available for each individual as required by state practice acts. Because the number and type of laws and regulations that may affect the operation of an HHA are continually expanding and changing, it is imperative that the HHA develop and maintain an active information network to keep abreast of the changes promulgated by legislative and regulatory bodies.

Meeting standard (b), factor (1) requires the agency to identify those individuals and entities that must be routinely disclosed to the State Agency at the time of the initial certification survey, for each survey, and at the time of any change in the ownership or management of the HHA. The need to communicate the required information to the State Agency on a timely basis should not be ignored. Policy statements relative to the management of the agency should specify that disclosure will occur as part of the survey process and whenever there is any change in the ownership or management of the agency and that updated information will be furnished to the secretary of Health and Human Services, via the State Agency, at intervals between recertification or within 35 days of a written request to do so.

Submitting the appropriate information to the State Agency in a timely basis requires full understanding of the terminology included in standard (b). A discussion of these terms follows.

As defined in §§420.201, 420.203, and 402.206, ownership interest means the possession of equity in the capital, the stock, or the profits of the HHA. A person with ownership or control interest is defined as one who:

- has an ownership interest totaling 5 percent or more in the HHA
- has an indirect ownership interest (i.e., any ownership interest in an entity that has an ownership interest in the HHA, including an ownership interest in any entity that has an indirect ownership interest in the HHA, equal to 5 percent or more in the HHA)
- has a combination of direct and indirect ownership interest equal to 5 percent or more in the HHA
- owns an interest of 5 percent or more in any mortgage, deed or trust, note, or other obligation secured by the HHA if that interest equals at least 5 percent of the value of the property or assets of the HHA
- is an officer or director of an HHA that is organized as a corporation

- is a partner in an HHA that is organized as a partnership

To determine whether the ownership interest exceeds the 5 percent reporting requirement and thus must be disclosed, the amount of indirect ownership is computed by multiplying the percentages of ownership in an entity and the HHA. For example, if A owns 10 percent of the stock in a corporation that owns 80 percent of the HHA, A's ownership in the HHA is 8 percent and must be reported. Conversely, if B owns 80 percent of the stock of a corporation that owns 5 percent of the stock of the HHA, B's interest equates to a 40 percent indirect ownership and need not be reported. When there is a need to determine applicability of disclosure for an individual who has ownership or control interest in any mortgage, deed or trust, note, or other obligation, the percentage of the obligation owned is multiplied by the percentage of the HHA's assets used to secure the obligation. For example, if X owns 20 percent of a note secured by 60 percent of the HHA's assets, X's interest in the provider's assets equates to 12 percent and must be disclosed. Conversely, if Y owns 30 percent of a note secured by 10 percent of the HHA's assets, Y's interest equals 3 percent and need not be reported.

The second factor in this standard requires the HHA to disclose the names and addresses of selected persons and/or organizations having a management responsibility for the HHA. This includes the officers and directors of the governing body of the HHA, any agent, or any managing employee. An agent is defined as any person who has been delegated the authority to obligate or act on behalf of the HHA. A managing employee is one who exercises operational or managerial control over, or directly or indirectly conducts, the day-to-day operation of the agency. Defined in this manner, a managing employee includes, but may not be limited to, a general manager, business manager, administrator, director, supervising physician, or registered nurse.

The third factor states that the agency must also disclose the names and addresses of any entity that is responsible for the management of the agency as well as the name and address of the chief executive officer and the directors of the entity.

There is one other requirement relative to information that must be disclosed by the HHA. §420.203, Disclosure of Hiring of Intermediary's Former Employees, requires the HHA to notify the secretary promptly if it, or its home office (in the case of a chain organization), employs or obtains the services of an individual who, at any time during the year preceding such employment, was employed in a managerial, accounting, auditing, or similar capacity by an agency or organization that currently serves, or at any time during the preceding year served, as a Medicare fiscal intermediary or carrier for the HHA. *Similar capacity* means the performance of essentially the same work functions as those of a manager, accountant, or auditor even though the individual is not so designated by title.

Standard (c) requires the HHA to act to ensure that mechanisms exist to monitor professional staff to verify that their performance meets applicable state practice acts as well as any internally or externally derived professional standards that are used by the HHA for the staff. These mechanisms should be identifiable in the agency's operational procedures and processes. The actions of the HHA relative to demonstrating compliance with this standard should be applicable to those personnel who provide service directly or via contractual arrangement as well as for personnel who, although employed by a facility, provide service to the facility-based HHA's patients.

§484.14—Condition of Participation: Organization, Services, and Administration

Organization, services furnished, administrative control, and lines of authority for the delegation of responsibility down to the patient care level are clearly set forth in writing and are readily identifiable. Administrative and supervisory functions are not delegated to another agency or organization, and all services not furnished directly, including services provided through subunits, are monitored and controlled by the parent agency. If an agency has subunits, appropriate administrative records are maintained for each subunit.

(a) Standard: Services furnished.

Part-time or intermittent skilled nursing and at least one other therapeutic service (physical, speech, or occupational therapy; medical social services; or home health aide services) are made available on a visiting basis in a place of residence used as a patient's home. An HHA must provide at least one of the qualifying services directly through agency employees but may provide the second qualifying service and additional services under arrangements with another agency or organization.

(b) Standard: Governing body.

A governing body (or designated persons so functioning) assumes full legal authority and responsibility for the operation of the agency. The governing body appoints a qualified administrator, arranges for professional advice as required under §484.16, adopts and periodically reviews bylaws or an acceptable equivalent, and oversees the management and fiscal affairs of the agency.

(c) Standard: Administrator.

The administrator, who may also be the supervising physician or registered nurse required under section (d) of this section, organizes and directs the agency's ongoing functions; maintains ongoing liaison among the governing body, the group of professional personnel, and the staff; employs qualified personnel and ensures adequate staff education and evaluations; ensures the accuracy of public information materials and activities; and implements an effective budgeting and accounting system. A qualified person is authorized in writing to act in the absence of the administrator.

(d) Standard: Supervising physician or registered nurse.

The skilled nursing and other therapeutic services furnished are under the supervision and direction of a physician or registered nurse (who preferably has at least 1 year of nursing experience and is a public health nurse). This person, or a similarly qualified alternative, is available at all times during operating hours and participates in all activities relevant to the professional services furnished, including the development of qualifications and the assignment of personnel.

(e) Standard: Personnel policies.

Personnel practices and patient care are supported by appropriate written personnel records. Personnel records include qualifications and licensure that are kept current.

(f) Standard: Personnel under hourly or per visit contracts.

If personnel under hourly or per visit contracts are used by the HHA, there is a written contract between those personnel and the agency that specifies the following:

(1) Patients are accepted for care only by the primary HHA.
(2) The services to be furnished.
(3) The necessity to conform to all applicable agency policies, including personnel qualifications.
(4) The responsibility for participating in developing plans of care.
(5) The manner in which the services will be controlled, coordinated, and evaluated by the primary HHA.
(6) The procedure for submitting clinical and progress notes, scheduling visits, periodic patient evaluation.
(7) The procedures for payment for services furnished under the contract.

(g) Standard: Coordination of patient services.

All personnel furnishing services maintain liaison to ensure that their efforts are coordinated effectively and support the objectives outlined in the plan of care. The clinical record or minutes of care conferences establish that effective interchange, reporting, and coordination of patient care do occur. A written summary report for each patient is sent to the attending physician at least every 62 days.

(h) Standard: Services under arrangements.

Services furnished under arrangements are subject to a written contract conforming with the requirements specified in paragraph (f) of this section and with the requirements of section 1861 (w) of the Act [(42 U.S.C. 1495x(w)].

(i) Standard: Institutional planning.

The HHA, under the direction of the governing body, prepares an overall plan and budget that includes an annual operating budget and a capital expenditure plan.

(1) Annual operating budget.

There is an annual operating budget that includes all anticipated income and expenses related to items that would, under generally accepted accounting principles, be considered income and expense items. However, it is not required that there be prepared, in connection with any budget, an item by item identification of the components of each type of anticipated income or expense.

(2) Capital expenditure plan.

(i) There is a capital plan for at least a 3-year period, including the operating budget year. The plan includes and identifies in detail the anticipated sources of funding for, and the objectives of, each anticipated expenditure of more than $600,000 for items that would, under generally accepted accounting principles, be considered capital items. In determining if a single capital expenditure exceeds $600,000, the cost of studies, surveys, designs, plans, working drawings, specifications, and other activities essential to the acquisition, improvement, modernization, expansion, or replacement of land plant, building, and equipment are included. Expenditures directly or indirectly related to capital expenditures, such as grading, paving, broker commissions, taxes assessed during the construction period, and cost involved in demolishing or razing structures on land, are also included. Transactions that are separated in time but are components of an overall plan or patient care objective are viewed in their entirety without regard to their timing. Other costs related to capital expenditures include title fees; permit and license fees; broker commissions; architect, legal, accounting, and appraisal fees; interest finance; or carrying charges on bonds, notes, and other costs incurred for borrowing funds.

(ii) If the anticipated source of financing is, in any part, the anticipated payment from Title V (Maternal and Child Health and Crippled Children's Services), or Title XVIII (Medicare), or Title XIX (Medicaid) of the Social Security Act, the plan specifies the following:

(A) Whether the proposed capital expenditure is required to conform, or is likely to be required to conform, to current standards, criteria, or plans developed in accordance with the Public Health Service Act or the Mental Retardation Facilities and Community Mental Health Centers Construction Act of 1963.

(B) Whether a capital expenditure proposal has been submitted to the designated planning agency for approval in accordance with section 1122 of the Act (42 U.S.C. 1320a-1) and implementing regulations.

(C) Whether the designated planning agency approved or disapproved the proposed capital expenditure if it was presented to that agency.

(3) Preparation and plan of budget.

The overall plan and budget is prepared under the direction of the governing body of the HHA by a committee consisting of representatives of the governing body, the administrative staff, and the medical staff (if any) of the HHA.

(4) Annual review of the plan and budget.

The overall plan and budget is reviewed and updated at least annually by the committee referred to in paragraph (ii)(3) of this section under the direction of the governing body of the HHA.

(j)   Standard: Laboratory services.

(1) If the HHA engages in laboratory testing outside of the context of assisting an individual in self-administering a test with an appliance that has been cleared for that purpose by the FDA, such testing must be in compliance with all applicable requirements of part 493 of this chapter.

(2) If the HHA chooses to refer specimens for laboratory testing to another laboratory, the referral laboratory must be certified in the appropriate specialties and subspecialties of services in accordance with the applicable requirements of Part 493 of this chapter.

The opening paragraph for this condition provides broad guidelines for the organization and administration of the HHA. Demonstration of compliance with the condition requires the HHA to have written materials that delineate the organization's structure and mechanisms for controlling and monitoring all aspects of the HHA's operation, whether it is freestanding, facility based, or a part of a state or local (city or county) health department. The agency may retain management services to strengthen its administrative proficiency, but decision-making responsibilities must remain within the HHA. It should be clear from the review of written materials to whom responsibility for administration and supervision is delegated and that responsibility for accepting patients for care and carrying out the treatment/interventions specified in the plans of care is reserved exclusively for the HHA. These responsibilities extend to and must be evident in branch offices operated by the agency, but they may be exercised differently in subunits. It should be noted that in the event that an HHA proposes to open a branch location, the State Agency must be notified. The notification must include how the proposed branch meets the definition of a branch office as found in 42 CRF 484.2 as well as a description of how the HHA intends to operate the branch. The HHA will receive written notification of whether the proposed location can be a branch or should be a subunit or independent HHA.

A subunit is defined as a semiautonomous unit under the same governing body as the parent agency that serves patients in a geographical area different from that of the parent agency. By virtue of the distance between the subunit and the parent agency, the former is judged incapable of sharing administration, supervision, and services on a daily basis with the parent agency and therefore must independently meet the conditions. A detailed discussion of characteristics that distinguish a branch office from a subunit is beyond the scope of this chapter. For further information, the reader is referred to Sections 2182 and 2184 of the *State Operations Manual* (Department of Health and Human Services, October 1993) and the state agency responsible for certification and survey activities.

Key to understanding the HHA's structure is the organizational chart. A current table of organization should be available that, at minimum, depicts the governing body, group of professional personnel, finance/budget committee, and all current positions, including positions filled by contracted personnel, as well as the relationships that exist among and between staff members, the governing body, and established committees. When applicable, the table of organization should depict the relationship between the HHA's main or home office and any branch office(s) and/or subunit(s) as well as the relationship with a parent agency or other controlling entity. More than one organizational table may be required to portray accurately the HHA and its relationships. The table(s) of organization should include a legend to define the types of relationships represented (supervisory, advisory, reporting, etc.). The document(s) should indicate the date of approval by the governing body. The table of organization should be reviewed against position descriptions to ensure that personnel, reporting, and/or supervisory relationships are consistent with those identified in the position descriptions.

Collectively, the written policy statements, procedures, guidelines, protocols, and other approved documents relative to the specific areas identified in the nine standards in this condition should clearly delineate the operational practices of the agency and the mechanisms for maintaining management accountability down to the patient care level. A discussion of the nine standards and the factors and elements in these standards follows.

To meet the intent of standard (a), the HHA must ensure that at least one of the qualifying services is provided by employees on an hourly or per visit basis. The term *qualifying service*, as used in this context, should not be confused with the same term used in a reimbursement sense. For Medicare reimbursement purposes, the patient must be admitted to the HHA to receive skilled nursing, physical therapy, and/or speech therapy. Consequently, these three services are known as primary or qualifying services. From a standard compliance standpoint, however, these three disciplines, as well as occupational therapy, medical social services, and home health aide services, are defined as qualifying services.

Health care facility–based agencies may utilize facility personnel to provide a qualifying service as direct employees, but the HHA must be able to demonstrate that this employee is available as needed during the agency's operating hours rather than at the discretion of the facility. Time records should be maintained for all personnel utilized in this manner.

Standard (b) addresses the function of the governing body. The bylaws exist as the document that codifies the governing body as the forum for setting the rules for the performance of the work of the HHA. At minimum, the bylaws, or an equivalent document, should specify the governing body's responsibility to appoint a qualified administrator, to maintain an advisory group of professional personnel, to adopt and subsequently review and revise the bylaws or an equivalent document to ensure that it is accurate, and to oversee the management and fiscal affairs of the agency. Minutes of governing body and committee meetings should provide evidence that the governing body receives sufficient information verbally and via written reports on a timely basis to enhance that body's ability to make decisions that contribute to organizational rationality.

Standard (c) requires the HHA to employ an individual who, subject to the approval of the governing body, develops, organizes, and manages the operation of the HHA by following established policies, procedures, and standards and rules of conduct. The administrator must meet the qualifications cited in the definition of administrator given in Subpart A: General Provisions, §484.2: Definitions, as well as any additional requirements set forth in the position description. Policies, procedures, and the position description should clearly convey the administrator's responsibility and commensurate authority, as delegated by the governing body, for organizational performance. A review of governing body, committee, and/or staff meeting minutes, reports, personnel records, public information materials, and similar sources should provide clear evidence that the administrator is fulfilling his or her mandated responsibilities. That the administrator ensures adequate staff education should be evident from a review of the continuing learning activities of those personnel utilized in the patient care and services program.

The person designated in writing to act in the administrator's absence should be qualified to do so. The individual should hold the requisite qualifications stated in the position description and be oriented to the administrator's role responsibilities. In the absence of the requisite qualifications, the governing body may waive this requirement to allow for the appointment of an individual to act on a temporary basis for the administrator. The decision to do so should be documented in governing body meeting minutes or some other document, such as a letter to the incumbent notifying him or her of the temporary appointment. It is necessary, however, that the incumbent meet the basic requirements set forth in the definition of administrator: to wit, be a licensed physician or registered nurse or have training and experience in health service administration and at least 1 year of supervisory or administrative experience in home health care or related programs.

Standard (d) specifies that the HHA must also employ a supervising physician or registered nurse to whom responsibility and authority are delegated for implementing the patient service program and for ensuring high-quality patient care in accordance with the HHA's purpose, objectives, philosophy, and policies. This responsibility is properly demonstrated through the execution of systematic processes for planning, coordinating, implementing, controlling, and evaluating those components that make up the patient service program. Specific activities for which the incumbent may be responsible or in which he or she may participate include, but may not be limited to, recruitment, selection, orientation, and evaluation of personnel; planning for new programs and/or modifications to existing programs; coaching staff for improved performance; developing and maintaining measurable standards of quality; and participating in strategic planning and decision making. Because a registered nurse usually fills this position, the term *supervising nurse* is used for the remainder of this chapter.

The supervising nurse must be readily available either on site or via a telecommunication system. The manner in which availability is demonstrated is a management decision. Nevertheless, it must be apparent that the supervising nurse is available to the HHA on a full-time basis. The position description, personnel record, or other source must identify the person authorized to act as the qualified alternate for the supervising nurse.

To meet the intent of standard (e), the HHA should have written policies that set forth the existing rules, regulations, benefits, and performance expectations for all personnel. Position descriptions should be established for each category of personnel that set forth the qualifications and duties required for the position. Personnel records must be maintained with materials that verify that each employee, including contracted personnel, possesses the requisite qualifications and that applicable personnel policies, such as health examination, orientation, and performance evaluations, are being followed. A copy of the professional license may be made if this is allowed by state law and agency policy. It is permissible to retain current professional licenses for all personnel in one separate file or a display case. It is recognized that some states prohibit copying of the professional license. In those states, the HHA must identify through the state licensing entity the accepted method(s) for documenting that personnel hold a current license. When a facility-based agency provides service using facility personnel, the credentials for these individuals should also be available.

Many agencies rail against the Medicare requirement to retain a current copy of the driver's license and automobile liability insurance for visiting personnel, citing the need to keep abreast of varying expiration dates as particularly troublesome. It is toward the elimination of one source of irritation and complaint that the reader is reminded that the conditions do not require the agency to maintain current drivers' licenses and automobile liability insurance; rather, in the absence of a state requirement, it is a requirement established by the organization. When such a requirement is established by the HHA, it must be met. It is possible to establish a policy that delineates the expectation that designated personnel will present evidence of a current driver's license and liability insurance at the time of hire, will keep these documents current and available for presentation at the request of the supervising nurse or other designated person, and will notify the HHA of any change in the status of the license without the attendant requirement that the HHA maintain evidence that these documents are indeed current.

Hourly or per visit contracts should be written with specificity to delineate clearly the manner in which the agency will meet the requirements in standard (f). For example, it is not sufficient simply to state that the agency will control, coordinate, and evaluate the services provided. The contract should identify the processes in place to control, coordinate, and evaluate the services. This includes the identification by title of personnel who are involved in these activities as well as any other relevant activities, such as the quarterly review of records, annual program evaluation, or other quality improvement initiatives. If payment for services is contingent upon the timely receipt of all required clinical record documentation or other materials, this should be stated in the contract. The contract must include a clause that allows the Controller General of the United States, the Department of Health and Human Services, and their duly authorized representatives access to the contractor's contract, books, documents, and records until the expiration of 4 years after the services are furnished under the contract when the cost or value of services is $10,000 or more over a 12-month period. The contract should also specify the terms and conditions for renewing and terminating the contract.

It is not necessary for a facility-based agency to have a contract with the facility for the use of facility personnel when these personnel provide care to the agency's patients during their usual hospital working shift. If the personnel provide care outside their usual shift, however, a contract would be necessary. The facility-based agency should develop a written agreement with the facility department or unit that specifies the arrangement that exists for the utilization and supervision of personnel and the provision of patient care. The HHA should maintain a current list of personnel who are available from a facility department.

Coordination of service is the focus of standard (g). At the risk of oversimplification, coordination is patient-focused, outcome-oriented planning and communication. Are the care providers, the caregivers, and the patient, to the extent possible, working in tandem to achieve a stated outcome? Are care providers' visits planned so as not to tire the patient? Are the occupational therapist's efforts to increase independence in activities of daily living (ADLs) supported by the activities of the home health aide to assist rather than perform selected ADLs for the patient? As an aside, effective communication is not one-way communication. Too often, it is assumed that all written communication must emanate from a registered nurse, either the nurse functioning as the primary nurse or the nurse's supervisor. All care providers should be oriented to their responsibility to document pertinent information that fosters the coordination of services. Patient conference minutes, case management notes, and other interdisciplinary communication tools are not the exclusive purview of the registered nurse. Coordination of services is an organizational imperative if positive outcomes are to be achieved in the most cost-effective and cost-efficient manner.

Policy statements and/or procedures should specify the responsibilities of identified direct service and/or supervisory personnel to ensure that coordination of services is a linchpin of patient care. That coordination of services is an active and ongoing process should be verifiable through a review of the clinical records and case conference reports (a copy or summary of case conferences should be retained in the clinical record). Such a review would demonstrate timely initiation of ordered and needed services or communication to the physician regarding the inability to provide the service(s) to afford the physician the option of obtaining the needed services from another source; personnel awareness of the goals for care established for each therapeutic discipline, as evident in the provision of treatments and interventions in a complementary manner; scheduling of visits to foster maximum participation of the patient in the plan of care; timely communication among personnel regarding the patient's response to treatment; any impediment(s) to full implementation of the plan of care and collaborative efforts to remove or minimize the impediment(s); and planning for the termination of service(s).

The record would also contain a succinct summary report to the attending physician at least every 62 days. It should be noted that the conditions refer to a 62-day period for the conduct of several activities; as a practical matter, this period may range from 60 to 62 days depending on the 2-month period covered. Subpart A: General Provision, §484.2: Definitions defines the summary report as "the compilation of the pertinent factors from a patient's clinical notes and progress notes that is submitted to the patient's physician." This pertinent information should be reported in a succinct, concise manner. Key words here are *pertinent*, *succinct*, and *concise*. Does the physician really need to know that the home health aide provided "personal care, hair and nail care, and food shopping" or that "RN supervises HHA every 2 weeks"? Why does the physician need to know "Blood obtained for PPT on 2/16/97 and transported to lab per order"? Does the physician take comfort in knowing "PT and OT continue to visit 2× wk"? Such statements are provider rather than patient focused and are of little value in assessing the patient's response, or lack thereof, to the interventions furnished.

The purpose of the summary report is to furnish the physician with information on which to base decisions about the efficacy of the plan of care and to make necessary modifications to the plan. If the summary is to serve this purpose, not only must it contain precise, objective information, but also it must be sent to the physician at the time the plan of care is developed for recertification. Some agencies send the 60-day summary report on a calendar basis or other 60-day time period established by the organization. Too often, this means that the physician receives the summary report several days or a week or more after the plan has been recertified. This practice effectively defeats the purpose of the summary report. It should be noted that the patient's condition may require a summary report to the physician at other than 60-day intervals, but these instances are infrequent. In such a situation, a progress note to the physician is generally more appropriate. Finally, a well-written summary report serves to support the organization's claim for reimbursement for the services rendered to date.

The summary report should answer questions such as: What does the physician need to know about the patient's condition and response to assess the effectiveness of the plan of care? In what measurable ways has the patient's condition changed as a result of the interventions provided? If the patient did not respond to a particular intervention, what changes were made in the plan of care, and what were the consequences? Does the patient's response over the past 62 days justify the request to continue service for another 62-day period? These or similar questions are designed to elicit information that fosters a descriptive portrayal of the patient's response to all the therapeutic interventions provided, to justify the HHA's claim for reimbursement, and, where appropriate, to support the need for continued care.

Standard (h) indicates that the content requirements for contracts arranged with groups or organizations for therapeutic services are the same as those specified in standard (f). Thus such contracts must address the areas cited in standard (f).

The focus of standard (i) is the agency's budget and capital expenditure plan. The HHA must have an annual budget that includes all anticipated income and expenses, consistent with generally accepted accounting principles, and a capital expenditure plan for at least a 3-year period when expenditures of more than $600,000 are anticipated for acquisition, expansion, or replacement of land, plant, building, and/or equipment. If a capital expenditure plan is necessary, it should conform to the requirements set forth in factor (2) of this standard.

Minutes of meetings or other written materials must document that the overall plan and budget is/was developed under the direction of the governing body by a committee that includes representatives of the governing body and the administrative staff. If the agency staff include physicians, a physician must also be represented on the committee. This standard does not require a physician member of the group of professional personnel to be represented on the committee. The dated minutes should document that the committee responsible for preparation of the budget meets at least annually, under the direction of the governing body, to update the annual plan and budget. Governing body minutes should document discussion, review, and approval of the annual plan and budget. For the facility-based HHA, it may be necessary to delineate the sequence of events that occur as a matter of course for the development of the annual budget for the facility to demonstrate how agency administrative representation is ensured when the budget committee exists as a standing committee of the facility's governing body.

Standard (j) requires the HHA to have evidence that it furnishes laboratory services in compliance with Part 493, Laboratory Services. For most agencies, obtaining a Clinical Laboratory Improvement Amendment (CLIA) waiver is sufficient to allow for the performance of certain tests that are waived. These tests are defined as simple laboratory examinations and procedures that are cleared by the FDA for home use, employ methodologies that are so simple and accurate as to render the likelihood of erroneous results negligible, or pose no reasonable risk of harm to the patient if the test is performed incorrectly. Examples of tests that may be performed under the CLIA waiver are as follows:

- dipstick or tablet reagent urinalysis (non-automated) for the following:
    1. bilirubin
    2. glucose
    3. hemoglobin
    4. ketone
    5. leukocytes
    6. nitrite
    7. pH

8. protein
9. specific gravity
10. urobilinogen

- fecal occult blood
- ovulation tests (visual color comparison tests for human luteinizing hormone)
- urine pregnancy tests (visual color comparison tests)
- erythrocyte sedimentation rate (nonautomated)
- hemoglobin–copper sulfate (nonautomated)
- blood glucose by glucose monitoring devices cleared by the FDA specifically for home use
- spun microhematocrit
- hemoglobin by single analyte instruments with self-contained or component features to perform specimen/reagent interaction, providing direct measurement and readout (e.g., HemaCue).

A discussion of the conditions and requirements that must be met by the HHA that furnishes a wider range of laboratory services is beyond the scope of this chapter. The reader is referred to Part 493, Laboratory Services. If the HHA furnishes laboratory services under arrangement, the HHA must ensure that the contracting laboratory meets the requirements of Part 493, Laboratory Services. The HHA should ensure that the referral laboratory is appropriately certified.

§484.16—Condition of Participation: Group of Professional Personnel

A group of professional personnel, which includes at least a physician and one registered nurse (preferably a public health nurse), and with appropriate representation from other professional disciplines, establishes and annually reviews the agency's policies governing the scope of services offered, admission and discharge policies, medical supervision and plans of care, emergency care, clinical records, personnel qualifications, and program evaluation.

At least one member of the group is neither an owner nor an employee of the agency.

(a) Standard: Advisory and evaluation function.

The group of professional personnel meets frequently to advise the agency on professional issues, to participate in the evaluation of the agency's program, and to assist the agency in maintaining liaison with other health care providers in the community and in the agency's community information program. The meetings are documented by dated minutes.

To meet this condition, there must be a committee composed of professionals who meet the stated representation requirements and actively function in an advisory and evaluation capacity. Additional representatives may be elected or appointed at the agency's discretion. The purview of the group of professional personnel includes the establishment and annual review of all policies governing the agency's patient care and service program, including program evaluation as well as evaluation of the qualifications of personnel utilized in the program. It is not necessary for the group to establish personnel qualifications or some types of policies when this responsibility is reserved for a higher authority. This frequently occurs in public health agencies operated by state, county, or city health departments. In this instance, the group should review these materials and make such recommendations as the group believes are appropriate. It should be noted that the governing body, having assumed full legal authority and responsibility for the operation of the agency, must approve or reject newly developed and/or revised policies and personnel qualifications. Facility-based agencies may have to involve additional personnel in the chain of command to the governing body or other established committees authorized to act for the governing body on these specific matters. The group is also responsible for ensuring that the annual program evaluation is completed, reviewed, approved, and subsequently submitted to the governing body.

It is the agency's responsibility to ensure that the group comprises individuals who are willing and available to participate on the committee. Agency bylaws or an equivalent document should provide for the election or appointment of members and for the replacement of members who are unable to participate actively on the committee. To ensure full representation at each meeting, it may be appropriate to have more than one representative for each required discipline. Should a member, particularly the physician member, not be present as planned, there should be documentation to establish that the member was afforded the opportunity for input regarding agenda topics and that his or her comments, concerns, or questions were subsequently communicated to the group.

Meeting minutes must document that the group has fulfilled its mandated responsibilities. Additionally, the minutes should document that, as necessary, the members, acting in an advisory capacity, provide guidance and technical assistance in their particular area of competence for the purpose of strengthening the agency's program. Furthermore, the minutes of the group's meetings should substantiate that the actions of the group are designed to ensure that the community served, broadly defined to include consumers, referral sources, physicians, and community organizations, is knowledgeable about and supportive of the work and objectives of the agency as evidenced by a willingness to use the agency's services.

Because of its mandated responsibilities, it is recommended that the group of professional personnel meet on a quarterly or semi-annual basis. It is questionable if an annual meeting is sufficient to keep the members informed of activities of the HHA, obtain professional advice on external and internal issues impacting the agency, and assure that this body functions effectively.

§484.18: Condition of Participation: Acceptance of Patients, Plan of Care, Medical Supervision

Patients are accepted for treatment on the basis of a reasonable expectation that the patient's medical, nursing, and social needs can be met adequately by the agency in the patient's place of residence. Care follows a written plan of care established and periodically reviewed by a doctor of medicine, osteopathy, or podiatric medicine.

(a) Standard: Plan of care.

The plan of care developed in consultation with the agency staff covers all pertinent diagnoses, including mental status, types of services and equipment required, frequency of visits, prognosis, rehabilitation potential, functional limitations, activities permitted, nutritional requirements, medications and treatments, any safety measures to protect against injury, instructions for timely discharge or referral, and other appropriate items. If a physician refers a patient under a plan of care that cannot be completed until after an evaluation visit, the physician is consulted to approve additions or modification to the original plan. Orders for therapy services include the specific procedures and modalities to be used and the amount, frequency, and duration. The therapist and other agency personnel participate in developing the plan of care.

(b) Standard: Periodic review of plan of care.

The total plan of care is reviewed by the attending physician and HHA personnel as often as the severity of the patient's condition requires, but at least once every 62 days. Agency professional staff promptly alert the physician to any changes that suggest a need to alter the plan of care.

(c) Standard: Conformance with physician's orders.

Drugs and treatments are administered by agency staff only as ordered by the physician. The nurse or therapist immediately records and signs oral orders and obtains the physician's countersignature. Agency staff check all medicines a patient may be taking to identify possible ineffective drug therapy or adverse reactions, significant side effects, drug allergies, and contraindicated medication and promptly report any problems to the physician.

At the risk of oversimplification, this condition requires the HHA to demonstrate how it will ensure that patients are accepted for care only after an analysis of externally and internally derived information supports an expectation that the patient will benefit from the agency's services and that care and services will be provided under the general supervision of the patient's physician in a manner consistent with the agency's established policies and procedures. The HHA must have written policies and procedures stating the process for accepting and evaluating referrals, designate those practitioners who may act as the patient's physician, specify the criteria that are considered in determining whether the patient may be accepted for care, and determine the manner in which the physician's orders may be communicated to the agency to ensure the prompt initiation of care. If the HHA accepts orders from a podiatrist, these orders must be within the podiatrist's scope of practice as defined in the applicable state practice act. Written policy/procedures should address the electronic transfer of physician's orders, mechanisms for the timely certification and recertification of the plan of care with authenticated and dated physician orders, and the procedures for receipt and countersignature of the physician's verbal order.

The agency's mechanism for conduct of the initial evaluation visit should ensure that the patient assessment is completed on a timely basis by staff holding the requisite skills to perform this activity. This has become critically important because of the more complex needs of an increasingly diverse home care population. The subsequent analysis of assessment data with interdisciplinary collaboration as warranted must be sufficient to determine the most appropriate course of care for the patient to achieve desired outcomes. Collectively, the HHA's processes should convey a sound understanding of the agency's obligations once the patient is accepted for care as well as recognition of the physician's responsibility for medical supervision.

The Health Care Financing Administration's (HCFA's) Form 485 (Home Health Certification and Plan of Treatment) is widely used as the plan of care, with HCFA Form 487 (Addendum to Plan of Treatment or Medical Update) being used to provide additional information as necessary. Agency policy should require the plan of care to contain the information specified in standard (a) with modification of the plan as necessary after completion of the initial evaluation visit by professional personnel. Policy statements should also require professional staff to collaborate with the attending physician to evaluate the patient's response to the plan of care and to modify the plan as needed throughout the course of care. The treatments and interventions ordered should be specified for each discipline with a visit frequency that is appropriate to meet the goals established for each therapeutic service. The goals or outcomes identified on the plan of care should be concise and reasonable considering the time-limited nature of the Medicare benefit. The clinical record should establish that, to the greatest degree possible, the goals were developed jointly with the patient or individual designated to act on the patient's behalf. The visit frequency may be ordered using a visit range. The review of clinical records, however, should verify that visit ranges are used to allow the staff to adjust visits readily to meet the patient's needs rather than to accommodate the ebb and flow of staff levels and patient census.

In sum, the plan of care should reflect an aggressive treatment program for the attainment of the highest possible level of independent functioning for the patient. It should exist as a dynamic rather than a static document, ever changing in reaction to the patient's documented responses. A review of the plan(s) of care in the clinical records must document that these requirements are met.

Standard (b) requires the review of the total plan of treatment as often as the severity of the patient's condition requires, but at least every 62 days. A perfunctory review is a disservice to the patient and frequently results in a plan of care that is a less than accurate prescription for care. Written procedures should require the professionals who have provided care to participate in this review to ensure that the plan is an accurate prescription for care vis-à-vis the patient's status. The agency should have written procedures to ensure the thoroughness and timeliness of this review. It is recommended that this review occur in conjunction with the continuing 62-day review of records required by §484.82 and discussed later in this chapter. The agency should also have established procedures to determine the accuracy of the plan of care when the patient is hospitalized during any certification period.

To demonstrate compliance with standard (c), HHA policy and procedure should require, and the clinical records should document, that care and services are provided only as ordered by the physician. Written policies should specify the necessity for a physician's order whenever there is a change in the plan of care, with the order being authenticated by the physician on a timely basis as identified in agency policy. This includes changes in the frequency of visits. After all, the attainment of the goals established for care is predicated on the provision of specified interventions at specified intervals; any change in this frequency in effect changes the plan of care and as such must be approved by the physician. To minimize the need to contact the physician each time there is a change in the visit pattern, consideration should be given to the use of visit ranges and a specified number of as-needed visits for identified potential problems that would necessitate additional visits.

As stated earlier in this section, all plans of care must be signed and dated by the physician. Policy statements should identify those professionals who may accept the physician's verbal order and require the physician's countersignature to be obtained as soon as possible. The phrase *as soon as possible* should be defined in writing by the HHA as within a reasonable time frame considering any applicable state law or regulation and/or accrediting body requirement.

Compliance with standard (c) requires that agency staff check the patient's medication regimen and promptly report any problems to the physician. There must be written policies relative to the administration and monitoring of drugs and biologicals. The clinical record must contain a current drug profile that identifies physician-ordered medications as well as any over-the-counter medication the patient is taking. At minimum, the profile should include the medication name, dose, route of administration, frequency, date ordered, and date discontinued. The profile should include the signature of the registered nurse(s) who initiates or updates the profile. Unless required by agency policy, it is not necessary for the physician to approve the patient's use of over-the-counter medication. The physician would be notified if the use of an over-the-counter medication is contraindicated or problematic, however.

Mechanisms should exist to ensure that monitoring of the patient's medication regimen occurs with a degree of regularity sufficient to recognize drug allergies or sensitivity, ineffective drug therapy, and/or adverse reactions and to implement promptly and appropriately actions for any untoward response. It is not unusual for the medication regimen to be altered by the physician during the course of care, but it is not necessary for agency staff to obtain written confirmation of the veracity of changes in the regimen that occur as a consequence of communication between the patient and the physician and/or the physician and the pharmacist. Certainly, the staff member would consult the physician if there are questions concerning a new or changed medication. The changes or additions should be noted on the medication profile in the clinical record and included in the plan of care when it is developed for recertification.

SUBPART C: FURNISHING OF SERVICES

§484.30—Condition of Participation: Skilled Nursing Services

The HHA furnishes skilled nursing services by or under the supervision of a registered nurse in accordance with the plan of care.

(a) Standard: Duties of the registered nurse.

The registered nurse makes the initial evaluation visit, regularly reevaluates the patient's nursing needs, initiates the plan of care and necessary revision, furnishes those services requiring substantial and specialized nursing skill, initiates appropriate preventive and rehabilitation nursing procedures, prepares clinical and progress notes, coordinates services, informs the physician and other personnel of changes in the patient's condition and needs, counsels the patient and family in meeting nursing and related needs, participates in inservice programs, and supervises and teaches other nursing personnel.

(b) Standard: Duties of the licensed practical nurse.

The licensed practical nurse furnishes services in accordance with agency policies; prepares clinical and progress notes; assists the physician and registered nurse in performing specialized procedures; prepares equipment and materials for treatments, observing aseptic technique as required; and assists the patient in learning appropriate self-care techniques.

This condition requires the HHA to have written policies that clearly designate the scope of skilled nursing services offered, including those services characterized as specialty nursing services; the manner in which these services are provided, supervised, and evaluated; and the mechanisms for ensuring that skilled nursing service is furnished in accordance with the plan of care and agency policies. Position descriptions, policy statements, and procedures should delineate the duties and performance expectations for the registered nurse and for the licensed practical nurse when this category of personnel is used for service. These duties should be consistent with state practice acts and should reflect current standards generally for professional nursing and specifically for nursing practice specialties. Agency policy should specify under what circumstances, if any, the initial evaluation visit may be made by a therapist instead of the registered nurse.

The clinical record must document the provision of skilled nursing care consistent with the plan of care and agency policy and procedures. The clinical record should demonstrate that the nurse understands the legal implications of clinical recording and documents accordingly (documentation is discussed further under §484.48, Condition of Participation: Clinical Records). Because the registered nurse is delegated the responsibility for coordination of services, the clinical record should document communication with the nursing staff and other providers to ensure that there is continuity of care among the nursing staff and the other disciplines involved with the patient. This is not to suggest that the responsibility to document interdisciplinary communication rests solely with nursing. Evidence to the contrary notwithstanding, the nurse is not endowed with an inalienable right to function as secretary for other members of the health team. Rather, it is the nurse's responsibility, often working in cooperation with the supervising nurse, to ensure that communication for coordination and evaluation of patient care does occur throughout the period when services are provided.

It should be clear from the review of clinical records that the difference between the registered nurse and the licensed practical nurse is recognized. The decision to assign the licensed practical nurse should be based on the patient's needs, not the HHA's need for a nurse to make a visit. The HHA that routinely assigns the licensed practical nurse to make visits without sound criteria for assignment does so at its own peril.

§484.32—Condition of Participation: Therapy Services

Any therapy service offered by the HHA directly or under arrangement is given by a qualified therapist or by a qualified therapist assistant under the supervision of a qualified therapist and in accordance with the plan of care. The qualified therapist assists the physician in evaluating level of function, helps develop the plan of care (revising as necessary), prepares clinical and progress notes, advises and consults with the family and other agency personnel, and participates in inservice programs.

(a) Standard: Supervision of physical therapist assistant and occupational therapy assistant.

Services furnished by a qualified physical therapist assistant or qualified occupational therapy assistant may be furnished under the supervision of a qualified physical or occupational therapist. A physical therapist assistant or occupational therapy assistant performs services planned, delegated, and supervised by the therapist; assists in preparing clinical notes and progress reports; and participates in educating the patient and family and in inservice programs.

(b) Standard: Supervision of speech therapy services.

Speech therapy services are furnished only by or under supervision of a qualified speech pathologist or audiologist.

This condition requires the HHA to establish written materials that govern the scope of each therapy service offered. The policies and related procedures should ensure that services are provided by or under the supervision of a qualified therapist. Policy statements should also specify the manner in which therapy services will be supervised, coordinated, and evaluated. The process for achieving these objectives should be congruous with the processes identified in any contractual arrangements for these services. Position descriptions should establish the requisite qualifications and duties for the therapist and assistant. These duties should include the functions identified in this condition and should be consistent with applicable state practice acts and professional standards. The manner in which therapy assistants are supervised should be defined in writing and be consistent with applicable state regulations and/or practice acts. For the speech therapist who is completing the clinical fellowship year, the HHA must define in writing how this individual will be supervised by a qualified speech/language pathologist. The position description and other related materials should ensure that the qualified therapist possesses the skills, knowledge, and ability to develop and implement in collaboration with the physician, as appropriate, a therapy program directed toward the attainment of measurable, functionally defined patient outcomes. A review of the clinical records must document that therapy services are provided consistent with the plan of care and with applicable policies and procedures.

The requirement that contracted therapists, and assistants if utilized, participate in inservice programs is frequently disregarded. At minimum, the HHA must be able to demonstrate that these personnel have attended inservice programs on Occupational Safety and Health Administration requirements and other applicable regulatory requirements. It is incumbent upon the HHA to be able to provide evidence that this requirement is considered in planning for and evaluating the provision of therapy service. The agency should maintain a record of the therapy staff's participation in continuing education activities, including inservice programs. Contracted providers should be held accountable for maintaining evidence of participation in inservice education.

§484.34—Condition of Participation: Medical Social Service

If the agency furnishes medical social services, those services are given by a qualified social worker or by a qualified social work assistant under the supervision of a qualified social worker and in accordance with the plan of care. The social worker assists the physician and other team members in understanding the significant social and emotional factors related to the health problems, participates in the development of the plan of care, prepares clinical and progress notes, works with the family, uses appropriate community resources, participates in discharge planning and inservice programs, and acts as a consultant to other agency personnel.

This condition requires the HHA to have written materials that clearly establish the scope of medical social services offered and the manner in which services will be provided, coordinated, supervised, and evaluated. Written policies/procedures, position descriptions, and contracts, if applicable, should specify the mechanisms that exist to ensure that the provision of medical social service meets the requirements in this condition as well as applicable state practice acts and professional standards. When social work assistants are utilized, policies, procedures, job descriptions, and contracts, if applicable, should specify the plan for providing supervision by a qualified social worker.

A review of clinical records should establish that the social service interventions are provided as ordered in the plan of care and that staff conform to agency policies when providing services. When indicated, the clinical record should document the social worker's efforts to assist other team members to understand the impact of social and emotional problems on the patient's ability to participate effectively in the plan of care. Where appropriate, the clinical records and/or case conference should also establish the social worker's involvement in discharge planning. The statement made earlier regarding the therapist's participation in continuing education activities, including inservice programs, is applicable to the social work staff as well.

§484.36—Condition of Participation: Home Health Aide Services

---

Home health aides are selected on the basis of such factors as a sympathetic attitude toward the care of the sick; ability to read, write, and carry out directions; and maturity and ability to deal effectively with the demands of the job. Aides are closely supervised to ensure their competence in providing care. For home health services furnished (either directly or through arrangements with other organizations) after August 14, 1990, the HHA must use individuals who meet the personnel qualifications specified in §484.4 for home health aide.

(a) Standard: Home health aide training.

(1) Content and duration of training.

The aide training program must address each of the following subject areas through classroom and supervised practical training.

(i) Communication skills.

(ii) Observation, reporting, and documentation of patient status and the care or service furnished.

(iii) Reading and recording temperature, pulse, and respiration.

(iv) Basic infection control procedures.

(v) Basic elements of body functioning and changes in body functioning that must be reported to an aide's supervisor.

(vi) Maintenance of a clean, safe, and healthy environment.

(vii) Recognizing emergencies and knowledge of emergency procedures.

(viii) The physical, emotional, and developmental needs of and ways to work with the populations served by the HHA, including the need for respect for the patient, his or her privacy, and his or her property.

(ix) Appropriate and safe techniques in personal hygiene and grooming that include—

(A) Bed bath;

(B) Sponge, tub, or shower bath;

(C) Shampoo (sink, tub, or bed);

(D) Nail and skin care;

(E) Oral hygiene; and

(F) Toileting and elimination.

(x) Safe transfer techniques and ambulation.

(xi) Normal range of motion and positioning.

(xii) Adequate nutrition and fluid intake.

(xiii) Any other task the HHA may choose to have the home health aide perform.

Supervised practical training means training in a laboratory or other setting in which the trainee demonstrates knowledge while performing tasks on an individual under the direct supervision of a registered nurse or licensed practical nurse.

(2) Conduct of training.

(i) Organizations.

A home health aide training program may be offered by any organization except an HHA that, within the previous 2 years, has been found

(A) Out of compliance with requirements of paragraph (a) or paragraph (b) of this section;

(B) To permit an individual who does not meet the definition of home health aide as specified in §484.4 to furnish home health aide services (with the exception of licensed health professionals and volunteers);

(C) Has been subjected to an extended (or partial extended) survey as a result of having been found to have furnished substandard care (or for other reasons at the discretion of HCFA or the state);

(D) Has been assessed a civil penalty of not less than $5,000 as an intermediate sanction;

(E) Has been found to have compliance deficiencies that endanger the health and safety of the HHA's patients and has had a temporary management appointed to oversee the management of the HHA;

(F) Has had all or part of its Medicare payments suspended; or

(G) Under any Federal or State law within the 2-year period beginning October 1, 1988—

(1) Has had its participation in the Medicare program terminated;

(2) Has been assessed a penalty of not less than $5,000 for deficiencies in Federal or State standards for HHAs;

(3) Was subject to suspension of Medicare payments to which it otherwise would have been entitled;

(4) Had operated under temporary management that was appointed to oversee the operation of the HHA and to ensure the health and safety of the HHA's patients; or

(5) Was closed or had its residents transferred by the State.

(ii) Qualifications for instructors.

The training of home health aides and the supervision of home health aides during the supervised practical portion of the training must be performed by or under the general supervision of a registered nurse who possesses a minimum of 2 years of nursing experience, at least 1 year of which must be in the provision of home health care. Other individuals may be used to provide instruction under the supervision of a qualified registered nurse.

(3) Documentation of training.

The HHA must maintain sufficient documentation to demonstrate that the requirements of this standard are met.

(b) Standard: Competency evaluation and in-service training.

(1) Applicability.

An individual may furnish home health aide services on behalf of an HHA only after the individual has successfully completed a competency evaluation program as described in this paragraph. The HHA is responsible for ensuring that the individuals who furnish home health aide service on its behalf meet the competency evaluation requirements of this section.

(2) Content and frequency of evaluations and of inservice training.
  (i) The competency evaluation must address each of the subjects listed in paragraphs (A)(1)(ii) through (xiii) of this section.
  (ii) The HHA must complete a performance review of each home health aide no less frequently than every 12 months.
  (iii) The home health aide must receive at least 12 hours of inservice training per calendar year. The inservice training may be furnished while the aide is furnishing care to patients.
(3) Conduct of evaluation and training.
  (i) Organizations.
    A home health aide competency evaluation program may be offered by an organization except as specified in paragraph (a)(2)(I) of this section. The inservice training may be offered by any organization.
  (ii) Evaluators and instructors.
    The competency evaluation must be performed by a registered nurse. The inservice training generally must be supervised by a registered nurse who possesses a minimum of 2 years of nursing experience, at least 1 year of which must be in the provision of home health care.
  (iii) Subject areas.
    The subject areas listed at paragraphs (a)(1)(iii), (ix), (x), and (xi) of this section must be evaluated after observation of the aide's performance of the tasks with a patient. The other subject areas in paragraph (a)(1) of this section may be evaluated through written examination or after observation of a home health aide with a patient.
(4) Competency determinations.
  (i) A home health aide is not considered competent in any task for which he or she is evaluated as unsatisfactory. The aide must not perform that task without direct supervision by a licensed nurse until after he or she receives training in the task for which he or she was evaluated as unsatisfactory and passes a subsequent evaluation with satisfactory rating.
  (ii) A home health aide is not considered to have successfully passed a competency evaluation if the aide has an unsatisfactory rating in more than one of the required areas.
(5) Documentation of competency evaluation.
  The HHA must maintain documentation which demonstrates that the requirements of this standard are met.
(6) Effective date.
  The HHA must implement a competency evaluation program that meets the requirements of this paragraph before February 14, 1990. The HHA must provide the preparation necessary for the individual to successfully complete the competency evaluation. After August 14, 1990, the HHA may use only those aides that [sic] have been found to be competent in accordance with §484.36(b).

(c) Standard: Assignment and duties of the home health aide.

The home health aide is assigned to a particular patient by a registered nurse. Written instructions for patient care are prepared by a registered nurse or therapist as appropriate. Duties include the performance of simple procedures as an extension of therapy services, personal care, ambulation and exercise, household services essential to health care at home, assistance with medications that are ordinarily self-administered, reporting of changes in the patient's condition and needs, and completion of appropriate records.

(d) Standard: Supervision.

The following requirements for supervision of the home health aides furnishing services to patients must be met.
(1) Home health aide services only.
  When only home health aide services are being furnished to a patient, a registered nurse must make a supervisory visit to the

patient's residence at least once every 60 days. Each supervisory visit must occur when the aide is furnishing patient care.

(2) Skilled nursing or physical, speech, or occupational therapy furnished.

When skilled nursing care or physical, speech, or occupational therapy is also being furnished to a patient, a registered nurse must make a supervisory visit to the patient's residence every 2 weeks (either when the aide is present to observe and assist or when the aide is absent) to assess relationships and to determine whether goals are being met. When only physical, speech, or occupational therapy is furnished in addition to home health aide services, a skilled therapist may make the supervisory visits in place of a registered nurse.

(e) **Personal care attendant: Evaluation requirements.**

(1) Applicability.

This paragraph applies to individuals who are employed by HHAs exclusively to furnish personal care attendant services under a Medicaid personal care benefit.

(2) Rule.

An individual may furnish personal care services, as defined in §440.170 of this chapter, on behalf of an HHA after the individual has been found competent by the state to furnish those services for which a competency evaluation is required by paragraph (b) of this section and that the individual is required to perform. The individual need not be determined competent in those services listed in paragraph (a) of this section that the individual is not required to furnish.

This condition sets forth the requirements that must be met when the HHA provides home health aide services. Specifically, the standards and factors in the condition specify those entities that may conduct a training and competency evaluation program, content areas for training and where that training may occur, the qualifications for instructors, the manner in which competency must be demonstrated and evaluated, and the requirements for the assignment and supervision of the home health aide.

For clarity, and to avoid repetition of the detailed information reported in the condition, the discussion of training and competency requirements is divided into the following subject areas: training, competency, and performance review requirements; instructors and evaluators; and inservice training. This section concludes with a discussion of the assignment, duties, and supervision of the qualified home health aide.

Training, Competency, and Performance Review Requirements

The agency must ensure that those individuals who provide home health aide services, either directly or via contractual arrangements, have successfully completed a state-established or other training program that meets the requirements set forth in standard (a) and a competency evaluation or state licensure program that meets the requirements set forth in standard (b) or a competency evaluation program that meets the requirements set forth in standard (b). The training program may be provided by any organization except a certified HHA that within the previous 2 years has been found out of compliance with standard (a), Home Health Aide Training, or standard (b), Competency Evaluation and Inservice Training.

If the HHA requires its home health aides to complete a training program, materials must be maintained that clearly establish that each home health aide completed a training program of appropriate length and content that was conducted by qualified instructors as defined in standard (a)(2)(ii) and discussed later in this section. These materials should make a clear distinction between what was taught in the classroom setting and what was taught during the supervised practical training. If the home health aide position description and/or the home health aide service policy statements require the aide to perform other tasks in addition to the basic skills specified in standard (a)(2)(iii), the manner in which these tasks will be taught and evaluated should also be documented.

To reiterate, it is imperative that the documentation of training be reported in detail because the determination that a training program did not meet the required specifications will result in a deficiency cited for standard (a), Home Health Aide Training. A deficiency for this standard prohibits the agency from conducting a training program for a 2-year period. If the deficiency is cited while a training program is in progress, the HHA may complete that program but may not begin another program for 24 months after receipt of written notice of the condition level deficiency.

Most of the admonitions stated for the training program are applicable to the competency evaluation as well. A competency evaluation must be completed successfully before the individual may provide service as a home health aide. The competency evaluation must encompass all the subject areas listed in standard (a)(1)(ii) through (xii). The candidate's competence in four task areas must be evaluated by observation of task performance with a patient or mock patient. The four task areas are, as cited in standard (a), home health aide training; (iii) reading and recording temperature, pulse, and respiration; (ix) appropriate and safe techniques in personal hygiene and grooming that include (A) bed bath, (B) sponge, tub, or shower bath, (C) shampoo (sink, tub, or bed), (D) nail and skin care, (E) oral hygiene, and (F) toileting and elimination; (x) safe transfer techniques and ambulation; and (xi) normal range of motion and positioning. The remaining subject areas may be evaluated through written examination, through oral examination, or after observation of the home health aide applicant with a patient. These areas are, as listed in standard (a), home health aide training; (i) communication skills; (ii) observation, reporting, and documentation of patient status and the care or service furnished; (iv) basic infection control procedures; (v) basic elements of body functioning and changes in body functioning that must be reported to an aide's supervisor; (vi) mainte-nance of a clean, safe, and healthy environment; (vii) recognizing emergencies and knowledge of emergency procedures; and (viii) the personal, physical, emotional, and developmental needs of and ways to work with the populations served by the HHA, including the need for respect for the patient, his or her privacy, and his or her property. As an aside, it should be noted that the competency evaluation for an individual who will be utilized to furnish personal care attendant services under the Medicaid personal care benefit may be limited to the evaluation of competency in those areas in standard (a)(1)(ii) through (xii) that the individual may be required to furnish.

Written materials should specify the method(s) used to test the home health aide applicant's competency in all the subject areas listed in standard (a)(ii) through (xiii). The tool(s) used to document competency should allow a reviewer to ascertain the specific tasks, ability, or knowledge area tested as well as the rating (satisfactory or unsatisfactory) attained by the person being evaluated. If competence is reported with a score, the score should be readily identifiable as either a satisfactory or an unsatisfactory rating. Furthermore, the materials should document that competency testing for standard (a)(iii), (ix), (x), and (xi) was performed with a patient or mock patient rather than a mannequin. An individual cannot be considered competent in any task for which he or she is evaluated as unsatisfactory. The HHA should establish in writing the mechanisms used to ensure that the individual who receives an unsatisfactory rating in any task does not perform that task except under the direct supervision of a licensed nurse until such time as he or she is evaluated again and receives a satisfactory rating. The method by which the aide subsequently attains the satisfactory rating should also be detailed in writing.

There is one other requirement germane to the training and competency of home health aides. The definition of *home health aide* in Subpart A of the conditions of participation, §484.4, Personnel Qualifications, states:

An individual is not considered to have completed a training and competency evaluation program, or a competency evaluation program, if since the individual's most recent completion of this program(s) there has been a continuous period of 24 consecutive months during none of which the individual furnished services described in §409.40 of this chapter for compensation.

As defined in §409.40, home health services means the following items and services:

- part-time or intermittent nursing care provided by or under the supervision of a registered professional nurse
- physical therapy, occupational therapy, or speech therapy
- medical social services provided under the direction of a physician
- part-time or intermittent services of a home health aide
- medical supplies (other than drugs and biologicals) and the use of medical appliances
- in the case of an HHA that is affiliated or under common control with a hospital, medical services provided by an intern or a resident under a teaching program as provided in §409.15

§409.42 sets forth conditions and requirements that must be met for the services identified in §409.40 and listed above to be covered by Medicare Part A. §409.15 specifies the criteria for interns and residents providing medical services as specified in (f) above.

The HHA must conduct a performance review of the home health aide no less frequently than every 12 months. The performance review interval and the individual(s) responsible for this review should be identified in the personnel policies or in other written material. In the absence of any state, statutory, or contractual requirements or the HHA's own policies, it is not necessary for the home health aide to complete a competency evaluation as all or part of the performance review.

Instructors and Evaluators

The training of the home health aides, including the supervised practical portion of the training, must be performed by or under the general supervision of a registered nurse who has a minimum of 2 years of nursing experience, at least 1 year of which must be in the provision of home health care. Under the general supervision of the qualified registered nurse, other individuals may function as instructors in the training program. These individuals include, but are not limited to, physical therapists, speech/language pathologists, medical social workers, psychologists, and registered dietitians. This general supervision is demonstrated through documented evidence of the qualified registered nurse's responsibility for the content and conduct of the training program.

The competency evaluation must be performed by a registered nurse. Inservice training must be provided under the general supervision of a registered nurse who has a minimum of 2 years of nursing experience, at least 1 year of which must be in the provision of home health care. The agency should maintain materials to document that the nurse(s) who function as instructors and evaluators hold the requisite qualifications. The qualifications of other professionals who participate in the training program should also be available.

Inservice Training

As stated in standard (b)(2)(ii), the home health aide must receive at least 12 hours of inservice per calendar year. To ensure that this requirement is met, it is recommended that inservice programs be scheduled at regular intervals throughout the year or during periods when the agency historically has a lower than usual census. Inservice programs should be designed to enhance the skills and knowledge required for successful performance or to introduce or review new or revised policies, procedures, and/or position descriptions. Of course, these new or revised materials will have been reviewed by the group of professional personnel.

Inservice training may be furnished while the aide is providing care to patients. If the HHA allows the inservice requirement to be met while the aide is furnishing patient care, there should be guidelines for staff to determine what may be taught in the patient care setting, who may provide the instruction, and how the learned task or skill is to be documented (for the purposes of meeting the inservice training requirement). As with other health care personnel, a record should be maintained of the aide's participation in inservice programs.

Assignment and Duties of the Home Health Aide

The HHA must ensure that the assignment of the home health aide to furnish care is based on the patient's need for personal care assistance identified, usually by the registered nurse, as part of the initial or a subsequent patient assessment. The home health aide furnishes care following the written instruction of the registered nurse or, where appropriate, the therapist. The instructions must specify not only what is to be done but how frequently it should be done. Because the home health aide is assigned to a patient to attain a specified outcome, in the majority of instances it is not appropriate for the designated tasks to be completed on an as-needed basis. It is assumed that the assigned tasks must be performed with some regularity if the desired outcome(s) is to be achieved. Throughout the course of care, the written instructions must be updated as frequently as necessary to ensure that the home health aide's duties are reflective of the patient's current needs.

There are numerous formats available to document the provision of home health aide service. Care should be taken, however, to ensure that the home health aide written instruction form is consistent with the format used by the home health aide to document the care furnished. Too often these formats contain different task definitions; therefore, it is difficult to ascertain that the aide has in fact completed all assigned tasks. An inability to establish clearly that the home health aide did indeed complete all the assigned tasks may present an area of risk for the HHA.

When the home health aide is expected to perform simple exercises as an extension of the therapy program, it is not sufficient to write on the assignment form "Exercises as per the therapist's instructions." The therapist must prepare written instructions for the exercises that the aide is to perform. A copy of the instructions should be available in the clinical record. It should be clear that the assigned exercises are not those that require the knowledge and skill of a therapist or therapy assistant. The HHA should have in place mechanisms to ensure that the home health aide who is assigned can competently perform the assigned duties as written by the registered nurse or therapist as appropriate.

A review of the assignment format and clinical record documentation should provide evidence that the patient's needs and the capabilities of the caregivers in the patient's support system as well as the capabilities of the aide were considered in the assignment of the aide and the duties to be performed. The goals or outcomes for the service should be evident. As noted earlier in this chapter, goals should be established for the services that are concise, realistic, and developed jointly with the patient or individual designated to act on the patient's behalf. The review of assignment formats should also document adherence to agency policies relative to the assignment and duties of the home health aide.

Supervision of the Home Health Aide

When home health aide service is furnished in conjunction with skilled nursing or physical therapy, occupational therapy, or speech therapy, the registered nurse must make a supervisory visit to the patient's residence at least every 2 weeks. When only physical therapy, occupational therapy, or speech therapy is being provided while the patient receives home health aide services, the supervisory visit may be made by a skilled therapist (not a therapy assistant) every 2 weeks at the patient's residence. (In this instance, although skilled nursing care is not being provided, the HHA has the option to require a registered nurse to make the home health aide supervisory visit every 2 weeks. Such a visit would be considered an administrative cost and could not be billed as a skilled nursing visit.) When only home health aide service is provided, a registered nurse must make a supervisory visit to the patient's residence at least every 60 days.

When home health aide service is provided in addition to skilled nursing, physical therapy, occupational therapy, or speech therapy, the supervisory visit may be made while the aide is present to observe and assist, as appropriate, or when the aide is absent to assess relationships and to determine whether the goals for care are met. Standard (d), Supervision does not specify a frequency interval for the presence of the home health aide when the supervisory visit is made; nevertheless, the HHA may want to specify such an interval in its policy to ensure that the registered nurse or therapist periodically supervises the aide while care is being provided. When home health aide service is the only service being provided, however, the registered nurse must make the supervisory visit when the aide is furnishing patient care.

Agency policy/procedure statements must set forth the agency's requirements regarding supervision of the home health aide. These requirements should be consistent with the requirements identified in standard (d), Supervision. At minimum, the policy statements should specify the professional(s) who may complete the supervisory visit, the frequency for supervision and any circumstance that affects the frequency of supervision (e.g., patient receiving home health aide service only), the focus or purpose of the supervisory visit, and the necessity to document the supervisory visit in the clinical record. It is not acceptable to conduct this supervision via telephone or in any setting other than the patient's residence.

The clinical record must clearly establish that the agency policy for supervision is being followed. The clinical records must contain written reports of supervisory findings. The supervisory visit notation should specify whether the aide was absent or present and should provide an objective assessment of relationships vis-à-vis the goals established for the service or the aide's performance of the assigned duties. Where applicable, the supervisory note or other format should document actions taken in response to information learned or observations made during the observation visit.

The HHA should institute mechanisms to ensure the routine comparative review of the format completed by the home health aide and the home health aide assignment format to ensure that the home health aide is completing each of the assigned duties. Often, the comparative review reveals that the home health aide performed duties that were not assigned, discontinued assigned duties, and/or did not perform all the assigned duties.

§484.38—Condition of Participation: Qualifying To Furnish Outpatient Physical Therapy or Speech Pathology Services

A HHA that wishes to furnish outpatient physical therapy or speech pathology services must meet all the pertinent conditions of this part and also must meet additional health and safety requirements set forth in §§405.1717 through 405.1719, 405.1721, 404.1723, and 405.1725 of this chapter to implement section 1861(p) of the Act.

§484.48—Condition of Participation: Clinical Records

A clinical record containing pertinent past and current findings in accordance with accepted professional standards is maintained for every patient receiving home health services. In addition to the plan of care, the record contains appropriate identifying information; name of the physician; drug, dietary, treatment, and activity orders; signed and dated clinical and progress notes; copies of summary reports sent to the attending physician; and a discharge summary.

(a) Standard: Retention of records.

Clinical records are retained for 5 years after the month the cost report to which the records apply is filed with the intermediary unless state law stipulates a longer period of time. Policies provide for retention even if the HHA discontinues operations. If a patient is transferred to another health facility, a copy of the record or abstract is sent with the patient.

(b) Standard: Protection of records.

Clinical record information is safeguarded against loss or unauthorized use. Written procedures govern use and removal of records and the conditions for release of information. The patient's written consent is required for release of information not authorized by law.

The clinical record maintained for each patient accepted for care must, at minimum, contain the information specified in the first paragraph. The record should also include any other documents as required by the HHA, such as the Patient Bill of Rights and consent forms. A review of the clinical records should establish that all required documents are in the record and that these documents are uniformly used and properly completed. The clinical record should be organized in a manner that provides for a chronology of events pertaining to interactions between the patient and members of the health team and that facilitates the incorporation, review, and retrieval of clinical record information. Collectively, the clinical recording documents must clearly establish the provision of physician-directed, coordinated, patient outcome–oriented care and concomitantly must substantiate the agency's claim for reimbursement and minimize the risk of exposure to liability through the documented provision of care in the amount, frequency, and duration ordered and in a manner that meets professional practice standards.

Although the description of the required content is self-explanatory, the need for and distinctions among the clinical note, progress note, and summary report should be clear to all service providers. These three clinical recording methods are defined in Subpart A, General Provisions. A clinical note is defined as "a notation of a contact with a patient that is written and dated by a member of the health team, and that describes signs and symptoms, treatments and drugs administered and the patient's reaction and any changes in physical or emotional condition." A progress note is defined as "a written notation, dated and signed by a member of the health team, that summarizes facts about care furnished and the patient's response during a given period of time." As noted earlier, a summary report is defined as "the compilation of the pertinent factors of a patient's clinical notes and progress notes that is submitted to the patient's physician."

Whatever the clinical recording system, every patient visit report should meet the definition of a clinical note. When clinical information is reported with a flowsheet format, the format should allow for the reporting of not only objective findings but also the patient's response to the intervention(s) furnished. As a general rule, a progress note is written at 30- or 60-day intervals; it should be prepared as frequently as warranted by the patient's condition or as specified in agency policy, however. The summary report is prepared and sent to the attending physician at least every 62 days during which the patient receives care. This report contains pertinent information ascertained from the clinical and progress notes. To ensure that the records are up to date, consideration should be given to the routine concurrent review of a random sample of the clinical records (this activity could be completed as part of the continuing review of clinical records required in condition 484.52, Evaluation of the Agency's Program).

Standard (a) requires the agency to have written policies for the retention of clinical records. The policies should be consistent with applicable state laws, including those pertaining to the retention of records of minors and the records of patients involved in litigation. The policy should recognize the need to retain the records in the event that the agency discontinues operations. Finally, the policies should ensure that, when a patient is transferred to another facility for continuing care, a copy of the record or an abstract is sent with the patient.

To meet the intent of standard (b), the agency must establish policies and attendant mechanisms ensuring that safeguards are in place to preserve and protect the clinical record yet meeting the need to have the records readily available for personnel who are caring for the patient. The policies should support the patient's right to confidentiality of medical records. Those individuals who may have access to the record should be identified, as should any restrictions on their access. When patient information is maintained via an automated system, mechanisms must be in place to limit access to this information. Policy statements should specify under what circumstances the clinical record, or parts thereof, may be removed from the protected environment maintained by the agency. When visiting staff are allowed to remove the clinical record or parts of the record from the agency, the agency should establish its expectation for the continued protection of the record. That the patient's consent is required for the release of information not authorized by law should be evident in written policies with supporting evidence in the clinical record. The content of any format used to obtain consent and procedures for obtaining this consent should include consideration of legal and ethical issues.

§484.52—Condition of Participation: Evaluation of the Agency's Program

The HHA has written policies requiring an overall evaluation of the agency's total program at least once a year by the group of professional personnel (or a committee of this group), HHA

staff, and consumers or by professional people outside the agency working in conjunction with consumers. The evaluation consists of an overall policy and administrative review and a clinical record review. The evaluation assesses the extent to which the agency's program is appropriate, adequate, effective, and efficient. Results of the evaluation are reported to and acted upon by those responsible for the operation of the agency and are maintained separately as administrative records.

(a) Standard: Policy and administrative review.

As part of the evaluation process, the policies and administrative practices of the agency are reviewed to determine the extent to which they promote patient care that is appropriate, adequate, effective, and efficient. Mechanisms are established in writing for the collection of pertinent data to assist in evaluation.

(b) Standard: Clinical record review.

At least quarterly, appropriate health professionals, representing at least the scope of the program, review a sample of both active and closed clinical records to determine whether established policies are followed in furnishing services directly or under arrangement. There is a continuing review of clinical records for each 62-day period that a patient receives home health services to determine adequacy of the plan of care and appropriateness of continuation of care.

This condition requires the HHA to conduct an overall evaluation of the agency's total program at least once a year. Those who may participate in the evaluation are identified in the condition. The objectives for the evaluation are to determine the extent to which the agency's program is appropriate (i.e., demonstrates the agency's mission and purposes), adequate (i.e., fosters attainment of the agency's goals and objectives), effective (i.e., significantly and positively affects those served by the agency), and efficient (i.e., demonstrates the most judicious use of financial, human, and information resources). Policy statements should ensure that the scope of the evaluation is sufficiently broad to achieve the evaluation objectives and to ensure that the written evaluation report, including findings and recommendations, is promptly reviewed by the advisory group of professional personnel or a committee acting for the group and is subsequently promptly submitted to the governing body and administrator for review and action. The agency should have a written plan for the evaluation that allows for the collection and review or analysis of information pertaining to the organization, activities, costs, and outcomes of the agency's programs.

Standard (a) requires a policy and administrative review. This review should be coupled with an analysis of personnel and patient service activity data to determine the degree to which the policies and administrative practices of the agency support the provision of high-quality patient care as defined with the agency's measures of quality. The mechanisms for collecting and compiling data (patient service, personnel, financial, etc.) to assist in the evaluation must be delineated in writing.

As part of the evaluation process, standard (b) mandates a review of a sample of open and closed clinical records on a quarterly basis. The review should be conducted by professionals representing the therapeutic services offered by the HHA during the quarter under review; other professionals may participate in the review at the agency's behest, however. The focus of the review is to ensure that services are provided in a manner that demonstrates compliance with professional practice acts, the plan of care, and the agency's written policies and procedures. The format used by the review should be designed to focus on these areas. It is not necessary that professionals conducting the review meet as a group, but the agency must be able to demonstrate that the time of the review of selected records does not exceed any 3-month period.

The findings from the review of clinical records should be summarized and reported in writing. The summary report should indicate the methodology for selecting the records, the num-

ber of records reviewed, and recommendations. The number of records should be sufficient to constitute a representative sample, but the condition no longer requires that a designated number of records be reviewed each quarter. Action plans for the short- and long-term correction of identified problems should be developed and implemented with appropriate follow-up to assess the effectiveness of the plan.

In addition to the quarterly review of records, standard (b) requires the review of the clinical record every 62 days that the patient receives home health services to determine the adequacy of the plan of care and the appropriateness of the continuation of care. Personnel responsible for completing this review should be identified in the position description or in procedures specifying how the review is to be accomplished. These procedures should ensure that the review is completed on a timely basis and that action is promptly taken whenever evidence of inadequacy or inappropriateness is found. This review should occur as part of the process to develop the plan of care for recertification and to aid in the preparation of the summary report.

The annual program evaluation and the quarterly review of clinical records should be part of the agency's comprehensive quality assurance program. These and other activities should provide objective data that can be used to define and measure quantitatively the quality of the care and services provided by the agency.

CONCLUSION

The Medicare-certified HHA must demonstrate compliance with conditions of participation on an ongoing basis regardless of organizational structure or design. To that end, the administrator must consistently act to ensure that the agency's policies, procedures, standards of practice, protocols, and other materials that delineate operational practices and expectations adequately and appropriately reflect the applicable requirements as set forth in the conditions of participation.

REFERENCES

Department of Health and Human Services (DHHS), Health Care Financing Administration. 1993, October. *State operations manual*. Provider certification transmittal no. 260, B-25. Washington, DC: HCFA.

Department of Health and Human Services, Health Care Financing Administration. 1989, August. 42 CFR Part 484. Medicare program: Home health agencies: Conditions of participation and reduction in recordkeeping requirements; interim final rule. *Federal Register* 54:33354–33373.

Department of Health and Human Services, Health Care Financing Administration. 1991, July. 42 CFR Part 484. Medicare program: Home health agencies: Conditions of participation. *Federal Register* 56:32967–32975.

Department of Health and Human Services, Health Care Financing Administration. 1991, September. 42 CFR Parts 409, 418, 484. Medicare program: Medicare coverage of home health services, Medicare conditions of participation, and home health aide supervision. *Federal Register* 56:49154–49172.

SUGGESTED READING

Department of Health and Human Services, Health Care Financing Administration. 1997. Medicare and Medicaid Program; Revision of the Conditions of Participation for Home Health Agencies and Use of the Outcome and Assessment Information Set (OASIS) As Part of the Revised Conditions of Participation for Home Health Agencies. *Federal Register,* 62 (46):11004–11035.

Department of Health and Human Sources, Health Care Financing Administration. 1997. Medicare and Medicaid Program; Use of the OASIS As Part of the Conditions of Participation for Home Health Agencies. *Federal Register*, 62 (46): 11035–11064.

Department of Health and Human Services, Health Care Financing Administration. 1993, January. 42 CFR Part 493. Medicare program: Laboratory services. *Federal Register*, 58.

Department of Health and Human Services, Health Care Financing Administration. 1992, February. 42 CFR Part 493. Medicare program: Laboratory services. *Federal Register*, 57.

CHAPTER 4

The Joint Commission's Home Care Accreditation Program

Maryanne L. Popovich and Richele C. Armstrong Schaffer

THE JOINT COMMISSION'S HOME CARE ACCREDITATION PROGRAM

The Joint Commission on Accreditation of Healthcare Organizations is a private, not-for-profit organization dedicated to improving the quality of health care provided to the public. This goal is realized through fulfillment of its roles as standard setter, evaluator, accreditation decision maker, and consultant. The Joint Commission is widely recognized for its dynamic leadership role in developing standards, and the survey and accreditation processes have been progressively updated to address the important changes and issues in the delivery of health services (Joint Commission, 1990). The Joint Commission believes that its standards should:

- focus on those functions and aspects of patient care that are essential to quality patient care
- provide a framework of guidance for accredited organizations and those seeking accreditation
- represent a consensus on the state of the art in expected organization performance
- state, to the extent possible, objectives or principles rather than specific mechanisms for meeting requirements
- be reasonable and surveyable

The original home care standards were developed over a 2-year period under the guidance of a national home care advisory committee. Several field reviews were conducted to obtain provider and consumer input into the draft standards, and 16 home care organizations participated in pilot testing before the standards were finalized. The first standards became effective June 1, 1988. Since then, there have been several revisions of the standards that have resulted in new standards manuals. These standards apply to both freestanding and hospital-based home care organizations, and they address the provision of various types of home care services. An organization is eligible to apply for a survey if it provides at least one of the following services in the patient's residence:

- Home health services are those services provided by health care professionals on a per visit or per hour basis to patients who have or are at risk of an injury, an illness, or a disabling condition or who are terminally ill and require short-term or long-term intervention by health professionals.
- Personal care and support services are those services provided on a per visit or per hour basis to meet the identified needs of patients who have or are at risk of an injury, an illness, or a disabling condition and who require assistance in personal care, activities of daily living, and maintenance and management of household routines.
- Pharmaceutical services are those services provided, directly or through contract with another organization, that procure, prepare, preserve, compound, dispense, and/

or distribute pharmaceutical products and monitor the patient's clinical status.

- Equipment management includes the selection, delivery, set-up, and maintenance of equipment to meet patients' needs and the education of patients in the equipment's use.
- Clinical respiratory services are those services provided by respiratory care practitioners to patients who have or are at risk of an injury, an illness, or a disabling condition or who are terminally ill and require short-term or long-term care intervention by health care professionals; such services are generally associated with the provision of equipment management services and may include, but need not be limited to, physical assessment, monitoring of vital signs, oximetry testing, and/or the administration of therapeutic treatments.
- Hospice includes an organized program that consists of services provided and coordinated by an interdisciplinary team at a frequency appropriate to meet the needs of patients who are diagnosed with a terminal illness and have a limited life span. The hospice specializes in providing palliative management of pain and other physical symptoms and meeting the psychosocial and spiritual needs of the patient and the patient's family or other primary care person(s). The program also includes a continuum of interdisciplinary team services across all settings where hospice care is provided, the availability of 24-hour access to care, utilization of volunteers, and bereavement care to the survivors, as needed, for an appropriate period of time.

THE HOME CARE STANDARDS

The survey and accreditation decision processes are based on an organization's demonstration of compliance with the standards in the *1997–1998 Comprehensive Accreditation Manual for Home Care* (CAMHC, Joint Commis-

sion, 1996). This standards manual is divided into two sections. Section 1 consists of five chapters that focus on an organization's important patient-focused functions. Section 2 includes six additional chapters that focus on important organizational functions that support how patient care is delivered. Although all the standards are considered important in the delivery of care or service, the following summary highlights key concepts and standards in each chapter.

Rights and Ethics

Standards in this chapter address the right of patients to make informed decisions regarding their care, including the right to formulate advance directives. The standards also require the organization to inform patients of their rights and to establish a mechanism for resolving patient complaints. In addition, the standards include requirements for an organizational mechanism to address ethical issues arising in the care of patients and for organizations to adopt ethical business practices.

Assessment

These standards set the expectations for an organization's processes related to patient assessment. The organization should collect relevant assessment data for every patient, analyze the data to determine the patient's needs, and make decisions regarding patient care and services. Assessment should occur at admission and then at appropriate points throughout the course of care or service. The standards also specify required elements for the assessment of several special populations, such as children and intrapartum women.

Care, Treatment, and Service

These standards set the requirements for processes that guide the care and services that patients receive. The standards require an organization to plan the services that each patient receives. The care planning process should identify the patient's problems and needs, care/treatment goals or expected outcomes, and the actions and interventions to achieve these goals.

The standards require that care be not only planned but implemented to meet the patient's problems and needs. In addition, the patient's response to care or service needs to be monitored throughout the course of care. The standards also require that care and services be provided in accordance with standards of practice.

Education

These standards relate to the educational needs of an organization's patients and their families. The standards require organizations to develop a systematic approach to patient education. An education program should help patients understand and cope with their health status and care options. Organizations should encourage patients and their families to be involved in care decisions and to learn care skills. The standards also identify specific topics that should be included in a patient education program.

Continuum of Care

These standards address the responsibility that an organization has to provide care and services in a continuous and coordinated manner that is appropriate for the patient's needs over the entire course of time that the patient is served by the organization. The standards require an organization to define its scope of services and only accept patients whose needs can be met by the organization. The standards set expectations for continuity of care from admission through discharge. The standards also expect the care to be coordinated with all care providers, both those within the organization and external care providers.

Improving Organization Performance

Standards in this chapter evaluate the organization's ability to monitor and improve the quality of its services through a planned and organizationwide approach. These standards require improvements to be planned and prioritized. The standards also address how processes are designed or redesigned; how and what data are collected, measured, and assessed; and how and when improvements are made. Whenever possible, the organization should consider staff and customer input as well as incorporate benchmarking and comparative data sources in its improvement activities.

Leadership

These standards address the authority and responsibilities of the organization's leadership, which includes the governing body, management, and supervisors. Leaders should provide the framework for planning, directing, coordinating, providing, and improving patient care and services. The standards look at the leadership role in setting the mission and priorities, strategic planning, budget approval, annual evaluation of the organization's performance as well as in resource and staff allocation. The standards require that the organization comply with applicable laws and regulations. Other standards address personnel and organizational management, development, implementation and review of policies and procedures, and development of written agreements. There are also several standards that relate directly to the role of the leaders in performance improvement.

Environmental Safety and Equipment Management

These standards address the organization's responsibility to provide care and service in a safe and effective manner. The organization should plan for and implement safety practices for both patients and staff. The organization needs to manage environments, including the patient's home, the home care organization's office, warehouses, pharmacies, and vehicles. The standards require an organization's program to consider fire safety, emergency preparedness, personal safety, basic home safety, and safe handling of medical gases and hazardous materials and wastes. In addition, the standards require an appropriate equipment management program, including routine and preventive maintenance, to ensure that the equipment used by patients and staff is safe and in working order and that equipment is appropriately set up in the home.

Management of Human Resources

The focus of these standards is the organization's need to provide adequate and appropriate staff to perform both organizational and patient care functions. The standards require the organization to define levels of experience, education, training, licensure, and qualifications for each category of staff. The organization should develop job descriptions for all staff. In addition, the organization needs to develop an education program for all staff that includes orientation and ongoing training for staff as well as an assessment of staff competence both at hire and on an ongoing basis. Depending on staff categories, the training needs and expectations may differ. Staff include direct staff, part-time and on-call staff, contracted staff, and hospice volunteers.

Management of Information

These standards look at the processes that an organization has in place to manage information. Information management should be planned and prioritized. The standards require that information be timely, accurate, and accessible. When appropriate, the organization needs to ensure that data are secure and confidential. In addition, these standards set the expectations for what should be included in the patient care record. The standards also identify data that are to be collected and aggregated into meaningful information and trended over time to support information sharing and communication to the appropriate individuals.

Surveillance, Prevention, and Control of Infection

These standards require an infection control program that includes the following specific processes: surveillance, identification, prevention, control of infections, and reporting. The program must include organizational policies and procedures addressing areas such as personal hygiene, precautions, aseptic procedures, communicable infections, reporting of patient and staff infections, and appropriate cleaning, disinfection, and/or sterilization of equipment and supplies. Policies and procedures should be based on infection trends and patterns, new scientific knowledge, and regulatory changes. The standards require that these policies and procedures be implemented across the organization. Data related to the infection control program should be collected, analyzed, and acted on when appropriate.

THE SURVEY PROCESS

Home care surveys are conducted by health care professionals who have both management and clinical experience in home care. The background of the surveyor and the duration of the survey are related to the type and volume of services provided. Agencies that provide intermittent or private duty nursing, home health aide, or homemaker services have a survey conducted by a home health nurse surveyor. Organizations providing home infusion therapy, including nursing as well as pharmaceutical services, are surveyed by a home health nurse and a pharmacist surveyor. Organizations providing only pharmaceutical products are surveyed by a pharmacist surveyor. Home medical equipment (HME) companies are surveyed by individuals with direct experience in owning or managing an HME business. If the supplier also provides clinical respiratory services, the surveyor is a respiratory care practitioner. A nurse surveyor will survey hospice services and, depending on the volume and scope of services, may be joined by a pharmacist and/or an HME surveyor. The duration of the survey is related to the types of services provided by the organization, the volume of patients/clients, and the organizational structure with respect to branch offices and contracted services.

The accreditation process is initiated when an organization submits an application for survey. Initial applications should be submitted at least 4 to 6 months before the requested month of the survey. Approximately 4 to 6 weeks before the survey, the organization is notified of the dates of the survey and the name(s) of the surveyor(s). The surveyors contact the organization 1 to 2 weeks before the survey to establish a tentative agenda for the survey. All surveys begin with an opening conference, in which surveyors summarize the purpose of the survey and how it will be conducted. At this time, they will review the proposed schedule of survey activities. This is also a time for key staff to be introduced to the surveyors.

At the end of each survey day, a short briefing is held with key managers. This meeting is designed for the surveyors and management staff to review the findings of the day, answer any questions, and review the schedule for the following day. An exit conference is planned for the last hour of the final day of the survey. This is the surveyors' closing statement and a time for the surveyors to identify all their findings. It is also an opportunity to discuss any findings, including recommendations, before the surveyors leave the site. The home care organization may decide who should attend this conference, but it is recommended that no more than six key management staff participate. In addition to the exit conference, the organization has the option to request a summation conference for all staff, in which the surveyors highlight the major findings of the survey.

An educational conference is also presented at some time during the course of the survey. The conference is led by one or more of the surveyors and is an opportunity for the organization to get consultation about an area related to the standards. The organization and surveyors should work together to find a topic that will be most beneficial for the surveyed organization.

The survey includes the following:

- management and governing body member interviews
- staff interviews (including hospice volunteers and contracted staff) from a variety of professional disciplines or job categories; the staff to be interviewed are selected by the surveyor(s)
- home visits to current patients; typically, a surveyor will visit two to three patients for each day of the survey (patients to be visited are selected by the surveyor and should reflect a variety of services provided)
- documentation review, including administrative, personnel, and clinical policies and procedures; orientation, inservice, continuing education, and competence assessment materials; governing body bylaws, charter, and/or articles of incorporation; governing body minutes; contracts; performance improvement materials; personnel records; a sample patient admission packet and patient education materials; promotional materials; equipment maintenance records; and pharmacy dispensing records
- random home care record review, including both current and discharged patients who represent a variety of diagnostic categories, services provided, branch offices (if applicable), and professional disciplines involved in the care
- review of equipment warehouse and delivery vehicles (when applicable)
- review of the pharmacy (when applicable)

For initial or focused surveys, the surveyors will evaluate that the standards have been met for a period of at least 4 months. On triennial resurveys, the surveyors may evaluate evidence of compliance over the previous triennial period; it is expected, however, that the organization will demonstrate compliance with the standards for a period of 12 months before resurvey. The CAMHC includes important policies regarding accreditation that home care organizations are expected to meet, the standards and their intents, guidelines that surveyors use to score compliance with the standards, examples of how an organization may choose to be in compliance with the standards, examples of how standards may be met, and the aggregation rules.

UNSCHEDULED, UNANNOUNCED, AND RANDOM UNANNOUNCED SURVEYS

Either an unscheduled or an unannounced survey may take place when the Joint Commission becomes aware of circumstances in an accredited organization that suggest a potentially serious standards compliance problem. The survey can either evaluate all the organization's services or be restricted to only those areas in which a serious standards compliance problem may exist.

On July 1, 1993, the Joint Commission began to conduct midcycle unannounced surveys of a random 5 percent sample of accredited organizations in each of the Joint Commission's seven accreditation programs. Random unannounced surveys are conducted for 1 day by one surveyor. The surveyor will direct his or her attention to the five performance areas that the previous year's national aggregate data identified as being most problematic for similar types of organizations. Results of random unannounced surveys can affect an organization's accreditation status. The Joint Commission absorbs all costs of conducting these unannounced surveys.

THE ACCREDITATION DECISION PROCESS

The accreditation decision for an organization is based on its demonstrated compliance with the standards in the CAMHC and is awarded for 3 years. Compliance with each standard is measured using a 1 through 5 scoring system. A score of 1 represents substantial compliance with a standard, and a score of 5

indicates no compliance. Scores of 3, 4, or 5 may result in a type I recommendation. If the organization receives a type I recommendation, the Joint Commission requires formal follow-up from the organization within a specified time frame. This follow-up may be in the form of a written progress report or a focused survey (where a surveyor will return to the organization to evaluate the standards that resulted in the type I recommendation). At the time of the follow-up, the organization must be able to demonstrate that it has corrected the identified deficiencies.

Upon completion of a survey, the surveyor returns his or her findings to the Joint Commission's headquarters, where staff review the documentation and scoring to ensure consistency in the interpretation of the standards and to recommend an accreditation decision. The Joint Commission awards the following categories of accreditation:

- accreditation with commendation
- accreditation with or without type I recommendation
- provisional accreditation
- conditional accreditation
- preliminary nonaccreditation
- not accredited

Accreditation with commendation is awarded to those organizations that receive an overall accreditation decision grid score of 90 or higher with no type I recommendations.

Accreditation may be awarded with or without type I recommendations. If accreditation is awarded with type I recommendations, the accreditation is contingent upon the agency addressing these recommendations within an identified time period, usually 6 months from the date of the accreditation award letter.

Under Track 1 of the Early Survey Policy (see below), provisional accreditation may be awarded to organizations after their first of two surveys. This survey will primarily focus on the organization's structural components, such as planning and policies and procedures. After the second survey, the provisional accreditation status will be changed to one of the other accreditation decisions.

Conditional accreditation is the decision made when the organization is not in substantial compliance with a majority of the home care standards but has been determined to be capable of resolving identified deficiencies. Conditional accreditation allows the organization 6 months to address the specific issues outlined in an approved plan of correction. After 6 months, a follow-up survey is conducted, and the survey findings will lead to a decision to accredit or not accredit the organization.

Preliminary nonaccreditation is assigned to organizations that are found to be in significant noncompliance with the home care standards or when accreditation is preliminarily withdrawn by the Joint Commission for other reasons (e.g., falsification of documents) before determination of the final accreditation decision.

Not accredited is the decision rendered by the accreditation committee when the survey findings indicate that the organization demonstrates minimal or no compliance with the majority of the standards and that it will take significant resources and time for the organization to correct these identified deficiencies. The organization may apply for another survey at a later date.

THE ACCREDITATION DECISION GRID

After the decision for accreditation, the organization receives an accreditation award letter, an official accreditation report listing any type I recommendations and corrective action that will need to be taken, any supplemental recommendations, and an accreditation decision grid. The grid is a one-page visual summary of key groupings of standards (which are called grid elements).

For standard specific scores to be turned into grid elements they need to be summarized or consolidated. This is achieved through the use of aggregation rules. Aggregation rules are formulas that do not average or sum standard specific scores but rather assign a weight to standards. Some standards carry more weight than others, such as those that directly affect patient care outcomes. For example, written policies relating to infection control weigh less heavily than the implementation of infection control procedures. Depending on the weight given to a specific standard or a grouping of related standards (e.g., information management planning or patient education), the grid element may receive a compliance score of 1 through 5. Scores of 3, 4, or 5 generally reflect a type I recommendation related to that grid element. The grid is used to determine the outcome of the accreditation decision. For example, an organization that receives a majority of scores of 4 or 5 on its decision grid will probably receive a decision of conditional accreditation or denial of accreditation. Exhibit 4–1 illustrates a blank 1997 accreditation decision grid.

EARLY SURVEY POLICY

Some organizations may choose to be surveyed under the Joint Commission Early Survey Policy. If an organization elects this survey option, it must be eligible and agree to two surveys. There are currently two early survey tracks to choose from.

On Track 1, the organization is eligible up to 2 months before operations begin. On the first survey, evaluation is limited to standards as they relate to structural components of the home care organization's clinical and administrative operations. Six months later, the organization receives a full survey, in which it is evaluated against all the standards, including implementation of its processes, policies, and procedures.

On Track 2, the organization must be in operation and have serviced at least ten patients by the time of the initial survey. The first survey is a full survey, but some standards are scored no lower than 3 because the required 4-month track record may not have been met. The organization will receive a decision of accreditation with type I recommendations. About 6 months later, the organization receives another full survey, including those track record requirements that

Exhibit 4–1   The Joint Commission's Home Care Accreditation Services Accreditation Decision Grid

Organization:_____   Survey Date: _____

Location: _____   Survey Type: _____

PATIENT-FOCUSED FUNCTIONS

Rights and Ethics	I	II	III	IV
Rights and Ethics				

Assessment	I	II	III	IV
Patient Assessment				
Assessment of Specific Patient Populations				

Care, Treatment, and Service	I	II	III	IV
Care-Planning Process				
Preparation and Dispensing				
Medication Administration				
Patient Medication Monitoring				
Nutrition Care				
Diagnostic Services				

Education	I	II	III	IV
Education Program Management				
Patient Education				
Education About Specific Care Issues				

Continuum of Care and Services	I	II	III	IV
Continuum of Care and Services				

ORGANIZATION FUNCTIONS

Improving Organizational Performance	
Plan and Design	
Measure	
Assess	
Improve	

Leadership	I	II	III	IV
Governance				
Operations				
Role in Improving Performance				

Environmental Safety and Equipment Management	I	II	III	IV
Environmental Safety				
Equipment Management				

Management of Human Resources	I	II	III	IV
Human Resources Management				

Management of Information	I	II	III	IV
Information-Management Planning				
Patient-Specific Data and Information				

Surveillance, Prevention, and Control of Infection	I	II	III	IV
Surveillance, Prevention, and Control of Infection				

Special Type I Recommendation(s)	

Summary Grid Score =	

Rating Scale:
  1 = Substantial compliance
  2 = Significant compliance
  3 = Partial compliance
  4 = Minimal compliance
  5 = No compliance
  N = Not applicable
  P = Defer to primary service
  C = Contracted service

1997 HCAS Grid—Effective: January 1997 © 1996

Legend:
  I   = Home health and/or personal care/support
  II = Equipment management and/or clinical respiratory therapy services
  III = Pharmaceutical services
  IV = Hospice services

Source: © 1997 HCAS Grid. Oakbrook Terrace, IL: Joint Commission on Accreditation of Healthcare Organizations, 1997. Reprinted with permission.

were not evaluated during the initial survey. The organization will probably continue with its original accreditation status unless serious compliance problems exist.

DEEMED STATUS OPTION FOR MEDICARE CERTIFICATION

For a home health agency to receive Medicare or Medicaid reimbursement, it must first be surveyed and certified by a state agency as complying with the conditions of participation set forth in the federal regulations developed by the Health Care Financing Administration (HCFA). If a national accrediting body, such as the Joint Commission, provides HCFA with reasonable assurance that a home health agency it accredits meets the federal conditions of participation, HCFA may deem that the home health agency meets certification requirements. This recognition is known as deemed status.

The Joint Commission first submitted its application to achieve such recognition for its home care accreditation program to HCFA in 1988. This application included a comprehensive comparison of the conditions of participation with the Joint Commission's home care standards as well as a detailed analysis of the accreditation decision-making process. As part of its review, HCFA also evaluated surveyor selection, training, and supervision; survey process methods; and the Joint Commission's general administrative policies and procedures. A final rule regarding deemed status for Joint Commission–accredited home health agencies was published in the *Federal Register* on June 30, 1993 and made effective September 28, 1993 ("Medicare and Medicaid Programs," 1993).

To ensure comparability between the federal certification and the Joint Commission evaluation processes, the Joint Commission agreed to several changes in its process for those home health agencies wishing to use accreditation for Medicare certification. Some changes are reflected in the standards and scoring guidelines of the CAMHC (Joint Commission, 1996). In

addition, the Joint Commission agreed to use the HCFA functional assessment instrument and certain sampling procedures for those home health agencies that wish to elect the deemed status option. Last, as required by law, any survey used for home health agency certification must be unannounced. Therefore, for those agencies interested in having the Joint Commission's evaluation serve in lieu of the state survey, the organization must elect the deemed status option, allowing the Joint Commission to conduct an unannounced survey. During an initial or regular triennial survey in which the organization takes the deemed status option, all applicable Joint Commission standards as well as the Medicare conditions of participation are surveyed. If a Joint Commission surveyor surveys the organization during the interim years of the triennial accreditation cycle, only those standards that are comparable with the Medicare conditions of participation are evaluated.

The alterations to the standards, scoring guidelines, and survey process do not change the fundamental intent of the Joint Commission accreditation approach but rather are designed to provide congruency with the related regulatory requirements and procedures. Accreditation is, and will remain, voluntary. Seeking deemed status is an option available to interested home health agencies, not a requirement. Agencies desiring Medicare approval may choose to be surveyed by an accrediting body, such as the Joint Commission, or by state surveyors. The Joint Commission award letters, decision reports, and decision grids make the distinction that an agency has elected the deemed status option and has undergone an annual unannounced survey for the purposes of satisfying certification requirements.

BENEFITS OF ACCREDITATION

Accreditation is a visible demonstration of an organization's commitment to providing high-quality care to the patients it serves. Some of the benefits of accreditation include the following:

- improved patient care by incorporation of standards that reflect maximum achievable expectations into daily practices
- provision of an objective, on-site evaluation based on nationally recognized standards
- individualized consultation and education by highly trained surveyors with experience in the home care field
- enhancement of community confidence, including discharge planners, consumers, case managers, and physicians who recognize Joint Commission accreditation
- reimbursement or recognition from third party payers that require accreditation

- enhanced team morale and pride in achieving accreditation
- improved risk management for the organization
- fulfillment of licensure requirements in some states

CONCLUSION

Accreditation represents an objective, rigorous evaluation by health care professionals using nationally recognized standards for the provision of home care services. Achieving accreditation signifies the commitment of the organization and its staff to continuous improvement in quality and performance.

REFERENCES

Joint Commission on Accreditation of Healthcare Organizations. 1990. *Committed to quality: An introduction to the Joint Commission on Accreditation of Healthcare Organizations*. 4th ed. Oakbrook Terrace, IL: Joint Commission.

Joint Commission on Accreditation of Healthcare Organizations. 1996. *1997–1998 Comprehensive Accreditation Manual for Home Care*. Oakbrook Terrace, IL: Joint Commission.

Medicare and Medicaid programs: Recognition of the Joint Commission on Accreditation of Healthcare Organizations standards for home care organizations. 1993. *Federal Register* 58:35007–35017.

CHAP Accreditation: Standards of Excellence for Home Care and Community Health Organizations

Theresa Sekan Ayer

The Community Health Accreditation Program, Inc. (CHAP) is the oldest organization accrediting community and home care agencies. It began providing this service in 1965 as part of the National League for Nursing (NLN), but in 1987 it was separately incorporated. The NLN provides various levels of support for CHAP with the primary goal of setting the highest possible standards for health care professionals working in home and community health services. Since its inception in the late 19th century, the NLN has been a strong advocate of measures that promote consumer health. The NLN's creation of a consumer-driven accreditation program more than 30 years ago demonstrated great foresight, anticipating the expansion of home and community care that would occur in the last half of this century.

CHAP is structured to demonstrate its commitment to quality and its belief that true quality can only be achieved by focusing on the needs of the consumer. CHAP is the only accrediting body in the nation that relies on standards of excellence to assess all areas of an organization: client satisfaction, risk management, fiscal viability, and overall strength of management. Most important, CHAP is the only accrediting body in the nation that has offered full public access to accreditation findings since its inception.

On May 29, 1992, the Department of Health and Human Services (DHHS) formally recognized CHAP's ability to ensure the quality of home health care services provided to Medicare and Medicaid clients by granting it deemed status for home health care (DHHS, 1992). Thus CHAP became the first private accrediting body to be given this distinctive authority. The term *deemed status* signifies that home health care agencies meeting CHAP's accreditation standards will be determined to have met the federal government's conditions of participation in the Medicare and Medicaid programs. CHAP was the first accrediting body, public or private, to implement the home health survey and certification provisions of the Omnibus Budget Reconciliation Act of 1987 (P.L. 100–203). In most areas, CHAP standards exceed the federal regulations.

The goal of this chapter is to give the reader an understanding of the benefits of accreditation, the key concepts related to CHAP accreditation, and an overview of the CHAP process. Integral to CHAP's accreditation process is its consultative nature. Holding firmly to its standards, CHAP takes the approach of improving the organization being reviewed. Also integral to this process is the strong focus on consumers as recipients of care. A basic CHAP tenet is the belief that both the provider and the recipient of care need to be directly involved in the development and evaluation of services. All CHAP standards and processes are organized to promote high-quality management and services that will result in positive/expected client outcomes in its accredited organizations.

PURPOSE OF ACCREDITATION

The process of accreditation promotes the coordination and integration of quality health care delivery by all disciplines. It fosters the best possible use of available health personnel and a climate for ongoing self-study and improvement. Accreditation distinguishes the excellent organization from its competition because peers from across the country have judged it as meeting high standards (Nassif, 1985). This process identifies for the consumer those agencies that have measurable quality indicators for structure, process, and outcomes.

BENEFITS OF ACCREDITATION

An organization must understand the value of accreditation to justify the commitment of the critical resources required to complete the steps of any accreditation process. Accreditation becomes an organizing concept to foster staff and organizational efficiency in care delivery. It is therefore important for all participants to understand the benefits of accreditation.

Benefits to Clients

Involving key clients in the process of accreditation helps them appreciate the complexity of an organization's functioning. The accreditation process clarifies to clients how services and programs are coordinated and how they relate to the organization's resources. Involving consumers in accreditation is a major, yet inexpensive, management initiative. Clients are fully aware of the products and services of the organization and have established an interpersonal relationship with the staff and management team. The interpersonal relationship that the organization strives to foster may

well help identify new or improved services or products.

Benefits to Staff

There are also benefits of accreditation that relate specifically to the organization's staff providing services. All types of organizations, from the most traditional to the most innovative, need to focus on securing a solid market for their services. All staff represent the first line of marketing and selling of an organization's services and products. "Our customers' perception of quality is in the hands of our people ... each daily interaction with a customer is critical. A positive interaction adds value—a negative experience can be devastating" (American Management Association, 1991, p. 14).

The accreditation process can help an organization define and develop a market in concert with professional practice standards. The accreditation process links the philosophy and expectations of the organization with the strength and potential of individual professionals. Accreditation also provides a mechanism for staff within a discipline and across disciplines to work collaboratively. The accreditation standards clarify roles and provide a mechanism by which all staff can share in the process of setting priorities within and among services and programs. Staff develop an organizationwide perspective on issues and can be less parochial in their vision. They see how the organization might evolve to better serve their clients and community while also improving its financial health.

Benefits to the Organization

As previously mentioned, it is essential that accreditation become a major benefit for the organization itself, separate from the benefits to clients and the staff who work for the organization. Accreditation must serve the organization. It must be a wise, acceptable investment from the point of view of both the individual providers of care and the management team, from the board of directors to the first-line managers. The process of accreditation can focus the organization's future development, if it commits to using the process proactively for continuous growth. It is an ongoing investment in improvement of services and in the integrity of the organization. Results range from enabling the organization to develop a visionary strategic plan and marketing strategy to developing continuing education programs specifically to meet evolving care technologies. Accreditation may also serve to foster business relationships among various corporations within a community. Organizations are continuously examining the potential for joint ventures and diversification of services within a community. Meeting national standards and developing a blueprint for quality services through the accreditation process ensure the organization's credibility in its promise of high-quality services.

Summary

The accreditation process is one that will demand continuous commitment to services and programs by all levels of staff within the organization. Benefits of accreditation developed by the organization demand an ongoing commitment of time and energy to improve organization functioning. The benefits of accreditation for the future productivity and fiscal solvency of the organization cannot be overestimated. When it becomes a "way of life," accreditation means continual quality improvement. Involvement of staff in the accreditation process results in improved services, decreased staff turnover, increased referrals, and increased staff productivity. The accreditation process can actually become a revenue generating source for the organization.

THE CHAP PHILOSOPHY AND VISION

The CHAP philosophy is founded on the basic principle that a voluntary commitment to excellence by home and community health organizations is the best way to ensure the availability of quality community-based health care services and products. This is essential as home and community health care becomes the centerpiece of the health care industry. It is CHAP's firm belief that any health care credentialing process should clearly separate excellent organizations and programs from those meeting only minimal safety standards, should be driven by consumer concerns, should be easily understood and administered, should evaluate the total system, and should be a participative and instructive process for the organizations seeking accreditation. In 1996, the CHAP Board of Directors developed a vision statement to confirm its belief in CHAP and its philosophy: "Creating the future: integrity, quality, and leadership in community health care. Really only one choice!"

THE CHAP MISSION AND PURPOSE

CHAP's mission is to provide leadership for enhancing the health and well-being of diverse communities. This is achieved through the development of standards of excellence that ensure the management of ethical, humane, and competent care in home, community, and public health settings. In addition, the development and dissemination of innovative products, services, and models of care and the creation of partnerships further promote this mission.

CHAP's purpose is to:

- develop and promulgate standards applicable to providers of home and community health care, whether individual or corporate, for profit or not for profit, public or private
- conduct evaluations of such providers and offer accreditation to those providers meeting or exceeding such standards, so that home and community health services may achieve a uniformly high standard
- provide an external, objective marker for an organization's public, demonstrating that it meets national standards of organizational strength and quality

- provide information to the public to assist individuals as they select home and community health services and providers

THE OBJECTIVES OF CHAP

CHAP's accreditation program was developed in response to fears and concerns by consumers about the quality of home care services. This vital consumer focus has been apparent in every aspect of CHAP's organization and function since its inception in the mid-1960s. CHAP's Board of Directors, which establishes broad policy, includes consumer representatives. Consumers also sit on CHAP's Board of Review, which makes the actual accreditation decisions. The content of the standards and the site visit process focus on excellence and quality through an unrelenting commitment to the consumer. The site visit reports are made available directly to the public.

The primary objectives of CHAP's innovative programs and research activities are to:

- develop and maintain state-of-the-art, consumer-oriented, national standards of excellence focusing on outcomes for the full range of services and products provided by home care and community health organizations
- identify home and community health organizations exhibiting excellence as measured by CHAP's standards
- stimulate continual improvement in the quality of home and community health care
- distinguish excellent community-based health care providers
- facilitate consumer access to accredited organizations
- assist accredited organizations in achieving and maintaining excellence
- stimulate innovation and creativity in home care and community health service delivery

- foster the long-term viability of accredited home care and community health service delivery
- ensure that purchasers and consumers have information readily available to make informed decisions regarding home care and community health services
- promote the development and dissemination of new knowledge in the field of home and community health care through ongoing research
- stimulate continuing growth and development of the home care and community health industry

THE GOVERNANCE OF CHAP

Consumers play an important role on CHAP's Board of Directors. This is a unique feature of CHAP among accrediting bodies in that it has been a vital component since CHAP's first board was convened. The first chair was Carolyne K. Davis, former head of the Health Care Financing Administration. The board includes experts in the field of quality improvement, representatives of business and insurance, home and community health providers, and individual consumers. Organizations that have been represented on CHAP's governing board include Ford Motor Company, the Health Insurance Association of America, the American Association of Retired Persons, the Pepsi-Cola Bottling Company, Nestlé, and Amtrak.

The CHAP Board of Review, the actual accreditation decision-making body, supports this consumer focus by including consumer representatives, health care experts, and all types of community health service providers. This ensures that those paying for and receiving care as well as those providing care are directly involved in determining the accreditation status of applicant organizations. This involvement ensures that the consumers' needs will be adequately met.

PUBLIC DISCLOSURE UNDER CHAP

CHAP firmly believes that consumers have the right to direct, immediate access to site visit findings for agencies from which they are contemplating purchasing services. One of the first actions taken by CHAP's Board of Directors was to adopt a policy of full public disclosure of accreditation reports directly to the public. CHAP was the first accrediting body to make this information available to the public. It is the only accrediting body that makes this information available for all the organizations it accredits, regardless of the service standards under which they are accredited. This is a marked departure from the procedures of any other accrediting body.

Upon request, whether via CHAP's toll-free number or in writing, CHAP provides consumers with an easy-to-read report containing basic information about the organization and its services and a summary of key findings of the organization's most recent site visit. The full board of review accreditation report is also available upon request. This is the actual report of the site visit findings submitted to the organization that details the standards that the organization has met or exceeded or has failed to meet and the specific actions that the organization is required to take to maintain accreditation.

EXPERT SITE VISITORS

CHAP's site visitors have a diverse range of pertinent experience and education. To ensure that CHAP's high standards are met and maintained, and to help participating organizations be viable for the long term, CHAP site visitors are experts in the areas of home and community health management as well as service delivery. The site visitors view themselves as consultants with the management team of the organization being visited. Their aim is to provide enlightened management practices in every aspect of organization operations, from marketing strategy, financial performance, and human resource

capabilities to strategic plans for new product lines to ensure future growth.

CHAP'S CONSUMER FOCUS FOR QUALITY IMPROVEMENT

CHAP standards require that a client satisfaction survey be completed for each program. In addition, evidence that the results of these surveys are incorporated into the program must be demonstrated to the site visitors. Not only do CHAP site visitors make home visits and talk with the clients, but they also telephone previously served clients who are willing to speak candidly about the services they have received.

KEY CONCEPTS IN CHAP ACCREDITATION: STANDARDS OF EXCELLENCE

CHAP is committed to setting and maintaining the highest standards in the industry, that is, CHAP Standards of Excellence, not merely minimum safety standards. CHAP's total commitment to consumer values is reflected throughout its standards, which identify the key attributes of organizations providing excellent care. CHAP accredits only those agencies capable of meeting these standards, which emphasize client outcomes and satisfaction, organizational management, and financial viability. CHAP Standards of Excellence for home and community health providers are blueprints for achieving excellence in every element of the home care business and were designed to reflect the ever-changing complexion of the industry. Four key principles form the framework for all CHAP standards:

1. The organization's structure and function consistently support its consumer-oriented philosophy, purpose, and mission.
2. The organization consistently provides high-quality services and products.
3. The organization has adequate human, financial, and physical resources effec-

tively organized to accomplish its stated purpose.

4. The organization is positioned for long-term viability.

These four principles form the basis for the Core Standards and all service-specific standards and are applicable to all home care and community health organizations and programs (for the convenience of Medicare-certified home health agencies, the standards are cross-referenced to the Medicare conditions of participation). The Core Standards, which cover general management, administration, and financial viability of the organization, are the same for all entities. These standards cover the following areas:

- educational qualifications and credentialing of all levels of management
- the organization's policies and procedures for public disclosure and client rights
- human resources management
- ongoing quality improvement mechanisms, including client satisfaction surveys and benchmarking, and the incorporation of the results into each program or service
- staffing patterns (appropriateness of workload for service delivery)
- contracts and agreements
- adequacy of financial controls and resources, including cash flow
- adequacy of financial information systems
- strategic planning and evaluation
- risk assessment and management
- marketing strategies and initiatives
- data collection and effective incorporation of data
- management information systems
- corporate climate and support of innovation

The service-specific standards, again based on the four key principles, have been developed for each of the following services:

- community nursing centers
- dialysis
- home care aide services

- home health–Medicare (professional and paraprofessional services)
- hospice services
- home infusion therapy
- home medical equipment
- pharmacy services
- private duty services
- public health services
- supplemental staffing

All service-specific standards address the following areas in the context of each service:

- overall program/service management
- qualifications, education, and supervision of professional staff
- qualifications, training, and supervision of paraprofessional staff
- quality improvement/utilization review activities
- level of client satisfaction through surveys and site visitor client interviews
- quality of clinical/service records
- client home visits
- staff interviews
- inter- and intraorganizational coordination of services
- client outcomes and benchmarking
- service/program planning and evaluation
- service/program fiscal viability
- infection control and safety
- service/program fostering of a climate of and direction for innovation

CHAP has established and refined a set of clear, consistent standards to suit the service mix of any particular applicant organization by combining the Core Standards with the service-specific standards. Each organization may then concern itself only with the set(s) of standards pertinent to its particular service mix. Home care and community health organizations that meet these standards demonstrate their commitment to the delivery of high-quality services and products while enjoying the unique benefits of CHAP accreditation.

EXAMPLE OF CHAP STANDARDS: OUTCOME MEASURES

Several years ago, CHAP incorporated outcome measures into its standards. How an agency makes a difference is a significant part of what the site visitors look for. To illustrate, CHAP's Core Standard CII states the overall principle that an organization must consistently provide high-quality services and products. Under the umbrella of this principle, Core Standard CII.6 requires an organization to ensure high quality by routinely assessing and measuring the adequacy, appropriateness, and effectiveness of services and products and by using the results to continually improve quality. Thirteen criteria support this standard; for instance, CII.6b requires that continuous quality monitoring of services include the evaluation of client outcome data. CII.6c requires that measurable program objectives be identified in terms of client outcomes (NLN/CHAP, 1997, pp. 24–25). These include, at a minimum, the group of clients who are the recipients of service, the expected behavior or result of service, the time frame for expected results, and the realistic percentage of clients who are likely to demonstrate expected outcomes within the specified time frame. As spelled out in the criteria, the site visitors look to see documentary evidence that the outcome objectives include the specified items, that each program has at least two client outcome objectives, and that the client outcomes are monitored.

BENCHMARKING

CHAP's commitment to accreditation with a strong consumer focus led to its development of outcomes management software for home care. It began with a $1.2 million grant from W.K. Kellogg Foundation, with which it conducted ground-breaking research that resulted in a system of benchmarks for home care across three broad areas: consumer, clinical, and organizational. In 1995, risk and financial management parameters were added. These five "pulse points," as they were named, became the software program *Benchmarks for Excellence in Home Care*. The original research included collective data from 2,006 consumers, 1,909 home care staff, and 138 managers and formed the basis for a national database.

Benchmark ratings are a powerful tool for assessing the strengths and weaknesses of an organization and for seeing where an organization stands in relation to the industry as a whole. These ratings can be used to drive internal quality improvement and to secure both industry and consumer recognition. Benchmark ratings highlight problem areas, so that quality improvement efforts can be directed where they are most needed. By providing a focused vision of what home care should provide, a benchmarking program gets everyone aiming at the same mark.

Benchmarking can assist in the accreditation process by helping an organization document its quality improvement efforts. Not only does benchmarking provide a quantifiable profile of services for reports to internal or external governing/oversight bodies, but it can also provide an invaluable comparative analysis of organizational outcomes among similar organizations. The requirement for benchmarking is increasingly being integrated into accrediting organization standards. Benchmarking can also provide organizations with the tools to monitor compliance with CHAP Standards of Excellence. Finally, benchmarking can assist in increasing consumer satisfaction, improve reimbursement, and increase contract procurement from managed care organizations.

THE ADVANTAGES OF CHAP ACCREDITATION

Among the advantages of CHAP accreditation are the following:

- customized clinical and management consultation to help an organization strengthen all facets of its operations
- increased efficiency and productivity

- systematic and comprehensive evaluation of an organization's performance from top to bottom
- a quality audit that ensures accountability to consumers and payers (insurance companies and businesses)
- a complete self-study review before an on-site accreditation visit
- the ability to market to consumers using the CHAP gold seal, which has been endorsed by major consumer groups
- access to payers requiring accreditation
- customized financial profiles
- participation in regional meetings of top managers of CHAP-accredited organizations
- assistance with local media
- involvement in developing and setting CHAP Standards and policies
- potential involvement in state-of-the-art national home care research and the ability to benefit from the findings of this research
- discounts on meetings, publications, and videos

OVERVIEW OF THE ACCREDITATION PROCESS

Accreditation by CHAP is accomplished through a simple four-step process: application and contract, self-study, site visit, and determination of accreditation status by the Board of Review.

Application and Contract

The completed application form, which includes a profile of the organization, is sent to CHAP with an application fee. The organizational profile allows CHAP staff to determine the applicable fees for each organization. Once the fees have been determined, CHAP will send a contract to the applicant organization outlining the specific elements of the accreditation fee. The contract covers the 3-year term of the accreditation cycle. The Core Standards, appropriate service-specific standards, and self-study guide are provided to the organization along with the contract.

Self-Study

The self-study guides an organization through a unique process of self-evaluation. The self-study is completed to prepare for the site visit, and it must be submitted to CHAP within 4 to 6 months of receipt of the contract. The self-study is a step-by-step guide to the self-assessment of administration, clinical services, and financial operations and is beneficial to any organization. The self-study allows the organization to compare itself with the CHAP Standards and become acquainted with the purpose of the accreditation site visit without having to purchase additional manuals. It addresses the clinical and business aspects of the organization by looking at the quality of services and products, the availability of resources, the fiscal viability of the organization, and its attention to consumers. Information from the self-study assists CHAP in planning for and conducting the site visit. When completed with input from all levels and types of staff, it reflects the collective vision of management, staff, and consumers.

Site Visit

CHAP evaluates the quality of home and community health organizations through unannounced site visits. Activities include home visits and telephone surveys to assess client satisfaction. CHAP requires agencies to perform regular client satisfaction surveys and to use the results to improve services.

Unannounced site visits are made by a team of trained site visitors specifically chosen for their specialized expertise. Visits average 4 or 5 days in length; the actual time for each organization is determined according to its size and complexity. The visits are designed to be a consultative, positive learning experience. On arrival, site visitors establish a schedule with the organization's management staff that includes a review of appropriate documents such as policies, board and management meeting minutes, and clinical records to ensure the quality of the organization's clinical services and products, the financial health of the organization, and its strategic plan. Considerable attention is given to interviews with staff, advisory committee members, and governing body members. Clients receive significant attention directly through interviews, home visits, and telephone surveys to ensure that the organization is committed to CHAP's consumer-oriented, outcome-based standards.

Findings of the site visitors are discussed at an exit conference. Consultation is always available from the site visitors regarding specific recommendations or areas in which the organization would like help. The consultation is always provided after the exit conference so that it does not interfere with the evaluation process.

Determination of Accreditation Status

The Board of Review, comprising community and home care administrators, consultants, and consumers from across the nation, evaluates the self-study and the site visit report and determines the accreditation status of the applicant organization, including any required actions, recommendations, or commendations. Once accredited, an organization receives annual unannounced site visits for the first 3 years of accreditation. The site visit interval may be as long as 36 months after the initial cycle for organizations with outstanding services and systems. In 1996 CHAP developed specific criteria for identifying organizations whose site

visits could be extended 24 to 36 months. These criteria will be implemented in 1997.

TYPES OF ORGANIZATIONS ELIGIBLE FOR CHAP ACCREDITATION

CHAP accreditation is available for all types of organizations, including nonprofit, proprietary, voluntary, government, facility based, and freestanding. That is, organizations providing health care services or products for the home or community sites are eligible for CHAP accreditation.

In 1996, CHAP added a special accreditation option for new home care organizations. This is called the JumpStart Option for accreditation. Under this option, start-up organizations, those in business for less than 2 years, can go through a streamlined accreditation process. The same standards must be met and the self-study must be completed, but in a more appropriate way for a start-up agency.

CONCLUSION

The decision by an organization to seek accreditation is a serious one. It demands commitment from management and staff at all levels because it is the path to continuous quality improvement. Initiatives and activities focused on internal improvements lead to results that affect the client positively, which is the ultimate goal of accreditation. Consumers and payers alike recognize that, when an organization has met rigorous national standards, it is more likely to have the consistent positive outcomes that consumers seek. The accreditation process provides a challenge to organizations to accept responsibility for their growth and development. Working through the accreditation process shows the standards to be more than abstract principles. The process, from application by the organization to the decision of the Board of Review, is one of continuous growth.

POSTSCRIPT

In 1997, the Foundation for Hospice and HomeCare merged with the National Association for Home Care (NAHC) and NAHC will be administering the Foundation's Program.

REFERENCES

American Management Association (AMA). 1991. *Blueprints for service quality: The Federal Express approach. AMA Management Briefing.* New York: AMA.

Department of Health and Human Services, Health Care Financing Administration. 1992, May. Medicare program: Recognition of the Community Health Accreditation Program standards for home care organizations. *Federal Register* 57:22773–22780.

Nassif, J. 1985. *The home health care solution.* New York: Harper & Row.

National League for Nursing (NLN) and Community Health Accreditation Program (CHAP). 1997. *Standards of excellence for home care organizations.* New York: NLN/CHAP.

SUGGESTED READING

Community Health Accreditation Program (CHAP). 1994. *In search of excellence in home care—Final report to W.K. Kellogg Foundation.* New York: CHAP.

Community Health Accreditation Program (CHAP). 1996. *Benchmarks for excellence in home care—Operator's tutorial.* New York: CHAP.

Zink, M.R. 1996. Home care accreditation with the Community Health Accreditation Program: Part II: The process. *Home Healthcare Nurse* 14:684–688.

CHAPTER 6

Accreditation by the Foundation for Hospice and Home Care, National HomeCaring Council

Ken Wessel

HISTORY

The National Council for Homemaker Services was incorporated in 1962 to promote high-quality homemaker services and to set standards for the field. The first set of standards was developed in 1965. In 1967, the National HomeCaring Council was cited in the *Federal Register* as the national standard-setting body for paraprofessionals. The training of homemaker–home health aides was a primary concern and led to the publishing of a training manual in 1967. That evolved into the *Model Curriculum and Teaching Guide for the Instruction of Homemaker–Home Health Aides*, first published in 1978 (Department of Health and Human Services, 1978). The accreditation program itself was developed in 1971. Initially, the process consisted of the review of self-study and other written documentation, but a comprehensive site visit survey was added in 1976. Over the years, this accreditation program became recognized in many states across the country, where it was designated as a requirement for participation in various Title III, Title XX, or Medicaid programs. In 1986, the National HomeCaring Council left New York and joined the Foundation for Hospice and Homecare in Washington DC. In 1994, the Council adopted the format of the home care aide standards and self-study (Foundation for Hospice and Homecare, 1994) to private duty nursing services. That accreditation option became available in 1995, and the first private duty nursing service was accredited through the National HomeCaring Council in 1996.

STRUCTURE

The National HomeCaring Council is a division of the Foundation for Hospice and Homecare with headquarters in Washington, DC. The accreditation program consists of two components. The Standards Committee is responsible for setting and reviewing standards to reflect current practice norms. The established standards are subject to approval by the Foundation Board. The Standards Committee meets periodically to keep up with the evolving field of home care.

The second component is the Accreditation Commission. This group consists of home care professionals, representatives of consumer groups, and volunteers. The Commission meets several times a year to review and make recommendations on accreditation applications. The Foundation Board can grant accreditation status based on these recommendations.

STANDARDS

Standards for home care aide and private duty nursing services are listed in Exhibit 6–1.

Exhibit 6–1 Standards for Home Care Aide and Private Duty Nursing Services

Home Care Aide Services

I.   There shall be a legally-constituted authority responsible for governance and performance.

II. There shall be compliance with legislation, which relates to prohibition of discriminatory practices.

III. There shall be responsible fiscal management.

IV. There shall be responsible personnel management including:
   A. Recruitment, selection, and retention of all personnel and;
   B. Written personnel policies, job descriptions, and wage scales established for each job category.

V.   Every Home Care Aide shall have received training for each task to be performed for the client.

VI. There shall be written eligibility criteria for service and written procedures for referral to other sources.

VII. There shall be supervision of the Home Care Aide service which shall ensure safe, effective, and appropriate care to each individual or family served.

VIII. There shall be an evaluation of all aspects of the service.

IX. There shall be ongoing interpretation of service to the community.

X.   There shall be a written statement of clients' rights and clear evidence that it is fully implemented.

XI. There shall be responsible management of safety in the care environment:
   A. To ensure the well-being of the patient and;
   B. To ensure the well-being of the caregiver(s).

Private Duty Nursing Services

(where different from above)

V.   There shall be professional case management services for all individuals and families served.

VII. There shall be professional registered nurse supervision of nursing personnel in the field to ensure safe, effective, and appropriate care to each individual or family served.

Courtesy of the Foundation for Hospice and Home Care, Washington, DC.

PROCESS

The accreditation process is the same for both home care aide and private duty nursing services. That process consists of application, self-study, a site visit, and Accreditation Commission review.

To be eligible to apply, the agency must have been in operation with the service to be accredited for at least 1 year. The agency must directly employ the direct service workers. All similar services in an organization are surveyed regardless of funding source. Application can be made by calling the National HomeCaring Council at (202) 547-7424.

The National HomeCaring Council selects two peer reviewers to analyze the self-study, perform a 2-day site visit survey of the agency, and submit a report to the Accreditation Commission. These reviewers have been trained by the Council and are always principals in home care agencies that have been accredited.

The first part of the self-study involves the applicant mailing questionnaires to a small sample of agency consumers. These questionnaires cover areas of customer satisfaction and clinical competence. They are returned directly to the National HomeCaring Council when completed and are reviewed by the two surveyors and the Commission.

The major part of the self-study consists of the applicant completing the 30-page self-study document. The document expands on the 11 standards and requires checking responses and narrative answers as well as listing supporting documentation being submitted by the agency. The Council suggests forming a broad-based committee among agency staff and board members to complete the self-study.

The completed self-study is forwarded to the National HomeCaring Council, and copies are sent to each peer reviewer for evaluation. They begin the completion of a reviewer's instrument that is used to score the self-study and the site visit survey. The lead reviewer will contact the agency when necessary to discuss any omissions or areas that need clarification. A site visit is scheduled, and the agency is asked to make a variety of board and staff members available for interviews.

During the 2-day site visit, the reviewers confirm documentation, evaluate selected personnel and case records, and interview staff and selected board members. The surveyors use this time to compare their analyses of the self-studies and resolve any contradictions that may have occurred. At the end of the site visit, the peer reviewers will conduct an exit interview with the agency director and give an overview of the findings. They will also submit a written report to the Commission that lists areas of concern as well as suggested commendations. The Commission staff will forward these written concerns to the agency and give the agency an opportunity to respond in writing before the meeting of the Accreditation Commission.

The Accreditation Commission will meet several times throughout the year to review agencies that have gone through this process. Whenever possible, one of the surveyors will present the agency to the Commission in person. Compliance with each standard is reviewed and voted on in turn. Each standard can be rated as noncompliance, partial conformity, substantial conformity, or full conformity. The Commission is assisted by numerical ratings in the reviewer's instrument. When all standards are rated, the results are evaluated in the aggregate, and an accreditation decision is made. Possible outcomes are to deny accreditation, postpone accreditation, grant provisional accreditation, or accredit. If information is missing and can be obtained by the next Commission meeting, postponement would be appropriate. Provisional accreditation could be granted if remedial action was required and could be anticipated within a specific time frame. These decisions are communicated to the agency along with final recommendations and commendations made by the Commission. An appeals process is in place for agencies that believe the standards were not properly applied.

The accreditation process operates on a 3-year cycle. Full self-studies and site visits are required at that interval. Interim reports are to be submitted midterm to ascertain whether there have been any substantive changes in the agency.

RECENT DEVELOPMENTS

In 1995, the home care aide self-study was computerized. The self-study can be completed and submitted on a floppy disk. Currently, this is only available for IBM-compatible computers using Microsoft *Word* for Windows.

In 1996, the Foundation for Hospice and Homecare began a dialogue with the Joint Commission on Accreditation of Healthcare Organizations. The goal of this initiative is to agree on protocols for reciprocity.

CONCLUSION

Voluntary accreditation by the National HomeCaring Council can help an agency demonstrate its administrative and clinical competence to the community as well as to state and local payer sources. It is an excellent quality improvement tool. The involvement of the board and all levels of staff in the process provides a team-building opportunity and essential information about current standards in the industry.

REFERENCES

Department of Health and Human Services. (DHHS). 1978. *Model curriculum and teaching guide for the instruction of homemakers–home health aides.* Publication No. HSA 80-5508. Rockville, MD: DHHS.

Foundation for Hospice and Homecare. 1994. *Self-study manual.* Washington, DC: National HomeCaring Council.

CHAPTER 7

Certificate of Need and Licensure

E. Michael Flanagan

At first glance, a health care entrepreneur's interest in home health as a business is understandable. The product to be furnished is readily identifiable and labor rather than material intensive. This means that the anticipated capital outlay for start-up costs should be minimal.

It is only when the entrepreneur confronts the complex and often confusing array of federal and state laws and regulations governing home health agencies (HHAs) that the hidden costs of establishing a home care program are realized.

This chapter discusses two aspects of this regulatory scheme: certificate of need (CON) and licensure. The impact of CON and licensure requirements on HHAs varies dramatically depending on the state in which the HHA operates.[1] It is important from the standpoint of marketing feasibility, however, to understand the specific requirements of the jurisdiction in which one plans to establish a home health program.

Finally, because many states have merged their state licensure function with their responsibilities concerning certification of new Medicare providers, some discussion of Medicare certification will be inevitable in this chapter, even though that topic is covered in more detail elsewhere in this book.

HHA CON REQUIREMENTS

Background

When Congress passed the National Health Planning and Resources Development Act of 1974,[2] it sought to rationalize the distribution of health services throughout the United States and to give individual states a legal mechanism to make prospective determinations of need for new health care services. These laudable objectives proved more problematic in practice than originally envisioned, and the 23 years since enactment of the law have seen the once energetically federal initiative become almost exclusively a creature of state law. Federal funding for health planning is virtually nonexistent today, and many states have repealed their CON laws and substituted more stringent licensure requirements for health care facilities.

The establishment of an HHA historically has required a limited capital expenditure. Moreover, the existence of CON requirements for HHAs in certain states has thus far failed to demonstrate a positive correlation between restricted market entry and lower costs per unit of service.[3] Consequently, a number of states have reconsidered the need to include HHAs in their CON laws, and at least four states (Texas, Tennessee, California, and Virginia) have eliminated HHAs from CON review in recent years.[4]

The increasing popularity of managed health care plans will probably convince more states in the future to eliminate HHAs from CON review because of the perceived natural constraints on the growth of HHAs due to capitation.

Impact on Feasibility Study

When someone decides to explore the possibility of entering the home health care market as a provider of services, essentially two options are available. The first is acquisition of part or all of an existing home health care business. The second is the creation of a new HHA that will compete for a share of the existing market. The presence of a CON law for HHAs in the state of intended operation is often the single most important determinant in deciding whether to go forward with the project in that state and under which option.

Some form of feasibility study is desirable for any prospective entrant into the home care business. The first consideration identified in a creditable feasibility study will be barriers to entry into the market. For example, some states (including Florida, Georgia, Alabama, Kentucky, and Mississippi) have at one time or another imposed moratoriums on the issuance of new HHA CONs. This would mean that the only opportunity for entry in these states would be the acquisition of an existing Medicare-certified HHA or establishment of a private pay HHA (i.e., an agency that provides no services to Medicare or Medicaid beneficiaries), if that is not a reviewable event under state law.[5]

A more recent barrier to entry has arisen within the past year because of federal government cutbacks in funding for state Medicare survey agencies. Some states, such as Illinois, performed virtually no new HHA provider surveys in fiscal year 1995 (ending September 30, 1995) because of the absence of funding. It is obvious that acquisition of an existing HHA under these circumstances would be preferable to waiting indefinitely for a new provider certification survey.

For all of the reasons set out above, if the state of operation in the new entrant's business plan is not predetermined, the existence of CON requirements could lead to the selection of a different state. Such a move is not without risk.

Selecting a Non-CON State

The selection of a non-CON state will have the immediate beneficial effect of eliminating the need for significant start-up costs for consulting, legal, and accounting expenses related to obtaining CON approval. On the other hand, absence of CON means that other competitors (including local hospitals) can invade the market at any time and steal away referral sources and valued employees.

Survival in such a competitive environment is difficult. Hospitals more than likely will have their own facility-based HHAs to capture their own home health referrals. At the same time, these hospitals will put pressure on their staff physicians to refer to the hospital-based agency. In addition, national chain home health providers are generally more active in these markets because their size allows them to endure the financial strains of longer start-up periods.

Thus the decision to pursue a non-CON state is not a panacea. In fact, certain state HHAs (Florida and Georgia, for example) have fought to preserve their state CON programs for HHAs motivated in large measure by their belief that CON is the only way to preserve the freestanding community-based HHA.

Acquiring an HHA in a CON State

Recognizing the difficulties of surviving in a non-CON state, it may be advisable to explore acquisition opportunities in a CON state.[6] In most CON states, the acquisition of an HHA's stock or a transfer of assets is considered a change of ownership. As such, unless the change of ownership is accompanied by a change in the scope of services or service area, it will be determined to be a nonreviewable event.[7]

It is often the case, however, that the state health planning agency will require notice of the change of ownership at some time in advance of the event.[8] Thus the recommended manner of proceeding is to identify the intended acquisition, negotiate the purchase offer, and then send a formal letter of intent to acquire the HHA to the state health planning agency. The letter should also request written confirmation that the acquisition is a nonreviewable event under the state CON law. Once the confirmation letter is received, the need to focus on CON issues is at an end unless a later modification of service or service area necessitates review.

If the acquisition entails simply a transfer of part or all of the existing agency's stock, the transaction might not even fall under the CON law's change of ownership rules. Thus, as in all potential CON matters, a careful review of the law and regulations could avoid unnecessary headaches.[9]

Obtaining a CON

This discussion is not for the faint of heart. Under the best of circumstances, obtaining a CON in a conscientiously regulated state can be a brutal affair involving intense political influence wielding and courtroom battles with established HHAs in the affected service area.

Based on experience, it can be anticipated that obtaining a CON will add $50,000 to $100,000 to agency start-up costs. This figure can rise significantly if an adversely affected HHA files suit to enjoin issuance of the CON. In one of the more famous CON wars, Johnson & Johnson waged a major campaign to obtain HHA CONs in Florida several years ago. The widely publicized assault on the state CON program ultimately brought the Florida Association of Home Health Agencies into the fray on the side of the state health planning agency. After having the regulatory basis upon which need determinations had been made in Florida since 1975 declared invalid,[10] Johnson & Johnson abandoned the effort, having spent approximately $3 million in a losing cause.

If you are still undaunted by the bleak prospects of obtaining a CON, then the first step to take would be to examine the CON law and regulations to determine whether there is any way

validly to claim entitlement to an exemption from the review requirement.

Exemptions may be available for a number of reasons based on your particular circumstances. We have already discussed the exemption based on change of ownership. Some states have so-called "grandfather" provisions in the CON law that exempt from review existing HHAs that have been providing home health services continuously in the state since a time before the effective data of the CON law. The "grandfather" provision that was a part of the Florida licensure law[11] until repealed in 1990 furnishes an excellent illustration of this type of exemption:

> Any home health agency operating and providing services in the state and having a provider number issued by the U.S. Department of Health, Education and Welfare on or before April 30, 1976 shall not be denied a license on the basis of not having received a Certificate of Need.[12]

Historically, Florida has administered its CON program on a district-by-district basis, each district comprising one or more counties. Because of this, HHAs that were Medicare certified and operational in the state before April 30, 1976 successfully used the "grandfather" provision to expand their service areas. By simply demonstrating to the state health planning office that it had seen one or more patients in the expansion district before the effective date, the HHA was able to obtain a determination that it would be exempt from review and able to serve that entire district as fully as any other preexisting HHA already serving the district.

Another exemption category applies to health maintenance organizations (HMOs) that seek to furnish home health services directly. Many states generally exempt HMOs from the coverage of their CON laws.[13] It is unclear, however, whether the exemption would apply to all services that the HMO furnishes directly.

Obviously, exemptions are exceptions to the rule that new HHAs must submit to CON review. If no exemption is available and acquisition is not feasible, it is important to have some understanding of the typical CON review process so that a strategy can be developed to ensure the best chance of a favorable outcome.

A Typical CON Review Process

All state CON laws differ in certain respects concerning the formalities of the review process, but I will attempt to outline a typical review sequence based on Maryland law.

The first step in the filing of a CON application is the submission of a letter of intent to the health planning agency.[14] If you are unfamiliar with the process generally, a telephone call to the agency would be advisable. Our experience indicates that health planning staff persons can be extremely helpful in guiding applicants through the maze of red tape that invariably accompanies CON actions.

The letter of intent is designed to alert the agency of an impending CON application. It usually includes the following information: a description of the proposed project, the nature and scope of new health services to be offered, the location of the project, and the estimated total project cost.[15] The letter of intent normally sets in motion a time period within which to file the CON application. Under Maryland law, the CON application must be submitted at least 60 days after the submission of the letter of intent, but the application must be received before the expiration of 180 days from the date of submission of the letter of intent.[16] If the application is received too early, it can be held over until the next review period after the expiration of the 60 days. If no application has been received by the expiration of the 180 days, the letter of intent is null and void, and the applicant must start over.[17] The time requirements vary from state to state, so that it is essential to know your particular state's rules.

It is also important to realize that a CON application takes a good deal of time and effort to complete and that the burden of proving entitlement to a CON rests squarely on the applicant. If you are serious about obtaining a CON,

it is advisable at this point to hire a consultant who specializes in completing and justifying CON applications. It is also a good idea at this time to start lining up whatever political assistance is available to you to begin the necessary lobbying effort to convince the state health planning agency of the need for a new HHA.

Once the application is submitted, the planning agency reviews it for completeness and assigns a docket number.[18] The agency will then notify the applicant in writing of the docketing and will also publish notice of the docketing in a newspaper of general circulation in the area of the proposed project.[19]

Some state planning programs (such as Maryland's) have routine review cycles into which similar applications are batched for the purpose of comparative review. In other words, if three new HHA CON applications are submitted in the same month, they will be assigned together to the same batching cycle, and their individual merits will be assessed in comparison with one another. Thus if only one new HHA is justified in the area, the best applicant of the three will be selected.

Parties that will be affected by the project (referred to in CON laws as interested persons or interested parties)[20] are entitled to request an evidentiary hearing to be conducted by the planning agency.[21] As a general rule, the hearing must be requested within a certain time period after the notice of docketing is published. The evidentiary hearing is conducted in a fashion similar to a courtroom trial, with counsel representing the parties, oral testimony including examination and cross-examination of witnesses, and a written report by the presiding officer with findings of fact and conclusions of law.[22] The final action of the evidentiary hearing is the issuance by the presiding officer of a proposed order, which will become final after the parties to the hearing have had an opportunity to file written objections and to give oral testimony before final action on the application.[23] The final order in most instances is a grant or denial of the application.

Another type of forum available to affected persons to comment on a proposed project is the public informational hearing.[24] Unlike the adversarial evidentiary hearing, the public informational hearing is more or less an open forum to provide the public with an opportunity to express its views on the project.

Regardless of whether the application is submitted to an evidentiary hearing or to comparative or individual review, its merits will be judged against certain parameters of need established by the state health planning program. These considerations will generally include the identification of a need for such a service in the state health plan,[25] the need of the population served or to be served (a supplemental analysis to the general need determinations included in the state health plan), the availability of less costly or more effective alternatives for addressing the unmet needs identified by the applicant, the immediate and long-term financial viability of the project, and the adequacy of staffing, community and professional support for the project.[26]

The decision of the planning agency concerning the application must be issued within a certain time period of docketing.[27] The planning agency can decide to grant the application, to deny it, or to grant it subject to specific conditions.[28] The decision must be in writing, setting forth the reasons for the action.

Assuming that the project has been approved either completely or with acceptable conditions, you might be lulled into thinking that your new HHA is home free. This, however, may be only the beginning of the ordeal. The final decision has created a new class of participants in the CON process called aggrieved parties. An aggrieved party is essentially an affected person who has been adversely affected by the final decision.[29] An aggrieved party (which obviously includes the applicant if the decision was a denial) has the right to request, upon a showing of good cause, a hearing for the purpose of reconsidering the final decision.[30] This reconsideration hearing must be requested within a short period of time after the date of the final decision

(normally within 15 days), and a reconsideration decision is considered a new final decision for purposes of appeal (and renewed requests for reconsideration hearings, etc.).

Finally, an aggrieved party that has not been able to show good cause for a reconsideration hearing or has not been satisfied by a reconsideration decision has the right to take a direct judicial appeal within a specified time frame of the date of the final decision.[31] The judicial appeal is normally made to the trial court level of the state court system, but the review of the case is normally limited to the record that has been developed in the administrative process. Furthermore, any decision at the trial court level may be appealed to the highest appellate level of the state courts and ultimately (carrying the process to its most sublimely ridiculous extent) to the U.S. Supreme Court if a sufficiently national issue can be demonstrated.

Summary

It should be clear from the tenor of the foregoing presentation that it is the opinion of this author that the CON process is an ineffective tool to ensure the appropriate distribution of health care resources. It is tedious, expensive, and ultimately incapable of preventing the granting of unnecessary projects to those with the will and financial and political backing to outlast the process. It is, however, a mandatory precondition to the establishment of a new HHA in 19 states and the District of Columbia. Thus if there is no alternative to submission to the CON process, then the foregoing information should prove useful.

HHA LICENSURE

Background

Because in states that have HHA licensure laws the license requirement is not used as a barrier to entry into the marketplace, there is no need to go into elaborate detail about the nuances of the licensure process. The political, practical, and economic realities of licensure are unambiguous: If the HHA meets certain conditions established by the state, it will be issued a license; if not, the HHA will not be permitted to operate until the conditions are met.

In some states, such as California, the licensure laws are so stringent and are enforced so rigorously that, from the standpoint of economic feasibility, they may constitute a barrier to the establishment of a new HHA. The California experience, however, is clearly the exception.

Of the 40 state licensure laws (including those of the District of Columbia) for HHAs, virtually all have requirements that track closely with the Medicare program's conditions of participation.[32] In fact, most states have unified their state licensure and Medicare certification functions into one office, which coordinates survey activities for both.

Before the Omnibus Budget Reconciliation Act of 1980, if an HHA was established in a state that had no HHA licensure law, the HHA was prohibited from participating in the Medicare program unless it had obtained status as a charitable organization under section 501(c)(3) of the Internal Revenue Code. This restriction was apparently based on the assumption that for-profit HHAs are inherently suspect without a state regulatory body in existence to police their operations. The 1980 legislation abolished such distinctions as a matter of federal law, but at least one state (New York) retained the restriction as a matter of state law until a few years ago.

State HHA licensure laws have generally been administered without much controversy, but it is important to understand your state's law (if any) so that potential problem areas can be anticipated.

Typical Licensure Law

Most states that have HHA licensure laws make it a criminal offense for anyone to operate an HHA without a license. In many instances, however, the licensure requirement applies only to those HHAs that intend to participate in the Medicare or Medicaid program. An HHA that is treating only private insurance or private pay patients will not be required to be licensed. Thus in these days of separate Medicare and private HHAs, it is important to know the coverage of your state's licensure law.

The licensure law sets out minimum operational standards for HHAs operating in the state that must be met at all times. An applicant for initial licensure must furnish certain minimal information to the licensing office on forms provided by the office, including the names and addresses of each officer and director of the HHA and of certain owners.[33]

Upon receipt of the application, the licensing office will schedule a survey to ensure that the HHA meets all requirements. The timing of the licensure survey in relation to the operational start-up of the HHA varies from state to state. It is important to make contact with the licensure office in advance of the survey to ascertain the level of activity the survey team is expecting to see by the date of the survey. Most states will not permit the HHA to see a patient before the license is issued. Others will expect to review a patient chart or two and thus will require some minimal visit activity before the licensure survey.

Essentially, the survey team will be seeking to determine that the key personnel of the HHA have the requisite skill level, that the required scope of services will be provided either directly or through contractual arrangements, that the HHA complies with all applicable state and federal laws, that the HHA has appropriate liability insurance to cover all employees and contractual indemnity to cover services provided under arrangement, and that the HHA has the requisite recordkeeping capability.[34]

If the HHA passes the survey, the state will issue a license for a 1-year period. Most states require that the annual application for relicensure be submitted well in advance of the expiration date (generally 60 days) so that any reinspection can be done and a new license issued before the expiration date. In at least one state (Florida), an administrative fine of $100 per day is levied against any HHA submitting its relicensure application less than 60 days before the expiration date.

If the HHA fails to meet licensure requirements, it will be denied a license. This decision is subject to appeal under the state's Administrative Procedures Act.

Finally, under certain circumstances the state can issue a provisional license (of normally 90 days in duration) to an HHA that is not in substantial compliance if the HHA has submitted an acceptable plan of correction to resolve the areas of noncompliance.[35]

Once the license is issued, it must be displayed in a place viewable by the general public.[36] If the HHA decides to relinquish the license voluntarily, or if it is denied, revoked, or suspended under administrative action, the HHA must provide requisite notice to the patients, their authorized representatives, attending physicians, and third party payers.[37]

The licensing agency has the right to investigate complaints and to ensure that the HHA is maintaining compliance with all licensure requirements including the governing authority of the HHA,[38] proper personnel,[39] staff supervision and training,[40] and the maintenance and safeguarding of clinical records.[41]

Some Legal and Practical Considerations about Licensure

Although licensure issues do not often arise as legal problems, some points about licensure in the context of CON and Medicare certification should be kept in mind.

As has already been mentioned, in CON states for HHAs, a CON or a formal exemption determination is a precondition to the issuance of a license. It is also true in many states, however, that the continuing viability of the CON is dependent on uninterrupted licensure. Thus if for some reason the HHA license is suspended or revoked, or if the agency ceases to operate for any period of time, the state, or more likely, a competing HHA could assert that the CON

has lapsed. It is important, therefore, that any licensure defects be rectified as soon as possible to avoid threatening the CON.

Licensure problems also seem to arise almost magically when an HHA is forced to fire one of its key employees. An unannounced inspection always seems to follow shortly on the heels of a terminated administrator. Accordingly, if it becomes necessary to fire a key employee, it is often wise to alert the licensure office that the action is pending and that you have taken appropriate steps to hire a qualified replacement. A preventive phone call could save you the aggravation of being visited by licensing inspectors carrying an order to show cause as to why the HHA should not be closed down for being improperly staffed.

Another problem with the license as it affects CON is the fact that health planning authorities look to the license to ascertain the HHA's service area. In states in which the service area is not clearly articulated in the CON, the counties or subdivisions listed on the HHA's license are looked upon as the best evidence of the HHA's service area. Thus whenever a licensure form needs to be completed that asks for any identification of service area (for example, single county or multicounty), to the extent that your answer is not clearly inconsistent with your CON approval, always select the most expansive definition.

Finally, it should be kept in mind that licensure is a precondition to Medicare certification, and although the two offices generally work closely together they do not always coordinate their efforts carefully enough. If a new HHA obtains Medicare certification before licensure is effective, or if licensure is lost for any period of time, the HHA will be forced to forfeit all payment for Medicare services furnished during the period without licensure.

CONCLUSION

If you are interested in becoming involved in the ownership and operation of an HHA, and you are still convinced after reading this chapter, press on. As the chapter indicates, there are often ways to circumvent the costly and time-consuming burdens of confronting the CON process head on. Licensure, on the other hand, must be faced, but it is not nearly so cumbersome or threatening a process. The important principle to keep in mind in dealing with CON and licensure issues is that anticipation and prevention of problems can save enormous headaches and expenses that come as a result of reacting to crises. Before you go flailing headlong into the regulatory process that encompasses home health care, establish a business plan, do a marketing feasibility study, retain competent advisors who are knowledgeable in the area, and develop a good working relationship with the government agencies that will determine your entitlement to CON and licensure. The game plan is to accomplish your objectives with the least possible expenditure of your resources. In the present home health care marketplace, there is no substitute for cost consciousness.

REFERENCES

1. At the present time, 39 states and the District of Columbia have CON and/or licensure requirements for HHAs. It should be noted, however, that not all states that have one requirement have the other. Thus 39 states and the District of Columbia have HHA licensure laws, and 20 states and the District of Columbia have HHA CON laws, but 3 of the HHA CON states (Vermont, Alabama, and West Virginia) have no HHA licensure laws. Furthermore, state legislatures are continually reviewing the need for such laws, particularly CON. Notably, the Florida legislature in 1992 reenacted the state licensure and CON laws by a narrow margin, but included a sunset provision in the new law that will cause it to expire on July I, 1997.

2. P.L. 93-641, 88 Stat. 2225 (January 4, 1975).

3. See generally Anderson, K.B., de Kass, D.S. (1986). *Certificate of need regulation of entry into home health care.* Washington, DC: Bureau of Economics.

4. Tennessee had repealed its CON requirements for HHAs but reinstated them after a rapid expansion of new HHAs in the state threatened to destabilize the entire industry. California has dropped its CON program in its entirety.

5. Most of the 21 CON states only require review if the HHA intends to seek reimbursement from the Medicare or Medicaid programs. Some jurisdictions, including Tennessee, West Virginia, and the District of Columbia, require CON review for all in-home services without regard to payment source.

6. Acquisitions of existing HHAs in non-CON states do occur when the purchaser is seeking to acquire an established patient base and/or goodwill.

7. See, for example, Md. Ann. Code section 19-115 (i)(2)(iii); COMAR section 10.24.01.03A(I).

8. *Id.*

9. We are aware of one instance in which a new entrant fought a long, costly, and ultimately successful battle to obtain a new HHA CON only to realize later that it would have been entitled automatically to a CON under the CON law's grandfather provision.

10. Florida had been using the so-called rule of 300 to make need determinations for new HHAs. The rule of 300 would prevent a new HHA from obtaining a CON unless it could demonstrate that all the existing agencies in the relevant market area had an average daily census of 300 patients. The rule was ultimately struck down by the Florida state courts as having been adopted without proper reliance on any empirical data justifying such a criterion.

11. Because in states having CON laws governing HHAs CON approval is a precondition to licensure, it is not uncommon that certain provisions in the licensure law will have a bearing on CON requirements. This is a point to bear in mind when determining whether to pursue CON.

12. Fla. Stat. Ann. section 400.,504 (1980). (Repealed by laws c. 90-319, § 10, effective July 3, 1990).

13. See, for example, Md. Stat. Ann. section 19-116 (1993 cumulative supplement).

14. See COMAR section 10.24.01.06C.

15. COMAR section 10.24.01.06C(2).

16. COMAR section 10.24.01.06C(4) and (6).

17. *Id.*

18. COMAR section 10.24.01.07A.

19. COMAR section 10.24.01.07A(6).

20. Under Maryland law, an interested person is defined as "an affected person who has made a written request to the Commission to receive copies of relevant notices concerning an application" (COMAR section 10.24.01.01-9(19)). An affected person includes, among others, the applicant, local health planning

authorities, consumers of health care services in the area of the project, existing health care facilities, insurers, and any competing applicants (COMAR 10.24.01101-1(B)(1)).

21. COMAR section 10.24.01.07C.

22. COMAR section 10.24.01.07E.

23. COMAR section 10.24.01.07F.

24. COMAR section 10.24.01.10

25. The state health plan is a document that sets present and projected need for the distribution of certain health care services and equipment throughout the state. Need is normally projected for a 5-year period.

26. COMAR section 10.24.01.07H.

27. See COMAR section 10.24.01.07K. In Maryland, the time period is 150 days if an evidentiary hearing is held and 120 days if not.

28. *Id.*

29. COMAR section 10.24.01.01-1B(2).

30. COMAR section 10.24.01.17.

31. COMAR section 10.24.01.18.

32. For a comparative illustration of the various state HHA licensure laws and key elements of Medicare conditions of participation, see *The "black box" of home care quality,* a report presented by the chair of the Select Committee on Aging, House of Representatives, 99th Cong., 2d sess. Prepared by the American Bar Association (August 1986).

33. See COMAR section 10.07.10.02B.

34. See COMAR section 10.07.10.04. Most licensure laws require HHAs to provide skilled nursing services and at least one of the following: physical therapy, occupational therapy, speech therapy, medical social services, or home health aide.

35. COMAR section 10.07.10.05.

36. COMAR section 10.07.10.07.

37. COMAR section 10.07.01.06.

38. See COMAR section 10.07.01.08.

39. See COMAR section 10.07.01.09.

40. See COMAR section 10.07.01.10.

41. See COMAR section 10.07.01.11.

CHAPTER 8

Professional Credentialing for Home Care/Hospice Personnel

Ann H. Cary

Agency administrators are constantly challenged to place well-qualified individuals in agency positions. Although the supply of and demand for well-qualified individuals never seem to be stable, the maldistribution of personnel in urban and rural areas poses an additional challenge to an agency's efforts. Rural agencies report unique problems in attracting and retaining top-notch personnel. There are several sources of guidelines from federal, state, and local jurisdictions as well as from organizations that promote agency accreditation. This chapter reviews these guidelines in discussing the minimum standards as well as distinctive credentials proposed for agency personnel. A discussion of the various certification and licensure options for the administrator is presented subsequently with a focus on the unique opportunities now available as a measure of distinction for the home health/hospice administrator.

Current guidelines and standards for administrators in home care can be found in the Medicare conditions of participation (COP) issued by the Department of Health and Human Services (DHHS, 1989, 1991). For agencies that operate under COP guidelines, the definitions provided in §484.14 provide that the administrator is a licensed physician, a registered nurse, or a person with training and experience in health service administration. The administrator should also have at least 1 year of administrative and

supervisory experience in either home health care or other health-related programs.

A second-level person in the agency who may have administrative responsibility for supervising skilled nursing and therapies is referred to as the supervising physician or registered nurse. COP guidelines suggest that this individual should have at least 1 year of experience and be a public health nurse. An individual representing this specialty is defined as a registered nurse who has graduated from a National League for Nursing (NLN) baccalaureate program or who has completed a post–registered nurse study program that includes public health nursing content approved by the NLN.

Although these federal regulations guide the directors, administrators, and supervisors in Medicare-certified agencies, other state and local requirements for agency licensure may present different guidelines. The trends in licensure and certification requirements for the agencies can only be determined by monitoring adaptations in state licensure laws for home health/hospice agencies.

In addition to the public regulations available to guide the standards of preparation and experience of the administrator, there are standards generated by professional organizations that represent personnel or accredit home health agencies. The Community Health Accreditation Program (CHAP), through its accreditation program, has established standards applicable to providers of home health care and community-based services (CHAP, 1993). Core standards for a home care agency indicate that the chief executive must have a master's degree in a health-related or business field and at least 2 years of administrative experience, or a bachelor's degree in a health-related field with a minimum of 5 years of administrative experience. Equivalent combinations of experience, education, and training may be substituted (C1.3b).

Standards also exist for the professional titled as a program administrator. The program administrator is a health care professional with relevant experience and educational preparation at the baccalaureate level and preferably a master's degree. The professional in this position is expected to have the knowledge, experience, and ability to administer effectively the professional services program (P1.3a).

The NLN has been accrediting home care organizations since 1965, and CHAP became a fully independent subsidiary of the NLN in 1987. CHAP accreditation standards address home care agencies, hospice programs, infusion therapy programs, home medical equipment (HME) programs, home pharmacy programs, public health nursing programs, and community nursing centers. The standards for program administrators for each of these programs vary, but minimally a baccalaureate degree, and preferably a master's degree, and relevant experience are required. The exception to this is the HME program administrator's requirement of 2 years of management experience with the education and knowledge to administer the program effectively (E1.3).

The Joint Commission on Accreditation of Healthcare Organizations initiated its voluntary accreditation program in 1988 for both community-based and hospital-based organizations offering home care services. Any organization providing one or more of the following direct or contractual services is eligible: equipment management, pharmaceutical, personal care or support, and home health services. The standards for the management of human resources (HR1 to HR7) indicate that the organizational leaders define the qualifications for all staff positions that are appropriate to the scope of care and services provided by the organization (Joint Commission, 1996).

As a point of interest, both CHAP and the Joint Commission announced a cooperative accreditation agreement whereby the Joint Commission will: recognize and accept the accreditation process, findings, and decisions of CHAP regarding home care organizations when surveying integrated health delivery systems and health plans. While CHAP and Joint Commission maintain unique approaches to accreditation, ... providers that are part of an integrated organization [can have the freedom to choose between them and] ... now can count on industry recognition regardless of their choices (NAHC, 1996c, p. 12).

The cooperative agreement announcement by CHAP and the Joint Commission promotes clarity in the acceptable standards for recognition of personnel occupying the administrator positions in accredited organizations and reduces unnecessary duplication of the accreditation requirements.

Standards of Home Health Nursing Practice is a publication issued by the American Nurses Association (ANA, 1986). Although the standards focus on the practice of home health nurses, they are relevant for nursing personnel in the field and in home health and hospice administration. Standard I states that, in the organization of home health services, the services are planned, organized, and directed by a master's-prepared professional nurse with experience in community health and administration (ANA, 1986). The ANA has published a *Statement on the Scope of Home Health Nursing Practice* (1992) for home health nurses that describes the philosophy, practice parameters, and ethical issues germane to home health care nursing practice. Both documents offer guidance in achieving excellence in care and may contribute to the focus of continuous quality improvement in the organization.

Although the National Association for Home Care (NAHC) does not establish standards for the administrators of their member home health agencies, the code of ethics adopted by the NAHC board addresses the ethical responsibility of an agency to hire qualified employees who are utilized at their level of competency (National Association for Home Care, 1982).

Standards for the qualifications of home care administrators can be found through public regulations and professional organizations. These standards change as the context of leadership needs in home care evolves. Additional standards for other personnel delivering care in the home health agency are also found in public regulations and professional standards criteria.

CURRENT GUIDELINES FOR NONADMINISTRATORS

A guide to the qualifications of personnel who deliver skilled nursing, therapies, or support to therapists was initially issued in 1985 by the Health Care Financing Administration and subsequently refined by the Omnibus Budget Reconciliation Act of 1987. Home health agencies are directed to utilize only individuals whose practices are congruent with professional standards in the specific health disciplines. The Health Care Financing Administration has issued the rules and regulations for home health aide training and competency requirements. The ANA has issued both standards (1986) and a scope of practice for home health nurses (1992). As Randall (1991) noted, however, there have been few nationally recognized home care certifications for personnel in home health nursing, home health therapies, or home-delivered medical social work. Therefore, agency-specific standards plus state practice acts have constituted major credentialing options for providers. It has only been since 1993 that two certification options for home health nurses have been

available from the American Nurses Credentialing Center (ANCC). Federal qualifying standards for nonadministrator personnel initially published in 1985 and amended in the document 42 CFR Part 484 in 1989 and 1991 include the following designations:

- Skilled nursing is provided by or through the direction of a registered nurse. The registered nurse must have graduated from an approved professional school of nursing and be licensed as a registered nurse in the state of practice.

- Licensed practical nurse standards require that the person be a licensed practical (vocational) nurse in his or her state of practice.

- Physician standards include holding a Doctor of Medicine, Doctor of Osteopathy, or Doctor of Podiatry and legal authorization to practice medicine and surgery in the current state of practice (§484.4; DHHS, 1989).

- Physical therapists need to maintain current licensure as physical therapists in their state of practice. The educational preparation, training opportunities, and qualifying examination criteria for those trained within and outside the United States are clearly described (§484.4; DHHS, 1989).

- Physical therapy assistant standards include state licensure to practice where applicable, experience, and proficiency examination demonstration. For exceptions see §484.4 (DHHS, 1989).

- Occupational therapist standards include any combination of graduation from an approved and accredited school, eligibility for the National Register Examination of the American Occupational Therapy Association, or the combination of experience and satisfactory grade performance on a proficiency examination. For exceptions see §484.4 (DHHS, 1989).

- Occupational therapy assistants must be certified as assistants by the American

Occupational Therapy Association or have 2 years of experience as an occupational therapy assistant and demonstrate a satisfactory proficiency score on examinations conducted, approved, or sponsored by the U.S. Public Health Service. For exceptions see §484.4 (DHHS, 1989).

- Social worker standards include a master's degree from a school of social work accredited by the Council on Social Work Education and 1 year of experience in a health care setting.
- Social work assistants must have a baccalaureate degree in social work or a related field and have had at least 1 year of social work in a health-related setting or a combination of 2 years of experience as a social work assistant and achievement of a satisfactory grade on a government-sponsored examination. For exceptions see §484.4 (DHHS, 1989).
- Speech-language pathologist or audiologist requirements include the necessary education and experience to obtain a certificate of clinical competence granted by the American Speech and Hearing Association or having met the educational requirements and currently accumulating the supervised experience necessary for certification.
- Home health aide personnel qualifications, training, and competency requirements have changed for the 1990s. Home health aides must have successfully completed a state-established or other type of program that meets the requirements specified in §484.36(a) and a competency evaluation or state licensure program that meets the requirements in §484.36(b) or (e). If an individual has not furnished services for a continuous period of 24 consecutive months after meeting the requirements, he or she will no longer be considered qualified. The training program requires a minimum of 75 hours of classroom and supervised practical training. Sixteen hours of classroom training must have

been completed before a minimum of 16 hours of supervised practical training. In addition, the home health aide must receive at least 12 hours of inservice training each calendar year (42 CFR, Part 484, 1991).

- Personal care attendants have also been addressed in the revised conditions of participation [§484.36(e)] in 1991. Standards and competency evaluation requirements for personal care attendants providing personal care services on behalf of a home health agency are the same as those for home health aides (42 CFR, Part 484, 1991).

The regulatory standards for nonadministrative personnel are diverse within titles and between professional and semiprofessional categories. Mechanisms for determining qualifications include licensure, certification, work and educational experience, proficiency examination grades, and competency training. As new therapies are included in reimbursement packages, standards for these specialists will need to be developed.

Concurrent monitoring and support for the maintenance and improvement of personnel capabilities are discussed in COP items relating to participation in inservice programs and orientation programs and to reviews of the currency of personnel employment requirements. Contract personnel are obligated by the agency to be held to the same qualifications as noncontract personnel (DHHS, 1989).

The CHAP standards for nonadministrative personnel are broad in nature. Employment qualifications and responsibilities are congruent with education and experience, provider needs, professional standards, and regulatory guidelines (CHAP, 1993). Joint Commission standards demand that home care personnel have qualifications and abilities equivalent to patients'/clients' needs and the skills necessary for the level of care required (Joint Commission, 1996). Both organizations promote standards for staff development in keeping with professional, licensure, or certification criteria.

CREDENTIAL OPTIONS UTILIZED BY HOME CARE ADMINISTRATORS

At present, there are multiple options for the home care administrator to obtain nationally recognized validation of professional administrative competency.

Nursing Administration Certification

The ANCC sponsors a two-level voluntary certification process for licensed registered nurses in administrative (nurse manager and executive level) positions (ANCC, 1997). Although applicants do not need to be ANA members, the first level of certification, certified nurse administrator (CNA), requires that the applicant hold a baccalaureate or higher degree in nursing. In addition, the applicant must have held a nurse manager or nurse executive position for the equivalent of 24 months, full time within the past 5 years, and have had 20 contact hours of continuing education applicable to nursing administration within the last 2 years. It is a requirement that a passing score on the written certification examination also be achieved.

The advanced level certification, certified nurse administrator, advanced (CNAA), recognizes the executive nurse's administrative tasks and functions. Requirements include a master's degree (if it is a nonnursing master's degree, the baccalaureate must be in nursing) and holding an executive position for 24 months within the last 5 years (congruent with published tasks listed for the advanced level). Additionally, 30 contact hours of continuing education applicable to nursing administration during the previous 2 years is required in the absence of a master's degree in nursing administration. A passing score on a written examination is required. Consultants and educators may apply for certification by meeting specific guidelines in the certification manual. Recertification is

obtained every 5 years either by providing evidence of continuing education or by obtaining a passing score on the examination.

In 1996, the ANCC initiated a third credentialing option for managers in home health care through certification as a clinical specialist in home health nursing (CS). A clinical specialist is described as proficient in planning, implementing, and evaluating programs, resources, services, and research for health care delivery to complex clients. Expertise in the process of case management, consultation, collaboration, and education of clients, staff, and other professions is also expected of this clinical specialist. Eligibility requirements include an active registered nurse license, a master's or higher degree in nursing, and practicing as a home health nurse for a minimum of 1,000 hours after conferral of a master's degree or having graduated from a clinical specialist in home health master's program in nursing (50 percent of graduate program clinical care can be applied to the 1,000-hour practice requirement). Additionally, the applicant must provide an average of 8 hours weekly of direct care or clinical management (ANCC, 1997). In the 22-year period since the ANCC's inception in 1975, more than 110,000 nurses have received all types of specialty certification through the ANCC.

Admission to the American College of Health Care Executives

The American College of Healthcare Executives (ACHE) is a voluntary professional society composed of members who have demonstrated career paths in health services administration. Affiliates of ACHE receive recognition through advancement in status as an associate, diplomate, and ultimately a fellow (FACHE). Each level has certain requirements for acceptance and recertification (ACHE, 1996). Admission as an associate is characterized by an initial commitment to health services administration. Eligibility requirements include a baccalaureate degree plus 3 years of health care experience, or a master's degree from a program accredited by the Accrediting Commission on Education for Health Services Administration, or any other master's degree plus 1 year of experience. Candidates must be employed full time in a health care management position, and one reference is required.

Diplomate status is the college's first credentialed status (ACHE-certified health executive), which confers recognition of the health management administrator's knowledge and capacity for competence in the field. It acknowledges leadership in the health care community as well as life-long learning. Applicants must be currently employed in a health care management position, must successfully pass an oral and written ACHE Board of Governors examination in health care management, and must have demonstrated leadership in civic/community activities and health care. Candidacy must be supported by references from two fellows or a diplomate and one other fellow. Evidence of having met 20 hours of category I or II continuing education is also required.

An application for advancement to fellow status can occur after the individual occupies diplomate status for 5 years. Eligibility requirements include a current position in health care management, leadership participation, and continuing education of 50 hours over the most recent 5 years, of which 25 hours must be in category I (ACHE education) programs. Three references from existing fellows of the College are required. Individuals who advance to the fellow status have successfully completed one of three activities: preparation of a thesis on a significant area of health care management, documentation of four case reports of real-life health care management problems in practice, or establishment and completion of a mentorship project with a promising junior executive/postgraduate fellow in their organization. Fellow status is reserved for those making distinctive contributions in the field of health care management. Opportunities are reserved for those holding fellow status to serve as an elected official of the College, serve on select committees, and administer the oral examination.

Recertification and reappointment opportunities vary: Fellows must be recertified every 10 years, diplomates must be recertified every 6 years, and associates must be reappointed every 6 years. The recertification/reappointment criteria include taking an examination or completing specified numbers of continuing education hours as well as providing evidence of participation in health care and community/civic affairs. For reappointment as an associate, references, continuing education, and community/health care affairs participation is required (ACHE, 1996). Individuals occupying home care management positions are eligible for application to the ACHE credentialing process.

NAHC Executive Certification

The most recent credentialing activity to validate the qualifications and practice of home care and hospice executives is the NAHC's Executive Certification Program. The NAHC program offers a comprehensive certification option designated by the certified home/hospice care executive (CHCE) credential. This credential is a trademark of NAHC and is limited to those who successfully complete the application, testing, and recertification process. The practice of home care and hospice executives is defined as follows:

> Home care and hospice executives set expectations; develop plans; and manage, assess, improve and maintain the organizations' activities. The areas of practice span finance, reimbursement, legal and regulatory issues; organization planning and management; human resources; quality and risk management; public relations and marketing; ethics and information management (NAHC, 1996a, pp. 2–3).

Requirements for certification (CHCE) include documentation of eligibility requirements, attestation to adhere to the NAHC code of ethics (1982), payment of fees, completion of application, and successful completion of the certification examination. Eligibility requirements vary (NAHC, 1996a):

- *Individuals with a master's degree*—Three years of home care and/or hospice experience
  1. *Executive level*—12 consecutive months full time within the last 3 years, or
  2. *Management level*—36 consecutive months full time within the last 4 years
- *Individuals with a bachelor's degree*—Four years of home care and/or hospice experience
  1. *Executive level*—18 consecutive months full time within the last 3 years, or
  2. *Management level*—30 consecutive months full time within the last 4 years
- *Individuals with an associate degree or professional licensure in a health-related field*: Five years of home care and/or hospice experience
  1. *Executive level*—24 consecutive months full time within the last 3 years, or
  2. *Management level*—36 consecutive months full time within the last 4 years.

For individuals achieving initial certification, recertification of the CHCE credential is required every 4 years by retesting or meeting continuing education and professional activity requirements.

The CHCE examination is composed of 170 questions, of which 150 are scorable and 20 are pretest questions. All questions are multiple-choice, four-option responses. The 20 pretest questions are not counted toward the candidate's score. Scaled scores on an examination range from 300 to 600, with the passing score being 500 (NAHC, 1996b). It is expected that the number of home care and hospice executives achieving the CHCE credential will grow rapidly as uniform standards and the value of continuous performance improvement in industry leadership become important to ensure protection of the public. In a purposeful survey of

home care administrators, the author found that, of those administrators who had administrative credentials, all the aforementioned methods were represented among them.

CONCLUSION

With home care services being provided in diverse and remote sites from the institutional setting, there are unique challenges in financial management, quality control, risk management, supervision and delegation methods, policy implementation, and organizational development. Reimbursement mechanisms place special demands on home care systems and their operations. The skills of providers are distinct and much more complex than simply moving the personnel from a hospital to a home care delivery mode, where independence and resourcefulness are critical to success. The evolution of integrated health care systems redefines the role and challenges of home and hospice executives daily.

The rationale for the creation of a certification process for administrators of home health and hospice goes beyond the assumption that the challenges to these executives reflect a diverse knowledge level. First, states are beginning to mandate certain credentials for administrators in home health agencies for their agencies to be licensed. Second, most other recognized delivery models (hospitals, nursing homes, and public health agencies) have some type of credentialing process in place to recognize the unique qualifications and knowledge of professionals in these respective systems. Certification is a profession's endorsement of these individuals. Home health and hospice administrators as an aggregate require a specific professional endorsement and unique opportunity. Third, home health administrators represent a diversity of educational backgrounds and professional and nonprofessional experiences. Parameters must be in place to offer boards, consumers, corporate headquarters, certifying agencies, and organizational personnel a measure of comparable worth in the credentials of administrators. Fourth, there is a new professional breed of health care manager known as the gatekeeper of health care: the physician administrator. Although the executive medicine/physician manager model is not currently in vogue for freestanding home health agencies, the experiences of sister health maintenance organization agencies and hospital-based agencies show that the competition for administrator positions in health care is intensifying with a newly prepared breed of physician manager.

As hospitals and multisystem entities move toward more fully integrated corporations, many income-producing ventures will emerge. By taking advantage of these opportunities, health care organizations will involve members of the medical staff in equity and management participation. One of the characteristics of a profession is its ability to regulate itself and to set its standards of practice. A certification process is a dimension that can build the image of home care administrators as professionals. This has the distinct advantage of administrators being recognized as professional peers by others who are distinguished in the health industry.

The unique certification process for administrators of home health and hospice agencies enhances professional distinction. In selecting certification options, many questions clarifying philosophy, sponsorship, eligibility, and impact arise. These questions reflect the issues inherent in designing, implementing, and evaluating a certification process that aims to recognize professional achievement and protect the public. Agency administrators can contribute to the caliber of the process by verbalizing suggestions and concerns, volunteering to serve on organizational committees implementing the process, validating with other professionals the successes and pitfalls of their own certification process, participating in feasibility studies as well as job analysis studies that can form the foundation for revisions, and challenging collegial creativity to generate ideas for measuring professional distinction. Although this idea may not be a popular one with all administrators, it offers the opportunity for self-regulation and a demonstration of skill and achievement not currently attributed in a standard way to home care administration. This avenue of change can create unparalleled opportunities for professional enhancement and recognition.

REFERENCES

American College of Health Care Executives (ACHE). 1996. *ACHE credentialing.* Chicago: ACHE.

American Nurses Association (ANA). 1986. *Standards of home health nursing practice.* Washington, DC: ANA.

American Nurses Association (ANA). 1992. *A statement on the scope of home health nursing practice.* Washington, DC: ANA.

American Nurses Credentialing Center (ANCC). 1997. *1997 Certification catalog.* Washington, DC: ANCC.

Community Health Accreditation Program (CHAP). 1993. *Standards of excellence for home care organizations.* New York: CHAP.

Department of Health and Human Services, Health Care Financing Administration. 1989. 42 CFR Part 484. Medicare program: Home health agencies: Conditions of participation and reduction in record keeping requirements; interim final rule. *Federal Register* 54:33354–44473.

Department of Health and Human Services. 1991. Conditions of participation: Home health aide services (§484.36–42 CFR Part 484). *Federal Register* 56:32967–32975.

Joint Commission on Accreditation of Healthcare Organizations. 1996. *The new 1997–98 comprehensive accreditation manual for home care.* Oakbrook Terrace, IL: Joint Commission.

National Association for Home Care (NAHC). 1982. *Code of ethics.* Washington, DC: NAHC.

National Association for Home Care (NAHC). 1996a. *Professional certification for home care and hospice executives: Candidates information handbook.* Washington, DC: NAHC.

National Association for Home Care (NAHC). 1996b. *Testing for professional certification for home care and hospice executives begins.* NAHC report No. 682. Washington, DC: NAHC.

National Association for Home Care. 1996c. CHAP and JCAHO announce cooperative agreement. *Home Care News*, September, p. 12.

Randall, D. 1991. Surveys of home health agencies. In *Health Law Trends*, Washington, DC: Arent, Fox, Kintner, Plotkin & Kahn.

CHAPTER 9

The Relationship of the Home Health Agency to the State Trade Association

Mary Kay Pera

An individual can satisfy basic needs for food and shelter, but he or she must have contact with other human beings to be complete. People joining together for a common purpose is the basis of institutions, trade, and professional associations. Group participation fulfills human needs; it stimulates economic activity and provides a way for people to work together for mutual benefit.

Modern associations have their roots in trade associations that existed thousands of years ago. Throughout the ages, people have banded together for mutual protection and advancement. In ancient Chinese, Japanese, and Indian civilizations, evidence exists of class trade groups that operated for the betterment of members. Trade groups in the Roman empire served regulatory protective functions and applied the concept of apprentice training. Seagoing Phoenician merchants protected their vessels from pirates by sailing together, and the Aramaeans formed large caravans to protect themselves from bandits while they transported goods over land.

Craft guilds and merchant guilds grew rapidly to serve an important function in society in general during the transition from ancient to medieval times. In England, the guilds-craft were formed to safeguard the rights of craftsmen and artisans and to set quality standards for their work. Guilds-merchants, associations of

traders and merchants, protected members and increased profits. Early guilds served important functions by encouraging new industries, improving processes, and promoting individual skill and training.

During early U.S. history, mercantilism was the dominant economic force. Carryovers from guilds existed particularly among craftsmen, and a degree of cooperation was found with colonial political authorities.

A parallel exists between the period of transition from medieval guilds to modern associations and the progress of civilization because education and prosperity became more widespread. Governments improved, inventions were ingenious, and communication and transportation became available to the masses rather than only to a privileged few.

Several associations existed in the United States before 1800, some of which are functioning today. Most associations of home health agencies, however, are comparatively young. As the home health industry has grown, individual agencies have experienced a need to join together to accomplish through the group what they could not alone.

ASSOCIATION STRUCTURE

The democratic process is epitomized in the organizational structure of most home health agency associations. Associations represent, protect, promote, and are a reflection of their members. The members are the foundation of any association. Ultimate decision making regarding rights and duties occurs at the membership level. The function of the association is to carry out the policies and programs that reflect the views of the majority of the membership. Members choose their leaders, who in turn set the policies of the association.

The leadership of the association is most often called the board of directors or board of trustees. The board is essentially the association's most important committee. These members are expected to be knowledgeable about the needs of the association and to use this knowledge to transact the business and supervise the affairs of the association so that its purpose may be achieved.

Officers are elected from the members of the board of directors either by the members of the board or by the membership, according to the policies of the association. The elected officers usually form the executive committee, which acts as a liaison and functions for the board between meetings.

Committees, which are usually appointed by the chief elected officer, represent the membership by providing input into the decision-making process and ensuring that all diverse interests of the membership are made known. The number, size, and type of committees vary according to the objectives of the association.

Staff members implement the policies and programs of the association. The chief staff person is hired by and reports to the board of directors through the executive committee.

The organizational structure of an association must allow for continued flexibility and responsiveness to member needs. Priorities change according to member needs. A strong, vital organization anticipates and accepts change.

WHAT ASSOCIATIONS DO

The reasons for the existence of home health agency associations are as numerous as the agencies themselves. Typically, however, there are some broad activities that an agency might expect from its association, depending on the availability of resources to support that agency.

The overwhelming majority of home health associations report some involvement in educational activities through sponsorship of seminars, workshops, and other programs. Many provide continuing education credits, awards, or certificates for completion of educational programs.

The majority also are involved with government relations programs. Action at the state and federal levels in both the legislative and the regulatory branches can affect the operation of the agency and the care that agency provides to patients. For example, a decision on Medicare by Congress, which is the Medicare agency's biggest payer, could alter significantly the provision of care by that agency.

The association opens the lines of communication, education, and persuasion between the association membership and the legislators and regulators. It becomes a two-way street. The association keeps members up to date on government action and the legislators and regulators informed about home health industry issues and concerns. At times, news from Capitol Hill is fast breaking. The association monitors events as they develop and disseminates information at once, placing the member agency at an advantage over the nonmember agency. Some associations have also formed political action committees through which the membership can support political candidates and incumbents who share their views.

One of the most valuable resources in association membership is the opportunity to meet colleagues in an informal setting and to exchange experiences. It is comforting to know "you are not alone" and helpful to learn what has worked and not worked for others. Many new ideas for resolutions to problems are spinoffs from ideas of others.

Communication is a key function of most home health agency associations. Through the newsletter, membership directory, annual report, position papers or other bulletins, and audio-video productions, associations disseminate information to the membership and/or the general public. Publicity and public relations activities are a part of the association's communications program, which members can often use as promotional material in their local areas.

Another program that is part of many home health associations is setting professional standards for home health agencies. The membership has a stake in each agency providing quality home health care. Through standardization of professional home health care, a direct short- and long-term benefit occurs to the members as well as the consumers they serve.

Some associations are also involved in collecting data about the home health industry, researching trends, and reporting outcomes. The ultimate test of an association's effectiveness, however, is not how many or what types of programs it offers but whether the association is meeting the needs and purposes of the membership.

GETTING THE MOST OUT OF MEMBERSHIP

The home health agency that is actively involved in its trade association is the agency that is likely to benefit most from membership. Involvement can take place at many different levels. Each agency must determine its reasons for belonging to the association and choose the appropriate level of involvement to meet those identified needs.

Participation at the board level requires the greatest amount of involvement in and commitment to the association. The board of directors is involved in policymaking, program planning, initiating change, and getting things done. A successful director is knowledgeable about home health, sensitive to the diverse needs of the membership, flexible, courageous, and, after deliberation, decisive on the issues. By virtue of election to the board, the member is recognized as a leader in the association, is on the cutting edge of the industry, and has the opportunity to affect the direction that the association and industry take.

Committees afford another major opportunity for involvement in the association. Committees are the backbone of the association and the means by which it functions. Service on a committee, which is generally for a year at a time, provides the members with a framework to bring issues before the association for consideration and action. The member with expertise in a given area is often welcomed on a committee that has a responsibility in that area. For example, the member with a strong background and interest in finance would be valuable to the association on the finance committee; a member with legislative or regulatory expertise could contribute to the association on a legislative committee.

An agency may choose not to participate on the board or a committee but remain involved in the association, deriving maximum benefits from membership. An involved association member has a number of important responsibilities. The member should:

- stay informed on the issues by reading all the information disseminated by the association
- learn to know the association's leadership and communicate individual issues and concerns to those people
- share experience with what has and has not worked and solicit experiences from others
- respond to requests for data on agency operations (every member's input is vital when the association is assessing industry-wide trends)
- ask questions (all questions are worth asking, no matter how insignificant they may seem)
- initiate requests for information (make the association accountable for responding to individual agency needs)
- attend educational programs (provide suggestions for additional, meaningful programs)

- respond to requests from the leadership for calls and letters to legislators (elected officials pay more attention when they hear from large numbers of constituents on a given issue)

The association can also be an invaluable resource in times of difficulty. An agency administrator may think that his or her agency is alone in facing a particular dilemma only to learn, upon calling the association, that many others are experiencing a similar difficulty. Even if the solution is not immediately found, it is comforting to know that you are not alone.

In approaching the association for assistance, there are certain steps that should be taken. First, identify the problem. Second, be specific about what you are requesting of the association. Third, supply supporting information, such as copies of correspondence, pertinent records, or details of what transpired while you were attempting to resolve the situation on your own. It is helpful to follow up any discussion of the sequence of events with a letter.

CONCLUSION

Membership in an association can yield substantial benefits to a home health agency. The collective wisdom of individual agencies is absolutely essential to compete in the complex health care environment. Individual agencies working alone can make progress, but it is the association with others of similar interest, the sharing of ideas and resources, and the discussion, modification, and filtration that can result in the greatest accomplishments. This, of course, is the essence of belonging to an association.

RESOURCE

American Society of Association Executives (ASAE)
ASAE Building
1575 I Street, NW
Washington, DC 20005-1168
(202) 626-2723
ASAE has a catalog of publications.

CHAPTER 10

The National Association for Home Care

Val J. Halamandaris

The National Association for Home Care (NAHC), the nation's largest and most broadly based organization representing home care professionals, is an aggressive advocate in Washington, DC. Committed to principles and activities designed to foster an environment where home care can thrive, the association works to support the dedicated efforts of home care providers who are helping Americans live dignified, independent lives regardless of age or physical ability. Its membership represents the full spectrum of the home care industry. Members benefit from comprehensive direct services designed to meet their specific needs.

NAHC is a trade association representing the interests of nearly 7,000 home care agencies, hospices, and home care aide organizations. Its members are primarily corporations or other organizational entities as well as state home care associations, medical equipment suppliers and other vendors, and schools. What these entities have in common is the provision of health care and supportive services on an outreach basis to the ill and infirm in their homes. NAHC also offers individual memberships. Increasingly, professionals such as social workers, nurses, and physical therapists who are employed by home care and hospice agencies and are interested in home care and hospice are joining one of the forums established by NAHC to serve the specific needs of these fields.

HOW NAHC WORKS

As the nation's voice for home care, NAHC presents a united front promoting trend-setting ideas, programs, and legislation on behalf of all those involved in home care, from the nurse, therapist, and home care aide to the patient and his or her family. The components of home care include skilled nursing, home care aide services, social work, therapy, physician services, adult day care, respite care, Meals-on-Wheels, transportation services, hospice, and many others. Because there are so many components of home care, NAHC retains a professional team of lobbyists, lawyers, policy specialists, and researchers, all of whom combine their efforts as watchdogs of this old-turned-new-again area of health care.

NAHC remains in close contact with the White House, Congress, the Health Care Financing Administration (HCFA), the Veterans Administration, and other government agencies; the courts; the state capitals; private enterprise, such as insurance companies, corporate executives, and benefits managers; as well as the rest of the established American health care system.

NAHC also nurtures a close, friendly relationship with the media, both local and national.

CODE OF ETHICS

NAHC has a tough code of ethics to which association members subscribe. NAHC's code of ethics has been copied or adapted by many state organizations. The code of ethics is shown in Exhibit 10–1.

NAHC's MISSION

NAHC's mission, like that of its members, can be summarized in the statement "We're bringing health care back home where it belongs." NAHC is dedicated to the proposition that Americans should receive the health care and social services they need in their own homes insofar as this is possible. NAHC

advances the proposition that senior citizens and other vulnerable groups should be assisted to live in independence through the intervention of home care services so that institutionalization is a last resort. NAHC seeks to reverse the current institutional bias that has led to hundreds of thousands, possibly millions, of fragile children and chronically ill seniors being placed in nursing homes or retained in hospitals when they could receive equal or better care at home. NAHC believes that home care and hospice keep families together and is devoted to doing anything in its power to preserve the sanctity of the American family.

NAHC's VALUES

NAHC's values, from which are derived its mission and specific objectives, include the development of a more caring society; the com-

---

Exhibit 10–1 NAHC's Code of Ethics

Preamble

The National Association for Home Care (NAHC) was founded with the intention of encouraging the development and the delivery of the highest quality of medical, social and supportive services to the aged, infirm and disabled.

In the process of bringing these essential services to the needy, the Association and its members seek to establish and retain the highest possible level of public confidence.

This Code of Ethics, adopted by the NAHC Board of Directors in September 1982, serves as a statement to the general public that the Association and its individual members stand for integrity and the highest ethical standards.

This Code of Ethics serves to inform members and the general public as to what are acceptable guidelines for ethical conduct for home care agencies and their employees.

It is inherent in the promulgation of this Code of Ethics that the Association and its members covenant to protect and preserve the basic rights

of their patients and to deal with them in an honest and ethical manner.

Finally, the Code of Ethics serves as notice to government officials that the Association expects its members to abide by all applicable laws and regulations. It is a precondition of membership in the Association that they do so and failure to comply will result in expulsion from membership in the Association in addition to other penalties prescribed by law.

The Code of Ethics is intended to serve as a guideline to agencies in the following areas:

A. Patient Rights and Responsibilities
B. Relationships to Other Provider Agencies
C. Responsibility to the National Association for Home Care
D. Fiscal Responsibilities
E. Marketing and Public Relations
F. Personnel
G. Legislative
H. Hearing Process

Courtesy of the National Association for Home Care, Washington, DC.

mitment to preserving the family unit; the preservation of the rights of the underprivileged, ill, and disabled; the protection of the environment; the promotion of wellness, health, and the universal right of access to the highest quality of health care for all; and the promotion of honesty, integrity, and quality.

NAHC's GOALS

NAHC has 15 goals that include serving as a unified voice for home care and hospice and providing direct services to its members. The specific goals and steps to achieve them are detailed below.

1. *Serve as the unified voice for the home care and hospice community* by making NAHC the information hub for hospice and home care services; disseminating NAHC's values and its broader mission to the general public, Congress, the media, community leaders, and trend setters; and broadening the scope of NAHC membership and representation to include nontraditional service providers, physicians, and organizations that provide specialized care.

2. *Provide direct needed services to the members* by conducting a "service audit" to identify the most and least valuable and effective services offered and to create new member benefits as indicated by member need; including as new benefits local marketing, advocacy, fundraising, and public relations as well as a professional placement service and a travel service; and expanding NAHC staff and resources to accommodate this growth.

3. *Heighten the political visibility of home care and hospice interests* by forming a grassroots political network and encouraging NAHC members to become involved, identifying key legislators at federal, state, and local levels and educating and honoring them; recruiting celebrities as spokespersons; and involving the

NAHC Board of Directors in these efforts.

4. *Influence the legislative, judicial, and regulatory processes with respect to issues of importance to hospice and home care* by exposing legislators to home care issues by taking them on home visits, visiting home care agency offices, and educating key legislative staff persons; providing financial support to key legislators; educating and supporting key regulatory contacts; including regulatory programs as part of the Policy Conference and setting up demonstration projects on regulatory issues; educating and supporting/honoring key judicial officials; and creating a forum of home care attorneys, using the Center for Health Care Law (CHCL) as the clearinghouse for home care and hospice case law.

5. *Sponsor research and gather and disseminate home care and hospice data* by establishing a National Center for Home Care and Hospice Research to act as a clearinghouse, to set national research and funding priorities, to create a home care and hospice library, and to gather all existing relevant data; generating private funds for home care and hospice research; and supporting grant requests from state associations for home care and hospice, universities, and provider organizations.

6. *Promote home care and hospice as central components of the health care delivery system* by commissioning public opinion surveys on patient satisfaction with home care, disseminating the results of these surveys, influencing educational curricula to make the home the primary setting for patient education, contacting and publicizing celebrities who have personal experience with home care and hospice, recruiting movie and television writers and producers to generate wider exposure for home care, and working

with special interest groups to incorporate home care information in their consumer education materials.

7. *Foster, develop, and promote high standards of patient care in home care and hospice services* by working with consumer groups to rewrite the Medicare conditions of participation; developing a model licensure law; working with universities and others to develop new standards to keep pace with medical technology and to develop an outcome-driven quality assurance program; disseminating and enforcing the NAHC code of ethics and developing an industry "seal of approval"; and encouraging home care agencies to seek accreditation and supporting "deemed status" for the Joint Commission on Accreditation of Healthcare Organizations and the Community Health Accreditation Program.

8. *Provide expert advice and assistance to members with respect to management, legal, and operational issues* by clearly defining the limits of NAHC's membership benefits and establishing a fee-for-service consulting service, providing members with a list of outside experts, developing workbook and audio-video packages of information, providing more management seminars, and continuing the certification program for home care executives.

9. *Disseminate information to the media and general public to promote the acceptance of home care and hospice services and to support caregivers who are family, neighbors, and friends (sometimes called the informal system of care)* by launching a national media campaign, building on National Home Care Month and National Hospice Month; developing a syndicated newspaper column and publishing books identifying home care's values and celebrating its heroes; developing programming for television and radio, including human interest pieces about home care

clients and caregivers, topics for talk shows, and subjects for sitcoms; publicizing opinion polls to show the public's preference for home care and to promote the values of home care, family solidarity, community service, and the development of a more caring society; and promoting home care as a valuable work setting to high schools and colleges.

10. *Expand private insurance and other third-party sources for financing hospice and home care services* by working to ensure that home care is a mandated benefit in state laws and national programs and is covered among employers who self-insure; developing a model home care and hospice insurance policy, a model long-term care insurance policy, and consumer information about how to select a good home care and hospice insurance policy; educating and recruiting state insurance commissioners; commending insurance companies whose policies cover home care services; and establishing a national case management company.

11. *Promote collaboration among national, state, and local organizations relating to home care and hospice services and issues* by working with the Long-Term Care Campaign and other coalitions to enact long-term care legislation based on home care, supporting state affiliates and developing a grassroots lobbying network at both state and national levels, and working with civic organizations to promote the broader values of home care.

12. *Initiate, sponsor, and promote educational programs* by presenting seminars and conferences on management issues, new technologies, legal issues, case management, hospice, private duty, and other non-Medicare issues and providing programming to assist state associations (e.g., workshops on how to lobby).

13. *Represent the interests of caregivers (nurses, home care aides, physicians, and*

therapists) who work in the home care field and encourage individuals to choose a career in home care and hospice services by preparing publications and videotapes to distribute to schools on home care and hospice as career choices; developing a program for home care organizations to "adopt" a school; taking children on home care visits; providing volunteer opportunities; helping create scholarship programs for those who work in home care; seeking funds to support federal and state job training programs in home care; encouraging home care organizations to provide improved employee benefits to all staff, such as health insurance and child care programs; and seeking an amendment to Medicaid allowing welfare recipients to retain health benefits if they work in home care.

14. *Protect the legal rights of hospice and home care beneficiaries, providers, and their employees* by increasing the staff resources in CHCL to create a forum of attorneys and establishing CHCL as the clearinghouse and coordinator of home care case law, preparing publications and audio-video presentations for both consumers and providers to help them understand their legal rights and obligations, working with state associations to create model legislation, and promoting CHCL with consumer groups and the media.

15. *Promote the independence of home care clients and seek their assistance to help shatter the myth that dependency is the necessary state for the aged and disabled in America* by supporting the growth of adult day and respite care services; supporting the development of in-home educational activities for chronically ill children, the disabled, and the sick elderly; identifying role models of active and successful elderly and disabled; and supporting intergenerational programs such as Foster Grandparents.

GOVERNANCE

Under its articles of incorporation, NAHC has four volunteer elected officers and one paid appointive. The bylaws create the appointive office of association president. NAHC's president is a member of the NAHC Board of Directors. The appointive office does not vote. All officers are elected and serve for a term of 2 years. The bylaws limit officers to no more than two consecutive elected terms.

The NAHC Board of Directors is made up of 25 members. Each of the 10 geographic regions of the United States elects 1 board member. The regions are as follows:

Region I, Connecticut, Maine, Massachusetts, New Hampshire, Rhode Island, and Vermont

Region II, New York, New Jersey, Puerto Rico, and the U.S. Virgin Islands

Region III, Delaware, the District of Columbia, Maryland, Pennsylvania, Virginia, and West Virginia

Region IV, Alabama, Florida, Georgia, Kentucky, Mississippi, North Carolina, South Carolina, and Tennessee

Region V, Illinois, Indiana, Michigan, Minnesota, Ohio, and Wisconsin

Region VI, Arkansas, Louisiana, New Mexico, Oklahoma, and Texas

Region VII, Iowa, Kansas, Missouri, and Nebraska

Region VIII, Colorado, Montana, North Dakota, South Dakota, Utah, and Wyoming

Region IX, Arizona, California, Hawaii, Nevada, American Samoa, and Guam

Region X, Alaska, Idaho, Oregon, and Washington

In addition, NAHC has 10 sections. Each elects its own representative to the board, as detailed below:

1. The official section consists of official agencies (city, county, or state health departments).
2. The voluntary section consists of visiting nurse associations and community-based voluntary agencies.
3. The proprietary section is made up of those agencies organized on a for-profit basis.
4. The institution-sponsored section comprises those agencies sponsored by and/or affiliated with a hospital, nursing home, or other institution.
5. The private, not-for-profit section is made up of those agencies whose incorporation status is nonprofit and privately held.
6. The home care aide section is for providers of home care aide services.
7. The hospice section is for providers of hospice services.
8. The state association section comprises the presidents and executives of the affiliated state associations for home care and hospice. When working as a body, the state association members form the Forum of State Associations, which recognizes NAHC as the official national organization representing home care and hospice.
9. The corporate section is comprised of multientity providers.
10. The pediatric section, which was established by the Board of Directors in 1991 to represent members in this fast-growing part of the home care industry.

The NAHC Board of Directors also includes five officers: chair, vice chair, secretary, treasurer, and president. Sectional or regional directors are responsible for presiding at their respective meetings and for bringing their constituents' concerns to the board's attention.

The Board of Directors is the chief policy-making body of the association and, through the programmatic budget, determines the organization's activities and their schedules and funding. The board develops and approves NAHC's legislative, regulatory, and hospice agenda each year, known as its Blueprint for Action.

COMMITTEES

NAHC has an Executive Committee consisting of four officers and three board members. It has the authority to exercise powers of the board between board meetings. The Finance Committee is comprised of 7 members. The NAHC treasurer is chair of this committee, which is charged with developing the NAHC budget and monitoring NAHC's financial affairs. The Membership Committee comprises 7 persons who advise the board and staff on membership recruitment and retention. The Bylaws Committee consists of 7 members and makes recommendations to the board on possible amendments to the bylaws. The Government Affairs Committee is made up of 7 members and helps develop legislative policy. Regulatory policy is developed by a subcommittee of the Government Affairs Committee. The Information Resources and Quality Assurance Committee, comprising 7 members, is responsible for data collection and education. The Annual Meeting Committee plans NAHC's largest event, generally held in October of each year. Finally, the Nominating Committee is made up of 10 members, representing each of NAHC's 10 sections, who are elected by the full NAHC membership each year. Its job is to select two candidates to run in opposition for each NAHC board position. The committee is balanced by auspice. It also chooses award winners.

In addition to these committees, NAHC has in the past created certain ad hoc committees, such as the Congressional Action Committee and the Long-Term Care Committee.

These committees have been highly successful. They have helped NAHC gather facts and establish and revise its policies. All committees issue reports and make recommendations to the entire NAHC board, which reserves to itself the power of making policy decisions.

COMMUNICATIONS AND INFORMATION DISSEMINATION

NAHC communicates with home care providers in a variety of ways.

Newsletters and Newspapers

The weekly *NAHC Report* gives NAHC members an in-depth understanding of specific legislative and regulatory issues and provides a medium for the communication of late-breaking news items related to NAHC positions.

Homecare News is NAHC's monthly newspaper to keep members informed about activities within NAHC as well as national, regional, and local news affecting the home care industry. It also serves as an information exchange among state associations.

Magazines

Caring addresses the interests and problems of infirm adults, fragile children, disabled persons, and those completing life with the principal focus on home and hospice care as a solution to many of these problems.

Electronic Communications and Information Services

NAHC maintains a full-featured World Wide Web site (http://www.nahc.org) to facilitate the gathering, analysis, and dissemination of information about home care on both a national and an international level to the home care industry and those interested in home care.

Education and Certification

NAHC provides education and fosters the dissemination of information through its meet-

ings. Each year the educational programs include the annual meeting, legal symposium and policy conference, and regional conferences.

Annual Meeting

The annual meeting provides for the dissemination and exchange of information relating to home care and hospice, encourages interaction among participants at educational and social events, and provides assistance with problem solving in clinical, professional, and management concerns for home care and hospice providers.

Legal Symposium and Policy Conferences

Educational programs are presented on pressing legislative and regulatory topics. The Legal Symposium is held in conjunction with the Policy Conference to provide attendees with information about the latest legal issues.

Regional Conferences

Educational conferences are held in each of the 10 regions of the country to promote and assist in the development and improvement of home care and hospice education and training programs for safe, effective, and efficient delivery of home care and hospice services.

Home Care Executives Certification

NAHC provides a certification program for qualified home care and hospice executives to recognize knowledgeable leaders in the industry.

DEPARTMENTS

CHCL

The CHCL preserves and protects the legal rights of fragile children, infirm adults, disabled persons, and those who are dying; preserves and protects the legal rights of NAHC, its members, and patients of home care and hospice programs in the community; educates NAHC members as to their legal rights and responsibilities; and increases access to the appropriate legal avenues as a means of ensuring enforcement of the rights of patients and the responsibilities of others. The CHCL provides initial generalized legal advice to members and fee-oriented services to members and nonmembers needing extensive individual legal representation. In addition, the CHCL provides counseling with regard to issues under the purview of NAHC's Regulatory Affairs Department in relation to federal regulations.

The CHCL actively explores and initiates legal action in concert with state associations to ensure fair and reasonable administration and reimbursement of Medicaid programs in each state. Educational activities include development of publications and presentation of an annual home care law symposium.

Government Affairs Department

This department initiates and works toward the enactment of legislation to meet the needs of all Americans, including home care as an acute and long-term care benefit. It advocates for the interests of NAHC members with respect to proposed federal legislation that affects or could affect the home care and hospice fields. The department also disseminates timely updates on legislative issues affecting the professions to NAHC members. It assists NAHC members in becoming involved in government relations and political action and organizes and coordinates their efforts, and it assists state associations, regions, and sections in crisis situations involving government affairs issues. It assists other organizations that have similar interests in forming coalitions targeted to achieve legislative results that are of mutual interest. Finally, this department heightens the political visibility of NAHC and its affiliate services and increases home care and hospice coverage by private insurance companies. Each year, the Government Affairs Department develops a Blueprint for Action that contains NAHC's positions on legislative issues and disseminates it to NAHC members, the media, the Executive Branch, and Congress.

Regulatory Affairs Department

The Regulatory Affairs Department preserves and protects the rights of fragile children, infirm adults, disabled persons, and the dying before regulatory agencies as well as the rights of NAHC, its members, and patients of home care and hospice organizations before these agencies. It educates NAHC members as to their rights and responsibilities before regulatory agencies and represents NAHC members and patients in their dealings with fiscal intermediaries, other third party payers, and regulatory bodies. This department reduces the paperwork burden and helps bring about greater efficiency in the health care system. It obtains HCFA's technical assistance to promote home care as a mandatory basic benefit, along with long-term care, in health care materials to empower home care agencies with information for grassroots efforts to promote home care services. Each year, in conjunction with the Regulatory Affairs Committee, the department develops a Regulatory Affairs Blueprint for Action and implements the Blueprint for Action plan recommendations.

Research Department

The Research Department develops and disseminates home care and hospice data and analyzes, coordinates, monitors, and promotes research related to hospice and home care services. Specific research objectives include continuing to work toward the development of a home care patient classification system and alternative payment system options; conducting research that will assist home care agencies and hospice organizations; carrying out home care and hospice literature searches; developing NAHC as a clearinghouse for all research; researching and publishing comparative data relating to the operation of hospices and home care organizations to establish some comparative standards; monitoring, analyzing, and reporting on various national quality assurance projects; and fostering the utilization of standard definitions for home care terminology.

AFFILIATE ORGANIZATIONS

In an effort to recognize the direction of the home care industry, NAHC has established affiliate organizations to provide a vehicle for communication and problem solving for unique types of providers.

Hospice Association of America

This program represents the interests of individuals and families in need of hospice services, promotes the concept of hospice with the media and public, and represents the interests of hospice providers.

Home Care Aide Association of America

This program establishes paraprofessional services as an integral part of home and hospice care within the organization, the industry, and relevant government agencies. It promotes national acceptance of a common title, standardized training, and a career ladder for home care and hospice paraprofessionals. Finally, it provides assistance to agencies in technical and programmatic areas in the development and administration of paraprofessional services.

Hospital Home Care Association of America

This program assists all providers with effective agency operations issues because hospital systems are currently in the process of reorganization. It also assists agencies with personnel management issues, information management,

billing, and regulatory compliance and in maintaining quality through programs that promote a customer satisfaction–driven philosophy, efficient and effective program management, and cost containment that helps agencies recognize costs for each service. Finally, it assists members with their efforts to influence legislation and national policy in the best interests of the entire home care field.

Proprietary Home Care Association of America

This program provides a forum within NAHC focusing on issues and concerns of special interest to proprietary home care providers. It enhances agency operations, promotes quality care and customer satisfaction, develops cost-effective strategies to compete in the health care marketplace, and represents the interest of proprietary providers before policymakers, the media, and the public.

World Homecare and Hospice Organization

This program, establishing a worldwide trade association for providers and professionals who deliver health and social services to clients in the home setting, shares information among service providers and their representative groups from nations around the world. It influences public policy in particular countries to improve public support and enhance home care services. This program also educates, trains, and assures quality among service providers to improve the quality of home care services across the globe, and it increases public awareness of and support for home care services around the world.

RESOURCE

National Association for Home Care
228 Seventh Street, SE
Washington, DC 20003
(202) 547-7424
NAHC has a catalog of publications.

PART III

Clinical Issues

CHAPTER 11

Self-Care Systems in Home Health Care Nursing

Joan Reynolds Yuan

If there was ever a time when nurses must be able to articulate what nursing is, it is now. In this time of cost containment, capitated rates, restructuring, and reengineering, nurses must be clear on when nursing is required. In this health care revolution, we cannot be locked into the Medicare illness model of home care. In a capitated system, keeping the person healthy is a priority and falls under the purview of nursing. According to Orem (1995), "a requirement for nursing in an adult is the absence of the ability to maintain continuously that amount and quality of self-care which is therapeutic in sustaining life and health, in recovering from disease or injury, or in coping with their effects" (p. 52). Because practice in a profession is based on theory, this chapter addresses systems of care based on Orem's nursing theory, its clinical applicability to home health care nursing, and its implications for nursing administration in a home health agency.

In the current cost-conscious environment, there are many changes occurring in health care and home health nursing. The role of the nurse as client advocate is crucial in the delivery of home health services. Of growing concern are the ability of the client to pay for care, the provision of adequate care, access to health services, and the developing tiers of care based on affluence and the reimbursement system (American Nurses Association [ANA], 1985).

Nurses are in a position to develop systems of care for people in the community based on health maintenance and promotion as well as ill care in the home. The *Guide for Community-Based Nursing Services* states "Consumers are moving from nearly total reliance on hospitals and other institutions to community-based services. This shift has been prompted by rising costs and diminishing resources, changing demographic patterns, and a rediscovery of the benefits, and perhaps the necessity, of self help" (ANA, 1985, p. 4).

Community health nurses have long practiced the concept of self-care. Since Lillian Wald conceptualized community health nursing at the turn of the century, self-care has been incorporated into the practice of this specialty. Home health care nursing is recognized as a unique and significant type of community-based nursing practice. The nurse generalist in home health care primarily provides care to individuals and families (ANA, 1986). Consumer involvement is important in the development of the plan of care in community health nursing because the goals and desired outcomes ultimately will be the responsibility of individuals (ANA, 1985).

Home health care nursing, a type of community-based nursing, focuses on the right and responsibility of the patient/family to be included in the planning of care. The Medicare condition of participation concerning patient rights (§484.10) mandates "The patient has the right to participate in the planning of the care. [The home health agency] must advise the patient in advance of the right to participate in planning the care or treatment and in planning changes in the care or treatment" (Department of Health and Human Services, 1989, p. 33369).

Orem's (1995) theory of self-care has significance for home health care. According to Orem, self-care is the practice of activities that are initiated and performed for oneself to maintain life, health, and well-being. Self-care requisites are descriptive of the kinds of purposive self-care that are required. Universal self-care requisites are common to all human beings adjusted for such factors as age, developmental state, and environment; examples are the maintenance of sufficient intake of air, water, and food.

Developmental self-care requisites are associated with developmental processes and conditions or events that affect development. These include the provision of care to prevent the occurrence of deleterious effects of certain conditions on human development. Health deviation self-care requisites exist for persons who are ill or injured, have specific forms of pathology, and are under medical treatment (Orem, 1995). Self-care agency is "the complex acquired ability to meet one's continuing requirements for care that regulates life processes, maintains or promotes integrity of human structure and functioning and human development, and promotes well-being" (Orem, 1995, p. 212). Dependent care agency is "the complex, acquired ability of mature or maturing persons to know and meet some or all of the self-care requisites of adolescent or adult persons who have health-derived or health-associated limitations of self-care agency, which places them in socially dependent relationships for care" (Orem, 1995, p. 242). Nurses must have the ability to view their patients as self-care and dependent care agents and to diagnose patients' abilities to engage in continuous and effective care.

Orem (1995) describes nursing, a helping art, as "the complex ability to accomplish or to contribute to the accomplishment of a person's usual and therapeutic self-care by compensating for or aiding in overcoming the physical or psychic conditions or disabilities that cause the person (1) to be unable to act, (2) to refrain from acting, or (3) to act ineffectively in self-care" (p. 119). The components of the nursing focus become the guides for nursing action. The self-care that the patient can or cannot manage and the reasons why are evaluated by the nurse when he or she selects among appropriate methods of helping. These methods include acting for or doing for another, guiding another, supporting another, providing an environment that promotes personal development, and teaching another (Orem, 1995).

Considering the concept that the nurse and/or patient can act to meet the patient's self-care requisites, three nursing systems have been identified: wholly compensatory, partly compensatory, and supportive-educative (Orem, 1995). The need for a wholly compensatory nursing system is identified when the patient is unable to engage in those self-care actions requiring self-directed and controlled ambulation and manipulative movement or is under the prescription to refrain from such activity. Three subtypes have been identified: persons who are unable to engage in any form of deliberate action, persons who are aware and may be able to make decisions about self-care but who cannot or should not perform actions requiring ambulation and manipulative movements, and persons who are unable to make rational judgments and decisions about self-care but who are ambulatory and may be able to perform some measures of self-care with continuous guidance and supervision (Orem, 1995). Frequently, the helping method utilized by the nurse in this system is acting and doing for another. The nurse must be able to design and manage effective care systems to meet the universal, developmental, and health deviation self-care requirements of these patients. This includes providing guidelines and supervising others who can contribute to the wholly compensatory care system (Orem, 1995).

In the partly compensatory system, both nurse and patient perform care measures or other actions involving manipulative tasks or ambulation. The distribution of responsibility varies with the patient's limitations in ambulation or manipulative activities, the knowledge and skill required, and the patient's psychological state. In this system, all five helping methods may be utilized (Orem, 1995).

The third system, supportive-educative, is used when the patient is able to perform or can and should learn to perform therapeutic self-care measures but cannot do so without assistance. Helping methods include support, guidance, provision of a developmental environment, and teaching (Orem, 1995).

Historically, the home health care nurse has cared for patients with many functional limitations in a way that would be considered wholly compensatory. Systems of care have been designed to include care provided by family, friends, and neighbors as well as by professional and ancillary staff. The number of patients in this population is growing at a time when society is unprepared to care for them. Because of changes in reimbursement, a frequently seen phenomenon is that patients are discharged home from the hospital quicker and sicker. This occurs at a time when many of the traditional supports are unavailable as a result of the increased numbers of women in the workforce outside the home, the migration of family members to other parts of the country, and the limited physical and financial resources of many of the young-old who are attempting to care for the old-old. Some of the patients in the wholly compensatory level have chronic problems, and third party payers will not reimburse for services provided. This is an area that must be addressed by the nursing administration. Is there an agency servicing the community that can provide home health aide, homemaker, and companion services that are affordable to the people in the community?

Many of the people currently being discharged home from the hospital have needs that must be addressed by highly skilled professionals. With advances in technology, patients are now at home with equipment such as ventilators. In many instances, family members will assume responsibility for the provision of care that was designed by the nurse in the wholly compensatory system. The home health care nurse is responsible for the coordination of services. Not only is this good nursing practice, but it is also mandated in §484.30 of the Medicare conditions of participation for Medicare reimbursement (Department of Health and Human Services, 1989). Services provided by the agency, such as physical therapy, occupational therapy, speech therapy, social services, and home health aide, must be coordinated. Services outside the agency, such as respiratory therapy, and the provision of specialized equipment must also be coordinated.

The nursing administrator should consider the special needs of the population in the community served by the agency. For example, some communities adjacent to a children's hospital may require private duty nurses for children home on ventilators. Although the structure of a nonprofit organization would not support this activity, a reorganization into various corporations could. Some patients in the wholly compensatory system are terminally ill and could benefit from hospice care. During the course of a terminal illness, a patient may shift from one system to another. This is affected by the reimbursement system. Although a patient is terminally ill and could benefit from nursing in a supportive-educative system, it is possible that these services would not be third party reimbursable because of strict interpretation of regulations such as homebound status. In these instances, other sources of reimbursement should be investigated.

Many of the patients seen at home by the home health care nurse are in a partly compensatory nursing system. Frequently, this skilled, hands-on care is reimbursed by third party payers. Patients who are receiving services in the home, such as intravenous therapy, are often able to participate in their care and can become independent in such activities as the administration of intravenous antibiotics. It continues to be the responsibility of the nurse to carry out such activities as monitoring the intravenous site for infection or infiltration and changing the catheter. Patients in this system may require multiple services. For example, a patient recovering from a cerebrovascular accident may be able to perform some self-care activities but, to become rehabilitated, may require extensive services including all the therapies. Other patients admitted to service in a home health agency are in a supportive-educative system. In this system, the patient's requirements for assistance relate to decision making, behavior control, and acquiring knowledge and skills (Orem, 1995). Changes in the patient's knowledge, understanding, or behavior should be documented. In this system, the nurse's role is frequently consultative. Some patients require information about the disease process, medication regimen, and safety factors in the home setting.

Preventive health care is an important area for home health care nurses. Three levels of prevention are recognized: primary, secondary, and tertiary. Primary prevention is required before the onset of disease and is directed to the promotion of integrity of structure and functioning and prevention of disease (Orem, 1995). Every person requiring nursing care has requirements at the primary level of prevention. Universal self-care and developmental self-care, when therapeutic, constitute prevention at the primary level (Orem, 1995). Home health care nurses

select, or assist the patient in selecting, methods for meeting self-care requisites that promote and maintain health and development and prevent specific disease (Orem, 1995). Secondary prevention is required after the onset of disease and is directed to the prevention of complications and prolonged disability. Tertiary prevention is appropriate when there is disability and limited functioning. It is directed toward bringing about effective functioning in accord with existing abilities. Health deviation self-care, when therapeutic, is health care at the secondary or tertiary level of prevention (Orem, 1995). Self-care measures are utilized to regulate and prevent effects of the disease, complications, and prolonged disability or to adapt functioning to compensate for the adverse effects of permanent dysfunction (Orem, 1995)

CONCLUSION

As we venture into a managed health care arena, let us be clear about the value of nursing. The value comes not only from managing health but from preventing disease. It is essential that the nursing administration of a home health agency be knowledgeable of the benefits of self-care and have the personnel necessary to design nursing systems. The self-care deficit theory can be utilized in the provision of care to those in the community who require skilled nursing services. Nursing administration must have a system in place to track the outcome of these nursing interventions provided through the nursing system design. This information will be crucial to survival in the health care revolution.

REFERENCES

American Nurses Association (ANA). 1985. *A guide for community-based nursing services.* Kansas City, MO: ANA.

American Nurses Association (ANA). 1986. *Standards of home health nursing practice.* Kansas City, MO: ANA.

Department of Health and Human Services. 1989. Conditions of participation for home health agencies. *Federal Register* 54:33354–33373.

Orem, D. 1995. *Nursing concepts of practice.* 5th ed. St. Louis, MO: Mosby-Year Book.

CHAPTER 12

Home Health Care Documentation and Recordkeeping

Elissa DellaMonica

Documentation is one of the ultimate challenges facing home health care administrators today. Changes in the health care environment have created a need for cost-effective, outcome-based systems of documentation. As hospitals aggressively work to decrease hospital length of stay, patients are being discharged "quicker and sicker." The increase in the acuity level of patients has necessitated clear, concise, accurate documentation with evidence of coordination of the multiple services needed to care for the patient.

This chapter presents home health care documentation and recordkeeping in their entirety. The regulatory bodies governing home health care, specifically the documentation requirements of the Medicare program, are addressed. Discussion includes the components of a clinical record, reasons for documentation, and current trends in documentation systems. Upon completion of this chapter, the reader will possess a basic knowledge of home health documentation and recordkeeping.

THE CHANGING HEALTH CARE ENVIRONMENT

As alluded to above, the delivery of health care is engulfed in an era of change. The 1980s were filled with numerous legislative and regulatory changes that had a major impact on the home care industry. The 1990s have seen the most dramatic changes with the conversion of Medicare patients to managed care, capitated risk contracts, and the proposed change in Medicare from cost reimbursement to prospective payment.

In 1982, the Tax Equity and Fiscal Responsibility Act was passed, which mandated that the Department of Health and Human Services (DHHS) institute the system of prospective reimbursement. The diagnosis-related group system of classification and reimbursement resulted in patients being discharged from hospitals in the acute or early recovery phase of an illness. The need for home care services increased because patients were discharged from hospitals requiring intensive levels of home care services. The industry as a whole realized significant increases in services and increasing Medicare expenditures at an average annual rate of 25 percent (National Association for Home Care [NAHC], 1991).

In 1985, the Health Care Financing Administration (HCFA) introduced the standardized plan of treatment forms commonly known as HCFA forms 485, 486, and 487 (DHHS, 1966). The introduction of these forms began a period of restrictive interpretation of the Medicare home health agency (HHA) manual. Throughout the country, agencies experienced an increase in medical and technical denials, all based on lack of supporting documentation.

Physician orders, progress notes, flow sheets, and assessment forms were closely scrutinized by the fiscal intermediary for homebound status, accuracy in completion of forms, and reasonable and necessary provision of services before agencies were reimbursed for skilled visits. The stringent interpretation of the existing regulations necessitated a dramatic increase in the need for perfect documentation.

In 1989, HCFA was forced to revise the Medicare HHA manual. The revisions were the result of the lawsuit brought by Representative Harvey Staggers and NAHC. The revisions resulted in a much less restrictive interpretation of the Medicare regulations, enabling nurses and other disciplines to provide medically needed home care services to homebound individuals. The fiscal intermediaries were no longer permitted to make a coverage decision based solely on the reviewer's general inferences about similar diagnoses; rather, decisions had to be based on objective clinical evidence regarding the patient's individual need for care (Harris, 1990).

With the rewrite of the Medicare HHA manual, home health agencies, through the mechanism of documentation, were now able to justify the need for more diverse, less restrictive home care services. Agencies could now provide case management services for patients requiring multidisciplinary management and evaluation of the care plan, venipuncture, and insulin administration for patients for whom there was no able or willing caregiver to administer the drug.

The importance of documentation cannot be stressed enough. The HHA manual revisions place even greater emphasis on the need for quality documentation. It is imperative that home health administrators recognize the impact of documentation on the continued viability of their organization.

REGULATIONS GOVERNING HOME HEALTH CARE DOCUMENTATION

All Medicare-certified home health agencies are governed by the Medicare conditions of participation (COPs; HCFA, 1989). An agency is certified as a Medicare provider based on the agency's compliance with the COPs. There are various COPs that govern home health care documentation. During the Medicare certification review site visit, all agencies must show that they are in compliance with the standards.

The COPs contain numerous standards that direct an agency's clinical record policy (HCFA, 1991). These are shown in Appendix 12–A. Agencies seeking Accreditation from the Joint Commission on Accreditation of Healthcare Organizations are required to comply with the Medicare COPs and the standards for home health care services as outlined in the Joint Commission's *Accreditation Manual for Home Care* (1996). Hospital-based HHAs are required to seek Joint Commission accreditation as part of the hospital's accreditation process. The *Accreditation Manual for Home Care* contains a listing of the standards as well as scoring guidelines that direct an agency in how to comply with the intent of the standards. This manual is highly recommended for those seeking accreditation. In addition, managed care companies are beginning to require accreditation as a stipulation for contracting.

The Community Health Accreditation Program (CHAP), under the auspices of the National League for Health Care, is the only independent accrediting body for home and community health organizations. CHAP accreditation is not mandatory, however. Agencies applying for CHAP accreditation must complete a self-study report verifying compliance with the standards as outlined in the manual. The self-study report is an intensive self-evaluation tool that addresses both business and clinical aspects of the organization (CHAP, 1993). The report is reviewed by an expert panel of administrators. A site visit by a few members of the panel is conducted to verify accuracy of the self-study report. An important component of the site visit consists of an extensive analysis of clinical documentation.

CHAP and Joint Commission standards were both developed to provide a means by which community health organizations could ensure excellence. HCFA issued regulations deeming agencies accredited by the Joint Commission (HCFA, 1993) and CHAP (DHHS, 1992) to meet the certification requirements for the Medicare program. Thus agencies that opt for deemed status are no longer subject to routine inspection by Medicare state survey agencies. The Joint Commission and CHAP surveyors are required to complete the Federal Functional Assessment Instrument as part of the unannounced periodic site visit.

CLINICAL RECORD POLICY

As previously stated, the prime source of funding for many agencies is Medicare. Hence the COPs are the primary tool with which agencies develop their documentation policies. Clinical record and documentation policies are a must for all HHAs. The clinical record policy addresses protection and retention of records, contents of the clinical record, requirements for the written plan of treatment, requirements for verbal orders, and record review policy. The clinical record policy is specific to the agency and describes the system of documentation that an agency is utilizing. The record policy is one that should be strictly adhered to because it will form the basis on which the documentation system is reviewed. During the Medicare certification process and the Joint Commission and CHAP review processes, an agency will be reviewed to verify compliance with its own policies (e.g., if the policy states that verbal orders will be signed and incorporated into the chart in 2 weeks, then it had better be done).

It behooves an administrator to develop a clinical record policy that does not place restraints on the agency. The policy should describe what is actually occurring in the management of the clinical record system. Time limits for return of forms from physicians should be avoided because forms are frequently lost or delayed in the physician's office or mail. Nevertheless, agencies should strive to get all verbal orders and plans of treatment signed and incorporated into the record within 1 to 2 weeks or according to state laws. All other agency forms, progress notes, and assessment forms should be incorporated into the record within 1 week.

An example of a clinical record policy is found in Appendix 12–B. The policy is specific to the agency because it describes the various forms that constitute the clinical record system. The policy clearly describes the agency's procedures for protection and retention of records. The policy indicates that the agency is in compliance with the Medicare COPs.

REASONS FOR DOCUMENTATION

During routine daily activities, a community health nurse spends approximately 35 percent of his or her time on documentation and 65 percent on patient care. For nurses, whose primary focus is the care of the patient, the amount of time spent on documentation seems to be counterproductive. Despite the frustrations felt by many community health nurses, the importance of documentation cannot be overemphasized.

Why do we document? There are many reasons, but the primary reason that comes to the mind of home health administrators is reimbursement. Documentation is the method through which the patient's need for home health services is presented (Jacob, 1985). Ineffective, poor documentation could jeopardize the financial stability of the organization. Medicare and other third party payers may require that documentation be submitted for review before reimbursing the agency. The documentation must objectively inform the reviewer and/or insurance case manager of the clinical status of the patient, inclusive of a description of the services being provided.

The plan of care is a universal form developed and distributed by HCFA. The forms are known as HCFA Form 485 (physician's plan of care), Form 486 (Medical Update and Patient Information), and Form 487 (Addendum; DHHS, 1966). The forms contain all the necessary data elements for a physician's plan of care as outlined in the COPs. The forms were developed to elicit specific information to enable the reviewer to make Medicare coverage determinations. Currently, the fiscal intermediaries no longer require that the physician's plan of care be submitted for review before paying the claim. The intermediary, however, can at any time request the plan of care as well as any other documents in the record. The reviewer will closely analyze the form for inconsistencies in the clinical picture (e.g., Is the diagnosis consistent with the treatment? Are there realistic and measurable goals? Is the care intermittent? Is the patient homebound? Do the clinical diagnosis, treatment, and services ordered support the statement on homebound status? Do the number of visits reflect overutilization of services?). If the reviewer detects any inconsistencies in the plan of care on comparison with the clinical notes, the determination may be made that the care was not reasonable and necessary, and the claim may be denied.

The Medicare fiscal intermediaries are conducting their review through a process called focus medical review (FMR). FMR is the process of targeting and directing medical review efforts on Medicare claims where there is the greatest risk of inappropriate program payment (DHHS, 1966). There has been a significant increase in the use of FMR as a result of concerns by the intermediary about overutilization of services. Through the process of FMR, the fiscal intermediary collects data from a variety of sources and conducts data analysis to identify practice patterns, aberrations, potential areas of overutilization, and patterns of noncovered services (NAHC, 1996). Although FMR is a process by which the fiscal intermediaries research and analyze data for aberrations, it is also the means by which reviewers determine whether services were reasonable and necessary. FMR is the current mechanism that Medicare uses for coverage decisions. The primary tool that is used in this review process is the clinical record, which is requested by the issuance of a computerized Form 488.

Aside from the physician's plan of care, Medicare and other third party payers frequently review progress notes, assessment forms, and verbal orders. Quality documentation should include observations written in both clinical and measurable terms (Jacob, 1985). This enables the reviewer and/or case manager to assess changes in the patient's condition. Descriptive, accurate documentation is essential to ensure reimbursement. As previously stated, the professional caregiver is directly accountable for reimbursement. It is only through the mechanism of documentation that an agency receives payment for services.

The second reason for documenting is to prove that quality care was rendered. In home care, the clinical record is the primary tool for assessing the quality and appropriateness of care. The clinical record is a mechanism of proof that the practitioner provided quality services. An agency evaluates for quality via the quarterly record review. The agency is responsible for developing criteria or standards on which to base the clinical record review. The criteria should be well defined and stated in measurable terms. The clinical record will be evaluated to verify compliance with the established criteria (see Chapter 24).

Good documentation reflects good care. If the required data do not appear in the clinical record, the quarterly record review may show deficiencies in the care provided to the patient. Remember: Care that is not documented is presumed not to have been done.

The third reason for documentation is to show evidence of coordination of services and continuity of care. Charting shows how several disciplines arrange for continuity and comprehensive care without duplication of services (Stanhope and Lancaster, 1984). The medical record gives members of the health care team a way to communicate with each other. This is accomplished through the formulation of discipline-specific care plans. Short- and long-range goals should be identified indicating expected outcomes for each discipline. These goals should be realistic, measurable, and achievable and should provide guidance in developing a discipline-specific care plan.

A care plan gives direction to patient care by showing all caregivers the goals that are established for a patient, and it gives clear direction for all caregivers to work toward achieving these goals. The plan of care and progress notes provide for continuity of care by informing other professionals of what has been accomplished in the care of the patient. It also informs the caregiver of the plans for future visits.

The coordination of services is documented in the progress note. As addressed in the Medicare COPs, all HHAs are required to show evidence of coordination of multiple services. This is accomplished by the performance and documentation of conferences. A multidisciplinary team conference must establish that there is effective interdisciplinary coordination of the plan of care. These conferences should include all disciplines involved in the care of the patient with reference to goals and expected outcomes.

There should also be evidence of coordination of services from administrative to supervisory clinical staff. Coordination between administrative and clinical staff is documented during patient care conferences and should include reference to the current status of the patient, changes in the plan of care, the ability to achieve the goals as stated in the plan of care, and plans for discharge. The administrative staff may also get involved in a clinical case conference when there is an issue that cannot be resolved at the clinical level. It is imperative that a progress note be documented with evidence of anticipated plans and expected outcomes.

During the Medicare certification visit and the Joint Commission and/or CHAP survey, the surveyor will request evidence of coordination of services at all levels. It behooves all agencies to monitor documentation of coordination of services closely as they are explicitly outlined in the COPs and the Joint Commission and CHAP standards.

The fourth reason to document is that it is a requirement of all professionals involved in the care of patients. Standards I through VI in *Clinical Nursing Practice* (American Nurses Association, 1991) addresses documentation as follows:

> *Standard I, assessment:* The nurse collects client health data.
>
> *Standard II, diagnosis:* The nurse analyzes the assessment data in determining diagnosis.
>
> *Standard III, outcome identification:* The nurse identifies expected outcomes individualized to the client.
>
> *Standard IV, planning:* The nurse develops a plan of care that prescribes interventions to attain expected outcomes.
>
> *Standard V, implementation:* The nurse implements the interventions identified in the plan of care.
>
> *Standard VI, evaluation:* The nurse evaluates the client's progress toward attainment of outcomes.

Good documentation also establishes the professional's and the agency's credibility. If a chart is poorly written and lacks appropriate terminology and measurable terms, it gives an unfavorable impression of the skill and knowledge of the professional caring for the patient (Jacob, 1985). Hence hospitals, physicians, and community agencies may be reluctant to refer patients.

The fifth reason for documentation addresses the liability issue. As previously stated, professional caregivers are required to show evidence of the care that was rendered. The Medicare COPs and the Joint Commission and CHAP standards all speak to the necessity of the physician's order before care is initiated and throughout the service period. Professional caregivers are required to report all changes in the patient's medical status to the physician. The caregiver may be held liable if there is no evidence of communication with the physician and no evidence of verbal orders to cover changes in the original plan of care.

Home health care workers are also accountable to the Medicare program in documenting provision of skilled services mandated by the federal regulations. An agency may be held liable for fraud and abuse if it cannot demonstrate through documentation that skilled services were provided to a homebound patient and that services were reasonable and necessary for the care of the client.

At all times, agencies must be prepared for an unannounced visit from the Medicare surveyor to certify an agency for participation in the Medicare program or an unannounced visit from the fiscal intermediary to conduct a coverage compliance review. The primary focus of these reviews is to conduct an intensive review of the client records to verify compliance with the federal regulations. State Medicaid reviewers may also conduct unannounced visits per the state statutory regulations. As of July 1993, the Joint Commission initiated unannounced surveys to ensure compliance with selected standards. It is imperative that home health administrators be aware of the quality and appropriateness of their staff's documentation because they are ultimately responsible for deficiencies that may be found.

THE KEY TO SUCCESSFUL DOCUMENTATION

The key to successful documentation lies in the caregiver's ability to paint a picture of the patient for the reviewer. This will enable the reviewer to understand the reason why services were rendered to the client. The reviewer's first introduction to the patient is the physician's plan of care. The plan of care must contain enough information to enable the reviewer to make a coverage determination. As discussed, agencies are using the standard Medicare certification and plan of care forms developed by HCFA. There are three separate pages to the HCFA forms. Form 485 is the actual plan of treatment and is the only form that must be sent

to the physician for signature. HCFA Form 486 is the medical update and patient information form. This form is a dual-purpose form. It is completed by the agency to provide Medicare with supplemental information that will enable the reviewer to make the coverage determination. It is also used as a summary/progress report that is sent to the physician every 62 days, a transfer abstract, and a discharge summary. HCFA Form 487 is an addendum for additional writing space to complete the forms.

There are a few key factors in completing the forms according to Medicare specifications. The diagnosis must be a clear diagnosis that conforms in terminology to that of the ninth revision of the *International Classification of Diseases* (ICD-9) published by the DHHS (Jones et al., 1993). The primary diagnosis listed should be the primary reason for which the patient is receiving home health services, which may be different from the primary diagnosis listed on the referral. Other diagnoses should be listed in order of importance. All diagnoses and surgical procedures should contain an ICD-9 code with date of onset and exacerbation. (A note of caution: Avoid chronic diagnoses such as Alzheimer's disease, for which there is a reasonable probability that skilled intervention will not effect a change in the patient's clinical status.)

The treatment orders should be listed per discipline. The orders must be clear and specific to the diagnosis, indicating frequency and duration. For example, ranges may be used when the stability of the condition is such that variations in frequency of treatment are required.

Orders for medication should include dose, frequency, and method of administration. New or changed drug status should be listed after the medication. This indicates to the reviewer the medications for which the patient will need instruction and review.

Goals, rehabilitation potential, and discharge plan should be specific to the diagnosis. The summary of clinical findings should include the clinical status of the client on admission to service and on recertification and the status of the patient over the last 62 days. The physician's signature must be original; a stamp of the physician's signature is not acceptable.

HCFA Form 486 (medical update and patient information) is an optional form to evaluate the effectiveness of care. Current Medicare regulations state that Form 486 need not be completed on a routine basis unless requested by the fiscal intermediary for review. Agencies are still required to complete a summary progress report that is sent to the physician every 62 days. Once an agency chooses to eliminate Form 486, it must make provisions to meet this Medicare COP.

In summary, the physician's plan of treatment is the reviewer's first introduction to the patient. It must show that services are coordinated and directed toward a common goal while summarizing the clinical status of the patient from the perspective of all the disciplines.

DOCUMENTATION OF SKILLED CARE

As previously stated, nurses, therapists, and social workers must document evidence that the patient is in need of skilled care. The initial evaluation is documented on assessment forms specific to each discipline. In addition to the assessment form, an agency may or may not require a clinical note. This initial evaluation documentation is important because it contains a brief description of the event or accident that rendered the patient homebound and in need of skilled services. The initial nursing note should contain pertinent findings of the nurse's physical assessment; identification of the need for instruction, observation, or treatment; review of medications, including a preliminary assessment of the patient's understanding of the purpose and signs and symptoms of reaction to the medication; identification of the need for home health aide services; identification of patient goals that are measurable and realistic; anticipated frequency and duration; and homebound status. Documentation includes that the patient has reviewed the bill of rights and has verbalized understanding of the bill of rights. There

must also be documentation addressing the existence of an advance directive. Instruction to the patient on how to formulate an advance directive is also recommended.

Per the 1996 Joint Commission standards, the initial visit should include documentation of a nutrition and safety assessment. The nutrition assessment forms the basis on which the nurse determines the patient's risk for nutritional problems. In addition, the safety assessment must address such things as fire safety, electrical safety, bed and mobility safety, bathroom safety, and medication safety. The use of patient teaching tools is required once a safety problem has been detected.

The physical therapy and occupational therapy evaluation notes should contain a gradient evaluation, which identifies the areas of deficiency; identification of short- and long-range goals; the specific therapy program to be initiated; the frequency and duration of visits; and evidence of homebound status. The speech pathologist evaluation should include the type of test used in the examination, the identified speech disorders, identification of patient goals that are realistic and measurable, the specific therapy program to be initiated, the frequency and duration of visits and a list of teaching tools given to the patient for practice and reinforcement, and evidence of homebound status. The social service evaluation should include the persons from whom pertinent information is elicited, the patient's participation or lack of participation in the discussion, the overall plan of action and actions to be initiated after the evaluation and before the patient is visited again, short- and long-range goals that are realistic and measurable, the frequency and duration of visits, and evidence of homebound status.

After completing the initial assessment/evaluation, which may or may not be done on a standard assessment/evaluation form, the caregiver is expected to document a clinical note. The clinical note is a dated, written notation by a member of the health care team on contact with a patient. The note contains a description of signs and symptoms, treatment and/or drugs given, the patient's reaction to the treatment, effects of medication, and changes in physical or emotional condition.

Documentation of instructions given to the patient must also appear in the clinical note. Instructions should be broken down to a specific drug, diet, treatment, or exercise. The use of patient teaching tools is highly recommended. Instructions should continue until the patient/family demonstrates the ability to perform the treatment independently or until the patient/family verbalizes understanding of, for example, medication side effects. Once the patient's understanding of the instruction is documented, further instructions do not constitute a need for ongoing skilled care. Remember: Be specific in your documentation of instructions, and do not repeat instructions once the client has become independent.

Skilled nursing observation and evaluation visits must be thoroughly documented. The nurse must show evidence of changes in the patient's clinical status with notification of the physician of changes that have occurred. Skilled observation and evaluation visits are usually covered as long as there are significant changes in the patient's clinical status. The nurse should attempt to chart negatively (e.g., describe in descriptive terms such things as the size, depth, and width of the wound; the color and odor of the exudate; the color of the sputum; the congestion of the lungs; the girth of the abdomen; responses to medications; and the severity of pain). Skilled observation and evaluation visits are important to the care of the client. To ensure reimbursement for these visits, the nurse must document all changes in the patient's status and all written changes by the physician on the plan of care (Engelbrecht, 1986).

Documentation of direct skilled care (e.g., catheter changes, treatments, or injections) is more simple because nurses are accustomed to documentation of specific tasks. Once again, nurses must be specific and describe the length and complexity of the treatment. The Medicare reviewer or case manager will be monitoring the complexity of the care to determine whether it could be done by a nonskilled caregiver (e.g., the family or home health aide). Treatments that require daily care over an extended period of time may not be covered because they may not meet the intermittent criterion.

Skilled nursing and therapy visits for management and evaluation of the care plan are reasonable and necessary. Case management is based on the concept that skilled personnel are needed to meet the patient's medical needs, promote recovery, and ensure medical safety even if the patient does not require skilled care.

All factors must be considered in documentation of management and evaluation of the care plan. Factors such as medications, diagnosis, safety, functional limitations, psychosocial issues, orders for multiple disciplines, goals, and rehabilitation potential must be identified. Documentation must demonstrate the relationship between symptoms and conditions creating a level of complexity that necessitates the intervention of a nurse or therapist. Specific goals must be identified addressing expected outcomes of case management services.

The skilled therapy clinical note should contain an assessment of the patient's clinical status from the therapist's viewpoint, an evaluation of progress or regression since the last visit, the specific therapy modality that was carried out during the visit, the response of the patient to the exercise/therapy during the visit, a statement indicating that the therapist is working toward accomplishment of goals, and a list of new problems that the therapist has discovered on the visit. The therapist's documentation must reflect the degree of motion lost and degree to be restored. Distances that the patient ambulated must be recorded in feet, and the degree of independence in transfer must be explicitly described. The speech pathologist must document the response of the client to therapy using percentages, degrees, number of repetitions, and the like.

As stated in the Medicare HHA manual, "Medical Social Service must contribute significantly to the treatment of the patient's medical condition" (DHHS, 1966, p. 15.11). The medical social service clinical note must contain a detailed description of the social problems that are affecting the patient and contributing to the instability of the disease process. The social worker is expected to describe how his or her intervention can improve the overall status of the patient. The documentation must contain the actual steps taken by the social worker to resolve the problem, the outcomes of the social worker's intervention, and plans for future intervention. Social service visits are generally provided at a maximum of one to three visits per patient. Clear, concise, explicit documentation is needed for coverage of medical social service visits.

In general, home health aides are not required to document in a narrative note. It is customary procedure for a home health aide to document on a worksheet outlining the home health aide's responsibilities. The nurse is expected to develop the home health aide plan of care that directs the aide's activities. The nurse is required to supervise the home health aide every 2 weeks and update the plan of care as needed. The supervision note should be included in a clinical note and must include instructions to the home health aide on the plan of care, the home health aide's understanding of the plan, and his or her ability to perform the necessary functions. The nurse should also include the plans for the future and anticipated plans for a change in aide schedule or discharge of aide service.

Another key issue for reimbursable documentation is homebound status. The reason that the patient is homebound must be discussed on admission and at least weekly thereafter. All disciplines involved in the care of the client should speak to the homebound status with a description of why the patient is homebound. Generalized weakness is not a reason for homebound status. Functional limitations should be clearly described and stated in measurable terms. One discipline must be careful to support another discipline's statement on homebound status. For example, nurses and home health aides must not make statements that are contradictory to the therapist's statements. For example, nurses and aides may indicate that the patient is ambulating without difficulty when the therapist is providing service for gait dysfunction. The nurse's statement may disqualify therapy services. Documentation of coordination via multidisciplinary case conferences will obviate this problem.

Remember: The key to successful documentation lies in the caregiver's ability to describe explicitly why the patient needs home health services and how home health services will improve the patient's overall clinical status. At the completion of your documentation, ask yourself: "Was the care I provided to this patient reasonable and necessary? Did I perform care that was ordered by the physician? Does the clinical note indicate that the patient was homebound? Did I improve the health status of the patient?" All these questions must be answered to ensure reimbursement.

CURRENT TRENDS IN DOCUMENTATION

Although the basic principles of documentation remain the same, there has been significant development of documentation systems. In this era of cost containment, HHAs are seeking more efficient, cost-effective means of documentation. In addition, Medicare and managed care insurers are requesting outcome data from agencies. An outcome, as defined by Shaughnessy and Crisler (1995), is a change in patient health status between two or more points in time. For the first time, professionals are requested to evaluate whether the services that were provided had a positive impact on the health status of the patient.

Designed specifically for HHAs, the Outcome and Assessment Information Set (OASIS) is a tool for measuring outcomes (Shaughnessy and Crisler, 1995). OASIS is used in addition to the assessment because it is not a clinical assessment tool. The tool is designed to measure physiological, functional, cognitive, emotional, and behavioral health. The tool is completed on admission, at follow-up points, and at discharge. It is anticipated that Medicare and other third party payers will require that the tool be completed on all patients because this will justify the need for home health services and thus payment for these services. From the agency's standpoint, outcomes analysis will be integral to a quality improvement program because it will form a basis on which to measure the quality and effectiveness of care.

CRITICAL PATHWAYS

Critical pathways are practice guidelines tailored to a specific patient population, such as patients with congestive heart failure. They are intended to promote the appropriate management of potential or defined health problems by providing a guideline for routine patient care. Unlike care plans, critical pathways provide a time frame for the completion of activities. In addition to providing staff with a clinical practice guideline, critical pathways may be used as a documentation tool. Because critical pathways are usually disease specific, variance reports are necessary to address deviations for patient/family goals, outcomes, and staff interventions (Spath, 1993). The critical pathway generally has a predetermined patient outcome that can easily be measured through variance tracking. The use of critical pathways in disease-specific management programs provides consistency and standardization to the clinical staff in the provision of care. Critical pathways are utilized by insurance case managers to assist them in the decision-making process regarding approval of services. As a documentation tool, critical pathways have their limitations because it is difficult to address all the patients' problems, so that staff must document extensively on variance reports.

COMPUTERIZED DOCUMENTATION

Perhaps the most exciting trend in home health documentation lies in the computeriza-

tion of the clinical record. Through the use of laptop computers, the clinical staff have the capability of documenting at the patient's home. Unlike paper charts, the computerized record allows the clinician to access the patient's record, so that all professional disciplines have current patient information. Generally, computerized documentation decreases the tedious redundancy of traditional charting because the clinician need enter patient information only once. This single data entry is sufficient to transfer the data to a variety of forms, such as the care plan and the physician's plan of treatment. Documentation of the clinical note is expedited because the nurse or therapist addresses the interventions previously identified on the care plan. Specific physician orders may also be carried forward from the physician's plan of care. At the completion of a day's documentation, the clinician takes the laptop home and connects it to his or her home phone line. At a preprogrammed time, the laptop transfers the patient data to the main server located in the central office. Later that night, the updated information is transferred back to the laptop. The following morning, the clinician has information about new referrals that he or she is expected to admit to service and current information about patients whom they are scheduled to visit.

In addition to improving the efficiency of staff, computerized documentation has numerous advantages. It forces standardization of documentation, thus improving the work of poor documenters. It enables the agency to customize its practice guidelines through the development of pop-up boxes or help screens that direct clinicians to select from a preapproved menu, thus improving patient care. It significantly improves multidisciplinary coordination of care and communication through the use of E-mail. Continuity of patient care is enhanced because all clinicians have access to current patient information. Linkage with insurance case managers is possible to ask for information about patient status. This could significantly decrease the amount of time spent on phone calls to insurance case managers, thus facilitating the precertification process. In addition, physicians may also query for patient information, which would facilitate the physician ordering process and decrease the number of phone calls to physicians.

MEDICAL RECORD DEPARTMENT

Our agency* utilizes a centralized filing system for storage of medical records. Active charts are kept in a Centrex circular file and shelf to allow for easy access. Discharged charts from the previous year are stored in a separate filing cabinet. All other discharged records are stored off the premises. Per agency policy, all charts must be kept for 7 years plus the age of majority. Charts are filed in numerical order utilizing a color-coded numbering system. This allows for quick identification of the clinical record. The department is staffed by a medical record coordinator and medical record clerks. The clinical staff are not permitted to access charts without completing a requisition slip. Staff may request a portion of the chart, the flow sheet, or the entire chart. Charts are not permitted to leave the office, but flow sheets and medication lists can to be taken to the patient's home. In general, staff are discouraged from handling the clinical records.

The agency has realized numerous benefits as a result of the tight controls on the medical record system. In general, charts are rarely misplaced or misfiled, forms are incorporated into the charts on a timely basis, and charts are maintained in proper order. The indirect benefits associated with a well-run medical record department are a decrease in the stress of visiting staff (because less time is spent on clerical activities), assistance to the supervisory staff when they are seeking patient information, a decrease in the time spent on quality record review (because charts are completed and forms are filed in order), improved efficiency in day-to-day operations of the clinical staff, and reassurance among the staff in knowing that the charts are ready for an unannounced survey by Medicare or the Joint Commission.

Clearly, the future of home care documentation lies in the computerization of the medical record. As previously discussed, this is accomplished through laptop technology that supports off-site entry of patient information. Administrators must keep abreast of the current technology because it may prove to be beneficial to the future of agency operations.

CONCLUSION

Quality reimbursable documentation requires the commitment of the entire agency. This commitment must encompass all levels of employees, from the chief administrative officer to the visiting staff to the clerical support staff. All levels of employees should be aware of their responsibilities in the documentation process. Administrators have as one of their primary responsibilities the education of the staff on the complexities of the documentation process and making them aware of the importance of documentation. In today's health care environment, documentation, completed accurately, timely, and efficiently, is the key to an agency's survival.

---

*Visiting Nurse Association of Eastern Montgomery County/A Department of Abington Memorial Hospital changed its name as of March 1997 and is now known as Abington Memorial Hospital Home Care.

BIBLIOGRAPHY

American Nurses Association (ANA). 1991. *Clinical nursing practice.* Washington, DC: ANA.

Community Health Accreditation Program. 1993. *Standards of excellence for home care organizations.* New York: National League for Health Care, Inc.

Department of Health and Human Services. 1966 (Reprinted 1971). *Medicare home health agency manual.* Washington, DC: Government Printing Office.

Department of Health and Human Services, Health Care Financing Administration. 1992. Medicare program: Recognition of the community health accreditation program standards for home health organizations. *Federal Register* 57:22773–22780.

Department of Health and Human Services. Health Care Financing Administration. March 10, 1997. Medicare and Medicaid Program; Revision of the Conditions of Participation in Home Health Agencies and Use of the Outcome and Assessment Information Set (OASIS) as part of the Revised Conditions of Participation for Home Health Agencies. *Federal Register* 62 (46):11004–11009.

Engelbrecht, L. 1986, March. Engelbrecht on documentation. *Home Health Journal,* p. 11.

Harris, M.D. 1990. The 1980s in review. *Home Healthcare Nurse* 8:10–12.

Health Care Financing Administration. 1989. 42 CFR Part 484. Medicare conditions of participation for home health agencies. *Federal Register* 54:33367–33373.

Health Care Financing Administration. 1991. 42 CFR Part 484. Medicare program: Home health agencies: Conditions of participation. *Federal Register* 56:32967–32975.

Health Care Financing Administration. 1993, June 30. Medicare and Medicaid programs: Recognition of the Joint Commission on Accreditation of Healthcare Organizations standards for home care organizations. *Federal Register* 58:35007.

Jacob, S.R. 1985. The impact of documentation in home health care. *Home Healthcare Nurse* 3:16–20.

Joint Commission on Accreditation of Healthcare Organizations. 1996. *1995 Accreditation manual for home care.* Oakbrook Terrace, IL: Joint Commission.

Jones, N., et al., eds. 1993. *International classification of diseases: Clinical modification.* 4th ed. Vols. 1–3. Alexandria, VA: St. Anthony's.

Medicare Home Health Agencies. Conditions of Participation. March 10, 1997. *Federal Register* 62 (46):11009–11035.

Medicare and Medicaid Program; Use of the OASIS as part of the Conditions of Participation for Home Health Agencies. March 10, 1997. *Federal Register* 62 (46):11035–11046.

National Association for Home Care (NAHC). 1991. *NAHC report: Dramatic home health and hospice spending increases testify to NAHC success in the courts and congress.* Washington, DC: NAHC.

National Association for Home Care (NAHC). 1996. *NAHC report: Providers experiencing the burdens of FMR.* Washington, DC: NAHC.

Shaughnessy, P., and K. Crisler. 1995. *Outcome based quality improvement.* Washington, DC: National Association for Home Care.

Spath, P. 1993. Critical paths: A tool for clinical process management. *Journal of the American Hospital Information Management Association* 64:56.

Stanhope, M., and J. Lancaster. 1984. *Community health nursing.* St. Louis: Mosby.

COP Standards Pertaining to HHA Clinical Record Policy

Subpart A: General Provisions

Clinical records shall be maintained on all patients, in order to participate as a home health agency.

A Clinical Note means a dated, written notation of a contact with a patient that is written and dated by a member of the health team and that describes signs and symptoms, treatment drugs administered and the patient's reaction and any changes in physical or emotional conditions.

484.10 COP: Patient Rights

The patient has the right to be informed of his or her rights. The HHA must protect and promote the exercise of these rights.

484.10 Standard: Notice of Rights

(1) The HHA must provide the patient with a written notice of the patient's rights in advance of furnishing care to the patient or during the initial evaluation visit before the initiation of treatment.

(2) The HHA must maintain documentation showing that it has complied with the requirements of this section.

484.10 (c) Standard: Right To Be Informed and To Participate in Planning Care and Treatment

(1) The patient has the right to be informed in advance about the care to be furnished, and of any changes in the care to be furnished.

  (i) The HHA must advise the patient in advance of the disciplines that will furnish care, and the frequency of visits proposed to be furnished.

  (ii) The HHA must advise the patient in advance of any change in the plan of care before the change is made.

(2) The patient has the right to participate in the planning of the care. The HHA must advise the patient in advance of the right to participate in planning the care or treatment and in planning changes in the care or treatment.

484.10 (d) Standard: Confidentiality of Medical Records

The patient has the right to confidentiality of the clinical records maintained by the HHA. The HHA must advise the patient of the agency's policies and procedures regarding disclosure of clinical records.

484.14 COP: Organization, Service, Administration

484.14(g) Standard: Coordination of Patient Services

All personnel providing services maintain liaison to ensure that their efforts effectively complement one another and support the objectives outlined in the Plan of Care. The clinical record or minutes of case conferences establish that effective interchange, reporting, and coordination of patient care [do] occur. A written summary report for each patient is sent to the attending physician at least every 62 days.

This standard establishes the agency's responsibilities in the coordination of services. There should be evidence in a clinical record of coordination [among] disciplines and coordination through the various levels of authority. Documentation of case conferences [is] an absolute must in all clinical records.

484.18 COP: Acceptance of Patients, Plan of Care, Medical Supervision

484.18(a) Standard: Plan of Care

The plan of care developed in consultation with the agency staff covers all pertinent diagnoses including: Mental status, types of service and equipment required, frequency of visits, prognosis, rehabilitation potential, functional limitations, activities permitted, nutritional requirements, medications and treatments, any safety measures to protect against injury, instructions for timely discharge or referral, any other appropriate items. If a physician refers a patient under a Plan of Care that cannot be completed until after an evaluation visit, the physician is consulted to approve additions or modifications to the original plan.

Orders for therapy services include the specific procedures and modalities to be used and the amount, frequency, and duration. The therapist and other agency personnel participate in developing the plan of care.

484.18(b) Standard: Periodic Review of Plan of Care

The total Plan of Care is reviewed by the attending physician and agency personnel as often as the severity of the patient's condition requires, but at least once every 62 days. Agency professional staff promptly alert the physician of any changes that suggest a need to alter the plan of care.

484.18(c) Standard: Conformance with Physician's Orders

Drugs and treatments are administered by agency staff as ordered by the physician. Nurse and therapist immediately record and sign oral orders and obtain the physician's countersignature.

Agency staff check all medicines a patient may be taking to identify possible ineffective drug therapy or adverse reactions, significant side effects, drug allergies, and contraindicated medications and report any problems to the physician.

484.48 COP: Clinical Records

A clinical record containing pertinent past and current findings in accordance with accepted professional standards is maintained for every patient receiving home health services. In addition to the plan of care, the record contains appropriate identifying information; name of physician; drug, dietary treatment, and activity orders; signed and dated clinical and progress notes; copies of summary reports sent to the attending physician; and a discharge summary.

484.48 (a) Standard: Retention of Records

Clinical records are maintained for five years after the month the cost report for which the records apply is filed with the intermediary, unless State law stipulates a longer period of time. Policies call for retention even if the agency discontinues operation. If the patient is transferred to another health facility, a copy of the record or abstract accompanies the patient.

484.48 (b) Standard: Protection of Records

Clinical record information is safeguarded against loss or unauthorized use. Written procedures govern use and removal of records and conditions for release of information not authorized by law.

Abington Memorial Hospital Home Care Policy for Clinical Records

PURPOSE: To maintain clinical records for all patients in a systematic, confidential manner.

RESPONSIBLE PERSONNEL: Executive director, director of professional services, clinical supervisors, medical record staff, visiting patient care staff.

OBJECTIVES: To maintain a complete record for each patient that provides a history and plan of care for the patient and provides a record of all care provided to the patient.

To provide a system for storage and maintenance of all records to protect the confidentiality of all information that meets all legal and regulatory requirements.

POLICY: A clinical record is maintained for each patient admitted in an individual folder filed in a color-coded, numeric system. Clinical records of current patients and closed records for the year are kept in house in protected files. All parts of the record remain in the office, except for the flow sheet, the medication list, and the master file input card, which may be taken on home visits. Records are retained for a minimum of 7 years in a protected area to safeguard against loss or unauthorized use. Records of minors are retained until the age of majority plus an additional 7 years.

Information from the clinical record will not be disclosed without the patient's consent, except as necessary to provide services and to obtain payment for those services or in response to a valid subpoena or court order.

The final responsibility for the patient records rests with the Executive Director and the Governing Body. If the organization is dissolved, the State Department of Health will be notified of the date of dissolution and the location of the records.

Source: Reprinted with permission of the Visiting Nurse Association of Eastern Montgomery County/A Department of Abington Memorial Hospital, Willow Grove, Pennsylvania.

PROCEDURE: *Action*

A. *Open records*

	Rationale

Action

A. *Open records*

1. A clinical record is initiated on every patient admitted for service, and a patient number is assigned. The same number is retained for patients readmitted.

2. Open records are filed numerically in the office on a central file maintained by the medical record staff.

Records are filed by a straight numeric system, color coded for each 100 records and for every 10 within the 100.

3. The contents of the clinical record containing past and current data are as follows:

   a. *Master file input data:* Contains appropriate identifying information and physician's name and telephone number.

     • Form is taken on home visits and becomes a permanent part of the record on discharge.
     • A duplicate copy of the form is kept in the clinical supervisor's folder while the patient is open to service.

   b. *Care plans*:
     • Are discipline specific: completed by nurse, physical therapist, occupational therapist, speech therapist, medical social worker.
     • Are completed on admission and readmission.

Rationale

1. Accurate information is captured for every patient upon admission, and a number is assigned for efficiency in filing all subsequent forms.

2. Central files by number and color code provide for optimum efficiency in filing and retrieving information. Central control of files maintains optimum standardization.

3. The clinical record contains all data on the patient to guide the care by all disciplines while the patient is receiving home care services.

PROCEDURE: *Action*   *Rationale*

- Include a current clinical assessment of the patient's status.
- Include a description of prob-
  lems/needs.
- Address   family/support   systems.
- Include patient goals.
- Include interventions specific to
  the patient:
  1) Nursing care plan
     (flow sheet)
     —Identifies problems
       based on nursing diagno-
       sis.
     —Utilizes flow sheets spe-
       cific to individual prob-
       lems.
     —If revised as needed
       based on patient/client
       status, may also include
       revisions to the plan in
       the clinical note.
  2) Home health aide plan of
     care
     —Is completed by the nurse
       when applicable.
     —Is reviewed and revised
       on an as needed basis.
     —Revisions to the plan are
       contained in the clinical
       note and communicated
       to the aide during the
       supervisory visit.
  3) Physical/speech/occupa-
     tional therapy evaluation
     and plan of care
     —Revisions to the plan are
       based on environment
       and patient/client health
       status.
     —Revisions to the plan are
       contained in the clinical
       note.
  4) Medical social service

PROCEDURE: *Action*   *Rationale*

        —Revisions to the plan are based on environment and patient/client health status.

        —Revisions to the plan are contained in the clinical note.

c. *Nursing assessment forms*:
- Contain pertinent family information.
- Contain pertinent past findings and a current clinical assessment of the patient's status.
- Are completed on admission and readmission.
- Contain a list of nursing diagnoses.

d. *Clinical notes*
- Current progress notes are dated and signed.
- Clinical notes are segregated on colored paper for ease in identification of disciplines.

e. *Physician's plan of treatment (POT)*
- The POT contains the specific services to be provided, including the type and frequency.
- The POT contains a summary report to the physician on admission and every 62 days thereafter.
- The POT is revised by agency personnel and reviewed by the attending physician once every 62 days.
- Additions or changes in the POT are confirmed with a verbal order.

f. *Patient authorization and release form*

g. *Medication list*
- Computerized form listing the name of the medication, dose, frequency and route, indications, side effects, and interactions.

PROCEDURE:　　*Action*　　　　　　　　　　　　　　　　*Rationale*

　　　　　　　　• Form is completed on admission and updated as needed.

　　　　h. *Discharge summary*
　　　　　　　　• Is completed by all disciplines.
　　　　　　　　• To include a summary of service from admission through discharge inclusive of goal attained. Summary sent to physician upon request.

　　　　i. *Written communications*
　　　　　　　　• Conference reports and reports to and from other participating organizations and to and from multidisciplinary professional personnel.

　　　　j. *Home health aide activity records* (when applicable)

　　　　k. *Patient discharge instruction sheet*
　　　　　　　　• Completed at time of discharge. Original to patient and copy in chart. Therapies include discharge instruction in the clinical note.

　　　　l. Patient bill of rights?
　　　　　　Signed copy.

4. All records are kept in a standardized file, and the filing sequence for active records is as follows:

　Left side (front to back)
　　　　a. Master file input card (at discharge)
　　　　b. Physician's orders—newest on top
　　　　　　1) Physical therapy, occupational therapy, speech therapy evaluation forms
　　　　　　2) Advance directive
　　　　c. Verbal orders
　　　　d. Family folder
　　　　e. HHA plan of care
　　　　f. Referral for services
　　　　g. Medicare termination letter (pink copy in chart)
　　　　h. Information release form
　　　　i. Miscellaneous forms:

4. Standardization increases efficiency of filing and retrieving information.

PROCEDURE: *Action*   *Rationale*

- Blue Cross Approval
- Laboratory reports
- Medicare questionnaires

j. Home health aide activity records (newest on top)

Right side (front to back)

a. Patient master update I (after discharge)

b. Problem list

c. Discharge summary (after discharge)

d. Progress notes (newest on top), color coded mount sheet per discipline:
   1) Yellow, nursing
   2) Pink, physical therapy
   3) Green, social service
   4) Gold, occupational therapy
   5) Blue, speech therapy

e. Flow sheet

f. Medication list

g. Nursing assessment

h. Social service assessment

5. Full-time visiting nurse staff tape and record notes and send tape with (pink) copy of the daily report sheet to the transcriptionist daily through interoffice mail. Other staff may tape notes depending upon the availability of a recorder.	5. Taping results of the visit increases efficiency of visiting staff and increases readability of the stored record.
6. The transcriptionist types the notes and returns them to the sender for reading and signature.	6. The signature of the professional staff person ensures accuracy of the typed note.
7. The professional staff send completed notes to the medical record staff for filing in the patient's record on a timely basis.	7. Filing by the medical record staff saves the time of the professional staff.
8. The medical record staff are responsible for maintaining all clinical record supplies in sufficient quantity.	8. Supplies are always available as needed.

B. *Reopening a previous admission*

1. The data of the previous admission are transferred to the right side of the file.	1. Having the data available from the previous admission is helpful in planning current care for the readmitted patient.

PROCEDURE: *Action*

Rationale

2. The divider is placed on the right side of the file with the tab labeled.

2. Having the data available from the previous admission is helpful in planning current care for the readmitted patient.

3. Subsequent filing sequence follows the current admission order as above.

3. Having the data available from the previous admission is helpful in planning current care for the readmitted patient.

C. *Discharged records*

1. When a patient is discharged, the order of the file remains the same.

1. The record is kept intact in case the data are needed for future admissions or other reasons.

2. The master file input card is placed on the left side.

2. The record is kept intact in case the data are needed for future admissions or other reasons.

3. The patient master update discharge form is placed on the right side.

3. The record is kept intact in case the data are needed for future admissions or other reasons.

4. The record is filed in the closed record file and kept there for the rest of the current year plus 1 year.

4. Closed records needing to be accessed are most often within this time frame of discharge.

5. Closed records for previous years are stored off the premises in storage that meets legal requirements.

5. Records are still available if needed but are not using valuable office space.

6. Records are retained for a minimum of 7 years. Records of minors are retained until the age of majority and an additional 7 years.

6. Patient records are retained to meet agency policy and state and federal statutes.

D. *Review and documentation of record*

1. All entries into the clinical record must be dated, authenticated, and titled. If the names appear once in the document, initials may be used. The following staff are authorized to make entries in and/or review the clinical record:
   • Executive director
   • Director of professional services
   • Clinical supervisors
   • Home care nurses

1. Documentation must be identified to meet legal requirements.

PROCEDURE: *Action*   *Rationale*

- Therapists (physical, occupational, speech)
- Home health aides
- Surveyors from licensing, certification, and accrediting bodies
- Professional Advisory Committee
- Volunteers (hospice)
- Volunteer coordinator (hospice)
- Physicians
- Home health aide clerk
- Therapy clerk
- Students
- Homemaker/home health aide supervisors
- Home health aides (HHA activity records only)
- Volunteer director
- Billing staff
- Medical record staff
- Pastoral care (hospice)
- Medical social worker
- Director of finance
- All transcriptionists

2. All entries recorded in the record must be legible and accurate. Errors are to be corrected but not obliterated. For errors noticed immediately, a line is to be drawn through the material and initialed, and *ME* (mistaken entry) is to be written above. For errors noted at a later date, the author must write "There is an error in my note of (date)." Then the note is rewritten at that point in the record, dated with the current date, and signed.

2. All data must be legally acceptable as to accuracy and legibility.

3. Only approved symbols and abbreviations are used in the clinical record, and there must be an explanatory legend available to personnel authorized to make entries and to read the entries.

3. Only approved symbols and abbreviations are used to prevent misinterpretation.

E. *Confidentiality of records*

1. The confidentiality of the clinical record will be maintained. Patients will be instructed to maintain confidentiality of any portion of the record that is left in the home (e.g., HHA plan of care or a flow sheet).

1. It is the responsibility of the department to maintain confidentiality of the clinical record.
Ensures compliance with COP 484.10 (d).

PROCEDURE: *Action*   *Rationale*

F. *Protection of records*

1. Authorized personnel, including students, volunteers, and cleaning service employees, have access to the Medical Records Department.

   1. Students are accepted upon recommendation of the educational facility. Selected volunteers are assigned to the department. Cleaning service staff are employees of Abington Memorial Hospital. Background information about personnel is contained in the Personnel Department.

2. The Medical Record Department is secured with locked doors and is fire protected with sprinklers.

   2. To ensure compliance with Medicare regulations.

3. Building complies with township codes with reference to fire regulations.

   3. The agency complies with local ordinances.

G. *Copying the clinical record*

1. In response to a subpoena, all portions of the record may be copied.

   1. Subpoenas mandate the release of information. Copies of the record are generally acceptable.

2. In response to a request from a government insurer and third party payer, clinical documents may be copied.

   2. Government regulations and third party insurers require release of clinical information to ascertain compliance with regulations and contract specifications also necessary for reimbursement.

3. Staff may copy any portion of the record to facilitate coordination of care.

   3. The staff maintain responsibility for the confidentiality for all copies.

4. Copies of the record must be discarded at the Visiting Nurses Association office.

   4. To ensure confidentiality of patient care documents.

5. Refer to policy 3:18-1, Release of HIV-Related Information.

   5. Must ensure compliance with Pennsylvania Act 148.

H. *Use of computer mail documentation*

1. The transmission of data via the Delta mail system is acceptable for entry into the clinical record.

   1. Allows for immediate access and retrieval of off-site data.

2. Home health aide schedules or changes will be accepted via the Delta mail system.

   2. Facilitates coordination of contracted home health aide services.

PROCEDURE: *Action*

3. The computerized printout of the change will be placed on a single sheet and signed by the individual who takes the message off the computer.

I. *Completion of record*

1. The home care record of a patient/client discharged from service is completed within 6 months.

Rationale

3. Provides for immediate notification to staff of home health aide changes.

1. The Medical Record Department reviews all discharge records for completeness.

COP 484.48
Origin date: 1/76
Revised date: 12/82; 1/86; 11/88; 2/90; 1/91; 8/91; 7/92; 5/94; 7/94
Approved by: Administration/Board/PAC
Originator: Administration
Distribution: Administration/Staff

CHAPTER 13

Computerized Clinical Documentation

Donna R. Baldwin

It is forecasted that the home care industry will invest more than $1.2 billion in information management technology by the year 2000 (Stern, 1996). A significant portion of these expenditures will involve computerized clinical documentation systems, which offer the potential to reduce costs, streamline paperwork, and improve organizational performance. Successful transition from manual charting to computerization, however, is not without challenges. The technology selected must both enhance current operations and enable the organization to prepare for the future. There is no "perfect" computer system, but through critical analysis home care organizations can choose the technology that is most congruent with their operations and can adapt the organizational environment to achieve maximum return on the investment.

DOCUMENTATION PROCESS

Documentation has been cited as one of the most frustrating aspects of home care nursing (Lynch, 1994). Home care nurses are generally more satisfied than nurses in other practice settings, but they are almost unanimous in identifying documentation as a major source of dissatisfaction (Baldwin and Price, 1994). Federal regulations, accreditation standards, and reimbursement procedures dictate the clinical data that must be recorded, and as a result documentation may account for up to 50 percent of the home care nurses' time (Westra and Raup, 1995).

Home care documentation is essentially a paper-driven system, which contributes to the nurses' frustration. Manual documentation is the established norm in health care and may be acceptable in an institutional setting where the patient and the clinical record are available at the same location. Home care, in contrast, is a mobile industry, with care being provided at multiple locations. Clinical data, recorded at the site of care delivery, must be transported to the office for filing, and staff must return to the office to access the clinical record. As a result, the paper-driven system can be both cumbersome and time consuming.

Manual documentation, although accepted, is not always effective in home care. The staff may provide high-quality care, but this is not necessarily reflected in the manual charting, which is often done after the fact. Clinicians habitually postpone charting until the end of the day, resulting in the loss of valuable information through inaccurate or incomplete recall. In addition, the multitude of forms required to meet specific data collection requirements contributes to the duplication of entries and results in a lack of consistency. Each form stands independent of the others, making it difficult to monitor the patient's progress and promote coordination of care.

Computerization has been proposed as the solution to frustration with documentation. Initial attempts were limited to billing software, however, which automated data entry to produce the plan of treatment. The growth and sophistication of claims submission packages simplified the billing process but did little to address the inadequacies associated with manual documentation.

DEFINING COMPUTERIZED CLINICAL DOCUMENTATION

Over the last few years, technology has been introduced in home care to computerize the recording of clinical data. A variety of options are currently available, but not all approaches address the entire scope of clinical documentation. To resolve the problems inherent in the manual process, a computerized system must contain three elements essential for timely, efficient, and effective clinical documentation. The most important requirement is that the computerized system be based on point-of-care entry of clinical data. Clinical staff must be able to enter clinical findings while in the patient's home. This is sometimes referred to as mobile computing because it involves the use of portable computers that are carried from one patient's home to another.

There has been a dramatic increase in the use of portable computers in home care, with almost 13,000 such devices currently being used by clinical staff (Grimm, 1996). Less than 5% of all home care visits involve computerized documentation, however, because many organizations have only implemented their systems for nursing (Pierce, 1995). Because of the reluctance to expand usage to all services providing care in the home, dual systems of documentation are in operation, which hampers care coordination. Therefore, to be completely effective, the computerized documentation systems must encompass all disciplines providing care for the patient.

Computerized documentation also requires that a clinical database be available to the field staff. The entry of clinical data can be automated, but the system will not promote consistency in documentation and enhance care coordination unless the field staff have access to the entire computerized record while at the site of care delivery.

IMPACT OF HEALTH CARE TRENDS ON DOCUMENTATION

The decision to computerize may be based on internal needs and deficiencies associated with the manual process, but health care trends relative to clinical documentation must also be considered. These external factors are the driving forces that affect the organization's information management requirements and contribute to both immediate and future needs.

Regulations and Standards

The most significant regulations affecting home care are the Medicare conditions of participation. These standards are fairly broad regarding patient care, but compliance is validated primarily by review of documentation. Although most computer documentation systems simplify compliance with current regulations, it has been predicted that the Health Care Financing Administration (HCFA) will begin to focus more on patient care outcomes rather than just compliance with care processes. Therefore, when a system is envisioned, both current and proposed regulatory requirements must be analyzed.

Federal regulations are of paramount importance, but state regulations are often more challenging. Commercial computerized documentation software is generic and may not assist the organization in complying with state regulations. In fact, the software may actually hamper compliance. A primary example is the fact that most commercial systems are designed for charting by exception, so that entry of clinical observations is only required when the clinician determines that the findings are not within normal limits. Some states, however, require complete documentation of clinical findings even if no problems are noted.

Accreditation standards for home care also place considerable emphasis on documentation. If the home care organization is accredited by either the Joint Commission on Accreditation of Healthcare Organizations or the Community Health Accreditation Program, such standards must be addressed when the computerization project is initiated. For example, Joint Commission-accredited organizations must ensure that the clinical documentation system will promote timely access to information, improve data accuracy, and maintain a balance of security of and ease of access to data (Joint Commission, 1995).

Outcome Measurement

Payers have always required documentation to support the services provided, but they are now beginning to expect quantifiable clinical data for outcome analysis. A major obstacle in obtaining such data is the lack of standardized terminology to document the care provided and the patient's response to care. Without uniform data definitions, each clinician records data independently, resulting in data that cannot be aggregated and compared. One set of uniform data definitions that is common in home care is *International Classification of Diseases* coding to classify diagnoses and procedures. With the advent of outcome measurement, however, the use of such codes will need to be expanded to the clinical staff. No longer will clinicians be permitted to record descriptions that are later coded by clerical staff; instead, clinical staff will need access to a comprehensive yet user-friendly coding program within the computerized documentation system.

Other uniform data definitions are not yet a reality. Much work has been done, but the issue is still controversial. The National Association for Home Care (NAHC) recognized the lack of uniform data definitions in 1993 and initiated a project to collect standardized, comparable home care data (NAHC, 1994). Sixty-four data elements have been defined, but most clinical elements have been deferred for further study. These include patient problems and interventions, which are a complex issue because of the lack of standardized nursing nomenclature. Instead of establishing one set of uniform data definitions, nursing has adopted four different classification schemes. These include the North American Nursing Diagnosis Association's (NANDA) nursing diagnoses, the Nursing Intervention Classification system, the Omaha System, and the Home Health Care Classification System. All approaches are recognized by the American Nurses Association and can be part of a computerized clinical documentation system.

Functional status has been recognized as a critical outcome indicator, but, as with nursing nomenclature, such measures have not been standardized. The Functional Assessment Instrument, used as part of the HCFA survey process, provides a rudimentary scoring system to measure activities of daily living. This classification system is used by most home care organizations and can be easily computerized. In contrast, some organizations have adopted the Functional Independence Measure to measure functional changes throughout the care continuum. Although this measurement tool is commonly used in other rehabilitation settings, it is not routinely included in computerized documentation systems for home care.

Although the request for outcome data was initially limited to private insurers, the need for outcome measurements will significantly increase once these measurements are mandated by HCFA. This shift toward clinical outcomes is the result of the 5-year study conducted by the Center for Health Policy and Services Research to develop outcome-based measures to quantify home care services (Shaughnessy et al., 1995). The resultant data collection tool, known as the Outcome and Assessment Information Set (OASIS), is currently being tested in a national demonstration project, and it is expected that

HCFA will propose the OASIS for the purpose of outcome monitoring as part of upcoming revisions to the conditions of participation. It is significant that the OASIS contains none of the nursing classification systems nor the most commonly used functional status measures. Instead, the OASIS stresses discipline-neutral measures relative to patient problems, interventions, and functional status.

Integrated Care Delivery

Patient care delivery needs to be integrated both internally and externally, and computerization must foster coordination both within the organization and throughout the continuum of care. Internal coordination requires access to information by all services providing patient care and is most effectively facilitated if all clinical documentation within the home care organization is incorporated into the computerized system. Consideration must also be given to the transfer of data between the clinical software and the billing and payroll programs because visit data may now be interfaced from the clinical documentation system for reimbursement and compensation purposes.

Hospital-based home care organizations and those that belong to a health care system require systems that enhance external integration of data with affiliated care providers. Therefore, the computerized clinical documentation system must have the ability to interface with other automated systems to analyze, predict, and effectively manage patients' health status across the continuum of care.

Reimbursement

Most computerized clinical documentation systems interact with billing programs that were designed based on the traditional Medicare fee-for-service model. Although such claims submission programs support retrospective reimbursement, they offer limited functionality for prospective payment or capitation. The advent of managed care requires the integration of

financial and clinical information so that the most cost-effective means of maintaining health status is determined and promoted. Therefore, both current and future reimbursement issues must be examined if the computerized clinical documentation system is to be linked to billing software.

FRAMEWORK FOR COMPUTERIZING DOCUMENTATION

Implementing computerized clinical documentation can be a project of immense proportions affecting virtually every area of operations within the home care organization. Because of the magnitude of the project, the technology selected must be congruent with the organization, and internal processes must be redesigned based on the enhanced information capabilities. The principles of project management offer a sound structure for technological implementation of a computerized clinical documentation system, but home care organizations that have pioneered such projects have identified issues critical to overall success.

Vision

A computerized clinical documentation system is a valuable tool by which the home care organization can improve information transfer processes. To align technology with operations, however, the organization must have a clear vision of information management expectations. A comprehensive needs assessment, based on both internal and external requirements for information, can serve as a foundation for formulation of goals to guide the organization throughout the computer implementation project. Typical needs and the corresponding goals are listed in Table 13–1.

Technology

Computerized documentation has become a reality in home care as a result of the technological advancements that complement the mobile

Table 13–1 Expectations of a Computerized Clinical Documentation System

Needs	Goals
Efficiency	Logical, effective, and efficient work flow Timely, consistent, accurate, and accessible documentation
Productivity	Reduction in paperwork Ability to increase visits made per clinician Reduction in rework
Cost effectiveness	Cost savings Cost avoidance Cost benefits
Staff satisfaction	Increased time for patient care delivery Continued staff retention
Management of information	Integrated, value-added system Effective use of resources
Quality improvement	Compliance with standards Ability to monitor and manage clinical outcomes

nature of the industry. The most significant impact was the introduction of portable computers to input and access data. Three different types of portable computers are currently available, and selection depends on the organization's needs, goals, work processes, and financial status. Each type of device has both strengths and limitations, as summarized in Table 13–2.

Application software is the computer program that facilitates the entry and transfer of clinical data. The majority of documentation programs permit data entry via a series of pop-up menus from which the desired options may be selected to verify the existence of a clinical finding. Because of the need to individualize documentation, some programs also offer the ability to enter free-form, narrative documentation. Application software once mandated the type of portable computer that could be used, but documentation programs have since been introduced that operate on more than one type of device.

Selection of technology begins with evaluation of the computer systems currently used within the organization. Although it may be more expedient to select the vendor supplying the organization's current billing system, this decision should be postponed until all available technology is researched. A review of the literature offers reports on product capabilities and vendor performance as well as anecdotal accounts of organizations that have computerized the documentation process. The published reports of successful implementation each identify a different computerized system, however.

The selection process is often based on financial considerations, but the least expensive technology may not be the most cost-effective technology. Financial justification requires in-depth analysis of potential cost savings through staff reduction, elimination of work processes,

Table 13–2 Comparison of Portable Computers

Device	Advantages	Disadvantages
Laptop or notebook computer	Data storage capabilities Ease of text entry Full-screen viewing	Weight/size Cost
Hand-held device	Weight/size Ease of transport Cost	Limited viewing screens Limited viewing capacity
Pen-based tablets	Ease of use Weight/size Ease of training	Cost Standardized pick lists Handwriting recognition unreliable

and better utilization of resources. The possibility of cost avoidance relative to additional equipment and cost benefits from increased staff efficiency also affect calculation of the actual financial expenditures.

An effective strategy in the selection of technology is a site visit to another organization that is an experienced user. By previewing the impact of the system on daily operations and the functionality of the technology, the capabilities of the computerized documentation system can be realistically evaluated. If detailed questions are prepared before the visit, the home care organization can obtain the information necessary to make an informed decision. Responses from the clinical, administrative, and information management staff at the site visit can also be instrumental in planning for computerization. Exhibit 13–1 offers a list of questions that may be asked during a site visit.

Commitment

The hardware and software may be key components of the computerized clinical documentation system, but commitment of the people within the organization is crucial to the success of the project. Involvement of the future users on the implementation team encourages commitment, and essential team members include staff from information systems and all clinical services. Operational areas such as utilization management, quality management, medical records, admissions, reimbursement, and employee compensation may also be represented on the team. If the project implementation team is formed as soon as the decision is made to investigate the possibility of computerizing documentation within the organization, team members can be vital in solicitation of input from staff regarding current needs and expectations and the development of realistic goals. Open communication and consensus decision making within the team further strengthen commitment to the project.

Human Factors

There is a tendency to focus on the technologic requirements associated with computerized documentation, but the ultimate outcome of the project is dependent upon the human factor: the clinical staff who will be using the system to input and access patient data. Because

Exhibit 13–1 Information To Be Obtained during a Site Visit

1. Does the processing unit have enough power and speed to support the software?	13. How is the clinical documentation system linked to billing and payroll?
2. What type of printer is used, and how many pages are printed daily?	14. How was training completed for the staff?
3. What brand of portable computers is used, and how much time has been devoted to repairs and maintenance?	15. What has been the impact of implementation on the management information services department?
4. What is the percentage of "failed" communications, and what are the reasons?	16. How have day-to-day operations changed within the organization since the system was implemented?
5. What types of standardized and customized reports can be generated by the system, and how are they used?	17. Who is responsible for printing, sorting, and filing paper forms?
6. Has there been a problem with collision of data?	18. What policies and procedures had to be modified based on the implementation?
7. How has security been established, and what privileges are given to clinicians?	19. Has the number of patient visits per clinician changed since implementation?
8. How are discipline addendums handled?	20. How has the implementation affected revenues within the organization?
9. What is the maximum caseload that can be stored on the portable computer?	21. What percentage of clinicians enter data at the point of care?
10. How is care coordinated within the organization, and how are recertifications prepared?	22. How has the quality of care improved?
11. Is there an electronic signature process, and how was it established?	23. What has been the effect of the implementation on staff morale?
12. How many referrals are received daily, and how do staff receive referral information?	24. Describe the major advantages and disadvantages of using the system.
	25. How could the organization further enhance operations based on the system?

implementation of a computerized clinical documentation system is a major change for the organization, preparations must be made to assist the staff in working through the change process. Clinical staff may accept the need for the change because of frustration with manual charting but still be hesitant to adapt to revised workflow processes. Therefore, proactive approaches must be implemented before actual installation of the computer system.

A critical area that must be addressed with staff is the entry of clinical data. Transcription usually refers to the entry of written data into a computer database. When a clinician jots down notes during a home visit and returns to the office to write them on the visit note form, however, this is also a form of transcription. Transcription may be acceptable with manual charting, but computerized documentation is based on data entry at the site of care delivery. If staff are not comfortable writing a visit note in the home, they will not adapt well to point-of-care data entry into a portable computer, and the full potential of the documentation system will never be realized. To address this issue, paper forms need to be revised to include checklists and prompts, and the expectation must be established that all visit notes will be completed at the site of care delivery. By the institution of point-of-care data entry with the manual system, the staff are better prepared for the eventual computerization of the process.

Acceptance of a computerized system by the clinical staff is also facilitated by familiarity with the data elements contained within the software. Many commercial computerized documentation systems offer a standardized package of textual data elements and coded options that can be selected by clinicians to enter clinical data. Because clinical staff may be unaccustomed to the standardized forced-choice options or may view the use of such options as "canned" documentation, some vendors allow customization of the options by the organization. Development of organization-specific options to be added to the software requires considerable time and effort on the part of the project implementation team but can be crucial in overall staff acceptance of the computerized documentation system.

The provision of education and training of the staff may significantly influence the outcome of the project. Vendors offer training as part of the installation package, but such training should be limited to the project implementation team members, who can then serve as trainers for the staff. Only by understanding the basic logic of the software and the capabilities of the system can team members develop an effective educational program based on how the computerized documentation system is to be used within the organization.

Two components essential to staff education are the practical aspects regarding use of a portable computer and use of the documentation software to input and access data. Various training methods may be used, depending on the type of portable computer selected and the complexity of the software. Most organizations, however, have found it beneficial to develop clinically based training programs, offer hands-on experience with the computer outside the clinical setting, and prepare step-by-step training manuals.

Workflow

Investments in computerized documentation technology offer the potential for effective processing of information. Nevertheless, the organization will not benefit from the enhanced capabilities unless the work processes associated with manual documentation are redesigned. The most profound effect on workflow within the organization will be computer entry of clinical data. Because the basic premise of computerized documentation is the entry of data at the site of care delivery, the need for data entry by clerical staff can be reduced and possibly eliminated.

The manner in which care is managed and provided by organizational staff may also be affected. Computerized documentation empowers the field staff to manage and coordinate patient care effectively, thus reducing the need for in-office coordinators or specially trained nurses to complete admission assessments and/or recertifications. Because the logical linking of data and the availability of prompts within the computer software promote data consistency and compliance with standards, the need for comprehensive in-office clinical record review is also decreased. As a result, the clinical practice model and the need for in-office support can be assessed and possibly redesigned based on enhanced technological capabilities.

EXAMPLE OF A SUCCESSFUL COMPUTER IMPLEMENTATION

Trinity HealthCare Services, serving the Memphis area in southwest Tennessee, was one of the first home care organizations to fully automate clinical documentation for all skilled services. As a Joint Commission–accredited, not-for-profit organization affiliated with a health care system, Trinity encompasses three areas of operations: a private-pay division, a home health agency, and a hospice. The initial project to computerize documentation focused on the home health agency, which is Medicare certified but offers services to a growing number of managed care patients. Agency staff include approximately 140 nurses, therapists, and social workers, who use portable computers to input and access clinical data. These skilled professionals, combined with 100 certified nursing assistants, make more than 300,000 visits annually to more than 2,000 patients.

In 1993, Trinity initiated the commitment to computerized documentation to alleviate staff frustration with documentation and paperwork.

The clinical practice model adopted by Trinity empowered the staff providing home services to manage and coordinate all aspects of patient care. The staff preferred this model to in-office case management, which they believed fostered task-oriented care. The associated responsibilities created a paperwork burden, however, and the staff desired computerization to facilitate documentation. Additional goals for computerization were identified through analysis of both current and future information management requirements.

Trinity selected *Clinical-Link*, a software product marketed by Delta Health Systems in Altoona, Pennsylvania, because of the architecture of the software, the inclusion of all disciplines in the documentation format, the ability to enter data by means of both forced-choice options and narrative entries, and the capability of interfacing data with the billing and payroll programs. Data are entered at the site of care delivery using subnotebook computers, which are commonly referred to as laptops. The staff prefer the laptops to other portable devices because of the full screen viewing, the ability to enter text data, and the large data storage capability. Complete computerized records for more than 60 patients can be maintained on each laptop because of the size of the hard drive. Data entry is simplified by the arrangement of forms within activities, as depicted in Figure 13–1. Portability of the laptop was not an issue because each device weighs approximately 3 lb, measures 5 by 7 in, and can operate on a fully charged battery for up to 8 hours.

Data are transferred between the laptops and the host computer via modem communications over telephone lines. Each laptop is equipped with an internal modem card, and the host computer receives data via 16 external modems. Data are automatically transmitted each night from the laptop to the host computer, also known as the server, at a preset time. Once the server processes all updated data, retransmission with each laptop is completed on a predetermined schedule. Only data for patients assigned to the laptop user are transmitted, however. Communications between the laptop and server can also be established on demand if the user needs to obtain additional assignments or patient data.

An additional module, consisting of a standardized nursing care plan based on NANDA diagnoses, was offered by the vendor, but the staff preferred the basic *Clinical-Link* structure. Clinicians complete discipline-specific assessments and care plans, but forms for documenting demographic information, diagnoses, medical history, and medications are shared. Pertinent data are then transferred to HCFA

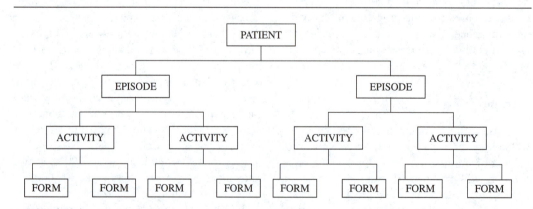

Figure 13-1 Organization of data within *Clinical-Link*.

Form 485, which serves as a comprehensive plan of care.

At the recommendation of the vendor, Trinity purchased an external library of drug information for inclusion in the documentation software. More than 9,000 medications are contained in the library, which supplies information such as the generic and brand names of the drug, appropriate uses, precautions or warnings, and potential side effects. Nurses can provide drug education while viewing the information on screen and by printing a hard copy of the information for the patient. The use of the drug library has promoted the identification of potential drug interactions and has standardized patient education relative to drug information.

Project Development

Trinity originally planned to limit computer implementation to 17 laptops. As recommended by the literature, additional laptops were to be slowly phased in over the next 3 to 5 years. When flow diagramming the work processes, however, the project implementation team discovered that partial implementation and the resultant parallel documentation systems would actually increase, rather than decrease, costs. Through extensive research, the implementation team prepared a proposal to justify the purchase of 123 additional laptop computers so that point-of-care computerized documentation could be implemented for all skilled services. This included all full-time and part-time nurses, physical therapists, speech therapists, occupational therapists, and social workers. Costs were justified through savings from the elimination of paid office time for the clinical staff, the reduction of data entry and support staff positions, and decreased printing costs, and the proposal was approved immediately before the installation in November 1994.

Education for in-office staff was conducted by a vendor representative, but the project implementation team, in conjunction with staff development personnel, designed the training program for the clinical staff. The training program consisted of 20 hours of instruction regarding use of the laptops, organization of data, entry and retrieval of data, and laptop communications, and the clinical staff attended training sessions in groups of eight each week until all laptops were assigned. Training manuals detailing the input of data based on agency operations were also developed and issued to users during the computer classes. Each staff member was expected to transition from paper forms within 6 weeks of completion of the training session. Full implementation of the computerized documentation system was achieved within 5 months of the installation. Exhibit 13–2 offers an overview of the training program.

Some organizations have reported difficulties with implementation of laptops as a result of staff unfamiliarity with computers and lack of typing skills. At Trinity, however, this was not a factor. The staff who had limited computer experience were attentive during the training sessions and found the software to be user-friendly. In contrast, the few staff members who were skilled in computers had greater difficulty because they were hesitant to accept the logic of the software program. To decrease the amount of typing necessary to enter data, the project team developed and added more than 3,000 textual and coded options to the system. Staff were encouraged to use the standardized options but were not restricted from entering additional text.

Security of Information

Because staff would have access to the database of Trinity's patients and their computerized records, security measures had to be implemented to protect the data and prevent unauthorized access. *Clinical-Link* has internal levels of security based on the privileges assigned to each user, and individual passwords are required to access the system. External levels of security, however, were developed by Trinity to protect the investment in the laptop computers.

Exhibit 13–2 Computer Implementation: Laptop
Training Program

Day 1 (8 hours)

Computer basics:
    Computer log-on
    Keyboard and function keys
    Organization of data

E-mail

Discipline assessment:
    Obtaining the assignment
    Selecting the patient
    Assessment activity
    Preparing the orders
    Ready for certification
    Assessment verbal order

Day 2 (8 hours)

Interim orders

Daily visit

Home health aide supervisory visit

Recertification:
    Determining patients requiring recertification
    Recertification activity
    Ready for recertification

Day 3 (4 hours)

Transfer process

Resume care

Discharge:
    Discipline discharge
    Discipline readmit
    Agency discharge

Laptop communications

When laptops were assigned, the users were required to sign an agreement specifying the care and use of the device. Exhibit 13–3 offers an example of Trinity's laptop agreement.

Clinical Record

Although clinical documentation has been computerized, an electronic clinical record is not yet a reality. Hard copies of the forms must be printed and filed in a paper record as each form is created and revised. The *Clinical-Link* system was designed so that the printed form could be reviewed and signed by the staff member who entered the data to validate the entry in the clinical record. Both HCFA and the Joint Commission, however, permit the use of a unique identifier or computer key to authenticate computerized entries for the clinical record if precautions are employed to ensure confidentiality and proper use of the identifier or key. Based on these standards, Trinity developed an agreement for all users to sign, stipulating that they would only use their assigned unique identifier to authenticate entries. The agreement is shown in Exhibit 13-4. As a result of the signed agreements, staff are not required to return to the office daily to sign the computer-generated forms, and this has greatly improved staff efficiency and acceptance of the computerized documentation system. During the implementation, however, written data had to be entered for staff who were not yet assigned laptops. When this occurred, the data entry staff used a special transcription identifier so that the form would be reviewed and signed by the primary author before being filed in the medical record.

The printing of the computer-generated forms was also an issue because of volume. After the nightly communications, by which data are transmitted to the host computer, up to 6,000 forms are printed that require a dedicated duplexing laser printer. Three additional laser printers are available for printing of reports and clinical forms on demand. Originally, forms were printed in batches based on the name of the primary author, and this required additional

Exhibit 13-3 Laptop Agreement

Trinity HealthCare Services
Home Health Agency
Clinical-Link Notebook Computer Agreement

As an employee of Trinity HealthCare Services Home Health Agency, I accept the assignment of *Clinical-Link* Notebook Computer (#_____). I understand that the Notebook is a component of the computer issued by the agency for documentation of clinical information. As a designated *Clinical-Link* Notebook computer user, I make the following agreements:

1. I agree to use the Notebook only for the purpose of documenting clinical information.
2. I agree to follow the instructions that I received regarding the care and use of the Notebook, including:
    a. transporting the Notebook only in the carrying case;
    b. preventing extensive exposure of the Notebook to temperature extremes;
    c. preventing exposure of the Notebook to water or other liquids;
    d. using a proper electrical outlet when connecting the Notebook to AC power; and
    e. never dissembling the Notebook.
3. I understand that, if the Notebook is damaged or lost due to willful neglect or willful abuse, I am financially responsible for repairs and/or replacement up to the full cost of the Notebook.
4. I agree that I will not load nor attempt to load any software programs to the Notebook.
5. I agree that I will perform Nightly Communications each day, unless an exception has been approved by the MIS Department, and I will perform Demand Communications as requested.
6. I agree to bring the Notebook issued to me, as well as additional equipment (e.g., modem, cables) to the MIS Department for maintenance inspection monthly and as requested.
7. In the event that my employment with Trinity HealthCare Services is terminated, I understand that I must return the Notebook to the MIS Department prior to or on my last day of employment.

Employee: _____ **Date:**_____

MIS Manager/Designee: _____ **Date:**_____

Courtesy of Trinity HealthCare Services, Memphis, Tennessee

---

sorting before filing in the clinical record. Updates to the software have since addressed this problem, so that all forms can now print alphabetically by patient name.

Evaluation

Monitoring of the project was ongoing, but evaluation of the effectiveness of the computerized documentation system was delayed until 4 months after full implementation. In August 1995, the outcome of the project was analyzed based on the preestablished goals of greater efficiency, increased productivity, cost effectiveness, staff satisfaction, improved management of information, quality improvement, and patient satisfaction.

Efficiency

Efficiency was initially measured in relation to the goal of timely, consistent, accurate, and accessible documentation. Computer entry of data at the point of care ensured that the documentation was timely and eliminated the need

Exhibit 13-4 Agreement for the Use of Unique Identifier

Trinity HealthCare Services
Home Health Agency

Agreement for Use of Unique Identifier for the Authentication
of Entries in the Computer Clinical Record

I acknowledge that, as an employee of Trinity HealthCare Services Home Health Agency, I have been authorized to make entries in the *Clinical-Link* computer system. I further acknowledge that I have been issued a unique identifier to be used when making clinical entries in *Clinical-Link*. I agree that I will keep the unique identifier confidential, and I will only use the unique identifier issued to me to authenticate entries in *Clinical-Link* for which I am the primary author.

To maintain security of the computer system for transcribed entries in *Clinical-Link*, I understand that any entries transcribed for me must be personally reviewed and authenticated by means of my handwritten signature and the date of review.

Employee: _____ **Date:** _____

Supervisor/Designee: _____ **Date:** _____

Courtesy of Trinity HealthCare Services, Memphis, Tennessee

---

for assessment and recertification information to be transcribed in the agency's database by clerical staff. There were problems with modem communications between the laptops and the host computer, but delays were no greater than with submission of written paperwork; furthermore, once the data were transmitted, they were immediately available for review. The consistency of documentation also improved as a result of on-screen prompts, the use of the coded and textual options within the software, and the ability to access prior assessments and clinical findings. Data were more accurate because software prompts required updating of the plan of care and generation of a physician's order before documentation of an intervention. This resulted in up-to-date plans of care, which significantly reduced the time required for the recertification activity. More important, the documentation was accessible so that current patient information was readily available and

staff could view assessments and visit notes entered by other disciplines.

Analysis of workflow patterns was also used to measure efficiency. During the implementation process, workflow was redesigned to eliminate redundancy and streamline operations. Duplication of paperwork was eliminated, work flowed more logically and effectively, and the computer became a valuable tool for review of records and retrieval of management information. For example, the tracking of outstanding assessments and recertifications required a full-time position with the complicated manual process but is now a completely automated process with the computerized system.

Because *Clinical-Link* contains a relational database, all activities must be completed timely to achieve efficient workflow. The software logic precipitated problems, however, if one discipline did not complete the recertification activity within the required time frame.

Some of the staff therefore were not pleased when the computer held them accountable for completing assigned tasks on a timely basis. Management was required to address such situations through the monitoring of computer-generated reports to ensure that efficient workflow was not impeded.

Overall, efficiency of the skilled disciplines improved with *Clinical-Link* because clinical data were integrated and accessible. Because of Trinity's decision for the nursing assistant services to continue manual charting, however, parallel documentation systems had to be maintained, which affected organizational efficiency. The skilled services prepare the nursing assistant plan of care using *Clinical-Link*, but the data have to be transmitted to the host computer and printed in the office and the form transported to the patient's home. Because nursing assistants do not have access to the computer, there are also delays in notifying them regarding newly admitted and discharged patients. It has been realized that greater efficiency could be gained by expanding computerized documentation to include the nursing assistant services, but it has been difficult to justify costs.

Productivity

During August 1995, a visit analysis was completed to determine the impact of computerization on staff productivity. At Trinity, the field staff are paid per visit, and before computer implementation each staff member was compensated for the 5 hours of office time required each week to complete paperwork. After the implementation, reimbursement for office time was eliminated because documentation could be completed in the patient's home. The results of the visit analysis revealed that computerization permitted each staff member to make up to two additional visits per day. The most significant finding, however, was the number of visits completed by the nurses performing the start of care assessments. Before computerization, these nurses typically completed no more than two assessments each day because of the amount of paperwork required. By August

1995, however, up to three assessments could be completed daily.

Productivity was also measured in terms of the time required for documentation because of the concern that the visit times would be significantly lengthened. Overall, the average visit time has increased less than 2 minutes. This may have been due to the fact that most of the staff were already accustomed to point-of-care data entry using the manual process. The length of a start of care assessment remained at approximately 90 minutes, but the majority of the documentation is now completed in the home, which allows patient participation in developing the plan of care. In contrast, the manual process required that most of the documentation be done in the office.

Documentation time in relation to the recertification process was significantly decreased. Before computerization, this activity required in-office time to review the clinical record and update the plan of care. Because *Clinical-Link* facilitates continual updating of the plan of care, the recertification activity now requires less than 15 minutes.

The reduction in rework has also enhanced productivity. Before computerization, extensive review was required to ensure that services were performed as prescribed and that the medication profiles were accurate. The prompts contained in the *Clinical-Link* system have decreased the problem with documenting orders because a physician's order can be automatically generated each time the plan of care is updated. Medication profiles are a required form for all nursing activities, and as a result accuracy has improved.

Cost Effectiveness

In the proposal for the additional laptops, the project implementation team projected a savings of $7.81 for each nursing visit within 6 months of full implementation. Comparison of financial data for October 1994 and August 1995 revealed that nursing costs had actually decreased by $12.69 per visit. During this 10-month time span, there were unanticipated expenditures, such as the purchase of additional printers and modems and the expansion of the information management department as well as the costs associated with training. The aggregate visit costs, however, were reduced by almost $5.00 per visit. Financial review since August 1995 has noted that aggregate visit costs have remained relatively unchanged.

Staff Satisfaction

In October 1994, the nursing staff at Trinity participated in a study to measure their levels of work satisfaction using the Work Characteristics Instrument as the data collection tool. Responses from the majority of the nurses revealed that, although they perceived their work as moderately to highly exciting, they viewed paperwork and documentation as the most frustrating aspects of their jobs. The survey was repeated in August 1995 to determine the impact of computerization on staff satisfaction. Results revealed that the overall levels of work satisfaction remained relatively unchanged, but the frustration with paperwork was replaced by technological concerns, such as unsuccessful modem communications. The study findings are presented in Table 13–3.

Work satisfaction was also measured in terms of retention. Other organizations that had implemented laptop computers had forewarned Trinity to expect up to a 10 percent turnover in clinical staff. As of August 1995, however, only one part-time therapist had resigned from Trin-

ity because of unwillingness to accept computerized documentation. This resignation was due, in part, to the procedure for completion of the recertification activity, and the procedure has since been revised.

The redesign of work processes could have affected in-office work satisfaction as a result of changes in job functions and workflow. The implementation team prepared for the reduction of positions through attrition, and as job functions changed there was a reallocation of assignments within the organization. This proactive approach was instrumental in maintaining staff satisfaction throughout the organization.

Management of Information

One of the goals at Trinity is effective use of resources regarding the management of information. This was partially accomplished with the improved access to current patient information, but effective use of resources to extract historical data was not achieved. *Clinical-Link*, like many similar products on the market, does not maintain a complete electronic record. To review and track previous data other than visit notes, interim orders, and communication documents, the paper records must still be retrieved.

To manage information effectively, Trinity sought an integrated system for the retrieval of information. Clinical data interface to the billing system to produce HCFA Form 485 and generate bills; visit data are interfaced to both the billing and payroll systems. Each system maintains a separate database, however, which must be accessed to extract information. Data can be transferred from one system to the other, but the actual interfacing of data between systems has been a challenge. Each system is written in a different programming language, and the data interface is not a completely automated system.

Quality Improvement

To ensure quality, there must be compliance with standards. Computerization has promoted

Table 13–3 Work Excitement Survey: Trinity HealthCare Service (Data Are Percentages)

Level of Work Excitement	October 1994	August 1995
Extremely excited	12	12
Very excited	21	19
Moderately excited	18	17
Somewhat excited	17	19
Not too excited	4	3
TOTAL	72	70

compliance with prompts to remind staff when a recertification activity is due, the ease of generating interim orders, and the ongoing revision of the plan of care. Computerized documentation has also facilitated on-screen review of records, so that the clinical record review process is more effective but less time consuming. Each supervisor completes a random review of visit notes weekly and offers immediate feedback to the staff member, which has resulted in a continual improvement of the quality of documentation.

An important aspect of our quality improvement process is outcome management. At this time, however, only coded data elements can be automatically extracted. As part of the *Clinical-Link* user group, Trinity has contributed input into the development of an additional module for the monitoring of clinical outcomes. Although the module is not yet available, Trinity has initiated outcome monitoring with the addition of the OASIS data elements to the forced-choice options within the system. Data extraction is not automated, however, and must be completed by means of on-screen review.

Patient Satisfaction

A major concern during computerization was the impact on patient care. Other organizations had reported that laptop computers interfered with the delivery of patient care, but feedback from the Trinity staff suggested the opposite. The staff reported that the use of the laptop promoted patient participation in the care planning process, which in turn increased interaction between the patient and staff. The results of the increased interaction have been evidenced by the responses to patient satisfaction surveys. Since implementation, patient satisfaction ratings have not decreased below 95.0 percent, and as of January 1996 they reached an all-time high of 96.1 percent.

CONCLUSION

Implementation of a computerized documentation system can enable the home care organization to manage clinical data in an accurate and efficient manner that enhances patient care. Organizational expectations must be aligned with technological capabilities, however, to realize the benefits of computerization. Organizations that have pioneered computerization of documentation demonstrate that success of the project also requires a detailed and well-executed plan, active involvement of staff, and the commitment of the entire organization.

REFERENCES

Baldwin, D., and S. Price. 1994. Work excitement: The energizer of home healthcare nursing. *Journal of Nursing Administration* 24:37–42.

Grimm, C. 1996. Today's hottest technology: Mobile computing. *Remington Report* 4:6–8.

Joint Commission on Accreditation of Healthcare Organizations. 1995. *Accreditation manual for home care.* Chicago: Joint Commission.

Lynch, S. 1994. Job satisfaction of home health nurses. *Home Healthcare Nurse* 12:21–28.

National Association for Home Care. 1994. Draft uniform data set for home care and hospice. *Caring* 14:10–75.

Pierce, C. 1995. The dawn of computer age for home care. *Health Data Management* 2:61–64.

Stern, E. 1996. Key management information strategies. *Remington Report* 4:10–13.

Shaughnessey, P., et al. 1995. Outcome-based quality improvement in home care. *Caring* 15:44–49.

Westra, B., and G. Raup. 1995. Computerized charting: An essential tool for survival. *Caring* 15:52–57.

CHAPTER 14

Implementing a Competency System in Home Care

Carol Clarke, Charlotte Banacki, and Margaret Golden

Competency assessment is absolutely essential for any organization. Employees must be qualified for each assignment. Before a home care agency can assign staff to care for a patient, it must be crystal clear that the staff person assigned has the competency and skill level to care for that particular patient. A competency system is an ongoing process that begins with the application process and continues through the employee's entire tenure with the agency. Quality improvement programs conducted on a regular schedule help monitor compliance with regard to competency.

Changes in health care, advances in medical technology, and changes in health care delivery systems make it imperative that agencies ensure up-to-date staff competencies. Managed care has had a major impact on home health. Patients are being discharged from the hospital after just a few days. Patients who were formerly kept in intensive care units are now receiving home care. These complex care issues add to the need to ensure ongoing competency. Leaders are faced with the overwhelming task of orienting ever-increasing numbers of new employees. In addition, they must also deal with "catching up" the documentation of competency for current employees. Whether a patient needs high-technology interventions or simply assistance with activities of daily living, he or she needs a competent employee caring for him or her.

Applicants to home care have increased. Staff are concerned about their positions in the hospital and are coming to home care. What they do not realize is that home health is not the same as working in the hospital because it requires different skills. Being a good hospital nurse does not guarantee that a person will be a good home care nurse. When you go to the home to deliver care, you are it. There isn't a coworker to turn to and ask "What do you think?"

Therefore, a critical assessment of competencies is a beginning point to determine which candidates are likely to succeed in home care. Excellent assessment skills and technical competence are absolutely essential. Good common sense and an understanding of norms help make the transition from the hospital to home care easier. Each agency establishes the competencies that are necessary to care for its patients. In addition, the agency must establish systems to validate these competencies. This chapter gives a detailed description of a competency system that works quite well for all levels of staff.

ORGANIZATIONAL ASSESSMENT

The best place to start is reviewing your scope of services. Are you an agency devoted to the care of certain groups of patients (e.g., hospice, acquired immunodeficiency syndrome, psychiatry, maternal–child, or high-technology

Exhibit 14–1 Performance Criteria in Job Descriptions

General terminology for certified home health aides (CHHAs)

Assists the patient with activities of daily living

Criteria-based measurable terminology for CHHAs

Competently assists patient in moving from bed to chair or wheelchair

Correctly prepares patient's meals according to plan of care

Dusts and vacuums the rooms the client uses

General terminology for staff RNs

Uses the nursing process

Criteria-based measurable terminology for staff RNs

Competently assesses and documents the patient's biophysical, psychosocial, safety, and educational needs

Designs a comprehensive nursing care plan that is consistent with the medical regimen to meet the patient's needs

Updates the nursing care plan as the patient's needs change, when the patient achieves goals, and/or a minimum of once a month

populations)? Do you primarily care for children, adults, or the elderly? Does your scope of care and services cover a broad range of patient groups? Be sure to include your most prevalent patient types in all your planning efforts.

Consider how many resources your agency is willing and able to devote to this project. At a minimum, it will take 6 months to put the basics in place. One year is more realistic because a competency system requires effective quality improvement and occurrence reporting processes. A team of supervisors and/or directors will need to devote time to initiate the project. After that, ongoing team effort will be required for planning, assessment, intervention, and follow-up.

Consider what the agency is willing to pay for. Will employees be expected to attend classes on their own time? Who will teach the orientation and continuing education classes? Will all or part of the learning be done through the use of self-study materials? Who will prepare these? Will you need to use a consultant to get you started? Will you need to subcontract out part of the project? Develop a preliminary budget, and meet with the executive director and/or owner of your agency before proceeding.

JOB DESCRIPTIONS

Job descriptions form the basis of any competency system. Have a group of leaders and staff pull out the current job descriptions and look at them critically. Are you using job descriptions tailored for your organization's needs, or are you using generic or hospital-based job descriptions? Is the content comprehensive enough to encompass your agency's scope of care and services? Do the competencies reflect current practice? Have you added new skills or services without updating job descriptions? If you do not have job descriptions tailored to your agency's needs, revisions will be required.

Are performance criteria written in general terms, or are they appropriately written in measurable terms, as outlined in Exhibit 14–1? Include a review of the qualifications, physical requirements, and working conditions listed in your job descriptions. Examples of qualifications, physical requirements, and working conditions for a registered nurse (RN) job description are outlined in Exhibit 14–2.

Exhibit 14–2 Qualifications, Physical Requirements, and Working Conditions for an RN Job Description

---

Qualifications

- Current state license as a registered professional nurse
- At least 1 year of experience as an RN within the past 3 years or documentation of a refresher course within the past year
- Able to meet health standards of employment
- Must maintain current cardio-pulmonary resuscitation certification
- Must successfully complete orientation examinations and competencies

Physical requirements

- Maintains physical capabilities to perform all work-related duties
- Ability to tolerate varied levels of stress

Working conditions

- Frequently handles sharp instruments and contaminated needles
- Cares for physically combative patients
- Potential exposure to hazardous substances (e.g., infections, chemotherapy agents)
- Potential exposure to infectious diseases
- Works in homes and neighborhoods of a variety of socioeconomic groups
- Frequent lifting of patients
- Emotional stress factor inherent in position

Consider having the group of leaders and staff who reviewed your job descriptions form a standing committee. Their responsibilities might include ongoing identification of new competencies and review of all care staff job descriptions at preset intervals. The National HomeCaring Council (1995a) standards for job description updates are as follows:[*]

> IVB-9: Job descriptions of personnel providing services in the home shall be reviewed at least every 3 years by a professional advisory committee composed of at least three professionals knowledgeable about the job requirements.

> IVB-3.1: The review date shall appear on the personnel policies and job descriptions.

SUPERVISOR COMPETENCIES

While you are reviewing job descriptions, be sure to review the competencies in the supervisors' job descriptions. The accreditation requirements of the Joint Commission on Accreditation of Healthcare Organizations (1996) for home care supervisor competence are as follows:[**]

> HR.3.2: The number and qualifications of individuals supervising care and service staff are appropriate to the scope of care and services provided by the organization.

You might be surprised to find out that, although your supervisors have excellent experience and are fully competent, their personnel files do not reflect these accomplishments.

---

[*]Courtesy of Foundation for Hospice and Homecare, Washington, DC.

[**]*Source:* © 1997–98 CAMHC, Oakbrook Terrace, IL: Joint Commission onAccreditation of Healthcare Organizations, 1997. Reprinted with permission.

Once identified, this problem is easily corrected. Have the supervisors submit copies of continuing education units from educational programs that they have attended. Successfully completed self-study modules are also acceptable. If they do not have these, simply choose programs and modules that are most appropriate to the scope of care and services that their roles encompass. If you cover high-technology cases, perhaps a local hospital will offer a preceptor experience in a critical care unit or the respiratory department.

Look carefully at the types of performance criteria outlined in the supervisors' job descriptions. The supervisors' leadership competencies are often not well defined. Exhibit 14–3 lists performance criteria that you might want to consider including in your agency's job descriptions.

APPLICATION PHASE

The prospective employee is required to complete an application and submit credentials to begin the competency evaluation process. Basic requirements include Social Security number, driver license number, I9, W2, and two references. Submission of the results of a current history and physical, purified protein derivative (PPD), chest radiograph (if PPD is positive), and rubella, rubeola, and hepatitis immunity is usually required to meet most agencies' health requirements. Proof of graduation from high school or a graduate equivalency degree is usually required for a certified home health aide (CHHA). Some agencies also require a criminal background check. Professional credentials complete the basic requirements for hire. These include an original copy of the RN or licensed practical nurse (LPN) certificate or CHHA certificate, basic cardiac life support certification, proof of graduation from an accredited nursing school (for nurses), and proof of 1 to 2 years of recent medical–surgical nursing experience (for nurses). Prospective employees are asked to present any other certifications that they have attained, including first aid, Heartsaver, American Nurses Association certifications, IV or PICC certifications, chemotherapy certification skills, and the like. Copies of continuing education units from continuing education courses and/or self-study modules are often required.

Keeping track of submitted requirements and credentials is a difficult task. Many agencies have paperwork tracked on various separate forms and computer databases. Exhibit 14–4 is a competency assessment form for RNs and LPNs that helps simplify this process. There is space for each criterion for identification of the date and person who verified the requirement or credential.

The second phase of the initial competency assessment involves written examinations. The

---

Exhibit 14–3 Performance Criteria for Supervisor Job Descriptions

- Facilitates professional growth and development of staff by coaching and providing orientation and continuing education classes.
- Demonstrates awareness of legal issues by tracking occurrences and taking appropriate steps to reduce risk.
- Effectively supervises and maintains safety standards in accordance with agency policies, to include fire, staff safety, patient safety, and emergency preparedness.

- Submits routine reports, evaluations, patient supervisory visit notes, and staff competency reviews within established time frames.
- Participates in the quality improvement process by identifying opportunities for improvement, completing studies, evaluating results, and taking actions to improve care and services.

Exhibit 14–4 Competency Assessment Form for RNs and LPNs

Employee: ID #: ☐ Initial Hire ☐ Re-hire		
Requirements/Credentials	Date verified	Initials
Application completed		
Social Security #:		
Drivers license #: Classification:		
I 9 ☐ Required ☐ Not required		
W 9 completed		
Reference #1 ☐ Sent/Date: Received: ☐ Written☐ Verbal		
Reference #2 ☐ Sent/Date: Received: ☐ Written☐ Verbal		
Malpractice insurance		
Interview completed ☐ Approved for hire pending completion of process		
Health records complete for: ☐ Physical		
☐ PPD		
☐ Chest X-Ray if PPD positive		
☐ Rubella		
☐ Rubeola or birth year:		
☐ Hepatitis immunization given ☐ Refused		
Criminal background check ☐ Sent/Date: ☐ Received/cleared		
Orientation ☐ Scheduled/Date: ☐ Attended/Date:		
Original New Jersey license ☐ RN☐ LPN #: Expir. Date:		
Photo ID completed		
Assignment preference form completed		
☐ One year general Medical Surgical Nursing experience, within past 3 years		
☐ Documented refresher course in the past year		
Certifications: ☐ CPR: Expir. Date:		
☐ IV Expir. Date:		
☐ First Aid Expir. Date:		
☐ ANA: Expir. Date:		
☐ Other: Expir. Date:		
☐ Other: Expir. Date:		
Continuing Education in the past 12 months		
Course: Date: CEU/Certificate		
☐		
☐		
☐		
☐		
☐		
☐		
Languages ☐ English ☐ Spanish ☐ Other:		

Courtesy of Clarke Health Care Consultants, Seminole, Florida.

purpose of the examinations is to test the applicant's basic cognitive knowledge. The primary examination should be a home care test that covers most of your agency's scope of care and services. For nurses, topics may include assessment, prioritization, care planning, safety, medications, clinical decision making, disease management, nutrition, and use of community resources. For CHHAs, observations, basic care modalities, safety, terminology, nutrition, reporting, and patient care are usually included on the test. Nurses whose assignments might involve specialty care are also asked to take examinations in high technology pediatrics, intravenous, maternal–child, chemotherapy, and the like to assess their competence. Each agency determines its own passing score; this is usually set at 80 to 85 percent.

All prospective employees are also asked to complete a self-assessment of their knowledge and skills in caring for adult and pediatric patients. They are asked to rate their ability as "independent," "needs review," or "never." This gives the nursing supervisor a baseline assessment of how the candidate rates his or her own competence. Two things are to be remembered when evaluating the self-assessment. First, the self-assessment represents a comprehensive list that covers most of your agency's scope of care and services. The particular candidate's assignments may never involve the full scope, so review this material in relation to the candidate's experience and possible future assignments. Second, individuals rate their competence based on their own perspective. Some candidates are overconfident and want to impress you. Others are more modest, and their ratings are consistently low. In the end, the only true measures of competence are the ratings done by your own validators. Exhibit 14–5 presents sample self-assessments for CHHAs and RNs/LPNs.

INTERVIEW PHASE

Once the applicant has completed the application process, he or she is scheduled for an interview. The interview phase further evaluates the candidate's degree of cognitive knowledge and clinical experience. After a brief period of socialization and review of the application, the interviewer presents the applicant with a case scenario. He or she then asks the applicant to identify key nursing care issues that require immediate interventions, to prioritize care, and to problem solve a variety of nursing issues. Examples of an RN scenario and a CHHA scenario are given below; naturally, you would design scenarios that represent cases prevalent in your scope of care and services.

> Mr. Jones is a 27-year-old patient with a diagnosis of human immunodeficiency virus, cytomegalovirus retinitis, dehydration, and dementia. You are assigned to administer Ganciclovir (DHPG) (300 mg in 100 mL 5 percent dextrose in water over 1 hour) via a Hickman-Broviac catheter. When you arrive at the house, Mr. Jones is upset. He cannot remember if he took his oral medications last evening or this morning. The house is in total disarray; there are dishes in the sink, clutter on the floor, and cups half-filled with juice all over the bedroom. Mr. Jones is unshaven and complaining of tingling of the extremities. Your assessment reveals blood pressure 100/60, heart rate 124 beat/min, respirations 24 per minute, temperature 101.4°F, and breath sounds clear. Mr. Jones has a reddened sacral area and dry skin. He does not remember if he ate breakfast. His roommate, Tom, is at work.

The interviewer asks the RN applicant to do the following:

- List four nursing diagnoses that pertain to this scenario.
- Identify four nursing issues that require immediate intervention.

Exhibit 14–5 Sample Self-Assessment Forms for CHHAs, RNs, and LPNs

CHHA Self-Assessment of Competency

Employee:_____ ID#_____ Date:_____

Knowledge/Skills	Adult			Children		
	Able to do	Need Review	Never did	Able to do	Need Review	Never did
Vital Signs:						
Temperature						
Pulse						
Respiration						
Blood Pressure						
Basic Care:						
Complete Bed Bath						
Bath Sponge, Tub or Shower						
Foot Care						
Mouth Care						
Hair Care						
Nail Care						
General Skin Care						
Decubiti Care (Bed Sore)						
Shampoo Sink, Tub or Bed						
Patient Positioning						
Toileting and Elimination						
Care of an Incontinent Patient						
Range of Motion						
Make Bed						
Patient Safety:						
Wheelchair						
Cane						
Walker						
Assist Patient Walking						
Transfer (bed to chair/wheelchair)						
Body Mechanics						
Patient Home Safety						
Special Care:						
Foley Catheter						
Condom Catheter						
Fractional Urines (S&A)						
Assist with Colostomy Care						
Knowledge of low salt diet						
Knowledge of low cholesterol (low fat) diet						
Knowledge of Diabetic Diet						

(continues)

Exhibit 14–5 (continued)

Knowledge/Skills	Adult			Children		
	Able to do	Need Review	Never did	Able to do	Need Review	Never did
Hoyer Lift						
Reinforce dressing						
Change simple nonsterile dressing						
Care of paralyzed patient						
Care of handicapped patient						
Care of retarded patient						
Care of psychiatric patient						
Care of autistic patient						
Care of elderly patient						
Care of confused patient						
Infection Control:						
Gloves						
Disposal of hazardous materials						
Universal Precautions						
Mask						
Gown						
Charting:						
Read and follow Aide Plan of Care						
CHHA Worksheet						
Activities of Daily Living:						
Dust and vacuum						
Wash dishes						
Clean kitchen, bedroom, bathroom						
Shop for patient						
Wash and iron clothes						
Prepare meals						
Communication with:						
Client						
Family/caregiver						
Health Care Team						
Supervisor						

continues

Exhibit 14–5 (continued)

RN and LPN Self-Assessment of Competency

Knowledge/Skills	Adult			Pediatric		
	Indep.	Need Review	Never	Indep.	Need Review	Never
Patient Status Assessment:						
Demographics, history						
Safety, Communication						
Neurological / sensory						
Cardiovascular						
Respiratory						
Communicable disease						
Musculoskeletal						
Gastrointestinal/nutritional						
Genitourinary						
Integumentary						
Pain, rehab, equipment						
Community resources						
Initiate Nursing Care Plan						
RN- Update Nursing Care Plan as patient achieves goals						
LPN- Assist RN in evaluating achievement of client goals						
Basic Nurses Note						
Document and report change in patient condition						
Patient & Family Teaching						
Discharge Planning						
Giving/Receiving Report						
Community Resource Referral						
IV Pumps:						
CADD PCA						
CADD TPN						
CADD PLUS						
QUEST 521/PLUS						
SIGMA 6000						
I-FLOW						
Gravity Control Device (Dial a flow)						
Venipuncture (Start IV):						
Peripheral						
Scalp Vein Needle (Butterfly)						

Courtesy of Clarke Health Care Consultants, Seminole, Florida.

- Prioritize Mr. Jones's care. What has to be done during this visit?
- Determine what information you must communicate to the physician, the agency, and Tom.
- What will you document in your note, and what other forms will you complete?

> Mrs. Smith is an 85-year-old patient. She weighs 92 lbs. At age 75, she broke her hip. Her diagnosis is heart failure. She wears glasses but often forgets to put them on. She is able to walk around by herself. When you arrive at the house one morning, the patient tells you that she fell on the way to the bathroom last night. You notice a new scatter rug in this bathroom. You also see that the patient is wearing new fancy slippers instead of her sneakers.

The interviewer asks the CHHA applicant to do the following:

- Identify what other observations should be made. This should include what you want to look at and what else you want to ask the patient.
- What safety measures should you institute right away?
- Is there anyone you should talk to about this?
- What will you document in your note?
- Are there any other forms or reports you should complete?

The interviewer rates the applicant's responses based on his or her clinical knowledge, ability to interpret and analyze data, ability to prioritize, and the interventions that he or she anticipates making. Separating the novice from the expert becomes quite easy. This technique also gives the interviewer an indication of how the applicant will think on his or her feet and, more important, whether he or she has common sense. If the prospective employee successfully completes the application phase, he or she is scheduled for the orientation program.

ORIENTATION

The orientation program must be interactive and include an evaluation of cognitive as well as clinical skills. The Joint Commission (1997–1998) has specific content requirements for orientation:[*]

> HR.4: All staff members are oriented to the organization and their responsibilities.

> HR.4.1: Personal care and support staff complete appropriate training before providing patient care.

The Joint Commission recommends including the following content in your orientation to meet the intent of these standards:

- the organization's mission, vision, and goals
- types of care or services provided
- the organization's policies and procedures, including those for advanced directives and death and dying
- confidentiality of patient information
- home safety, including bathroom, fire, environmental, and electrical safety
- safety issues in the home care organization, including fire prevention and security
- emergency preparedness
- appropriate action in unsafe situations
- infection prevention and control, including personal hygiene, aseptic procedures, communicable infections, precautions, and cleaning, disinfection, and sterilization of equipment and supplies
- storage of, handling of, and access to supplies, medical gases, and drugs
- equipment management, including safe and appropriate use of equipment
- identification, handling, and disposal of hazardous or infectious materials and

---

[*]*Source:* © 1997–98 CAMHC, Oakbrook Terrace, IL: Joint Commission on Accreditation of Healthcare Organizations, 1997. Reprinted with permission.

wastes in a safe and sanitary manner and according to law and regulation

- tests to be performed by the staff
- screening for abuse and neglect
- referral guidelines, including guidelines for timeliness
- care or services provided by other staff members to facilitate coordination and appropriate patient referral
- community resources
- care or service responsibilities
- other care responsibilities

In addition to meeting the requirements above, it is important to include the following topics in the orientation:

- patient rights and responsibilities
- employee availability (promptness, leaving early, relief, work week, on-call procedure, no call/no show)
- employee discipline
- time slips
- dress code
- credentialing and employee requirements for hire and throughout employment
- competency assessment procedures and ongoing competency requirements
- ethics
- occurrence reporting
- adverse drug reactions (nurses only)
- physician orders (nurses only)
- medication administration (nurses only)
- staff safety
- client consent
- drug-free workplace
- nursing process (observation or assessment, developing and updating or following care plans, progress notes and documentation tips; this section is tailored to the participant: RN, LPN, or CHHA)
- client and caregiver education
- quality improvement
- communication skills
- nutrition

At first look, this content might seem to encompass too many topics. If you want to end up with a well-informed, cooperative, competent employee, however, this is a worthwhile investment of time and effort.

There are several useful methods for presenting the orientation materials. First, hold orientations in comfortable, well-lit rooms. Two rooms are preferable: one for lectures and examinations and the other for a skills laboratory. Each participant is given a complete outline of the content to be discussed. The use of a continuous format, with agency forms, job descriptions, and policies included, works the best. A combination of lecture, discussion, demonstration, return demonstration, case studies, and role playing helps these adult learners hear, see, feel, and practice.

COMPETENCY ASSESSMENT

To test competence, your agency can use a pre–post orientation examination in class and actually test the prospective employees' competence on basic cognitive and technical skills in the laboratory. Exhibit 14–6 is an example of an RN/LPN competency assessment, and Exhibit 14–7 is an example of a CHHA competency assessment. In both cases, these forms are initiated in orientation and completed during the orientation phase in the home.

As discussed previously, competency assessments need to be tailored to your agency's scope of care and services. For example, if you have more high technology than is represented in Exhibits 14–6 and 14–7, you would include the equipment you use. In either case, be careful to choose the specific knowledge and skills in which the employee must be competent before he or she is assigned to a patient alone. Be realistic, not idealistic, when determining your basic requirements. Applicants who do not have any home care experience should be given an opportunity for a preceptor experience. This can be as in-depth and intensive as required. The experienced nurse guides the new applicant through the entire process. Elements of a preceptor experience for an RN include the following:

Exhibit 14–6 RN and LPN Competency Assessment

Employee: _____ ID#: _____ □ RN □ LPN □ Initial orientation □ Re-orientation □ Other: _____

| Knowledge/Skill | Competent | Needs Improvement | | Method | | | | | | | Initials | Retest | |
	Date	Date	Comments	Obsrv Class Date	Obsrv Home Date	Exam Date	Score	Verbal Date	SLP Date			Date	Initials
Home Care exam													
Orientation exam													
Pediatric exam													
High Tech exam													
IV exam													
ASSESSMENT													
Demographics, history													
Safety, Communication													
Neurological/sensory													
Cardiovascular													
Respiratory													
Communicable disease													
Musculoskeletal													
Gastrointestinal/nutritional													
Genitourinary													
Integumentary													
Pain, rehab, equipment													
Community resources													
BASIC NURSING SKILLS													
Care plan													
Follows basic care plan													
Documenting care													
Client/caregiver education													
Basic IV care													
Hyperalimentation													
Foley care													

continues

Exhibit 14–6 (continued)

Knowledge/Skill	Competent	Needs Improvement		Method							Initials	Retest	
				Obsrv Class	Obsrv Home	Exam		Verbal	SLP				
	Date	Date	Comments	Date	Date	Date	Score	Date	Date			Date	Initials
Tube feeding													
Communication clients													
Communication supervisor													
Univ. prec./Infection control													
Safe: Transfer													
Ambulation													
Home environment													
Body mechanics													
CARE PRIORITIES for FIRST ASSIGNMENT:													
Adult													
Geriatric													
Pediatric													
Psychiatric													

Validators: Initials_____ Signature/title_____ Initials_____ Signature/title_____

Initials_____ Signature/title_____ Initials_____ Signature/title_____

☐ Requirements and credentials complete   Signature/title_____   Date:_____
☐ Required competencies complete for assignment   Signature/title_____   Date:_____

Courtesy of Clarke Health Care Consultants, Seminole, Florida.

Exhibit 14–7 CHHA Competency Assessment

Employee: _____   ID#: _____   □ Initial orientation   □ Re-orientation   □ Other: _____

Knowledge/Skill	Competent	Needs Improvement		Method							Initials	Retest	
				Obsrv Class	Obsrv Home	Exam		Verbal	SLP				
	Date	Date	Comments	Date	Date	Date	Score	Date	Date			Date	Initials
CHHA Home Care exam													
Orientation exam													
MANDATORY TASKS													
Read and record temperature													
Take and record pulse													
Take and record respiration													
Bed bath													
Sponge, tub and shower bath													
Shampoo													
Nail care													
Skin care													
Oral hygiene													
Toileting and elimination													
Positioning													
Safe: Transfer													
Ambulation													
Home environment													
Body mechanics													
Range of motion													
Communication clients													
Communication supervisor													
Body functions and change in condition													
Observe, report, and document client status													
Universal precautions													

continues

Exhibit 14–7 (continued)

Knowledge/Skill	Competent Date	Needs Improvement Date	Comments	Method Obsrv Class Date	Obsrv Home Date	Exam Date	Exam Score	Verbal Date	SLP Date	Initials	Retest Date	Retest Initials
Maintain clean and healthy environment												
Recognize and react to emergency situation												
Physical, emotional, and developmental needs												
Respect for patient privacy and property												
Adequate nutritional intake												
CARE PRIORITIES FOR FIRST ASSIGNMENT:												
Adult												
Geriatric												
Pediatric												
Psychiatric												
Follow plan of care												

Validators: Initials _____ Signature/title _____   Initials _____ Signature/title _____

         Initials _____ Signature/title _____   Initials _____ Signature/title _____

☐ Requirements and credentials complete   Signature/title _____   Date: _____

☐ Required competencies complete for assignment   Signature/title _____   Date: _____

Courtesy of Clarke Health Care Consultants, Seminole, Florida.

- patient status assessment
- initiation of nursing care
- updating the care plan
- basic nursing notes
- documentation of changes in patient condition
- client and caregiver education
- discharge planning
- giving/receiving reports
- community resources
- laboratory value interpretation
- communication with client, caregiver, physician, and supervisor

An LPN preceptor experience would entail the following elements:

- documentation of the client's physical assessment and findings
- implementation of the nursing plan of care
- assisting the RN in evaluating achievement of client goals
- reinforcement of client instructions from the RN or physician
- basic nursing notes
- documentation of changes in patient condition
- giving/receiving reports
- communication with client, caregiver, and RN supervisor

If you are planning to use preceptors, be sure to test their competence to precept, too. This usually requires a class outlining responsibilities and competency testing. Role playing is an effective way to ascertain what and how the preceptor will teach. It is important for the preceptors to teach only agency policies. Include the documentation of preceptor competence in the preceptors' personnel files.

At the end of the orientation program, you have a good sense of the new employee's competence. You will also have a basis for making appropriate assignments. The level of the new hire's competence will guide you in planning for additional supervision, if it is necessary.

SIGN-OFF

At the culmination of the orientation phase, a final sign-off is required. All persons validating requirements, credentials, and competencies must sign the competency assessment forms. In addition, a final sign-off for the requirements and credentials outlined in Exhibit 14–4 and the competencies outlined in Exhibits 14–6 and 14–7 is required. This is the final check before the new hire is assigned to care for a patient independently.

ONGOING ASSESSMENT OF COMPETENCY

The fact that the new employee met all your initial requirements for credentials and competencies does not guarantee that he or she will still be competent next month, when he or she is assigned to a new case, or when new equipment or policies are introduced. A good next step, therefore, is the supervisor visit. This is the ideal time to check the employee's competency. Exhibits 14–8 and 14–9 are forms that can be used to document the patient's satisfaction with the employee's performance and the supervisor's evaluation of the employee's competence. These forms can be used on every supervisor visit and also when the supervisor opens a new case with the employee.

For each performance criterion, the supervisor rates the employee as "competent" or "needs improvement." If the employee does need improvement, there is space provided to outline what he or she needs to improve as well as to review his or her behavior, knowledge, or skill and to write comments. You will note there are blanks under performance criteria for additional knowledge and skills required on a particular case. So, if the patient has a tracheostomy, needs suctioning and has a ventilator you would enter it and validate the employee competency. These spaces can be used for a variety of topics that meet your agency's or the individual patient's needs. The supervisor then determines

Exhibit 14–8 RN and LPN Competency Review

RN and LPN Competency Review

Employee:_____ Client:_____ Date:_____

Client Observation of Employee

Prompt □   Late □   Respects Rights: Yes   □   Needs Improvement □
Communication: Good □ Needs Improvement □ Quality of Care: Good □ Needs Improvement □

Comments: _____

_____

Competency Review

Performance	Competent	Needs Improvement	Reviewed	Comments
Dress Code, ID, Hygiene				
Initiative				
Psychosocial/Communication				
Knowledge: Diagnosis/Regime				
RN: Care Planning/Updating				
RN: Achievement of Goals				
LPN: Physical Assessment				
LPN: Contributes to Care Plan				
Implements Care Plan				
Organizing/Prioritizing				
Medications				
Occurrence Reporting				
Univ. Prec/Infection Control				
Equipment Maintenance				
Coordinating Service				
RN: Discharging Planning				
Documents client/caregiver educ.				
Safe: Transfer/Amb./Environment				
Body Mechanics				
Wound Care				
IV Care				

Client's needs are being met by the employee: Yes □   No □

Comments: _____

_____

□   Review policy:_____   □   Attend class:_____
□   SLP:_____   □   Meet with Director of Patient Services

Employee Signature_____Supervisor_____

Courtesy of Clarke Health Care Consultants, Seminole, Florida.

Exhibit 14–9 CHHA Competency Review

CHHA Competency Review

Employee:_____ Client:_____ Date:_____

Client Observation of Employee

Prompt ☐   Late ☐   Respects Rights: Yes   ☐ Needs Improvement ☐
Communication: Good ☐ Needs Improvement ☐ Quality of Care: Good ☐ Needs Improvement ☐

Comments: _____

_____

Competency Review

Performance	Competent	Needs Improvement	Reviewed	Comments
Dress Code				
ID Available				
Personal Hygiene				
Initiative				
Attitude				
Psychosocial/Communication				
Client Diagnosis/Needs				
Follows Plan of Care				
Prioritizes Duties				
Completes Worksheet				
Occurrence Reporting				
Safe: Transfer				
Ambulation				
Home Environment				
Body Mechanics				
Client Nutrition				
Universal Precautions				
Range of Motion				

Client's needs are being met by the employee: Yes ☐   No ☐

Comments: _____

_____

_____

_____

☐   Review policy:_____   ☐   Attend class:_____
☐   SLP:_____   ☐   Meet with Director of Patient Services

Employee Signature_____Supervisor_____

Courtesy of Clarke Health Care Consultants, Seminole, Florida.

whether the patient's needs are being met by the employee.

To complete this process the supervisor makes an overall comment about his or her assessment of the employee's competence. Check-off boxes are provided on the forms shown in Exhibits 14–8 and 14–9 to guide the employee in taking actions to improve performance. These include which policy to review, which self-learning package to complete, what class to attend, and whether the employee should meet with the director of patient services. Both the employee and the supervisor sign the form. The employee is given a copy, and one copy is filed in the employee's personnel file.

QUALITY IMPROVEMENT PROGRAM

Ongoing competency assessments of RNs, LPNs, and CHHAs are an integral part of the quality improvement program. Statistically valid samplings of these reviews are analyzed. It is even better if you document right on a computer program so that all the results can be compiled. The leadership team can then evaluate competency across RN, LPN, and CHHA groups. The analysis will point out what knowledge and skills most frequently need improvement. It will also reveal the special competencies that are most frequently required.

OCCURRENCE MONITORING

Occurrence monitoring statistics should be reviewed by the agency's leaders on a monthly basis. They, too, reveal valuable information about competency. Look for trends that point to possible employee competence issues. These include errors in care or treatment, falls, injuries, infections, admissions to the emergency department or hospital, complaints, decubiti, inadequate client and caregiver education, and the like.

CONTINUING EDUCATION

The leader's evaluation of the quality improvement and occurrence monitoring data forms the basis for planning continuing education programs to improve employee competence. Also used is the supervisor's knowledge of new equipment, new technology, changes in patient mix, mandatory requirements, and employee requests. Each of these criteria points out competence issues that have already appeared or those that are likely to appear. Quarterly planning sessions help keep your agency on the cutting edge of competence training.

Take the example of a quality improvement study involving admissions to the emergency department and the hospital. In this scenario, you note an increase in both types of admissions every year during flu season. Further investigation reveals that only 20 percent of the elderly patients you serve had flu shots and that 35 percent of the patients who developed flu were admitted for lengthy hospital stays for pneumonia. Your search also led you to the realization that your staff did little patient education about how to prevent flu. In addition, only 25 percent of the CHHAs assigned to these elderly patients even reported the onset of flu to their supervisors.

This scenario plays out in many communities. This type of fact finding gives the agency an excellent opportunity to improve patient care. Classes and/or self-learning programs can be set up to improve employee competence in patient education about preventing flu and responding to the early symptoms of flu. Sharing the improvements realized the next year will help reinforce the employees' positive response to competency training.

METHODS

Several options are open to you when planning continuing education to improve staff competency. Traditionally, classes are offered on a regular basis. To enhance the effectiveness of classes, consider using role playing, demonstrations, case studies, and hands-on practice. Competency testing should be tied to all classes with pre–post tests, verbal testing, and return demonstrations. Also use an evaluation form to determine the employee's evaluation of the effectiveness of the educational offering. Another widely used method is self-learning modules. These work especially well with nurses. A post test must be part of the module. In all cases, a minimum passing score must be set. Employees who fail the test should be given the opportunity to study and retake the test.

The agency will need to communicate competency requirements clearly to the employees. Each person must be aware of his or her quarterly and annual requirements. Compliance in meeting job category and personal competency requirements must be tracked and shared with employees.

POLICIES AND PROCEDURES

Do you have multiple policy and procedure books? Do your staff know what is in them? Where are the policy books kept? If your agency is like most others, the policies are kept in the administrator's or supervisor's office. How can the employees follow policies that they do not know about?

Several solutions can help improve employees' competence related to policies. First, pertinent policies should be part of the orientation. Second, general policies relating to most patient care should be kept in the back of the patient's chart in the home. These include occurrence reporting, medication administration, patient safety, and equipment maintenance, among others. Policies specific to a particular patient are brought to the home by the supervisor and put into the back of the chart; examples include policies relating to ventilators, tracheostomies, suctioning equipment, gastric tubes, and the like.

This system gives the employees a quick reference. Staff caring for the patient are required to initial all policies in the chart. You can also systematize how you release policies. For example, all policies could be approved by the leadership committee and then released to staff with paychecks. Staff would be responsible for reading and comprehending all releases and would be required to sign a form verifying that they received a specific group of policies, know that they are responsible for reading and comprehending them, and will ask their supervisor if they have any questions. Some policies could be released in a self-learning module so that post tests could be included.

PERFORMANCE EVALUATIONS

Employee competence is assessed on a more formal basis at the end of the probation period and on an annual basis. The National HomeCaring Council (1995b) standards for written evaluations are as follows:

> IVA-2.5: A written evaluation is performed at least by the first 6 months of employment based on the job requirements.

> VII-3: The nursing supervisor shall do an annual performance review of nursing personnel. The review should be signed and dated by the supervisor and the employee.

The performance evaluation should include every performance criterion listed in the job description. In preparing the performance evaluation, the supervisor uses the competency assessments made during supervisory visits, the employee's compliance in completing ongoing competency requirements, and the employee's competence in reading, comprehending, and signing off on policies. On the form shown in Exhibit 14–10, the employee is rated as E (exceed) if performance far exceeds position requirements and established standards and is sustained at that level. A rating of C (competent) is given if performance meets necessary position requirements and established standards. This employee achieves position requirements in a fully competent manner. The

Exhibit 14–10 Portion of LPN Performance Evaluation

LPN PERFORMANCE APPRAISAL

Performance Criteria	Achievement			Comments	Performance Improvement Plan
	E	C	N I		
Maintains standards of Nursing care and implements the policies and procedures established by the agency.					
Performs physical assessments consistent with standards of Nursing Practice.					
Observes and documents patient's biophysical, psychosocial, and educational needs to assist the RN in patient assessment and care planning.					
Consistently follows the Nursing Plan of Care for the client developed by the RN.					
Accurately documents implementation of the client's plan of care.					
Reinforces instructions given to the patient by the physician and registered nurse and refers new needs for instruction to the registered nurse.					
Supervises and coaches the client and his/her family members in giving care.					
Demonstrates the ability to communicate effectively with the client and his/her family members.					
Consistently reports appropriate changes in the client's condition to the Nursing Supervisor.					
Administers and documents client's selected prescribed medication competently under specific policies and procedures.					
Demonstrates competence in performing all treatments per MD and RN plan of care.					
Consistently adheres to universal precautions, aseptic techniques, and infection control policies.					

Courtesy of Clarke Health Care Consultants, Seminole, Florida.

employee receives a rating of NI (needs improvement) when performance does not meet the requirements of the position and established standards. Written comments and a performance improvement plan are required for all performance criteria rated as NI. Employees must improve their competence in these areas to continue employment.

CONCLUSION

Developing a competency system involves establishing standards, hiring appropriate staff, orienting new employees, assessing ongoing competency, tracking data, and implementing systems to improve performance for both individuals and groups. This process is vital to the survival of any organization that wants to provide high-quality care and services.

REFERENCES

Joint Commission on Accreditation of Healthcare Organizations. 1996. 1997–1998 Comprehensive accreditation manual for home care. Oakbrook Terrace, IL: Joint Commission.

National HomeCaring Council. 1995a. *Private duty nursing interpretation of standards*. Washington, DC: Foundation for Hospice and Homecare.

National HomeCaring Council. 1995b. *Self-study manual*. Washington, DC: Foundation for Hospice and Homecare.

CHAPTER 15

A Patient Classification Outcome Criteria System

Elizabeth A. Daubert

This chapter provides a detailed description of the rehabilitation potential patient classification system. It also indicates that administrators of home care agencies were interested in identifying and developing patient classification systems that emphasized the importance of outcomes of patient care as early as the 1970s. Community-based home health agencies, such as visiting nurse associations, official public health nursing agencies, and hospital-based home care programs, have long grappled with the task of developing reliable, valid ways to measure the quality of services they provide. For the most part, past efforts have been confined to ensuring that a high level of quality care is rendered by periodically evaluating the agency's organizational and management structure and by maintaining a method of record review. These quality assurance activities can and do produce indicators concerning the quality of care provided to patients and families, but neither provides objective evidence to answer an equally important question: What difference did agency service make in a patient's health status?

With increasing frequency, real and potential consumers of service, federal and state legislators and regulators, and third party payers are asking for hard data that home health service does, indeed, make a difference in a patient's health status. The answer to this question lies in the development of an assurance tool that has the capacity objectively to evaluate patient outcome, the status of a patient at the time of discharge from agency service. An outcome measurement module is a must for any good quality assurance program.

Outcome measures, using medical diagnosis or acuity level or for a specific health discipline, are fairly common in acute and long-term care facilities. The use of outcome-oriented systems in home health agencies, however, is still the unusual rather than the usual case. Designing a system that will provide objective evidence of the quality of care provided by home health care agencies is not an impossible task, but two problems identified by Aydelotte (1973) immediately appear: the difficulties in describing the effect of care that an agency hopes to achieve, and the problems of identifying the specific population(s) served by a home health care agency.

Attempts to define outcome criteria for each home health discipline or according to medical diagnosis are fraught with problems, for several reasons. For example, five of the six traditional home health services—nursing, social work, physical therapy, speech therapy, and occupational therapy—are independent disciplines, which means that each service functions with complete autonomy in a patient situation. Therefore, the efforts of each discipline are distinct and measurable. The sixth discipline, however, home health aide service, is neither an independent discipline nor autonomous. Instead, it is a totally dependent discipline because it always functions as a supplement or extension of nursing, physical therapy, or speech therapy service. To write measurable outcome criteria, each service discipline must be able to stand alone in a service setting; each must be independent. Also, the ultimate measure of patient outcome is not which service or mix of services is provided. Rather, the final measure of the effectiveness of service is the outcome, the actual functioning level of a patient at the time of discharge from service. This is the reason why it is not practical for a home health agency to use outcome criteria according to each discipline provided.

It is equally impractical or ineffective to use patient diagnosis as a basis for developing outcome criteria for an agency-based home health program. It might be feasible if all patients within an agency's population had only one diagnosis, but the average patient admitted to an agency's illness service program has three or more diagnoses. When one deals with a patient population with multiple diagnoses, using outcome criteria based upon patient diagnosis becomes an impractical, unwieldy approach. Such a method would mean that not one set but multiple sets of outcome criteria would have to be applied in each patient situation. The paperwork alone would be time consuming and cost prohibitive.

The pitfalls of using either the service discipline approach or a medical diagnosis approach can be avoided by classifying patients by groups according to each group's rehabilitation potential. Of greater value, the intent of such a system is met because the characteristic that is measured is the outcome, the end result of the care. The following is an example of an outcome measurement system that has the proven capacity to measure patient outcome, the status of a patient at the time of discharge from home health agency service.

THE PATIENT CLASSIFICATION OUTCOME SYSTEM

The patient classification outcome (PCO) system, developed in 1977, is a formal method of measuring patient outcome based upon classifying all patients admitted to an agency's home health care program, regardless of the number of diagnoses per patient or the mix of agency services given, into one of five patient groups according to each patient's rehabilitation potential. Each of the five patient groups is specifically defined to provide clarity and uniformity for assignment of patients to a particular group. In addition, each group has an identified ultimate program objective and a separate set of subobjectives. All service program objectives, both ultimate objectives and subobjectives, are based upon the premise that the terms *service program objectives* and *patient care goals* are synonymous. Justification for such a conclusion is based upon the following definitions:

- *Goal*: an aim; the end toward which effort is directed.
- *Objective*: an aim, or end of action; a goal.

For each patient group, a specific ultimate program objective and a separate set of program subobjectives have been identified. Each ultimate program objective and set of subobjectives applies to all six home health care service components (nursing, home health aide, physical therapy, speech therapy, occupational therapy, and social work). Finally, each set of program objectives becomes the criteria, or standards, that are used to judge the effectiveness of an agency's home health care program in meeting the health needs/problems of its patient population. All applicable subobjectives for each patient group must be met to verify that the ultimate goal has been accomplished for each patient.

PATIENT GROUPS AND OBJECTIVES

A delineation of the five patient groups as well as a set of corresponding objectives, both ultimate objectives and subobjectives, is as follows.

Patient Group I

These are patients with acute, nonchronic, episodic type disease or disability (e.g., wound infection, fracture, pneumonia, poor nutritional habits, gastrointestinal disorder, uncomplicated surgical procedure, gestational diabetes, gestational hypertension, etc.) who will return to pre-illness level of functioning.

- *Ultimate program objective for group I*: Either the patient will achieve complete recovery from illness or the patient's immediate health need/problem that prompted admission to service (e.g., proper use of crutches, walker, etc. or need to learn correct technique for dressing change) will be eliminated.
- *Program subobjectives for group I*
  1. Patient will demonstrate capacity to return to pre-episodic level of functioning.
  2. Patient will demonstrate the ability to manage independently his or her personal care needs.
  3. Patient/family will demonstrate the ability to assume responsibility for any ongoing medical supervision.
  4. If indicated, patient/family will demonstrate an understanding of the prescribed diet.
  5. If indicated, patient/family will demonstrate an understanding of the prescribed medication regimen.
  6. If indicated, patient/family will demonstrate the ability to perform independently prescribed treatments/exercises.
  7. If indicated, patient/family will demonstrate knowledge of important safety measures.
  8. If indicated, patient/family will demonstrate knowledge of available community resources.

Patient Group II

These are patients with early-stage chronic disease or disability (e.g., cardiac disease, diabetes, cerebrovascular accident [CVA] with no residual or slight hemiparesis, chronic obstructive pulmonary disease [COPD], arthritis, hypertension, etc.) who are experiencing an acute episode of illness but have the potential for returning to their pre-episodic level of functioning.

- *Ultimate program objective for group II*: Patient/family will manage chronic health problem(s) without ongoing agency service.
- *Program subobjectives for group II*
  1. Patient will demonstrate capacity to return to pre-episodic level of functioning.
  2. Patient/family will demonstrate the ability to manage independently the patient's personal care needs.
  3. Patient/family will demonstrate the ability to assume responsibility for maintaining ongoing medical supervision.
  4. If indicated, patient/family will demonstrate an understanding of the prescribed diet.
  5. If indicated, patient/family will demonstrate an understanding of the prescribed medication regimen.
  6. If indicated, patient/family will demonstrate the ability to perform independently prescribed treatments/exercises.
  7. Patient/family will recognize signs of significant physical or emotional changes as well as the need to communicate these changes to the appropriate health care provider.
  8. If indicated, patient/family will demonstrate an understanding of the restrictions imposed by the illness or disability.
  9. If indicated, patient/family will demonstrate knowledge of important safety measures.

10. If indicated, patient/family will demonstrate knowledge of available community resources.

Patient Group III

The criteria for these patients are as follows: Patients with intermediate stage chronic disease or disability who, even though a return to pre-illness level of functioning is not possible, will have the potential for increasing their level of functioning and will eventually function without agency service(s); *or* patients with advanced stage chronic disease or disability who do not have the potential for increasing their level of functioning but who, because of assistance provided by a family member, will eventually function without agency service(s). Examples are cardiac disease, CVA with hemiparesis, arthritis, congestive heart failure, amputation of a limb, diabetes with blindness, and the like.

- *Ultimate program objective for group III*: Patient will be rehabilitated to his or her maximum level of physical, emotional, and social functioning, and patient/family will manage chronic health problem(s) without continued agency service(s).
- *Program subobjectives for group III*
  1. Patient/family will demonstrate the ability to manage independently chronic health problem(s).
  2. Patient/family will demonstrate some improvement in ability to function independently.
  3. Patient/family will demonstrate the ability to manage independently the patient's personal care needs.
  4. Patient/family will demonstrate the ability to assume responsibility for maintaining ongoing medical supervision.
  5. If indicated, patient/family will demonstrate an understanding of the prescribed diet.

6. If indicated, patient/family will demonstrate an understanding of the prescribed medication regimen.
7. If indicated, patient/family will demonstrate the ability to perform independently prescribed treatments/exercises.
8. Patient/family will demonstrate the ability to recognize signs of significant physical or emotional change as well as the need to communicate these changes to the appropriate health care provider.
9. If indicated, patient/family will demonstrate an understanding of the restrictions imposed by the patient's illness.
10. If indicated, patient/family will demonstrate knowledge of important safety measures.
11. If indicated, patient/family will demonstrate knowledge of available community resources.

Patient Group IV

These are patients with advanced-stage chronic disease or disability (e.g., advanced heart disease, neurological problems, severe arthritis, organic brain syndrome, fractures, gastrointestinal disorder, CVA with residual hemiplegia, cancer, pernicious anemia, etc.) who can only be maintained at home because of ongoing agency service(s).

- *Ultimate program objective for group IV*: Patient will be maintained at home as long as possible with ongoing agency service.
- *Program subobjectives for group IV*
  1. Patient will receive agency service at the level and intensity needed and within the normal limits of the agency to provide such service.
  2. Patient/family will demonstrate the ability to manage the patient's personal care needs with or without agency assistance.

3. Patient/family will demonstrate the ability to assume responsibility for maintaining ongoing medical supervision.

4. If indicated, patient/family will demonstrate an understanding of the prescribed diet.

5. If indicated, patient/family will demonstrate an understanding of the prescribed medication regimen.

6. If indicated, patient/family will demonstrate the ability to perform prescribed treatments/exercises.

7. Patient/family will demonstrate the ability to recognize signs of significant physical or emotional change as well as the need to communicate these changes to the appropriate health care provider.

8. If indicated, patient/family will demonstrate an understanding of the restrictions imposed by the patient's illness.

9. If indicated, patient/family will demonstrate knowledge of important safety measures.

10. Complications and regression will be prevented insofar as possible.

11. If indicated, patient/family will demonstrate knowledge of available community resources.

Patient Group V

These are patients with an end-stage illness (e.g., terminal COPD, cancer, renal failure, cardiac disease, cirrhosis, etc.).

- *Ultimate program objective for group V:* Patient will be maintained at home during the end stage of illness for as long as possible with agency service.
- *Program subobjectives for group V*
  1. Patient will receive agency service at the level and intensity needed and within the normal limits of the agency to provide such service.

2. Patient/family will demonstrate the ability to manage the patient's personal care needs with or without agency assistance.

3. Patient/family will demonstrate the ability to assume responsibility for maintaining ongoing medical supervision.

4. If indicated, patient/family will demonstrate an understanding of the prescribed diet.

5. If indicated, patient/family will demonstrate an understanding of the prescribed medication regimen.

6. If indicated, patient/family will demonstrate the ability to perform prescribed treatments/exercises.

7. Patient/family will demonstrate the ability to recognize signs of significant physical or emotional change as well as the need to communicate these changes to the appropriate health care provider.

8. Patient's pain/discomfort will be controlled to the extent possible.

9. Patient/family will receive emotional support as needed.

10. Patient/family will be allowed to express feelings about dying.

11. Patient/family will receive assistance as needed to prepare for death.

12. If indicated, patient/family will demonstrate knowledge of important safety measures.

13. If indicated, patient/family will demonstrate knowledge of available community resources.

14. If indicated, family will receive support during the mourning period.

PATIENT ADMISSION

Every patient admitted to an agency's home health program, even if it is a second or third admission, should be assessed and entered into one of the five patient groups. This process usually begins after the initial visit but no later than the third home visit. At that time, the primary caregiver (nurse or therapist) matches the patient's medical diagnosis(es), all identified health needs/problems presented by the patient/family, and the primary caregiver's assessment of the patient/family rehabilitation potential to the typology, or definition, and set of objectives for each patient group. The patient group that fits the patient situation is then selected. Second, the primary caregiver indicates the selected patient group in the goal section of the patient's record. Because the ultimate program objectives and patient care goals are the same, the objective for the selected group then becomes the long-term program service goal toward which all subsequent action is directed, regardless of the mix of disciplines supplying service to that patient. Third, the primary caregiver records all applicable subobjectives listed for that particular patient group in the patient's care plan. Because the applicable subobjectives are considered minimum goals, the patient care plan will also contain additional action goals tailored to the individual situation.

For example, Mr. A, a 68-year-old married man with a 7-year history of atherosclerotic heart disease and a 1-year history of diabetes mellitus (controlled by daily insulin and a prescribed diet), was referred for agency service upon hospital discharge after a partial colectomy that was performed to remove benign polyps. After surgery, Mr. A developed a secondary wound infection that was subsequently incised and drained. Mr. A was referred to the home health agency for monitoring of his wound and instruction for him and his wife in daily dressing changes of the draining wound. During the first home visit, the primary nurse thought that Mr. and Mrs. A were of average intelligence and that both seemed willing to learn the dressing procedure. Mr. A's insulin injection technique was assessed as safe and adequate, but his understanding of the need for daily urine testing and diabetic foot care was limited. In addition, he was not adhering to a 2-g sodium-restricted, low-cholesterol, 1,800-calorie diabetic diet. In assessing his rehabilitation potential, the primary nurse judged Mr. A as hav-

ing the capacity, with Mrs. A's assistance, eventually to manage his chronic health problems without ongoing agency service. By matching the above patient data with the definition and the set of objectives for each patient group, the primary nurse selects group II as the appropriate one for Mr. A. To enter Mr. A into the system, the primary nurse selects the appropriate patient group, indicates it on the care plan, and incorporates and customizes all applicable subobjectives listed for a group II patient in the patient action plan portion of the record. Had Mr. A needed the involvement of any special therapy services, such as physical/speech/occupational therapy or social work, the primary nurse would have discussed the selection of the patient group with the involved therapist(s) or social worker.

The terminology used in the statement of each subobjective does not stipulate that the patient/family will do, will accept, or will adhere to the stated action (e.g., patient/family will follow prescribed diet). Rather, each stated subobjective specifies that a patient/family will demonstrate an understanding of, an ability to, or knowledge of. The rationale for such terminology is based upon two factors. First, besides the provision of therapeutic care, a major function of every professional caregiver is to teach, to give patients/families the knowledge they need either to lessen or to eliminate their presenting health needs. Second, it is beyond the realm of the community-based professional caregiver actually to modify, much less control, patient/family behavior. It is essential that all patient care personnel who use this system have a clear understanding and acceptance of this principle. At the same time, however, it is recognized that some patient/family members will indeed modify their behavior as the result of the primary caregiver's teaching regimen. Whenever behavior modification is evident, a brief, concise description of the modified behavior should be documented in the patient record (e.g., patient/family verbalized all elements of prescribed diet, and weekly food intake chart substantiated fact).

As ongoing service is provided, the patient record must contain documentation that subsequent action was taken on each applicable subobjective as well as a description of the patient/family response. Furthermore, all applicable subobjectives must be attained to determine upon discharge from service that the program goal was accomplished. Each time a patient is discharged from an agency service, a discharge summary form is completed. Included on this form is specific information such as patient name, length of service, diagnosis(es), service program goal, goal accomplishment, reason for discharge, total visits made by each discipline, cost of each service discipline, payment source, and total cost of all services provided. The original copy is forwarded to the agency's statistical department, and the carbon copy is placed in the patient's record (Exhibit 15–1).

ADVANTAGES

Besides accomplishing the development of a method to identify and measure patient outcome, its primary purpose, the PCO system has several other advantages.

Saves Staff Time and Reduces Paperwork

The PCO system saves staff time and reduces paperwork because it reduces recording time. It also helps professional patient care staff with decision making and visiting of long-term service goals for each patient. In addition, each set of subobjectives serves as a helpful guide, or checklist, for staff to use for organizing their thinking as they develop patient care plans. Finally, the discharge summary form also reduces recording time.

Expands an Agency's Statistical Information System

Statistical data compiled by most agencies are usually limited to a breakdown of patient population by geographical location, age, race, sex, primary diagnosis, and payment source.

Because the PCO system provides a breakdown of patient population according to patient groups based on each patient's rehabilitation potential, the system also gives an agency access to descriptive data that more precisely define the specific health needs and rehabilitation potential of its patient population. The system can be used by agencies of any size because the data can be collected either manually or by computer.

Assists an Agency in Establishing Measurable Objectives for Its Home Health Program

Because the system has the capacity to collect data concerning the number of patients, according to patient group, who fell in the "goal accomplished" as well as the "goal not accomplished" categories, an agency can use these data to determine measurable objectives for its illness service program. For instance, in one agency where the system was operational for several years, the system's annual statistical report form produced the findings for the 1985 service year shown in Table 15–1.

Agency personnel can use these percentage figures as a basis for establishing measurable objectives for the illness service program for each service year. Depending upon circumstances, agency personnel might adjust the prior year's data either upward or downward when setting measurable objectives for each patient group for the upcoming service year.

Assists an Agency in Assessing the Delivery of Service

By providing objective evidence concerning the degree of effectiveness of its services in the population served, an agency will know its success and failure rate. For example, the system will generate on an ongoing basis a breakdown of the number of patients in each group for whom the service goal was accomplished (the success rate) and the number of patients in each

Exhibit 15–1 Discharge Summary Form

NURSE/THERAPIST COMPLETES BOXED AREAS □ ONLY; ALL OTHER AREAS TO BE
COMPLETED BY CLERICAL STAFF

Pt. Name _____ Town_____ C.T._____
      Last   First   No.   No.

Patient Number_____

First VNA Visit ___/___/___Last VNA Visit ___/___/___Total Length of Service_____ days (Circle
                                                                      months one)

Primary Dx._____ | Total Number of Dx. |_____
        Code

Payment Source: Primary_____Secondary_____
                          Code   Code(s)

| SERVICE PROGRAM GOAL | (Check one)

□ Group I—Will eliminate health problem/need.

□ Group II—Will learn to independently manage continuing health problem(s).

□ Group III—Will learn to function at maximum level.

□ Group IV—Chronically ill patient will be maintained at home with VNA assistance.

□ Group V—Patient with end-stage terminal illness will be maintained at home as long as possible.

| SERVICE GOAL ACCOMPLISHED | (Check one) □ Yes □ No

| REASON FOR DISCHARGE | (Check one box *ONLY*)

□ Service program goal accomplished   □ Pt. moved

□ Pt. hospitalized   □ Refused to obtain MD appointment

□ Pt. admitted to a nursing home   □ Refused continued service

□ Pt. died at home   □ Obtained service from another source

□ Refused to provide financial data   □ Cont'd service need H.H. aide; no payment source

Total Visits Made: _____   _____   _____   _____   _____   _____
                  Nsg.   P.T.   Soc. W.   Sp. T.   O.T.   HHA hrs./visits
                                                                   (delete one)

Cost of service: $_____ $_____ $____ $_____ $_____ $_____
                      Nsg.   P.T.   Soc. W.   Sp. T.   O.T.   HHA

TOTAL COST OF ALL SERVICES: $_____

Upon completion, the white copy is forwarded to the statistical clerk, the pink copy is filed with the
patient's record, and the yellow copy is forwarded to the billing department.

Table 15–1 Sample Annual Statistics

Group	Goal Met	Goal Not Met
I	84.3%	15.7%
II	85.8%	14.2%
III	76.8%	23.2%
IV	82.5%	17.5%
V	89.8%	10.2%

group for whom the service goal was not attained (the failure rate). For the latter, the system also provides a breakdown of the reasons why the service goal was not accomplished (e.g., patient hospitalized, patient died, patient/family refused continued service, etc.). Such data can help an agency assess its current methods of delivering service and plan corrective action where needed. For instance, if there is an inordinate number of "patient/family refused continued service" reasons, an examination of these patient records may uncover specific weaknesses in the agency's current method of delivering service. Subsequent action can then be taken to strengthen or eliminate these areas of deficiency. Alternatively, if many patients are discharged because their continuing need is for home health aide service only but they cannot afford to pay for ongoing aide service and no third party coverage exists to pay for continued service, these data could be used to validate the need for funding from sources such as United Way, private foundations, or municipal and state governments. The result might be expansion of the agency's home health aide service with additional funds.

Helps Forecast Future Staffing Patterns

These data can also be used to estimate future staffing needs and appropriate use of various kinds of patient care personnel. For example, if the number of patients admitted to group IV shows a steady increase each year, then an agency might adjust its staffing ratio by employing greater numbers of home health aide personnel and fewer professional staff.

Provides Data Concerning the Mix of Personnel and the Cost of Service

The system has the capacity to produce descriptive information related to the average mix of service personnel and the subsequent cost by patient group and/or patient primary diagnosis. This information can be used by the agency in interpreting its service to the community and to third-party payers.

VALIDATING RELIABILITY

The fact that the primary caregiver enters a patient into the system upon patient admission and, at the time of patient discharge from service, determines whether the service program goal was accomplished or not accomplished might be considered a weakness, a major flaw in the system. Therefore, to eliminate this concern and in so doing ensure the reliability and validity of the system, the following criteria should be added to an agency's method of record audit: service program goal, documentation regarding subobjectives, and the discharge summary. The addition of these items will ensure that the record contains evidence to substantiate that at the time of discharge the correct patient group was selected. Also, if the primary caregiver indicated that the goal was accomplished, then the action plan, service record, and narrative portion of the record should contain evidence that the appropriate actions were listed and taken on each applicable subobjective identified for the selected patient group and that the record contains a description of the patient/family change in knowledge, understanding, and behavior that occurred during the course of service. By the addition of the above criteria to an agency's record audit process, the need to establish a separate system to monitor the reliability and validity of the system is avoided.

CONCLUSION

The PCO system is operational and working well in several agencies in various areas of the United States. It has proved to be a valid method to identify and measure patient outcomes. The secondary benefits derived from its use have helped improve the efficiency and effectiveness of agencies' home health care programs. This PCO system is registered with the U.S. Copyright Office. Therefore, before reproduction or use of part or all of this system, permission must be obtained from its creator, Elizabeth A. Daubert.

The staff at the Visiting Nurse Association of Eastern Montgomery County/A Department of Abington Memorial Hospital in Willow Grove, Pennsylvania purchased the rights to use this PCO system in the mid-1980s. The Visiting Nurse Association has used a modification of this system and nursing diagnoses to identify and evaluate clinical and financial outcomes of home health care (Harris et al., 1985; Harris, 1994).

REFERENCES

Aydelotte, M. 1973, July. Quality assurance programs in nursing: Definitions and problems. Paper presented at the Connecticut Hospital Association Workshop, Hamden, CT.

Harris, M. 1994. Clinical and financial outcomes of patient care. In *Handbook of home health care administration*, ed. M. Harris, 289–308. Gaithersburg, MD: Aspen.

Harris, M., et al. 1985. A patient classification system in home health care. *Nursing Economics* 3:276–282.

SUGGESTED READING

Bailit, H., et al. 1975. Assessing the quality of care. *Nursing Outlook* 23:152–159.

Bloch, D. 1975. Evaluation of nursing care in terms of process and outcome; issues in research and quality assurance. *Nursing Research* 24:256–263.

Daubert, E.A. 1977. A system to evaluate home health care services. *Nursing Outlook* 25:168–171.

CHAPTER 16

Classification:
A Tool for Managed Care

Donna Ambler Peters

The idea of patient classification is not new. It can be traced back to the beginning of modern day nursing, when Florence Nightingale placed the most acutely ill patients in a ward nearest the nurse's desk and the least ill farthest from the desk (Giovannetti and Thiessen, 1983). Today, the end product of the grouping of patients is known as a patient classification system, which has been used in nursing to calculate staffing needs and, more recently, to cost out nursing services.

As popular as patient classification systems are, however, other classifications are also used in the profession of nursing. Classification of nursing diagnoses, for example, has been stimulated by the convening of national conferences on the classification of nursing diagnoses in the early 1970s and the more recent formation of the North American Nursing Diagnosis Association (NANDA) to develop, refine, and promote a taxonomy of nursing diagnoses. Although the NANDA taxonomy is popular, this chapter discusses the Omaha System because it is a nursing diagnosis taxonomy specific for community health. The chapter examines the concept of classification as it applies to patient classification systems and nursing diagnoses. It discusses how a nursing diagnosis taxonomy can be used for clinical management of a home health agency and can be incorporated into a patient classification system for administrative man-

agement of an agency. By focusing clinical and administrative management on defined groups, an agency can be in a better position to deal with the emerging trend of managed care.

CLASSIFICATION THEORY

Scientific inquiry has two major objectives: to describe a particular phenomenon in the world, and to establish the general principles by which the phenomenon can be explained and predicted. To develop the explanatory and predictive principles, scientifically useful concepts are required. These useful types of concept formations are procedures of quantitative ordering, comparative ordering, and classification (Hempel, 1952).

The classificatory concept depicts a characteristic that any object in the domain under consideration must either have or lack. It is an either-or situation. Ordering concepts, on the other hand, attribute a value to each item in the domain, providing a gradation of the characteristics. Stated another way, the characteristics used in an ordering concept are criteria of precedence and coincidence, whereas the characteristics used in a classification concept are criteria for class membership. The value of the characteristics in an ordering concept may be numerical, giving a quantitative ordering (relative values), or simply ordinal. These concept formations are explained by the theory of classificatory procedures and systems (Hempel, 1965; Sokal, 1974).

In a patient classification system, the class to be divided is patients, and the subclasses are groups of patients with a need for a particular kind of care. In actuality, the concept used is a comparative ordering because the amount of care required falls on a continuum rather than in the dichotomy of requiring care or not requiring care. The characteristics used for placing a patient at the appropriate level on the continuum are usually critical indicators of care that depict greater or lesser needs for care. The greater the needs for care, the higher the level at which the patient is placed. In usage, however, the procedure has been called a classification.

In a nursing diagnosis taxonomy, the class to be divided is nursing diagnosis, and the subclasses are the signs and symptoms that a patient may exhibit. These essential characteristics determine membership in the subclass (i.e., the patient either has the diagnosis or does not have it). The subclasses are not on a continuum, and there is no value (either relative or numerical) assigned to any of the diagnoses. Thus this procedure is defined as a classificatory concept rather than a comparative ordering, which is used by patient classification systems. In addition, because it is the class of nursing diagnoses that is being divided and not patients, as in a patient classification system, a patient having more than one nursing diagnosis may appear in more than one category (i.e., patients are not placed in mutually exclusive categories).

PATIENT CLASSIFICATION SYSTEMS

A patient classification system is a "generic term used to describe a variety of methods for grouping or categorizing patients according to their perceived requirements for nursing care" (Giovannetti and Thiessen, 1983, p. 1). Categorization can be based on natural classifications (patient characteristics) or artificial classifications (critical indicators of care). Classification is done either by rating patient characteristics simultaneously and placing them in a category (prototype design) or by rating the patient on several separate critical indicators of care and combining these ratings to provide an overall rating that determines the category into which the patient is placed (factor evaluation; Abdellah and Levine, 1978; Bermas and Van Slyck, 1984; Giovannetti, 1979).

There are three basic elements in a patient classification system: a procedure for grouping patients that includes the frequency of classification and the means of reporting these data, a quantification of the nursing care resources associated with each category of care, and a method for calculating staffing for required nursing hours. Such a system can be used to monitor productivity levels, to predict and justify staffing needs in the budgetary process, and to provide a basis for nursing charges (Alward, 1983). It must be emphasized, however, that such a system justifies cost only and cannot justify the care.

Logically, it is reasonable to expect that staffing levels based on a patient classification system will have a positive relationship to the quality of care. In practice, however, three problems are evident: The existence of a patient classification system does not guarantee adequate staff, there is no guarantee that nurses will or can perform in the manner described in the system, and the staffing levels obtained by a patient classification system represent only the quantitative aspect of the complex system of patient care (Brown, 1980; Giovannetti and Thiessen, 1983; Sienkiewicz, 1984).

NURSING DIAGNOSIS TAXONOMY

A nursing diagnosis taxonomy is simply the classification of nursing diagnoses. The nursing diagnoses that make up the taxonomy could be derived either deductively or inductively. To be derived deductively, a distinct group of actual and potential health conditions that are amenable to nursing intervention must exist. Currently, however, there is no consensus on the definitions of these conditions; rather, several models exist, each providing a different orientation to nursing. Nursing diagnoses derived inductively are based on a description of clients' health problems as they are encountered in practice. Developing a taxonomy of these diagnoses is one way of describing the domain of nursing and thus communicating the nature of that service both to other nurses and to those outside the profession, such as patients, other professionals, auditors, and legislators (Roy, 1975). Watson (1994) has gone so far as to state "If we fail to clarify nursing practice within a nursing paradigm, we are . . . on our way out" (p. 86).

A nursing diagnosis taxonomy for community health nursing was developed by the Visiting Nurse Association of Omaha (Simmons, 1980). This taxonomy is consistent with the general and comprehensive practice of community health nursing, which includes the following tenets: It is not limited to a particular age or diagnostic group; it is continuing, not episodic; it uses a holistic approach for health promotion, health maintenance, health education, coordination, and continuity of care; it recognizes the influence of social and ecological issues; and it utilizes the dynamic forces that influence change (American Nurses Association, 1974; Simmons, 1980).

The 44 nursing diagnoses included in the taxonomy were arrived at empirically from the practice of the community health nurses employed by the visiting nurse agency. The diagnoses are organized by the four broad domains addressed by community health nurses: environmental, psychosocial, physiological, and health-related behaviors. Each diagnosis is described by a list of signs and symptoms, that is, general statements condensed from assessment data that are patient specific and are used to arrive at the problem label (diagnosis). For example, one of the problem labels in the health-related behaviors domain is nutrition. There are eight descriptors or signs and symptoms for this problem label, one of which is "weighs 10 percent more than average." The problem may be referenced as

health promotion, potential, or deficit/impairment/actual. The patient may be defined as an individual or family (Martin et al., 1986). For example, if a person were more than 10 percent overweight as a result of poor personal eating habits, this would be an actual individual problem. If the person were dependent on the family to buy, prepare, and bring the food to the bedside, however, the problem would be a family problem. If this same person were currently at an appropriate weight but the family were feeding the patient an extreme number of calories for the patient's activity level, this would be a potential family problem.

The Omaha System not only provides nursing diagnoses and specific descriptors for each diagnosis but also includes a problem rating scale for outcomes and an intervention scheme. The problem rating scale is a 5-point Likert type scale that measures the concepts of knowledge, behavior, and status for each identified problem. It provides an evaluation framework for monitoring patient progress on each problem throughout the patient's admission. The intervention scheme is used in conjunction with the problem rating scale. The scheme is an organized framework of nursing activities designed to address specific nursing problems using four broad categories of interventions: health teaching, treatments, case management, and surveillance (Martin and Scheet, 1991).

CLINICAL MANAGEMENT

Patient classification systems, by definition, are more of an administrative tool than an aid to clinical management. Some improvement in nursing care plans and chart documentation has been seen where classification data are obtained from these documents. The critical indicators of care used in patient classification systems are inadequate criteria for evaluating the quality of care received, however, until a relationship between these indicators and the progress of the patient's condition has been established (Aydelotte, 1973). Furthermore, the tasks, activities, and categories of nursing work found in the systems do not reflect the nature and full character of nursing practice.

Using a classification of nursing diagnoses, however, directly focuses on the care of the client. Nursing diagnosis is the pivotal factor in the nursing process, which is central to community health practice and all nursing actions. Structurally, the nursing process is adapted from the scientific approach to solving problems. It consists of four steps: assessing, planning, implementing, and evaluating. The end point of the assessment stage is the nursing diagnosis. If there is no nursing diagnosis, then there is no reason to continue to the other components of the process.

Using a nursing diagnosis taxonomy inductively derived from community health practice actually defines that practice. Therefore, because the Omaha System defines community health care, when used correctly it provides for the planning, organizing, and prioritizing of that care. It allows for the sifting and sorting of information in an organized fashion. It actually provides a building block of care; the more difficult and time consuming the case and the more extenuating the circumstances, the more problems will be identified from more domains. By identifying the subsequent problems, the nurse is able to communicate in a logical, concise way to his or her superiors, auditors, payers, and others that this is a difficult case and more time is needed.

It is the classification of the nursing diagnoses that facilitates the organizing and prioritizing of care. The physiological domain, for example, generally provides the structure for those nursing interventions that are closely aligned with the medical regimen. As any nurse working in home health care knows, however, it is those problems that are often the easiest to handle. The diagnoses under the other three domains are the ones that are often the most difficult and time consuming. For example, the definition of the health-related behaviors domain states that these problems require personal motivation on the part of the client,

thereby indicating that resolution of the problem may be more difficult (Simmons, 1980).

Utilizing the Omaha System to show the sequencing of care allows nurses to define and document adequately the complexity of care inherent in these other domains. For example, a patient with tuberculosis may be referred to an agency for monitoring and streptomycin injections. The nurse may begin by using the diagnosis of "respiration: impairment" (physiological domain) to follow the patient's physiological state. Upon assessment, however, it is found that the patient is not taking his medication regularly and is also consuming an excessive amount of alcohol. The diagnosis of "prescribed medication regimen: impairment" (health-related behavior domain) may then be added and a care plan developed to inform the patient of the consequences of not taking the medication and of mixing the medication with alcohol. On subsequent visits the situation may be no better, so that interventions are revised to include family counseling and the involvement of other community agencies. Eventually it is decided that the underlying problem is really alcoholism, and a third diagnosis, "substance use: actual" (also from the health-related behaviors domain), is identified and a relevant plan of care developed. Thus there is a clearly sequenced description of what was done in this case and how it required both changes in interventions and subsequent identification of additional nursing diagnoses from another domain. Additionally, the use of the problem rating scale provides the guide posts to evaluate whether the interventions made a difference in the patient's condition.

Furthermore, when this sequencing of care is done in advance for defined groups of patients, it becomes a standardized approach to care. This standardized approach can be called a critical path (defined as a predetermined sequencing and timing of care activities, including nursing, therapies, and medical interventions, through an expected course of care toward an expected outcome) for care that can be examined and compared over time or with other approaches. Critical paths were used by the National Aeronautics and Space Administration space program for activities that were time sensitive toward achievement of the overall goal; they began to be used in health care in the early 1970s. They have become popular today with managed care and the increased importance of meeting outcomes within a designated number of visits. Critical paths provide staff with guidelines for best practice (i.e., which activities or interventions lead to the best outcomes). Other benefits include standardization of documentation of care, delineation of role responsibility for each discipline involved in care (which also provides for greater interdisciplinary collaboration), improved resource management through comprehensive care planning, and a tool for teaching new staff and students how to care for a specific patient condition.

Most important, critical paths can be a valuable tool for quality improvement. In fact, without tying critical paths to the continuous quality improvement program, an agency may not see an improvement in outcomes or a reduction in costs. The key is the documenting, collecting, analyzing, and reporting of variances from the critical paths, or variance management (Schriefer, 1995). Both positive and negative variances are critical to identifying what works and what needs improvement. Analysis of the variations can be used to revise the critical path, encourage clinical practice to be consistent with the critical path, identify changes to length of stay and resource use, and utilize aggregated data for financial and care analyses (Coffey et al., 1995).

Not all patients can be grouped into critical paths; therefore, for these patients case management is more appropriate. Even for these cases, however, the Omaha System can improve quality within an agency. This scheme makes the nurse ask critical questions, such as: What data do I need to make a comprehensive assessment? Why am I visiting this case? Do I need to continue visiting? Is this a problem I can do something about, or is it best handled by another discipline or another agency? It also forces

agency administration to examine policy to determine whether there are existing policies or procedures that impede the team concept of care or hamper efficient patient-oriented care. For example, in one agency, usual procedure was to refer cases to the social worker using a referral form. The social worker did not have access to the patient chart. It became apparent, after implementation of the Omaha System, that the social worker needed not only access to the chart but also more intimate communication with the nurse because both often were working on the same patient problem and a common (supplemental) plan of care.

The building block for successful quality improvement programs and for successful competition within a managed care environment is data. The way to powerful data is documentation. Documentation improves with the use of the Omaha System because the scheme provides objective terminology rather than subjective descriptions and because it provides a unifying and organizing framework for care and therefore also for documentation. In an exploratory study done in New Jersey to determine the effectiveness of the Omaha System in improving the community health nurse's ability to identify patient health problems, it was found that, after nurses used the scheme for 6 months, there was an overall improvement in charting of patient information. This study involved three test agencies and four control agencies. Test agency staff members were educated in the use of the Omaha System; control agencies were not. Data were gathered using both pretesting and posttesting of staff and auditing of discharged patient charts. The charts were scored as a percentage of criteria met for each step in the nursing process. From pretest to posttest audits, an average net change for the experimental group, which implemented the Omaha System, over the control group, which did not implement it, was 11 percent (Cell et al., 1984).

The Omaha System was originally designed to be used with any documentation system used by an agency, whether problem oriented or narrative, based on flow sheets or encounter forms, or structured in any other way for a given agency (Simmons, 1980). In practice, however, it has been found that most agencies, at minimum, change their assessment forms at the time of implementation so that the information is organized using the four domains. It is also usually discovered that the assessment information required for using the Omaha System is more comprehensive than that found on the agency's current form. Therefore, the form is upgraded to become more comprehensive.

Improving documentation in community health is important because current documentation is redundant, not standardized; lacks the key aspects of care; and is expensive to retrieve for any type of analysis. Therefore, information that is needed for guiding practice, setting professional standards, fulfilling payer and surveyor requirements, benchmarking, establishing outcomes, and setting health care policy is missing (Raup and Westra, 1996). Furthermore, inadequate common denominators in charting have made it difficult for researchers to collect data across agencies. Thus it is difficult to generalize research findings to the industry at large.

The Outcome and Assessment Information Set (OASIS) has recently been released by Medicare to provide for standard outcome and assessment data across agencies (Shaughnessy and Crisler, 1995). Raup and Westra (1996) state that OASIS is easily integrated with the Omaha System and that, combined, they provide a comprehensive assessment care plan and evaluation of patient care. They meet the multiple demands for data and offer the clinical data necessary to shape future policy.

Once the language for community health care is standardized, it can then be more readily communicated from one nurse to another, to supervisors, to the patient, to other health workers, and to surveyors and payers. Finally, there is a way to remove the stereotype that home health care nurses only teach individuals with diabetes to give themselves insulin, insert Foleys, or remove fecal impactions on Friday afternoons. Providing hospital discharge coordinators, staff nurses, and others with a list of the 44 nursing diagnoses in the taxonomy helps them understand home health care nursing. Thus it is easier for these people to discern what type of patient is appropriate to refer for home care. Also, the standard nomenclature provided in the Omaha System means the same thing to everyone reading the chart, which facilitates both communication and understanding. No longer do supervisors and auditors have to peruse thick charts, trying to identify and evaluate the care rendered. Instead, use of the standard diagnoses, interventions, and outcomes allows anyone to follow the professional caregiver's movement through the problem-solving process.

ADMINISTRATIVE MANAGEMENT

Patient classification systems are valuable management tools for staffing, budgeting, monitoring productivity, costing, and program planning. Historically in home health care, however, classification has been more for the purpose of quality management than for resource allocation or costing. This is expected because the Medicare law of 1965 ensured optimal payment to all providers and makes no effort toward cost containment. The law, however, was accompanied by certification regulations that set forth standards for quality aimed at limiting participation in the program to those facilities that provide at least minimum care (Kurowski, 1980; Mundinger, 1983). Thus the motivation for enhancing quality was greater than the motivation for efficient use of resources. Today, with the evolution of managed care, the picture is different. With home health care agencies caring for more patients, sicker patients, and more high-technology patients and at the same time facing restrictive managed care agreements, efficient resource allocation and costing of services are of paramount importance. In response to this pinch in financial resources, some research has been done in home health care to discover possible critical indicators of care for a patient classification system that will predict resource consumption (Ballard and McNamara,

1983; Hardy, 1984; Sienkiewicz, 1984). What is needed, however, is the use of a nursing diagnosis taxonomy as the basis for categorization of patients. Such a taxonomy already exists in the form of the Omaha System, and this taxonomy defines the essence of home health care. Following are some advantages in using such a taxonomy.

Patient classification systems are used for program planning. The Omaha System provides the necessary information as a management tool for program planning. Analysis of specific nursing diagnoses addressed by nurses within a given agency allows the agency to devise and revise its programs systematically according to patient and community needs (Simmons, 1980). It gives the agency the necessary data to interface with other community agencies and leaders for solving suprasystem problems, such as identifying nutritional needs of patients that are not being met by the local food program. Ideally, categorization of patients would also link quality care to the reimbursement or costing of care, although current patient classification systems are limited in their ability to accomplish this.

The Omaha System as a nursing diagnosis taxonomy for community health both defines reimbursable nursing care under Medicare (facilitation of the medical treatment plan) and provides for a holistic assessment of the patient (Pankratz, 1985). Thus it provides for high-quality nursing care at home while at the same time surviving this world of regulation and cost containment. To prove the viability of this state-ment, a small, unpublished pilot study was done by this author in 1985 on 41 Medicare patient records in two separate home health agencies to determine whether the goals associated with the identified nursing diagnoses were being achieved under current Medicare law. Charts were selected from the total patient population for 1984 from these two agencies. Criteria for chart selection included Medicare payment, normative discharge (i.e., improved health status), nursing as the primary service used, and inclusion of the nursing diagnosis "integument: impairment." This diagnosis was used as a tracer. The findings indicated that proper use of the Omaha System for planning, documenting, and evaluating care allowed the attainment of 96 percent of the predetermined patient outcomes before the patient was discharged. Unfortunately, the study also showed that often the scheme was not being used at its maximum, resulting once more in inadequate documentation of home health care activities (Table 16–1).

Patient classification requires the use of critical indicators of care or essential characteristics. The Omaha System has been evaluated for its contribution to the essential characteristics that have an effect on nursing workload. In another unpublished study, it was hypothesized that the quantity of nursing care demanded would be a function of the patient's living arrangements and support system, age, sex, ability to perform activities of daily living, prior source of care, presence of surgical intervention, and nursing diagnosis. All the variables except the nursing

---

Table 16–1 Nursing Diagnoses Identified and Outcomes Met by Agency A (Visiting Nurse Association) and Agency B (Hospital-Based Agency)

Agency	Problems Identified	Problems Not Identified	Outcomes Met at Discharge[*]	Outcomes Not Met at Discharge[*]
A (n = 102)	76 (74.5%)	26 (25.5%)	64 (84.2%)	12 (15.8%)
B (n = 61)	41 (67.2%)	20 (32.8%)	39 (95.1%)	2 (4.9%)
Both (complete charts available)	27 (16.6%)		26 (96.0%)	

[*]Could not be determined for unidentified problems.

diagnosis had been measured in previous studies. This study consisted of 68 patient records from two home health agencies. The records were drawn from the total patient population of these agencies for 1984 using a random numbers table. The inclusion of nursing diagnoses with the variables from previous studies helped account for 41.9 percent of the variance in registered nurse visits. Ballard and McNamara (1983), who did not use nursing diagnoses, were only able to explain 31.9 percent of the total variance. In addition, the only variables to enter the regression equation for intensity of nursing visits (number of nursing visits to length of service) were nursing diagnoses. This may indicate that certain problems identified by nurses are especially predictive when one is examining the intensity of service rendered to a patient. Such a finding is important because reimbursements and technological reforms have led to more intense services being provided to home care patients.

Another study (Martin and Scheet, 1985) also indicates that the classification of nursing diagnoses may be an important way of examining the costs of home health care. This study found that the number of nursing diagnoses and race were significant in predicting length of agency service. Hays (1992) found not only that nursing diagnoses were a predictor of direct hours of nursing care but also that the use of potential and health promotion nursing diagnoses in the Omaha System increased the amount of prediction. Thus there is significant evidence that nursing diagnoses play an important part in the provision of home health care and in allocating resources (money and personnel) for that care. A nursing diagnosis taxonomy per se, however, cannot be used as a patient classification system because it categorizes nursing diagnoses, not patients. In a nursing diagnosis taxonomy, patients cannot be placed into mutually exclusive categories. In addition, a nursing diagnosis taxonomy uses the classificatory concepts of class membership, whereas a patient classification system uses the ordering concepts of precedence and coincidence. For example, a patient

to be classified in a patient classification system would be evaluated using established critical indicators of care and then would be placed into a level based on the importance or weight of the critical indicators connected with that patient's care. Nursing diagnoses within a taxonomy, however, could be used as the critical indicators of care for placing a patient into a level.

Work has been done on incorporating the Omaha System nursing diagnosis taxonomy into a patient classification system. The Community Health Intensity Rating Scale (CHIRS) was developed by expert groups of community health nurses based on 15 community health parameters inductively derived from the Omaha System. These parameters (Table 16–2) represent content areas of the four domains (environmental, psychosocial, physiological, and health-related behaviors) identified in the Omaha System.

CHIRS also utilizes the nursing process as the organizational structure within each parameter to provide for the definition of the patient's nursing requirements by both essential characteristics and critical indicators of care (i.e., assessment and evaluation steps reflect essential characteristics, and planning and implementation steps reflect critical indicators of care). Essential characteristics for each parameter are noted in Table 16–2. Critical indicators of care for all parameters are nursing diagnoses, other disciplines involved in care, discharge plan, teaching/guidance, monitoring/measurements, referral/coordination, and treatments/care. Incorporating the nursing process necessitated a prototype method of classification to avoid the artificial separation of actions (assessment, planning, implementation, and evaluation), which in reality are not separated. The scale delineates four categories or levels of care (minor, moderate, major, and extreme). Thus it includes four patient profiles for each of the 15 parameters, one profile to illustrate the extent of nursing input required for patient care within each level. Each profile includes several elements that define the steps of the nursing process for that level. For example, in the

Table 16–2 CHIRS Parameters

Parameter	Essential Characteristics
Environmental Domain	
Finances	Financial resources, employment, health insurance, money management
Physical environment/safety	Residence/living conditions, utilities, sanitation, neighborhood, pets, access to commercial services
Psychosocial Domain	
Community networking	Knowledge of resources, availability/use of resources, emergency plan
Family system	Family, family process/roles, caregiving system, social network, interpersonal relationships
Emotional/mental response	Adjustment/coping, emotional state, cultural attitudes, spiritual beliefs, mental status
Individual growth and development	Early development, sense of self, spiritual growth, adaptation to aging
Physiological Domain	
Sensory function	Sensory perception, pain/discomfort
Respiratory and circulatory function	Airway, breathing, cardiovascular status, tissue perfusion, endurance
Neuromusculoskeletal function	Consciousness, orientation, communication, speech, physical mobility
Reproductive/sexual function	Peripartum, sexual organs/menses, sexual practices
Digestion/elimination	Ingestion, assimilation, metabolism, bowel function, bladder habits, renal function
Structural integrity	Skin integrity, immune response
Health-Related Behaviors	
Nutrition	Food selection/preparation, diet, intake, eating, weight
Personal habits	Personal hygiene, exercise regimen, sleep habits, smoking, substance use
Health management	Engagement, technical skill, medications

parameter of nutrition, one of the elements in the assessment part of this parameter is weight, as addressed under the nursing diagnosis of nutrition in the Omaha System. This element is defined over the four levels as follows:

level 1, within normal limits for height

level 2, greater than 10 percent above or below ideal weight

level 3, greater than 25 percent above or below ideal weight

level 4, morbid obesity/severe emaciation

In scoring the tool, one rating is made for each parameter by selection of the appropriate patient profile. The overall rating is then calculated using an implicit integration of the ratings assigned to each parameter (Peters, 1988). Initial use of this scale on 560 cases from two different agencies significantly identified four subgroups in regard to the amount of their nursing requirements (Peters, 1988). This was supported in a second study of 237 cases in a third agency (Hays, 1992). In the original study, CHIRS explained 6 percent of the variation in amount of care provided by a nurse (Peters, 1988). In the second study, which was done using a revised CHIRS, the amount of variation explained was 10 percent (Hays, 1992).

CHIRS has been tested with several different community health groups, including patients with acquired immunodeficiency syndrome, high-risk prenatal clients and high-risk infants, high-technology and home care clients, and the homeless, and it is currently being adapted for use by school health nurses. In a study of 133 public health nursing clients from a midwestern city/county health department, a composite measure of nursing service was developed, called nursing effort, to capture nursing services that were provided both during and outside visits. This measure included the number of nursing visits, number of telephone calls to and on behalf of the client, and number of not home/not found visits. Use of this measure of nursing effort significantly increased the amount of variance explained by CHIRS (Hays, 1995). This indicates that CHIRS recognizes the time spent outside home visits and validates efforts such as phone calls, coordination activities, and other activities of indirect care. This is important because innovative interventions offered under managed care, such as electronic interventions and telephone visits, change the amount of direct contact in the home (Peters and Hays, 1995). Because CHIRS recognizes activities beyond direct care, it may prove to be a useful tool in measuring and costing services provided.

One means by which managed care is postulated to achieve cost savings is by focusing health care services to meet the needs of specific types of consumers or conditions. A secondary analysis of three data sets from these CHIRS studies found that the salient parameters varied depending on the population, indicating that home care is delivered to widely diverse groups and that aggregating data that may appear to go together may obscure important, unique information. No one parameter was significant across all three data sets. Furthermore, of the 12 salient parameters among the three study samples, only half were from the physio-logical domain, the domain that drives the medical model. Thus it seems that the medical model is insufficient to account for the care needed by community health clients (Hays et al., 1996). This is important information for agencies as they determine what care is appropriate to provide to their clients and who are the best practitioners to provide that care. Recognizing which parameters are important for their caseload assists agencies in determining the expertise and abilities needed by staff and what education and credentials are required.

CONCLUSION

Use of a nursing diagnosis taxonomy is valuable in defining, organizing, directing, and communicating home care. It provides the basis for quality and clinical management of care. Its use as a management tool for staffing and costing is limited, however, because it does not place patients into mutually exclusive categories. Nevertheless, research studies indicate that such a taxonomy does provide useful information in allocating resources.

A patient classification system (CHIRS) has been developed that incorporates the Omaha System taxonomy and categorizes patients into four levels of care. This system has the potential to measure costs and determine staffing levels as well as to address the qualitative issues of care. More work needs to be done, but the Omaha System and CHIRS provide agencies with valid and reliable tools for the clinical and administrative management of home care.

Quality improvement, outcomes benchmarking, and cost of care are some of the important activities that can be enhanced at the agency level. Perhaps even more important, however, is the opportunity for recognition of the value of home care's contribution to the health of the community. A standardized language and a comprehensive unit of service for costing are two of the products that will allow home care to find its place at the managed care table.

REFERENCES

Abdellah, F., and E. Levine. 1978. *Better patient care through nursing research.* 2d ed. New York: Macmillan.

Alward, R. 1983. Patient classification schemes; the ideal vs. reality. *Journal of Nursing Administration* 13:14–19.

American Nurses Association (ANA) 1974. *Standards of community health nursing practice.* Kansas City, MO: ANA.

Aydelotte, M.R. 1973. *Nurse staffing methodology.* DHEW Publication No. (NIH) 73-433. Washington, DC: Government Printing Office.

Ballard, S., and R. McNamara. 1983. Quantifying nursing needs in home health care. *Nursing Research* 32:236–241.

Bermas, N., and A. Van Slyck. 1984. Patient classification systems and the nursing department. *Hospitals* 58:99–100.

Brown, B.I. 1980. Realistic workloads for community health nurses. *Nursing Outlook* 28:233–237.

Cell, P., et al. 1984. Implementing a nursing diagnosis system through research: The New Jersey experience. *Home Healthcare Nurse* 2:26–32.

Coffey, R.J., et al. 1995. Extending the application of critical path methods. *Quality Management in Health Care* 3:14–19.

Giovannetti, P. 1979. Understanding patient classification systems. *Journal of Nursing Administration* 9:4–9.

Giovannetti, P., and M. Thiessen. 1983. *Patient classification for nurse staffing: Criteria for selection and implementation.* Edmonton, Alberta: Alberta Association of Registered Nurses.

Hardy, J.A. 1984. A patient classification system for home health patients. *Caring* 3:26–27.

Hays, B.J. 1992. Nursing care requirements and resource consumption in home health care. *Nursing Research* 41:138–143.

Hays, B.J. 1995. Nursing intensity as a predictor of resource consumption in public health nursing. *Nursing Research* 44:106–110.

Hays, B.J., et al. 1996. *The utility of CHIRS parameters in predicting resource consumption among community health nursing client populations: A secondary analysis.* Unpublished manuscript.

Hempel, C.G. 1952. *Fundamentals of concept formation in empirical science.* Chicago: University of Chicago Press.

Hempel, C.G. 1965. *Aspects of scientific explanation and other essays in the philosophy of science.* New York: Free Press.

Kurowski, B.T. 1980. *A cost-effectiveness analysis of home health care: Implications for public policy and future research.* PhD diss., University of Colorado, Denver.

Martin, K.S., and N.J. Scheet. 1985. The Omaha system: Implications for costing community health nursing. In F.A. Schaffer (Ed.), *Costing out nursing: Pricing our product* (pp. 197–206). New York: National League for Nursing.

Martin, K.S., and N.J. Scheet. 1991. *The Omaha system.* Philadelphia: Saunders.

Martin, K.S., et al. 1986. *Client management information system for community health nursing agencies: An implementation manual.* Rockville, MD: Division of Nursing, Department of Health and Human Services.

Mundinger, M.O. 1983. *Home care controversy: Too little, too late, too costly.* Gaithersburg, MD: Aspen.

Pankratz, J.D. 1985. *Serving two masters? Professional standards of care and reimbursable care.* Paper presented at the First National Symposium on Home Health Care, Ann Arbor, MI.

Peters, D.A. 1988. Development of a community health intensity rating scale. *Nursing Research* 37:202–207.

Peters, D.A., and B.J. Hays. 1995. Measuring the essence of nursing: A guide for future practice. *Journal of Professional Nursing* 11:358–363.

Raup, G., and B.L. Westra. 1996. *Alternate approaches to outcomes data—what provides value?* Paper presented at the Eleventh National Symposium on Home Health Care, Ann Arbor, MI.

Roy, C., Sr. 1975. A diagnostic classification system for nursing. *Nursing Outlook* 23:90–94.

Schriefer, J. (1995) Managing critical pathway variances. *Quality Management in Health Care* 3:30–42.

Shaughnessy, P.W., and K.S. Crisler. 1995. *Outcome-based quality improvement: A manual for home care agencies on how to use outcomes.* Washington DC: National Association for Home Care.

Sienkiewicz, J.I. 1984. Patient classification in community health nursing. *Nursing Outlook* 32:319–321.

Simmons, D.A. 1980. *A classification scheme for client problems in community health nursing* (DHHS Publication No. HRA 80–16). Washington, DC: Government Printing Office.

Sokal, R. 1974. Classification: Purposes, principles, progress, prospects. *Science* 185:1115–1123.

Watson, J. 1994. Have we arrived or are we on our way out? *Image* 26:86.

SUGGESTED READING

Peters, D.A. 1995. Outcomes: The mainstay of a framework for quality care. *Journal of Nursing Care Quality* 10:61–69.

Peters, D.A. 1992. A new look for quality in home care. *Journal of Nursing Administration* 22:21–26.

CHAPTER 17

Analysis and Management of Home Health Nursing Caseloads and Workloads

Judith Lloyd Storfjell, Carol Easley Allen, Cheryl E. Easley

BACKGROUND

Management of nursing productivity is critical to the financial viability of home health services agencies because nursing wages are usually the largest single budget item, often representing more than half the entire budget. Under fee-for-service payment (payment per visit), the focus of nursing productivity management has been increasing the number of nursing visits per day or month. As reimbursement methodologies shift to case rates and capitation, home visit efficiency is still essential, but the amount of nursing intervention required to accomplish a specific outcome may be even more important. In other words, it is increasingly necessary to monitor and control the number of visits per case as well as the number of visits per day. Coupled with this shift in reimbursement is an increasingly diverse client mix that includes not only highly acute cases but also more long-term cases.

To meet this challenge successfully, home care managers need to establish and monitor nursing productivity standards. These standards, however, have to take into account the type and complexity of care required by the client.

PURPOSE OF THE EASLEY-STORFJELL CASELOAD/ WORKLOAD ANALYSIS INSTRUMENTS

The Easley-Storfjell Instruments for Caseload/ Workload Analysis (CL/WLA) were designed to give home care nursing managers tools to plan, monitor, and evaluate nursing activities simply and effectively. They have been used successfully throughout the United States and Canada by a variety of home health and community health agencies since 1977. Their continuing use is due largely to their flexibility and adaptability to various types of settings and clients as well as their ease of use and acceptance by both managers and nursing staff. The following criteria were used in the development of these management tools:

- *Facilitate the supervisory process.* The chief purpose is to assist clinical managers in assignment of cases, to identify caseload problems and patterns, and to provide a format for supervisory conferences and discussions with staff. By periodic, joint review and rating of cases, a caseload and workload analysis can be combined easily with other nurse supervisor activities.

- *Be simple to use.* CL/WLA was kept extremely simple so that it would be easily understood by all levels of personnel. Rather than taking extra time from a busy manager's schedule, these instruments should reduce the amount of supervisory time required. Although they are presented here in a manual format, a number of organizations have incorporated them into computer applications.
- *Be flexible.* CL/WLA can be used with a variety of staffing patterns, including teams and individually managed caseloads. In addition, they can be adapted for use in many types of community health agencies and for various professionals who carry caseloads, including therapists, social workers, and case managers.
- *Include complexity, time, and intervention measures.* These three variables are seen as the key indicators for appropriate staffing and productivity planning.
- *Provide summary reports.* CL/WLA can be summarized by individual, team, office, district, or agency.
- *Be compatible with other tools.* Although the information obtained from CL/WLA is valuable in its own right, it can be augmented by data derived from other analyses, including activity-based costing and management, cost reports, and time studies.
- *Provide management information.* Some management uses of CL/WLA include projecting and evaluating staffing needs and monitoring trends. Findings can be compared with established standards or indicators.

DESCRIPTION OF THE CL/WLA PROCESS

There are two major components of the CL/WLA process: caseload analysis, which involves summarizing the characteristics of individual cases (or clients) carried and/or managed by an individual nurse; and workload analysis, which involves summarizing all activities required of the nurse, including caseload responsibilities. Home health nursing visits vary according to three critical dimensions: the number of visits required to provide care (time), the type of interventions used by the nurse during the visit, and the difficulty or complexity of the care provided.

Therefore, CL/WLA provides a description of a nurse's caseload according to time, type of intervention, and complexity of care factors. Both time and complexity are divided into four levels of intensity according to the frequency of visits and six difficulty of care variables. The third dimension, nursing interventions, is incorporated into the complexity scale.

There are five major activities (or interventions) that a nurse performs during a home visit:

1. assessing the client, environment, and plan of care (using clinical judgment)
2. teaching the client and caregivers
3. providing direct physical care to the client (technical tasks)
4. providing psychosocial support to the client and caregivers
5. coordinating care with other entities and persons (managing the case)

These five interventions are combined with an acuity measure (number of nursing problems) to form a patient classification system. This system has been shown to be both reliable and valid in grouping home care clients according to the complexity (difficulty) of their nursing care needs (Albrecht, 1991). It has also been used successfully independent of the CL/WLA process as a method for measuring complexity of care and to document the major home care nursing interventions (assessment, teaching, physical care, psychosocial support, and coordination/management).

The Easley-Storfjell process for analyzing caseload and workload consists of four steps:

1. Each case is analyzed to predict the number of visits required to accomplish estab-

lished goals and to determine the complexity of nursing care required.

2. Time and complexity ratings are charted on a visual graph.
3. Time for noncaseload work requirements or duties is calculated.
4. Findings are summarized, and the number of required visits is compared with the number possible according to the workload analysis.

INSTRUCTIONS FOR USE OF CL/WLA INSTRUMENTS

Specific instructions for completing the four steps outlined above follow.

Step 1

Complexity and number of visits are seen as the most important variables in assessing the level of nursing care required and the amount of work time needed. Therefore, these two factors are assessed separately.

The amount of time required is assigned a rating from 1 to 4 according to the following scale:

1, 1 visit or fewer per month
2, 2 to 3 visits per month
3, 1 to 2 visits per week
4, 3 to 5 visits per week

This scale can be adjusted by the individual agency according to actual patterns of visit intensity.

Complexity of care (difficulty) is determined by using the patient classification system, which is based on assessing six variables—the five nursing interventions and one severity of illness (acuity) indicator:

A, clinical judgment required (assessment needs)
B, teaching needs
C, physical care needs (technical procedures)
D, psychosocial support needs
E, coordination and care management needs

F, number and severity of problems

The complexity variables have also been assigned four categories on a 4-point scale from minimal complexity (1) to very great complexity (4). Descriptions of the nursing care requirements for each criterion or level of complexity are shown in Exhibit 17–1. These complexity levels may also be correlated by the agency with its typical levels of nursing practice and ancillary support.

It is often found that the best way to rate cases is through a joint conference between the clinical manager and the staff nurse. This process offers an opportunity for a generalized caseload review and specific planning for each case. During this conference, more accurate information regarding the current status of the client can be obtained, and care plans and goals can be identified. At the same time, the cases are listed on the caseload analysis roster (Exhibit 17–2) along with the ratings for time and complexity. Space also is provided for recording the length of time a case has been open, the appropriate program area or the client's diagnostic category, and the total number of visits required during the current month.

Step 2

The time and difficulty ratings are then charted on the caseload analysis graph (Exhibit 17–3) to obtain a graphic representation of the entire caseload. This chart, more than any other portion of the CL/WLA, has been beneficial in assisting the individual nurse in "visualizing" his or her caseload by depicting both the complexity and the time requirements of the entire caseload. The average number of monthly visits required by the caseload can also be calculated on this form if it was calculated on the caseload analysis roster.

Step 3

Home health nurses usually have other work responsibilities in addition to their caseload

Exhibit 17–1   CL/WLA Guidelines

TIME DETERMINATION

1. Monthly or less; only 1 visit
2. Biweekly
3. 1–2 times per week
4. 3–5 times per week

COMPLEXITY DETERMINATION

Assign the highest numerical categorical rating (most difficult) in which the case meets two or more of the criteria.
Based on:

A. Clinical judgment/assessment
B. Teaching/education needs
C. Physical care
D. Psychosocial needs
E. Coordination/management
F. Number and severity of problems

1. **Minimal**
   A. Requires limited judgment, use of common sense, observation of fairly predictable change in patient status
   B. Requires basic health teaching
   C. Requires no or simple maintenance care
   D. Requires ability to relate to patients and families
   E. Requires limited involvement of only one other provider/agency
   F. Few or uncomplicated problems

2. **Moderate**
   A. Requires use of basic problem-solving techniques, ability to make limited patient assessments
   B. Requires teaching related to common health problems
   C. Requires basic rehabilitation or use of uncomplicated technical skills
   D. Requires use of basic interpersonal relationship skills
   E. Requires limited involvement of two other providers/agencies
   F. Several problems with limited complexity

3. **Great**
   A. Requires use of well-developed problem-solving skills enhanced by comprehensive knowledge of physical and social sciences, ability to make patient and family assessments
   B. Requires teaching related to illness, complications and/or comprehensive health supervision
   C. Requires use of complicated technical skills
   D. Requires professional insight and intervention skills in coping with psychosocial needs
   E. Requires extensive involvement of at least one other provider/agency or coordination of several providers/agencies
   F. Several complicated problems

4. **Very Great**
   A. Requires use of creativity, ability to initiate and coordinate plan for patient or family care, use of additional resources and increased supervisory support, ability to make comprehensive patient and family assessment
   B. Requires teaching related to unusual health problems or teaching/learning difficulties
   C. Requires knowledge of scientific rationale that underlies techniques, ability to modify care in response to patient/family need
   D. Requires ability to intervene in severe psychosocial problems
   E. Requires extensive coordination of multiple providers/agencies
   F. Numerous or complicated problems requiring augmentation of the knowledge base

Exhibit 17–2   Caseload Analysis Roster

Name _____ Position _____ Date _____

Case Number/Name	Days/Weeks Open	Priority/ Program/ Diagnosis	Complexity Rating	Time Rating	Total Visits Required This Month
1.					
2.					
3.					
4.					
5.					
6.					
7.					
8.					
9.					
10.					
11.					
12.					
13.					
14.					
15.					
16.					
17.					
18.					
19.					
20.					
Totals					
Averages					

Exhibit 17–3   Caseload Analysis Graph

Name_____ Position _____ Date _____

Complexity

	1	2	3	4	Total Cases
4					
3					
2					
1					
Total Cases					

(Vertical axis label: **Time**)

Codes		
Time	**Complexity**	**Based On**
1: Monthly; One Visit	**1:** Minimal	**A:** Clinical Judgment (assessment)
2: Biweekly	**2:** Moderate	**B:** Teaching Needs (education)
3: One-Two Times per Week	**3:** Great	**C:** Physical Care
4: Three-Five Times per Week	**4:** Very Great	**D:** Psychosocial Needs
		E: Coordination
		F: Number & Severity of Problems

requirements. These assignments and duties also require a commitment of time. The time allocation worksheet (Exhibit 17–4) facilitates the calculation of the time needed for the range of duties that constitute the nurse's total workload. The following specific areas are included on the form:

- personal adjustments (vacation, sick time, holiday or paid days off)
- supportive activities (supervisor conferences, continuing education, committees, staff meetings)
- special assignments (teaching classes, hospital liaison, preceptoring)
- field activities (clinics, community meetings, committees)

Here again, because of the flexibility designed into the system, organizations can modify this tool to provide a realistic representation of their specific workload components.

When the time needed for non–client-related activities is subtracted from the total paid time, the time that remains for client-related activities (caseload duties) can be determined. This includes the time actually spent in the home with clients and time for travel to and from home visits, documentation of care provided, and coordination of care activities.

The information generated from the analysis of individual nurses' workloads can be grouped by team or department. Aggregate workload data are valuable in assessing workload requirements and allocating time for part or all of the nursing staff. By analysis of staff time, it is possible to document staffing needs and to adjust non–client-related work assignments.

Step 4

Finally, the caseload and workload time requirements are summarized on the top portion of the caseload/workload summary (Exhibit 17–5). The number of home visits that each nurse can make is calculated by dividing the total time available by the average time needed for a home visit. The average time per visit can

be determined by doing an actual time study or using organizational productivity standards. If either of these is not available, several studies have shown that an average home visit, including visit support time, often averages about 90 minutes (Storfjell, 1989a). The number of home visits required by the caseload can then be compared with the number of visits possible based on the workload requirements. By subtracting the average number of home visits required by the caseload from the number of visits possible based on available time, a determination can be made easily regarding the reasonableness of caseload requirements.

IMPLICATIONS

Analysis of nursing workloads and caseloads using the CL/WLA approach has implications for home health administrators, managers, and nursing staff as well as the home health industry as a whole.

Administrative Uses

It is important for home health managers to be able to project staffing needs and costs as well as to evaluate utilization of nursing staff. By compilation of data on comprehensive nursing resource demands, staffing needs can be compared with the use of time and the types of services being delivered (Allen et al., 1986).

Through repeated analyses, trends in service delivery can be ascertained. Data provided by workload trends for the entire organization may be used to determine or justify budgetary allocations for nursing staff. In addition, comparisons can be made between service trends and established goals and priorities.

CL/WLA differs from other productivity methodologies because it takes into account the complexity of nursing care required as well as time requirements. The impact of the case complexity as a cost driver can be studied, and case rates can be estimated by type of care adjusted for complexity. This approach to productivity measurement and management meshes well

Exhibit 17–4　Time Allocation Worksheet

Name _____**Position** _____ **Date**_____

Time Available (Monthly, Yearly)	_____

Time Utilization

1. Personal Adjustments:	Hours	Totals
a. Annual Leave/Holiday	_____	
b. Other_____ _____	_____ _____	_____

2. Supportive Activities:		
a. Supervisor/Nurse Conference	_____	
b. Staff Meetings	_____	
c. Continuing Education/Workshop	_____	
d. Committees	_____	
e. Other_____ _____	_____ _____	_____

3. Special Assignments:		
a. Classes	_____	
b. Hospital Liaison	_____	
c. Field Advisor	_____	
d. Other_____ _____	_____ _____	_____

4. Field Activities (Community Service):		
a. Committees/Meetings_____ _____	_____ _____	
b. Clinics		
c. Other_____ _____	_____ _____	_____

Total Scheduled Time	
Time Available for Home Visits, Consultation, Documentation, and Follow-Up	

Exhibit 17–5   Caseload/Workload Summary

Name _____ Position _____ Date_____

	Total	Average
A. Caseload		
1. Total cases	_____	_____
2. Time factor	_____	_____
3. Complexity factor	_____	_____
4. Total required H.V.'s	_____	_____
5. Average weeks open	_____	_____
6. Program categorical analysis (*priority/program/diagnosis*) _____ _____ _____ _____	_____ _____ _____ _____	_____ _____ _____ _____

	Monthly	Yearly
B. Time (monthly, yearly)		
1. Total time available	_____	_____
2. Scheduled time	_____	_____
3. Time available for H.V.'s	_____	_____
4. Time per home visit	_____	_____
5. Number of H.V.'s possible (*divide 3 by 4*)	_____	_____
6. Number of H.V.'s required by caseload	_____	_____
7. Number of H.V.'s to new referrals	_____	_____
8. TOTAL required H.V.'s	_____	_____
9. Excess H.V.'s required (*8 larger than 5*)	_____	_____
10. Additional H.V.'s possible (*5 larger than 6*)	_____	_____
11. Average mileage (*optional*)	_____	_____

with activity-based costing and management approaches. The CL/WLA tools can be modified to reflect the agency's standard activities and processes. Periodic reviews and updates can be entered into the activity-based costing and management models, and a more precise calculation of costs of products and activities can be tracked.

Clinical Manager Uses

CL/WLA allows clinical managers to base hiring decisions on projections of the nursing care demands of the overall agency's caseload and workload. The complexity profile of a caseload may indicate a need for a particular type of nursing staff, which will obviate underutilization of nursing skills. In this way, nursing costs can be managed effectively based on actual data that justify the budgetary requirements of nursing staff mix.

Because time utilization is individualized by assessment of all the workload activities for each nurse, many of the pitfalls encountered by assigning average productivity standards to specific individuals are avoided. If an individualized productivity monitoring tool is desired, the number of visits required by the caseload and the number of visits possible according to the workload analysis can be calculated easily on a monthly basis and compared with actual performance.

In addition to general staffing uses, the tools are especially beneficial for supervising individual nurses, especially for evaluating and adjusting individual case assignments. A concentration of high-complexity (social or medical) cases may signal a nurse's need for additional training or support, whereas a caseload complexity rating lower than the nurse's skill level may be the key to restlessness or low moral. Staff development needs can be identified from both individual and aggregate data. For example, if a particular nurse has a high percentage of clients with a certain diagnosis, continuing education in that area might be important.

The average length of time for which cases are open should alert the clinical manager to those nurses who either carry cases too long or close them too quickly. In addition, because initial visits are usually longer than repeat visits (Storfjell, 1989b), nurses with few visits per case may need to have lower productivity standards than nurses with more visits per case. The manager can monitor individual or aggregate productivity data by making a few adjustments to the forms to record and monitor the caseload at regular intervals. This allows the establishment of individual productivity standards based on the specific workload requirements of each nurse.

CL/WLA is also useful when cases are transferred to another nurse or in the orientation of new staff or managers. As home care organizations increase their use of part-time staff and team nursing to improve scheduling flexibility, it is even more important to have a readily available method of allocating cases among a varying group of nursing staff at any given time. The time and complexity ratings provide this capability. The most beneficial use of the CL/WLA process, however, continues to be for providing a framework for clinical managers and direct care providers to communicate and plan client care, including identifying the type of intervention needed, its complexity, and the time required.

Staff Uses

This systematic analysis allows nurses to organize their activities, streamline caseloads, and obtain a realistic picture of workload demands and expectations, all of which lead to greater efficiency, more appropriate time utilization, and increased cost effectiveness. Individual staff members can benefit when a realistic caseload and workload have been defined and goals for service delineated.

Industry Uses

Standards for nursing care based on professional ideals and goals must be established in home care. The model of care that will be recognized in home care nursing will be critically influenced by the patient classification system and the overall dimensions of the workload that are deemed appropriate by those private and public organizations that fund home care services. In addition to facilitating supervision, assisting staff with time management, and providing pertinent data for administrators, the Easley-Storfjell CL/WLA instruments can provide the home care industry with the data necessary to support resource utilization while demonstrating efficiency in management of personnel and finances. The patient classification system standardizes client complexity variables and also provides standard nursing interventions that can be used for quantification of nursing care in research endeavors.

CONCLUSION

Home health care nursing managers are increasingly being required to manage and document the type and quantity of services provided by the agencies that employ them and to reduce costs while increasing or maintaining service quality. The Easley-Storfjell CL/WLA instruments provide a more refined method of analyzing the home health nurse's caseload and workload, thus providing valuable management information for use by administrative, supervisory, and direct service personnel. The reliability and validity of the tools have been demonstrated, but, even more important, experience has shown them to be practical and extremely useful in various types of community health agencies.

REFERENCES

Albrecht, M.N. 1991. Home health care: Reliability and validity testing of a patient classification instrument. *Public Health Nursing* 5:124–131.

Allen, C.E., et al. 1986. Cost management through caseload–workload analysis. In *Patients and purse strings: Patient classification and cost management*, ed F. Shaffer, 331–446. New York: National League for Nursing.

Storfjell, J.L. 1989a. Home care productivity: Is the home visit an adequate measure? *Caring* 8:60–65.

Storfjell, J.L. 1989b. How valuable are nurses' skills? A case for fair pricing in home health care. *Nursing and Health Care* 10:310–313.

CHAPTER 18

The Home Health Care Classification of Nursing: Diagnoses and Interventions

Virginia K. Saba

To develop a method to assess and classify home health Medicare patients to predict their need for nursing and other home care services as well as their outcomes of care, data on actual measures of resources employed were used to predict resource requirements. A national sample of 646 home health agencies, randomly stratified by staff size, type of ownership, and geographic location, participated in the study. The home health agencies collected data on 8,961 newly discharged cases using a specially designed abstract form. Each case represented a patient's entire episode of home health care from admission to discharge.

HOME HEALTH CARE COMPONENTS

The 20 home health care components (HHCCs) shown in Exhibit 18–1 provide the framework for the classification and coding of nursing diagnoses and nursing interventions. They were empirically developed to categorize, process, and statistically analyze the data for the two variables from the study patients. An HHCC is defined as a category that represents a functional, physiological, psychological, or behavioral home health care pattern. Each HHCC represents a unique category used to assess patient care requirements and to measure resources used and patient outcomes.

DEVELOPMENTAL STRATEGY

The HHCC nursing diagnoses and nursing interventions were designed for the computer processing and analysis of the study data. As part of the study protocol, two open-ended questions were included on the abstract form to

Exhibit 18–1 HHCC Framework

A. Activity component
B. Bowel elimination component
C. Cardiac component
D. Cognitive component
E. Coping component
F. Fluid volume component
G. Health behavior component
H. Medication component
I. Metabolic component
J. Nutritional component
K. Physical regulation component
L. Respiratory component
M. Role relationship component
N. Safety component
O. Self-care component
P. Self-concept component
Q. Sensory component
R. Skin integrity component
S. Tissue perfusion component
T. Urinary elimination component

Source: Reprinted by permission of the National Association for Home Care, from *Caring* magazine, Vol. XI, No. 3, March 1992. Not for further reproduction.

collect: nursing diagnoses and/or patient problems, and nursing services. The narrative answers consisted of statements collected from records of the study patients for the entire episode of home health care. The first question included all nursing diagnoses or patient problems assessed by the primary nurse as the major reasons why the patient needed home health care. Also collected was the disposition of each nursing diagnosis or patient problem on discharge. The second question included all skilled nursing services, significant treatments, activities, and interventions provided by the nurses during the episode.

At that time there did not exist a classification or coding scheme specific to home health care for either nursing diagnoses or nursing interventions. Initially the narrative text collected from the first 1,000 patients was entered into a computerized database to determine common terms. By using permuted key word sorts, like terms were sorted and clustered. Examples of groupings follow:

- nursing diagnoses: alteration in comfort, alteration in pain, and alteration in comfort due to pain were clustered as comfort alteration.
- nursing interventions: instruct wound healing and teach wound care were clustered in two ways: instruct and teach were clustered because teach and instruct became synonyms and wound healing and wound care were clustered as wound care.

Hundreds of other key word sorts were analyzed. The terms for the nursing diagnoses and nursing interventions were not only sorted separately but also matched together by patient. By using this technique, the research staff developed a tentative list of approximately 200 discrete nursing diagnoses and 800 discrete interventions. After further testing and refinement, the two classification and coding schemes were finalized and used to code the two questions.

NURSING DIAGNOSES

All nursing diagnoses and/or patient problems were collected for an entire episode of home health care for each study patient. They were assessed by the primary nurse as requiring nursing services.

A nursing diagnosis (North American Nursing Diagnosis Association [NANDA], 1990) is "a clinical judgment about individual, family, or community responses to actual or potential health problems/life processes. Nursing diagnoses provide the basis for selection of nursing interventions to achieve outcomes for which the nurse is accountable."

Classification Strategy

The nursing diagnosis statements were coded using an adapted version of the Nursing Diagnosis Taxonomy 1 (Fitzpatrick et al., 1989). The taxonomy was expanded and modified to include other home health diagnostic conditions. It resulted in a classification scheme consisting of 145 nursing diagnoses (50 two-digit major categories divided into 95 three-digit subcategories). This was used to code the 40,361 nursing diagnoses and/or patient problems collected from the study patients.

Expected Outcomes

Expected outcomes were considered outcome measures of home health care and were also collected for the nursing diagnoses. The patients' nursing diagnoses were evaluated by the primary nurse on discharge from home health care. They were coded using one of three conditions: improved, stabilized, and deteriorated.

NURSING INTERVENTIONS

All nursing interventions were collected for the entire episode of home health care. They included not only the 28 Health Care Financing Administration (HCFA) skilled treatment codes (HCFA, 1977) but also the coded narrative statements collected from the open-ended question.

A nursing intervention is defined as a nursing service, significant treatment, intervention, or activity identified to carry out the medical and nursing order. Patient services are usually initiated as medical orders by the referring physician and are reviewed by the primary nurse on admission. As part of the admission assessment, the primary nurse also identifies the nursing orders based on the nursing diagnoses or patient problems, and together they form a plan of care for the patient.

Classification Strategy

The classification strategy for the narrative statements included not only the development of the nursing intervention categories and subcategories but also a suffix to code the type of nursing intervention action.

In testing and examining the data, it was noted that there were generally two aspects to a nursing service statement: the service itself and the action modifying it. Four different types of nursing actions appeared over and over again: assessment, direct care, teaching, and management of nursing services. A strategy using different codes to depict these four types of actions reduced the list of nursing interventions and simplified the coding process.

The nursing actions are categorized as follows:

- assess: collect and analyze data on health status
- direct care: perform a therapeutic action
- teach: provide knowledge and skill
- manage: coordinate and refer

The final classification scheme consisted of 160 nursing interventions (60 two-digit major categories divided into 100 three-digit subcategories). This was used to code the 80,283 nursing services, the largest volume of nursing services ever collected on patients receiving home health care.

CODING FRAMEWORK

The nursing diagnoses and nursing intervention classification schemes also required a coding framework to facilitate computer processing. Using the format of the 10th revision of the *International Classification of Diseases,* a five-character alphanumeric code was developed (World Health Organization, 1990).

The code consisted of an alphabetic character in the first position for the HHCC, followed by two numeric digits for the major category, followed by two decimal digits, the fourth for a subcategory and the fifth for the modifier.

The modifiers were different for each of the two classifications. For nursing diagnoses the modifiers were used to code the expected outcome on discharge as follows: code 1 for improved, code 2 for stabilized, and code 3 for deteriorated. For nursing interventions the modifiers were used to code the type of action as follows: code 1 for assess, code 2 for direct care, code 3 for teach, and code 4 for manage.

Nursing Diagnoses

The nursing diagnosis coding scheme uses the five-character alphanumeric code. A nursing diagnosis can be coded with or without an expected outcome (Figure 18–1).

Nursing Interventions

A similar five-character code is used for the nursing interventions coding scheme, but the type of action is included as a suffix using the fifth digit (Figure 18–2).

ANALYSIS

The study data were analyzed using a variety of statistical methods. Frequency distributions were tested and analyzed to develop appropriate groupings that were statistically significant and could be used for the analytical models.

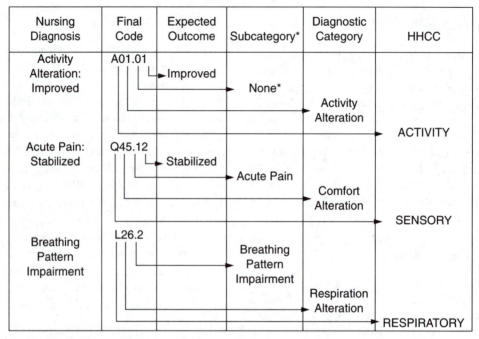

*Insert zero for none or blank.

Figure 18–1 Examples of nursing diagnoses with and without expected outcome codes.

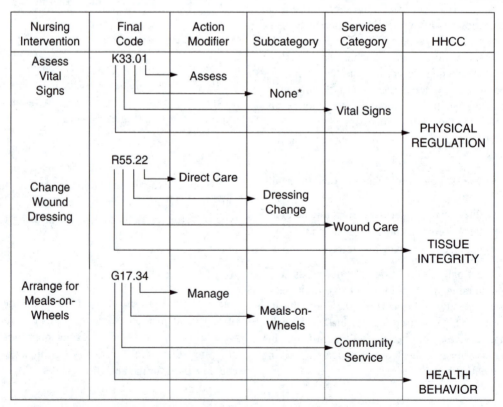

*Insert zero for none or blank.

Figure 18–2 Examples of nursing interventions with types of action codes.

Nursing Diagnoses

Several different groupings of nursing diagnostic categories were tested to determine which were the most relevant and the best predictors of home health care requirements. NANDA's 9 human response patterns (NANDA, 1990), Gordon's 11 functional health patterns (1982), and other groupings such as 10 physiological body systems were used. It was determined, however, that the 20 HHCCs were the most relevant groupings and the most usable for the statistical analyses. They were determined to be highly predictive of resource requirements (Exhibit 18–2) for the nursing diagnosis HHCC and coding scheme.

Nursing Interventions

The nursing interventions were considered critical measures of the actual resources used. The groupings that were tested and analyzed to determine the most relevant ones included using the detailed list of 60 major categories, four types of nursing intervention actions, and combinations of both. It was determined that the 20 HHCCs were the most relevant and most usable for measuring the actual resources provided (Exhibit 18–3) for the nursing interventions and coding scheme (Saba et al., 1991).

Both schemes are being used in computer-based HHCC systems.

IMPLICATIONS

The classification of home health care nursing diagnoses and interventions using the 20 HHCCs as its framework provides a new structure for classifying and coding home health care. These classifications are based on clinical knowledge and empirical data and provide an analytical model for measuring and evaluating home health care.

They offer a new approach for structuring the patient record, documenting the process of care, and determining resource requirements. In addtion, they can be used as the data dictionary for including clinical practice elements into computerized information systems. The classifications can contribute to the knowledge base on nursing and other related services for the home health care industry.

The next step is to use these schemes to document current home health nursing practice modalities. In this way, deficiencies can be determined and refinements made. Other research and practice settings, such as ambulatory care and long-term care facilities, may also find the classification of home health care nursing diagnoses and interventions useful.

Exhibit 18–2 Home Health Care Classification (HHCC) of Nursing Diagnoses and Coding Scheme: 50 Major Categories and 95 Subcategories

I. **CODING STRUCTURE**
- HHCC: first alphabetical code A to T
- Nursing diagnosis major category: second/third digit 01 to 50
- Nursing diagnosis subcategory: fourth decimal digit 1 to 9
- Discharge status/goal: fifth digit 1 to 3 (use only one: 1, improved; 2, stabilized; 3, deteriorated)

II. **50 NURSING DIAGNOSIS MAJOR CATEGORIES AND 95 SUBCATEGORIES**

  A. Activity component
  01 Activity Alteration
    01.1 Activity intolerance
    01.2 Activity intolerance risk
    01.3 Diversional activity deficit
    01.4 Fatigue
    01.5 Physical mobility impairment
    01.6 Sleep pattern disturbance
  02 Musculoskeletal Alteration

  B. Bowel Elimination Component
  03 Bowel Elimination Alteration
    03.1 Bowel incontinence
    03.2 Colonic constipation
    03.3 Diarrhea
    03.4 Fecal impaction
    03.5 Perceived constipation
    03.6 Unspecified constipation
  04 Gastrointestinal Alteration

  C. Cardiac Component
  05 Cardiac Output Alteration
  06 Cardiovascular Alteration
    06.1 Blood pressure alteration

  D. Cognitive Component
  07 Cerebral Alteration
  08 Knowledge Deficit
    08.1 Knowledge deficit of diagnostic test
    08.2 Knowledge deficit of dietary regimen
    08.3 Knowledge deficit of disease process
    08.4 Knowledge deficit of fluid volume
    08.5 Knowledge deficit of medication regimen
    08.6 Knowledge deficit of safety precautions

      08.7 Knowledge deficit of therapeutic regimen
  09 Thought Processes Alteration

  E. Coping Component
  10 Dying Process
  11 Family Coping Impairment
    11.1 Compromised family coping
    11.2 Disabled family coping
  12 Individual Coping Impairment
    12.1 Adjustment impairment
    12.2 Decisional conflict
    12.3 Defensive coping
    12.4 Denial
  13 Post-Trauma Response
    13.1 Rape trauma syndrome
  14 Spiritual State Alteration
    14.1 Spiritual distress

  F. Fluid Volume Component
  15 Fluid Volume Alteration
    15.1 Fluid volume deficit
    15.2 Fluid volume deficit risk
    15.3 Fluid volume excess
    15.4 Fluid volume excess risk

  G. Health Behavior Component
  16 Growth and Development Alteration
  17 Health Maintenance Alteration
  18 Health-Seeking Behavior Alteration
  19 Home Maintenance Alteration
  20 Noncompliance
    20.1 Noncompliance of diagnostic test
    20.2 Noncompliance of dietary regimen
    20.3 Noncompliance of fluid volume
    20.4 Noncompliance of medication regimen
    20.5 Noncompliance of safety precautions
    20.6 Noncompliance of therapeutic regimen

  H. Medication Component
  21 Medication Risk
    21.1 Polypharmacy

  I. Metabolic Component
  22 Endocrine Alteration
  23 Immunologic Alteration
    23.1 Protection alteration

  J. Nutritional Component
  24 Nutrition Alteration
    24.1 Body nutrition deficit

continues

Exhibit 18–2   continued

24.2 Body nutrition deficit risk
24.3 Body nutrition excess
24.4 Body nutrition excess risk
K. Physical Regulation Component
25 Physical Regulation Alteration
    25.1 Dysreflexia
    25.2 Hyperthermia
    25.3 Hypothermia
    25.4 Thermoregulation impairment
    25.5 Infection risk
    25.6 Infection unspecified
L. Respiratory Component
26 Respiration Alteration
    26.1 Airway clearance impairment
    26.2 Breathing pattern impairment
    26.3 Gas exchange impairment
M. Role Relationship Component
27 Role Performance Alteration
    27.1 Parental role conflict
    27.2 Parenting alteration
    27.3 Sexual dysfunction
28 Communication Impairment
    28.1 Verbal impairment
29 Family Processes Alteration
30 Grieving
    30.1 Anticipatory grieving
    30.2 Dysfunctional grieving
31 Sexuality Patterns Alteration
32 Socialization Alteration
    32.1 Social interaction alteration
    32.2 Social isolation
N. Safety Component
33 Injury Risk
    33.1 Aspiration risk
    33.2 Disuse syndrome
    33.3 Poisoning risk
    33.4 Suffocation risk
    33.5 Trauma risk
34 Violence Risk
O. Self-Care Component
35 Bathing/Hygiene Deficit
36 Dressing/Grooming Deficit
37 Feeding Deficit
    37.1 Breastfeeding impairment
    37.2 Swallowing impairment
38 Self-Care Deficit
    38.1 Activities of daily living alteration

38.2 Instrumental activities of daily
    living alteration
39 Toileting Deficit
P. Self-Concept Component
40 Anxiety
41 Fear
42 Meaningfulness Alteration
    42.1 Hopelessness
    42.2 Powerlessness
43 Self-Concept Alteration
    43.1 Body image disturbance
    43.2 Personal identity disturbance
    43.3 Chronic low self-esteem disturbance
    43.4 Situational self-esteem disturbance
Q. Sensory Component
44 Sensory Perceptual Alteration
    44.1 Auditory alteration
    44.2 Gustatory alteration
    44.3 Kinesthetic alteration
    44.4 Olfactory alteration
    44.5 Tactile alteration
    44.6 Unilateral neglect
    44.7 Visual alteration
45 Comfort Alteration
    45.1 Acute pain
    45.2 Chronic pain
    45.3 Unspecified pain
R. Skin Integrity Component
46 Tissue Integrity Alteration
    46.1 Oral mucous membranes impair-
    ment
    46.2 Skin integrity impairment
    46.3 Skin integrity impairment risk
    46.4 Skin incision
47 Peripheral Alteration
S. Tissue Perfusion Component
48 Tissue Perfusion Alteration
T. Urinary Elimination Component
49 Urinary Elimination Alteration
    49.1 Functional urinary incontinence
    49.2 Reflex urinary incontinence
    49.3 Stress urinary incontinence
    49.4 Total urinary incontinence
    49.5 Urge urinary incontinence
    49.6 Urinary retention
50 Renal Alteration

Source: Adapted from North American Nursing Diagnosis Association (NANDA, 1992). NANDA Nursing Diagnoses: Definitions and Classification 1992–1993, Philadelphia, PA: NANDA.

Exhibit 18–3 Home Health Care Classification (HHCC) of Nursing Interventions and Coding Scheme: 60 Major Categories and 100 Subcategories

I. **CODING STRUCTURE**
- HHCC: first alphabetical code A to T
- Nursing intervention major category: second/third digit 01 to 50
- Nursing intervention subcategory: fourth decimal digit 1 to 9
- Type of nursing action: fifth digit 1 to 4 (use only one: 1. assess; 2, care; 3, teach; 4, manage)

II. **60 NURSING INTERVENTION MAJOR CATEGORIES AND 100 SUBCATEGORIES**

A. Activity Component
01 Activity Care
  01.1 Cardiac rehabilitation
  01.2 Energy conservation
02 Fracture Care
  02.1 Cast care
  02.2 Immobilizer
03 Mobility Therapy
  03.1 Ambulation therapy
  03.2 Assistive device therapy
  03.3 Transfer care
04 Sleep Pattern Care
05 Rehabilitation Care
  05.1 Range of motion
  05.2 Rehabilitation exercise

B. Bowel Elimination Component
06 Bowel Care
  06.1 Bowel training
  06.2 Disimpaction
  06.3 Enema
07 Ostomy Care
  07.1 Ostomy irrigation

C. Cardiac Component
08 Cardiac Care
09 Pacemaker Care

D. Cognitive Component
10 Behavior Care
11 Reality Orientation

E. Coping Component
12 Counseling Service
  12.1 Coping support
  12.2 Stress control
13 Emotional Support
  13.1 Spiritual comfort
14 Terminal Care

  14.1 Bereavement support
  14.2 Dying/death measures
  14.3 Funeral arrangements

F. Fluid Volume Component
15 Fluid Therapy
  15.1 Hydration status
  15.2 Intake/output
16 Infusion Care
  16.1 Intravenous care
  16.2 Venous catheter care

G. Health Behavior Component
17 Community Special Programs
  17.1 Adult day center
  17.2 Hospice
  17.3 Meals-on-Wheels
  17.4 Other community special program
18 Compliance Care
  18.1 Compliance with diet
  18.2 Compliance with fluid volume
  18.3 Compliance with medical regime
  18.4 Compliance with medication regime
  18.5 Compliance with safety precautions
  18.6 Compliance with therapeutic regime
19 Nursing Contact
  19.1 Bill of rights
  19.2 Nursing care coordination
  19.3 Nursing status report
20 Physician Contact
  20.1 Medical regime orders
  20.2 Physician status report
21 Professional/Ancillary Services
  21.1 Home health aide service
  21.2 Medical social worker service
  21.3 Nurse specialist service
  21.4 Occupational therapist service
  21.5 Physical therapist service
  21.6 Speech therapist service
  21.7 Other ancillary service
  21.8 Other professional service

H. Medication Component
22 Chemotherapy Care
23 Injection Administration
  23.1 Insulin injection
  23.2 Vitamin B_{12} injection
24 Medication Administration
  24.1 Medication actions
  24.2 Medication prefill preparation

continues

Exhibit 18–3 continued

24.3 Medication side effects
25 Radiation Therapy Care
I. Metabolic Component
26 Allergic Reaction Care
27 Diabetic Care
J. Nutritional Component
28 Gastrostomy/Nasogastric Tube Care
  28.1 Gastrostomy/nasogastric tube insertion
  28.2 Gastrostomy/nasogastric tube irrigation
29 Nutrition Care
  29.1 Enteral/parenteral feeding
  29.2 Feeding technique
  29.3 Regular diet
  29.4 Special diet
K. Physical Regulatory Component
30 Infection Control
  30.1 Universal precautions
31 Physical Health Care
  31.1 Health history
  31.2 Health promotion
  31.3 Physical examination
  31.4 Physical measurements
32 Specimen Analysis
  32.1 Blood specimen analysis
  32.2 Stool specimen analysis
  32.3 Urine specimen analysis
  32.4 Other specimen analysis
33 Vital Signs
  33.1 Blood pressure
  33.2 Temperature/pulse respiration
34 Weight Control
L. Respiratory Component
35 Oxygen Therapy Care
36 Respiratory Care
  36.1 Breathing exercises
  36.2 Chest physiotherapy
  36.3 Inhalation therapy
  36.4 Ventilator care
37 Tracheostomy Care
M. Role Relationship Component
38 Communication Care
39 Psychosocial Analysis
  39.1 Home situation analysis
  39.2 Interpersonal dynamics analysis

N. Safety Component
40 Abuse Control
41 Emergency Care
42 Safety Precautions
  42.1 Environmental safety
  42.2 Equipment safety
  42.3 Individual safety
O. Self-Care Component
43 Personal Care
  43.1 Activities of daily living
  43.2 Instrumental activities of daily living
44 Bedbound Care
44.1 Positioning therapy
P. Self-Concept Component
45 Mental Health Care
  45.1 Mental health history
  45.2 Mental health promotion
  45.3 Mental health screening
  45.4 Mental health treatment
46 Violence Control
Q. Sensory Component
47 Pain Control
48 Comfort Care
49 Ear Care
  49.1 Hearing aid care
  49.2 Wax removal
50 Eye care
  50.1 Cataract care
R. Skin Integrity Component
51 Decubitus Care
  51.1 Decubitus stage 1
  51.2 Decubitus stage 2
  51.3 Decubitus stage 3
  51.4 Decubitus stage 4
52 Edema Control
53 Mouth Care
53.1 Denture care
54 Skin Care
  54.1 Skin breakdown control
55 Wound Care
  55.1 Drainage tube care
  55.2 Dressing change
  55.3 Incision care
S. Tissue Perfusion Component
56 Foot Care
57 Perineal Care

continues

Exhibit 18–3   continued

T. Urinary Elimination Component	60 Urinary Catheter Care
58 Bladder Care	60.1 Urinary catheter insertion
58.1 Bladder instillation	60.1 Urinary catheter irrigation
58.2 Bladder training	60.2 Urinary catheter irrigation
59 Dialysis Care	

REFERENCES

Fitzpatrick. J.J., et al. 1989. Translating nursing diagnosis into ICD code. *American Journal of Nursing* 89(4):493–495.

Gordon, M. 1982. *Manual of nursing diagnosis.* New York: McGraw-Hill.

North American Nursing Diagnosis Association (NANDA). 1990. *Taxonomy I: Revised 1992.* St. Louis: NANDA.

Saba, V.K., et al. 1991. *Final report: Develop and demonstrate a method for classifying home health patients to predict resource requirements and to measure outcomes* (HCFA Pub. No. 17-C-98983/3). Washington, DC: Unpublished.

Health Care Financing Administration (HCFA). 1977. *Medicare home health agency manual* (HCFA Pub. No. HIM11). Washington, DC: HCFA.

World Health Organization (WHO). 1990. *Final draft proposal for the tenth revision of the international classification of diseases (ICD-10).* Geneva: WHO.

CHAPTER 19

Nursing Diagnoses in Community Health Nursing

Carol Ann Parente

THE CONCEPT

The concept of nursing diagnoses may initially strike the community health administrator as more appropriate for clinical use. After all, of what use is an alteration in skin integrity at budget time? The definition and application of nursing diagnoses would definitely seem more valuable to those who provide direct patient services and their immediate supervisors. The nursing diagnosis concept, however, may prove to be valuable indeed to the administrative team, as demonstrated in this chapter. Discussions of nursing diagnoses in recent literature generally focus on their clinical uses and benefits. This chapter, however, discusses the concept, process, and effects of nursing diagnoses from a community health administrative perspective.

Nursing diagnosis represents the continuing steps in the profession's attempts to define its scope and science. Controversy has swirled around the concept since its inception. The debate continues today regarding the appropriateness of identified diagnoses (Jacoby, 1985), the taxonomy selected (Lunney, 1982), and even the idea of diagnoses made by nurses (Shamansky and Yanni, 1983). Some investigators (Sherwood et al., 1988) take issue with specific diagnostic labels, such as *noncompliance* and *knowledge deficit*. Mitchell (1991) proposes that ethical dilemmas surrounding the diagnos-

tic process negate the usefulness of nursing diagnoses and in fact may undermine professional growth.

Proponents focus on the value of a common language, which offers nursing a minimum data set across practice settings and a theoretical and pragmatic foundation for eventual direct reimbursement of nursing activities (Gordon, 1987). More recently, Carpenito (1995b) cites nursing diagnoses as leading to a clearer identification of the body of nursing knowledge, promoting greater accountability and ultimately greater professional autonomy.

In spite of the debate, or perhaps because of it, the concept of nursing diagnoses has continued to gain acceptance and widespread use since the first National Conference on Classification of Nursing Diagnoses, which was convened in St. Louis in the early 1970s. The concept has become well entrenched at all levels of education and in various fields of practice. Indeed, the American Nurses Association (ANA), in its social policy statement of 1980, described nursing as "the diagnosis and treatment of human responses to actual and potential health problems" (ANA, 1980a, 9). In 1995, the ANA's social policy statement cited "the application of scientific knowledge to the processes of diagnosis and treatment" as an essential feature of contemporary nursing practice (ANA, 1995, 6). The ANA's *Standards of Community*

225

Health Nursing Practice further elaborates on nursing diagnoses as being derived from health status data and leading to subsequent goals and interventions (ANA, 1986). The ANA clearly sees the nursing diagnostic process as a key nursing function that is vital to providing quality professional nursing care. In addition, many state nurse practice acts now include the nursing diagnosis as part of the defined functions of the professional nurse.

Nursing diagnoses evolved over several paths during the 1970s and 1980s. The most commonly accepted format emerged from the North American Nursing Diagnosis Association (NANDA). This group evolved from the National Conference Group on Classification of Nursing Diagnoses. The NANDA diagnosis list may be used by nurses in all clinical fields. Over the years since the first National Conference on the Classification of Nursing Diagnoses in 1973, the list of diagnoses has been revised slowly. Current diagnoses represent the series of conferences and refinements since the first NANDA conference. From the original list of 34, the number of nursing diagnoses has grown to 123 (Carpenito, 1995b). Considering the number of medical diagnoses available, it is clear that we are still making our first steps in this area.

Classification of nursing diagnoses in the NANDA system makes use of nine broad human response categories: exchanging, communicating, relating, valuing, choosing, moving, perceiving, knowing, and feeling. Nursing diagnoses in these categories range from the physiological (e.g., altered nutrition in the exchanging category) to the spiritual (e.g., spiritual distress) and the psychosocial (e.g., ineffective individual coping). Diagnoses related to activities of daily living are found within the moving category; sensory input and self-concept diagnoses are located in the perceiving category. Knowledge deficit is a diagnosis under knowing, and the feeling category includes diagnoses such as pain, anxiety, and grieving (Carroll-Johnson, 1991).

Nursing diagnoses differ, however, from our medical colleagues' diagnostic categories by defining actual or potential human responses to health problems (Gordon, 1976) rather than describing specific disease or illness states. Furthermore, the ninth NANDA conference described nursing diagnoses as including individual, family, or community response to actual or potential health problems or life situations (NANDA, 1992). The relationship of nursing diagnoses to medical diagnoses may in one sense be demonstrated in the problem-etiology-symptom format of nursing diagnoses as described by Gordon (1982). Here, the nursing diagnosis is the problem or first part of the diagnostic statement. The etiology, second in the statement format, is shown in relationship to the problem and is often (but not always) the medical illness or treatment. Resulting symptoms form the last part of the diagnosis and further individualize the nursing diagnosis to reflect a specific patient's problem. An example is as follows: alteration in nutrition, less than body requirements related to chemotherapy resulting in anorexia, and taste changes. The relationship of the nursing diagnosis to the medical diagnosis is one that must be considered carefully by the community health administrator in these days of close scrutiny by third party payers for reimbursable services.

Another nursing diagnosis group is of particular interest to community health administrators and nursing staffs. The Omaha Visiting Nurse Association (Simmons, 1980), under a 1977 contract with the Division of Nursing, Human Resources Administration, Department of Health and Human Services (DHHS), defined and tested a patient diagnostic and classification scheme. Four domains of nursing endeavor (environmental, psychosocial, physiological, and health behaviors) were defined, and related diagnoses were elaborated. The diagnostic categories resemble the NANDA list in some areas and define other diagnoses with more direct community health impact, such as income and sanitation deficits. The structure of the diagnosis scheme, now known as the Omaha System, is somewhat similar to the NANDA format. The Omaha diagnosis is listed first and is individualized for a particular patient by the use of modifiers, which are specific for each diagnosis. The Omaha System was structured initially to be computerized, further enhancing its usefulness to the community health administrator. This built-in computerization allows the administrator to maximize the information available about an agency's population.

The home health care components (HHCCs; Saba, 1992) represent an adaptation of the NANDA taxonomy I and include classification and coding of both nursing diagnoses and interventions gathered from a national sample of 646 home health agencies. Twenty HHCCs were derived from the data to categorize nursing diagnoses and interventions (Saba, 1992). Diagnoses and interventions are coded under each HHCC as discharge status/goals for diagnoses and actions are coded under interventions. This integration of diagnosis, intervention, and outcome is designed for computerization and retrieval of data that are useful for administrators.

Some authorities (Campbell, 1978; Lunney, 1982) suggest variations on the diagnostic taxonomy in response to patient and nursing needs. Of particular concern are the areas of wellness care and the independent versus interdependent actions of the nurse. Most NANDA diagnoses indicate a problem with the patient's health and/or his or her response to health. The Omaha System does address wellness or health behaviors to some extent. Unfortunately, wellness care is not fully addressed by the diagnostic labels, and equally unfortunately it is not reimbursable in the current third party payer environment. Recently, participants at NANDA conferences have developed axes such as unit of analysis (i.e., individual, family, and community), age group, wellness, and illness to be included in taxonomy II of NANDA and to give further dimension to nursing diagnoses. Kelley and colleagues (1995) recently proposed a trifocal model of nursing diagnoses that includes not only the existence of an identified problem

(e.g., a risk or high risk of a particular nursing diagnosis) but also an opportunity for enhancement. This allows the nurse to identify and intervene in an area to promote the patient's health and wellness. The authors suggest that the label "opportunity for enhancement" would facilitate classifications along the illness-wellness axis. These axes may give the community health nurse, researcher, and administrator the opportunity to address the wellness and community issues previously lacking in the NANDA system. Additionally, the NANDA nursing diagnoses have been proposed for inclusion in the next revision of the *International Classification of Diseases* (Carroll-Johnson, 1991). This proposal could have far-reaching implications for community health administrators through enhancing international nurse communications and further validating nursing services, including wellness activities, for reimbursement.

Controversial, too, is the independent response of the nurse in treating certain diagnostic categories (e.g., the NANDA-approved impaired gas exchange). Many of the physiologically based diagnoses are considered to have interdependent responses that are based on both medical and nursing orders (Kim, 1985). Some argue that nurses do not even have the tools to assess such diagnoses (Jacoby, 1985). Gordon's (1995) diagnostic manual clearly suggests medical referral in cases in which a nurse suspects an interdependent diagnosis (e.g., impaired gas exchange). Carpenito (1995b) describes a list of "collaborative" problems as potential complications attached to medial diagnoses (e.g., potential complication: peripheral vascular disease). These problems occur in association with a given pathology and would require both medical and nursing interventions to achieve patient goals. This particular area is less problematic to the community health administrator because the current atmosphere dictates a signed physician's order to cover any nursing activities. When the legislative climate changes to allow direct reimbursement for nursing activities, these interdependent diagnoses may present an administrative challenge.

THE PROCESS

Now that we have described the concept of nursing diagnoses, how do we establish the diagnosis? A larger question also remains: What conceptual framework would give focus and definition to the diagnostic process? To respond to the first question, Gordon (1982) notes that nursing diagnosis is both a label and an action. Diagnosis therefore requires a nursing knowledge base and skill in application of the nursing process. The second question may prove to be more difficult to answer clearly in that no one unified framework has been established for the profession. Consideration must then be given to the nursing agency's and the individual nurse's philosophy and the framework that most closely corresponds to it.

The nursing process involves the methodical examination, definition, and solution of the patient's health problems in relation to nursing. More traditionally, the process is defined as assessment, planning, intervention, and evaluation. The ANA model practice act statement (1980b) inserts the diagnostic step directly after assessment in its discussion of the nursing process. The step-by-step nature of the nursing process and the placement of the nursing diagnosis within it help define and organize the patient's care needs for the staff nurse regardless of the complexity of that patient's problems.

Clearly, the nursing diagnosis is established within the nursing process. The staff nurse, after the initial assessment of the patient, defines problems (the diagnosis) that may be addressed by nursing interventions and may reflect the instructions of the medical regimen, such as knowledge deficit related to a 2-g sodium diet. The diet in the example is prescribed by the physician, and the nurse's evaluation shows that the patient in some way lacks the information to select that diet appropriately. For those nurses who are unfamiliar with the diagnostic categories and their defining characteristics, several pocket-size manuals are available to help clarify and select appropriate diagnoses (Gordon, 1995; Jaffe et al., 1993; Kim et al., 1987; NANDA, 1992; Sherwood et al., 1988). By following the definition of the nursing diagnosis, the nurse can proceed to plan and implement interventions based on the problem and the goals set by the patient and nurse. The final step in the process is the evaluation of the effectiveness of the interventions and the overall plan. This step guides the nurse in revision or adaptation of the plan to meet the patient's needs most effectively.

Selection of a particular diagnosis is based on analysis of the patient's nursing assessment data. The focus and definition of the nursing assessment come from a conceptual framework. A variety of frameworks are available for the clinical nurse's examination. Some popular nursing frameworks include Roy's adaptation model, Roger's life process conceptual framework, Neuman's behavioral systems, and Orem's self-care agencies (Riehl and Roy, 1980). Many agencies and certainly many individuals use an eclectic approach, some combination of a formalized framework and unspoken concepts that guides their practice. An additional factor in considering a practical conceptual framework for an agency is the demand of third party payers because, although the patient may have an adaptive or self-care problem, that diagnosis may not represent a reimbursable nursing activity.

Regardless of the framework selected, the nursing assessment must consider all aspects of the patient's care needs. Gordon (1995) suggests a functional approach and considers 11 health patterns that are necessary for a complete assessment in any framework: health perception/health management, nutritional-metabolic pattern, elimination pattern, activity-exercise, cognitive-perceptual pattern, sleep-rest pattern, self-perception/self-concept, role relationship pattern, sexuality-reproductive pattern, coping-stress-tolerance pattern, and value-brief pattern. The sample nursing assessment shown in Exhibit 19–1 contains functional elements as

Exhibit 19–1   Sample Nursing Assessment Form

Pt. #_____ Pt. Name _____

T_____ P_____ R_____ BP_____ BP (standing prn) _____ Wt _____ Ht _____

Pt's major health concern/goal: _____

_____

Hx of present illness:_____

_____

Medical/surgical hx: _____

_____

Code: WNL = within normal limits   P = protein   N = not assessed
            DNA = does not apply   + = positive   − = negative

Assessment	Code	Describe or Measure
1. *Skin*		
a. Color		
b. Condition		
c. Temperature		
d. Turgor		
e. Nails		
f. Rash		
g. Lesion/Ulcers		
2. *Eyes*		
a. Vision		
b. Condition		
c. Last Eye Exam		
d. Glasses		
3. *ENT*		
a. Teeth and Gums		
b. Dentures		
c. Throat		
d. Tongue		
e. Hearing		
f. Hearing Aid		
4. *Resp. System*		
a. Aids		
b. Chest Config.		
c. Auscultation		
d. Breathing Pattern		
e. Cough Pattern/Secretions		
f. Smoking History		
5. *Cardiovascular*		
a. Rhythm		
b. Cap. Refill/Pedal Pulses		
c. Pain/Palpitations		
d. Pacemaker		
e. Edema		

	RT	LT	
Pedal			
Ankle			
Calf			

Assessment	Code	Describe or Measure
6. *Reproductive*		
a. Appearance of Breasts		
b. Breast Self-Exam		
c. Appearance of Genitalia		
d. Discharge/Secretions		

continues

Exhibit 19–1   continued

Assessment	Code	Describe or Measure
7. *Urinary*		
a. Continence		
b. Freq./Dysuria		
c. Color/Character		
d. Incontinence Mgt.		
e. Foley Size/Type/Last Chg.		
8. *G.I.*		
a. Abdominal Configuration		
b. Abd. Pain/Tenderness/ Distention		
c. Bowel Sounds		
d. Bowel Habits: Continence		
Date Last BM		
Laxative Use		
e. Nausea/Vomiting/Other Symp.		
f. Nutrit. Status/Recent Wt. Chg.		
g. Difficulty Chewing/Swallowing		
h. Appetite		
i. Diet		
9. *Neuro*		
a. Pupils		
b. LOC/Orientation		
c. Fainting/Dizziness		
d. Spasticity/Paresis		
e. Paresthesias (Numbness/ Tingling/Burning)		
f. Coordination/Balance		
g. Seizures/Tremors		
h. Speech		
i. Pain		
10. *Musculoskel*		
a. Posture		
b. Deformities/Amputations		
c. Contractures		

Assistance						Comments
11. *ADLs*	*Indep*	*Min*	*Mod*	*Max*	*Unable To Do*	
a. Toileting						
b. Personal Care						
c. Meal Prep.						
d. Eating						
e. Transfers						
f. Dressing						
g. Ambulation						
h. Stairs						
i. Household Activities						
j. Laundry						
k. Telephone						
l. Assistive Devices						
m. Sleep						
n. Money Management						

Exhibit 19–1   continued

Assessment	Code	Describe or Measure
12. Psychosocial		
a. Behavior		
b. Affect		
c. Habits (Drug/ETOH)		
d. Language		
e. Literacy		
f. Learning Ability		
g. Religious Affiliation		

13. Family/Environment
   a. Family Composition

   b. Physical Environment

   c. Caregiver: Name

                 Relationship

                 Age

                 Health Prob.

                 Learning Abil.

Problem/Nursing Diagnosis

#	Date	

Date_____RN Signature_____

Source: Reprinted with permission of the Visiting Nurse Association of Eastern Montgomery County, Department of Abington Memorial Hospital, Willow Grove, Pennsylvania.

suggested by Gordon (1995) as well as physical assessment and historical data.

Once selected, the nursing diagnosis can be documented in a variety of ways. Particularly useful is the problem-oriented method of charting, which allows the nurse to address each problem separately and systematically. First described by Weed (1971), the problem-oriented method contains four main components: a problem list, a defined database, initial and revised plans, and progress notes. For our purposes, the nursing diagnoses are the problems listed, and the previously discussed nursing assessment is the database. Goals or expected outcomes are listed with the problems and diagnoses, and detailed plans are established on the physician's order forms or plans of treatment. Progress notes are formulated using the SOAP method (subjective, objective, assessment, and plan). In this format, subjective data represent the patient's point of view, objective data are the evidence collected by the professional, assessment is the professional's analysis of both the subjective and the objective data, and the plan outlines the steps needed to deal with the assessment and the overall problem or diagnosis.

Flow sheets or some other abbreviated form of documentation, such as checklists, may be used with a narrative description of the nursing diagnoses and the subsequent nursing interventions. Depending on the agency's documentation policies and third party demands, the nurse may document every visit on the flow sheet and record a narrative only when changes occur or as mandated by the agency. This combination may prove to be time saving for the community health nurse while also preserving a graphic flow of the patient's needs. Parameters necessary to measure the patient's progress and the effectiveness of the nursing interventions may be defined individually on the flow sheet for each patient according to his or her diagnoses.

Standardized flow sheets, which reflect parameters necessary to assess and intervene in specific diagnostic categories, can also be established. The standardized flow sheets may be designed to promote a minimum level of nursing care expected by the agency for a certain diagnosis. Items found on the flow sheets may include physical data, such as vital signs, measurements of a wound, or peripheral edema; instruction needs, such as insulin administration and diet instructions; psychosocial data, such as affect; and treatment needs, such as wound dressing changes or catheter changes. Individualization of the patient's care needs to reflect his or her own nursing diagnosis, etiology, and symptoms may be accomplished if the standardized flow sheets have ample space for the nurse to document the patient's specific requirements (Exhibit 19–2). In this manner, the nurse may overcome the tendency to fit the patient to the diagnosis rather than fit the diagnosis to the patient. Standardized flow sheets may be designed by the agency staff based on their documentation requirements and care plans related to specific nursing diagnoses. Parameters are formatted according to the nursing process and may be adapted from a variety of sources, including clinicians, staff members, nursing texts, and nursing care plan manuals.

Many recent projects also identify and classify nursing interventions that can be used as parameters in standardized charting. The National Intervention Classification project, the HHCCs, the International Classification in Nursing Project, and the Omaha System are among many classifications of interventions at various levels of development that may correlate with nursing diagnoses (Snyder et al., 1996). The Agency for Health Care Policy and Research (AHCPR), established by Congress in 1989, has examined both traditional medical and variations of nursing diagnoses, such as urinary incontinence and pressure ulcer treatment (Bergstrom et al., 1994; Fantl et al., 1996). AHCPR guidelines may also be incorporated into standardized charting formats to reflect current national standards for selected problems. Several nursing investigators have also developed a series of nursing care plans for home care agencies based on nursing diagnoses; these may also serve as reference points for

Exhibit 19–2 Standardized Flow Sheet: #9 Pain R/T

PT. # _____ NAME _____ PG. _____

PARAMETERS/INTERVENTIONS	DATE																												
GOAL																														
ASSESSMENT																														
Location of Pain																														
Type																														
Intensity																														
Onset/Duration																														
Associated Symptoms																														
Alleviated by																														
Aggravated by																														
Rest/Activity Patterns																														
Mental Status																														
INSTRUCTION																														
Side Effects of Analgesics: Sedation, Nausea, Constipation																														
Comfort Measures																														
INTERVENTION AS INDICATED																														
Pain Control: Method																														
Med Dose																														
Frequency																														
Relief																														
Breakthrough Pain																														

Intensity Scale (0–5 Scale)
0 = No Pain   5 = Excruciating Pain

C = Care; D = Disc.; E = Eval.; N = Narrative; DNA = Does Not Apply; NA = Not Assessed; IB = Instr. Begun; IC = Instr. Contd.; S = Supvsn.; U = Unchgd; + = Yes; – = No standardized flow sheet parameters (Carpenito, 1995a; Gould and Wargo, 1987; Walsh et al., 1987). The use of standardized flow sheets in conjunction with a nursing diagnosis taxonomy may further contribute to the establishment of outcomes in relation to a quality assurance program.

Computer programs have been designed to provide nurse-friendly formats for individualized clinical information systems for nursing diagnoses and plans of care. Much of this work has been done in acute care settings, but with advancements in portable hardware technologies, including laptop and notebook computers, the home care arena is showing an expansion in automation of nursing diagnosis–related plans of care (Hannah et al., 1987). These computerized clinical information systems will eventually replace the paper standardized flow sheets currently in use. For data to be retrieved from computerized systems, a standard or structured language must be used. Nursing diagnoses lists approved by NANDA, the Omaha System, or the HHCCs or adapted by a particular agency (Exhibit 19–3) should help staff avoid confusing or chaotic terminology that prohibits data collection. The inclusion of a nursing diagnosis format in management information systems will additionally link clinical and financial data for community health administrators (Martin et al., 1992). This link will take on increasing importance in the era of health care reform in providing information about costing out of nursing services and utilization of resources.

THE EFFECTS

The effects of nursing diagnoses may be evident in many facets of community health nursing, including administration, clinical practice, and associated research. This is not to say that there are no problems with nursing diagnoses. The taxonomy is often awkward, whether the NANDA system, the Omaha System, or another system is used. In addition, even though there has been almost two decades of work on the taxonomy, the language of nursing diagnoses

can and will change as nursing further refines the lists and explores the range of its professional practice. Defining characteristics for the diagnoses may not always be clear to the practicing staff nurse, and there may be some resulting confusion as to the choice of an accurate and appropriate diagnosis (Dalton, 1985). The concurrent assessment and documentation scheme for nursing diagnoses may be cumbersome initially for staff unaccustomed to the concepts of nursing process and diagnosis. Conversion to a nursing diagnosis system will require considerable staff development efforts. Although more recently educated nurses may find the process easy, older nurses may be unsure and may need guidance from both development and supervisory staff in selection and documentation of a nursing diagnosis. There are also possible legal considerations in nursing diagnoses, such as inaccurate diagnoses or misdiagnoses resulting in improper nursing treatment. In actuality, nursing diagnoses represent the labeling of problems that nurses normally treat; therefore, nurses would be held accountable for their actions whether or not the label or diagnosis is attached (Gordon, 1982).

For the clinical nurse, the advantages of nursing diagnoses include the standardization of the language used to communicate within the profession. The communications link of nursing diagnoses aids community health nurses in validating their practices for themselves, their peers, supervisors, and third party payers. For the community health nurse, the stresses of independent home care and the many documentation requirements associated with third party payers can contribute to a burnout problem (Marvan-Hyam, 1986). The nursing diagnosis, which clearly shows the nurse's professional assessment, goals, and interventions, may increase professional self-worth. This may be accomplished by helping the nurse view the nursing process as a proactive problem-solving technique rather than merely reactively carrying out the physician's orders. The use of nursing diagnoses in an agency's documentation system can also help clarify communications among

Exhibit 19–3   Sample Nursing Diagnosis List

Type	Seq	Text
SNPB	1	AGEN
SNPB	2	#18 Fluid Volume Deficit
SNPB	3	#24E Altered Health Maint: Impaired Bone Density
SNPB	4	#27J Knowledge Deficit: Chemotherapy
SNPB	5	#29 Noncompliance
SNPB	6	#33 Altered Oral Mucous Membranes
SNPB	7	#38 Self-Bathing—Hygiene Deficit
SNPB	8	#51 Risk for Activity Intolerance
SNPB	9	#55 Risk for Fluid Volume Deficit
SNPB	10	#73 Health-Seeking Behaviors
SNPB	11	#82 Total Self-Care Deficit
SNPB	12	#83 Self-Dressing—Grooming Deficit
SNPB	13	#85 Self-Toileting Deficit
SNPB	14	RESP
SNPB	15	#2 Ineffective Airway Clearance
SNPB	16	#7 Ineffective Breathing Pattern
SNPB	17	#21 Impaired Gas Exchange
SNPB	18	#107 Inability To Sustain Spontaneous Ventilation
SNPB	19	#108 Dysfunctional Ventilatory Weaning Response
SNPB	20	CV
SNPB	21	#8 Decreased Cardiac Output
SNPB	22	#19 Risk Fluid Volume Deficit
SNPB	23	#20 Fluid Volume Excess
SNPB	24	#24A Altered Health Maint: Cardiac
SNPB	25	#24B Altered Health Maint: HTN
SNPB	26	#48 Altered Tissue Perfusion
SNPB	27	GI
SNPB	28	#4 Constipation
SNPB	29	#5 Diarrhea
SNPB	30	#6 Bowel Incontinence
SNPB	31	#27E Knowledge Deficit: GI Bleed
SNPB	32	#21I Knowledge Deficit: Ostomy
SNPB	33	#78 Colonic Constipation
SNPB	34	#79 Perceived Constipation
SNPB	35	GU
SNPB	36	#24K Altered Health Maint: Renal Disease
SNPB	37	#49 Altered Urinary Elimination Pattern
SNPB	38	#59 Functional Incontinence
SNPB	39	#60 Reflex Incontinence
SNPB	40	#61 Stress Incontinence
SNPB	41	#62 Total Incontinence
SNPB	42	#63 Urge Incontinence
SNPB	43	#72 Urinary Retention

continues

Exhibit 19–3   continued

Type	Seq	Text
SNPB	44	ENDO
SNPB	45	#27A Knowledge Deficit: Diabetes
SNPB	46	NEURO/PAIN
SNPB	47	#1 Activity Intolerance
SNPB	48	#9 Pain
SNPB	49	#10 Impaired Verbal Communication
SNPB	50	#24C Altered Health Maint: CVA
SNPB	51	#27D Knowledge Deficit: Bedbound
SNPB	52	#28 Impaired Physical Mobility
SNPB	53	#53 Chronic Pain
SNPB	54	#57 Hyperthermia
SNPB	55	#67 Impaired Swallowing (Uncompensated)
SNPB	56	#68 Risk for Altered Body Temperature
SNPB	57	#69A Ineffective Thermoregulation
SNPB	58	#77 Risk for Aspiration
SNPB	59	#81 Risk for Disuse Syndrome
SNPB	60	#86 Dysreflexia
SNPB	61	#87 Sensory Overload Effects
SNPB	62	#109 Risk Peripheral Neurovascular Dysfunct.
SNPB	63	NUTR
SNPB	64	#27M Knowledge Deficit: Enteral Feedings
SNPB	65	#30 Altered Nutrition: Less Than Body Requirements
SNPB	66	#31 Altered Nutrition: More Than Body Requirements
SNPB	67	#32 Altered Nutrition: Risk for More than Body Requirements
SNPB	68	#84 Self-Feeding Deficit
SNPB	69	SAFE
SNPB	70	#25 Impaired Home Maintenance Management
SNPB	71	#26A Risk for Injury
SNPB	72	#35 Risk for Infection
SNPB	73	#74 Risk for Poisoning
SNPB	74	#75 Risk for Suffocation
SNPB	75	#113 Altered Protection
SNPB	76	SKIN
SNPB	77	#42 Pressure Ulcer
SNPB	79	#43 Risk for Impaired Skin Integrity
SNPB	79	#70 Impaired Tissue Integrity
SNPB	80	#110 Impaired Skin Integrity
SNPB	81	PSYCH
SNPB	82	#3 Anxiety
SNPB	83	#11 Ineffective Coping (Individual)
SNPB	84	#12 Family Coping: Compromised
SNPB	85	#13 Family Coping: Disabling
SNPB	86	#14 Family Coping: Potential for Growth
SNPB	87	#15 Diversional Activity Deficit
SNPB	88	#16 Altered Family Processes
SNPB	89	#17 Fear (Specify Focus)

continues

Exhibit 19–3 continued

Type	Seq	Text
SNPB	90	#22 Anticipatory Grieving
SNPB	91	#23 Dysfunctional Grieving
SNPB	92	#36 Powerlessness
SNPB	93	#37 Rape Trauma Syndrome
SNPB	94	#39 Self-Esteem Disturbances
SNPB	95	#40 Sensory Deprivation
SNPB	96	#41 Sexual Dysfunction
SNPB	97	#44 Sleep-Pattern Disturbance
SNPB	98	#45 Social Isolation
SNPB	99	#46 Spiritual Distress (Distress of Human Spirit)
SNPB	100	#47 Altered Thought Processes
SNPB	101	#50 Risk for Violence
SNPB	102	#52 Impaired Adjustment
SNPB	103	#56 Hopelessness
SNPB	104	#64 Unilateral Neglect
SNPB	105	#65 Altered Sexuality Patterns
SNPB	106	#66 Impaired Social Interaction
SNPB	107	#71 Post-Trauma Response
SNPB	108	#80 Fatigue
SNPB	109	#88 Decisional Conflict
SNPB	110	#89 Chronic Low Self-Esteem
SNPB	111	#90 Situational Low Self-Esteem
SNPB	112	#91 Body Image Disturbance
SNPB	113	#92 Personal Identity Disturbance
SNPB	114	#93 Altered Role Performance
SNPB	115	#95 Parental Role Conflict
SNPB	116	#96 Rape Trauma Syndrome: Compound Reaction
SNPB	117	#97 Rape Trauma Syndrome: Silent Reaction
SNPB	118	#98 Defensive Coping
SNPB	119	#99 Ineffective Denial
SNPB	120	#100 Caregiver Role Strain
SNPB	121	#101 Risk for Caregiver Role Strain
SNPB	122	#102 Risk for Self-Mutilation
SNPB	123	#103 Relocation Stress Syndrome
SNPB	124	#104 Ineffective Management of Therap. Regimen
SNPB	125	#111 Depression
SNPB	126	IV
SNPB	127	#27C Knowledge Deficit: IV Therapy
SNPB	128	#27K Knowledge Deficit: Central Venous Access Device
SNPB	129	MATERNAL/CHILD
SNPB	130	#24F Altered Health Maint: Pregnancy
SNPB	131	#24G Altered Health Maint: Hyperbilirubinemia
SNPB	132	#24I Altered Health Maint: Asthma
SNPB	133	#24 Altered Prenatal Health Maintenance
SNPB	134	#26B Risk for Injury R/T Drug/Alcohol Withdrawal
SNPB	135	#27F Knowledge Deficit: Post Partum Care/Breast Feeding

continues

Exhibit 19–3   continued

SNPB	136	#27G Knowledge Deficit: Post Partum Care/Lactation Suppression
SNPB	137	#27H Knowledge Deficit: Infant Care
SNPB	138	#27I Knowledge Deficit: Apnea Monitor
SNPB	139	#34 Altered Parenting (Specify Education)
SNPB	140	#54 Altered Growth and Development
SNPB	141	#69 Ineffective Thermoregulation R/T Prematurity
SNPB	142	#76 Ineffective Breastfeeding
SNPB	143	#76A Ineffective Breastfeeding: Breast Engorgement
SNPB	144	#76B Ineffective Breastfeeding: Sore Nipples
SNPB	145	#76C Ineffective Breastfeeding: Flat Inverted Nipples
SNPB	146	#94 Risk for Altered Parenting (Specify)
SNPB	147	#105 Interrupted Breastfeeding
SNPB	148	#106 Ineffective Infant Feeding Pattern

*** End Of Report ***

Source: Reprinted with permission of Visiting Nurse Association of Eastern Montgomery County, A Department of Arlington Memorial Hospital, Willow Grove, Pennsylvania.

staff members when many nurses are needed to see an individual patient, for instance during weekend or vacation coverage. The nursing diagnosis can help clarify priority problems, and when standardized flow sheets or computerized care plans are used the covering nurse can quickly and confidently follow the primary nurse's care plan as outlined by the selected parameters or interventions. Nursing diagnoses can also facilitate communication between the community and our acute and long-term care colleagues to promote continuity of the patient's care. The transition from hospital to home and home to independence or other care mode may be eased if the nursing diagnoses are clear and the goals or expected outcomes are well defined.

Nursing diagnoses and expected outcomes also may be included in the process of development of critical pathways. Critical pathways, which are time lines of multidisciplinary activities, plans, and outcomes, describe care for patients in an episode of illness for a specific diagnosis-related group (DRG), such as total hip replacement. Nursing diagnoses for a majority (75 percent) of patients in a DRG could be included in the critical pathway of patients as they move through an illness (Carpenito, 1995a).

In addition, the use of the nursing diagnosis may assist in a peer review process (Warren, 1983). The practice of diagnosing and treating competently can be evaluated by peers reviewing a nursing record that includes a database. For supervisory staff, the use of a nursing diagnosis taxonomy by clinical nurses can assist them in evaluating nursing competence and accountability. The supervisor may review the nurse's competence via joint home visits, patient care conferences focusing on nursing diagnosis selection and treatment, or chart review. Areas of staff concern may be identified by both staff and supervisors and converted into staff development programs as appropriate. The usefulness of nursing diagnoses clinically is perhaps most crucial when one considers third party reimbursement. This issue is clearly valuable to the community health nurse and administrator considering the Medicare regulation stipulating reimbursement for skilled nursing services (DHHS, 1996). Nursing diagnoses can, within the Health Care Financing Administration's constraints regarding time, homebound status, and patient response or progress, assist in documenting areas where nursing contributes significantly to the patient's care and hence is more likely to be considered skilled.

In addition to the benefits of diagnoses for the clinical staff, distinct advantages accrue to the community health administrator from the use of nursing diagnoses within the agency. The administrator may identify many valuable statistics for the provision of cost-effective, quality care based on the staff's use of the nursing diagnoses. As an example, these statistics may show length of service per diagnosis and cost per diagnosis. How long is the mean service period for the patient with an alteration in skin integrity? How much does it cost to care for the average patient with an alteration in mobility? What other services are required for a person with a self-care deficit? What are the most frequently occurring diagnoses for the agency's population base? Analysis of the accumulated data could prove useful in considering the impact of prospective payments in home health care, in planning services and community programs, and in planning staff expansions or reductions. Chapter 27 demonstrates how one agency is using data reflecting the staff's nursing diagnoses and a patient classification system (Harris et al., 1987).

A sound quality improvement program may also be an outcome of nursing diagnosis use. Reviewers can identify the appropriateness of the diagnoses and the accompanying goals, interventions, and outcomes as documented in the chart. The consistency of a nursing diagnosis taxonomy such as the Omaha System or the NANDA system helps clarify the patient's problems even though the reviewer may see only a "paper patient." The clear identification of the goals and outcomes related to the diagnosis helps the quality assurance process determine the effectiveness of the available nursing services and the nurse's coordination of services required by the patient. A utilization process may also be facilitated by nursing diagnosis statistics gathered on length of service per diagnosis, number and frequency of visits, and number of disciplines involved per diagnosis.

Nursing research could be encouraged within the clinical practice and administrative fields to seek refinements of the diagnostic taxonomies and standardization of interventions and to develop levels of acuity of nursing intensity. These and other research efforts may prove valuable to the community health administrator who seeks to retain an edge in the competitive home health care market.

REFERENCES

American Nurses Association (ANA). 1980a. *A social policy statement*. Kansas City, MO: ANA.

American Nurses Association (ANA). 1980b. *The nursing practice act: Suggested state legislation*. Kansas City, MO: ANA.

American Nurses Association (ANA). 1986. *Standards of community health nursing practice*. Kansas City, MO: ANA.

American Nurses Association (ANA). 1995. *Nursing's social policy statement*. Washington, DC: ANA.

Bergstrom, N., et al. 1994, December. *Pressure ulcer treatment clinical practice guideline* (Quick Reference Guide for Clinicians No. 15). Rockville, MD: U.S. Department of Health and Human Services, Public Health Service,

Agency for Health Care Policy and Research. AHCPR Pub. No. 95-0653.

Campbell, C. 1978. *Nursing diagnosis and interventions in nursing practice*. New York: Wiley.

Carpenito, L.J. 1995a. *Nursing care plans and documentation*. Philadelphia: Lippincott.

Carpenito, L.J. 1995b. *Nursing diagnosis: Application to clinical practice*. Philadelphia: Lippincott.

Carroll-Johnson, R.M., ed. 1991. *Classification of nursing diagnosis: Proceedings of the Ninth Conference*. Philadelphia: Lippincott.

Dalton, J. 1985. A descriptive study: Defining characteristics of the nursing diagnosis "cardiac output, alterations in: decreased." *Image* 17:113–117.

Department of Health and Human Services, Health Care Financing Administration. 1996, April. *Health insurance manual* (HIM II Revisions 277). Washington, DC: Government Printing Office.

Fantl, J.A., et al. 1996, March. *Managing acute and chronic urinary incontinence* (Quick Reference Guide for Clinicians No. 2, 1996 Update). Rockville, MD: U.S. Department of Health and Human Services, Public Health Service, Agency for Health Care Policy and Research. AHCPR Pub. No. 96-0686.

Gordon, M. 1976. Nursing diagnosis and the diagnostic process. *American Journal of Nursing* 76:1276–1300.

Gordon, M. 1982. *Nursing diagnosis: Process and application*. New York: McGraw-Hill.

Gordon, M. 1987. Issues in nursing diagnoses. In *Classification of nursing diagnoses. Proceedings of the Seventh Conference*, ed. A.M. McLane, 17–20. St. Louis: Mosby.

Gordon, M. 1995. *Manual of nursing diagnosis*. St. Louis: Mosby–Year Book.

Gould, E.J., and J. Wargo. 1987. *Home health nursing care plans*. Gaithersburg, MD: Aspen.

Hannah, K.J., et al., eds. 1987. *Clinical judgment and decision making: The future with nursing diagnosis*. New York: Wiley.

Harris, M., et al. 1987. Tracking the cost of home care. *American Journal of Nursing* 87:1500–1502.

Jacoby, M.K. 1985. The dilemma of physiological problems: Eliminating the double standards. *American Journal of Nursing* 85:281–285.

Jaffe, M.S., and L. Skidmore-Roth. 1993. *Home health nursing care plans*. St. Louis: Mosby.

Kelley, J., et al. 1995. A trifocal model of nursing diagnosis: Wellness reinforced. *Nursing Diagnosis* 6:123–128.

Kim, M.J. 1985. Without collaboration, what's left? *American Journal of Nursing* 85:281–284.

Kim, M.J., et al. 1987. *Pocket guide to nursing diagnosis*. St. Louis: Mosby–Year Book.

Lunney, M. 1982. Nursing diagnosis: Refining the system. *American Journal of Nursing* 82:456–459.

Martin, K., et al. 1992. The Omaha System, a research based model for decision making. *Journal of Nursing Administration* 22:47–52.

Marvan-Hyam, J. 1986. Occupational stress of the home health nurse. *Home Healthcare Nurse* 4:18–21.

Mitchell, G. 1991. Nursing diagnosis: An ethical analysis. *Image* 23:101–103.

North American Nursing Diagnosis Association (NANDA). 1992. *NANDA nursing diagnoses: Definitions and classification*. St. Louis: NANDA.

Riehl, J.P., and C. Roy, eds. 1980. *Conceptual models of nursing practice*. New York: Appleton-Century-Crofts.

Saba, V. 1992. The classification of home health care nursing diagnoses and interventions. *Caring* 11:50–57.

Shamansky, S.L., and C.R. Yanni. 1983. In opposition to nursing diagnosis: A minority opinion. *Image* 15:47–50.

Sherwood, M.J., et al. 1988. *Determining nursing diagnosis through assessment*. Baltimore: Williams & Wilkins.

Simmons, D.A. 1980. A classification scheme for client problems in community health nursing. Washington, DC: Government Printing Office. DHHS Pub. No. HRA 80-16.

Snyder, M., et al. 1996. Defining nursing interventions. *Image* 28:137–141.

Walsh, J., et al. 1987. *Manual of home health nursing*. Philadelphia: Lippincott.

Warren, J.J. 1983. Accountability and nursing diagnosis. *Journal of Nursing Administration* 17:34–37.

Weed, L.L. 1971. *Medical records, medical education and patient care*. Cleveland: Case Western Reserve University Press.

SUGGESTED READING

Ballard, S., and R. McNamara. 1983. Qualifying nursing needs in home health care. *Nursing Research* 32:236–241.

Carnevali, D., and M.D. Thomas. 1993. *Diagnostic reasoning and treatment decision making in nursing*. Philadelphia: Lippincott.

Carroll-Johnson, R.M., and M. Paquette, eds. 1994. *Classification of nursing diagnosis: Proceedings of the tenth conference*. Philadelphia: Lippincott.

Daubert, E. 1979. Patient classifications systems and outcome criteria. *Nursing Outlook* 27:450–454.

Giovannetti, T. 1979. Understanding patient classification systems. *Journal of Nursing Administration* 9:4–9.

Hardy, J. 1984. A patient classification system for home health patients. *Caring* 3:26–27.

Harris, M., et al. 1985. A patient classification system in home health care. *Nursing Economics* 3:276–282.

Kim, M.J., and A.M. McLane, eds. 1984. *Classification of nursing diagnoses, proceedings of the Fifth National Conference*. St. Louis: Mosby.

Kim, M.J., and D.A. Morita. 1982. *Classification of nursing diagnosis (third and fourth national conferences)*. New York: McGraw-Hill.

McLane, A.M., ed. 1987. *Classification of nursing diagnosis*. St. Louis: Mosby.

National League for Nursing (NLN). 1974. *Problem-oriented systems of patient care*. New York: NLN.

Sienkiewicz, J. 1984. Patient classification in community health nursing. *Nursing Outlook* 32:219–221.

Visiting Nurse Association (VNA) of New Haven. 1980. *Patient classification objective system methodology manual*. New Haven, CT: VNA of New Haven.

CHAPTER 20

Maternal–Child Health Program

Louise A. Harmer

The establishment and maintenance of a maternal–child health (MCH) home care program represent a holistic process. The client, the family, and the environment are to be considered in the home care planning as much as the diagnosis and prognosis. Although pediatric home care programs have developed in two ways, intermittent skilled care and continuous care, it is not within the scope of this chapter to discuss continuous care pediatric home care. Rather, this chapter discusses intermittent skilled nursing visits provided to the pediatric population, including high-risk infants, young children, and teenagers with a wide range of diagnoses and special needs. In addition intermittent home care services are offered to the pregnant woman to prepare her for delivery and early discharge and/or to manage high-risk prenatal conditions. Currently, the legislative process has increased the hospital length of stay for postpartum women to 48 hours after vaginal delivery and 96 hours after cesarean delivery (National Association for Home Care, 1996). When postpartum women and their infants are encouraged to leave the hospital early (12 to 36 hours after vaginal delivery and 72 hours after cesarean delivery), it is imperative that a home care follow- up plan be established. Early discharge programs have taught us that this is a safe and cost-effective process when provision is made for physical assessment of the mother and infant and for ongoing instruction in self-care and infant care.

That home care is a viable alternative to prolonged hospitalization for the pediatric client has been documented in the literature for several years, and home care is now considered the standard of care. Intervention by a community health nurse will promote optimal health for the families of high-risk infants (Jacknick et al., 1983) and will assist families through the transition from hospital to home (Speakman, 1981). With cost containment and health care reform, health care providers are pressured to provide care in less expensive environments. Several alternatives to lengthy hospitalization have been identified, including educating parents and providing home care services with the aid of visiting nurses. In addition, it is the home care nurse who helps family members recognize problems when they are unable to articulate their concerns (Kemper, 1994). A team effort that involves a community plan for systematic visits to the home maintains and enhances the physician's role in the plan for the family and has the priceless advantage of making available an understanding, experienced person to carry out the plan and report back. In addition, the community health nurse shares intimate knowledge of the social and economic problems of the family and is able to monitor the home environment (Wilson, 1978).

The primary goal of discharge planning for the high-risk infant is ensuring a safe and smooth transition from the high-technology hospital environment to a home setting in which adequate support systems are in place. The successful discharge plan is one that matches the infant's needs with appropriate resources and ensures that there are no delays in service or fragmentation or duplication of services (Mujsce and Nelson, 1992). Intervention after hospital discharge is recognized as important in helping prevent failure to thrive, child abuse, and accidents as well as in improving the developmental level of the child (Brooten, 1983).

Administrative considerations in the development of an MCH home care program include funding and staffing issues. Despite the fact that home care significantly lowers the hospital length of stay and therefore the overall costs of managing chronically ill and disabled children or high-risk pregnancies, government and private insurance may pay only a portion of the actual home care expenses. In addition, many families in the childbearing and child-rearing age categories are uninsured or underinsured. Therefore, any reimbursement received may be but a portion of the actual cost. In addition, the operation of a quality MCH department requires the addition of staff who are knowledgeable and experienced in managing the needs of MCH clients and their families. The addition of advanced practice nurses enhances the department staffing because these nurses provide consultation, research, education, and support to other staff members.

Staffing in the MCH department is not limited to nurses; medical social workers, developmental therapists, home health aides, and other support personnel need to be matched to the needs of the clients. Other support personnel may include the home health equipment company or in-home volunteers who can assist with child care and companionship for other children in the family. Thus effective home care management is directly linked to the commitment of the home care staff and their support of the family. With a combined knowledge of adaptation theory, nursing process, and crisis theory on the part of home care nurses, the quality of human experience can be effectively influenced by nursing intervention.

The Roy adaptation model for nursing practice views the individual as a biopsychosocial being in constant interaction with a changing environment (Roy, 1980). The model is based on the premise that, to respond positively to environmental changes, people must adapt. Adaptation is a function of the stimulus presented, and the level of adaptation is determined by focal, contextual, and residual stimuli. Roy's model directs the goal of nursing toward bringing about an adapted state in the patient and family that frees them to respond to other stimuli. Health and illness are inevitable dimensions of human life and are viewed as a continuum (Roy, 1980). Intervention in the home is individualized and needs to be adjusted to changes in the infant's or child's condition and the needs of the family.

To provide adequate health care in the home, one must consider the individual's environment and remember that the individual's needs are not limited to the presenting symptoms of the illness. The nursing process identifies individuals and groups of individuals as open systems, affecting and being affected by their internal and external environments (Turner, 1974). In other words, the nursing process is the operational framework for nursing practice to carry out actions with and for the clients, be they individuals, families, or communities. It utilizes the functions of assessment, intervention, and evaluation and demands that judgments be made by the nurse. The nurse decides what evidence to gather, how to analyze it, and what conclusions can best be drawn from it (assessment). Once the assessment process is initiated, the nurse can decide with the client what goals are desirable and attainable and how they can be achieved (intervention). Interventions are then evaluated for effectiveness. If determined to be ineffective (evaluation), they can be reassessed, and the cycle begins again.

The concept of crisis as a conceptual approach to family nursing was identified in 1974 by Hall and Weaver. Individuals entering the health care system may be faced with a new, different, and difficult situation. Anxiety distorts their perceptions, and their situational supports may be few or nonexistent. Because of their accessibility to families, nurses are in a position to offer intervention aimed at prevention, support, or therapy. Development of realistic plans for the future of the child is almost impossible until the parents are able to work through their feelings of anger, grief, disappointment, and fear (Schroeder, 1974). Without a doubt, caring for a high-risk infant or chronically ill child creates increased responsibility for the family and especially for the primary caregiver. The assumption of full responsibility for infants and children with special needs can be facilitated by the intervention of the community health nurse and/or advanced practice nurse. These health professionals can ease the transition from hospital to home through direct patient and family contact and by adapting principles of health care to the home situation. In addition, appropriate teaching strategies and timely, suitable intervention enhance the family's understanding and ability to master complex tasks.

Among the many benefits of pediatric home care, children do better at home, and there is improved compliance with the treatment plan. Chronically ill and high-risk infants show improved health and well-being with fewer complications of the primary diagnosis. In addition to being a cost effective means of providing acute care, pediatric home care is an excellent way to heal our children in an environment conducive to normal growth and development (Bock, 1986).

GOALS OF PEDIATRIC HOME CARE

Children survive premature birth and devastating illness, and families are taking an active part in the health care of their children. As a result, more extensive care is being provided at home than was previously thought possible. Management of the pediatric home care client is as diverse as there are diagnoses, ages, and developmental levels of clients and differences in environmental and family support systems. One thing that does remain stable is that, as the time for hospital discharge approaches, the nurse–parent relationship undergoes change. As parents are taught and master unfamiliar caretaking tasks, the nurse assumes the role of a "health care resource for the parents and the parents become a caretaking and informational resource for the nurse. Through this process, parents regain their sense of control" (Cagan, 1988, 275). It is this relationship that is continued and fostered in home care. The parents are in control again, and the nurse offers the reassurance and guidance needed for successful management of the home care plan.

The goals of the pediatric home care program (Bock, 1986) include the following:

- Facilitate the transition from hospital to home and community.
- Stabilize the child in the home environment.
- Determine the child's and family's continuing needs, and make appropriate referrals to community agencies.
- Coordinate the interdisciplinary plan of care.
- Monitor the parents' level of comprehension and ability to assimilate the child's needs into the daily routine of the family.

Facilitate the Transition from Hospital to Home and Community

The initiation of home care can be an exciting, joyful time as well as a time of much apprehension. Ideally, the parents have had opportunity to problem solve and become familiar with the patient's needs before discharge. Many clients will require complex care and may need ongoing treatment, such as special medications, apnea monitors, oxygen, feeding tubes, or other specialized equipment.

Durable medical equipment and supplies must be suitable for pediatric clients, and adapting the home environment to the needs of the child can be a real challenge. Equipment should be centrally located so that the child can be incorporated into the family circle as much as possible. Location of the equipment often requires creative planning because several rooms may be used during the course of the day (e.g., the dining area, the recreation area, and the child's sleeping area). In addition, excursions from the house may involve additional planning to make the trip successful. Other factors that need to be thought through include other children, household pets, and safety factors.

The home care nurse helps individualize the child's and family's treatment plan to their specific needs. In addition, the home care nurse can educate the family about other options and community resources that may be utilized in the management of the child's care. The telephone company, the power company, and community emergency systems may need to be notified of the client's condition and specific equipment needs. Emergency telephone numbers and written instructions, including a list of medications, should be posted by each phone in the house.

Stabilize the Child in the Home Environment

As much as the home environment is considered conducive to healing and normal growth and development, environmental stress may be a critical factor in the maintenance of physiological balance. Initially, some clients may make rapid progress in the home environment, while others may deteriorate (Block, 1989). The home care nurse evaluates the client's progress by weight check, observation of the feeding process, systems review, and physical assessment. In addition, medications, including dosage, side effects, and route of administration, are evaluated for tolerance and scheduling. Medication dosages will be affected by weight changes and improvement in the client's condition and need to be monitored closely.

The home care nurse also evaluates the environment for possible sources of stress, physical, emotional, or psychosocial. For example, physical stressors, such as passive smoke, strong chemical odors, and household pets, may interfere with recovery or compromise respiratory status. Emotional stress, such as a high level of anxiety or fear of loss of the child, may interfere with bonding or the ability to perform some of the child's care. Psychosocial stressors, such as inadequate financial resources or a dysfunctional family system, will interfere with the primary caregiver's ability to provide appropriate care for the child.

Determine Continuing Needs

Knowledge of all community resources and public health services available to the family is important in the management of the individual client and family. Many resources are location specific, but federal programs insure case management and early intervention services. Collaboration between the local MCH office and other agencies is intended to ensure effective linkage of services at the community level. A variety of services are available and range from center-based programs to home based services. In addition, there are a variety of financial resources and emotional support programs available to the families. The home care nurse can assist the family in identifying and utilizing appropriate resources. High-risk neonatal follow-up clinics offer collaborative, multidisciplinary evaluations and anticipatory guidance, supplemental services, and linkage to other health care resources for emotional support and educational programs.

Public Law 99-457, the Education of the Handicapped Act amendment of 1986, provides funding for comprehensive, family-oriented systems of service for children from birth through age 2 years who have (or are at risk because of) disabilities or developmental delays. This law is a series of amendments to the earlier Education for All Handicapped Children Act of 1975 (P.L. 94-142), which mandated free and appropriate education in the least restrictive environment for all handicapped youngsters between the ages of 5 and 21 years. This was the beginning of mainstreaming and brought handicapped children out of the shadows and into the mainstream of society (Blackman, 1991). The original Act gave the states the option of lowering the age at which children become eligible for early intervention services to 3 years. The amendments extended services to all handicapped preschool children, and educational services where extended to provide developmental support for infants from birth to age 3 years, thereby supporting the extension of appropriate early intervention programs directly to neonatal intensive care unit graduates. That early recognition and remediation programs were frequently successful in the prevention of chronic developmental disabilities was finally recognized and funded.

Children who qualify for early intervention services are broadly defined, and each state has been given the task of defining the terms *at-risk* and *developmental delay* for eligibility criteria for individual programs. Therefore, all children who exhibit delays in meeting age-appropriate expectations in the areas of affective, cognitive, communicative, perceptual-motor, physical, or social development to an extent that they require special help on a regular basis to function in an adaptive manner should be referred for evaluation and placement in early intervention services. The home care nurse helps the family recognize the need for additional services as well as understand the benefit in utilizing the services and provides the knowledge to access the program.

Coordinate the Interdisciplinary Plan of Care

The nurse is the coordinator for the child's and family's plan of care and ensures that all health team members understand and follow the specific treatment plan. The home care team members may include, but are not limited to, the nurse and community physician, therapists (physical, occupational, and speech), the medical social worker, home health aides, volunteers and pastoral care workers, and the equipment company. The team is as diversified as the child's and family's needs. Open lines of communication and team conferences enhance the delivery of service. In addition, many insurance carriers are adding a case management component to their insurance benefits, and this person becomes an objective member of the home care team.

Monitor the Parents' Level of Adaptation

One component of home care that makes it successful is recognition of the family's or caregiver's role in the home care program and the needs of the family. No matter how complicated or straightforward the child's care is, the primary caregiver needs recognition for the job that he or she is doing and time with significant others and other family members. Interventions to modify the environment and decrease personal stress includes strategies to decrease stressors, maintain and/or increase resources, change inaccurate beliefs, and help parents help their children (Austin, 1990).

To decrease stress in the early stages of the illness, the nurse must provide accurate, basic information about the condition, its treatment, and expected outcome. Later, as the illness and its impact become clearer, the nurse gives more in-depth information and explores with the parents their fears, concerns, and guilt feelings. Offering information about other parents' fears and concerns provides an opportunity for them to recognize that their own feelings are normal, and they will be more comfortable expressing their concerns about the impact of the illness on their child and family (Austin, 1990).

Utilizing resources includes individual, family, and extrafamily strengths and coping mechanisms. Individual resources include the person's own self-esteem and ability to care for the child. Appropriate family resources are defined as stability, cohesion, effective communication, role flexibility, shared values, and mechanisms to handle differences and conflict. Social support is found in the extrafamily resources (e.g., relatives, friends, work associates, and organizations). The nurse functions as a facilitator, helping the family problem solve, identify sources of support, and develop positive attitudes about accepting help.

It is possible to change negative attitudes to positive ones because attitudes are composed of feelings associated with beliefs (Austin, 1990). The home care nurse is the educator and can provide new information that will counter erroneous beliefs. New information, or the same information presented differently, demystifies the condition, and the parents can be encouraged to explore the positive aspects of the chronic condition. As a result, the family is strengthened and unified.

PRENATAL AND POSTPARTAL HOME CARE PROGRAM

Home care also benefits the new family because the nurse facilitates the problem-solving and decision-making processes necessary for successful management of the pregnancy and postpartum care. Planning for the birth begins early in the pregnancy as families begin to gather material resources and equipment needed for the newborn and to educate themselves about pregnancy, delivery, and parenting.

As early discharge becomes an acceptable option for the healthy family, ongoing education and home care follow-up become essential components of the plan of care. Preparation for early discharge should begin prenatally with assessment of the family's knowledge base and readiness to learn as well as the support system available to the new mother once she is discharged. Prenatal contact with the home care nurse by visit or telephone provides for identification of potential problems and establishes the relationship for the postpartum home visits.

When a pregnancy becomes high risk, requiring modification of activities of daily living, home care services benefit the client and family. The nurse is able to monitor maternal and fetal well-being, coordinate use of support services, instruct the client to monitor her contractions and follow the treatment plan recommended by her physician, and recommend community and family resources to help her stay on bedrest and still manage her household.

Currently, legislative processes are in place to ensure two to four maternity hospital days after delivery and encourages home follow-up of mother and infant. Patients may be discharged earlier at the physician's discretion. Postpartum early discharge is defined as 6 to 36 hours (1 day) after uncomplicated vaginal delivery or about 72 hours (3 days) after uncomplicated cesarean delivery. Home care follow-up of early discharge is medically necessary, provides for an all-systems assessment of both mother and newborn, allows an opportunity for family members to ask questions pertaining to the status of both mother and infant, and provides an opportunity for evaluation of the parent–infant interaction. The home evaluation also provides an opportunity for assessment of family dynamics and support systems, and the need for referral to community programs.

Independent of the length of hospital stay for postpartum recovery, complications and problems with the infant and mother will require additional home care intervention. The problems or complications can be classified as physical, psychosocial, or educational. The mother's physical complaints may include signs and symptoms of infection, hypertension, edema, pain, or constipation. Variations of normal infant assessment most commonly include breastfeeding or bottle-feeding difficulties, jaundice, and excessive loss of weight. Psychosocial problems include poor self-esteem, emotional swings and depression, sleep deprivation, inadequate material resources, and lack of adequate support. Additional education about the normal postpartum recovery process and infant care as well as contact with the physician can resolve many of these discomforts or abnormalities.

For some jaundiced infants, home phototherapy is the appropriate treatment. The home care nurse is responsible for instructing the parent or family about signs and symptoms of the complications of hyperbilirubinemia. In addition, the nurse coordinates the infant's care, provides daily assessment of infant status, draws blood for measurement of bilirubin levels, and reports daily progress to the physician. Treatment usually is completed in about 3 to 4 days, and the family and infant have benefited from the additional bonding and prevention of rehospitalization.

CONCLUSION

The MCH home care program draws from a group of clients who are as diverse as their diagnoses, ages, and developmental levels and as different as their environmental and family support systems. Intervention using a holistic approach is the basic ingredient of the successful management of an MCH home care program. When the nurse uses nursing interventions that incorporate adaptation theory, nursing process, and crisis theory, the benefits of home care are realized as the child begins to thrive and show improved health and well-being and is incorporated more and more into the family circle. The five goals of pediatric home care described in this chapter give the child back to the parents and allow the parents to regain their sense of control. The nurse's role facilitates transition to the home, stabilization in the home environment, referral to appropriate programs, coordination of the home care team, and assessment of the parents' needs. The nurse–parent relationship changes over time, and the nurse assumes the role of a health care resource person for the parents as the parents become the caretaking and informational resource for the nurse.

Pediatric home care is here to stay. Current economic considerations are a major factor in the development of pediatric home care as it becomes increasingly attractive to providers, insurance carriers, the government, and patients (Schuman, 1990). The challenge of the 1990s to pediatricians is to reduce unnecessary hospitalization for the benefit of the children, their families, their physicians, third party payers, and health care reformers. Despite legislative pressure for extended length of stay for maternity patients, early discharge of the postpartum patient with home care follow-up is a safe and more comfortable option for some families. Management of postpartum clients and infants at home is beneficial to the entire family because it enhances bonding with extended family members and is effective in keeping costs to a minimum.

REFERENCES

Austin, J.K. 1990. Assessment of coping mechanisms used by parents and children with chronic illness. *MCN* 15:98–102.

Blackman, J.A. 1991. Public Law 99-457: Advance or albatross? *Contemporary Pediatrics* 8:81–95.

Block, C., et. al. 1989. Homecare for high risk infants the first year. *Caring* 8:11–17.

Bock, R.H. 1986. Pediatric home health care, *Focus* 6:5–7.

Brooten, D. 1983. Issues for research on alternative patterns of care for low birthweight infants. *Image* 15:80–83.

Cagan, J. 1988. Weaning parents from intensive care unit care, *MCN* 13:275–277.

Hall, J.E., and B.R. Weaver. 1974. Crisis: A conceptual approach to family nursing. In *Nursing of Families in crisis*, eds. J.F. Hall and B.R. Weaver. 3–9. Philadelphia: Lippincott.

Jacknick, M., et al. 1983. Evaluating public health follow-up of the high risk infant. *MCN* 8:252–256.

Kemper, K. 1994. Is this hospitalization really necessary? *Contemporary Pediatrics* 11:43–56.

Mujsce, D., and N. Nelson. 1992. High risk follow-up. In *Primary pediatric care*, 2d ed., R.A. Hoeckelman, 509–517. Philadelphia: Mosby.

National Association for Home Care (NAHC) 1996. *Baby discharge* (NAHC Report No. 679) Washington D.C. NAHC.

Roy, C. 1980. The Roy adaptation model. In *Conceptual models for nursing practice*, 2d ed., eds. J.P. Riehl and C. Roy, 179–188. New York: Appleton-Century-Crofts.

Schroeder, E. 1974. The birth of a defective child: A cause for grieving. In *Nursing of families in crisis*, eds. J.F. Hall and B.R. Weaver, 158–170. Philadelphia: Lippincott.

Schuman, A.J. 1990. Homeward bound: The explosion in pediatric home care. *Contemporary Pediatrics* 7:26–54.

Speakman, K. 1981. The art of health visiting. *Nursing Mirror* 10:33–34.

Turner, M.N. 1974. Nursing process: An operational framework for nursing practice. In *Nursing of families in crisis*, eds. J.F. Hall and B.R. Weaver, 10–32. Philadelphia: Lippincott.

Wilson, J.L. 1978. Pediatric perceptions: The public health nurse—A neglected resource. *Pediatrics* 51:206–209.

SUGGESTED READING

Department of Public Welfare. 1983. *Procedural safeguards for children in early intervention services*. Commonwealth of Pennsylvania, Offices of Mental Health and Mental Retardation. Harrisburg, PA.

Dickason, E. et al. 1990. *Maternal infant nursing care*. Philadelphia: Mosby.

Harris, M., et al. 1985. Agency profile: Development of the pediatric home care program. *Caring* 4:82.

Hutchins, V. 1988. *Linkages* (Bureau of Maternal and Child Health and Resources Development Workgroup Report). Rockville, MD: Health Resources and Services Administration.

Ludwig, M.A. 1990. Phototherapy in the home setting. *Journal of Pediatric Health Care* 4:304–308.

McFadden, E. 1991. The Wallaby phototherapy system: a new approach to phototherapy. *Journal of Pediatric Nursing* 6:206–208.

Richards, D. 1991. Perinatal education to improve birth outcomes. *Home Healthcare Nurse* 9:35–39.

Roberts, I. 1976. Research and health visitor. *Health Visitor* 49:354–357.

Zerwekh, J. 1991. Tales from public health nursing: True detectives. *American Journal of Nursing* 10:30–36.

CHAPTER 21

High-Technology Home Care Services

Vincent C. DiTrapano and James J. Williams

The introduction of the prospective payment system and its wide acceptance by other insurance payers has brought a tremendous shift of complex home care services needs to the community. *High-technology home care* has become an acceptable term to describe many comprehensive home services. The term *high technology* can be intimidating and at the same time misleading. The high technology of yesterday has become the routine of today as new and more sophisticated therapies have been added to the service model. Nonetheless, *high-technology home care* has become the catch term to describe a wide variety of services and capabilities.

Most high-technology services can be divided into three basic categories: (1) those in which a pharmaceutical agent is delivered to the patient, such as intravenous drugs, antibiotics, or pain medication, (2) respiratory therapy, such as ventilators and apnea monitors, and (3) nutritional services, such as total parenteral and enteral nutrition. Most additional therapies can be placed into one of these three categories.

Acceptance by the medical community, the insurance carriers, and the patients of home care as an alternative to institutionalized care is making demands on home care administrators to develop these capabilities. In an effort to meet the community's needs and to maintain viability in the growing health care market, home care administrators must respond to the complex technological demands of caring for the seriously ill patient in the home setting.

This chapter discusses the issues to be addressed by those considering development of high-technology services. A review of the rapid progress that has led to the emergence of high-technology care in the community reveals that the quick acceptance of innovative health care, advances in life-support technology, and the institution of medical cost-containment programs have prompted many home health agencies to explore new, advanced levels of home care.

The challenge to the home health agency is to meet the demand for a new level of care that now exists in the home. This care requires a high degree of competency, accountability, and cost effectiveness. Any agency venturing into these waters must be willing to invest the time, the money, and the energy in innovative program development and the necessary clinical staff development. It will take strategic planning for the home care agencies to meet the needs of high-technology therapies in the community. Ensuring successful high-technology therapies will require a commitment from the administration of the home care agency, resources (both financial and operational), and acceptance by personnel of these therapies.

THE PLANNING PROCESS

The first step in the development of these capabilities is the planning process. There are six basic criteria that are part of this planning:

1. set objectives
2. plan a market or service analysis
3. determine service capabilities
4. develop staff
5. develop a financial plan
6. establish and implement a timetable

Set Objectives

The objectives set must be reasonable and attainable. The agency must decide exactly what role it will play in the provision of high-technology services. Is the agency to be the coordinator of services, taking the leadership role and managing the other disciplines (pharmacy, distribution, and reimbursement) in the provision of the services, or is the agency simply interested in providing the nursing capabilities and having someone else be the coordinator? This is an important consideration. If the agency wishes to provide only nursing, then the strategies that are employed from that point on are different from the strategies needed if the agency wishes to be in the business.

As a coordinator of services, it will be the agency's responsibility to develop or subcontract with the other disciplines to be able to provide the services adequately. In addition, the agency as the coordinator must then be ready and willing to market those services to health care professionals. As a nursing subcontractor to another company that maintains the coordinator role, however, the agency must concentrate all its energies on developing the clinical skills of its personnel. There is a significant difference, and it must be given careful consideration. The objectives that are set from that point on are related to that initial decision.

Other objectives to be considered are as follows. A decision must be made as to which therapies the home care agency is willing to

support. Will it be pharmacy-related products? Is there a role for the agency in provision of respiratory services and nutritional services? What will the agency's relationship be with other providers of services? Many home care companies are looking for a home care agency with which they can subcontract nursing services. There is also the opportunity for a home care agency simply to be a subcontractor to a home care company.

Plan a Market or Service Analysis

The next step in the planning process is a market or service analysis. High-technology home care is a mature market. In almost every section of the country, there are people able to provide these services. Before entering this market, the home care agency should (actually, must) do a thorough analysis of what service capabilities exist. If one is simply going to duplicate services that already exist, it will be much more difficult for a start-up operation. Many agencies will start by finding a niche in the marketplace. Specialization in pain management or nutritional therapies will give the agency a cautious entree into the marketplace.

Determine Service Capabilities

After setting objectives and completing a market analysis, the agency must next determine its service capabilities. When a decision has been made as to what home care capabilities the agency is interested in providing, a thorough research into the requirements to provide that service is necessary. It may mean a subcontractor relationship with a pharmacy provider. It may mean having a separate category of nursing clinician capabilities. It may mean having reimbursement specialists either as part of the staff or under contract. One document that would be an excellent resource at this stage of the developmental process is the *1997–98 Comprehensive Accreditation Manual for Home Care*

(Joint Commission on Accreditation of Healthcare Organizations [Joint Commission], 1996). This manual will allow the agency administrator to review exactly what services and specialized personnel are going to be needed to provide therapy successfully.

Develop Staff

After service capabilities are determined, the next step in the planning process is the educa-

tion of the staff of the agency. It may be that in the agency both professional and nonprofessional personnel exist and that retraining or a specialized training process is necessary. If that is not the case, then recruitment of specialized professional and nonprofessional employees will be necessary. The development of role descriptions and performance appraisals will be part of the staff development process (Exhibit 21–1).

Exhibit 21–1 Position: Nurse Clinician/Home Care

Reports to: Regional Nursing Service Manager

Tasks

1. Provides primary case management for patients receiving infusion therapy.
2. Performs initial assessment for client when referred for home infusion therapy to determine appropriateness of patient for therapy and to assess learning needs.
3. Assesses home environment for storage areas and preparation and administration facilities for safe infusion therapy.
4. Assists referral source in planning patient care to ensure a smooth transition to home therapy.
5. Works in conjunction with pharmacy and other members of the infusion therapy staff to plan process for implementation of service.
6. Provides patient/caregiver education related to infusion therapy.
7. Performs ongoing assessment of clinical status of each patient to determine needs/problems or change in status related to infusion therapy.
8. Provides ongoing documentation as established in accordance with Joint Commission guidelines relative to client assessments, interventions, and response to therapy. Communicates verbally and in writing, as dictated by policy, with patient's physician and other disciplines involved in the plan of care.
9. Provides consultative patient care or support in collaboration with another nursing agency.

10. Initiates and manages, as a primary case manager or as a consultant, peripheral therapy, peripherally inserted control catheter (PICC), and Landmark catheters (as credentials allow).
11. Manages central venous catheters and ports.
12. Manages enteral and parenteral therapies, pain management, hemotherapy, IV antibiotics, hydration, and the related technology required to deliver these therapies.
13. Participates in on-call program as directed by immediate supervisor.
14. Participates in activities that promote professional growth and offer opportunities to maintain expertise in clinical specialty.

Results

- 90% to 100% of home health quality assurance thresholds met
- nursing report submitted to regional nursing services manager weekly
- 100% client satisfaction
- positive work spirit

Procedures

- consistent application of company policies and procedures
- communicates with nursing service manager weekly
- consistent application of nursing practice
- confidentiality

Source: Courtesy of Vitalink Pharmacy Services.

Develop a Financial Plan

To be successful, an agency must have an adequate and well-thought-out financial plan. Entree of a home care agency into the high-technology market is not without risk. It is a competitive market, one in which reimbursement expertise has become an art. A well-thought-out financial plan that completely encompasses the financial investment the agency must make is critical. Outside professional help would be beneficial for the novice.

Once that has been developed, the next step is actually to make the decision. The agency now has a clear set of objectives and a complete understanding of what its niche in the market will be. There is an understanding of what service capabilities will need to be developed to provide these services successfully. There is an understanding of the people, professional and nonprofessional, who will be dedicated to providing these services. A financial plan stating the initial investment and payoff to support the plan has been completed, and the program has the support of the administration and the acceptance of the professional staff.

Establish and Implement a Timetable

Once the decision has been made, a timetable should be developed and implemented. The implementation of the timetable will be based on all the considerations discussed previously. It is also suggested that a periodic review of the progress that the agency is making in regard to the plan and a modification of the timetable, if necessary, be performed. The danger is to rush in too quickly and not be prepared. A well-thought-out plan with a flexible implementation schedule will ensure the greatest degree of success.

DELIVERING HIGH-TECHNOLOGY SERVICES

The process for delivering high-technology services consists of seven steps:

1. the intake process or procedure, often called the patient entry process
2. the acceptance criteria as established by the agency
3. the consent to therapy as documented by the patient
4. the documentation policy
5. the coordination of pharmacy and/or equipment needs
6. the admission package
7. the care plan

The Intake Procedure

The intake procedure begins with giving the initial referral to a qualified person in the order-entry or admissions department. The responsibility of that department is to collect an accurate patient database.

Exhibit 21–2 is an example of a database form used in patient entry. The information gathered is used to do an insurance verification, documenting what will be paid for, what the deductible or the coinsurance requirements to the patient will be, and what documentation and forms will be necessary to provide smooth payment terms. The database information is shared with the following:

- pharmacy, to determine things such as drug availability and capability, equipment needs (pump, pole), drug stability, and prescription verification
- nursing, to evaluate issues such as nursing role and involvement, care plan development, and visitation schedule
- distribution service, for delivery coordination
- billing department, to generate an invoice and delivery receipt and to notify the responsible party

A proper intake procedure is vital to a successful outcome. Often this coordination must be done in a short period of time, sometimes only a couple of hours. Today many discharge planners are aware of the complexity of high-

Exhibit 21–2 Patient Information Referral Data

Patient Name _____   Primary Caregiver_____

Address _____   Address _____

Phone _____   Phone _____

Date of Birth _____   Relationship to Patient _____

REFERRAL INFORMATION

Referral Source _____   Contact _____

Address _____   Phone _____

Attending Physician _____

Address _____   Phone _____

Nursing Agency _____   Contact _____

Address _____   Phone _____

INSURANCE INFORMATION

Current Payer Status _____   Social Security Number _____

Medicare #—A _____   B (if applicable) _____

D.P.A. # _____

Insurance:

    Identification # _____

    Name of Carrier _____

    Address of Carrier _____

    Phone _____

    Contact _____

Private:

    Responsible Party _____

    Address _____

    Phone _____

Miscellaneous Comments:_____

_____

_____

Person Completing Form: _____   Date: _____

Source: Courtesy of Vitalink Pharmacy Services.

technology therapy. The real complexity is often the coordination of the discharge itself.

Determining eligibility can be based on input from multiple disciplines within the home care agency. The eligibility will be based on financial criteria, clinical criteria, and logistics. Exhibit 21–3 is an example of an initial patient assessment.

Once the determination for eligibility has been made, the referral source must be made aware and a timetable for discharge established. It is imperative at this point that a determination be made as to the proper person to bill. This could be either the patient or a responsible party with legal responsibility over that patient.

The communication within the home care agency, or between the home care agency and other providers of service to the patient, is critical at this point. Proper discharge to high-technology home care requires coordination of activities and supply delivery among nursing, the physician, the hospital discharge planner, the pharmacy, the equipment provider (if the equipment provider is not the pharmacy), the distribution or delivery piece, and the reimbursement piece. Needless to say, if all those disciplines are located at different sites, the coordination of their activities and the timetable for delivery are important.

Also, an accurate assessment of the patient's supply and/or equipment needs must be made. This will often be done by the home care agency, based on the type of therapy being provided; by the physician, based on his or her prescription requirements; and by the family, based on their logistical needs.

Considerations such as back-up pumps, waste or contaminated waste disposal, and on-call requirements need to be given thought at this time. Also, the pharmacy's responsibility at this juncture is to confirm the prescription needs with the physician. It is important to understand that the prescription as written in the hospital may be different from the prescription written for the patient upon discharge to the home. A pharmacist experienced in home care and high-technology therapies can be invaluable in help-

ing determine a prescription that will allow the greatest ease of administration in the home.

Acceptance Criteria

The next aspect in the delivery of high-technology services is for the home care agency to adopt acceptance criteria for each therapy that it is interested in offering. This will assist the members of the home care agency team in aligning with what is acceptable in terms of providing services. Exhibit 21–4 gives examples of acceptance criteria that could be established for the provision of a number of services.

Consent to Therapy

The third step in the patient entry procedure is to obtain a consent to therapy. The consent to therapy is important because it gives legal authority to the agency to provide the therapy. In addition, it documents the patient's understanding of the treatment, its purpose, and the risks involved in the event of a potential adverse or unfavorable consequence (Exhibit 21–5).

Once therapy has been established, then the responsibilities of all these disciplines and the coordination and successful completion of therapy are imperative. The importance of the distribution and delivery component of high-technology therapies cannot be overstated. The delivery personnel are responsible for the timeliness of the delivery, the completion of the order, and the set-up of equipment. Other than the nurse, the delivery person is the most visible person to the home care patient. If this delivery person exhibits a cordial, confident nature, it will go a long way in helping the patient have confidence in the delivery of these services.

Documentation Policy

The most important aspect of providing high-technology nursing services by any nursing agency will be the development of a sound and responsible documentation policy. The purpose of the documentation policy should be to facilitate the smooth transition of patients from the acute care setting to the home care environment.

There are many reference sources for the development of such a policy, including the Joint Commission, the Centers for Disease Control and Prevention, the Intravenous Nurse Society, and the American Society for Parenteral and Enteral Nutrition. The pharmaceutical policies as stated by these specific organizations can be used as parameters to develop the individual policy for the agency.

The documentation policy of the agency will require the development of some specific forms, including the following:

- A monitoring form will assist the nurse in monitoring the patient's status at home. It can be used to communicate with the physician after a home care visit.
- A progress report is used when any contact is made by the home care agency with the patient, the physician, or a caregiver. This progress report should document telephone or actual communication that takes place. It is important that the entries be complete, dated, and signed. The progress report should be treated as any inpatient progress report of any patient's hospital record.
- The physician's care plan is another form that should be developed. The objective of the physician's care plan is to ensure physician awareness of an agreement with the course of therapy directed. Exhibit 21–6 is an example of a physician's plan of treatment or plan of care form that might be used.
- The individualized nursing care plan form can be either standardized or individualized. Such forms are used after a thorough patient assessment to identify individual patient needs is completed. This becomes an integral part of the ongoing plan of treatment and identifies the care to be rendered by the nurse.

- A problem list is used to assist in the development of a care plan for an individual home care patient.
- The initial patient assessment form provides a tool to assist the nurse in obtaining a thorough assessment of home patients, including environmental, psychosocial, and psychological factors.

Among the environmental issues that should be considered are those specific family members who also live in the household and their relationship to the patient. The living area that the patient will occupy, be it the bedroom or the living room, and the specifics related to that room must be assessed. The home environment should be examined in terms of cleanliness, safety, possible interference with the equipment that is going to be supplied, stairs, any pets that might be in the house, and personal hygiene issues related to the environment as it relates to patient care.

In addition, specific utility needs have to be addressed to ensure a working phone, an adequate water supply, and the like. One issue that is frequently encountered is the availability of an appropriate electrical outlet to allow the utilization of pumps required in the patient's therapy (every experienced home care nurse or delivery person will have an adequate supply of electrical adaptors to apply a three-prong plug in a two-prong outlet).

Psychosocial considerations are also considered during the environmental assessment. Who is the primary caretaker, and what is the primary caretaker's relationship to the patient? Is there a secondary caretaker, and what is this person's relationship to the patient? How many hours per day will the individual have the caretaker's assistance, and at what times of the day will the caretaker be available? How do the caretaker and the rest of the family react to the patient's therapy, and what is their emotional status? This is particularly important for patients who are receiving pain management for terminal illnesses.

Exhibit 21–3 Patient Assessment and Medical History

Name _____

Address _____

City _____   State _____   ZIP Code _____

S.S.N. _____   D.O.B. _____   Age _____ Sex _____

Occupation _____

Attending Physician _____

   Address _____

   City _____   State _____   ZIP Code _____

Primary Caregiver _____

   Address _____

   City _____   State _____   ZIP Code _____

Relationship to Patient _____

History

Date _____   T _____   P _____   R _____   B.P. _____

   Allergies _____   Ht. _____   Wt. _____

Diagnosis: Primary _____

             Secondary _____

             Chief Complaint _____

Medical History _____

_____

_____

_____

_____

_____

_____

_____

_____

Social History _____

_____

_____

_____

_____

_____

continues

Exhibit 21–3 continued

Medications

	NAME	ROUTE	DOSAGE	FREQUENCY
1.				
2.				
3.				
4.				
5.				
6.				
7.				
8.				
9.				
10.				

Review of Systems

1. H.E.E.N.T.

Head __ No Problem   Ears __ No Problem
__ Headaches   __ Earaches
__ Facial Pain   __ Drainage
Eyes   __ No Problem   __ Tinnitus
__ Burning/Pain   __ Hearing Loss
                            R __ L __
__ Redness   Mouth __ No Problem
__ Glaucoma   __ Loss of Taste
__ Cataracts   __ Difficulty Chewing
__ Discharge   __ Dentures
__ Diplopia   Throat __ No Problem
__ Vision Loss   __ Hoarseness/Voice
                               Change
__ Contacts/Glasses   __ Dysphagia
OTHER _____
_____
_____

2. CARDIOPULMONARY

LUNG SOUNDS
                            __ Normal Sounds
__ No Problem   __ Abnormal Sounds
OTHER _____
_____

CHEST
__ No Problems   __ Cough
__ Wheeze   __ Sputum
__ Asthma   __ Smokes
__ S.O.B.   □ At Rest   □ w/Activity
OTHER_____
_____

3. CARDIOVASCULAR

__ No Problem
__ Pacemaker
__ Orthopnea
__ Cyanosis __ Peripheral __ Central
__ Palpitations
__ Cardiac Limitations
__ Chest Pains
Location _____ Severity _____
Duration _____ Management _____
__ Hypotension
OTHER _____
_____
_____
_____
_____

4. PERIPHERAL CIRCULATION

LOWER EXTREMITIES
__ No Problem   __ Phlebitis
__ Stasis Ulcer   __ Amputation
__ Varicose Veins
__ Edema
__ Temperature
__ Color
OTHER _____
_____

UPPER EXTREMITIES
__ No Problem
__ Numbness or Tingling
OTHER_____
_____

continues

Exhibit 21–3 continued

5. GASTROINTESTINAL

__ No Problem   __ Nausea/Vomiting

__ Jaundice   __ Excessive Gas &/or

__ Hernia   Distention

__ Bleeding   __ Hemorrhoids

__ Diarrhea   __ Pain/Tenderness

__ Ulcer   __Constipation

__ Ostomy_____

Diet _____

Appetite_____

Recent Wt.   Gain ___ Loss ___ Amount _____

6. GENITOURINARY

__ No Problem   __ Burning

__ Frequency   __ Ileoconduit

__ Nocturia   __ Pain

__ Urgency   __ Incontinent

__ Catheter

     Type/Size _____

     Frequency of Change_____

OTHER _____

_____

7. REPRODUCTIVE

__ No Problem

OTHER _____

_____

8. BREAST

__ No Problem   __ Mastectomy

__ Lumps   __ Discharge

__ Dimpling   __ Pain/Tenderness

OTHER _____

_____

9. ENDOCRINE

__ No Problem   __ Hyperthyroidism

__ Diabetes   __ Hypothyroidism

__ Goiter   __ Hypoglycemia

OTHER _____

_____

10. MUSCULAR/SKELETAL

__ No Problem

__ Arthritis

__ Weakness _____

    Grip Strength   R ___ L ___

__ Spasticity

__ Joint Mobility/R.O.M. _____

__ Prosthesis

__ Pain

OTHER _____

_____

11. NEUROLOGICAL

__ No Problem

__ Orientation-   Person □ Yes   □ No

                 Place   □ Yes   □ No

                 Time   □ Yes   □ No

__ Level of Consciousness _____

__ Vertigo

__ Syncope

__ Pupil Reaction- R _____ L _____

__ Seizures—Describe _____

__Abnormal Motor Function (e.g., coordination, paralysis, tremor)

__ Speech Abnormalities (e.g., aphasia, slurring)

__ Poor Balance

OTHER _____

_____

12. PSYCHOSOCIAL

__ No Problem   __ Uncooperative

__ Anxious   __ Depressed

__ Relaxation/Hobbies _____

__ Habits (Alcohol/Drugs) _____

__ Motivation _____

__ Family Dynamics _____

_____

OTHER _____

_____

13. PAIN

__ No Problem

__ Location _____

__ Frequency _____

__ Intensity _____

Response to Relief Measures _____

_____

OTHER/DESCRIBE _____

_____

14. SLEEP PATTERNS

__ No Problem

__ Insomnia _____

__ Recent Changes _____

OTHER _____

_____

continues

Exhibit 21–3 continued

15. INTEGUMENTARY
Skin   Skin Turgor
☐ Clear and Intact   ☐ Rash   ☐ Good   ☐ Fair   ☐ Poor
☐ Pruritus   ☐ Bruises
Wound/Decubitus
   Location _____   Drainage _____
Measurement/Stage _____
Comments _____
Venous/Enteral Access Site
   Venous Access Site
   ☐ Clean and Dry   ☐ Edema   ☐ Erythema   ☐ Drainage   ☐ Tenderness   ☐ Blistering
   ☐ OTHER _____
Enteral Tube Size
☐ Clean and Dry   ☐ Edema   ☐ Erythema   ☐ Drainage   ☐ Tenderness   ☐ Excoriated
☐ OTHER _____
16. ENVIRONMENTAL ASSESSMENT
Home Access _____
Transfer Safety
   Bathroom _____
   Barriers_____
Additional Support Services
   ____ PT   ____ Speech   ____ Other
   ____ OT   ____ Home Health Aide
MISCELLANEOUS COMMENTS _____
_____
_____
_____
_____
_____
_____
_____
_____
_____
_____
_____
_____
_____
_____
_____
_____

Assessment Completed By _____Title _____Date _____

Source: Courtesy of Vitalink Pharmacy Services.

Exhibit 21–4 Examples of Acceptance Criteria

Enteral Feedings

1. The patient should be medically stable and not in need of in-hospital treatment. The patient should require only intermittent observation and evaluation.
2. The patient should have, as determined by the attending physician, medical problems such that the use of enteral feeding in the home or nursing home is appropriate.
3. The patient should have a primary physician who will monitor the enteral feeding and be responsible for interactions with the clinical laboratory. Nursing support services should be available and should be able to respond to requests within an acceptable period of time.
4. Except in unusual circumstances, there should be a second person (caregiver) who is willing to be actively involved in learning and managing the proposed therapy.
5. The patient and/or caregiver should be emotionally and physically capable and willing to use the supplies and equipment to administer the therapy. They should be able to complete successfully an acceptable training program. Adequate training time should be available.
6. The patient's environment should be suitable for antibiotic therapy. There should be proper lighting, proper electrical outlets, adequate plumbing and refrigeration, and a telephone should be readily available.
7. The patient or other responsible person should be able to comprehend any financial responsibilities incurred in association with the therapy.
8. Any patient who does not meet the above criteria but is felt to require enteral feedings to maintain his or her health status must be presented to the patient care conference to determine eligibility.

Type of tube should be a consideration in home therapy. Strongly recommend use of a gastrostomy or percutaneous endoscopic gastrostomy tube for administration of all home enteral therapies. Risk of aspiration is greatly reduced with the use of these tubes. Use of a nasogastric tube is not recommended.

Hydration

1. The patient should be medically stable and not in need of in-hospital treatment. The patient should require only intermittent observation and evaluation.
2. The patient should have, as determined by the attending physician, medical problems such that the use of hydration therapy in the home or nursing home is appropriate.
3. The patient should have a primary physician who will monitor the hydration therapy and be responsible for interactions with the clinical laboratory. Nursing support services should be available and should be able to respond to requests within an acceptable period of time.
4. Except in unusual circumstances, there should be a second person (caregiver) who is willing to be actively involved in learning and managing the proposed therapy.
5. The patient and/or caregiver should be emotionally and physically capable and willing to use the supplies and equipment to administer the therapy. They should be able to complete successfully an acceptable training program. Adequate training time should be available.
6. The patient's environment should be suitable for hydration therapy. There should be proper lighting, proper electrical outlets, adequate plumbing and refrigeration, and a telephone should be readily available.
7. The patient or other responsible person should be able to comprehend any financial responsibilities incurred in association with the therapy.
8. Any patient who does not meet the above criteria but is felt to require hydration therapy to maintain his or her health status must be presented to the patient care conference to determine eligibility.

Antibiotic Therapy

1. The patient should be medically stable and not in need of in-hospital treatment. The patient should require only intermittent observation and evaluation.
2. The patient should have, as determined by the attending physician, medical problems such

continues

Exhibit 21–4 continued

that the use of antibiotic therapy in the home or nursing home is appropriate.

3. The patient should have a primary physician who will monitor the antibiotic therapy and be responsible for interactions with the clinical laboratory. Nursing support services should be available and should be able to respond to requests within an acceptable period of time.

4. Except in unusual circumstances, there should be a second person (caregiver) who is willing to be actively involved in learning and managing the proposed therapy.

5. The patient and/or caregiver should be emotionally and physically capable and willing to use the supplies and equipment to administer the therapy. They should be able to complete successfully an acceptable training program. Adequate training time should be available.

6. The patient's environment should be suitable for antibiotic therapy. There should be proper lighting, proper electrical outlets, adequate plumbing and refrigeration, and a telephone should be readily available.

7. The patient or other responsible person should be able to comprehend any financial responsibilities incurred in association with the therapy.

8. Any patient who does not meet the above criteria but is felt to require antibiotic therapy to maintain his or her health status must be presented to the patient care conference to determine eligibility.

Total Parenteral Nutrition (TPN)

1. The patient should be medically stable and not in need of in-hospital treatment. The patient should require only intermittent observation and evaluation.

2. The patient should have, as determined by the attending physician, medical problems such that the use of TPN in the home or nursing home is appropriate.

3. The patient should have a primary physician who will monitor the TPN therapy and be responsible for interactions with the clinical laboratory. Nursing support services should be available and should be able to respond to requests within an acceptable period of time.

4. Except in unusual circumstances, there should be a second person (caregiver) who is willing to be actively involved in learning and managing the proposed therapy.

5. The patient and/or caregiver should be emotionally and physically capable and willing to use the supplies and equipment to administer the therapy. They should be able to complete successfully an acceptable training program. Adequate training time should be available.

6. The patient's environment should be suitable for TPN therapy. There should be proper lighting, proper electrical outlets, adequate plumbing and refrigeration, and a telephone should be readily available.

7. The patient or other responsible person should be able to comprehend any financial responsibilities incurred in association with the therapy.

8. Any patient who does not meet the above criteria but is felt to require TPN therapy to maintain his or her health status must be presented to the patient care conference to determine eligibility.

Type of access is extremely important. Recommend central line in most instances (i.e., Hickman, Broviac, Mediport, or P.I.C.C.) for administration of home hyperalimentation.

Pain Management

1. The patient should be medically stable and not in need of in-hospital treatment. The patient should require only intermittent observation and evaluation.

2. The patient should have, as determined by the attending physician, medical problems such that the use of pain management in the home or nursing home is appropriate.

3. The patient should have a primary physician who will monitor the pain management therapy and be responsible for interactions with the clinical laboratory. Nursing support services should be available and should be able to respond to requests within an acceptable period of time.

4. Except in unusual circumstances, there should be a second person (caregiver) who is willing

continues

Exhibit 21–4 continued

to be actively involved in learning and managing the proposed therapy.

5. The patient and/or caregiver should be emotionally and physically capable and willing to use the supplies and equipment to administer the therapy. They should be able to complete successfully an acceptable training program. Adequate training time should be available.

6. The patient's environment should be suitable for pain management therapy. There should be proper lighting, proper electrical outlets, adequate plumbing and refrigeration, and a telephone should be readily available.

7. The patient or other responsible person should be able to comprehend any financial responsibilities incurred in association with the therapy.

8. Any patient who does not meet the above criteria but is felt to require pain management therapy to maintain his or her health status must be presented to the patient care conference to determine eligibility.

IV Chemotherapy

1. The patient should be medically stable and not in need of in-hospital treatment. The patient should require only intermittent observation and evaluation.

2. The patient should have, as determined by the attending physician, medical problems such that the use of IV chemotherapy in the home or nursing home is appropriate.

3. The patient should have a primary physician who will monitor the IV chemotherapy and be responsible for interactions with the clinical laboratory. Nursing support services should be available and should be able to respond to requests within an acceptable period of time.

4. Except in unusual circumstances, there should be a second person (caregiver) who is willing to be actively involved in learning and managing the proposed therapy.

5. The patient and/or caregiver should be emotionally and physically capable and willing to use the supplies and equipment to administer the therapy. They should be able to complete successfully an acceptable training program. Adequate training time should be available.

6. The patient's environment should be suitable for IV chemotherapy. There should be proper lighting, proper electrical outlets, adequate plumbing and refrigeration, and a telephone should be readily available.

7. The patient or other responsible person should be able to comprehend any financial responsibilities incurred in association with the therapy.

8. Any patient who does not meet the above criteria but is felt to require IV chemotherapy to maintain his or her health status must be presented to the patient care conference to determine eligibility.

Would not begin home chemotherapy until patient has received an initial course of therapy in a controlled environment (i.e., hospital or outpatient clinic), and then under the supervision of a certified chemotherapy nurse.

Source: Courtesy of Vitalink Pharmacy Services.

Exhibit 21–5 Consent Agreement

Patient Name _____

Address _____

City _____ State _____ ZIP _____

Phone _____ S.S.N. _____

I.   I/We understand that by signing this Agreement, I/We authorize *Agency Name* to perform upon me (or patient indicated above) the following procedure:

_____

_____

_____

_____

_____

II.   I have been informed of the purpose for the above procedure, including the possible complications and treatment alternatives.

III.   I have received and read the instruction sheet and am aware of how to contact the agency should any problems occur.

IV.   I release *Agency Name* from any responsibility for adverse effects or consequences unless those effects/consequences result from negligence in the performance of care.

V.   I understand that I can revoke this consent at any time, either orally or in writing.

VI.   My signature on this form certifies that I have read and understand the above consent and that the procedure has been fully explained to me.

VII.   I understand that I or a family member will assume responsibility for maintaining and monitoring the therapy in the home.

_____   _____

Witness   **Patient Signature or Responsible Party**

_____   _____

Witness   Relationship to Patient

I have fully explained the purpose of the therapy as well as the risks, consequences, and possible complications and alternative treatments available to the patient.

_____   _____

Date   Signature of Nurse

Source: Courtesy of Vitalink Pharmacy Services.

Exhibit 21–6 Physician's Treatment Plan

Patient Name_____

Address _____

City _____   State _____   ZIP _____

Phone _____

Primary Caregiver _____   Relationship to Patient_____

   Address _____

   City _____   State _____   ZIP _____

   Phone _____

Nursing Agency

Name_____

Primary Care Nurse _____

   Address _____

   City _____   State _____   ZIP _____

   Phone _____

Primary Diagnosis _____

Secondary Diagnosis _____

Allergies _____

Medication Order

Medication _____   Dose_____

   Route _____   Frequency _____

Duration of Therapy_____

IV Therapy Order

_____

_____

_____

Duration of Therapy

_____

_____

_____

continues

Exhibit 21–6 continued

MEDICATION PATIENT IS PRESENTLY ON

Medication	Dose	Frequency	Rate

_____

_____

_____

_____

_____

_____

_____

_____

_____

_____

LABORATORY STUDIES ORDERED   FREQUENCY TO BE DRAWN

_____

_____

_____

_____

_____

_____

_____

☐ Call Reports to Me Directly   ☐ Send Reports to My Office

Patient Name_____

MENTAL STATUS	FUNCTIONAL LIMITATIONS	PHYSICAL LIMITATIONS
☐ Alert	☐ None	☐ None
☐ Oriented	☐ Speech	☐ Ambulation
☐ Confused	☐ Mental	☐ Aphasic
☐ Depressed	☐ Amputation	☐ Dyspnea
☐ Anxious	☐ Paralysis	☐ Respiratory _____
	☐ L Side ☐ R Side ☐ Other	☐ Endurance
	☐ Hearing	☐ Bowel/Bladder Incontinence
	☐ Blind	☐ Diabetic

continues

Exhibit 21–6 continued

ACTIVITIES PERMITTED
☐ No Restrictions   ☐ Independent   ☐ Complete Bedrest
☐ Bathroom Privileges   ☐ Transfer Bed/Chair   ☐ Other
☐ Weight Bearing   Partial   ☐ L   ☐ R
Assistive Devices   ☐ Cane   ☐ Wheelchair   ☐ Walker   ☐ Crutches   ☐ Other _____

Orders for Services and Treatments

Yes	No		Yes	No	
☐	☐	Skilled nursing visits frequently	☐	☐	Insert a:
☐	☐	Teach administration of therapy:	☐	☐	☐ Short Line☐ Midline☐ Long Line
☐	☐	☐ Antibiotic☐ Chemo☐ Hydration	☐	☐	Placement: _____
☐	☐	☐ Pain Mgt.☐ Other: _____	☐	☐	X-Ray:☐ Yes☐ No
☐	☐	Instruct on administration of:	☐	☐	Perform nutritional assessment every: ___
		☐ Lipids☐ TPN	☐	☐	Apply dressing of choice
☐	☐	Teach/assess for untoward reactions to	☐	☐	Rotate peripheral site every 48–72 hours
		therapy			and PRN with catheter of choice
☐	☐	Teach/assess/monitor:☐ IV☐ Enteral Site			Other: _____
☐	☐	Teach/assess/monitor vital signs, nutri-	☐	☐	Assess and inspect peripheral IV catheter
		tion, hydration			site more frequently if left in place
☐	☐	Teach/assess/monitor IV/Enteral dress-			longer than 72 hours; rotate site at first
		ing change			sign of any complication with catheter of
☐	☐	Teach/assess/monitor central catheter			choice
		self-care management	☐	☐	Provide 24-hour on-call service, follow-
☐	☐	Teach handwashing, aseptic technique,			up, monitoring, routine status
		injection cap change			reports
☐	☐	Teach self-care monitoring, trouble-	☐	☐	Provide discharge summary to physician
		shooting, management of complica-			and patient/caregiver discharge instruc-
		tions			tions. Anticipated discharge date: _____
☐	☐	Obtain vital signs each visit	☐	☐	Notify physician of any adverse reaction to
					therapy.
			☐	☐	Other: _____

Comments: _____

_____

_____

___ I certify that the above home health services are required and authorized by me. This patient is
    under my care and in need of skilled nursing and/or therapy services. I will review the plan of
    treatment per the agency's policy.
___ I recertify this patient for the above needed home health services, skilled nursing, and/or therapy services.

Physician Name _____   ID # _____

  Address _____

  Phone _____

_____   _____
Date   Physician Signature

_____   _____
Date   Primary Nurse Signature

Source: Courtesy of Vitalink Pharmacy Services.

Considerations about patients themselves include the following: What is their mental status? Are they oriented? Are they anxious? How anxious are they? What is their emotional response to the treatments that they've received before discharge to the home? What is their ability to learn? Has there been any history of substance use (e.g., alcohol, tobacco, or drugs), and what has been the frequency and history of their use? Psychosocial considerations are related to the assessment of the patient's disease and relevant medical history.

Other forms that could be considered part of the documentation policy are the following:

- A discharge summary form could be used to provide a summary to the physician of a course of therapy after a patient is discharged to the home.
- The patient medication record is used to facilitate compliance with the patient's medication schedule; it is particularly useful for IV antibiotics and total parenteral nutrition.
- A client flow sheet is used to allow the caregiver or the patient to record data and to facilitate patient monitoring by the nurse. This form particularly involves the patient and caregiver and the rendering of care. It can be a valuable tool to the home nurse if supporting documentation is done between visits.
- The patient/family teaching record (Exhibit 21–7) is useful in documenting the specific procedures that have been taught. It can serve as an evaluation of the patient's response as well as his or her ability to provide self-care.

Coordination of Pharmacy and/or Equipment

The coordination of pharmacy and/or equipment needs is the next procedure for delivering high-technology therapies. As stated, the pharmacy and equipment provider may be the same or different organizations and may or may not be part of the home care agency structure.

In most home care environment scenarios, the disciplines of pharmacy, nursing, and medicine are located remotely from one another, working from separate sets of forms and documentation procedures and frequently separate sets of priorities relating to the timely delivery of the pharmaceutical. The greater the coordination of activity between pharmacy and nursing, the greater the chance of success. Pharmacy should be a part of weekly reviews or clinical conferences wherein specific patient issues are discussed. Pharmacy should be part of the flow of information from physician care plans or nursing care plans. In general, the involvement of the pharmacy, and specifically the pharmacist, in the overall treatment and clinical issues related to specific patients is essential to the delivery of high-technology home care services. Finding an interested pharmacy provider willing to do this can be difficult.

The Admissions Package

On admission, patients should receive a packet of information dealing with areas of service that would be important to them. They should receive a statement of ownership, a copy of their rights and responsibilities, a statement of how the system works, a statement of ways to deal with problems, specific drug information related to their therapy, and teaching brochures dealing with their particular therapy. The contents of the admission package should also include a description of the services being provided, a training manual for the therapy, a letter describing their financial responsibility, and a consent to therapy form. The nurse clinician responsible for a given patient will take an active role in the development of these documents as well as in their explanation and execution with the patient.

Exhibit 21–7 Patient/Family Teaching Record for IV Therapy

Patient Name _____

Key: I—Verbalizes Understanding 2—Performs with Supervision 3—Performs Independently 4—See Additional Comments

Content	Pt. Response	Content	Pt. Response
I. PURPOSE		**III. TERMINATING INFUSION**	
—States purpose of IV therapy		—Closes roller clamp on tubing	
—Names IV therapy and possible side effects		—Removes tape securing tubing to arm	
—Verbalizes expected duration of therapy		—Withdraws needle from INT cap	
II. ADMINISTRATION		—Removes needle from end of IV tubing using aseptic technique	
—Names times for infusing medicine		—Replaces with sterile capped needle	
—States frequency for tubing changes		—Cleanses INT cap with _____ anti-septic solution	
—Inspects supplies checking:		—Flushes IV catheter with ____ mL of NSS	
Packaging		—Cleanses INT cap with _____ antiseptic solution	
Solution			
Labels		—Flushes IV catheter with _____ mL of heparin (____ unit/mL)	
—Inspects infusion site for redness, swelling		—Stores supplies until next infusion time	
—Brings medication to room temperature		**IV. CARE AND STORAGE OF SUPPLIES**	
—Cleans work area		—Stores medication in freezer/refrigerator/room temperature	
—Washes hands before all procedures			
—Gathers appropriate supplies		—Describes thawing and warming procedure for medication	
—Spikes bag using aseptic technique			
— Primes tubing to expel air		—Stores infusion supplies in a safe, clean area	
—Attaches needle to tubing using aseptic technique		—Describes purpose of and use of sharps disposal container	
—Cleanses INT cap with ____ aseptic solution		—Identifies situations in which solutions are not to be used	
—Flushes IV catheter with ____ mL of NSS		—Identifies situations in which supplies are not to be used	
—Cleanses INT cap with _____ antiseptic solution		**V. MONITORING**	
—Hangs medication 3 ft above infusion site		—Identifies possible side effects of medication infusion	
—Inserts needle into INT cap to connect medication for infusion		—Identifies the need for IV restart:	
		—Phlebitis	
—Tapes needle and tubing to arm to prevent disconnecting		—Infiltration	
		—Leaking	
—Adjusts flow rate using roller clamp on tubing		—Describes the course of action to be taken if complication occurs	
—Regulates flow rate at ____ mgtts/min		—Correctly identifies person(s) to be called re problems:	
—Keeps arm (if peripheral site) below heart		—IV therapy nurse	
—Monitors flow rate during infusion		—Physician	
—Pump:		—Visiting nurse	
—Places tubing in pump		—Ambulance	
—Sets rate at ____ mL/hour		—Identifies regular supply delivery day and time	
—Connects set to ____ access device			
—Keeps pump plugged into outlet when not ambulatory			
—States reason for alarms and demonstrates procedures for troubleshooting alarm conditions			

Initials _____ Name _____

Initials _____ Name _____

Initials _____ Name _____

Additional Comments: _____

_____

Source: Courtesy of Vitalink Pharmacy Services.

The Care Plan

The final phase of the process for delivery of high-technology therapies is the development of a care plan. The objective of the care plan is to ensure awareness and agreement of all parties involved in the course of therapy for the patient (see Exhibit 21–6).

CONCLUSION

It is possible to provide a myriad of safe high-technology services to patients in their homes. Home health agency administrators need to be cognizant of the numerous issues that need to be addressed to provide a successful program. The challenge is to meet the demand for this new level of care, which requires a high degree of competency, accountability, and cost effectiveness. Time, dollars, staff, and energy must be invested to achieve successful patient outcomes.

REFERENCE

Joint Commission for Accreditation of Healthcare Organizations. (1996). *1997–98 Comprehensive accreditation manual for home care*. Oakbrook Terrace, IL: Author.

CHAPTER 22

Discharge of a Ventilator-Dependent Child from the Hospital to Home

Andrea Gendelman and Zoe Ann Kinney

Katie is a bright 5-year-old girl who attends kindergarten. She is a little different from her classmates in that she is wheelchair bound and requires mechanical ventilation. Katie spent her first 9 months of life in a pediatric intensive care unit, where she was successfully weaned to requiring nighttime ventilation and subsequently was discharged to home. This case study illustrates the safe and successful discharge of the ventilator-dependent child from the hospital to home.

The polio epidemics of the 1940s through the 1950s spurred medical advances in mechanical ventilation. With these advances, neonatology and pediatric critical care medicine evolved, becoming adept at treating critically ill infants and children. Some of the infants and children who survive the acute stages of an illness continue to have complex medical problems and disabilities, with an increasing number being dependent on sophisticated technological support, such as mechanical ventilators. Traditionally, children who required this level of support remained in intensive care units, an environment incongruous with normal growth and development. Long-term hospitalization of technology-dependent children is no longer an option as a result of policymaking and reimbursement strategies that limit length of stay and health care expenditures. Home care of the technology-dependent child provides cost-effective care in an environment conducive to meeting the developmental and psychosocial needs of the child and family.

Katie was delivered at full term after an uncomplicated pregnancy, born with an L1-2 myelomeningocele with Arnold-Chiari malformation. She underwent posterior fossa compression and had multiple medical problems, including hydrocephalus necessitating placement of a ventriculoperitoneal shunt, upper airway obstruction requiring a tracheostomy at 2 weeks of age, apnea requiring full ventilatory support, and paraplegia. Over the course of a 9-month hospitalization, Katie's condition stabilized, and she demonstrated continued growth and development.

Katie's mother, Ms. M., a single parent and now mother of two, actively participated in Katie's well-infant care shortly after birth. As Katie's condition improved, her mother began learning how to care for her more complex needs. As Katie was successfully stabilized, her mother expressed interest in taking her daughter home. The medical staff recognized that the intensive care unit was not conducive to Katie's further growth and development and felt that she would be an acceptable candidate for home care.

The decision to discharge a ventilator-assisted child to home is intricate. Not every child and/or family is appropriate for home care. The child must be medically stable, as demonstrated by a stable airway, baseline oxygen requirements that do not fluctuate, blood gases that remain within medically acceptable limits, and positive gains on the growth scale. Commensurately, the parents must display the desire and ability to learn to successfully manage the care of the ventilator-assisted child.

Once a family has been identified as appropriate for home care, a discharge plan is formulated. This is accomplished with the input of the following people: the parents, primary physician, primary nurse, social worker and/or discharge coordinator, respiratory therapist, and developmental therapists. This team must consider closely all aspects of the child's care to provide a smooth transition from the hospital to home.

FUNDING FOR HOME CARE

Determining the funding for home care is often the most complex and time-consuming aspect of the discharge process. Katie was covered by her mother's private insurance policy. The policy reimbursed for a maximum of 120 days of patient hospitalization and had a $500,000 major medical benefit. The 120 inpatient days were exhausted, and the remaining 5 months of hospital costs were paid via the major medical portion of the policy. At an average cost of $60,000 per month, $300,000 of the major medical benefit was used for her hospitalization. The remaining $200,000 was targeted for home care.

The social worker contacted the case manager of the insurer to ensure that the remaining major medical funds would be available for home care coverage. Because Katie would have exhausted more than half her major medical funds by her discharge date, the social worker sought a secondary, long-term funding course. An application was submitted to the state Medicaid waiver program for Katie. The waiver program in her state provides reimbursement for the home care of a predetermined number of technology-dependent children. The reimbursement covers durable medical equipment (DME), supplies, and up to 16 hours of nursing care per day depending on the severity of the child's medical needs. The waiver program deems a child eligible for medical assistance regardless of parental income and assets.

The social worker also filed an application for Katie to the Ventilator Assisted Children/Home Program (VAC/HP), a program funded by the Commonwealth of Pennsylvania. The VAC/HP would provide supportive and advocacy services via a case coordinator once Katie was home. The program's administrator would remain available to the discharging institution for assistance with the discharge process.

TEACHING PLAN

The teaching plan for the family can be devised and implemented concurrent with negotiating for home care funding. Ms. M. identified one back-up caregiver to assist in Katie's care in the event that Ms. M. was not available for Katie. Ms. M. and the back-up caregiver completed an extensive teaching plan, which covered:

- anatomy of the respiratory system
- the child's diagnosis as it related to the tracheostomy and mechanical ventilation
- signs and symptoms of infection
- care of the tracheostomy
- pulmonary toilet
- emergency care of the artificial airway
- cardiopulmonary resuscitation
- administration of medications and nutritional supplements via nasogastric tube
- physical and occupational therapy exercises
- operation and maintenance of the ventilator and associated equipment

Before discharge, Ms. M. and the secondary caregiver were required to spend at least 24 consecutive hours in the hospital providing all Katie's care. During the education process, the hospital social worker met with the primary nurse and the respiratory therapist to compile a list of necessary equipment and supplies for home.

SELECTION OF A DME VENDOR

Once the lists of equipment and supplies were complete, the social worker and Ms. M. reviewed the selection of a DME provider. While interviewing possible vendors, the family should consider the following questions:

- Does the vendor guarantee 24-hour service?
- What is the vendor's proximity to the home?
- What is the vendor's response time to service and emergency calls?
- What is the vendor's experience with the population of ventilator-assisted children?
- Will the vendor accept the funding mechanism's reimbursement as payment in full?
- Is the vendor Medicaid certified in the state in which the family resides?

Ms. M. interviewed and identified a DME vendor. The vendor was given an itemized list of the necessary equipment and supplies for Katie. The equipment to be used at home, including the ventilator and its external battery, cascade humidifier, and pulse oximeter were delivered to the hospital's biomedical department to be evaluated for safety and proper functioning. Before discharge, Katie was placed on the equipment for 1 week to familiarize the mother and caregivers with it and to assess further its safety and performance.

The day before discharge, the vendor delivered and set up all the equipment in Katie's home; disposable supplies sufficient for 1 month were provided. The respiratory therapist reviewed with the mother and home care staff the equipment's maintenance and function. On the day of discharge, the respiratory therapist was present in the home to assess Katie's adaptation to the equipment.

One aspect of the discharge plan that can be easily overlooked is the possible purchase of equipment. Katie's physicians determined that she would require mechanical ventilation for an extended period of time. As a cost-saving measure, the social worker negotiated with the insurer to purchase one complete set of equipment along with the service contract. The rationale behind the purchase of equipment is that the rental of the ventilator alone for 1 year will exceed its purchase price.

HOME NURSING CARE

A major component of home care for a ventilator-assisted child is nursing care. The parents, with insight from the child's physician and social worker, must determine the amount and type of nursing care to be used at home. This will vary because each family is unique in its composition and obligations (parents' careers, other dependents, and the intricacy of the child's care).

Katie's sister was 6 years old, and her mother worked full time. Katie was on the ventilator 12 hours per day and required pulmonary toilet at least every 4 hours. A nursing time study performed in the hospital demonstrated that Katie needed at least 16 hours of direct nursing care per day as well as continuous monitoring. Ms. M. chose to utilize the 16 hours of nursing care per day with one day shift and one night shift. Katie's mother worked a full 8-hour day, Monday through Friday, and had a half-hour commute to work. Ms. M.'s friend and neighbor elected to care for Katie for the hour each day that the nurse and Ms. M. were not available.

Home nursing care for a ventilator-assisted child can be provided by a registered nurse, a licensed practical nurse, and in some cases a home health aide. Because of the complexity of Katie's care, the medical staff recommended that registered nurses and licensed practical nurses should provide her care at home. Taking into consideration the long-term plan for Katie's home care funding, the discharge team suggested that Ms. M. choose a Medicaid-certified nursing agency. This would ensure consistency of care for Katie when the funding mechanism changed from the major medical benefit to the state Medicaid waiver program.

Selecting a nursing agency can be a difficult task for a family, but with guidance and support from experienced hospital personnel the family can feel confident in making an informed decision. The social worker assisted Ms. M. in interviewing nursing agencies. Together they outlined a list of considerations that were important to Ms. M.:

- the nursing agency's experience with the pediatric ventilator-dependent population
- the agency's ability to staff the case to the family's satisfaction
- the experience and qualifications of the agency's nurses
- the agency's policies on notification of and coverage for call-outs and vacations
- the agency's philosophy of nursing care
- the family's ability to maintain autonomy in caring for the child at home

After interviewing four nursing agencies, Ms. M. selected one she felt would best meet the family's needs.

For the discharging institution and the family to be assured that the home care nurses are competent in providing the patient care, it is beneficial that as many of the home care nurses as possible be trained by the patient's primary nurse before discharge. It is important that there be an established teaching plan with specific objectives to promote consistency and maximum benefit from the teaching sessions. Katie's nursing case manager and four home care nurses were trained at the hospital.

HOME ASSESSMENT

Before discharge, it is essential to assess that the child's home environment is safe and appropriate. This is best accomplished with a home visit by the social worker and the primary nurse. The visit also provides an opportunity to assist the family in developing concrete plans for the child's care at home. The family may need guidance with decisions such as where physi-

cally to locate the child and her necessary equipment. Ms. M. lived in a small, two-bedroom house with her 6-year-old daughter, and she had initially planned for Katie to share the room with her sister. The nurse/social work team suggested that the rarely used dining room be converted into a room for Katie. This would afford her sister privacy and the ability to sleep through the night undisturbed by Katie's care. A representative from the DME provider visited the home to assess its electrical capabilities and to determine whether additional outlets were necessary.

DEVELOPMENTAL NEEDS

A complete home care plan for the ventilator-assisted child addresses his or her developmental needs. During the child's hospitalization, he or she will most likely be evaluated by the physical, occupational, and speech therapists. If they recommend continued therapies for the child at home, it is advisable to obtain the prescriptions for the therapies and to register the child for those services in the community before discharge.

It was recommended that Katie receive physical, occupational, and speech therapies each once a week for at least the first 6 months she was home. The social worker informed the case worker for the County Office of Mental Health/Mental Retardation of Katie's history, developmental needs, and therapy recommendations. The case worker agreed to schedule an appointment with the family once Katie was at home for the assessment and evaluation of speech, physical, and occupational therapies.

EMERGENCY RESOURCES

Last, Ms. M. received assistance in compiling a list of emergency resources. The social worker notified the gas, electric, and phone companies as well as the police, fire, and rescue squad that a child on life support equipment was being discharged into the community. Katie was identified as a priority by each of these service providers in the event of an emergency or interruption of services. Katie's primary nurse suggested that Ms. M. keep a card by every phone, listing emergency telephone numbers and pertinent information about Katie's medical condition. Ms. M. elected to have a phone placed in Katie's room as an added safety measure.

THE HOME NURSING CARE PLAN

The week before discharge, the nursing agency's case manager met with Ms. M. and Katie's primary nurse to develop the home nursing care plan (Table 22–1). The social worker, primary nurse, and agency case manager addressed with Ms. M. the realities of home care for a family with a ventilator-dependent child.

Ms. M. and her family may experience many new stressors during the first few months of Katie's homecoming. Two of the most frequently identified stresses of home care are the disruption in family life style and the lack of privacy due to the constant flow of personnel through the home. Some families manage this by organizing the home in such a manner that the child's care, and therefore the nursing personnel, are confined to certain areas in the home. For example, if nursing personnel care for the child during the night, the child's room is optimally located distant from the family bedrooms. This will foster a maximal degree of privacy for the parents and isolate the rest of the family from the disturbance of the frequent alarms.

Another life-style change that families often experience is a sense of social isolation and alienation from friends and family. Parents are unable to partake in social activities because they are often confined to the home to care for their child. Friends and relatives may feel inadequate to assist the parents in caring for their family. It can be difficult for parents to alter nursing shifts or arrange for a skilled caregiver to watch the child when they wish to attend a social event.

Management issues may create added stress on the family. Once the child is home, the role of patient advocate is transferred from the inpatient primary nurse to the parent(s). It is the responsibility of the parents to communicate with the home care nurses, physicians, case managers, therapists, and so forth to ensure the safety and welfare of the child. Parents may feel overwhelmed with providing the day-to-day care and coordinating services. To alleviate some of this stress, some families have learned to delegate responsibilities as part of their management strategy. A primary nurse or night nurse may be given the job of taking inventory and reordering supplies.

Cost containment within the home care setting should be addressed with the family before discharge. In the hospital, disposable items are used once and discarded to reduce the risk of contamination and the incidence of nosocomial infections. During the daily routine, hospital personnel give little thought to the cost of those items. Families with limited home care funds do not have that luxury. Educating the family and other caregivers about supply costs, cleaning, disinfection, and reuse of certain supplies can greatly affect the expenditure of home care dollars.

While discussing fiscal matters, it is important to emphasize the financial implications that the home care setting will have for the family. Uncovered nursing shifts may necessitate that a parent remain at home, therefore missing work and possibly losing wages. Also, the family's utility bills can be expected to increase once the technology-dependent child is home. It is not unusual for the electricity bill to double. Some families have benefitted from enrolling in their local electric company's budget payment plan.

The homecoming of a ventilator-dependent child may have a great impact on siblings. Often the child has been hospitalized for a long period of time, and the siblings may not identify the child as a brother or sister. Also, the demanding nature of the child's illness and care may leave a sibling feeling jealous and neglected. These feelings may be exhibited as

Table 22–1 Home Care Plan

Problem	Goals	Assessments	Interventions
Alteration in respiratory status secondary to tracheostomy and need for mechanical ventilation.	Katie will have a patent airway and adequate respiratory function. Katie will eventually be weaned from respiratory support during the day.	Observe Katie for signs of respiratory distress: Restlessness Nasal flaring Retractions Cyanosis Tachypnea Check ventilator settings (rate, inspiratory pressure, oxygen, dial volume, alarms).	1. Maintain patient #2 Portex tracheostomy tube at all times: • Suction every 2 hours and as needed. • Provide humidification via ventilator. • Change tracheostomy tube weekly (Wednesdays). 2. Maintain ventilator settings as ordered. Maintain humidifier temperature at 30°–34°C. Empty H_2O traps as needed. 3. When going outside on a trip, always take emergency travel bag. Should include: • Tracheostomy tube with strings • Endotracheal tube • Portable suction • Resuscitation bag • K-Y jelly • Saline • Scissors and hemostat
Potential for respiratory infections secondary to tracheostomy.	Katie will be free of respiratory infections and atelectasis.	Assess breath sounds every 4 hours. Observe for signs and symptoms of respiratory infection: change in amount, color, odor, consistency of secretions; decreased aeration; fever; chest congestion; fatigue.	1. Follow good handwashing technique. Always wash hands before tracheostomy care. 2. Daily tracheostomy care: • Clean tracheostomy site with water (half strength peroxide if crusted). • Change tracheostomy dressing twice daily and as needed. • Change tracheostomy strings every morning and as needed. • Change tracheostomy tube weekly (Wednesdays) with sterile technique and two caregivers. 3. Chest percussion every 4 hours while awake. Instilled 1–2 mL normal saline as needed for thick secretions. 4. Maintain clean technique during suctioning: every 1–2 hours while awake, every 4–6 hours while asleep. 5. Change disposable ventilator tubing every 3 days (on night shift). 6. Change and disinfect cascade humidifier and non-disposable ventilator parts every 3 days (night shift).
Alteration in growth and development secondary to diagnosis and prolonged hospitalization.	Katie will increase her developmental skills and reach age-appropriate developmental milestones.	Assess developmental skills.	1. Encourage Katie to be independent: Allow her to feed herself, assist in dressing herself. 2. Follow posted daily schedule for activities. 3. Provide play time and encourage development skills. • Gross motor: Encourage full use of upper extremities. Provide passive range of motion exercises to lower extremities, follow prescribed leg and foot splint schedule.

continues

Table 22–1 continued

Problem	Goals	Assessments	Interventions
			• Fine motor: Encourage use of crayons, blocks, etc.
			• Speech: Encourage Katie to vocalize around tracheostomy. Katie knows some sign language.
			4. Speak to Katie about her environment. Introduce new things she has not had the opportunity to experience while in the hospital. Follow through on speech therapist recommendations.
			5. Katie will receive physical, occupational, and speech therapy each once per week.
Alteration in nutritional status secondary to poor oral intake and new environment.	Katie will gain weight.	Weigh weekly.	1. Provide high-calorie, high-protein meals with three snacks at 10 a.m., 2 p.m., and bedtime.
			2. Allow Katie to eat with the family, sitting at the table in highchair. Provide favorite foods.
			3. Encourage Katie to use a cup. Do not give her a bottle until after meals.
Potential alteration in family functioning secondary to child's prolonged hospitalization and complex needs.	Katie will become an active family member. The M.s will be an intact family unit.	Assess family for signs of stress.	1. Allow time for individual attention to Katie and her sister by mother.
			2. Encourage Katie and her sister to play together.
			3. Provide time for Ms. M. to go out by herself.
			4. Provide time for family to socialize as a unit.
			5. Allow Katie's sister to participate in Katie's care.
			6. Maintain familiar routines for children.

anger, depression, somatic complaints, behavior disorders, nightmares, and general disequilibrium. Parents, relatives, and health care professionals can assist the sibling(s) in adjusting to the myriad changes that the home care setting brings by including them whenever appropriate in activities and care, patiently answering their questions, displaying genuine interest in their own activities and achievements, allowing the siblings to spend time together, avoiding displacement of the siblings from their own bedrooms, and maintaining continuity of familiar routines.

CONCLUSION

Our experience has shown that, with careful planning, thorough education of the parents and caregivers, and coordination of community resources, a safe and successful discharge for the ventilator-assisted child can be accomplished.

PART IV

Quality Assessment and Improvement

CHAPTER 23

Performance Improvement

Nancy L. Bohnet

Performance improvement (PI) in home care has evolved from a long series of efforts to monitor and evaluate quality of patient care services. Providers of health care have long been interested in monitoring the quality of patient care services. Around the turn of the century, implicit review was used to investigate morbidity and mortality rates after certain medical procedures or inpatient stays. The next development was audits of the medical record: Specific criteria were established and defined, and a standard of expected compliance was determined. Closed records were reviewed for compliance with the predetermined standard, and results were reported to the organization's leaders. This process had no priority setting for problem resolution.

The next evolution, quality assurance through monitoring and evaluation, has occurred in a planned and systematic manner over the past 10 years. An organization's scope of care is determined by identification of the types of services provided and the types of patients served. Aspects of care are identified and include referral, care planning, treatment procedures, administration of medications, and discharge planning. Clinical indicators are developed and thresholds for evaluation established; if the threshold is not reached, there is no problem. The most common source used to obtain data is the patient record. If the threshold is reached, an opportunity for improvement occurs. Corrective action is taken, and after an appropriate time interval compliance with the indicator is again evaluated. If the problem is resolved, the cycle is finished; if not, a new plan for resolution is developed.

Although this system is clearly an improvement over chart audits, there are some basic deficits in the process. The establishment of thresholds needs to be realistic and reasonable. For example, a threshold of 85 percent or 90 percent might be set unless a clinical event would result in serious difficulties or death, such as administration of the wrong drug or extravasation of a vesicant chemotherapeutic agent. The tacit understanding, therefore, is that 10 percent or 15 percent of the time it is all right not to comply with the indicator. In addition, priorities are not established for correction of problems.

Over the last decade, several things have happened that have paved the way for PI in home care. Cost containment strategies, including prospective payment, capitation, and managed care, have shifted health care from institutions to the home. As home care has grown, organizations have faced increased scrutiny and demands for accountability. There is a need to examine outcomes as well as those elements that improve patient care while being cost effective. The degree to which a home care organization carries out its key processes and functions will influence its outcomes (Joint Commission on Accreditation of Healthcare Organizations, 1995). Experts such as J. Edwards Deming (Walton, 1986), Juran (1988), and Crosby (1984) have promoted quality in American industry for more than a decade. Deming's 14 points for the provision of quality products/services, Juran's quality trilogy (quality planning, quality control, and quality implementation), and Crosby's 14 steps for top-down quality management are all adaptable to health care in general and home care specifically.

All the experts agree that an organization must understand its key functions and processes, measure quality, and build quality into the functions and processes. A home care function is a group of processes with a common goal; a process is a series of goal-directed activities (Joint Commission, 1995). For example, patient assessment is a function, whereas obtaining the information about the patient's medication profile is a process. Leadership is a function within an organization, and driving the quality improvement activities is a process.

For an organizational philosophy of quality to be implemented, the leaders must be 100 percent committed to it (McLaughlin and Kaluzny, 1990). Leaders are responsible for setting the tone for a nonpunitive, respectful environment. Education must be provided to help employees understand improvement techniques and statistical measurements. Those who are to investigate processes and devise ways to improve them must be given the opportunity to do so. Leaders have to be involved at all levels of PI by understanding organizational processes and providing resources for improvement activities in terms of time, people, and information systems. A different type of leadership is required for PI, one that understands that people must work together both within and across departments and that the people who do the work are in the best position to offer improvement suggestions. Therefore, staff from the entire organization must be involved in improvement activities (Bohnet, 1995). Not only must the

leaders understand the importance of organizational commitment, they must educate the next level down, one level at a time, until every employee has a basic knowledge of PI. Improving quality increases productivity because less time is spent redoing, repairing, and inspecting. When processes are studied, unnecessary and redundant steps can be eliminated, resulting in streamlining (Berger, 1991). Thus not only are money and time saved, but productivity is improved and customers are better satisfied. Overall, improved quality provides an organization with a competitive advantage (Berger, 1991).

INITIATION AND IMPLEMENTATION

There are several stages in putting a PI program in place. The first stage, initiation, requires the leaders to study the principles of PI, to educate the managers under them, to identify key functions of the organization, and to develop a quality vision statement. This vision will help everyone understand the commitment to quality and will serve as an organizational guideline during the transition to and actual adoption of PI (Bohnet et al., 1993).

The next stage is implementation, whereby management establishes priorities for examining certain key functions that can be improved. Project teams are chosen, and the work begins. Teams need some education about PI (e.g., teamwork and quality improvement tools). Teams must understand the goal for their group's work and should have basic guidelines for productive meetings. Every group should have a leader who understands the process being investigated as well as a facilitator. The leader prepares and distributes an agenda (an essential item) for each meeting, and the facilitator keeps the meeting on track and on time, also reminding the group of its stated goal and progress toward it. Minutes must be taken for each meeting to record discussions, assignments, and progress. They serve also as a review for the next meeting. Each meeting should be evaluated by the leader and facilitator, and then the next meeting's agenda can be prepared (Lynn, 1991; Scholtes, 1988). The first projects undertaken should be relatively simple and quickly implemented. This early win strategy will help gain employee buy-in and familiarize the teams and leaders with the PI process.

In addition to education about PI principles and philosophy, PI tools must be taught to the team as needed. Basic tools used to identify, analyze, and solve problems include brainstorming, multivoting, cause-and-effect diagrams, flow charts, run charts, control charts, histograms, and Pareto charts.

Brainstorming

This technique enables all team members to generate as many ideas as possible in a short period of time as to the causes of or solutions to a problem. Guidelines are as follows (Joint Commission, 1993b):

1. Allow two to three minutes for the group members to gather their thoughts in silence.
2. State that no idea is to be criticized.
3. Have the group members give their thoughts in a predetermined order; these are listed on a flip chart (no comments are made by anyone).
4. Clarify the list to make sure that ideas are clearly understood by all. The team will

have a varied list that is not refined but full of possibilities.

Multivoting

The team that has generated a list of possibilities can sort it out into groups of similar ideas. Sometimes topics can be condensed by grouping three or four similar ideas into one. Team members are asked to vote on only three to five items that are deemed to be most pertinent to the problem. One or two items receiving the most total votes can receive further attention (Joint Commission, 1991).

Cause-and-Effect Diagrams

This type of diagram helps teams picture a large number of possible causes of a specific outcome (Figure 23–1). An example of the use of this tool would be listing the causes of infection at discharge among patients receiving intravenous antibiotics at home (Figure 23–2). Listed at the top of the diagram are the main causes of the outcome. Subcauses can branch off main causes—these further identify the result or outcome (Joint Commission, 1993b); in this example, the outcome is a poor one.

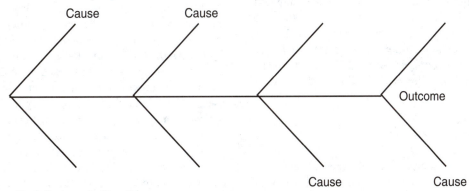

Figure 23–1 Cause-and-effect diagram.

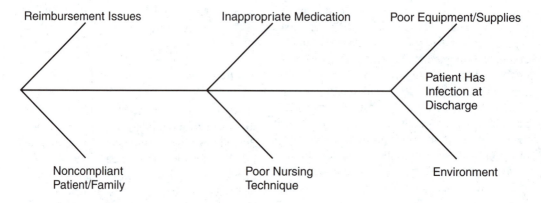

Figure 23–2 Application of a cause-and-effect diagram to a specific problem.

Flow Charts

Processes must be understood to be improved. Flow charts depict sequential steps in a process. This enables a team to identify redundancies and misunderstandings and guides the team in creating a more systematic and efficient process. For example, a patient is admitted to home care as illustrated in Figure 23–3. Simple shapes are used for different aspects of the process: ovals for start and end, diamonds for decisions, rectangles for steps, and circles for holding the process and proceeding no further.

Run Charts

This type of tool allows a team to look for patterns or trends over time. It has an x axis (horizontal), which indicates a time or sequence, and a y axis (vertical), which indicates a unit of measurement (Joint Commission, 1993b). Patterns of referrals from a particular hospital are depicted in Figure 23–4 as an example.

Control Charts

These are run charts with the mean and one to three standard deviations above and below the mean calculated and with upper and lower lim-

its determined (Joint Commission, 1991). These limits show whether a process is in statistical control. The run chart for referrals becomes a control chart with the necessary calculations (Figure 23–5).

Histograms

The histogram is a vertical bar graph that displays variations in data. The x axis displays frequency, and the y axis displays classes or ranges of data. Frequent patient diagnoses in a home care organization are shown as a histogram in Figure 23–6.

Pareto Charts

The histogram becomes a Pareto chart when the data are arranged in descending order from left to right for the events being studied (Joint Commission, 1991). If the home care organization wishes to develop patient teaching tools for the most common diagnoses, a Pareto chart is useful. The Pareto chart shown in Figure 23–7 indicates that 57 percent of all patients have congestive heart failure and diabetes. This indicates the need to concentrate on those areas first and that more than half the patients in home care will benefit from the work involved in generating patient education materials.

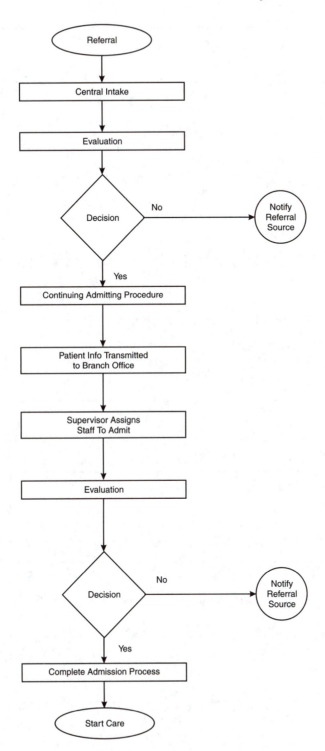

Figure 23–3 Flow chart for admission to home care.

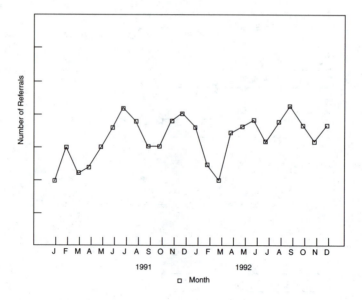

Figure 23–4 Run chart for referrals from a particular hospital.

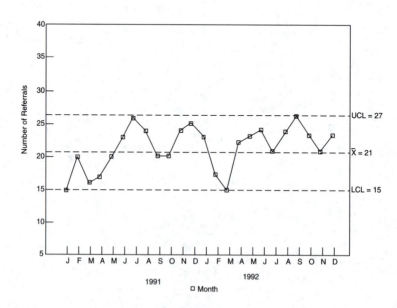

Figure 23–5 Control chart for referrals from a particular hospital.

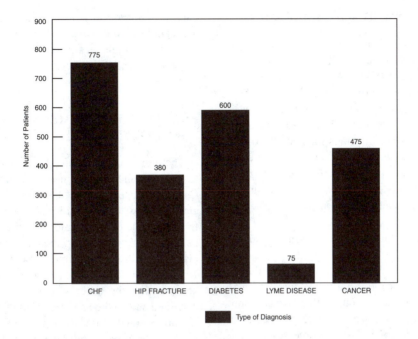

Figure 23–6 Histogram showing diagnoses of patients admitted to home care, 1992. CHF, congestive heart failure.

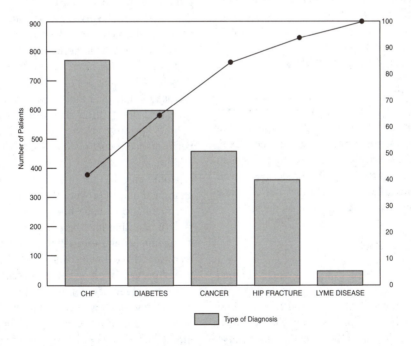

Figure 23–7 Pareto chart showing diagnoses of patients admitted to home care, 1992. The line indicates the cumulative percentage of the total patients per diagnosis. CHF, congestive heart failure.

VARIATION AND BENCHMARKING

An important consideration when one is analyzing data is variation. There is variation in every aspect of the things we do as well as in nature. All variation is caused: A person's weight goes up or down daily, as does his or her performance. If there is a lack of understanding of variance, several things happen: People are blamed for problems that are not there, purchases of unnecessary equipment are made, time is wasted looking for trends that are not there, and needless actions are taken (Nolan and Provost, 1990).

Variation is due to either common cause or special cause (Nolan and Provost, 1990). Common cause variation is the ever-present fluctuation in processes. Special cause correlates with something happening out of the ordinary: snow storms, tornadoes, lack of staff, new competition, or closure of a referral source, for example. Variation may also be due to tampering or making unnecessary adjustments to compensate for common cause variation. Regular, systematic patterns and long-term trends may also result in variation, which is known as structural variation. It is essential to understand variation and to distinguish among its causes (Joiner and Gaudard, 1990).

PI also utilizes benchmarking as a technique (McLaughlin and Kaluzny, 1990). A process that is done the best by another organization (health care or industry) is used as the model standard for performance. Learning how an organization carries out its process so well makes it possible to emulate that performance by matching what that organization does.

ACCELERATION

After two to three processes are examined when people are beginning to understand PI, acceleration occurs. At this stage, a cultural change slowly takes place within the organization. People begin to believe that they have good ideas for improvement, that they can make a real difference, and that almost any process can be improved. It is exciting at this stage to see people taking ownership of problem solutions. Most employees truly want to do a good job and are delighted that their input results in improvement.

PROCESS MEASUREMENT AND IMPROVEMENT

There are many systems devised for process assessment and improvement: the PDCA cycle (plan, do, check, act), FOCUS (find, organize, clarify, understand, select [or solution]), and the five-stage plan (understand the process, eliminate errors, remove slack, reduce variation, and plan for continuous improvement; Scholtes, 1988). Regardless of the method employed, it is obvious that the process must be completely dissected and studied before a plan of correction is implemented. After a sufficient time period elapses, the process must be studied to determine whether it has been improved, has stayed at an improved level without slipping, or has other improvement opportunities. A systematic approach to PI involves measurement, analysis, action, and review (Joint Commission, 1993b).

Measurement is important in PI. The guesses and estimates that often determine management decisions become obsolete. Measurement and the use of statistical tools have several benefits: increased observation accuracy and conclusion validity, priority setting, and establishment of performance benchmarks (Joint Commission, 1993a).

Home care is rich in processes that may be examined and improved. Referrals, admissions, documentation, and billing are aspects of patient care that may be problematic. Reducing redundancies and errors helps increase productivity and drive down costs. Other areas that can be improved include management/billing of supplies, inventory control, billing, and delivery. Obtaining signed orders and laboratory results is important and may not be done in a timely manner. The delay may result in tardy billing or patient record discharge. Staff issues may also be improved, such as weekend and holiday rotation and on-call nursing coverage. Potential problem areas of patient care include care planning, treatment procedures, medication administration, infection control, and care coordination (Bohnet et al., 1993).

CONCLUSION

PI must be driven by top management personnel, who must understand an organization's key processes. It involves workers across departments and necessitates the use of tools and statistics. It will work in health care as well as it has in industry. As home care organizations attempt to serve patients better and compete more effectively, many will design or redesign their services to be more efficient, to be attentive to customer expectations, and to improve patient outcomes (Joint Commission, 1994). Total quality will be the way to differentiate among health care organizations. Prices will be equal, so that the quality and value of service will distinguish organizations. This means that quality can no longer be delegated to an individual or department but must become inherent within the organizational philosophy (Gillem, 1988).

REFERENCES

Berger, C. 1991. *Quality improvement through leadership and empowerment: A business survival handbook.* Harrisburg, PA: MILRITE Council.

Bohnet, N. 1995. Continuous quality improvement in home care. In *Core curriculum for home health care nursing,* ed. K. Morgan and S. McClain. Gaithersburg, MD: Aspen.

Bohnet, N., et al. 1993. Continuous quality improvement: Improving quality in your home care organization. *Journal of Nursing Administration* 23:42–48.

Crosby, P. 1984. *Quality without tears: The art of hassle-free management.* New York: McGraw-Hill.

Gillem, T. 1988. Responding to the consumer's demand for the best value health care. *Journal of Nursing Quality Assurance* 2:70–78.

Joiner, B., and M. Gaudard. 1990. Variation, management and W. Edwards Deming. *Quality Progress* 23(5):29–37.

Joint Commission on Accreditation of Healthcare Organizations. 1991. *An introduction to QI in health care.* Oakbrook Terrace, IL: Joint Commission.

Joint Commission on Accreditation of Healthcare Organizations. 1993a. *The measurement mandate.* Oakbrook Terrace, IL: Joint Commission.

Joint Commission on Accreditation of Healthcare Organizations. 1993b. *Using tools in a health care setting.* Oakbrook Terrace, IL: Joint Commission.

Joint Commission on Accreditation of Healthcare Organizations. 1994. *Forms, charts and other tools for performance improvement.* Oakbrook Terrace, IL: Joint Commission.

Joint Commission on Accreditation of Healthcare Organizations. 1995. *Framework for improving performance: A guide for home care and hospice organizations.* Oakbrook Terrace, IL: Joint Commission.

Juran, J. 1988. *Juran on planning for quality.* New York: McGraw-Hill.

Lynn, M. 1991. Deming's quality principles: A health care application. *Hospital and Health Services Administration* 36:111–120.

McLaughlin, C., and A. Kaluzny. 1990. Total quality management in health: Making it work. *Health Care Management Review* 15:7–12.

Nolan, T., and L. Provost. 1990. Understanding variation. *Quality Progress* 23(23):70–79.

Scholtes, P. 1988. *The team handbook.* Madison, WI: Joiner Associates.

Walton, M. 1986. *The Deming management method.* New York: Putnam.

CHAPTER 24

Quality Assessment/Performance Improvement: An Administrator's Viewpoint

Marilyn D. Harris

In the 1990s, current quality concepts and efforts are expressed in terms of total quality management, continuous quality improvement, and performance improvement (PI). The Visiting Nurse Association (VNA) of Eastern Montgomery County/Department of Abington Memorial Hospital has adopted the PI initiative and has initiated departmentwide teams to identify and facilitate needed systems changes to attain specific goals. Quality assessment/performance improvement (QA/PI) activities that address structural and process components of the overall QA/PI process are in place with the ultimate goal of improvement in patient outcomes. This chapter describes several of these structural and process criteria that have enabled the VNA to evaluate patient care from both financial and clinical perspectives.

Quality assurance (QA) is a term that is heard frequently in health care. What does it mean? How is it accomplished? The *American College Dictionary* defines the word *quality* as "a character with respect to excellence, fineness or grade of excellence." *Assurance* is defined as "the understanding or making certain; a positive declaration intended to give confidence." Combining these two definitions, QA can be thought of as the process of making certain or guaranteeing that high-quality care will be provided to clients, which will instill confidence in the product or service provided.

In spite of this definition, Meisenheimer (1985) states that QA is an elusive, if not a frequently misunderstood, concept. As noted earlier, QA activities are just one aspect of the larger QA/PI concept. QA is a proactive set of policies and activities utilized to evaluate the patient care delivery scope and quality. The recommendations from this evaluation usually result in stronger enforcement of a procedure or a change of procedure (Ruane, 1994). A QA program in a home health agency is necessary for multiple reasons: to monitor and evaluate client care; to identify, hire, and retain the appropriate level of personnel to meet clients' needs; to meet standards established by the Medicare conditions of participation (COPs), accrediting bodies, professional organizations, and the agency; to speak to risk management issues; and to address and resolve identified problems.

It is necessary to utilize multiple structure, process, and outcomes criteria; to identify and measure the grade of excellence; and to have confidence in the overall procedure and final results. The agency must define what is to be measured; how measurement will be accomplished, by whom, and when (daily, monthly, or annually); and what is to be done with the identified outcomes, or what information will be shared with whom (e.g., feedback to staff, the board of directors, the professional advisory committee, funding sources, and regulatory agencies). The format for this feedback must be clearly designed so that data can be displayed in an understandable and useful manner.

There must be administrative support to accomplish the primary goal of providing quality health care services in the home. Support must also be demonstrated through the provision of whatever time, dollars, and personnel are necessary to measure the degree of attainment of this goal. This type of support is a critical element of the QA process in the 1990s because more attention must be given to containing and reducing costs while continuing to provide high-quality care to patients.

NEEDS AND EXPECTATIONS FOR SURVIVAL AND GROWTH

Quality is usually viewed from the perspective of client care. What is quality care? What is quality care provided in the home setting? How and by whom is it evaluated? To have a complete picture, myriad vantage points must be considered.

The Consumer's Viewpoint

Today's consumers—our patients and their families—are asking questions about their home care services. These questions concern coverage of services and financial issues. One reason is that some consumers are being asked to pay a higher portion of health care costs through increased deductibles or coinsurance or to assume all payment for noncovered services. This may include home health aide service, which is considered a patient responsibility by some third-party payers.

Patients or their families may define quality as having the nurse, therapist, or aide arrive at the home before noon to provide care. They may equate quality with having their personal preference for a particular caregiver honored. Quality may also be measured from the perspective of what is wanted and expected for a positive outcome rather than what is needed.

Another criterion used to measure quality may be who is responsible for payment of the bill. Patients who personally pay for services may perceive quality differently from those who perceive services as being free (i.e., paid for by insurance).

To elicit and appreciate the patient's perception of care, a discharge questionnaire (Exhibit 24–1) is sent to a random selection of VNA patients or families each quarter. Questionnaires are also sent to all patients in a selected population, such as our hospice program. This selection process allows for two viewpoints: that of an independent reviewer, and that of the patient or family. Discrepancies, if any, are noted, followed up by the supervisor, and resolved through discussion with those responding to the questionnaire, the reviewer, and the VNA staff.

In today's health care environment, patients and families are frequently expected to participate in the care process. This is especially true in the case of hospice care, intravenous therapy, and care of ventilator-dependent clients of all ages. Data from the American Association of Retired Persons (1987) indicate that family members provide 80 percent of the care needed by older relatives. This causes concern among employers, who are confronted with consequent absenteeism and stress-related illnesses. It also raises the issue of quality of care. Not only may families be incapable of meeting the responsibility to perform high-technology procedures on a 24-hour basis, but they may be trying to do so without what they perceive to be adequate training and support even though they have been taught and demonstrated a specific procedure.

The Third-Party Payer's Viewpoint

Third-party payers may define quality in terms of a specified time frame, such as the provisions of home care services to a subscriber over a predetermined amount of time and with a specific number of visits based on a medical diagnosis. In reality, the expected progress or outcome does not always occur within these time frames. When expected outcomes do not

Exhibit 24–1 Discharge Patient Questionnaire

1. What services were provided?
   ____ Nursing   ____ Occupational Therapy
   ____ Home Health Aide   ____ Speech Therapy
        (personal care)   ____ Physical Therapy
   ____ Social Worker   ____ Dietitian

2. Was the service what you expected it to be? _____

3. VNA personnel considered my family's special needs.

Poor	Fair	Satisfactory	Very Good	Excellent
1	2	3	4	5

4. I was satisfied with the personnel.

Poor	Fair	Satisfactory	Very Good	Excellent
1	2	3	4	5

5. Were there other services you would have liked us to provide?_____

6. Instructions provided by VNA personnel related to my health care needs were clear.

Poor	Fair	Satisfactory	Very Good	Excellent
1	2	3	4	5

7. Questions were answered adequately.

Poor	Fair	Satisfactory	Very Good	Excellent
1	2	3	4	5

8. This service helped me achieve my health care goals.

Poor	Fair	Satisfactory	Very Good	Excellent
1	2	3	4	5

9. Would you use this service again? _____

10. Would you recommend this service to others?_____

11. What suggestions would you make to improve the service? _____

_____

_____

12. Additional comments:_____

_____

_____

Signature: _____   Date: _____

Source: Reprinted with permission of the Visiting Nurse Association of Eastern Montgomery County/Department of Abington Memorial Hospital, Willow Grove, Pennsylvania.

occur within a given time frame and payment for additional visits is not available to home care providers, it seems that the payer's definition of quality is measured in terms of dollars saved rather than patient services or outcomes. Professionals in any home health agency, not to mention those writing for the industry journals, can provide case studies that demonstrate the dichotomy between medically needed services and services for which there is available reimbursement. These discrepancies are also noted in cases that are heard by administrative law judges.

One of the home care standards in the *1997–98 Comprehensive Accreditation Manual for Home Care* (Joint Commission on Accreditation of Healthcare Organizations, 1996) mandates that agencies address the issue of precipitous discharge of patients. One indicator of this important aspect of care is that before discharge from VNA service, patients for whom third-party reimbursement has been denied will be offered care options. The chart must document that instructions have been given to the patient and/or family about options for continued care that are available, such as:

- ongoing VNA skilled care on a fee-for-service basis or as able to be provided within the financial and clinical capability of the organization
- transfer to a different level of care
- linkage with other community resources that can meet the continued need

One-hundred percent of the records of VNA patients who are discharged with a reason of "visits exhausted" are reviewed as part of the monthly QA/PI process, and any identified problem is brought to the attention of the nurse, supervisor, and administration through the reporting process.

The Legislative and Regulatory Viewpoint

Policymakers at both state and national levels are interested in supporting the quality of care concept while saving dollars overall on specific programs. Prospective payment demonstration projects for home care, capitation systems, and the current Medicare cost limit system are examples of existing and future dollar-saving proposals.

Halamandaris (1985) states that the general perception in Congress is that diagnosis-related groups have been a success, at least enough of a success that Medicare should continue to move in the direction of a prospective payment system for nursing homes, home health agencies, and perhaps even physicians. The federal budget reconciliation bill signed by President Reagan on December 22, 1987 required the secretary of the Department of Health and Human Services to conduct a demonstration of prospective payment for home health care. Such demonstration projects are now in process. Home health administrators need to be aware of and involved in this type of project and monitor its progress. Alternative payment methods are going to increase rather than decrease in importance in the future. The intensity of the review process to which home health agencies are subjected will continue; regulations will escalate.

In 1987, home health agencies became subject to another review process related to QA. Congress had mandated in 1986 that peer review organizations (PROs, successors of professional standards review organizations) conduct QA reviews on home health agencies and skilled nursing facilities ("Review Responsibilities," 1985). Section 9353(c) of the Omnibus Budget Reconciliation Act of 1986 (amended Section 1153) required PROs to respond to all written Medicare beneficiary complaints received after August 1, 1987 concerning the quality of care provided by skilled nursing facilities, home health agencies, or hospital outpatient departments. Although the PRO review process has changed, PROs continue to respond to patient complaints. Additional information about the PRO process is presented in Chapter 64.

The Professional's Viewpoint

From the professional's viewpoint, quality care usually means providing services in the amount needed for the client to become independent or return to a pre-illness level of functioning. The professional goal often seems to be in direct conflict with the funding source's goals related to payment for service. Home care nurses and other professionals share frustration with, and concern over, the current home care reimbursement climate. Medical and technical denials of care, the limited number of authorized visits for which payment is available through some insurers, and the lack of time available to deliver high-quality care in the stated time frames are continuing to challenge home care professionals of all disciplines. Professionals, guided by their personal value systems and their commitment to attaining the standards of care established by professional organizations, may experience disillusionment with the current health care system.

The Viewpoint of Accrediting and Certifying Agencies

The site visitor from an accrediting or certifying body may equate quality with having all administrative and clinical documentation completed on a timely basis, meeting all standards at an acceptable level, achieving high patient satisfaction, and achieving positive patient outcomes. Certification is necessary for Medicare or Medicaid dollars. The certification process indicates that an agency has met minimum standards to ensure client safety. The Medicare COPs must be adhered to for an agency to participate in these federally funded programs. Although the time frame for site visits has changed (Tirone, 1996), an agency must be prepared for an unannounced visit at any time.

Accreditation is a voluntary process. The standards include not only the basic COP standards but also standards designed by the accrediting body that are more stringent than the COP standards. Since 1993, both the Community Health Accreditation Program (CHAP) and the Joint Commission have been granted deemed status (refer to Chapters 4 and 5 for detailed information about each program).

There are many ways in which the overall quality of programs and services can be improved when an agency undergoes a comprehensive review. Both CHAP and the National HomeCaring Council (NHCC; see Chapter 6) currently require home health, homemaker/home health aide, and/or private duty nursing agencies to complete a self-study report. This provides an opportunity for the reviewer to examine the agency with a magnifying glass. The report provides needed information for the site visitors and serves as an educational tool for board members who volunteer their time to serve, acquainting them with the agency's expectations and the roles and responsibilities of providers and consumers. It is an excellent source for orienting individuals joining the agency and is also a ready reference for staff, who frequently refer to it when writing proposals. Although the Joint Commission does not require the detailed written self-evaluation study, the same process must be completed in-house to meet the standards and prepare for the site visit. The concern of the board and staff for quality of patient care is expressed through an accreditation program such as CHAP, the Joint Commission, and the NHCC.

The Viewpoint of the Home Health Agency

From an agency's perspective, quality of care issues assume an added dimension. In addition to the previously mentioned issues, all of which are crucial to survival, important considerations include the types and quality of staff needed to provide services, the agency's financial and legal liability for patient care when payment is denied by third-party payers, and analyses of the financial impact of all these issues on agency operations and survival.

EVALUATING CLINICAL AND FINANCIAL DATA TO IMPROVE QUALITY OF CARE

Home health agencies have been required for years to identify costs incurred by each discipline. This is usually done in relationship to the Medicare cost report. Because prospective payment for home care is not finalized, administrators must be able to merge clinical and financial data to determine the outcomes of these aspects of a QA/PI program. The two main questions to be asked and answered are these: Was quality care provided from a clinical viewpoint? Was quality care provided from a financial viewpoint?

Ehrat (1987) states that in the absence of generic indicators of quality, each nursing organization must develop valid items or criteria that can measure quality care in the provider institution. The quality assurance/improvement (QAI) policy, the annual program evaluation policy, and the quarterly record review for nursing and home health aides were designed by the VNA to include an evaluation of both clinical and financial data related to patient care as well as overall administrative issues, such as program evaluation; the time frame for each activity is identified in the QAI calendar (Appendix 24–A). All these activities are components of the VNA's overall annual PI plan.

From the mid-1980s through the fiscal year ending June 30, 1996, clinical and financial outcomes were addressed through the use of a patient classification system (PCS; Exhibit 24–2) and nursing diagnoses (refer to Part III of this book). Beginning July 1, 1996, the VNA implemented a computerized clinical documentation system. This system incorporates some elements of the Outcome and Assessment Information Set (OASIS; Shaughnessy and Crisler, 1995), which will result in a change in the use of the PCS that the VNA has used for the past 10 years. A PCS can be used to identify the levels of care that the patient requires. Nurses select the one category or level of care that best

describes that patient's long-range goal. Standardized flow sheets for each of the five levels of care list the long-range goal and the subobjectives that must be addressed from a clinical perspective. Standardized flow sheets for the nursing diagnoses approved by the North American Nursing Diagnosis Association itemize the parameters that must be addressed for clients with a specific nursing diagnosis. These are considered short-term goals.

The outcomes of clinical care must be quantified so that clinical and financial data can be statistically analyzed manually or via computer. It is important to build as many aspects of the evaluation process as possible into the daily or monthly data collection process. In addition to the evaluation of client care through a PCS, clinical care is evaluated through record review and physician and patient/family evaluations of the quality of care provided. Once the clinical data have been quantified through the use of an accepted PCS, additional statistical and financial data can be analyzed to answer the second question noted earlier: Was quality care provided from a financial viewpoint?

Ehrat (1987) states that quality care issues become more focused as length of stay (LOS) and patient mix patterns change. In reality, both these factors affect financial outcomes. When clinical outcome data are available by multiple PCSs (e.g., rehabilitation potential, nursing diagnoses, major disease category, *International Classification of Diseases* codes, etc.), several probing questions can be answered: Was quality care provided when the patient fell within the average charge for this category of patient? Did the patient with a high (or low) cost, a long (or short) LOS, or a large (or small) number of visits receive quality care compared with the average client? If so, what affected the cost or LOS?

When one is evaluating financial factors, it is important to remember that any of the above-mentioned variables (e.g., LOS, number of visits, etc.) may result in decreased productivity with a resulting decrease in overall dollars to

Exhibit 24–2 Abbreviated Description of PCS*

Group I   *Recovery.* The patient will return to preillness level of functioning.

Sample subobjectives:
Patient/family will demonstrate ability to perform independently prescribed treatments/ exercises.
If indicated, patient/family will demonstrate knowledge of important safety measures.

Group II   *Self-care.* The patient is experiencing an acute illness but has the potential for returning to preepisodic level of functioning.

Sample subobjectives:
Patient/family will demonstrate ability to assume responsibility for maintaining ongoing medical supervision.
If indicated, patient/family will demonstrate understanding of restrictions imposed by the illness or disability.

Group III   *Rehabilitation.* The patient will eventually function without agency services.

Sample subobjectives:
Patient/family will demonstrate ability to assume responsibility for maintaining ongoing medical supervision.
If indicated, patient/family will demonstrate ability to perform independently prescribed treatment/exercises.

Group IV   *Maintenance.* The patient will remain at home as long as possible with ongoing agency services.

Sample subobjectives:
If indicated, patient/family will demonstrate understanding of prescribed diet.
If indicated, patient/family will demonstrate knowledge of important safety measures.

Group V   *Terminal.* The patient will be maintained at home during the end stage of illness as long as possible with agency services.

Sample subobjectives:
Patient/family will receive emotional support as needed.
Patient/family will receive assistance as needed to prepare for death.

*This PCS is adapted from the patient classification/objective system of the VNA of New Haven. The VNA of Eastern Montgomery County has purchased the right to use this system. Copyright © Elizabeth A. Daubert.

---

the agency based on the current per visit reimbursement system. The patient mix, including high-technology patients who may require longer visits and increased and more detailed documentation, cannot be ignored. The issue of productivity is addressed later in this chapter as well as in other chapters. The findings of the combined evaluation of clinical and financial outcomes have been described elsewhere (Buck and Harris, 1987; Harris et al., 1987).

ANALYZING RESOURCES

Among the major concerns of administrators are the quantity and quality of human and financial resources available to them as they fulfill their obligation to assess and improve patient care.

Human Resources

The quality of an agency's programs and services depends on its having a qualified and adequate staff to provide care. To ensure the development of competent individuals with a strong and flexible scientific base for practice, home care agencies must collaborate with educational institutions.

Service/Education Collaboration

The partnership between education and service must reflect congruence among philosophies of education, that is, what constitutes an appropriate learning experience to achieve the student's goals and objectives while maintaining the integrity of the home care agency (Appendix 24–B). Opportunities must be agreed upon that foster leadership and management skills and allow students from all disciplines to come to understand the process of caring for clients and their families in a cost-effective manner. By collaborating with expert home care providers and faculty, students will be socialized to function autonomously and will be sensitive to current socioeconomic and political environments. Faculty knowledgeable in professional and regulatory standards must promote involvement in QA/PI activities such as the following:

- nursing and multidisciplinary chart reviews
- reimbursement review sessions
- admission and discharge planning meetings
- use of employee evaluation methods
- design and analysis of patient/family satisfaction questionnaires
- development of standards of care

- certification and accreditation standards

Collaborating and confronting the issues of quality education will produce competent practitioners who can assess the needs of intellectually and culturally varied patients and families, establish goals for outcomes, and determine successful interventions. Students who can think critically, who exhibit self-confidence and leadership abilities, who understand the business environment, and who willingly accept social responsibilities will emerge with a competitive advantage as "high-tech, high-touch" practitioners.

Employment Criteria

Because patients require various types and levels of care, the home health agency must utilize personnel with different educational preparations. It is a given that competent professionals and support personnel provide care in accordance with a physician's plan of care, agency policy, and the individual patient's needs. To accomplish this, the agency's board and administration must establish personnel policies that address employment criteria, staffing patterns, and other factors that contribute to quality care.

Employment criteria must be established and adhered to for all levels of personnel. Job descriptions should be available to staff during the interviewing process and must include all expectations for performance. The current requirements of professional and government organizations for professional and support personnel must also be included. Once an individual is hired, a copy of the job description or the employment letter should be signed by the employee to confirm understanding of and agreement to the expectations; it should then be placed in the individual's personnel file.

Support personnel who are involved in direct care to clients, such as home health aides, must complete or show evidence of having completed an approved training program and must be competency evaluated to meet the Medicare COP standards. It is important to consider the quality factor because it is related to the other support staff (e.g., the receptionist and billing personnel) who are indirectly involved in patient care but are vital when quality is evaluated by patients and payers. The patient's first experience with the agency is usually with the receptionist or intake nurse. This interaction frequently determines whether there are positive or negative expectations regarding other agency personnel. A patient's perception of quality begins at this stage in the process of care.

Staffing Patterns

Closely related to employment criteria is the identification of the level of professional needed to carry out the mission of the agency. Does the agency require an individual practitioner who is licensed and also certified in specialty areas such as pediatrics, oncology, geriatrics, and psychiatry? Does this certification have to be granted at the state or national level? Administrators must be familiar with the many certifying organizations and know what level of professional is needed to meet state and federal certification and accreditation requirements ("1996 Career Guide," 1996; Fickerssen, 1985; National Association for Home Care, 1996; Wilson, 1996). Another factor to be considered is whether additional financial remuneration will be available if there are additional credentials. Unless financial or other rewards are clearly evident, employees may not perceive certification as important.

In many home health agencies, there is a limited number of high level positions because of the size of the agency. To retain staff, it may be necessary to consider a method of encouraging, recognizing and rewarding those individuals who continue to provide direct care. Del Bueno (1982) describes a clinical ladder as a hierarchy of criteria intended to provide a means for evaluating and developing professional nurses who provide direct care to clients. Although most published material addresses clinical ladders in acute care settings, Whitney and Jung (1987) describe a clinical ladder program specifically for a home health agency and include four lev-

els of clinical nurse performance standards. Administrators must be involved with staff in identifying performance standards for each level, assigning a dollar value to the achievement of stated goals, and describing how nurses move from one level to another.

Staff productivity is important in home care because the current reimbursement basis is the cost per visit. Multiple factors affect the productivity of staff. Travel-related variables include weather, detours, traffic, and distance between patients. Client-related variables include the client's living arrangements and learning abilities, the levels of care required on specific visits, conferences, and telephone time. Work-related variables include student assignments, staff meetings, documentation of client care for professional and reimbursement purposes, and the agency's reporting requirements.

Staffing patterns in home care have changed. In the past, home health care was attractive to many nurses because it provided a 9-to-5 job. This is no longer the case. Home health agencies must have staff available to accept calls and make visits 24 hours a day, 7 days a week to meet the needs of patients and families and to remain competitive. Administrators are exploring new staffing patterns, such as full-time night call, flex time to accommodate heavy or light client census or acuity levels, and separate staff for weekends and visits after hours. Each of these alternatives has to be assessed from a quality standpoint. Questions to be asked concern the level of patient care required, the qualifications of staff who apply for on-call positions, and whether full-time staff should take on-call duty because they may be most familiar with the agency's caseload, systems, and so forth. The cost of each method of staffing must be analyzed and justified.

Staffing with full-time employees has benefits related to continuity of care as well as staff availability and competence in the many procedures now required by patients. Fluctuating caseloads within agencies and the shortage of professional and support personnel, however, have resulted in alternative staffing patterns.

The use of part-time or relief staff and a flex-time staffing pattern is now familiar to most home health agency administrators. Contracting agencies that have experienced home care nurses are also used to provide needed services to patients for cost effectiveness. The advantages and disadvantages of various staffing patterns and their impact on the quality of patient care and staff productivity are discussed in other chapters.

Peer Review

Peer review is another important administrative process that is part of the overall QA/PI program in a home health agency. Reasons for reviewing clinical records include the following:

- meeting the Medicare COP standards
- determining whether an agency's policies and procedures are being followed
- identifying unmet patient/family needs
- identifying individual and group trends related to the provision of care
- maintaining professional standards
- sharing findings with staff as a basis to maintain or improve the quality of care

Although this time-consuming process is sometimes considered just more paperwork, there are multiple benefits, including the knowledge that services are provided by competent staff in a safe and cost-effective manner.

Inservice or Continuing Education

To keep abreast of changes in professional practice and to meet the Medicare COPs, accreditation standards, and Occupational Health and Safety Administration regulations, inservice education and training are critical components of home care practices and administrative planning. Responsibility for participation in educational offerings belongs jointly to the agency and its professionals. Mechanisms must be established by which professionals can share information with colleagues. Program summaries (Exhibit 24–3) should be kept by the individual responsible for educational func-

tions and placed in employee files for performance appraisal purposes, advancement, and promotion.

Summary

In short, all the issues related to human resources—recruitment and retention, job descriptions, verification of credentials such as licensure and certification, assignment and supervision of staff, orientation, inservice training, continuing education, ongoing performance evaluations, career ladders, and productivity monitoring—contribute to the home health agency administrator's confidence that quality care is delivered to patients.

Financial Resources

Although administrators must be concerned with the delivery and measurement of the quality of care that clients receive, they must also be concerned with the cost effectiveness of the agency's programs and services. There is a cost associated with the time, materials, and personnel needed to reach stated goals. One of the questions to be considered is whether quality of care has been sacrificed to achieve a balanced budget.

Tonges (1985) states that in a cost-containment atmosphere providers must either lower their standards or find ways to provide quality care more economically. Administrators must find ways to be more cost effective because health care providers must not lower standards of care. This requires providers to examine ways to decrease costs (e.g., alternative payment schemes for staff, such as per case, per visit, or on the basis of contracts, instead of traditional salaried or hourly patterns). It also requires a thorough review of line items in the budget. Providers also need to use teaching tools specific to the agency's unique client population to assist and augment the teaching done by the professionals. There must be an increased emphasis on help provided by the family, volunteers, and other support personnel. The report published by Arthur Andersen & Com-

Exhibit 24–3 Education Program Summary

Program Title: _____

Date: _____ Type of Program: Orientation: _____ Mandatory Program: _____

Time: _____ Inservice: _____ Continuing Education: _____

In-House Program: _____ In-State Program: _____ Out-of-State Program: _____

Program in Response to Monitoring and Evaluation Deficiency: Yes: _____ No: _____

Name of Presenter(s): _____

Summary of Program Content: _____

_____

_____

Assessment of Program Content: _____

Utilization of Information Gained from Program: _____

Enhanced Practice: _____ How? _____

Met Expectations of: HHC Agency: _____ Accrediting Agency: _____

Credentialing Agency: _____ Other: _____

Program Information Shared: No _____ N/A _____ Yes (How?): _____

_____

ATTACHMENTS: Attendance Sheets;
Program
Brochure/Materials

_____

(Signature/Position, Person Completing Form) (Date)

Source: Courtesy of Claire Meisenheimer.

pany and the American College of Health Care Executives (Umbdemstock, 1987) indicated that 90 percent of the combined panels of health care executives, physicians, nurses, and trustees participating in the study agreed that by 1995:

- acceptable definitions of quality health care would be developed
- providers would be better able to measure the quality of the care that they provide
- providers would monitor and report on the quality of their health care services
- regulators would use this information in connection with licensure

The findings also indicated that more than 70 percent of the panel:

- anticipated that payments for health services would be based at least in part on quality measures
- believed that providers would sacrifice quality of care for financial viability
- believed that future capitation systems would sacrifice quality of care for financial viability

Some of the projections for the year 1995 were realized. In light of these realities, it is imperative that administrators use all available resources to analyze the costs and benefits of providing quality health services in the home and find ways to achieve the goal of quality patient care.

Smeltzer (1985) states that cost analysis considers all resources, including personnel and materials as well as client contributions and other contributions received from inside and outside the organization. Cost benefit analysis requires that direct and indirect costs and benefits (or results) be expressed in monetary terms. Costs include not only the time and salaries of personnel at all levels but also expenditures for computer programming and equipment, monthly servicing, supplies, building maintenance, and volunteer time (translated into dollar amounts) that may be associated with the QA/PI program.

There are many benefits of a QA/PI program. To a Medicare-certified agency, it means continued federal funding because the results of the program reflect that outcomes are patient focused and that there is satisfaction with the quality of care provided. Other third-party payers are also requesting a copy of an agency's QA/PI program, and sometimes a copy of the annual evaluation of the program's outcomes, as one aspect of the evaluation process when selecting contractors. The ability of an agency's administrator to document that quality care is provided by the staff, as evidenced through various trending and tracking methods, may result in added contracts for the agency, which may enhance the agency's financial position.

As far back as 1978, Partridge discussed community health administration in a cost containment era: "In the face of mushrooming pressures, constituencies, and complexities, we have but three alternatives: (1) we can muddle on with our unsatisfying, uneven, national performance; (2) we can succumb; or, (3) we can emerge into a tomorrow we helped fashion" (p. 10). As we progress into the 21st century, home health administrators must help ensure quality care for home care patients. We can do no less.

CONCLUSION

The home health agency's administrator has an important role in the agency's QA/PI program. The administrator must:

- be accountable for quality patient care
- commit time, dollars, personnel, and space to the overall process
- remain knowledgeable about QA/PI requirements
- make changes when necessary (e.g., follow through on findings and recommendations)
- work with the governing body to recruit and retain sufficient qualified staff through sound personnel policies, competitive salaries, and good working conditions

- solicit consumer input into the evaluation process
- provide support and encouragement at all levels of the agency's activities

Quality care is the result of having a philosophy, qualified staff, sound and safe policies and procedures, and performing evaluation and following through on findings with corrective actions. Agency and professional standards must be addressed. Accreditation, certification, and licensure standards for the agency must be maintained. Professional licensure and certification, orientation, inservice training, and continuing education are all necessary to provide high-quality care in a changing health care environment. Many of the activities related to the provision of quality care, such as collaborating with educational institutions to provide clinical experiences and orientation, inservice training, and continuing education for all staff, involve a commitment of dollars, time, and personnel from the administrator. "Quality is an achievable, measurable, profitable entity that can be instilled once you have commitment and understanding and are prepared for hard work" (Crosby, 1980, 6).

REFERENCES

American Association of Retired Persons (AARP). 1987. *Caregivers in the workplace.* Washington, DC: AARP.

Buck, J., and M. Harris. 1987. Costing home health care. *Home Healthcare Nurse* 5:17–29.

1996 career guide. 1996. *American Journal of Nursing.* 96:19–25.

Crosby, P. 1980. *Quality is free: The art of making quality certain.* New York: Mentor.

Del Bueno, D. 1982. A clinical ladder? Maybe. *Journal of Nursing Administration* 12:19–22.

Ehrat, K. 1987. The cost–quality balance: An analysis of quality, effectiveness, efficiency, and cost. *Journal of Nursing Administration* 17:6–13.

Fickerssen, J. 1985. Getting certified. *American Journal of Nursing* 85:265–269.

Halamandaris, V. 1985. The future of home care in America. *Caring* 10:4–11.

Harris, M., et al. 1987. Cost containment: Relating quality and cost in a home health care agency. *Quality Review Bulletin* 13:175–181.

Joint Commission on Accreditation of Healthcare Organizations. 1996. *1997–98 Comprehensive accreditation manual for home care.* Oakbrook Terrace, IL: Joint Commission.

Meisenheimer, C., ed. 1985. *Quality assurance: A complete guide to effective programming.* Gaithersburg, MD: Aspen.

National Association for Home Care. 1996. *Candidate information handbook: Professional certification for home care & hospice executives.* Washington, DC: National Association for Home Care.

Partridge, K. 1978. *Community health administration in a cost-containment era.* New York: National League for Nursing.

Review responsibilities of utilization and quality control peer review organizations. 1985. *Federal Register,* 50, 42 CFR, 446.7–476.143.

Ruane, N. 1994. Program evaluation. In *Handbook of home health care administration,* ed. M. Harris, 269–283. Gaithersburg, MD: Aspen.

Shaughnessy, P., and K. Crisler. 1995. *Outcome-based quality improvement.* Washington, DC: National Association for Home Care.

Smeltzer, C. 1985. Evaluating program effectiveness. In *Quality assurance: A complete guide to effective programs,* ed. C. Meisenheimer, 157–167. Gaithersburg, MD: Aspen.

Tirone, A. 1996. *Intervals between standard surveys for home health agencies.* Rockville, MD: Health Care Financing Administration.

Tonges, M. 1985. Quality with economy: Doing the right thing for less. *Nursing Economics* 3:205–311.

Umbdemstock, R., ed. 1987. *The future of healthcare: Changes and choices.* Arthur Andersen & Co. and the American College of Healthcare Executives.

Wilson, J. 1996. National certification for home care nurses: Bird by bird. *Home Healthcare Nurse* 14:817–821.

Whitney, D., and J. Jung. 1987. A clinical ladder program for home health nurses. In *Third National Nursing Symposium on Home Health Care: Book of abstracts and presentation outlines,* ed. L. Daniel. Ann Arbor, MI: University of Michigan.

SUGGESTED READING

Aguayo, R. 1991. *Dr. Deming: The American who taught the Japanese about quality.* New York: Simon & Schuster.

Crosby, P. 1984. *Quality without tears. The art of hassle-free management.* New York: McGraw-Hill.

Crosby, P. 1989. *Let's talk quality.* New York: McGraw-Hill.

Deming, W. 1986. *Out of the crisis.* Cambridge, MA: MIT Press.

Joint Commission on Accreditation of Healthcare Organizations. 1993. *Quality improvement in home care.* Oakbrook Terrace, IL: Joint Commission.

Juran, J. 1989. *Juran on leadership for quality. An executive handbook.* New York: Macmillan.

Keystone Peer Review Organization (KePRO). 1996, April 26. *KePRO Provider Bulletin.* Harrisburg, PA: KePRO.

Kirsch, A., and S. Donovon. 1992. The journey to quality improvement in home care. *Caring* 11:46–51.

Policies and Forms for Evaluation of Clinical and Financial Data

QUALITY ASSESSMENT AND IMPROVEMENT POLICY

PURPOSE: To systematically evaluate the quality of care rendered to individuals, families, and the community, in order to improve the quality of the care provided, and to assure proper utilization of services.

RESPONSIBLE PERSONNEL: Nurses, Therapists, Social Workers, Members of the Professional Advisory Committee (PAC), Supervisors, Administrators, and Community Members

OBJECTIVES:
1. To assess and evaluate the quality and appropriateness of care.
2. To identify deviations from standards.
3. To address and resolve identified problems.
4. To recommend methods to improve care.

POLICY: As we strive for excellence in the provision of care, the organization is committed to the development and implementation of a quality assessment and improvement program. The multifaceted program encompasses an ongoing evaluation of structural, process, and outcome criteria. To ensure quality-effective, cost-effective services (within available resources) to individuals, families, and the community, we subscribe to compliance with both internal and external standards. (Conditions of Participation, Joint Commission, ANA, NAHC.)

PROCEDURE:

Action	*Rationale*
A. Quarterly Record Review	
1. *Quarterly Periods*	1. Quarterly reports assess the services provided to substantiate adherence to agency policies, internal, and external standards of services for maintenance of optimal care, safety, and adequate supportive services. C.O.P. 484.52 (b).
a. *1st Quarter* May-June-July (Quarterly report due by 3rd Thursday in September).	
b. *2nd Quarter* Aug.-Sept.-Oct. (Quarterly report due by 3rd Thursday in December).	
c. *3rd Quarter* Nov.-Dec.-Jan. (Quarterly report due by 3rd Thursday in March).	
d. *4th Quarter* Feb.-March-April (Quarterly report due by 3rd Thursday in June).	

PROCEDURE: *Action*   *Rationale*

Annual report due 3rd
Thursday in June.

2. The computer system generates a quarterly summary report which provides a numerical list of individuals serviced by all disciplines during the quarter. Based on these data, 10% of the records to a maximum of 50 per discipline per quarter are chosen. If the number is less than 10 cases per discipline for the quarter, all records for that discipline will be reviewed.

3. Records for review are selected randomly from the quality assurance review list, the visit register, and/or the active and discharged chart files.

4. Recording of individual record findings and recommendations on quality assurance/assessment forms are implemented with 3 weeks notice as follows:

   a. Nursing and HHA: Nursing staff, supervisors, nurse volunteers.
   b. Physical therapy: Physical therapists—no one will review their own record.
   c. MSS: Review with neighboring home care agency.
   d. Speech Pathology: Review by speech contractor.
   e. Occupational Therapy: Alternate between contractors.

5. A summary of findings and recommendations is recorded in:

   a. Committee quarterly minutes and PAC minutes.
   b. Annual report to PAC at end of 4th quarter as part of agency's program evaluation.

   Rationale: 5. This summary complies with Medicare Conditions of Participation.

6. A summary of findings is presented to staff members.

   Rationale: 6. The staff use the summary report to identify areas of strengths and weaknesses, then recommend and initiate action for the enhancement of care.

PROCEDURE: *Action*   *Rationale*

B.Discharged Patient Questionnaires

1. Each month, discharged patient question-naires are mailed to 10% of the patients/families listed on the discharged patient computer list.

2. The QAI supervisor reviews each ques-tionnaire. If a problem area is identified, it is addressed with the appropriate em-ployee and supervisory staff, if indicated. Compliments to individuals are shared with individual and supervisory staff when indicated.

3. The QAI supervisor tallies the results of the survey and prepares a summary report for the executive director. These summa-ries may be utilized in the overall agency evaluation.

C.Unsolicited Letters

1. Unsolicited patient, family, community group letters are read and analyzed. Praise and/or problems are directed to and addressed with the appropriate persons by the QAI supervisor. Comments that the writer shares about services and/or per-sonnel are reviewed and taken into con-sideration to praise employees and/or address and correct cited problems.

D.Annual Physician Questionnaires

1. On an annual basis, questionnaires are mailed to physicians whose patients require a recertification of a plan of treat-ment during a 62-day cycle. Any neces-sary follow-up is directed by the QAI supervisor.

E.Utilization Review

1. Utilization is linked to the quality of ser-vices. Utilization of services is evaluated during the quarterly review process. Refer to Utilization Review Policy, #3.15.

Rationale column:

1. These questionnaires pro-vide data to evaluate patient satisfaction with services provided.

2. This review provides for fol-low-up on patient responses.

3. This summary is utilized in the overall program evalua-tion.

1. The patient has the right to direct comments concerning quality of care to the organi-zation.

1. These questionnaires en-courage physician input as to their perception of the qual-ity of services, since a physi-cian who perceives the organization as providing quality care is more apt to refer his or her patients for services.

1. This review ensures proper utilization of all disciplines and services.

PROCEDURE: *Action*   *Rationale*

F.Annual Program Evaluation

1. The Professional Advisory Committee, administration, and staff are involved in the evaluation process as detailed in the Annual Program Evaluation Policy, #1.14. Within 90 days of the close of the fiscal year, representatives from the PAC meet to complete the necessary worksheets. A summary evaluation is presented to the PAC.	1. Annual evaluation is required by Medicare C.O.P. 484.52 to assess the extent to which the program services are appropriate, adequate, effective, and efficient.

G.Evaluation of Clinical Competence

1. Hiring practices are in accordance with C.O.P. 484.4.	1. To meet C.O.P. 484.4 from a structural perspective. Clinical competence and education are necessary to provide quality care.
2. Copies of licenses, when applicable, are on file. Certification, where applicable (i.e., ANA certification for community or home health nurse), is encouraged.	2. To meet C.O.P. 484.4 from a structural perspective. Clinical competence and education are necessary to provide quality care.
3. Each employee/volunteer is oriented to his/her roles and responsibilities.	3. To meet C.O.P. 484.4 from a structural perspective. Clinical competence and education are necessary to provide quality care.
4. Continuing education is linked to the quality assessment and improvement program to ensure that training is commensurate with quality care needs.	4. To meet C.O.P. 484.4 from a structural perspective. Clinical competence and education are necessary to provide quality care.
5. Licenses are verified on all physicians ordering home care services.	5. To meet C.O.P. 484.4 from a structural perspective. Clinical competence and education are necessary to provide quality care.
6. Physician management of home care patients will be evaluated on a periodic basis and for selected cases.	6. This evaluation will be done by a subcommittee of the PAC.

PROCEDURE: *Action*   *Rationale*

H.Monitoring and Review of Patient Outcome

1. Services are goal oriented. Outcomes are addressed through the use of a patient classification system and nursing diagnoses. Staff must quantify goal attainment. Financial and clinical goal attainment data are available on a monthly basis through the Management Information System printouts. Data are analyzed on a periodic basis. Results are shared with appropriate staff members.

1. These steps evaluate goal attainment and ensure that quality care was rendered.

I.Incident Reports

1. Any staff involved in an incident must complete an incident report and submit it to the Director of Professional Services. Trends identified are given to the QAI supervisor for further study and follow-up.

1. Trends in reportable incidents are a quality assurance/ risk management concern and should be studied and acted upon.

J.Assessment of Important Aspects of Care

1. Refer to Quality Assessment and Improvement plan for important aspects of care.

1. Ongoing and systematic assessment of important aspects of care and quality indicators is conducted to identify and resolve problems in structure, process, or outcome.

COP 484.16; 484.52
Joint Commission
Origin date: 11/87
Revised date: 9/88; 9/89; 8/93
Approved by: Administration/Board/PAC/AMH QAI Committee
Originator: Administration
Distribution: Administration/Staff/Contractors/PAC/Volunteers

Program Evaluation

PURPOSE: To establish a process for program evaluation.

RESPONSIBLE PERSON: Professional Advisory Committee's subcommittee for evaluation, Executive Director, and Administrative Staff

OBJECTIVES: To carry out an annual program evaluation to assess the extent to which the program provides patient care that is appropriate, adequate, effective, and efficient, and to determine any areas needing improvement. To provide a means to identify and plan for improvements needed.

POLICY: The program evaluation subcommittee of the Professional Advisory Committee, facilitated by the Executive Director, conducts an annual evaluation of the policies and administrative practices of the organization. The subcommittee prepares a written report which is presented to and approved by the Professional Advisory Committee. The approved report is submitted to the Board of Trustees through the hospital's Executive Vice President.

PROCEDURE:

Action	*Rationale*
1. The PAC chair appoints the subcommittee.	1. This allows for representatives of the various disciplines to perform the evaluation.
2. The Executive Director or designee prepares the following documents for the committee:	2. This permits the committee to gain a comprehensive view of the program and work efficiently.

a. Quarterly and annual statistics.
b. Narrative report prepared by the Executive Director.
c. Policy and procedure manual.
d. Clinical record review summaries for the past year.
e. Financial budget.
f. Summary results of ongoing programs for patients and staff.
g. Other material requested by the committee.

PROCEDURE:

Action	*Rationale*
3. The evaluation subcommittee reviews the material using a standardized format and drafts a summary report for review and action by the Professional Advisory Committee.	3. The PAC carries approval authority for this evaluation report.
4. After approval by the PAC, the report is submitted to the Governing Body (through the hospital's Executive Vice President) for approval and kept on file.	4. This report is needed for regulatory survey visits.
5. Recommendations are reviewed by the administrative staff and incorporated into the organization's plan for action for the coming year.	5. The ultimate purpose of an evaluation is to identify areas of improvement and to implement actions to accomplish same.

COP: 484.52
Origin date: 7/79
Revised date: 8/88; 8/89; 1/96
Approved by: Administration/Board/PAC
Originator: Administration
Distribution: Administration/Board/PAC

Courtesy of Visiting Nurse Association of Eastern Montgomery County/Department of Abington Memorial Hospital, Willow Grove, Pennsylvania.

Quality Assurance—
Quarterly Record Review

NURSING (HOME HEALTH AIDE)

Client Name: _____   Date of Review: _____

Client Case No.: _____   Present Quarter: _____

Primary Nurse Name: _____   Months Included: _____

Status of Record: Active _____   _____

              Discharged_____   _____

Signature of Reviewer

Services Involved:

	YES	NO	N/A	Comments
I. Assessment				
A. Does the clinical record include assessment of physical, psycho-social, and environmental needs of patient/family?				
B. Was the nursing assessment form updated upon each new plan of treatment or each past hospital-ization?				
C. Were nursing diagnoses based on assessment factors?				
D. Did the primary nurse select the correct patient group on admis-sion?				
E. If the patient's status changed, was the patient group changed accordingly?				
II. Planning				
A. Were client goals stated?				
B. Were the nursing parameters specific to the identified nursing diagnoses/problem?				
C. Was the plan of treatment (orders) current and signed by physician?				
D. Was the POT completed in accordance with agency policy?				

311

	YES	NO	N/A	Comments
E. Were signed verbal orders obtained to cover any change in the plan of treatment?				
III. Implementation				
A. Was the frequency of nursing visits based on the assessment of the client's needs?				
B. Was the service provided consistent with the care plan?				
C. Does the record contain evidence that the applicable subobjectives in the patient classification/objectives system were being acted upon?				
D. Did the nurse request consultative services of other disciplines when needed?				
E. Did the nurse regularly supervise the performance of the HHA/LPN?				
F. HHA consistent with client's needs?				
G. Did the nurse demonstrate evidence of his/her coordination of all services?				
H. Did the nurse hold conferences/joint visits with other services when appropriate?				
I. Did the nurse notify the physician/other team members of any significant changes in the client's status?				
J. Were service reports legible, dated, and signed?				
K. Did service reports include: 1. Adequate information regarding the client's current condition?				
2. Specific treatments/instructions given?				
3. The date of the next visit?				
L. Were the following forms present and updated according to agency protocol: 1. Authorization and Release Form?				

	YES	NO	N/A	Comments
2. Medicare Termination letter?				
3. HHA Plan of Care?				
4. Family Information Sheet?				
M. Does the record contain evidence that medications were checked for significant side effects and indications?				
N. In the opinion of the reviewer, were services: Appropriately utilized?				
Overutilized?				
Underutilized?				
IV. Evaluation				
A. Were patient/family responses to nursing intervention documented?				
B. Were necessary modifications in the care plan made based on the nurse's evaluation?				
C. If discharged from nursing service: 1. Was discharge a logical development of the care plan and client goals?				
2. Does the record contain a description of the patient/family change in knowledge, understanding, and/or behavior as the result of the nurse's intervention?				
3. Was there evidence of the client's goals having been met?				
4. Was the discharge summary present and accurately completed?				
5. Were the nursing diagnoses on the discharge computer summary consistent with those on the problem list?				
6. Were the service codes (group # and goal attainment) listed on the discharge computer summary consistent with the evidence found in the record?				

	YES	NO	N/A	Comments
7. Was the physician notified of client's discharge?				
V. Joint Commission: Medication Management Patient/significant other was instructed in all new medications within 4 weeks.				
A. Indication				
B. Dosage				
C. Frequency				
D. Route				
E. Adverse Reactions				
F. Drug Interactions				
VI. AHCPR: Urinary Incontinence in Adults				
A. Was the genitourinary system assessed?				
B. Was a problem with incontinence/ retention identified?				
C. Was a nursing diagnosis made related to incontinence/retention?				
D. What was the number of the nursing diagnosis, e.g., 72, 49?				
E. Was referral to incontinence/ retention specialist, e.g., Golden Horizons, urologist offered?				
F. Was referral made to incontinence/retention specialist, e.g., Golden Horizons, urologist?				
G. Is Foley present?				
H. If Foley present, does patient meet following guidelines for Foley catheter: Patient has urinary retention and is:				
1. Severely impaired for whom bed and clothing changes are disruptive				
2. Grade III or IV decubitus ulcer				
3. Terminally ill				
I. If patient does not meet guidelines, was patient informed of increased risk of morbidity, e.g., U.I.I., urosepsis, and mortality?				

	YES	NO	N/A	Comments
VII. AHCPR: Prevention/Treatment of Pressure Ulcers				
A. Is Braden Scale completed on chart for nursing admissions after 12/1/95?				
B. What is Braden Score number?				
C. If patient is at risk (Braden score < 14), is nursing diagnosis related to a risk factor present?				
D. 1. If patient is at risk, did a pressure ulcer breakdown develop during this SOC?				
2. If patient developed a pressure ulcer, did they have an able and willing caregiver?				

Courtesy of Visiting Nurse Association of Eastern Montgomery County/Department of Abington Memorial Hospital, Willow Grove, Pennsylvania.

QAI CALENDAR

Fiscal Year	Jan	Feb	Mar	Apr	May	June	July	Aug	Sep	Oct	Nov	Dec
Utilization Review and Record Review	X	X	X	X	X	X	X	X	X	X	X	X
Record Review Summary			X			X			X			X
Annual Record Review Summary						X						
Patient Questionnaires Mailed	X	X	X	X	X	X	X	X	X	X	X	X
Patient Questionnaires Followed Up	X	X	X	X	X	X	X	X	X	X	X	X
Analyze Unsolicited Letters	X	X	X	X	X	X	X	X	X	X	X	X
Physicians' Questionnaires Mailed	X											
Assessment of Important Aspects of Care	X	X	X	X	X	X	X	X	X	X	X	X
Evaluation of Clinical Competence	X	X	X	X	X	X	X	X	X	X	X	X
Monitoring and Review of Patient Outcomes	X	X	X	X	X	X	X	X	X	X	X	X
Incident Report Follow-Up	X	X	X	X	X	X	X	X	X	X	X	X
Annual Agency Evaluation									X			

Courtesy of Visiting Nurse Association of Eastern Montgomery County/Department of Abington Memorial Hospital, Willow Grove, Pennsylvania.

Field Agency Agreement

The University of Pennsylvania School of Nursing and _____,
mutually agree to the following plan for clinical experience until further notice. This agreement is
cancelable on 30 days written notice by either party.

I. The _____ will provide clinical experience for students, and supervision will be provided by the School of Nursing faculty. Supervision applies primarily to undergraduate students and/or as specifically agreed upon by the Agency and School of Nursing representative.

Responsibilities

A. University of Pennsylvania School of Nursing
1. Will be responsible for the selection and planning of student learning experiences in consultation with appropriate clinical staff.
2. Will be responsible for the instruction, guidance, and evaluation of students' activities in patient care.
3. Will inform the Agency of the approximate number of students who will be having experience in nursing.
4. Will assume the responsibilities of familiarizing itself with the policies and facilities of the Agency before the instruction of students in the clinical laboratory.
5. The University of Pennsylvania carries malpractice insurance, which covers students during course-related clinical experience in an agency, in the minimum amount of $1 million. If proof of coverage is required, please send a written request of same to Assistant Director, Office of Risk Management, 423 Franklin Building, University of Pennsylvania, Philadelphia, PA 19104-6205, with a copy of the executed agreement.

B. Agency
1. Will serve as a clinical laboratory in which nursing students may be assigned for educational experience.
2. Will provide staff time for planning with the SCHOOL faculty for student learning experiences.
3. Will provide staff time for the orientation of the SCHOOL faculty to the Agency's facilities and policies.
4. Will provide conference room space for faculty and students.
5. Will provide emergency medical care within the scope of its ability for the nursing students in the event of injury or illness. Worker's compensation and disability and professional liability insurance will not be provided by Agency (see item II below).

II. Students will be responsible for completing physical examinations and laboratory studies as may be required by the Agency. Students are responsible for carrying their own health insurance, and, in the event of injury in the Agency, their insurance will cover the cost.

III. Publications: No material relative to this field experience may be published without the mutual consent of the Agency and the University of Pennsylvania. Neither party shall use the names, logos, trademarks, or names of employees or students of the other party in any publicity, advertising, publication, or other communication without prior consent of the other.

IV. The Trustees of the University of Pennsylvania, intending to be legally bound, hereby indemnify and save harmless the Agency from and against any liability for personal injury, professional liability, or property damage resulting directly and solely from negligence in the clinical practice of the School's students of nursing and will reimburse your Agency for any costs incurred in defending litigation resulting directly and solely from such negligence.

V. The _____, intending to be legally bound, hereby indemnifies and saves harmless the University of Pennsylvania from and against any liability for personal injury, professional liability, or property damage resulting directly and solely from negligence in the clinical practice of the Agency's personnel and will reimburse the Trustees of the University of Pennsylvania for any costs incurred in defending litigation resulting directly and solely from such negligence.

VI. _____

_____

_____

Signed: _____ Agency Officer

Agency:_____

Date: _____

Signed: _____ Dean, School of Nursing

for   the Trustees of the University of Pennsylvania

Date: _____

Courtesy of University of Pennsylvania School of Nursing and the VNA of Eastern Montgomery County/Department of Abington Memorial Hospital, Willow Grove, Pennsylvania.

CHAPTER 25

Quality Planning for Quality Patient Care

Marilyn D. Harris and Joan Reynolds Yuan

Home care in the 1990s presents many challenges for administrators, caregivers, and patients. It is an era characterized by an aging population, high cost of health care, high-technology care, consumers who are disgruntled with the health care system, organizations grappling with a changing environment, an increased number of case management programs, and resultant fiscal constraints. How do the administrators of a home care organization ensure that quality health care services are being provided, and why should they care? Nursing is a key service in most skilled home care organizations. Nursing, being an art as well as a science, is known for its caring function. Caring has been described as nursing's central moral ideal (Pater and Gallop, 1994). This professional care and caring must be evident in the design and implementation of the quality program and the quality assessment/performance improvement (QA/PI) plan.

A quality program may be shaped by the Juran (1989) trilogy of processes: quality planning, quality control or quality assurance in nursing peer review activities, and quality improvement. Quality planning refers to the activity of developing products or processes required to meet customers' needs. Quality control (quality assurance) is a process that evaluates quality performance, compares actual performance with quality goals, and acts on the

differences. Quality improvement is a process of raising quality performance to unprecedented levels.

Deming (1982) writes in response to the question "How do you go about improving quality and productivity?" that "Best efforts are essential. Unfortunately, best efforts, people charging this way and that way without guidance of principles, can do a lot of damage. Think of the chaos that would come if everyone did his best not knowing what to do" (p. 19). Deming advises that a constancy of purpose needs to be created toward the improvement of products and services. It is the responsibility of the leaders to identify areas that need improvement.

Although quality improvement is a process that utilizes scientific tools, quality planning or choosing quality improvement projects involves not only science but caring. Some quality programs are designed with a heavy emphasis on inspection of areas that may have no relevance to the customer. Quality programs in some home care organizations take on the shape of the CIA or the KGB and achieve what? The development of a quality plan is not for the paper chase. In an attempt to ensure the quality and appropriateness of care, the quality program must have clinical relevance and be meaningful to the customer. Often in nursing, it has been said that things would change if the Congressperson's mother were the recipient of care. This idea can be applied to the design of a quality plan. Quality takes on a different dimension when it makes a difference in the care provided. We should ask this question when the quality plan is designed: "Would I want my mother to receive care from this organization, and how can I make sure that she would receive what she needs?"

The quality plan that is designed with care and a constancy of purpose must be meaningful and workable. For example, the administration must be committed to the measurement of patient outcomes. The quality plan could include measurement of outcomes by a patient classification such as the rehabilitation potential patient classification system (RPPCS; Daubert, 1979; Harris, 1994) that is used at the Visiting Nurse Association of Eastern Montgomery County/Department of Abington Memorial Hospital (VNA). To ensure interrater reliability in this system, the accuracy of the classification within RPPCS is determined at the same time that the quarterly record review of a random selection of records is completed by the VNA staff as one aspect of the Medicare record review process. The measurement of a patient's goal attainment on discharge from VNA service provides the home health agency's administrative staff with data that can be used to improve patient care. If a positive outcome was not obtained from a risk management perspective, several questions could be asked. Were the standards of the state's peer review organization for home health agencies met? If not, why not? If the anticipated outcomes goal was for the patient to be rehabilitated but the patient died, other questions to be answered are: Was the patient terminally ill? If so, why wasn't the patient reclassified into the terminal care category of care, and why weren't the specific terminal care parameters as defined by the RPPCS addressed? Additional questions that could be asked relate to the level of personnel providing care, including their educational preparation and clinical skills. Effective July 1996, some changes were made in the VNA's clinical docu-

mentation system to accommodate the implementation of a computerized clinical system and to incorporate some elements of outcome-based quality improvement (Shaughnessy and Crisler, 1995).

Consumers can share their thoughts on caregivers, attitudes, and perceptions of competency through formal questionnaires or unsolicited letters, but organizations cannot depend on consumers to identify technical problems. Administration has an important role in the structure of the quality program. Crosby (1984) states that senior management is 100 percent responsible for problems with quality and their continuance. The American Nurses Association (ANA, 1991) states that organized nursing services are obligated to provide effective nursing care to society and that a QA/PI program is necessary to determine the degree to which the provision of nursing care complies with standards. These criteria are as follows:

- A written plan exists for the ongoing monitoring and evaluation of nursing care.
- Nurses participate in the monitoring and evaluation of nursing care in accordance with established professional, regulatory, and organizational standards of practice.
- Actions are taken to resolve problems and improve care; these activities are documented and evaluated for effectiveness.
- The QA/PI program itself is periodically evaluated to determine its effectiveness.
- The QA/PI program is an integral part of the risk management and quality assurance effort of the organization as a whole.
- Recipients of nursing care have the opportunity to express their satisfaction and perceptions of the quality of care they have received.

The ANA code for nurses standard 8 (1985) states that the nurse participates in the profession's efforts to implement and improve standards of nursing. This standard addresses the nurse's responsibilities to the public and the profession. Some of the provisions include the nurse's responsibilities to monitor standards in daily practice and to participate actively in the profession's ongoing efforts to foster optimal standards of practice at the local, regional, state, and national levels of the health care system.

The collection and analysis of nursing data are essential components of managing and providing high-quality home health care in the 1990s. There is a role for each member of the staff of the agency in this process in data collection, development of protocols, or involvement in the implementation of newly published guidelines and protocols. It must be remembered that data collection represents more than just statistics. There is the human side of data collection, the actual benefits to patients and their families as a result of these findings. This aspect of the QA/PI process is brought to life through the words of Doris Schwartz, author of *Give Us To Go Blithely* (1995). Schwartz was honored in 1994 with the Lillian D. Wald Spirit of Nursing Award. In a letter reflecting on her many experiences, Schwartz (1994) recalls that one of her former students talked with her at this awards ceremony and reminded her that she taught epidemiology. The former student related that she hated the idea of math because she did not see its relevance to patient care. What this student remembered Schwartz stating was "We can all rejoice in the statistics that show that infant deaths in our district were reduced last year by six-tenths of a percent, but as caregivers, we need to remember that no mother ever lost six-tenths of a baby." These words put statistics into perspective and present the reality associated with what would otherwise be only numbers.

Too often, quality planning, quality assurance, and quality improvement take second place to putting out the fires. It seems prudent to utilize scarce resources to plan, monitor, and design mechanisms to improve the organization's performance. Administration must be committed to establishing a system to track, evaluate, and improve care. Quality as conformance to requirements is therefore specific and lends credence to the need to meet professional standards (e.g., the ANA's standards for home

health [1986]) and to conform to and implement these standards as well as Agency for Health Care Policy and Research (AHCPR) guidelines (Department of Health and Human Services [DHHS], 1992a, 1992b, 1992c).

Quality improvement is receiving increased attention at the national level. Section 2 of the Joint Commission on Accreditation of Healthcare Organizations' *1997–98 Comprehensive Accreditation Manual for Home Care* (1996) is titled "Improving Organization Performance." It states "The goal of the improving organization performance function is that the organization designs processes well and systematically measures, assesses, and improves its performance to improve patient outcomes" (p. 267). This section of the manual focuses on a framework for improving functions. The characteristics of what is done and how it is done are called dimensions of performance. Essential processes include design performance, measurement performance, assessment, and performance improvement (PI). This approach does not leave anything to chance or subscribe to the attitude "I'll do it when I have time!" Administrative commitment, professional and support staff, time, and dollars are required to have a successful program.

The Health Care Financing Administration released a draft of proposed revisions to the home health agency Medicare conditions of participation (COPs) that includes a separate COP titled "Quality Improvement" (Rak, 1994). The COP states that the home health agency must develop, implement, and maintain an effective, continuous quality improvement program that reflects the complexity of its organization and services. There are two draft standards that list specific criteria on current clinical practice guidelines and professional practice standards applicable to patients in home care, measures of staff performance, patient rights, and satisfaction measures.

PI must be an integral part of home health care each day; this can be accomplished through various methods. During a recent presentation at the annual meeting of the National Association for Home Care, one of the speakers noted that it is not unusual for 10 years to elapse from the introduction of national standards to their implementation. In light of the AHCPR guidelines that have been published, would you want your Congressperson's (or your) mother to receive home health care through an agency that implemented the guidelines in 1 to 2 years or that waited 10 years or more?

The AHCPR was established in 1989 by Congress to improve the quality and effectiveness of health care and access to care. At the VNA, each staff nurse received a copy of the AHCPR guidelines for urinary incontinence in adults (DHHS, 1992a, 1992b, 1992c) immediately after they were published in 1992, plus several other guidelines. In 1994, a PI indicator was included in the PI plan, and a PI team was formed to examine the issues of urinary incontinence and Foley catheter use among patients admitted for home care because urinary incontinence is prevalent in American adults. Also, Foley catheters used for incontinence management are a significant source of urinary tract infections, sepsis, and mortality.

The first phase of the VNA's PI effort was the attainment of 100 percent compliance with all instructions related to the care of a Foley catheter for all patients with an indwelling catheter. After this goal had been attained for a 6-month period, the next phase was put in place to assess each patient to determine whether he or she meets the AHCPR guidelines for use of a Foley catheter. This phase included ongoing educational programs for all nursing staff, development of an improved history and physical assessment form (which includes space to record the results of dipstick urinalysis), development of a refined standardized flow sheet for documentation and patient teaching tools, and mailing of an informational letter to all staff and nonstaff referring physicians to advise them of the VNA's process to implement the national guidelines for urinary incontinence. This notice to the physicians of the VNA's plans was vitally important because their assistance and cooperation are needed in providing patient and family

education when a Foley catheter is requested by the patient or family in an attempt to control incontinence but is not the treatment of choice for numerous reasons. Data collection at the VNA during 1994 for this population showed that the VNA sample closely mirrored the national data. Based on these VNA data, the administrative staff are able to measure goal attainment for those VNA patients who meet the AHCPR guidelines during each year.

It is important to document improvements and positive outcomes for the VNA patients. It is also beneficial to benchmark against other home health agencies. Benchmarking (Mecon Associates, 1994) is a tool or technique that provides for the identification and comparison of various measures among similar organizations. Departments can compare performance and practices against those of departments or organizations that have similar characteristics and are identified as best performers. Davis (1994) states that benchmarking opens windows to new ideas and ways of doing business. It highlights the gap between what is and what is possible.

Since 1994, staff at the VNA have been involved in an annual benchmarking process as one of the hospital's departments. The administrative staff of each department are asked to identify costs, productivity, and statistics by cost centers for their department. These data are shared with the outside benchmarking organization, which inputs data into its national database. After the accuracy of these reports is verified, a report is generated that lists other home health care and hospice departments/organizations nationwide that are similar in characteristics and are identified as best performers. The administrative staff review these reports, identify gaps and opportunities for improvement, and develop written questions that are shared with those home care and hospice agencies across the country that agree to share their information. This process provides for follow-up telephone calls among agency administrative staff to explore answers to specific questions that help clarify or explain variations in costs, staffing, visit time, and productivity. Once these relationships have been established, there can be sharing of clinical as well as administrative information.

There must be a constancy of purpose to ensure that home health care patients receive quality care. Nursing leaders are obligated to design a quality plan that will measure outcomes and ensure that certification, accreditation, and national, state, professional, and agency standards and guidelines are met. There must also be a commitment to improved quality of care when standards are not met or when there are opportunities to raise the standards

after comparison with the performance of other home care agencies through the benchmarking process.

The development of a quality plan and the related QA/PI activities is vital to quality patient care. This quality focus must also be the very essence of the home health agency's business plan to meet the needs of the myriad customers, who include physicians and third-party payers as well as patients and families. Quality planning for quality patient care will enable administrators to face and meet the multiple challenges in the competitive environment that exists in the 1990s.

REFERENCES

American Nurses Association (ANA). 1985. *Code for nurses with interpretative statements*. Kansas City, MO: ANA.

American Nurses Association (ANA). 1986. *Standards for home health nursing practice*. Kansas City, MO: ANA.

American Nurses Association (ANA). 1991. *Standards for organized nursing service*. Washington, DC: ANA.

Crosby, P. 1984. *Quality without tears. The art of hassle-free management*. New York: Plume.

Daubert, E. 1979. Patient classification systems and outcome criteria. *Nursing Outlook* 27:450–454.

Davis, R. 1994. *Total quality management for home care*. Gaithersburg, MD: Aspen.

Deming, W. 1982. *Out of the crisis*. Cambridge, MA: MIT Press.

Department of Health and Human Services (DHHS), Public Health Service, Agency for Health Care Policy and Research. 1992a. *Urinary incontinence in adults. Clinical practice guidelines* (AHCPR Pub. No. 92-0038). Rockville, MD: DHHS.

Department of Health and Human Services (DHHS), Public Health Service, Agency for Health Care Policy and Research. 1992b. *Urinary incontinence in adults. A patient's guide* (AHCPR Pub. No. 92-0040). Rockville, MD: DHHS.

Department of Health and Human Services (DHHS), Public Health Service, Agency for Health Care Policy and

Research. 1992c. *Urinary incontinence in adults. Quick reference guide for clinicians* (AHCPR Pub. No. 92-0041). Rockville, MD: DHHS.

Harris, M. 1994. Clinical and financial outcomes of patient care. In *Handbook of home health care administration*, ed. M. Harris, 298–308. Gaithersburg, MD: Aspen.

Joint Commission on Accreditation of Healthcare Organizations. 1996. *1997–98 Comprehensive accreditation manual for home health*. Oakbrook Terrace, IL: Joint Commission.

Juran, J. 1989. *Juran on leadership for quality. An executive handbook*. New York: Free Press.

Mecon Associates. 1994. *Mecon peer operations benchmarking database service*. San Ramon, CA: Mecon.

Pater, E., and R. Gallop. 1994. The ethic of care: A comparison of nursing and medical students. *Image* 26:47–51.

Rak, K. 1994, November 21. *Home health line, quality improvement*, pp. 1–8.

Schwartz, D. 1995. *My Fifty Years in Nursing: Give Us To Go Blithely*. New York: Springer.

Schwartz, D. 1994, March 16. Personal letter.

Shaughnessy, P., and K. Crisler. 1995. *Outcome-based quality improvement*. Washington, DC: National Association for Home Care.

CHAPTER 26

Program Evaluation

Nancy DiPasquale Ruane and Joseph W. Ruane

Program evaluation measures effectiveness, a major concern of home health agencies. It is used to measure the status quo and to project future changes and anticipated agency responses. External and internal constraints and supports influence program evaluations. Information gathering and analysis provide a basis for rational decision making.

DEFINITIONS AND CHARACTERISTICS

Program

A program is a structured set of activities organized to accomplish a goal. It pursues a comprehensive goal with multifaceted objectives utilizing various levels of human potential and resources. A program activates a prearranged plan of operation, which acts as an outline of the work to be done by the organization. The viability and progress of a program rely on the effectiveness of its evaluation.

Evaluation

Evaluation is the process of assessing qualities or characteristics of an individual, an intervention, a program, or an agency as the basis for making a judgment. The emphasis in evaluation is collecting data designed to delineate the relevant, identifying features of factors under study.

It involves a systematic process of determining the extent to which the objectives are achieved. Evaluation starts with quantitative measurement and goes beyond it to include qualitative description and judgment.

The effectiveness of evaluation can be promoted by attention to the following points:

- Evaluation is a process of analysis.
- Evaluation is a means to an end and not an end in itself.
- Evaluation is a method of gathering and processing evidence that may indicate a need for improvement.
- Evaluation clarifies goals and expected outcomes.
- Evaluation is a process of determining the extent to which goals and objectives are met.
- Evaluation is a system of quality control that determines the effectiveness of the program.
- Evaluation must be focused on utilization to identify what changes must be made to ensure the effectiveness of the program (National League for Nursing [NLN], 1974).
- Evaluation must be credible.
- Evaluation will stimulate ideological, ethical, and political discussion.

An evaluation has a sponsor. This is the person or organization that requests the evaluation and is responsible for its completion. In a home health agency, the sponsor may be the governing body, fulfilling the mandate of certification and accreditation bodies as well as its desire to provide quality services. There is always an audience for an evaluation. Evaluation needs will not go away. Evaluation has become part of the tools of government. Contracts for program assessment will continue to need well-trained researchers (Miller, 1991). More often, federal and state governments and foundations request evaluations for accountability or for new program funding.

Of course, the findings and recommendations are reported to the sponsor, but there are other recipients of the information. The audience varies and may include the program managers and staff, the recipients of the program services, prospective consumers, special interest groups, professional peer groups, and the community served by the agency (Herman et al., 1987).

Evaluation may be formative or summative. Formative evaluation assesses how well the program is going. It is used throughout the duration of the program for the primary purpose of improving the program operation. Formative evaluation helps determine whether the program is moving toward its goals and objectives. It differs from summative evaluation in timing and audience, which is usually the program management and staff. The emphasis is improvement as the program continues. Summative evaluation focuses on assessing the achievement of the goals and objectives of the program. It is done annually, at other specified intervals, or at the conclusion of the program period. Summative evaluation determines whether the goals and objectives of the program have been attained, and it gives feedback for future planning. It looks at the total impact of the program (Breckon, 1982).

Program Evaluation

Program evaluation is a set of methods, skills, and individualized interpretations used to determine the necessity, compliance, and rele-vance of an agency's goals and activities. It provides a basis for rational decision making for the future. Program evaluation without sensitive adaptation results in sterile critiques and recommendations without vision.

Program evaluation involves conducting systematic research within an agency to acquire information that can be fed back to enhance the agency's functioning. It is applied research involving problem solving and strategic action (Rothman, 1980). Evaluation research differs from basic research; the latter produces or verifies theories and knowledge and is not aimed at prescribing a solution to a problem. Program evaluation entails such inquiries as needs assessment, agency mission, statement and beliefs, descriptive information about quality of services delivered and client outcomes, and cost analysis. Comparative use of evaluation research can lead to meaningful theory and build upon it.

ISSUES

Relationship to Planning

Program evaluation is part of the cycle of program development. The cycle begins with the planning phase, moves through the implementation phase, and is followed by the review or evaluation phase. This last phase of program development is linked directly into the planning phase, at which point the cycle is reviewed. Figure 26–1 illustrates this cycle. Planning for program evaluation must be incorporated during program planning so that data needed for evaluating program outcomes will be available when the time comes for the actual evaluation (Clark, 1992).

Program evaluation is reactive evaluation for proactive planning. It is like a "mirror image of planning in that it is the process of looking back upon action, making judgment about it in order to provide the necessary information for planning for the future" (Blum, 1979, 542). Program evaluation acts as a comet in the heavens. A

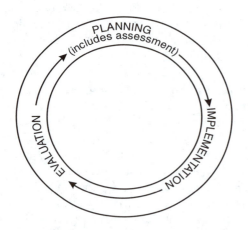

Figure 26–1 Cycle of program development. The cycle starts with the planning phase and moves to the implementation phase, then to the evaluation phase, and then back to the planning phase, at which point the cycle starts again. *Source:* Copyright © Nancy D. Ruane.

comet, with energy from its source, has momentum and gains speed as it is propelled through space to fulfill its purpose in the universe. Program evaluation gathers and analyzes data from the program's activities and propels the findings into the future to plan for progressive development. This concept is depicted in Figure 26–2, which also illustrates the context and purpose of program evaluation.

Accountability

Program evaluations are conducted to describe and assess the effects of program activity. This information is essential because the agency, through its governing body, is accountable to the community that it serves. Accountability includes the quality and extent of the services provided and the funds used to finance the services. In proprietary agencies, the stockholders constitute another group that expects accountability. An effective program evaluation can establish accountability to all its stakeholders.

Relationship to Quality Assurance

Home health care is familiar with accountability. It is the common denominator for quality assurance and program evaluation. Both processes are evaluative in nature and are essential to the existence, growth, and development of an agency. Program evaluation focuses on examining the achievement of the outcome of a set of objectives, activities, and services. This examination leads to recommendations, which feed directly into the planning process. Quality assurance is a proactive set of policies and activities utilized to evaluate the scope and effectiveness of patient care delivery. The recommendations from this evaluation usually result in stronger enforcement of a procedure or a change of procedure to improve quality of care.

INFLUENCES ON PROGRAM EVALUATION

External Influences

Although program evaluation is designed to assess the appropriateness, adequacy, effectiveness, and efficiency of an agency, it is affected by forces over which it has little or no control. These forces may be characteristics of the climate of the industry, the population served by the agency, rules and regulations imposed by legislation, and third-party payers (see Figure 26–2).

Industry

The climate of the industry is influenced by numerous factors. Home health agencies have proliferated overwhelmingly since the late 1970s, especially in those states that do not require a certificate of need. This has placed agencies in adversarial positions with each other. This climate provides support for performing program evaluation, however, and is a strong influence in urging agencies to go through this process. In addition to the increasing number of agencies, managed care systems,

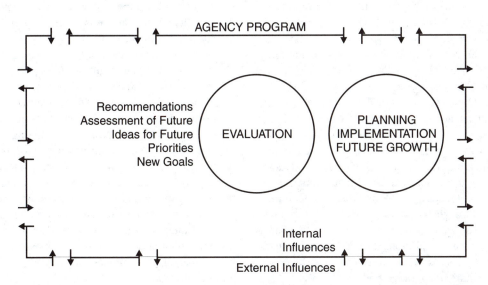

The agency program is an open system that has internal and external influences. The internal influences are contained within the boundary of the agency and affect the program evaluation process. The agency program output crosses over the boundary into the community, usually local but sometimes national. The external influences lie beyond the agency boundary and affect the agency program and its evaluation by crossing over the boundary.

Internal Influences	*External Influences*
Agency philosophy and goals	Patient population
Management	Demographics
Staff	Health status and needs
Policies	Economic status
Procedures	Demand for service
Management information system	Market competition
	Legislation
	Industry trends
	Third-party payers
	Home health associations
	Managed care programs

Figure 26–2 Context and purpose of program evaluation. *Source:* Copyright © Nancy D. Ruane.

the economic forecast, and future trends of the industry must be researched and understood because their effect is unavoidable.

This force in the industry has prompted some agencies to go beyond the minimum criteria imposed by Medicare. Many agencies utilize the accreditation services of the National League for Nursing through its Community Health Accreditation Program (CHAP) or the Joint Commission on Accreditation of Healthcare Organizations. For hospital-based home health agencies, accreditation by the Joint Commission is not optional because the home health agency is part of the hospital organization. Medicare criteria for program evaluation require the assessment of organizational structure and process. CHAP and the Joint Commission, through recent revisions, have expanded the evaluative emphasis to include standards that concern quality health care outcome statements. This shift requires agencies seeking accreditation by these bodies to reflect these standards in their programs.

In addition to the above accrediting organizations, there are other industry associations that develop codes of ethics and standards for their membership. Membership in these organizations is voluntary, and the codes and standards are developed by the markets. Nevertheless, the codes and standards do influence the programs of the member agencies by establishing guidelines for quality programs. Indirectly, these guidelines influence the nonmember agencies because they establish informal criteria that are accepted by the industry.

Population Served

The population served by the agency influences the services offered. The demographics, health status, health needs, and socioeconomic levels of the people served by the agency all affect the type and amount of services that will be utilized by the community. Careful monitoring of population shifts, health statistics, and the economy of the region is absolutely necessary and, therefore, is an item to be considered in program evaluation. The reliable use of social indicators permits comparison with other communities and societies.

Rules and Regulations

The mandates imposed by rules and regulations of legislation and third-party payers are the strongest influences on program evaluation. Many states require licensure before an agency can provide any home health services (Warhola, 1980). In some states, only certified home health programs are required to be licensed. The licensing agency is usually the state government. The licensing criteria require the agency to have program evaluation policies and procedures. The state health department evaluates these programs at specified intervals. Usually the agency must complete a self-study report and experience an on-site visit. The criteria used for this internal report mandate that at least organizational structure and process evaluation be completed. This process is in itself a program evaluation.

The third-party payers view program evaluation as a vital indicator of the agency's functioning. Program evaluation is required by Medicare, Medicaid, and Blue Cross, and most commercial insurers use the Medicare certification criteria as a standard for measuring the acceptability of an agency for reimbursement eligibility. Therefore, for an agency to be eligible for reimbursement and to survive as a provider, program evaluation must be included in its policies.

Internal Influences

Influences that the agency develops or can usually control still have an impact on program evaluation. This group of influences includes the agency's philosophy and goals, the quality of its staff, the expertise of its management, and the system of managing all patient information within the agency (see Figure 26–2).

Philosophy and Goals

In the development of an agency, the philosophy and goals, or mission statement, are created initially to give substance to the project. From this statement, the agency's founders draw the ideas and direction for the programs. The objectives and policies for the implementation of the programs emanate from the ideas. Directed by the objectives and policies, the program managers guide the staff's activity to provide services. The program objectives, along with the mission statement, give direction to the evaluation because they are included in the criteria used to measure program effectiveness.

Staff

The quality of the members of the staff affects program evaluation because the staff are actors in the performance of the program activity. Inadequately prepared, undereducated staff can lead to ineffectiveness of programs and may become a threat to the program's quality. Control of the quality of the staff begins with the job advertisement, continues through the selection process, and is maintained through employer evaluation and staff development.

Management

The expertise of management influences program planning and implementation as well as program evaluation. The quality of management is essential not only to maintain the program's effectiveness but also to ensure that the programs are properly planned. Ineffective managers lead to ineffective leadership and ineffective functioning of staff. The program goals will not be achieved, as the evaluation will reveal.

Management Information System

The patient information system is vital to program evaluation. It represents a significant portion of the information that is gathered for analysis in the evaluation process. Therefore, the lack of accuracy and other characteristics of the system influence program evaluation. Tracking of the information can be done by computer or by hand. In either case, the information must become part of the system and monitored at certain checkpoints for accuracy so that quality and comprehensiveness of care can be demonstrated. For example, effective

evaluation must take into account the withdrawals and additions to the patient population; only an accurate system can measure such variations.

DEVELOPMENT OF A PROGRAM EVALUATION SYSTEM

Since the beginning of the home health care movement, evaluation has been an integral part of the fundamental principles and practices of the industry. Evaluation areas are numerous and can be endless. There are relevant issues that must be considered and heeded in approaching evaluation. Investigative areas are selected according to their influences on patients, home health agency management staff, and the community served by the agency. The focus of the evaluation is also dictated by those regulatory and accreditation bodies that set standards for the industry.

Relevant Issues

By law, the Medicare regulations require certified home health agencies to evaluate their programs. The section on evaluation states that the agency must have written policies requiring an overall evaluation of the agency's total program at least once a year. The evaluation must be completed by the professional advisory group of the agency or a committee of that group along with the home health agency staff and consumers. The professional advisory group includes at least one registered nurse (preferably a public health nurse) and one physician as well as appropriate representation from the other professional disciplines that administer the scope of services. Overall policy, administrative, and clinical record reviews are included.

The aim of the evaluation is to assess the extent to which the agency's patient service delivery is appropriate, adequate, effective, and efficient. Each policy and administrative practice and its effect on patient care is reviewed. A report of the evaluation is presented to the governing body for action. The report is maintained as a part of the administrative record.

The agency must have established written mechanisms for the collection of data to assist the evaluation. The data may include numbers of patients receiving each service offered, sources of referral, number of patient visits, criteria for admissions, reasons for discharge, total staff days for each service offered, and number of patients not accepted (with reasons). If other data are available, they may be included because they will broaden and strengthen the statistical picture presented. This section also addresses the clinical record review, which is accomplished through quality assurance and utilization review (see Chapter 24). The Medicare conditions of participation serve as the basic structure upon which an evaluation program for home health agencies can be built (Stuart-Siddal, 1986).

The Joint Commission is a private, nonprofit organization whose purpose is to encourage the attainment of uniformly high standards of institutional health care. Its manual notes that one of its roles is that of evaluator. All hospital-based agencies are required to have Joint Commission accreditation. Other home health agencies may choose to request it. The Joint Commission standards require that the program's policies and procedures be reviewed annually and revised as necessary. The time of the last review and/or revision must be indicated. The evaluators are the individuals who are representative of the home care services provided. At least one physician and one registered nurse are among the evaluators. The specific inclusion of a physician as a reviewer is unique to this evaluation.

Through CHAP, the home health agencies participate in a voluntary accreditation process that aims to evaluate and improve the agency's services. To qualify for accreditation, the agency must complete a self-study report and experience an on-site visit (NLN, 1993). The CHAP criteria require annual program evaluation. The evaluation includes the assessment of program services and practice policies, the quality of care delivered by each discipline, the pop-ulation served, the services and visits provided, and the client/patient outcomes.

The agency must have an overall program evaluation plan that includes strategic planning and marketing, organization and administrative review, programs and service, and staffing policies and practices. This plan should indicate the frequency of each evaluation and the person or group responsible as well as the purpose of the evaluation. CHAP places responsibility for implementing the evaluation on the governing body for the professional advisory group. This annual review prevents the typical demise of reports (i.e., their being ignored and forgotten, left to collect dust on some bookshelf; Babbie, 1995).

Another mechanism that has a part in controlling the quality of care is licensure. Some states have assumed the responsibility for mandatory regulation. The regulations vary from state to state. The criteria are similar to the criteria for Medicare certification, with minor variations in each state. Generally, states establish agencies composed of a majority of professionals to set the guidelines for licensure. This process gives the states a means to revoke a license and therefore to prevent an agency from continuing in the provider role if compliance with criteria is not demonstrated (Spiegel, 1983).

Considering the nature of the home health care setting, the program evaluation is a mechanism utilized to ensure the delivery of quality care. It is difficult and costly to do comprehensive on-site evaluation of the care as it is being delivered. Other methods of evaluation involving staff and patients are employed to ensure the high quality of certain aspects of the agency's program. The staff participate in evaluating home visits, conducting surveys of other agencies in the area, opinion polling of patients and referral services, and making descriptive reviews and comparative evaluations. Usually the patients are involved in evaluation by answering opinion or attitude polls and by commenting on care received at specific times by specific health professionals.

Areas To Be Evaluated

Program evaluation has four areas of concern: organization, activities, outcomes, and costs. These areas are also known as structure, process, outcome, and fiscal evaluation. Structure deals with the administrative organization, the facilities and equipment, scope of services, the qualifications and profiles of the professional personnel, the characteristics of the patient population, and the policies and procedures governing patient care. Process involves the activities that are planned to occur in the program. Outcomes refers to the program or patient objectives in relation to their attainment. The fiscal area focuses on costs and cost accountability (Dever, 1980).

Structure may be considered an input measure of the quality of services based on the number, type, and quality of the resources used in the production of the services. Structure is an indirect measure because it does not consider the activities or actual result. Because of this, structure may be considered an inferior area to evaluation (U.S. House of Representatives, 1976). Structure and its relationship to process and outcomes have sufficient support, however. Donabedian (1978) supported the evaluation of structure on the assumption that, when an agency has good structure, good care will follow. CHAP, in its accreditation program, pays particular attention to the achievement and maintenance of an efficient, effective management structure in the delivery of quality care. Therefore, the evaluation of structure continues to be a relevant area of focus.

Process is an indicator of the quality of care used to assess the activities of the multidisciplinary team and the programs in the management of patients. Process measurement documents the activities that make up a program and the flow of these activities. The specific activities are directed by the agency mission and the policies and procedures that evolve from it. Generally, such measures study the degree of conformity with standards and expectations that are established by the peer groups and leaders of the professions (U.S. House of Representatives, 1976).

Outcome measures the quality of care in which the standard of judgment is the attainment of a specified result. The outcome of patient care is measured by the parameters set by the health professionals providing the care. These professionals are guided by the standards of their professions and are directed by the agency mission, policies, and procedures (U.S. House of Representatives, 1976).

Fiscal evaluation looks at planned and actual expenditures. The planned or budgeted expenditures are compared with the actual expenditures. Another aspect to be examined is whether the actual activities occurred as a result of the expenditure of the resources. Actual costs and possible alternative costs are considered. This evaluation may also involve the study of bookkeeping, billing, banking policies, procedures, and systems.

The sources of information for program evaluation are the patient and family or significant other, the patient's clinical record, the analysis of patient statistics, the administrative and organizational documents, community statistics, and financial records and reports. The patients and their families or significant others can influence the program by choosing to accept or deny services. They also play a significant part in the accomplishment of outcomes by cooperating with health professionals. Assessing the patient's reactions, feelings, and judgments about the program is important to the evaluation of both process and outcome. The opinions of the patient and family can be evaluated by surveys or questionnaires, which are mailed or used in telephone contact. Concrete cost estimates cannot be provided because several factors affect cost, namely cost per respondent associated with the type of method, sample size, length of the questionnaire, time frame in which the data are needed, personnel wages, and other situational conditions (Dillman, 1978; Dillman et al., 1974).

The use of the clinical record as a source of information for program evaluation has been reported in the literature since the 1960s (Helbig et al., 1972). The clinical record reveals information about process and outcome. Along with the analysis of patient statistics, which reveals, at minimum, reasons for admission and discharge, amount and types of services, number of visits, and patients' diagnoses, the evaluator can report a significant amount of information to the governing body.

The documents related to the administration and organization of the agency give the evaluator information from the agency's philosophy and objectives about the most specific patient care policy. Their information forms the framework upon which the program is built and can reveal much about the program's quality. The statistics that describe the community served by the agency are important to the evaluator in developing recommendations. Without knowledge of community needs, it is difficult to recommend changes and plans for the future. Financial records and reports assist the evaluator in realizing the cost effectiveness of the program. Cost accountability is as much a reality as professional accountability. Sufficient information about fiscal evaluation is included in every program evaluation, so that the governing body can make the correct decisions about future programs.

EVALUATION MODELS

To ensure a well-organized evaluation study, an evaluation model is used. Models reinforce conclusions drawn by the evaluator. Without a model, the information presented after an evaluation may be misinterpreted. Typically, the program evaluations performed by home health agencies are summative evaluations. This type of evaluation is associated with the use of a model (Fitz-Gibbon and Morris, 1987). The summative evaluation, described earlier in this chapter, is the focus of the following discussion and illustration.

Systems Model

The systems model of evaluation focuses on the process as a working model or social unit capable of achieving a goal. This model is concerned with attaining objectives, coordinating the functioning of units, maintaining resources, and adapting to the environment. The systems model examines other aspects in addition to the goal. Recognizing that organizations have multiple goals, this model considers a single goal attainment in relation to its effect on other goals in the system.

The variables that are described and evaluated are the input, the throughput, and the output. Input refers to characteristics and conditions of the people and the resources. Throughput refers to human and nonhuman resources and processes. Output refers to the product of the system (Baker and Northman, 1979; LaParta, 1975; Schulbert et al., 1969; Stanhope and Lancaster, 1988). The systems model is comprehensive because it considers more elements and describes their interaction with each other.

Structure-Process-Outcome Model

The structure-process-outcome model of Donabedian (1978) was designed primarily for medical care. Because it is applicable to the broader areas of health care, today it is a popular method. The definitions of structure, process, and outcome were presented earlier in this chapter. The rationale of structure evaluation is based on the concept that good care is dependent upon good administration, organization, facilities, and providers. Donabedian (1978) believed that, through review of the patient record and direct observation of care, an evaluative judgment can be made. The activities performed by the provider of care can be labeled good and competent when viewed in the context of a certain patient. Although outcome usually refers to the attainment of a goal for patient recovery, it is also used to convey changes in health status, health-related knowledge, attitude, and behavior. The tracer method, based on the premise that health status and care can be evaluated by viewing specific health problems called tracers, is a structure-process-outcome model that uses the results in comparative research (Stanhope and Lancaster, 1996).

Goal Attainment Model

The goal attainment model refers to a method for assessing the effectiveness of a program by measurement of the predetermined goals. The components of the goal attainment model are developing objectives, deciding how to measure the objectives, collecting information, assessing the effects, and analyzing and interpreting data. Shields (1974) developed an example of the goal attainment model. For each goal, the evaluator examines the categories of wherewithal, structure, operations, and outcomes.

Wherewithal refers to resources, materials, equipment, and physical facilities. Structure includes the organizational framework or the administrative structure, lines of authority, committee linkages, and patterns of communication. Operations pertain to processes and procedures for carrying out program goals. Outcome refers to the level of attainment of a goal (Shields, 1974). Effectiveness is directly concerned with goal attainment (Miller, 1991). The criteria applied to outcomes are effectiveness (the attainment of purpose), efficiency or cost effectiveness, and control (whether unexpected events were associated with the program). The evaluation process is applied to each goal in the program (Stanhope and Lancaster, 1988).

Planned versus Actual Performance Model

The planned versus actual performance model compares preprogram-targeted objectives with the actual program performance. Realistic goals are established for the evaluation criteria. The establishment of realistic goals is an important issue. The model assumes that the goals that are established are the best available indicators of the actual accomplishments. It can be used widely and regularly once a plan for program evaluation is developed (Dever, 1980).

Summary

The systems model, structure-process-outcome-model, goal attainment model, and comparison of planned and actual performance model described here are the most practical ones for a home health agency to use. Each of these designs may be applied with limited resources and minimal personnel. As a home health agency management tool, program evaluation must demonstrate its worth. The expected results of program evaluation are benefit increase and cost reduction (fiscal evaluation), increase in efficiency and productivity (structure evaluation), improvement in effectiveness (process evaluation), and documented change in health behavior and status of patients (outcome evaluation).

PROGRAM EVALUATION TOOLS

An evaluation tool or instrument is used to identify the information to collect and provides the evaluation criteria. There are numerous tools in the literature for conducting a program evaluation (Bulaw, 1986; Herman et al., 1978, 1987; Kosecaff and Fink, 1982; NLN, 1990). A review of these tools for the purpose of selection is time and cost effective. A program evaluation tool is a worksheet that indicates those areas to be evaluated, the time of evaluation, the rationale for the evaluation, and the evaluator.

In designing or selecting a tool, the following guidelines provide direction for evaluation (Dever, 1980; Kosecaff and Fink, 1982):

- How well did the program achieve its goals or outcomes?
- Were the program's activities implemented as planned?
- How effective were the activities in achieving the goals?
- Does the program have any unintended adverse or beneficial effects?
- Are the quantity and scope of service provided sufficient to meet the needs of the program participants?

- How quickly does the program respond to requests for service?
- Are patients discharged from the program prematurely?
- Do the patients, families, or significant others who use the program consider it satisfactory?
- What did the program cost?
- How did social, political, and regulatory factors influence the program's development and impact?
- How well was the program managed?
- What is to be changed in the program in the immediate future and in the long-term plan?

In addition to the above guidelines, the following criteria assist in ensuring that the assessment by the tool will be valid, accurate, and complete:

- The tool provides useful information about the program that justifies the collection, analysis, and presentation of the data.
- The tool addresses the aspects of concern of the governing body and regulatory agencies.
- The sources of data requested by the tool are sufficiently reliable. There are no biases, exaggerations, omissions, or errors that will cause the tool to become inaccurate or misleading.
- The tool enables the data to be collected and analyzed in time for the deadline.
- The tool does not restrain the evaluator from obtaining required information.
- The cost requirements for utilization of the tool can be met by the agency.
- The information that the tool produces can be interpreted clearly as desirable or undesirable (Dever, 1980).
- The tool has validity. Each criterion in the tool is based on expert judgment, past experience, and data from research.

COLLECTION OF INFORMATION

After one considers the development or selection of a tool for program evaluation,

thought is given to collecting information or data. This involves numerous and important techniques. In the selection of the correct technique for a program, the following factors should be considered. First, the technique should be acceptable to the governing body and management staff; be technically sound to collect data that are reliable, valid, and targeted to evaluation criteria; provide the best data that the budget can afford; and allow sufficient time for collection and analysis of the data before the deadline (Kosecaff and Fink, 1982).

The major methods and strategies that are utilized to collect information are as follows:

- review of the organization of the agency
- critical review of administrative philosophy, goals, objectives, and documents
- clinical record review for quality and utilization of services (the quality assurance and utilization review committee reports may be used, or the evaluator may review a sampling of clinical records)
- patient care policies and procedures review and evaluation using the current literature of the multidisciplinary health professions as a resource
- review of the goals and objectives of each program for attainment and relevance
- critical review of personnel policies, job descriptions, professional qualifications, and activities
- reports of the Medicare survey, state licensing consultants, or accreditation agencies
- recommendations from the agency committees
- results of patient opinion surveys and patient letters of appreciation and complaint
- results of referral source opinion surveys
- compilation of any patient statistics that can be acquired from the agency information system
- analysis of the proposed and actual budget and the cost report

PROGRAM EVALUATION REPORT

The report is the official record of the program evaluation. The audience of the report should be considered so that the style of writing will be understood. The evaluation findings should be communicated in a comprehensible way without compromising any qualitative and quantitative details.

A clear and logical evaluation report increases the credibility of the information presented. The report should include the following:

- an introduction, which briefly describes the program(s) being evaluated, the participants conducting the evaluation, and the approach to the evaluation
- the evaluation model and evaluation tool description, including any limitation (attach a copy of the tool if possible; if not, give some sample items and present information about the reliability and validity of the tool)
- a summary of all activities performed in the collection of data and what sources were used
- the results of any analysis that was done to arrive at answers to the evaluation criteria (use graphs and other visual presentations where applicable)
- the evaluation findings, the answers to the evaluation questions, and the evaluator's interpretation of the findings (it is important to point out the strengths and weaknesses of a program and to report the limitations of the findings)
- the recommendations and modifications for the program (prioritize the recommendations so that they may be incorporated readily into the plan)
- a report on the sequence of events in conducting the evaluation and recommendations for future evaluation (this may be appended to the report for the governing body and the management team)

A summary or brief overview of the evaluation report explains the purpose of the evaluation and lists its major recommendations and conclusions. It contains enough detail to be usable and believable but is easy to read. The summary may be placed at the beginning of the evaluation as an introduction. Because the summary may be more widely circulated and read than the complete report, it should be prepared carefully.

The evaluation report may begin with a section devoted to background information concerning the program. A description of the development of the program and its purpose sets the evaluation in context. The amount of detail presented is dependent upon the audience's degree of familiarity with the program (Fitz-Gibbon and Morris, 1987; Kosecaff and Fink, 1982).

It is important to emphasize here that the recommendations of the evaluation report must be communicated effectively to the persons responsible for plan development. The evaluation of a program is one of the ways in which the planners get a sense of how their ideas are being implemented. The relevance of what was planned in the past has a significant influence on what is planned for the future. Communication of evaluation findings, so that the planner or planning committee has a better comprehension of program effectiveness, is a vital step in the evaluation process (Blum, 1979).

The evaluator(s) can go one step further and present questions about the future to the planners as part of the section on recommendations. These questions can address such subjects as population shifts; prospective payment programs; changes in federal, state, or local regulations regarding health care delivery; consumer movements; and occurrence of a disaster.

SYSTEMATIC APPROACH TO PROGRAM EVALUATION

A program comes into being because an individual, a committee, or other group of concerned persons has an idea for a service that is needed by the community. The idea's creator visualizes a set of goals that, when taken collectively, become the program. The next phase in the development of the program, after the idea is conceptualized, is the stating of goals. Planning and evaluation are continually interfacing. The evaluative process, which begins operation at the outset of the program, is similar to the planning process in the development of the program.

The first step in the evaluative process is to look at the goals of the program. The goals must be clear, specific, and measurable. They should be people oriented. They must address program outcomes. The next step in the evaluative process is to clarify goals. Any goals that are not measurable, people oriented, or stated in outcome terminology should be rewritten. It may be necessary to change the stated measurement in the goal to be more realistic or relevant. The process then moves on to goal activation, or the implementation of the goals. At this time, the activities of the program are being performed, and the patients are receiving the services. The measurement of the goal effect follows. At this stage, the goal effect is measured through patient statistics and utilization review data. The final step in the evaluative process is the evaluation of the program. This is the judgment concerning the attainment of the program goals.

The planning for program evaluation is also part of the program plan. It is similar to the evaluative process but is more direct, specific, and task oriented. The steps in planning for program evaluation are as follows (Stanhope and Lancaster, 1988):

1. Identify people as evaluators. Usually program personnel, professional advisory board members, and consumers are included.
2. Conduct preliminary meetings to discuss the evaluation's purpose. A decision is reached to do the evaluation in a specific time period. A time line is drawn to indicate who will evaluate each section of the program in the time indicated.
3. Review the literature (this is done by the evaluators who are external to the program).

4. Determine the methods of conducting the evaluation. What evidence is needed to measure the program outcomes?
5. Conduct the evaluation.
6. Determine what committee or individual will write the program evaluation report after receiving recommendations from the evaluators.
7. Determine who will compose the planning group, who will carry out the recommendations for change, and how the change will be accomplished.
8. Present the evaluation report to the governing body, planning group, and community groups. The recommendations are emphasized so that they are not ignored but are received and implemented if possible.

OPERATIONAL CONSIDERATIONS IN PROGRAM EVALUATION

Even though the principles of evaluation are known, a critical aspect of evaluation should be considered. The present climate of the home health industry embodies cost containment. Everyone is seeking to prove cost effectiveness in the delivery of home care services. The federal government has awarded grants to studies to develop cost-effective care techniques, such as prospective payment systems. It may be erroneous to concentrate solely on dollars, however. Although containment is important, we must remember that care of human beings is at least equally important.

Benefits of the Program Evaluation

The central benefits of a program evaluation are the judgments concerning the attainment of the goals of the program. Through evaluation, the program managers and governing body can determine whether the program's purpose is being fulfilled. The feedback, which gives information about goal attainment, also verifies that the program is effective. This knowledge assists the decision makers in planning for future allocation of funds. Competent monitoring or evaluation of the program enables the decision makers to determine whether the achieved goals can be met in a more cost-effective manner.

Fiscal accountability may be another benefit derived from program evaluation. Funds given to operate a program must be spent for the purposes for which they are given. The accountability for the funds requires more than simple auditing of accounting records. The funding agency may take an alternative approach to monitoring; namely, if certain milestones (structure, process, and outcome) are achieved within the stated budget, it is assumed that the money given to the agency has been used appropriately (Alkin and Solman, 1983).

Evaluation can make contributions to the store of knowledge about the program, certain professional activities, and consumer needs. This information can be used to market the program through direct marketing and public relations efforts. It can provide a basis of comparison from which to judge the relative quality of good practice. Accumulated information from many evaluations can serve as a basis for conclusions about what sorts of programs work best.

Program evaluation is an intelligent response to controversy. An accumulation of strong data can resolve a situation beset by diverse opinions. Evaluation also persuades people to pay attention to data concerning what home health agencies are doing. It is the best response to the individuals who continuously push new ideas without substance. Innovations must be tried, but if health professionals never find out which ones are worthwhile, home health agencies will deliver care with a fad-oriented mentality. Each time an evaluation is conducted, additional people acquire evaluation skills. As more people in home health agencies become familiar with evaluation methods, they will be able to collect information and distinguish valuable, effective innovations from ineffective fads (Herman et al., 1987).

Cautions on Evaluation

Much work over the past 30 years has taught us to be cautious in interpreting results of evaluation research or program evaluations. The many stakeholders—program administrators, professionals, evaluators, legislators, directors, consumer advocates, and others—all may view results differently. Evaluators have gradually come to understand the need to use multiple methods in evaluation. The quality of knowledge increases with critical public scrutiny of it (Shadish et al., 1990). The focused evaluation of single agencies, such as those providing home health care, moves us closer to meaningful evaluations and program improvement.

Special Implementation Considerations

The organization of the home health agency may present specific circumstances that directly influence program evaluation. Most home health agencies have only one site. In these agencies, some decentralization is necessary. In such situations, the decentralization is not merely physical. The home health personnel who work in the site offices and neighborhoods are in the best position to know the problems, needs, and resources of the area served by the site office. Therefore, the personnel from that home health agency site, under the direction of the site administrator, should have the responsibility and the authority for determining and carrying out the details of the daily operations and activities. They function, of course, within the overall agency philosophy, goals, and policies. Capable leaders are placed in the administrative positions for the decentralized units. They administer their local programs to the maximum extent feasible.

Program evaluation in the one-site agency is conducted without difficulty because everything to be evaluated is centralized. In the multisite agency, the planning is more tedious. The governing body of a multisite agency has two operations. The first is to evaluate the total agency as one site. With this plan, the evaluator(s) must coordinate the data so that each site is represented in the evaluation of each goal in the program. This approach is difficult to coordinate and requires meticulous attention to ensure accuracy. If the governing body chooses to evaluate each site individually, the evaluator's task is less complicated. Also, this approach will enable the agency to do comparison evaluation studies. These studies will yield valuable information about the differences and similarities in the program as it is delivered to different communities. Program evaluation in a multisite agency is a challenge to the most seasoned evaluator. The information that this eval-

uation yields can be so rewarding, however, that it negates the frustrations of the experience.

Program Evaluation Tool Formats

There are numerous approaches to presenting a program evaluation tool. Appendix 26–A gives a few approaches. Each format attempts to assess the extent to which the home health care agency's program is appropriate, adequate, effective, and efficient. These formats may be modified as necessary to meet the objectives of the evaluator or evaluation team.

REFERENCES

Alkin, M., and L. Solman. 1983. *The costs of evaluation*. Beverly Hills: Sage.

Babbie, E. 1995. *The practice of social research*. 7th ed. Belmont, CA: Wadsworth.

Baker, F., and J.E. Northman. 1979. Evaluation of a school mental health clinic. In *Program evaluation in the health field*, vol. 2, eds. H.C. Schulbert and F. Baker. New York: Human Sciences Press.

Blum, H. 1979. *Planning for health*. New York: Human Sciences Press.

Breckon, D.J. 1982. *Hospital health education*. Gaithersburg, MD: Aspen.

Bulaw, J.M. 1986. *Administrative policies and procedures for home health care*. Gaithersburg, MD: Aspen.

Clark, M.J. 1992. *Nursing in the community*. East Norwalk, CT: Appleton & Lange.

Dever, G.E.A. 1980. *Community health analysis*. Gaithersburg, MD: Aspen.

Dillman, D.A. 1978. *Mail and telephone surveys*. New York: Wiley.

Dillman, D.A., et al. 1974. Increasing mail questionnaire response: A four state comparison. *American Sociological Review* 39:744–756.

Donabedian, A. 1978. The quality of medical care. In *Health care regulation, economics, ethics, and practice*, ed. P.H. Abelson. Washington, DC: American Association for the Advancement of Science.

Fitz-Gibbon, C., and L. Morris. 1987. *How to design a program evaluation*. Newbury Park, CA: Sage.

Helbig, D., et al. 1972. The care component core. *American Journal of Public Health* 62:540–546.

Herman, J. et al. 1978. *How to measure program implementation*. Beverly Hills: Sage.

Herman, J., et al. 1987. *Evaluator's handbook*. Newbury Park, CA: Sage.

Kosecaff, J., and A. Fink. 1982. *Evaluation basics*. Beverly Hills: Sage.

LaParta, J.W. 1975. *Health care delivery system: Evaluation criteria*. Springfield, IL: Thomas.

Miller, D.C. 1991. *Handbook of research design and social measurement*. 5th ed. Beverly Hills: Sage.

National League for Nursing (NLN). 1974. *Faculty-curriculum evaluation. Part II* (Pub. No. 15-1530). New York: NLN.

National League for Nursing (NLN). 1990. *Self study report for home care organization*. New York: NLN.

National League for Nursing (NLN). 1993. *Self study report for home care organization*. New York: NLN.

Rothman, J. 1980. *Using research in organizations*. Beverly Hills: Sage.

Schulbert, H.C., et al. 1969. *Program evaluation in the health field*. New York: Behavioral Publications.

Shadish, W.R., et al. 1990. *Foundations of program evaluation: Theories of practice*. Beverly Hills: Sage.

Shields, M. 1974. July. An evaluation model for science programs. *Nursing Outlook* 22:448.

Spiegel, A.D. 1983. *Home health care*. Owings Mills, MD: National Health Publishing.

Stanhope, M., and J. Lancaster. 1988. *Community health nursing*: Third edition. St. Louis: Mosby.

Stanhope, M., and J. Lancaster. 1996. *Community health nursing*: Fourth edition. St. Louis: Mosby.

Stuart-Siddal, S. 1986. *Home health care nursing.* Gaithersburg, MD: Aspen.

U.S. House of Representatives, Committee on Interstate and Foreign Commerce, Subcommittee on Health and the Environment. 1976. *A discursive dictionary of health care.* Washington, DC: U.S. Government Printing Office.

Warhola, C.F.R. 1980. *Planning for home health services* (DHHS Pub. No. [HRA] 80-14017). Washington, DC: U.S. Government Printing Office.

Formats for Presenting Program Evaluation Tools

Format 1

Evaluation Area with Outcomes	Outcome Met YES NO	Corrective Action Needed	Suggested Frequency and Month
A. Administration 　1. The governing body maintains relevant articles of incorporation			Once a year July
B. Organization 　1. The chief executive officer (CEO) keeps the operating chief (OC) up to date			Once a year July
C. Patient Care Policies 　1. All patients who fit the admission criteria received care from the agency			Twice a year March September
D. Nursing Services (etc.)			Annually

Continue this format until all areas that are to be evaluated are completed.

Source: Copyright © Nancy D. Ruane.

FORMAT 2

Activity with Outcomes	Evaluation Frequency	Responsible Group/Person	Outcome Met YES NO
A. Organizational Structure	Annually	Governing Body or Ad Hoc Committee	
1. Articles of Incorporation	Annually		
2. Bylaws: The governing body reviews the bylaws annually	Annually		
3. Agency Philosophy: The governing body and staff review the philosophy annually	Annually		
B. Financial Management	Monthly	Finance Committee	

Continue this format until all areas that are to be evaluated are completed.

FORMAT 3

Activity with Outcomes	Minimum Frequency	Responsible Body/Person	Comments
A. Organizational Structure 1. The CEO manages the day-to-day operation of the agency	Yearly and prn	Board of Directors	
B. Administrative Policies	Monthly and prn	Board of Directors	
C. Financial Management 1. The controller prepares for the preparation of monthly financial statements	Monthly	Finance Committee	
D. Community Assessment	Annually	Program Coordinator	
E. Program Services	Quarterly	Professional Advisory Committee, Program Coordinator	

Continue this format until all areas that are to be evaluated are completed.

FORMAT 4

Evaluation Area: List Outcomes under Category	Frequency	Responsible Committee/Person	Outcome Met YES NO
Organization and Administration			
A. Organization Chart The CEO keeps the OC consistent with the agency operation	Annually	Board, CEO	
B. Philosophy and Goals	Annually	Board	
C. Administrative Policies	Annually and prn	Board, CEO	
D. Administrative Procedures	Annually and prn	Board, CEO	
E. Community Needs	Annually	Board, CEO, Consultant	
F. Financial Management	Monthly	Board and Finance Committee	
Program and Services			
A. Program Services	Annually	Board, CEO, Professional Advisory Board	
B. Practice Policies		Procedures Committee	
C. Quality Assurance/ Utilization Review (QA/UR)		QA Committee, UR Committee	

Continue this format until all areas that are to be evaluated are completed.

FORMAT 5

Evaluation Area with Outcomes under Each Category	Frequency	Responsible Body/Person	Outcome Met YES NO	Comments
Structure				
A. Organization The CEO keeps the OC consistent with agency operation	Annually Annually	Board Professional Advisory Board		
B. Administrative 1. Policies: All patients who meet criteria receive care from the agency 2. Procedures	Annually			
C. Community Needs	Annually			
D. Facilities 1. Equipment	Annually			
E. Staff	Annually			
Process				
A. Program Services Skilled Nursing HHA PT OT MSS	Twice a year	CEO Director of Professional/ Patient Services Staff		
B. Utilization of Services	Four times a year	CEO, Professional Advisory Board		

Continue this format until all areas that are to be evaluated are completed.

CHAPTER 27

Clinical and Financial Evaluations of Patient Care

Marilyn D. Harris

The Visiting Nurse Association (VNA) of Eastern Montgomery County/Department of Abington Memorial Hospital is a nonprofit, hospital-based, Medicare-certified home health agency and hospice. It is accredited with commendation by the Joint Commission on Accreditation of Healthcare Organizations. During fiscal year (FY) 1996, the staff made approximately 130,000 home health visits. The agency has an average of 600 admissions and 500 discharges each month and approximately 1,100 patients on service each month. The hospice program provided approximately 10,000 benefit days, most of which were routine days. The professional staff include registered nurses; certified pediatric and adult nurse practitioners; clinical nurse specialists; physical, occupational, and speech therapists; and medical social workers. Home health aides and volunteers are available for both programs. Additional disciplines are available for the hospice program. Specialty areas of nursing include psychiatry, pediatrics, enterostomal therapy, and genitourinary (continence management) therapy. Contract services supplement staff during peak times or in selected practice areas.

PATIENT CLASSIFICATION SYSTEM: BACKGROUND AND SIGNIFICANCE

The Tax Equity and Fiscal Responsibility Act of 1982 dramatically changed the way hospitals are reimbursed for inpatient care. Hospitals are paid a flat, illness-specific amount that is set prospectively. The rationale for a prospective payment mechanism is to encourage hospital efficiency and thereby reduce Medicare costs. The Health Care Financing Administration has been charged with developing strategies that will reduce Medicare costs for home health services.

Thus the area of methodological research in nursing that has received a great amount of attention has been patient classification systems (Ballard and McNamara, 1983; Daubert, 1979; Giovannetti, 1979; Hardy, 1984; Harris et al., 1987; Martin and Scheet, 1992; Saba, 1992a, 1992b; Saba and Zuckerman, 1992; Saba et al., 1991; Sienkiewicz, 1984; Wilson, 1992). This is not surprising because the purpose of these instruments is to respond to the variable nature of demand for nursing care in a variety of settings through assessment of patients' requirements for nursing care. Nursing administrators are confronted with the task of ensuring provision of quality care, which requires adequate staffing, appropriate staff mix, and the maintenance of staff with sophisticated skills to meet patients' needs. These conditions must be realized under government regulations, present economic conditions, public scrutiny, and budget constraints. It is therefore essential for the nurse executive to utilize tools that can address these issues. One such tool is the rehabilitation potential patient classification system (RPPCS).

Daubert (1979) described and implemented the RPPCS in a community health agency. Daubert's method is copyrighted and was developed as one component of a quality assurance program to evaluate patient outcomes. Daubert's system offers five client categories describing the characteristics of clients assigned to each category. Each category has a set of subobjectives that are considered minimum goals. In this system, the subobjectives must be met for the ultimate problem objectives to be achieved. The VNA has collected statistical and/or financial data by multiple classification systems for several years. These include referral source, municipality, major disease category (MDC), VNA of New Haven's RPPCS category (Daubert, 1979), total number of cases, nursing diagnosis (ND), and *International Classification of Diseases* (ICD-9) code. A variety of data are generated through our management information system: total charge per case and per case by discipline, average length of stay, average number of visits by case and by discipline, and RPPCS, ND, and MDC.

Based on the assumption that reimbursement for home care services will change from a per visit system to another, currently undetermined system in the future and that NDs rather than medical diagnoses influence the level and amount of services that home care patients require, the administrative staff were interested in including the identification of the charge by ND. The staff were also interested in identifying those NDs that occur most frequently and those that are included within each of the five goals of the RPPCS and the 23 MDCs.

ND DATA COLLECTION

This project was initiated in July 1985. The first month was used to finalize the computer program with our computer service. Data collection began in August 1985.

Currently, the VNA's statistical and financial data are collected on a daily basis. The forms used for this purpose are shown in Appendix 27–A. The visiting staff complete a daily report form. Initial data for all new patients are input into the management information system via a patient master update (PMU) form. Any changes, additions, or deletions to service are input via PMU form II. The use of the PMU II allows the agency to calculate charges by length of stay by discipline. To collect data by ND, an ND discharge summary is used. The top portion of the form includes information relevant to total agency service: agency name, date on which the form was completed, patient name and number, patient status, discharge reason, date of discharge, service codes (goal on admission and goal attainment on discharge for the RPPCS), and start of care date. The remainder of the form lists the NDs (Gordon, 1995) used by the staff. The staff are asked to indicate the percentage of total time spent on each ND and the start and stop dates for each diagnosis.

To assign a dollar value to each diagnosis, the total charge of nursing service must be divided by some method. At the beginning of the project, the following options were discussed:

- Charge is to be divided equally among all NDs.
- Charge is to be divided by a percentage of the time spent on each diagnosis by total case. Staff nurses will assign the percentage of time to each diagnosis on discharge. This will be subjective.
- Charge is to be divided by the percentage of time spent on each visit (although this would be the most accurate in theory, it could be the least accurate in practice; for example, staff could forget to identify ND service codes on each visit given all the other documentation that has to be done to meet billing, legal, and agency standards).

Administration chose the second option because the primary nurse is the person who can assign a percentage to each diagnosis in relationship to the total care provided during the patient's length of stay with the VNA.

The VNA staff use a problem-oriented record system based on NDs. Each problem must be addressed and a notation made in the clinical record at the time it is resolved or when the patient is discharged from agency service. At the beginning of the project, there was discussion regarding the assignment of a quantifying goal to each ND. Although this would be ideal, it was decided that the VNA would benefit more by using goals identified by RPPCS rather than one for each problem based on an ND. To identify specific individuals with specific NDs and to identify charges associated with these NDs, patient names and numbers were built into the data collection system for internal quality assessment/performance improvement (QA/PI) purposes.

For the current study, all patients admitted to and discharged from nursing service were included in the data collection. The purposes of the study were to document the charge for care by ND, to identify NDs within the RPPCS and MDC, to identify the average length of stay on VNA service, and to identify the average number of visits per case by ND. At any time, 3 years of cumulative data are included in the computer printouts.

DEVELOPMENT OF STANDARDIZED FLOW SHEETS

Before the study began, several preliminary steps were taken, including the development of standardized flow sheets (SFSs), general assessment sheets for each group in the RPPCS, and corresponding discharge summaries. These SFSs encourage documentation of quality care delivered for a specific group of patients with a specific ND by outlining the parameters to be addressed. The use of SFSs also encourages efficiency when one is documenting care. Nurses write a narrative for each patient visit to meet the needs of third-party payers. Preprinted flow sheets reduce the time required to complete charting. The development of SFSs was also in response to staff's request for this type of charting format.

The flow sheets were originally developed by three nurses: the director of professional services, a nurse practitioner, and the nursing supervisor responsible for the VNA's QA/PI program. These individuals read the relevant literature and drew on their experiences in community health nursing. The staff provided feedback on the completeness and practicality of the flow sheets developed by these managers. The director of professional services, supervisors, nurse practitioners, and selected staff nurses developed additional SFSs for such areas as psychiatric and pediatric diagnoses. As of June 1996, changes were in process as the agency transitioned from a manual to a computerized clinical documentation system and incorporated components of Shaughnessy and Crisler's (1995) outcome-based quality improvement tool.

A general assessment flow sheet was developed for each of the five groups in the RPPCS (see Appendix 27–A). This provided a method to measure the overall outcome objectives. These five groups also represented the patients' long-range goals. Initially, a pilot study was conducted with four of the staff nurses. The results of this pilot showed that the patients in the study had been placed in the correct group 90 percent of the time. Current findings continue to meet this threshold.

The ND flow sheets were developed at the same time that the general assessment sheets were done. Initially, 15 of the most commonly used NDs were selected. At present, approximately 40 ND flow sheets are available for staff. The flow sheets were developed with emphasis on the primary nurse's ability to individualize care for each patient. Nurses complete blank flow sheets for NDs for which SFSs are not yet available.

Objective data such as breath sounds, diet, and safety as well as subobjective data from the RPPCS are on the general assessment sheet. Data specific to a particular problem are on the ND flow sheet. Some duplication is unavoidable, however. For example, blood pressure appears on both the general assessment RPPCS form and the altered health maintenance ND flow sheet. In the future, duplication will be eliminated through the use of the computerized documentation system, which is programmed to recognize unique data elements.

The agency utilizes a problem-oriented record system. The NDs are the problems. As mentioned above, there are flow sheets for the five patient groups in the RPPCS. Patients are entered into one of these groups on admission to the agency. A standardized discharge summary is used for each of the five patient groups. The subobjectives appropriate for each group match those on the flow sheets. On discharge, the nurse uses this checklist to indicate whether the patient or family has demonstrated an increase in knowledge and understanding or has undergone a behavior change. Goal attainment (outcome) is noted as none, moderate, or maximum. This form is completed in duplicate, and one copy is sent to the patient's physician upon request.

Evidence must be presented in the body of the record to substantiate the identified outcome. The nurse must address each ND by recording the specific outcome and the date on which it occurred. When a problem is not resolved, the nurse records the status and date of discharge from agency service. Since 1992, the clinical outcomes for the RPPCS have included data from all disciplines. When therapy service continues after nursing service has been discontinued, the therapy supervisor is responsible for reviewing the discharge summary form to ensure that the outcome data for therapy are consistent with the nursing outcomes and that the correct level of goal attainment has been recorded.

STAFF EDUCATION

Formal orientation of staff to the new system and forms through lectures, slides, and overheads was done before the start of the study. A manual was distributed to each nurse that included sample forms, case studies, and charting guidelines. The educational process also included practice sessions in classifying patients into the correct group. There were general discussions, questions, and answers. These sessions were done in both large and small groups by the administrative and supervisory staff. This educational process is now part of the orientation to the agency for all professionals.

QA/PI

The correct identification of the RPPCS and ND for each patient is included as one aspect of the VNA's QA/PI program. When the patient is not placed in the correct category on admission, the discharge summary cannot be completed because the categories do not coincide. This patient's chart receives additional review at the time of the record audit if the admitting medical diagnosis does not qualify the patient for a specific group in the classification system.

Several check points are built into the QA/PI program to ensure accuracy. On admission, each chart is reviewed by the clinical supervisor to determine that the nurse has selected the correct group. Any change from this original grouping must be discussed with the supervisor. The master file input cards are reviewed for gross errors by the supervisors on admission. The PMU forms are reviewed on discharge from service.

The QA/PI program includes a quarterly review of a random selection of both open and closed records. This random selection procedure is programmed into our computer system. The review format includes questions that have been brought before an expert panel to establish validity. Recommended changes are incorporated into the review checklist.

A maximum of 50 nursing records are reviewed each quarter based on the number of patients who receive nursing service. One hundred records were reviewed during the 6-month study period; agreement was 98 percent. During each subsequent quarterly record review cycle, agreement has ranged from 96 percent to 100 percent. Based on this finding plus the overall results of the record review process, the management staff have determined that the data are valid.

DATA ANALYSIS

At the end of the pilot project, 6-month data (August 1985 to January 1986) were analyzed. Five hundred forty-one patients were discharged during this time period. The number of NDs per patient ranged from 1 to 6 (average, 1.8). In 1986, the VNA identified 50 NDs to be used by the staff. Thirty-one were identified during data collection. In 1991 there were 99 NDs on the approved list, and in 1993 there were 109 NDs. Fifty were used by the staff in 1991 and 55 in 1993. As of June 30, 1991, there were 7,868 patients in the study (3-year cumulative data) with an average charge of $866 per ND. As of June 30, 1993, there were 9,872 patients in the study with an average charge of $1,007 per ND. As of June 30, 1996, there were 15,487 patients in the study with an average charge of $911 per ND.

Analysis by ND

The five most frequently identified NDs in 1986 were altered health maintenance, knowledge deficit, self-bathing/hygiene deficit, impaired skin integrity, and ineffective breathing pattern; these represented 62 percent of all diagnoses identified by the staff (Table 27–1). In FY 1993, the same 5 NDs were identified 76 percent of the time. At the end of FY 1996, the same five NDs were identified 81 percent of the time. One reason for this finding may be that the NDs used are physiologically based and are identified as Medicare-reimbursable diagnoses.

The charge per ND is included on the monthly printout. Each diagnosis may be only a percentage of the total charge for care for a patient, depending on the number of NDs identified for that patient. The five most expensive NDs during FY 1996 are listed in Table 27–2. Table 27–3 lists the NDs with the highest number of visits. It is interesting to note that several of these NDs were also among the most expensive and most frequently identified.

Analysis by ICD-9 Code

At times, more in-depth studies have been done. In 1991, with the help of a graduate student who completed a summer internship program at the VNA, we were able to analyze the *International Classification of Diseases* (ICD-9) code prevalence for the five most common NDs. The purpose of this project was to determine whether one or more ICD-9 codes represented a significant proportion of all codes within each of the five most common NDs for all active patients for the month of June 1991 at the VNA. The summaries generated by the VNA's information system provided the total number of patients in each ND category and an individual listing of each patient in numeric order by ND code number. The individual listing included the ICD-9 code assigned to each patient. These codes were also presented in numeric order within each ND code.

After the five most common NDs were identified, the ICD-9 codes within them were listed in numeric order by the first three digits. The frequency of each ICD-9 code within the ND was then determined from the individual listing. The result of this process was a breakdown of

---

Table 27–1 Percentage of Total NDs of the Five Most Frequently Identified NDs, by FY

FY 1986	FY 1991	FY 1993	FY 1995	FY 1996
62%	77%	76%	75%	81%

Table 27–2 Five Most Expensive NDs (June 30, 1996)

ND*	Cost
Activity intolerance (6)	$1,535
Impaired skin integrity (85)	1,080
Self-esteem disturbance (6)	903
Potential for impaired skin integrity (85)	874
Altered health maintenance (4,519)	793

*Numbers in parentheses indicate number of patients with ND

the five most common NDs by ICD-9 code and a listing of the frequency of each ICD-9 code within the ND. The frequency of each ICD-9 code was then divided by the sum of the frequencies of all codes within the ND. The resulting numbers provided the percentage of the total frequency in the diagnosis represented by each ICD-9 code. For example, ND-27, knowledge deficit, was the most common ND in June 1991. There were 2,087 individually listed knowledge deficit diagnoses in that month, and within those ND-27 diagnoses there were 281 different ICD-9 codes (by first three digits only). The only ICD-9 code to occur 209 times or more (10 percent of 2,087 or greater) was v24, postpartum care and examination, which occurred 294 times (14 percent of the ND-27 total of 2,087 individual listings).

The percentages indicated that none of the ICD-9 codes had a strong association with any of the five NDs. Only 7 codes represented 10 percent or more of the total for any diagnosis, and no code exceeded 23 percent of the total. Additionally, none of the 7 codes representing 10 percent or more of one ND achieved that level of representation in another ND. Those ICD-9 codes representing at least 10 percent of all codes within an ND are presented in Table 27–4.

Analysis by RPPCS

The VNA uses RPPCS to identify goals on admission to home care services and to quantify goal attainment on discharge. The administrative staff can determine the percentage of patients within each of the five classification categories and the percentage of goal attainment within each group (Table 27–5). For this study, the total number of visits by rehabilitation goal was also analyzed. Patients in the maintenance (group 4) level of care, followed by the rehabilitation (group 3) patients, were the most costly to staff. Overall, the average charge per case for the 2,988 patients for FY 1991 was $2,041 with an average of 20 visits during a length of stay of 27 days. In FY 1993, there were 3,494 patients with an average charge of $2,321 per case for an average of 22 visits during a 29-day length of stay. In FY 1996 there were 5,387 patients with an average charge of $1,686 per case for an

Table 27–3 NDs with Highest Number of Visits (June 30, 1996)

ND	Number of Cases	Number of Visits
Self-esteem disturbance	6	23
Activity intolerance	6	19
Impaired skin integrity	3,074	17
Potential for impaired skin integrity	85	16
Self-bathing/hygiene deficit	3,732	15
Functional incontinence	19	14
Altered urinary elimination pattern	806	13

Table 27–4   ICD-9 Codes Representing 10% or More of All Codes within an ND

ICD-9 Name	ICD-9 Code	ND	ND Code	ICD-9 Percentage
Heart failure	428	Altered health maintenance	24	23
Chronic airway obstruction	496	Ineffective breathing pattern	7	20
Pneumonia, organism unspecified	486	Ineffective breathing pattern	7	15
Postpartum care and examination	v24	Knowledge deficit	27	14
Acute myocardial infarction	296	Altered health maintenance	24	12
Chronic ulcer of skin	707	Impaired skin integrity	42	12
Malignant neoplasm of trachea, bronchus, and lung	162	Ineffective breathing pattern	7	12

Table 27–5   Clinical Outcomes in Home Health Care: Goal Attainment Data, June 30, 1996

Goal	Outcome*	Number of Cases	Percentage of Goal	Percentage of Total
Recovery	1		98	
		3,414		
	2	69	2	
	3	2	0	
Subtotal		3,485	100	24
Self-care	1	95	80	
	2	27	20	
	3	0		
Subtotal		122	100	1
Rehabilitation	1	7,833	73	
	2	3,020	26	
	3	72	1	
Subtotal		10,925	100	69
Maintenance	1	112	50	
	2	135	50	
	3	1	1	
Subtotal		248	100	2
Terminal	1	247	35	
	2	455	64	
	3	5	1	
Subtotal		708	100	4
TOTAL		15,487		100

*1, attained all goals; 2, attained some goals; 3, attained no goals.

average of 16 visits during a 24-day length of stay.

Analysis by MDC

The total number of visits and charges by MDC was analyzed. Four of the VNA's most frequently identified MDCs corresponded to four of the five most frequently identified MDCs in the Commonwealth of Pennsylvania (Pennsylvania Department of Health, 1995). In Pennsylvania, the five most frequent MDCs in 1995 were circulatory, respiratory, endocrine, neoplasms, and musculoskeletal.

CONCLUSION

In the 1990s, there is increased emphasis on the identification and measurement of patient-focused outcomes to meet certification, licensing, accreditation, professional, and agency standards. The clinical outcomes of care are important for all these reasons. It is also imperative that administrators analyze financial outcomes of care in preparation for a different payment system in the future.

Clinical and financial data by ND, RPPCS, MDC, and ICD-9 code have been identified for one VNA. Comparisons have been made for data from FY 1986, 1991, 1993, and 1996. Similarities over time could be a function of the current reimbursement system (i.e., Medicare plan of care and billing forms for patients with these problems are less likely to raise questions on medical review or audit by a fiscal intermediary). They could also mean that nurses are identifying but not documenting other NDs.

Administrators must always keep alert to proposed changes in reimbursement methods for home care services. Agency administrators must concentrate on establishing and measuring the outcomes of patient care to meet certification and accreditation standards. They must also select a patient classification system that meets their needs and begin to document the cost and charges associated with care by a method other than the per visit basis. This will enable administrators to determine what changes need to be made to continue to provide quality home health care services when Medicare and other payers changes from a per visit basis to another method of payment in the future.

REFERENCES

Ballard, S., and R. McNamara. 1983. Quantifying nursing needs in home health care. *Nursing Research* 32:236–241.

Daubert, E. 1979. Patient classification systems and outcome criteria. *Nursing Outlook* 27:450–454.

Giovannetti, T. 1979. Understanding patient classification systems. *Journal of Nursing Administration* 9:4–9.

Gordon, M. 1995. *Manual of nursing diagnosis 1995–1996*. St. Louis: Mosby–Year Book.

Hardy, J. 1984. A patient classification system for home health patients. *Caring* 3:26–27.

Harris, M., et al. 1987. Relating quality and cost in a home care agency. *Quality Review Bulletin* 13:175–181.

Martin, K., and N. Scheet. 1992. *The Omaha System. Application for community health nursing*. Philadelphia: Saunders.

Pennsylvania Department of Health. 1995. *Annual statistics from the 1995 annual registration data collection report—Home health agencies*. Harrisburg, PA: Commonwealth of Pennsylvania.

Saba, V. 1992a. Home health care classification. *Caring* 11:58–60.

Saba, V. 1992b. The classification of home health care nursing diagnoses and intervention. *Caring* 11:50–57.

Saba, V., and A. Zuckerman. 1992. A new home health classification method. *Caring* 11:29–34.

Saba, V., et al. 1991. A nursing intervention taxonomy for home health care. *Nursing and Health Care* 12:296–299.

Shaughnessy, P., and K. Crisler. 1995. *Outcome based quality improvement*. Washington, DC: National Association for Home Care.

Sienkiewicz, J. 1984. Patient classification in community health nursing. *Nursing Outlook* 32:219–221.

Wilson, A. 1992. Patient functional assessment tools and integration of OCS into nursing documentation. In *Outcomes concept systems: A guide to the measurement of patient outcomes*, ed. A. Wilson, 4–34. Harrison, NY: Wilson and Associates.

Data Collection Forms and Flow Sheets

Daily Report Form

Daily Report

Employee Number _____

BATCH NUMBER _____

NAME _____

WEEK-DAY _____

DATE _____

On Duty _____ A.M.

On Duty _____ P.M.

Off Duty _____ A.M. TOTAL _____

Off Duty _____ P.M.

Personal Car Mileage

Start _____

Finish _____

Total _____

	Regular
25	Vacation
26	Personal
27	Sick
28	Holiday
29	Make Up
30	Other

PATIENT NUMBER	PATIENT NAME		VR	VISIT CHARGE	ALLOW	TOTAL CHARGE	PAYER OVR	START TIME	FINISH TIME	VISIT TIME	NONVISIT TIME		R/X 1	R/X 2	MA PROC CODE	MILES
	LAST	FIRST									HOURS	CODE				
TOTALS																

continues

Daily Report Form continued

Visit Reason Codes (VR)
A Nursing
B Physical Therapy
C Speech Therapy
D Occupational Therapy
E Medical Social Service
F Home Health Aide
H Assessment
M HHA Supervision
P Not Home
Q Non-Visit Time
R Non-Chargeable Visit

Non-Visit Time Codes
01 Visit Travel Time
02 Office Time
05 EPSDT
06 Team Management
07 Travel Difficulties
08 Staff Meetings
09 Bereavement Visit
10 Education
11 Record Review
12 Observation
13 Evaluation - Not Opened
14 Liaison
15 Travel to Office
16 MSW Office Consultation
18 Montg Co Health Dept Education
19 Community Health Education
22 Hospice Activity

Payer Codes
10 Medicare
29 Medical Assistance
38 Independence Blue Cross
41 Self Pay
42 Veterans
43 Private Insurance
45 US HealthCare
49 Other

Time Conversion

Minute	Decimal
6	.10
12	.20
15	.25
18	.30
24	.40
30	.50
36	.60
42	.70
45	.75
48	.80
54	.90
60	1.00

RX Codes
01 IV
02 Hospice Non-Benefit
03 HHA Supervision
06 Prenatal Admission Visit
07 Routine Admission Visit
08 Beeper Visit
09 BID Visit
50 TAPP Follow up Visit
51 TAPP Home Assessment Visit
99 Visit Approval

Source: Reprinted with permission of the Visiting Nurse Association of Eastern Montgomery County/Dept. of Abington Memorial Hospital, Willow Grove, Pennsylvania.

PMU Form and ND Discharge Summary

PT. #_____ NAME_____ STATUS [4]

	Last	**First**

D/C Reason [ ]   D/C Date___/___/___ Service Codes_____/_____

Group#/Goal Attainment#

1. Died
2. Visits Exhausted
3. Normal
4. Hospital   SOC DATE ___/___/___
5. Moved
6. Other   SIGNATURE_____DATE_____
7. Nursing Home

NURSING DIAGNOSIS		% OF CARE	START DATE	CLOSE DATE
1	Activity Intolerance			
2	Ineffective Airway Clearance			
3	Anxiety			
4	Constipation			
5	Diarrhea			
6	Bowel Incontinence			
7	Ineffective Breathing Pattern			
8	Decreased Cardiac Output			
9	Pain			
10	Impaired Verbal Communication			
11	Ineffective Coping (Individual)			
12	Ineffective Family Coping: Compromised			
13	Ineffective Family Coping: Disabling			
14	Family Coping: Potential for Growth			
15	Diversional Activity Deficit			
16	Altered Family Processes			
17	Fear			

NURSING DIAGNOSIS		% OF CARE	START DATE	CLOSE DATE
18	Fluid Volume Deficit (Actual X1)			
19	Potential Fluid Volume Deficit			
20	Fluid Volume Excess			
21	Impaired Gas Exchange			
22	Anticipatory Grieving			
23	Dysfunctional Grieving			
24	Altered Health Maint. a) Cardiac; b) HTN; c) CVA; d) Other			
25	Impaired Home Maintenance Management			
26	Potential for Injury			
27	Knowledge Deficit: a) Diabetes; b) General			
28	Impaired Physical Mobility			
29	Noncompliance			
30	Altered Nutrition: Less than Body Requirements			
31	Altered Nutrition: More than Body Requirements			
32	Altered Nutrition: Potential for More than Body Requirements			

continues

Source: Reprinted with permission of the Visiting Nurse Association of Eastern Montgomery County/Dept. of Abington Memorial Hospital, Willow Grove, Pennsylvania.

	NURSING DIAGNOSIS	% OF CARE	START DATE	CLOSE DATE
33	Altered Oral Mucous Membranes			
34	Altered Parenting			
35	Potential for Infection			
36	Powerlessness			
37	Rape Trauma Syndrome			
38	Self-Bathing–Hygiene Deficit			
39	Self-Esteem Disturbance			
40	Sensory-Perceptual Alteration: Input Deficit			
41	Sexual Dysfunction			
42	Impaired Skin Integrity			
43	Potential for Skin Integrity			
44	Sleep Pattern Disturbance			
45	Social Isolation			
46	Spiritual Distress (Distress of Human Spirit)			
47	Impaired Thought Processes			
48	Altered Time Perfusion			
49	Altered Urinary Elimination Pattern			
50	Potential for Violence			
51	Potential Activity Intolerance			
52	Impaired Adjustment			
53	Chronic Pain			
54	Altered Growth and Development			
55	Fluid Volume Deficit (Actual X2)			
56	Hopelessness			
57	Hyperthermia			
58	Hypothermia			

	NURSING DIAGNOSIS	% OF CARE	START DATE	CLOSE DATE
59	Functional Incontinence			
60	Reflex Incontinence			
61	Stress Incontinence			
62	Total Incontinence			
63	Urge Incontinence			
64	Unilateral Neglect			
65	Altered Sexuality Patterns			
66	Impaired Social Interaction			
67	Impaired Swallowing			
68	Potential for Altered Body Temperature			
69	Ineffective Thermoregulation			
70	Impaired Tissue Integrity			
71	Posttrauma Response			
72	Urinary Retention			
73	Health-Seeking Behaviors			
74	Potential for Poisoning			
75	Potential for Suffocation			
76	Ineffective Breastfeeding			
77	Potential for Aspiration			
78	Colonic Constipation			
79	Perceived Constipation			
80	Fatigue			
81	Potential for Disuse Syndrome			
82	Total Self-Care Deficit			
83	Self-Dressing–Grooming Deficit			
84	Self-Feeding Deficit			

PMU Form continued

NURSING DIAGNOSIS		% OF CARE	START DATE	CLOSE DATE
85	Self-Toileting Deficit			
86	Dysreflexia			
87	Sensory-Perceptual Alteration: Input Excess			
88	Decisional Conflict			
89	Chronic Low Self-Esteem			
90	Situational Low Self-Esteem			
91	Body Image Disturbance			
92	Personal Identity Disturbance			
93	Disturbance in Role Performance			
94	Potential for Altered Parenting			
95	Parental Role Conflict			
96	Rape Trauma Syndrome: Compound Reaction			
97	Rape Trauma Syndrome: Silent Reaction			

NURSING DIAGNOSIS		% OF CARE	START DATE	CLOSE DATE
98	Defensive Coping			
99	Ineffective Denial			
100	Caregiver Role Strain			
101	High Risk for Caregiver Role Strain			
102	High Risk for Self-Mutilation			
103	Relocation Stress Syndrome			
104	Ineffective Management of Therap. Reg. (Indiv.)			
105	Interrupted Breastfeeding			
106	Ineffective Infant Feeding Pattern			
107	Inability To Sustain Spontaneous Ventilation			
108	Dysfunctional Ventilatory Weaning Response			
109	High Risk-Peripheral Neurovascular Dysfunc.			

PMU Form II

EMPLOYEE NAME _____

PT. #_____ **Name**_____ **Date** _____

Discipline		ICD-9 Code	Date Soc Begins	Date Soc Ends	Remarks
Nursing	1				
P.T.	2				
Speech	3				
O.T.	4				
M.S.S.	5				
HHA	6				
Office	7				

Remarks: 1 = Discharge; 2 = Hospital Admission; 3 = Diagnosis Change

Source: Reprinted with permission of the Visiting Nurse Association of Eastern Montgomery County/Dept. of Abington Memorial Hospital, Willow Grove, Pennsylvania.

General Assessment: Intermediate/Advanced Chronic Rehabilitation

PT. # _____ NAME_____ PG_____

PARAMETERS/INTERVENTIONS		Date	Date	Date	Date	Date	Date
Vital signs	BP						
	P						
	R/T						
Breath sounds	RUL						
	RML						
	RLL						
	LUL						
	LLL						
Assess edema prn							
Assess nutrit. status/appet.							
_____Diet instruction							
Demonstrates understdg–diet							
Eval. elim. patterns							
Assess/instruct meds. regimen: indic, dose, freq, route, SE, inter (per med list)							
Demonstrates understdg–meds							
Assess ability-perform							
Treatment_____							
Treatment instruction							
Demonstrates ability to do treatments							
Assess/instruct safety in home							
Demo knowledge of safety							
Assess emotional status/coping mechanisms							
Provide emotional support							
Recog phys/emotional chgs Communicates chgs to app prof							
Assess/instruct re:							
_____ Restrictions							
Demo understdg restrictions							
Notify pt of change in POC							
Next RN/MD visit							
Brth sounds Advent sounds	RN SIG						
1. Full 0. None 1. Rales							
2. Diminished 2. Ronchi 3. Wheezes							
3. Absent 4. Friction rub							

C = Care; D = Disc.; E = Eval.; N = Narrative; DNA = Does Not Apply; NA = Not Assessed; IB = Instr. Begun; IC = Instr. Contd.; S = Supvsn.; U = Unchgd.; + = Yes; − = No

continues

Date	Date	Date	Date	Date	Date	Date	Date	Date

Source: Reprinted with permission of the Visiting Nurse Association of Eastern Montgomery County/Dept. of Abington Memorial Hospital, Willow Grove, Pennsylvania.

Sample SFS: Impaired Skin Integrity/Potential for Impaired Skin Integrity

PT. # _____ NAME_____ PG. _____

PARAMETERS/INTERVENTIONS	Date	Date	Date	Date	Date	Date
GOAL						
WOUND ASSESSMENT						
SITE:_____ Grade						
Length/Width/Depth (cm)						
Color						
Surrounding Tissue						
Pain						
Drainage: Amount/Odor						
Color/Consistency						
Photograph						
Healing/Response to Rx						
INSTRUCTION						
Positioning						
S&S of infection						
INTERVENTION AS INDICATED						
Prevention Measures/Equipment						
Wound Care						
Codes	RN SIG					
Gr. 1—Red, unbroken						
Gr. 2—Break in epidermis						
Gr. 3—Subcut. tissue, necrotic						
Gr. 4—Muscle, bone exposed						

C = Care; D = Disc.; E = Eval.; N = Narrative; DNA = Does Not Apply; NA = Not Assessed; IB = Instr. Begun; IC = Instr. Contd.; S = Supvsn.; U = Unchgd.; + = Yes; − = No

Date	Date	Date	Date	Date	Date	Date	Date	Date

Source: Reprinted with permission of the Visiting Nurse Association of Eastern Montgomery County/Dept. of Abington Memorial Hospital, Willow Grove, Pennsylvania.

Nursing Discharge Summary: Intermediate/Advanced Chronic: Rehabilitation

PATIENT. # _____ NAME_____ DATE_____

Ultimate Objective: Patient will be rehabilitated to maximum level of physical, emotional, and social functioning; patient/family will manage chronic health problems without continued VNA service. To achieve this objective, positive patient outcomes must be evidenced. A positive patient outcome indicates that the patient/family has demonstrated an increase in knowledge and understanding or has had a behavior change. Ultimate objective attainment is determined by demonstrating that applicative subobjectives were met/nursing problems were resolved.

Subobjectives	*Assess*	*Instruct*	*Outcome*
Diet			
Med. Regimen			
Treatments/Exercises			
Safety Measures			
Medical Supervision			
Recognizes Physical/ Emotional Change			
Communicates Change to Approp. Profess.			
Restrictions Imposed by Illness			

Goal Attainment Code:

_____#1 Maximum: All applicable subobjectives were met/nursing problems were resolved.

_____#2 Moderate: Less than 100% of the applicable subobjectives/nursing problems were resolved.

_____#3 None: None of the applicable subobjectives was met/nursing problems was resolved.

Codes: DNA = does not apply; + = yes; − = no

Summary of Services

_____

_____

Problems (include O/A per nsg. dx.)

_____

_____

_____

Physician Notified of Discharge: Mail [   ]   Phone [   ] Signature: _____

Source: Reprinted with permission of the Visiting Nurse Association of Eastern Montgomery County/Dept. of Abington Memorial Hospital, Willow Grove, Pennsylvania.

CHAPTER 28

Critical Pathways

M. Kelly Cooke and Theresa M. Brodrick

Colossal changes in the delivery of traditional health care services have occurred rapidly over the last decade. With alterations in the very fabric of provider payment, skyrocketing health care costs, and innovations in medical technology, successful patient care as an effective strategy to control costs is imperative. Case management and managed care have emerged as cost-effective designs aimed specifically at obtaining desired patient outcomes (Bower, 1992). Early evidence suggests that the critical pathway, introduced as a tool to enhance managed care, can significantly improve multidisciplinary communication and coordination of patient activities in addition to controlling costs.

Case management, which encapsulates managed care and the critical pathway, has been an essential component of home care service for more than a century. Traditionally, the visiting nurse was the case manager. Assuming responsibility for the home management of patient care, nurses provided medical services under the direction of the physician. Today, in the acute and chronic care settings, case management has evolved as a means to ensure continuity across the patient's entire health care continuum. By addressing the entire episode of an illness, case management bridges many stages of life and all clinical settings. While strongly supporting multidisciplinary communication, this framework provides an avenue for continuous improvement in quality (Zander, 1990). Managed care also focuses on patient outcomes within fiscally responsible time frames and oversees care at a specific period during a patient's illness. Qualities specific to managed care include its highly differentiated settings and unit-based operations (Bower, 1988). Zander (1985) introduced critical pathways into acute care nursing practice in the mid-1980s as a mechanism to improve quality while decreasing hospital length of stay. The pathway identifies key events that must occur while care is provided to produce maximum quality at minimum costs. Just as traditional health care has evolved over the last few years, pathway development has evolved to reflect an integrated care delivery system. This chapter explores development and utilization of critical pathways in the home health setting and discusses the implications for improving quality of care.

PATHWAY DEVELOPMENT

Derived from a term in computer technology, the critical pathway identifies a particular progression of events that may include physician orders and multidisciplinary standards of practice. Each step in the pathway process must be completed in sequence before one proceeds to the next step. A deviation is a variance or detour

365

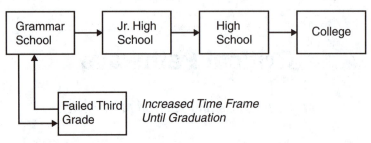

Figure 28–1 Critical Path Deviation

from the pathway, which increases the period allotted to achieve specific goals. Rectifying the detour allows the patient to resume course, as Figure 28–1 illustrates.

Expanding beyond a single episode of illness, some pathways encompass and standardize the care provided between various settings. Telephone contact, physician office visits, skilled nursing facility services, and home care services are often integrated into a common pathway. Protocols that address the patient's condition over time eliminate problems with fragmentation and duplication of service. A standard format is utilized across all settings and includes guidelines, transitional planning, and expected outcomes of care (Tichawa, 1996).

Because pathways focus on sites of care and/or timelines, days, weeks, or visits generally represent effective measurements to gauge the outcome of care rendered. Pathways will differ because patient protocols and physician orders vary greatly. The nurse should view the pathway as a unique version of the nursing care plan that incorporates standing orders (Zander, 1988). Experts recommend that agencies include the pathway form as part of the permanent medical record, but some risk managers believe that this may create a legal liability for the agency. The pathway describes care for 50 percent to 75 percent of patients in a specific diagnosis-related group (DRG; McKenzie et al., 1989). Listing the DRG on the actual pathway tool may assist the agency in computerization and data collection. The *International Classifi-cation of Diseases* (ICD-9) codes on the pathway ideally should match the codes on Health Care Financing Administration forms and form UB-92. Continuous quality improvement and utilization review activities based on actual pathway results clearly trend and measure patient outcomes or results of the care provided by agency personnel.

High-volume cases lend themselves well to pathway development. One specific diagnosis or DRG is chosen to begin the process. Goodwin (1992) suggests that staff review a sample of cases to decide the following:

- Which particular cases or DRGs occurred most frequently?
- Which nursing interventions occurred most frequently?
- When during care did these interventions occur?

Employees develop time frames, interventions, and expected patient outcomes for the pathway after careful case and record review. The pathway should contain realistic goals and interventions and reflect care that is specific to the agency.

It is best to design a pathway by using key professional personnel, available resources, and a multidisciplinary approach. Integrated pathways, which address patient conditions over various times and settings, should incorporate staff from several sites and include transition planning and outcomes (Tichawa, 1996). Standards of care, in particular Agency for

Health Care Policy and Research standards, as well as agency policies and procedures and the population of patients served are crucial elements to consider when one is designing a critical pathway. The structure of the model must fit the agency's mission and goals (Zander, 1993). Although derived from standard nursing interventions, pathways must allow for individualization because changes in the plan of care often occur based on the clinician's skilled assessment. Initially piloting a pathway for 3 to 6 months enables the organization to make revisions as appropriate. Evaluation of pathway effectiveness should occur as part of the agency's continuous quality improvement activities. The annual program evaluation should also generally address the effectiveness of each pathway over the course of the year.

Personnel should document patient information such as name, medical record number, start of care date, and ICD-9 code on the pathway form. Each nurse documenting on the pathway must include his or her initials, signature, and title. Because the pathway may replace the nursing care plan, a section should be left for individualization. The clinician also needs a blank section to document other findings, so that additional physician orders and nursing interventions can be written directly on the form. As the agency refines the tool, multidisciplinary interventions are also incorporated at the discretion of the nurse. The nurse initials a particular column on the pathway form to show interventions and outcomes that have occurred. Notations on the pathway should also indicate what has not occurred. Clinicians are responsible for reporting this information on the variance tracking tool and clinical note if appropriate.

VARIANCE ANALYSIS

Critical pathway tools are grids that depict patient and staff behavior against a timeline for a specific patient population. When expected patient outcomes do not occur within the time prescribed, variances result. Positive variances occur when patients progress toward outcomes

faster than anticipated. Negative variances occur when there is a time delay in attaining patient outcomes (Zander, 1993).

Zander (1989) developed three broad categories to classify variance according to causality as follows:

1. variances caused within the system
2. variances caused by the practitioner
3. variances caused by the patient

Most home health agencies already have continuous quality improvement activities in place. These three variance groupings help the organization identify problems and refine the processes needed to improve quality. Variances caused by the system describe pathway detours directly related to provider system problems. These variances are most commonly found in the acute care setting. An example of a home care system variance is a nurse not performing wound care within the specified visit as a result of a tardy delivery of supplies. The variance investigation by the clinician later reveals that the supply company is mailing soft goods instead of driving them to patients' homes. The tracking tool provides early identification of this problem, and the agency can promptly correct it.

Because of the nature of patient care in the home, variances caused by the practitioner are also common in the home health setting. For example, a newly diagnosed diabetic patient is ordered to have a blood sample drawn by the nurse for glucose analysis during the first week of service. This activity is inadvertently omitted by the practitioner, and the patient's dosage of insulin is not adjusted correctly. The practitioner has created a delay in the desired patient outcome by not following the plan of care.

Patient variances relate directly to the patient; that is, failure to meet the timeline for expected patient outcomes is due solely to patient variables. For example, a patient with acquired immunodeficiency syndrome requires teaching about symptom control on the third visit. The nurse is unable to instruct the patient because of pain management problems. The patient's uncontrolled pain creates a delay on the pathway. Patient variances most commonly occur in the community health setting.

Analysis of pathway variance is essential to improving the quality of service that the agency offers. Variance review should occur on each visit and formally at regular intervals. The clinician records the variance on a tracking sheet while concurrently noting the patient outcome due to treatment in the progress note (Zander, 1993). If the occurrence does not result in a time delay affecting the visit pattern or patient outcomes, recording it as a variance is not necessary. Variance tracking sheets should not be considered part of the permanent medical record (Zander, 1989). Institutions often use colored paper for the variance tracking form to remind medical record staff to remove them from the chart before permanent filing.

The variance tracking form enables the clinician to document the progress of problems related to staff behavior and patient outcomes. Initial and ongoing staff education ensures that variance data are accurate and reliable. Staff will record few variance data if they view the variance tool as a policing mechanism (Zander, 1993). Tracking tools, when structured correctly, provide the agency with just the correct amount of data. Therefore, it is important that the pathway reflect 75 percent of the general population studied. According to Zander (1993), when pathways reflect patterns of care for 80 percent of the population, variances occur 20 percent of the time. Concurrent and retrospective review is important in tracking variances.

Variance information provides a strong database for improving quality. Data related to agency readmission rates and the outcome of patient teaching can be helpful when one is measuring agency cost and quality of service. Systems problems, trends, and weaknesses can lead the agency to much needed policy and procedure changes. Concurrent and retrospective variance review creates a dynamic process for system checks and balances that ultimately result in an improved health care product (Zander, 1993).

GUIDELINES FOR PATHWAY UTILIZATION

The registered nurse who admits the patient selects the critical pathway. On the first visit, the clinician individualizes and modifies the pathway based on physician orders and patient needs. In cases of multiple diagnoses or sites, the nurse should merge several pathways and make one patient-specific pathway according to agency policy. Changes to the pathway after the first visit are considered variances. The pathway, reviewed with the patient and family before the start of care, encourages client participation. Some agencies provide the patient with a patient pathway tool that mirrors the critical pathway but is written in lay terms. This strategy improves communication with the patient regarding his or her care and enhances patient satisfaction. After reviewing the patient pathway and participating in the plan of care, the patient assumes shared responsibility for the outcomes of his or her treatment.

Pathways should be kept with the nurse in the field or in the home care record for easy access. During each visit, the nurse should review each patient's progress on the pathway and identify and document variances. The clinician documents all variances on the variance tracking sheet and channels this information to the appropriate personnel for quality assessment and improvement purposes.

The nurse completes a variance tracking sheet with the patient's name and ICD-9 code for every patient pathway. This is always done, even if a variance does not occur, for statistical purposes. The individual responsible for data collection eliminates this procedure after refining the tool when data collection reveals no further problems. Empowering visiting staff to problem solve effectively with pathway use eliminates variance recurrence. For maximum effectiveness, agency management supports the visiting nurse when he or she develops and carries out a plan to correct negative variances. Agency administration and team members should use the corrective action plans implemented by nurses when setting up quality controls. Using critical pathways during patient conferences and team meetings enhances communication and fosters attainment of favorable patient outcomes.

SAMPLE PATHWAY

A sample critical pathway for a home care patient with congestive heart failure (CHF) is presented in Exhibit 28–1. Because the agency that developed the tool found that 80 percent of patients with CHF require 6 weeks of service, that time frame is utilized. Blank lines should be incorporated throughout the form to allow for individualization by the nurse. Some agencies find it helpful to have the case managers hand write time lines when developing the pathway tool until data collection is complete. Many organizations also preprint nursing activities and diagnoses and have the nurse initial all those that apply. Arrows are used to indicate those activities or interventions that occur over several weeks of service. Exhibit 28–2 represents a patient pathway, which is given to the patient and discussed on admission. The patient pathway is not an essential component of the critical pathway but often aids in patient communication, enhances customer satisfaction, and increases patient participation in the plan of care. An example of a variance tracking tool is presented in Exhibit 28–3. The tracking form highlights the data that home care agencies collect to improve quality. Organizations should base their pathways on practices, policies, and procedures specific to their agency and the population served.

BENEFITS OF PATHWAY USE

Pathways tend to decrease fragmentation of services when agencies complement staff with part-time or temporary nurses and enhance continuity between institutions. The contribution of part-time and temporary nurses improves with pathway use because documentation is outcome oriented. The clinician requires less time to give a report or to catch up on what occurred previously. Nurses can decide quickly what has occurred in the plan of care and what needs to occur to move a patient toward a specific outcome. Job satisfaction improves because the clinician can see how his or her contributions fit into the patient's total care (Bower, 1992).

According to Bower (1992), the critical pathway stimulates the creation of new or refined services. Agencies routinely conduct concurrent research vis-à-vis variance tracking to identify the most appropriate method of care delivery. Variances used to improve quality continuously address issues such as whether an intervention should be done differently or during a different visit. Staff participation is also helpful when the agency is exploring ways to improve the utilization of service.

When reviewed with the patient, the pathway lends itself well to improving self-care capabilities (Bower, 1992). The patient is an active participant in his or her plan of care. Patient education may help decrease agency readmission rates and enable proper utilization of service. Finally, the pathway helps improve patient satisfaction. By discussing expectations of service on the first visit, the nurse gives the patient the opportunity to verbalize concerns about his or her care before interventions take place.

Conservation of nursing time is an indirect benefit of pathway use (Bower, 1992). The tool is easy for staff to follow, helps prevent redundancy of services, and provides for shorter, more efficient reports. The pathway can replace all or parts of the nursing teaching flow sheets, care plans, and nursing progress notes, thereby streamlining documentation. Easily identified, individualized nursing interventions, goals, and treatments reflect reimbursement requirements and governing body regulations. Less documentation in the clinical note occurs because the nurse documents the patient's response to the therapeutic interventions provided. Supplying new staff with a copy of the pathway also simplifies orientation. New personnel are exposed to tasks and job expectations in a structured, systematic manner (Zander, 1987).

Exhibit 28–1 CHF Pathway

PATIENT NAME: _____   MEDICAL RECORD NUMBER: _____   SOC DATE: _____   ICD 9 #4280 NSG

DX/PROBLEM
1. Alteration in cardiac output related to CHF.
2. Lack of knowledge related to home care service, diet and medications.
3. Self care deficit related to fatigue and activity intolerance.
4. _____

	WEEK 1	INT	WEEK 2	INT	WEEK 3	INT	WEEK 4	INT	WEEK 5	INT	WEEK 6	INT	Outcome Met Y N
Patient Outcomes	Pt will state s/s CHF. Pt will accurately state dosage & medication schedule. Pt will maintain safe home environment. Pt will understand home care services as evidenced by participation in the plan of care. Other:___						Pt's fluid balance & weight will stabilize.		Patient adheres to diet. Pt will have adequate cardiac output. Pt will state activity allowances & restrictions within threshold of cardiac limitations.		Pt will resume responsibility for self care with (circle) minimal/ moderate/maximum assistance. Pt accurately states purpose & side effects of meds. Pt accurately identifies s/s to report to MD.		
Teaching/ Patient Activities	Instruct pt on s/s CHF & home safety guidelines. Teach pt how to take radial pulse. Begin medication instruction; have pt state dosage & schedule of medications.		Have pt record weekly daily weights (circle). Instruct in proper diet & hydration.		Discuss pulmonary, toilet & breathing exercises. Have pt keep diet log.		Discuss risk factors: alcohol, smoking, weight & ↑ cholesterol. Instruct in energy conservation, task simplification & planned rest periods. Discuss activity intolerance & fatigue.		Have pt discuss which risk factors he/ she can ↓.				

continues

Exhibit 28–1 continued

	WEEK 1	INT	WEEK 2	INT	WEEK 3	INT	WEEK 4	INT	WEEK 5	INT	WEEK 6	INT	Outcome Met Y N
Nursing Activities	Review MD orders & patient pathway. Review Advance Directives & emergency on call system. Instruct pt in Bill of Rights. Assess medications in the home to ensure all are present as ordered, & pt knowledge related to same. Assess level of tolerance for ADLs & physical activities. Assess coping skills, psychosocial needs & provide emotional support PRN.		Assess recall of medication instruction.		Review weights as recorded by pt.		Review diet log.				Close to home care service. Review discharge instructions.		
Treatments and Diagnostics	Cardiopulmonary assessment VS, temperature, BP, lung auscultation (including history of cough, orthopnea, diaphoresis). Inspect LEs for swelling &/or breakdown. Weekly daily weights (circle) Weekly daily LE measurements (circle) Other: _____ Record findings on clinical note												

continues

Exhibit 28–1 continued

	WEEK 1	INT	WEEK 2	INT	WEEK 3	INT	WEEK 4	INT	WEEK 5	INT	WEEK 6	INT	Outcome Met Y N
Referrals and Consults	PT OT ST HHA MSW (circle) Area on Aging: Y N Date ___ Other ___												
Home Safety and DME	Does home environment detract from implementation of plan of care? Y N DME in home: Y N List ___ Other ___		Assess home safety. Address areas as appropriate. Other: ___										
Discharge Planning	Initiate discharge planning. Discuss length of service.						Discuss discharge plan. Inform pt that there are approximately 2 more weeks of service.		Remind pt 1 more week of service.		Arrange for follow up with Dr. ___ on ___		
Other													

Initial: ___ RN Signature: ___ Initial: ___ RN Signature: ___ Initial: ___ RN Signature: ___ Initial: ___ RN Signature ___ Initial: ___ RN Signature: ___ Initial: ___ RN Signature: ___ Initial: ___ RN Signature: ___

Exhibit 28–2 Patient Pathway for CHF

	Week 1–3	Week 4–6	Week ___
Nursing Activities	Your nurse will: • review doctor's orders with you. • ask to see your medications and begin instruction. • assess your activity tolerance. • review your diet and fluid intake.	Your nurse will: • review your diet log and weights. • assess your recall of medication instruction.	
Pt. Activities/Education	Teach you how to check your pulse, and instruct you about your diet and fluid intake. Ask you to weigh yourself and record it. Teach you about your activities to prevent fatigue. Ask you to keep a diet log.	The nurse will teach you risk factors of CHF, such as smoking, drinking, and high cholesterol foods. She will also teach you signs & symptoms of CHF to report to your physician.	
Treatments	The nurse will listen to your heart & lungs and assess weight and blood pressure. Assess your feet and ankles for swelling and measure them. Take your vital signs: pulse, respirations & temperature.	Same treatments as week 1–3. Nurse visits less frequently as your condition improves.	
Home Safety	Review home safety guidelines. Assess the safety of your home environment. Check all the medical equipment in your home to ensure proper working order. Review agency on-call & emergency system.	As you improve, you will resume responsibility for self-care in a safe manner to prevent any injuries.	
Discharge Planning	Please ask any questions if there is something you don't fully understand about your care.	Prepare you for discharge from home visits. Review all discharge instructions. Arrange a follow-up appointment with your doctor.	

Exhibit 28–3 Variance Tracking Tool

Quality Assessment and Improvement Tool Pathway: DRG _____

Date	Week of Service	Variation	QA&I Code	Reason	Action Taken	Int.

Patient Reasons
11: Patient Complication
12: Patient Request
13: Social/Family Issues
14: Knowledge Deficit
15: Alteration in LOC
16: Other

Practitioner Reasons
21: Incomplete Data
22: Practitioner Preference
23: Delay
24: Other

System Reasons
31: Delay of Service
32: Service Not Available
33: Delay of Procedure/Test
34: Delay Obtaining Results
35: Lack of Equipment
36: Other

Job satisfaction for clinical and management staff improves with the use of pathways because a positive work environment cultivates cooperation throughout the organization and among various sites. Communicating the patient's progress to the multidisciplinary team ensures that organized, efficient care occurs (Bower, 1992). Conservation of nursing time also correlates positively with enhanced job satisfaction. Performing criteria-based evaluations is no longer a problem for the supervising nurse. With the pathway framework, nursing staff are formally accountable for the outcomes specified on the tool (Zander, 1991). Empowering the staff nurse as case manager enhances autonomy and allows the supervisor more time to focus on team development and mentoring.

COST VERSUS QUALITY

Our present economy challenges home health agencies to structure visits promoting cost-effective care within the appropriate length of stay. With capitation and third-party reimbursement, pathways provide a strong framework for visit utilization. Under the present Medicare guidelines, agency reimbursement is based on the number of visits. Care provided must be medically necessary and approved by the fiscal intermediary. Agencies are paid for the actual visits that they provide. Visits on the pathway are increased or decreased as a result of patient need, denials, readmission rates, and the like. Other insurers reimburse agencies utilizing capitated rates because reimbursement under this arrangement is fixed per patient. The pathway provides the mechanism to produce the desired clinical patient outcome while controlling costs. To enhance fiscal health, visit volume is generally limited, and the agency nurse must carefully plan to provide the optimal level of care within the desired number of patient visits. Critical pathways provide a tool to ensure the most cost-effective quality care possible.

Although pathways provide collaborative guidelines for skilled clinical interventions, barriers to implementation exist. The system may require a general change in philosophy. Ongoing staff training and development must occur. Because home health patients frequently are admitted to service from the acute care setting with multiple diagnoses, staff must combine and revise pathways based on several DRGs. Failure to meet goals may increase patient length of stay. Often, it is difficult to get some members of the multidisciplinary team to support a new service product. Although pathways may enhance the general quality of care, more research is necessary to document actual cost savings in the home health setting.

The critical pathway lends itself well to the monitoring and evaluation activities that agencies perform to measure quality. By clearly defining the scope of patient care and services rendered, the nursing activities with the greatest impact on patient care are easily targeted. Based on the variance tracking data collected, high-volume, high-risk, and problem-prone areas are continuously addressed.

Pathways measure the documentation of time frames, behaviors, and processes affecting the delivery of patient care. This activity enables the agency to gauge the results of action taken in terms of patient outcome. Pathways allow for explicit, objective measures of quality. Variances reflect the structure, process, and outcomes of care. Because regulating bodies require that agencies address all the services rendered in terms of patient outcomes, many managed care companies and third-party payers presently utilize pathways. This methodology is perfect for the home health setting.

CONCLUSION

Home health agencies need to continue to expand their pathways to include multiple sites and episodes of patient illnesses so that the process for managing care can be continuous and standardized. Third-party payers, surveying organizations, and many managed care companies strongly focus on patient goals and the desired outcome of patient care when measuring quality. Pathways provide the formula necessary to govern utilization of professional services based on patient need. Agencies should develop pathways specific to their norms and the clientele served.

Home care reimbursement is transitioning to provide payment for patient outcomes of care rather than patient visits. The pathway will enable the organization to link costs with actual care given. Because all providers will be competing within the managed care environment, the pathway will ensure a systematic, quality-driven approach.

REFERENCES

Bower, K. 1988. Managed care: Controlling costs, guaranteeing outcomes. *Definition* 3:1–3.

Bower, K. 1992. *Case management by nurses*. Washington, DC: American Nurses Association.

Goodwin, D. 1992. Critical pathways in home healthcare. *Journal of Nursing Administration* 22:35–40.

McKenzie, C., et al. 1989. Care and cost: Nursing case management improves both. *Nursing Management* 20:30–34.

Tichawa, U. 1996. The pathway project bridging care across the continuum. *Focus on Geriatric Care and Rehabilitation* 9:1–8.

Zander, K. 1985. Second generation primary nursing. *Journal of Nursing Administration* 15:18–24.

Zander, K. 1987. Critical paths: Marking the course. *Definition* 2:1–4.

Zander, K. 1988. Nursing case management: Strategic management of cost and quality outcomes. *Journal of Nursing Administration* 18:23–30.

Zander, K. 1989. Managed care: Integrating QA in everyday practice. *Definition* 4:1–2.

Zander, K. 1990. Differentiating managed care and case management. *Definition* 5:1–2.

Zander, K. 1991. What's new in managed care and case management. *New Definition* 6:1–2.

Zander, K. 1993. Quantifying, managing, and improving quality part IV: The retrospective use of variance. *New Definition* 8:1–3.

SUGGESTED READING

Cohen, E. 1991. Nursing case management, does it pay? *Journal of Nursing Administration* 21:20–24.

Faherty, B. 1990. Case management, the latest buzzword: What it is and what it isn't. *Caring* 9:20–24.

Falconer, J., et al. 1993. The critical path method in stroke rehabilitation: Lessons from an experiment in cost containment and outcome improvement. *Quarterly Review Bulletin* 19:8–16.

Hoyer, R. 1990. Case management and the payor: Where are we and where do we go from here? *Caring* 9:4–12.

Kralovec, T., et al. 1991. The application of total quality management concepts in a service line cardiovascular program. *Nursing Administration Quarterly* 15:1–8.

Luttman, R. 1993. The critical path alone does nothing to improve performance. *Quality Review Bulletin* 19:142–143.

Sinnen, M., and S.M. Mackinnon. 1991. Coordinated care in a community hospital. *Nursing Management* 22:38–42.

Strong, A., and N. Sneed. 1991. Clinical evaluation of a critical path for coronary artery bypass surgery patients. *Progress in Cardiovascular Nursing* 6:29–37.

CHAPTER 29

Outcome-Based Quality Improvement

Peter W. Shaughnessy and Kathryn S. Crisler

Home health care represents one component of the health care continuum. The largest single component of home health care comprises services covered by Medicare. This component of Medicare has been growing rapidly, and concerns with both the cost and quality of home care have increased along with Medicare expenditures. Between 1990 and 1995, the number of Medicare beneficiaries receiving home health care almost doubled (from 1.9 million to 3.6 million), and annual visits per person served grew equally dramatically (from 36 to 70). The combined effect was to increase total Medicare home health visits from 70 million to 252 million and Medicare home health expenditures from $3.9 billion to $16.0 billion (Prospective Payment Assessment Commission, 1996).

As home health care visits and expenditures grow, the importance of objectively assessing the impacts of care increases correspondingly. Payers are interested in the quality of care received relative to what is being paid. Although quality of health care can be examined from the perspectives of structure, process, or outcome, there is increasing emphasis on the outcomes of care, corresponding to the interest in exactly what happens to patients' health status as a result of receiving care. In addition to payer interest, accreditation and certification programs, such as the Joint Commission on Accreditation of Healthcare Organizations and the Community Health Accreditation Program of the National League for Nursing, as well as state and federal government certification agencies have become progressively more outcome oriented. Equally important, home care agencies are increasingly concerned with measuring their own performance relative to other providers or standards. This combination of factors has fueled a powerful movement toward outcome measurement in home care.

This chapter focuses on the work conducted by the Center for Health Services and Policy Research at the University of Colorado Health Sciences Center. The research that led to the development of the outcome-based quality improvement approach described here was developed for home health care over nearly a decade with several million dollars in funding from the Health Care Financing Administration (HCFA) and the Robert Wood Johnson Foundation. The resulting outcome measure system and its application for performance improvement constitute a methodology termed outcome-based quality improvement (OBQI) in home care. The measure system was developed predominantly for Medicare beneficiaries. The resulting measures pertain to all adult patients, however, and measures for younger populations as well as specific subgroups of patients can be developed in the future.

The focus of the OBQI approach is patient outcomes that occur over a home health care episode. The purpose of the original research was to develop valid and reliable measures of patient outcomes that could be precisely quantified and compared across home health agencies and patients. Subsequent sections of this chapter describe the outcome measures and discuss incorporating the measures into an OBQI system at both agency and national levels.

The evolution of the outcome measure system and the performance improvement approach based on the measure system has involved a number of separate but integrated activities (Shaughnessy, 1991; Shaughnessy et al., 1994a, 1995b, 1996). These have included comprehensive reviews of outcome measures and related papers, documents, and articles published in the research literature and the provider and clinical literature as well as reviews of outcome measures in use or under development by individual agencies or groups of agencies (i.e., in their formative stages). A number of clinical panels have been convened to review the outcome measures and approaches at regular intervals.

A variety of data sources were examined for potential information about outcome measurement. Outcome measures were specified first, and data items needed to measure outcomes were developed thereafter. Extant sources of information for such data items were examined, including clinical records, claims or billing data, and other administrative data. After an extensive examination of such data sources, we concluded that it would be necessary to develop a new data set to measure properly the outcomes that had been specified. Several hundred home care agencies throughout the United States participated in the developmental efforts over a period of several years, including various types of research investigations, data item refinement (including validity and reliability testing), and both demonstration and evaluation projects (Crisler et al., 1994; Powell et al., 1994; Shaughnessy et al., 1994a, 1995b).

The system described here is currently under consideration by the Medicare program for national implementation in the context of the home health agency survey and certification program. The overall plan is to incorporate outcomes into the certification process, so that agencies that are performing adequately or above average in terms of outcomes will receive relatively little survey/certification/regulatory review, with such review focusing predominantly on agencies for which outcomes are inadequate. For such agencies, regulatory activities can be targeted on those areas where outcomes are inferior. The overall system described here is therefore intended for application by individual home health agencies and by purchasers of home care who wish to assess what is happening to patients/clients as a result of their financial investment.

TYPES OF OUTCOMES

The fundamental definition of a patient level outcome is a change in health status between two or more time points. In the current OBQI system, this is the basic or anchoring definition of an outcome. It is termed an end-result outcome because it reflects change in patient health status over the course of time, which is the focal point of health care provision. The two time points that are typically used to gauge outcomes in home care are start of care (SOC) and discharge. Health status, as noted above, is broadly defined, encompassing physiological, functional, cognitive, mental, and social health. Illustrations of end-result outcomes include improvement in ability to ambulate between admission and discharge, decline in dyspnea between admission and 120 days after admission, stabilization or no change in pain interfering with activities between 60 and 180 days, and improvement in ability to manage oral medications between admission and discharge. The third illustration demonstrates that it is not necessary to consider SOC and discharge as the only two follow-up points that define outcomes.

A second type of outcome used that is under development for future use in OBQI is termed an instrumental outcome (or intermediate-result outcome). An instrumental outcome is a change in patient's (or informal caregiver's) behavior, emotions, or knowledge that can influence a patient's end-result outcomes. Illustrations of instrumental outcomes include change in compliance with the treatment regimen, knowledge of self-care, signs and symptoms to report to the physician, informal caregiver strain, patient or family satisfaction with care, and motivation to improve. These are termed instrumental outcomes because, although they are outcomes in their own right, their (non)attainment can influence the (non)attainment of end-result outcomes. Instrumental outcomes are critical in home care but are more difficult to measure than end-result outcomes and therefore are not in widespread use in OBQI at the present time. It is anticipated that as additional research and developmental efforts focus on such outcomes, however, they will be used more widely in OBQI in the home care field.

The third type of outcome is utilization outcomes, which refer to utilization of non–home care services that reflects a (typically substantial and untoward) change in health status over time. Illustrations of utilization outcomes include hospital admission, nursing home admission, and emergent care. These are also termed proxy outcomes because they are often (but not always) surrogates for untoward or negative health status changes in patients. Such outcomes have the redeeming feature that they are more straightforward to measure, although statistical risk adjustment is often of paramount importance in comparing such outcomes across different groups of patients.

An outcome measure is a quantification of an outcome. Under the assumption that the outcome under consideration is an end-result outcome, an outcome measure is a quantified change in patient health status between two or more time points. The change referred to in this case is intrinsic to the patient (e.g., the provi-

sion of a cane or walker is not intrinsic to the patient and is therefore not an outcome). The change can represent improvement, stabilization, or worsening. Objective measures are superior to subjective measures in that, when one is quantifying outcomes, specific, reliable, and objective health status scales should be used for end-result and instrumental outcomes, and precise information about health care use should be used to measure utilization outcomes.

A wide variety of outcomes and outcome measures were specified in the developmental research that underpins OBQI. Over time, these were culled, modified, or refined from different vantage points, including clinical relevance, reliability, specificity, practicality, utility for quality improvement purposes, and minimization of statistical redundancy. Efforts are ongoing to remedy various constraints and limitations of the system as well as to improve measures and develop new ones. Because the initial objectives focused on specifying outcome measures, all data items followed from the outcome measures. That is, OBQI data items were not first specified and then used to determine which measures would be possible. The primary focus was outcome measures that could be integrated to form a system that would be valid and practical for OBQI, with all other considerations (including data items) being secondary to this purpose.

DATA ITEM SET

The set of data items used in the OBQI system is termed the Outcome and Assessment Information Set (OASIS). It was tailored to home care after investigation of the appropriateness of using data items from other fields (such as the Functional Independence Measure data set in the rehabilitation field and the Minimum Data Set in the nursing home field; Fries et al., 1994; Granger et al., 1993, 1995; Hawes et al., 1995; Morris et al., 1990; State University of New York at Buffalo, 1993, 1995). Extensive modifications of these data sets would have been necessary to adapt them properly to home care; in addition, several of the items did not necessarily provide the information needed to measure the outcomes needed for home care. Nevertheless, the OASIS data set is continuing to undergo refinement, as is the scope of the OBQI home care measure system. The first release of the 79-item OASIS occurred in August 1995 as a special supplement to the National Association for Home Care's *NAHC Report* (NAHC, 1995). This was termed OASIS-A and will be followed by subsequent releases that will be termed OASIS-B, OASIS-C, and so forth.

OASIS is not intended to be a comprehensive assessment instrument. Rather, it is a set of data items that are essential for measuring or risk-adjusting outcomes in the home care field. It is strongly recommended that OASIS items be embedded within the comprehensive assessment instrument of each home care agency that uses the OBQI measure system, replacing those items in current assessment instruments that address similar concepts. Adding the OASIS items to an existing assessment instrument will create substantial redundancy because almost all OASIS items correspond to analogous, but typically less precise, items that are already

used for comprehensive assessment (in addition to this redundancy, adding similar items serves only to increase an already substantial documentation burden in home care).

To measure outcomes, because these have been defined as changes in health status, it is necessary to collect OASIS data items at 60-day intervals until and including time of discharge. Further specifics are available in other research documents and the OBQI manual written for home care agencies wishing to implement OBQI (Shaughnessy et al., 1995a).

TWO-STAGE CONTINUOUS QUALITY IMPROVEMENT SCREEN

The general framework for OBQI is the two-stage continuous quality improvement (CQI) screen depicted in Figure 29–1. This schematic shows the overall OBQI approach. The sequence of events on the left side of the figure constitute the first-stage screen, and those on the right side constitute the second-stage screen. In the conduct of the two-stage CQI screen, data must be collected at the above-mentioned intervals for all adult patients.

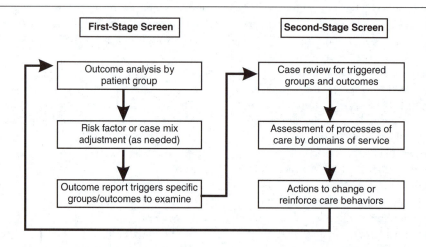

Figure 29–1 Two-Stage CQI Screen. *Source:* Adapted from Figure 4 of P.W. Shaughnessy, K.S. Crisler, R.E. Schlenker, A.G. Arnold, A.M. Kramer, M.C. Powell, and D.F. Hittle. Measuring and assuring the quality of home health care. *Health Care Financing Review* 16(1):35–67, Fall 1994.

The first-stage screen consists of outcome analyses by patient groups. This step entails computing outcome measures from the OBQI outcome measure system on a condition-by-condition basis using quality indicator groups (QUIGs). Although there are a number of ways to stratify patients into groups, the QUIG classi-fication system given in Exhibit 29–1 has been developed for initial use and subsequent refine-ment for OBQI applications (Kramer et al., 1990; Shaughnessy et al., 1995a). It consists of 25 (potentially overlapping) patient conditions for which outcome measures have been speci-fied. After outcome measures are computed

---

Exhibit 29–1 Description of QUIGs and Examples

Acute conditions

1. Acute orthopedic conditions (e.g., fracture, amputation, joint replacement, degenerative joint dis-ease)
2. Acute neurological conditions (e.g., cerebrovascular accident, multiple sclerosis, head injury)
3. Open wounds and lesions (e.g., pressure ulcers, surgical wounds, stasis ulcers)
4. Terminal conditions (e.g., palliative care for malignant neoplasms, advanced cardiopulmonary dis-ease, end-stage acquired immunodeficiency syndrome [AIDS])
5. Acute cardiac/peripheral vascular conditions (e.g., congestive heart failure, angina, coronary artery disease, hypertension, myocardial infarction)
6. Acute pulmonary conditions (e.g., chronic obstructive pulmonary disease, pneumonia, pulmonary edema)
7. Acute diabetes mellitus[*]
8. Acute gastrointestinal disorders (e.g., gastric ulcer, diverticulitis, constipation with changing treat-ment approaches, ostomies, liver disease)
9. Contagious/communicable conditions (e.g., hepatitis, tuberculosis, AIDS, *Salmonella* infection)
10. Acute urinary incontinence/catheter[*]
11. Acute mental/emotional conditions (e.g., anxiety disorder, depression, bipolar disorder)
12. Oxygen therapy[*]
13. Intravenous/infusion therapy[*]
14. Enteral/parenteral nutrition (e.g., total parenteral nutrition, gastrostomy/jejunostomy feeding)
15. Ventilator therapy[*]
16. Other acute conditions[*]

Chronic conditions

17. Chronic dependence in living skills (e.g., meal preparation, housekeeping, laundry)
18. Chronic dependence in personal care (e.g., bathing, dressing, grooming)
19. Chronic impaired ambulation/mobility (e.g., ambulation, transferring, toileting)
20. Chronic eating disability[*]
21. Chronic urinary incontinence/catheter use[*]
22. Chronic dependence in medication administration[*]
23. Chronic pain[*]
24. Chronic cognitive/mental/behavioral problems (e.g., Alzheimer's disease, confusion, agitation, chronic brain syndrome)
25. Chronic patients with caregiver present[*]

[*]Example not given because QUIG name is sufficient to define the condition.

Source: Adapted from Table 3 of P.W. Shaughnessy, K.S. Crisler, R.E. Schlenker, A.G. Arnold, A.M. Kramer, M.C. Powell, and D.F. Hittle. Measuring and assuring the quality of home health care. *Health Care Financing Review* 16(1):35–67, Fall 1994.

using the OASIS data set, risk adjustment is undertaken and outcome reports are produced for specific QUIGs of relevance to the agency (termed focused outcome reports) and for all adult patients (termed a global outcome report).

The production of outcome reports is the culmination of the first-stage screen. Using these reports, agency staff can determine which outcomes are inferior and which are exemplary. The outcomes on which the agency staff elect to focus for purposes of subsequent review are called target outcomes and constitute the focal point of the second-stage screen. A variety of activities can be undertaken as part of the second-stage screen, but all activities involve investigating care provided for purposes of reinforcing those care behaviors that produce exemplary outcomes or remedying problems in care behaviors that produce inferior outcomes. This usually entails record review for the triggered outcomes to determine specific activities in care provision (e.g., assessment, care planning, intervention, or care coordination/referral) that should be reinforced or remedied. The second-stage screen culminates with a written plan of action specifically targeted at changing or reinforcing care behaviors that produce certain outcomes. The plan of action entails specifying what will be done, how it will be done, who will undertake the activities necessary to change care behaviors, when it will be done, and how the process of implementing change will be monitored. The effectiveness of the second-stage screen, including the final plan of action, can then be assessed by virtue of continued data collection and review of outcome reports for the next period of time. This permits agency staff to determine whether outcomes targeted for improvement have in fact improved and whether those targeted for reinforcement have remained the same or improved. The heart of the CQI process, therefore, is producing outcome reports on a regular basis that can be used to monitor outcomes of care and assess whether changes introduced to remedy problems have improved outcomes and whether reinforcement activities implemented to maintain exemplary or superior outcomes have done so.

SAMPLE OUTCOME REPORT

Figure 29–2 contains an excerpt from a hypothetical outcome report for an individual home care agency. It displays results for two improvement measures (from among several such measures) that pertain to orthopedic patients.

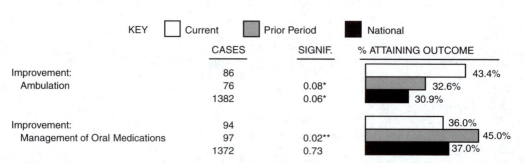

*The probability is 10% or less that this difference is due to chance, and 90% or more that the difference is real.

**The probability is 5% or less that this difference is due to chance, and 95% or more that the difference is real.

Figure 29–2 Excerpt from Agency Level Outcome Report for Orthopedic Patients (Hypothetical). *Source:* Adapted from Figure 5 of P.W. Shaughnessy, K.S. Crisler, R.E. Schlenker, A.G. Arnold, A.M. Kramer, M.C. Powell, and D.F. Hittle. Measuring and assuring the quality of home health care. *Health Care Financing Review* 16(1):35–67, Fall 1994.

Orthopedic conditions constitute one of the QUIGs. Improvement measures that correspond to end-result outcomes, such as improvement in ambulation or improvement in management of oral medications (as indicated in Figure 29–2), are constructed from health status scales at two points in time. In this case, the outcome measures correspond to change in ambulation status or ability to manage oral medications between SOC and discharge. The results indicate that 43.4 percent of orthopedic patients improved in ambulation during the current reporting period (most recent year) for the agency compared with 32.6 percent of orthopedic patients for the agency's prior period (preceding year) and 30.9 percent of patients from a national benchmark sample. Eighty-six orthopedic patients contributed to the outcome results in the current reporting period, 76 contributed from the prior period, and 1,382 contributed from the national benchmark sample. The comparison between the current and prior period outcomes resulted in a statistically significant difference between the two means (i.e., 43.4 percent versus 32.6 percent; $p = .08$). The comparison with the national benchmark sample is significant at $p = .06$. An analogous statistical interpretation pertains for improvement in management of oral medications. The outcome reports routinely contain asterisked, double asterisked, or nonasterisked items depending on whether the statistical significance occurs at the .10 level, the .05 level, or not at all (i.e., $p > .10$), respectively. (The p-values correspond to the significance level of a dichotomous indicator of agency versus reference group in a multivariate logistic regression model using several risk factors as well as this dichotomy. Each outcome measure requires its own risk model. The test used for significance of the coefficient of this dichotomy (actually the odds ratio) is a type of chi-square test.)

CURRENT OBQI DEMONSTRATION PROGRAMS

In the context of various demonstration programs, approximately 160 agencies are pres-ently implementing and formally maintaining OBQI approaches that employ OASIS and the aforementioned system of outcome measures. In addition, a number of other home care agencies throughout the United States are beginning to implement OBQI under the auspices of state associations, state governments, provider chains/corporations, provider coalitions, and even individual providers. One of the more important OBQI demonstration projects is the national Medicare OBQI demonstration program that is funded by HCFA. This large-scale test of the prototype OBQI system that will be used under Medicare involves 50 agencies from 26 states. It began in 1995 and will continue until 1999, with three rounds of data collection and outcome (and cost/resource consumption) reporting. Annual outcome reports are being produced for the 50 participating agencies in 1997, 1998, and 1999. All agencies are collecting OASIS data for their adult home care patients. Outcome reports are risk adjusted, and the two-stage screen described previously is being implemented for each of the three rounds of outcome reports.

An analogous project was implemented in New York state in 1996. This project involved 22 home care agencies from New York, will further test the OBQI system in terms of personal care, and will entail at least two if not three rounds of data collection and outcome reporting before a final decision is made for statewide implementation in New York. A Colorado OBQI pilot project involving three agencies has been in place since 1993. Also, because HCFA is planning to use OBQI in the context of its national quality assurance and improvement program, HCFA's per episode prospective payment demonstration (involving 91 agencies from California, Texas, Illinois, Florida, and Massachusetts) is using OBQI to monitor and ensure the quality of home care (Abt Associates, 1995; Goldberg and Schmitz, 1994).

The purpose of the three-agency OBQI pilot in Colorado was to gain experience with OBQI in its initial stages. Funded by the Robert Wood Johnson Foundation, the goal was to implement primary data collection in three separate agencies using an initial data set that was later changed considerably, eventually becoming the OASIS after a series of iterations. The three agencies were provided selected types of outcome reports and were allowed to conduct their second-stage screens in any manner they wished. Our goal was to monitor how the three agencies might implement the OBQI approach rather than direct how they might do so. As a result of the demonstration (which still continues), we have substantially modified the entire OBQI process in a variety of ways. The data collection approach and methodologies are much more structured. Data items have become more specific, and outcome reporting entails more precise risk adjustment. A specific set of activities is now recommended for the second-stage screen. This approach is being further refined in the context of the national Medicare quality assurance demonstration mentioned above and is documented in the OBQI manual mentioned earlier.

A number of practical issues have arisen in our initial OBQI work, resulting in a series of tips and practical pointers that can now be provided to agencies interested in implementing OBQI on their own (as well as those participating in the large-scale demonstrations mentioned above). For example, we have learned that it is important not to permit providers of care simply to carry data items forward from SOC to follow-up points by providing information only about those items that they believe have changed. This creates an incentive to minimize time spent collecting data at follow-up and inaccurately results in relatively few changes in patient status between admission and follow-up. When providers of care reassess health status at follow-up time points, considerably more changes are detected than if they are allowed to carry forward SOC health status items by default. The outcome reports for two pilot agencies were used to improve or change outcomes (demonstrated by subsequent outcome reports and reflected by substantial changes at the agency level that in turn had an effect on outcomes).

CONCLUSION

We are at a unique point in the evolution of home care in the United States. A convergence of factors is occurring, both internal and external to the industry, that will guide and even reshape the provision of home care over the next decade (Riley, 1989; Weissert et al., 1988). Home care probably will move in the direction of per episode prospective payment, increased penetration by managed care organizations, outcomes monitoring and management, and greater standardization of care processes. Over the next several years, progressively more comprehensive analyses of the cost and effectiveness of home care will be conducted between and among different types of home care providers and relative to other types of care (Hedrick and Inui, 1986; Kenney and Dubay, 1992; Kramer et al., 1997; Murdaugh, 1992). An essential ingredient for all such applications is a carefully and systematically derived set of data items that can be used to characterize the health status and care needs of home care patients at SOC and at regular time points thereafter, including discharge. Patient-level information about volume of services (visits) by discipline will also be essential for such analyses.

Therefore, as home care continues to grow and evolve, it should and will be analyzed more carefully in terms of its costs and benefits. As discussed at the outset of this chapter, a framework is needed that enables us to integrate cost and effectiveness issues in home care so that decisions and refinements in the provision of home care can be made at the levels of individual patients/clients, home care agencies, and our home care delivery system, including integrating home care with other types of health care. In this regard, we first need a framework for concurrently evaluating the effectiveness of home care.

The outcome analyses and reports presented in the previous section constitute the basic component of this framework. Such reports can provide information at the agency level and at the system level about the effectiveness of home care. The framework should permit us to analyze outcomes (i.e., effectiveness) for different types of patients/clients, that is, according to different types of patient/client conditions or impairments, age groups, payer sources, and the like.

Above all, we should adhere to the principle that this effectiveness framework must be useful and of practical value to individual home care agencies, not simply to payers or regulators. Without serving the needs of home care agencies in a practical sense, system level reporting and monitoring activities will sink under their own weight. On the other hand, if an effectiveness monitoring (i.e., outcome monitoring) framework is of direct value for purposes of clinical management, quality improvement, case mix monitoring, cost monitoring, and meeting regulatory and other fiscal requirements, the information and reporting system is likely to be diligently and accurately maintained by home health agency staff.

REFERENCES

Abt Associates, Inc. 1995. *National home health agency prospective payment demonstration: Phase II: Procedures manual for home health agencies.* Cambridge, MA: Abt Associates.

Crisler, K.S., et al. 1994. *Objective review criteria for abstracting data for clinical record review of home health care,* vol. 3. Denver: University of Colorado Health Sciences Center, Center for Health Services Research.

Fries, B.E., et al. 1994. Refining a case-mix measure for nursing homes: Resource utilization groups (RUG-III). *Medical Care* 32:668–685.

Goldberg, H.B., and R.J. Schmitz. 1994. Contemplating home health PPS: Current patterns of Medicare service use. *Health Care Financing Review* 16:109–130.

Granger, C.V., et al. 1993. Performance profiles of the Functional Independence Measure. *American Journal of Physical Medicine and Rehabilitation* 72:84–89.

Granger, C.V., et al. 1995. The Uniform Data System for Medical Rehabilitation: Report of first admissions for 1993. *American Journal of Physical Medicine and Rehabilitation* 74:62–66.

Hawes, C., et al. 1995. Reliability estimates for the Minimum Data Set for nursing home resident assessment and care screening (MDS). *Gerontologist* 35:172–178.

Hedrick, S.C., and T.S. Inui. 1986. The effectiveness and cost of home care: An information synthesis. *Health Services Research* 20:851–880.

Kenney, G.M., and L.C. Dubay. 1992. Explaining area variation in the use of Medicare home health services. *Medical Care* 30:43–57.

Kramer, A.M., et al. 1990. Assessing and assuring the quality of home health care: A conceptual framework. *Milbank Quarterly* 68:413–443.

Kramer, A.M., et al. 1997. Outcomes and costs after hip fracture and stroke: A comparison of rehabilitation settings. *Journal of the American Medical Association* 277:396–404.

Morris, J.N., et al. 1990. Designing the national resident assessment instrument for nursing homes. *Gerontologist* 30:293–307.

Murdaugh, C. 1992. Quality of life, functional status, patient satisfaction. In *Patient outcomes research: Examining the effectiveness of nursing practice*: *Proceedings of a Conference* (Pub. No. NIH-93-3411). Washington, DC: U.S. Department of Health and Human Services, Public Health Service, National Institutes of Health.

National Association for Home Care (NAHC). 1995. Medicare's OASIS: Standardized outcome and assessment information set for home health care. *NAHC Report* (special supplement no. 625, August 11, 1995). Washington, DC: NAHC.

Powell, M.C., et al. 1994. *Technical appendices to the report on measuring outcomes of home health care,* vol. 2. Denver: University of Colorado Health Sciences Center, Center for Health Services Research.

Prospective Payment Assessment Commission (ProPAC). 1996. *Medicare and the American health care system. Report to Congress.* Washington, DC: ProPAC.

Riley, P.A. 1989. *Quality assurance in home care.* Washington, DC: American Association of Retired Persons.

Shaughnessy, P.W. 1991. *Shaping policy for long-term care: Learning from the effectiveness of hospital swing beds.* Ann Arbor, MI: Health Administration Press.

Shaughnessy, P.W., et al. 1994a. Measuring and assuring the quality of home care. *Health Care Financing Review* 16:35–68.

Shaughnessy, P.W., et al. 1994b. *Measuring outcomes of home health care, vol. 1*. Denver: Center for Health Policy Research.

Shaughnessy, P.W., et al. 1995a. *Outcome-based quality improvement: A manual for home care agencies on how to use outcomes*. Washington, DC: National Association for Home Care.

Shaughnessy, P.W., et al. 1995b. Outcome-based quality improvement in home care. *Caring* 14:44–49.

Shaughnessy, P.W., et al. 1996. Home health care: Moving forward with continuous quality improvement. *Journal of Aging and Social Policy* 7:149–167.

State University of New York (SUNY) at Buffalo. 1993. *Guide to the Uniform Data Set for Medical Rehabilitation (adult FIM^{SM}) version 4.0*. Buffalo, NY: SUNY–Buffalo.

State University of New York (SUNY) at Buffalo. 1995. *Getting started with the Uniform Data System for Medical Rehabilitation (adult FIM^{SM})*. Buffalo, NY: SUNY–Buffalo.

Weissert, W.G., et al. 1988. Past and future of home- and community-based long-term care. *Milbank Quarterly* 66:309–388.

CHAPTER **30**

Evaluating the Quality of Home Care Services Using Patient Outcome Data

Marilyn D. Harris and Michael Dugan

Patient outcome data are an increasingly important component of the evaluation of the home care services provided to patients. The Health Care Financing Administration (HCFA) is developing quality indicators (QI) for home health care that reflect changes in functional and health status. Initially, HCFA will use the indicators to guide the frequency of surveys in different agencies and to target the survey to the areas of greatest concern in each agency. In the longer run, however, the indicators will make a greater contribution to quality by allowing agencies to monitor and improve patient care and allowing HCFA to give agencies objective data on their relative performance. Two examples of quality indicators are the percentage of patients showing improvement in ambulation and the percentage of patients readmitted to an acute care hospital (Jencks, 1995). Barbara J. Gagel (1995) of HCFA's Health Standards and Quality Bureau (HSQB) states that HCFA is refocusing its attention, away from the structures and processes of health care, to outcomes and to expectations and strategies for improvement. This will be accomplished through revising the conditions of participation for home health agencies, reinforcing an outcome-based focus through revised survey procedures and developing QIs that focus very heavily on patient outcomes rather than on the organization and activities of the provider.

The National Medicare Quality Assurance and Improvement Demonstration (MESA) project that is now under way at the Colorado Center for Health Policy and Services Research includes 50 home health agencies that will implement and maintain a systematic approach to collecting outcome-related data and to improving quality using outcome findings. This large-scale demonstration program will be a prototype of the national program to be implemented by Medicare over the next several years (Shaughnessy and Crisler, 1995). Shaughnessy and Crisler define a patient-level outcome as a change in patient health status between two or more time points. These authors point out that the change can be positive, neutral, or negative and that the change can occur either as a result of the care provided or the natural progression of disease and disability. They describe three types of outcomes:

> **End-Result Outcome** is a change in patient health status between two or more time points.
>
> **Intermediate-Result Outcome** is a change in patient's (or information caregiver's) behavior, emotions, or

Source: Reprinted with permission from M.D. Harris and M. Dugan, Evaluating the Quality of Home Care Services Using Patient Outcome Data, *Home Healthcare Nurse*, Vol. 14, No. 6, pp. 463–467, © 1996, Lippincott-Raven Publishers.

knowledge that can influence the patient's end-result outcomes.

Utilization Outcome is a type of health care utilization that reflects (typically, a substantial) change in patient health status over time. Examples of this type of outcome are an admission to a hospital, nursing home or emergent care during the home care stay.

The authors also refer to a global outcome that pertains to all patients (analysis of hospitalization rates for all patients admitted to a home care agency in a given year) or a focused outcome such as a change in ambulation ability for orthopedic patients.

Medicare's OASIS: Standardized Outcome and Assessment Information Set for Home Health Care (Shaughnessy et al., 1995) was published in 1995. The OASIS data set that HCFA is expected to propose for purposes of outcome-based quality improvement by Medicare (as part of the new Conditions of Participation) has been under development for several years and was published in draft form. A second draft or revision of the OASIS will be available in 1997. The final version will be released in two or three years, after sufficient experience with the draft versions of the data set has accrued (Shaughnessy et al., 1995). A footnote to this publication states that "HCFA is not imposing this draft data set on any agency. An agency's decision to use OASIS-A is entirely voluntary." The data collection is completed on admission, at 60-day intervals, including the time of discharge from home care. These data are used to document patient outcomes. One data element addresses outcomes relevant to emergent care and/or reason for hospitalization.

The Tax Equity and Fiscal Responsibility Act of 1982 (Peer Review Improvement Act of 1982) established the Utilization and Quality Control Peer Review Organization (PRO). Home health agencies (HHAs) became subject to PRO review when Section 9393(c) of the Omnibus Budget Reconciliation Act of 1986

amended Section 1154(a)(14). The HHA reviews are many times the result of intervening care provided by the HHA between two hospital admissions occurring within 31 days of each other (Harris, 1993; Harris and McDonald, 1991).

One focus of the Visiting Nurse Association of Eastern Montgomery County (VNA)/Department of Abington Memorial Hospital's (AMH) Quality Assessment/Performance Improvement (QA/PI) program during 1995 was to identify the patients who were rehospitalized at AMH after an initial hospital discharge to home care services. A database was compiled using characteristics of the targeted patients as well as data from all AMH utilization encounters for these patients. The goal of the project was to uncover any trends shared by a significant majority of recidivist patients as compared with the entire VNA population as the baseline in order to improve patient outcomes. The sample size was 45 patients who met the following criteria:

- initial hospital discharge between January 1 and May 31, 1995
- rehospitalization required within 31 days of discharge
- hospitalized exclusively at AMH
- received home care services from the VNA between hospitalizations

PROCEDURE

The VNA Master Patient List for fiscal year 1995 was used to determine the population for the specified time period. The sample was selected using the stated criteria. All relevant information was obtained from individual patient records. The hospital's computer system provided specific diagnostic and AMH encounter information that was incorporated into the patient database.

Data analysis was completed by using the *t* test with .05 level of significance. Clinical analysis of the diagnoses was completed by the Director of Performance Improvement/Education. Interviews were conducted with representatives from the VNA, AMH Discharge Planning, Admissions and the Management Information Systems departments during the course of the project for reasons of clarification and/or explanation of procedures.

FINDINGS

Age

The age of a patient in need of a repeat hospitalization was significantly higher than that of the average VNA patient. The mean age of all VNA patients was approximately 54 years; the mean age of patients in the sample was 77.3. Approximately one-third of the VNA admissions during the study were for the early-discharge maternity program, which accounts for the mean age of 54 years.

Figure 30–1 shows the differences between the VNA population and the sample. The recidivist group had the highest percentage of its population between the ages of 60 and 100. Over one-third of the sample patients were between the ages of 76 and 85. The same age group comprised only 19 percent of the total population. Though the effect on the total population mirrors that of the sample group, it does so on a smaller scale. The implication is that the advanced age of a hospitalized VNA patient often necessitates further acute care within a short period of time.

Insurers

The most significant difference in this grouping was that Medicare insured a much larger proportion of patients from the recidivist sample than the total population. All other recidivist

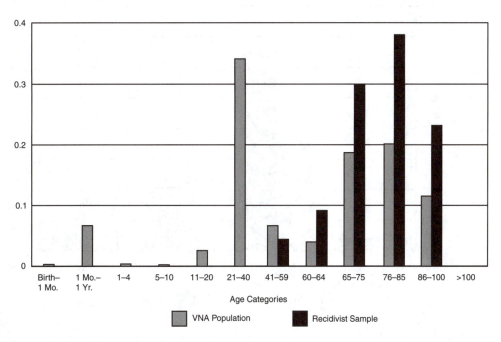

Figure 30–1 Age Differences between VNA Population and Recidivist Sample. *Source:* Reprinted with permission from M.D. Harris and M. Dugan, Evaluating the Quality of Home Care Services Using Patient Outcome Data, *Home Healthcare Nurse*, Vol. 14, No. 6, pp. 463–467, © 1996, Lippincott-Raven Publishers.

insurers were proportionally less than the VNA population, with private insurers having the largest disparity (17 percent of sample; 6.7 percent of population). Although approximately 29 percent of patient visits are through managed care programs, Medicare managed care constituted a small percentage of VNA insurers and the majority of the privately insured clients were under the age of 65.

Figure 30–2 underscores the age discrepancy noted. A majority (66.7 percent) of all recidivist patients had Medicare as their primary insurance compared to only 39 percent of the population.

Sex, Race, and Lifestyle

The recidivist group had proportionally more males, blacks, and those who lived alone than in

the VNA population (see Figure 30–3) although these results should be cautiously considered. There is no statistically significant disparity between the sample and the population, using a .05 level of significance, though these results do pass a .1 significance level test.

AMH Encounters

A survey of all AMH encounters was completed for the recidivist group for the period of time between January 1 and June 31, 1995. This was done to get a clear understanding of the entire health care utilization that was required by this segment of the population for a six-month period. The categories of encounter sites included: Emergency/Trauma Center, Out-Patient (OP) Clinic, Inpatient, Gastro-Intestinal Procedure Unit, OP–AMH Health Center, Same

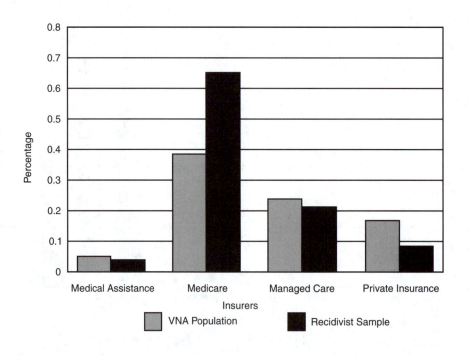

Figure 30–2 Insurer Differences between VNA Population and Recidivist Sample. *Source:* Reprinted with permission from M.D. Harris and M. Dugan, Evaluating the Quality of Home Care Services Using Patient Outcome Data, *Home Healthcare Nurse*, Vol. 14, No. 6, pp. 463–467, © 1996, Lippincott-Raven Publishers.

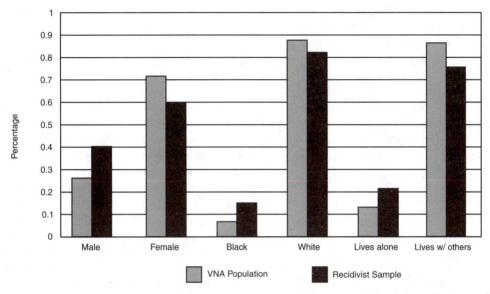

Figure 30–3 Sex, Race, and Lifestyle Differences between VNA and Recidivist Sample. *Source:* Reprinted with permission from M.D. Harris and M. Dugan, Evaluating the Quality of Home Care Services Using Patient Outcome Data, *Home Healthcare Nurse*, Vol. 14, No. 6, pp. 463–467, © 1996, Lippincott-Raven Publishers.

Day Procedure, OP–Central Registration, Rehab Medicine, OP–Medical Plaza, and OP–Psychiatry. During a 6-month period, the average recidivist patient had 2.91 inpatient admissions and 1.91 encounters with all other AMH facilities.

VNA Visits

The number of VNA visits and number of hours spent with the patient between hospitalizations vary widely. No comparative data were measured against this level of utilization.

Diagnoses

An analysis of patient diagnoses was completed for the first and second hospitalizations, as well as for the VNA admission. The first hospital admission diagnoses were reviewed and compared with the diagnoses on admission to the VNA and on readmission to the hospital in order to identify one of two relationships: 1) a causal or symptomatic relationship of an early

diagnosis to the two other later diagnoses; or 2) an identical diagnostic classification occurring through the two episodes of acute care and the one episode of home care.

There was a unifying diagnostic "thread" running through only 35.6 percent of all the patients in the recidivist sample. Sixty-four point four percent of the sample patients had one and sometimes two diagnoses that were dissimilar to the original hospital admitting diagnosis. The assumption is that, in almost two-thirds of the recidivist cases, there was no recurring disease or disorder that was being inadequately addressed through inpatient or VNA treatment. Often, very dissimilar maladies were experienced by an individual in a short period of time.

Patients Who Expired following Readmission to the Hospital

The incidence of death of recidivist patients during the study period was 4 out of 45. Translated yearly, the mortality rate would be 17.8

percent. The mortality rate of the VNA total population for the same year was much lower (4.2 percent). The recidivist patient was over four times more likely to die than the general VNA population over the course of the year. The VNA records for these four patients were reviewed by the director of performance improvement/education at the VNA and revealed the following profiles on admission to VNA service:

A 72-year-old male with malignant neoplasm of the lung.

A 77-year-old female with multiple myeloma, open wound, and pleural effusion.

An 87-year-old male with compression fracture of the spine, pneumonia.

An 87-year-old female with congestive heart failure and renal failure.

The home care services provided to these patients met the PRO home health standards and no quality of care issues were identified during internal record reviews.

Length of Stay (LOS)

The first hospitalization length of stay for the recidivist patients was more than a day longer than the average LOS for all Medicare patients at AMH during the same time frame.

Summary of Study

The VNA patients in need of repeat hospitalizations were older and sicker than the average VNA patients. There was no evidence that the patients had been treated ineffectively by either the hospital or the VNA. The advanced age, multiple diagnoses, and increased mortality rate of these patients point to the same conclusions. The patients are experiencing overall body system breakdown that is consistent with the last months of life. Each progressive level of deterioration

required a coinciding therapeutic response, resulting in increased AMH encounters.

IMPLICATION FOR HOME HEALTH CARE NURSES

So what does OASIS with its emphasis on patient outcomes (and other proposed outcome-based regulations) do for the field nurse besides adding to the mountain of paperwork already being done (Carr, 1996)? Carr suggests that OASIS will improve the continuity and consistency of the care process and help to define the home health care nurses' ability to define clearly what our care accomplishes. In the future, one agency's outcome data can be compared with aggregate outcome data. Home health care nurses constantly seek ways to provide high-quality care in a cost-effective manner based on professional standards, to meet expectations, of patients and families, and to achieve positive patient outcomes. Positive patient outcomes are as important to home health care nurses as they are to HCFA, the PRO, certification and accreditation surveyors.

In the future, it is expected that home health care nurses will provide fewer visits to more patients as the number of individuals who enroll in Medicare managed care programs continues to increase. New and enhanced technologies including the use of electronic home monitoring devices (Joyce, 1994; Sanders, 1995; Spurck et al., 1995) will become an everyday occurrence in the 21st century as home health care nurses work with other professionals to provide high-quality care and seek to maintain patients in their homes rather than in the more costly acute care setting.

Acknowledgment

The authors thank Joan Reynolds Yuan, MSN, RNC, Director of Performance Improvement and Education at the Visiting Nurse Association of Eastern Montgomery County/ Department of Abington Memorial Hospital, for her assistance in the analysis of clinical data.

BIBLIOGRAPHY

Carr, P. 1996. Get ready for OASIS. *Home Healthcare Nurse* 14:61–62.

Gagel, B. 1995. Health care quality improvement program: A new approach. *Health Care Financing Review* 16:15–23.

Harris, M. 1993. The peer review organization process revisited. *Home Healthcare Nurse* 11:67–68.

Harris, M., and M. McDonald. 1991. The peer review organization. *Home Healthcare Nurse* 9:37–42.

Jencks, S. 1995. Measuring quality of care under Medicare and Medicaid. *Health Care Financing Review* 16:39–54.

Joyce, M. 1994. HMOs turn to home health firms to monitor patients. *Philadelphia Business Journal* 13:5B, 13B.

Sanders, J. 1995. Telemedicine challenges to implementation. *The Remington Report* 3:34–39.

Shaughnessy, P., and K. Crisler. 1995. *Outcome-based quality improvement*. Washington, DC: National Association for Home Care.

Shaughnessy, P., et al. 1995. *Medicare's OASIS: Standardized outcome and assessment information set for home health care*. Washington, DC: National Association for Home Care.

Spurck, P., et al. 1995. The impact of wireless telecommunication system on time efficiency. *Journal of Nursing Administration* 25:21–26.

CHAPTER 31

Implementing the Agency for Health Care Policy and Research Urinary Incontinence Guideline in a Home Health Agency

Diane K. Newman, Carol Ann Parente, and Joan Reynolds Yuan

Urinary incontinence (UI), the involuntary loss of urine, is a frequently seen diagnosis in home patients requiring skilled nursing care. Preliminary data from a survey of 8,400 home and hospice health agencies indicate that genitourinary conditions were among the 20 leading first-listed diagnoses for patients added to their caseloads (Strahan, 1994). UI is a leading diagnosis for homebound individuals and first in total charges to Medicare for nursing services per person served (Ruther and Helbing, 1988). In a study of low-income, elderly individuals receiving publicly funded home care services, 23 percent were incontinent of urine and generated greater costs because of paraprofessional and other supportive care (Baker and Bice, 1995). These data indicate that UI is common among home care populations. Homebound individuals, by definition, either cannot leave their homes or do so with considerable difficulty as a result of a temporary or chronic disability (Strahan, 1994). The combination of decreased functional ability and UI is a particular challenge to professional and nonprofessional caregivers. The magnitude of the problem of caring for incontinent homebound individuals will no doubt increase as the absolute number of aged persons increases and as maintenance of dependent, elderly persons at home becomes more common. Home care agencies will need to address this common and costly problem. This chapter outlines one home health agency's approach to the problem of UI that spanned a 4-year period.

MANAGING UI IN THE HOMEBOUND

In 1992, the Agency for Health Care Policy and Research (AHCPR) released a clinical practice guideline on UI in adults (AHCPR, 1992). This report highlights the prevalence and costs of UI while indicating that the problem is underdiagnosed and undertreated by health care clinicians. This guideline was updated in 1996 (Fantl et al., 1996). This guideline notes that UI is predominantly seen in elderly women. This is of significance in that women make up the majority of the older population, represent a larger proportion of the total population at each higher age, and report higher rates of physical disability. Both guidelines make recommendations for application and management of indwelling Foley catheters, but the 1996 AHCPR publication gives specific recommendations for the use of catheters for the management of UI (Exhibit 31–1). The guideline also notes that indwelling catheter use in the homebound patient is common and requires paraprofessionals for activities of daily living and supervision by a registered nurse. The use of indwelling

Exhibit 31–1 AHCPR Recommendations for Use of an Indwelling Catheter

- Indwelling catheters may be recommended as a supportive measure for patients whose incontinence is caused by obstruction and for whom other interventions are not feasible.
- Indwelling catheters are recommended for selected incontinent patients who are terminally ill or for patients with pressure ulcers as short-term treatment.
- Indwelling catheters are recommended in severely impaired individuals in whom alternative interventions are not an option and when a patient lives alone and a caregiver is unavailable to provide other supportive measures.

Source: Adapted from Fantl, JA, Newman, DK, Colling, J, et al. "Urinary Incontinence in Adults: Acute and Chronic Management" Clinical Practice Guideline, No 2, 1996 Update, Rockville, MD: US Department of Health and Human Services. Public Health Service, Agency for Health Care Policy and Research, AHCPR Publication No. 96-0682. March 1996.

catheters increases the overall cost of home care.

CATHETER USE IN THE HOME

Prevalence studies of indwelling catheter use have been conducted in acute care hospitals and nursing homes, but actual catheter use in home care is not well documented. A recent publication from the Centers for Disease Control and Prevention reported characteristics of the 1994 National Home and Hospice Care Survey (Day, 1996). In that survey, 12 percent of elderly men and 7 percent of women had an ostomy or an indwelling catheter. Another survey questioned 471 agencies from 45 states concerning long-term indwelling catheter use, associated costs, and nursing practices (ConvaTec, 1996). The majority of agencies responding managed more than 16 Foley catheters per month; the national average is 28 per month. The most frequently occurring diagnoses of these patients were urinary retention (UR), UI, and neurogenic bladder. Bladder spasms (37 percent), catheter blockage (48 percent), and leakage (48 percent) were the most frequently occurring problems necessitating unscheduled patient visits for almost half these agencies (46 percent). Chronic urinary tract infection (UTI) was reported as a problem in most patients, with one to two episodes occurring per year. Almost 70 percent of the agencies reported that Foley catheter

patients were covered by Medicare insurance. Based on available information about catheter use in the home, use of these devices increases overall costs and contributes to nursing care problems and increased visits.

CURRENT NURSING RESEARCH ON UI IN THE HOMEBOUND

Unfortunately, evaluation tools are not mandated for home care agencies providing skilled nursing visits. Thus identification of UI depends on the quality of continence questions included in each agency's nursing assessment and on the skill and knowledge of the nurse. Alternatives to indwelling catheters are not offered or chosen because there are few studies that have focused on the outcome of specific alternatives. In the area of assessment and behavioral management of UI among homebound individuals, research has been performed on the successful use of pelvic muscle rehabilitation augmented with bladder training and biofeedback therapy for cognitively intact home care subjects (Rose et al., 1990). Twenty-one elderly homebound patients were visited and treated with a combination of behavioral therapies by continence nurse practitioner specialists. Improvement in weekly incontinence episodes was 78 percent from the baseline rate. Two case studies were reported of severely disabled but cognitively intact homebound individuals who were successfully treated with biofeedback-assisted pelvic muscle exercises (McDowell et al., 1994). Another study reported a program implemented in a home health agency that involved the use of pelvic muscle exercises for the treatment of urge incontinence (Flynn et al., 1994). Incontinence episodes per week were reduced by a mean of 82 percent. The investigators concluded that using pelvic muscle exercises resulted in both a clinically and a statistically significant decrease in UI among these patients. Currently, there are several studies being performed using a variety of treatment modalities for both cognitively impaired and cognitively intact homebound persons living in both urban and rural areas.

Although behavioral treatments have undergone limited study in this population, management of persons with long-term intractable UI has not been studied. These individuals tend to be frail elders who have cognitive or physical impairments and are not appropriate candidates for other treatments, such as surgery, pharmacological therapy, toileting schedules, and pelvic muscle exercises. Information regarding the most effective and efficient method to optimize continence in this population is lacking. Internal and external catheters, absorbent products, and collection devices represent an integral part of home care nursing of incontinence and are frequently used.

ONE AGENCY'S UI DILEMMA

In 1991, the Visiting Nurse Association of Eastern Montgomery County (VNA) identified UI (altered urinary elimination) as being consistently among the top 10 diagnostic categories for the past years, although UI might not be clearly identified as the problem etiology. A typical management strategy for the incontinent home care patient would be placement of an indwelling Foley catheter. Frequently, the patient with UI was maintained with the catheter for life. The presence of a catheter in the patient meant the continuation of skilled nursing services, home health aide services, and

Medicare-covered catheter supplies. The catheter also meant that the patient was at increased risk for catheter-related problems, from simple blockage and leakage to serious infection, sepsis, and death. The AHCPR guideline notes that bacteriuria develops in most persons within 2 to 4 weeks of catheter insertion (Warren et al., 1988). Cases of sepsis and death due to severe UTI have been reported. Other complications associated with indwelling catheters include obstruction secondary to encrustation, leakage, unprescribed removal, pain, bladder spasms, urethral erosion, stones, epididymitis, urethritis, periurethral abscess, chronic renal inflammatory changes, fistula formation, hematuria, and urinary leakage. There is no standard management of indwelling catheters, but the usual practice is to change indwelling catheters every 30 days.

IDENTIFICATION OF CATHETER-RELATED PROBLEMS

In 1991, the VNA had identified problems with several catheter maintenance patients who required frequent after-hours visits for catheter leakage and obstruction. At that time, based on physician orders, the staff nurses were still teaching patients and their families to irrigate catheters in an attempt to clear blockage and regain patency. These catheter-related problems were believed to be secondary to lack of adequate hydration. Controversy ensued as various members of the staff debated the merits of irrigation for catheter blockage and leakage. The AHCPR UI guideline notes that there is no benefit from catheter irrigation because bladder irrigation of catheters may actually damage bladder mucosa (Thompson et al., 1984). The VNA decided to be proactive and sought the advice of a continence nurse practitioner specialist to assist the agency with developing protocols to address catheter-related problems. The continence nurse practitioner specialist was a panel member of the 1992 AHCPR guideline and the cochair of the panel for the 1996 version.

To implement this protocol, changes were made to documentation tools, flow sheets, and staff instruction guides. It was believed that these tools and instructions were contributing to the recurring catheter-related problems. In addition, the continence nurse practitioner specialist was brought on as a consultant to provide staff consultation, direct patient care, and expert opinion on the problem of UI and catheter-related problems. The VNA staff referred patients to the continence nurse practitioner specialist if the complexity of the case necessitated the specialist's expertise or if the patient would benefit from behavioral training, including biofeedback therapy (Exhibit 31–2). The AHCPR guideline recommends that a person with an indwelling catheter should be periodically reassessed to determine whether a voiding trial or bladder retraining program might be effective in eliminating the need for the catheter. The continence nurse specialist developed a protocol for catheter removal and bladder retraining that was utilized in the VNA patient population (Exhibit 31–3).

Quality Assessment and Improvement Plan

Based on the 1992 AHCPR UI guideline, the VNA adopted recommendations in the form of a quality assessment improvement (QAI) plan. The initial indicator developed was "The patient/caregiver will be instructed in the care of the Foley catheter." Monitoring of the indicator was initiated. Specific instructions for the patient and caregivers regarding catheter use included the following:

- cleansing around the urethral meatus with soap and water at least once daily
- fluid intake of 1,500 mL minimum (if no fluid restriction)
- securing the catheter through anchoring
- positioning of the drainage bag
- emergency removal of the catheter
- emptying of the drainage bag every 8 hours
- maintenance of the closed system

The results of the first 3 months of evaluation were not promising. All instruction items fell below 100 percent compliance except cleansing around the meatus. Maintenance of a closed system was not documented at all. The results of this evaluation led to immediate corrective action. The flow sheet used by the nursing staff to document the care of a patient with an alteration in urinary elimination related to Foley catheter use was revised to eliminate reference to irrigation, and instruction on maintaining a closed system was inserted. These cues or parameters on the VNA flow sheets set the standards for the care given to the patient during the home visit, and it was hoped that clarifying the parameters would lead to improved compliance with the QAI plan.

In addition to the flow sheet adaptations, nursing rounds were held for the staff in July 1993 with the VNA's adult nurse practitioner and the continence nurse practitioner specialist as moderators. Case studies were presented focusing on both catheter management and continence management alternatives. The presentation also included distribution of copies of the 1992 AHCPR guidelines on UI in adults. Copies of the clinical guidelines, quick reference guidelines, and patient guidelines were made available to all clinical nursing staff. The subsequent QAI record reviews showed gradual improvement in compliance with the indicator on instruction in maintenance of a closed system, with 100 percent compliance occurring between May 1994 and January 1995.

Concern about catheter maintenance and continence management continued among the VNA administrative and supervisory staff. Although a closed system became part of expected VNA practice, there were still no standards established regarding the use of catheters for incontinent patients, including discussions of alternative management options and risks of complications due to the use of the catheter. Therefore, it was concluded that standards should be expanded to include a comprehensive nursing approach to the problem of UI and to reduce catheter-related problems through the formation

Exhibit 31–2 Behavioral Interventions

Type	Toileting Programs			Pelvic Muscle Rehabilitation	
	Scheduled Toileting/Habit Training	Prompted Voiding	Bladder Training	Pelvic Muscle Exercises	Biofeedback
Definition	• Timed scheduled voiding • Habit training scheduled to match patient's voiding habits • Caregiver dependent	• Scheduled voiding that requires prompting from caregiver • Caregiver dependent	• Systematic ability to delay voiding through the use of urge inhibition • Active rehabilitation and education techniques	• Planned, active exercises of pelvic muscles to increase periurethral muscle strength • Active rehabilitation and education techniques	• Method that uses electronic or mechanical instruments to display information about neuromuscular and/or bladder activity, particularly with pelvic muscle exercises. Can be used in association with other programs • Active rehabilitation and education techniques
Target population	• Cognitively impaired • Functionally disabled • Incomplete bladder emptying • Caregiver dependent	• Functionally able to use toilet or toileting device • Able to feel urge sensation • Able to request toileting assistance • Availability of caregiver	• Cognitively intact • Ability to discern urge sensation • Cognitively able to understand or learn how to inhibit urge • Able to toilet themselves or with assistance	• Able to identify and contract pelvic muscles • Compliance with instructions	• Ability to understand analogue or digital signals using auditory or visual display • Motivated persons who are able to learn voluntary control through observation of the biofeedback • Health care provider who can appropriately assess the UI problem and provide behavioral interventions

Source: Adapted from Fantl, JA, Newman, DK, Colling, J, et al. "Managing Acute and Chronic Urinary Incontinence," Clinical Practice Guideline, Quick Reference Guide for Clinicians, No 2, 1996 Update, Rockville, MD: US Department of Health and Human Services. Public Health Service, Agency for Health Care Policy and Research, AHCPR Publication No. 96-0686. March 1996.

Exhibit 31–3 Procedure for Bladder Retraining of Catheter-Dependent Patients

1. Obtain physician order for catheter removal and bedside cystometrogram (CMG). A bedside CMG may be indicated to determine the ability of the bladder to fill, store, and evacuate urine. The CMG will allow evaluation of the presence of urge sensation and unstable (hyperactive) bladder. Equipment used is either a 50-mL syringe and sterile water or an intravenous bag and tubing.

2. Start the patient on a broad-spectrum antibiotic before or at the time of catheter removal.

3. Disconnect the catheter from the drainage tube. Instill sterile water into the bladder in 25-mL increments in supine or sitting position until the patient experiences an urge to void. The patient is asked to report first sensation of bladder fullness ("I'm starting to feel like I have to go"). The patient is asked to report the strong or "must" urge, which occurs at bladder capacity ("I really have to go, I can't hold it anymore"). If leakage of water occurs around the catheter or the catheter is expelled during the CMG, this may indicate the presence of involuntary bladder contractions.

4. Once the patient experiences the "must" or strong urge, remove the catheter, and have the patient attempt to void. Check for postvoid residual urine (PVR) volume. PVR should be checked within 5 to 10 minutes after voiding by either catheterization or performance of an ultrasound of the pelvis to locate bladder volume. PVRs of less than 50 mL are normal. Repetitive PVRs ranging from 100 to 200 mL or higher are considered evidence of inadequate emptying.

5. Place the patient on a timed voiding schedule, every 2 hours during waking hours.

6. Monitor the patient for PVRs for two consecutive days.

7. Teach the patient pelvic muscle exercises and bladder retraining if appropriate.

Source: Adapted with permission from D.K. Newman, Continence Technology, Access to Continence Care and Treatment, © 1995, D.K. Newman.

of a quality improvement (QI) team, which was established in early 1994 to incorporate the AHCPR guidelines into VNA practice and to teach nursing staff to identify the problem of UI within their patient base.

Implementing the QI Team Approach

The QI team at the VNA consisted of members of both clinical and supervisory staffs. The QI team included the director of QI, a clinical supervisor, three staff nurses, and the adult nurse practitioner. To establish a smooth working relationship and awareness of the problem, the team members were initially educated about both the problem of UI and QI concepts and tools. Once the team was established, the members developed the following mission statement to guide their subsequent activities:

The QI team will identify and evaluate the VNA's patient population with UI/UR, collect and analyze data related to UI/UR management, and make recommendations to implement the AHCPR guidelines within the limits of patient choice and home care practice. Patients with recognized UI/UR will have education and referral for UI/UR management according to the AHCPR guidelines.

The team identified limitations to the implementation of the AHCPR guidelines, including patient reluctance to disclose incontinence and refusal to follow through on nursing suggestions to manage incontinence by alternative means. From a professional perspective, the nursing staff and attending physicians may have been unaware of the AHCPR guidelines on incontinence. No additional personnel would be assigned to evaluate and/or manage incontinent patients for the nursing staff, and full evaluation of the incontinent patient (e.g., pelvic examination) would not be within the scope of all home care nurses. UI management strategies, however, included toileting programs, bladder retraining, and the use of devices and products.

QI Team Process

The process of the QI team fell into place with literature review and discussion at the regularly scheduled meetings. To collect data related to the current practices regarding UI/UR, additional record review questions were developed specific to the assessment of the genitourinary tract, diagnosis and management of incontinence, and/or management of a Foley catheter (if present). These questions were added to the routine quality assessment record review conducted quarterly at the VNA. Baseline data collection on the VNA population showed Foley catheters to be present in 5 percent to 7 percent of the VNA population between November 1993 and April 1994. The problem of incontinence was noted during random record review in 22 percent of the VNA population. This was consistent with the AHCPR estimate of incontinence occurring in 15 percent to 30 percent of the population older than 60 years. Although the problem of incontinence may have been noted in the nursing record, the issue may or may not have been further addressed by the nursing staff during the home care length of service. For instance, a patient whose primary diagnosis was a fractured hip may have been noted to be incontinent of urine in the nursing assessment, but no nursing diagnosis was made related to altered urinary elimination by the primary nurse because the standardized flow sheet (care plan) for that problem at the VNA deals mostly with Foley catheter use, and the patient did not have an indwelling catheter. Without a nursing diagnosis and related flow sheet (care plan), the

patient's care related to UI was haphazard, ranging from direct intervention by the primary nurse, to referral to the continence nurse practitioner specialist, to ignoring the problem completely.

UI Flow Chart

Once the team secured firm data related to the extent of the problem at the VNA and evaluated the current practices, they designed a flow chart of the expected nursing practice related to the care of the incontinent patient and documented the expected barriers to care. These discussions focused on the patient and professional limitations that needed countering to maximize successful transition to implementing the AHCPR guidelines. Some of the problems identified by the QI team were inconvenience for the patient and family, who were used to Foley placement once a month to manage incontinence. This was not surprising. A study of caregivers of community-dwelling, chronically ill older persons found that 75 percent of those who cared for incontinent family members felt that maintaining continence was burdensome. The burden was related to time spent in providing care, the patient's immobility, and lack of social supports (Flaherty et al., 1992). Another factor was physician and nurse reluctance to alter the plan of care because of lack of knowledge of alternative management. The QI team also consulted with the continence nurse practitioner specialist periodically to keep her informed of their activities related to incontinence and to seek information about strategies to improve patient care.

Staff nurses on the team were uncomfortable with making an accurate incontinence diagnosis, so the QI team developed a history form, assessment tool, and bladder record for the nursing staff to identify specific types of incontinence (see Appendix 31–A). Precise assessment and history information was listed to guide the staff nurse in making an appropriate nursing diagnosis related to incontinence. This was paired with a new flow sheet for incontinence, which allowed the nurse to focus more specifically on the parameters to manage incontinence, including precipitating factors such as diet, fluid intake, and bowel patterns. The QI team also incorporated new teaching plans for incontinent patients into VNA practice. The education tools covered bladder training, a diet and fluid guide, pelvic floor exercises, and the steps in clean intermittent catheterization.

Targeted Staff Education

The final steps toward implementation of the AHCPR guidelines for incontinence were accomplished by the QI team through education efforts. The members of the QI team and the VNA's continence nurse practitioner specialist held a staff inservice to acquaint the nursing staff with the AHCPR guidelines, agency expectations for catheter use, and the new incontinence assessment tool and flow sheet. The new education tools were also presented. The VNA also sought the support of the agency's professional advisory committee and the hospital's chief of staff to help in the implementation of changes in the usual home care practices for catheters and incontinence management. An educational memo for the agency's referring physicians was distributed to alert the professional community to the AHCPR guidelines regarding incontinence and the VNA's quality initiatives for catheterized and incontinent patients.

The QI team then set into motion the current important aspect of care: monitoring compliance with the revised catheter/incontinence management expectations. The VNA's current expectation is 95 percent compliance with the AHCPR guideline criteria for use of Foley catheters, including urinary retention not otherwise

managed and grade 3 or 4 decubitus ulcers, terminal illness, severe impairment, and postsurgical intervention. Patients who do not meet the criteria are informed of the risks of indwelling catheters, and consent is secured for continued use of the catheter.

Since the implementation of the user-friendly tools (flow sheets, assessment form, and teaching tools), specific incontinence diagnoses and hence interventions have been identified 59 times. Although indwelling Foley catheters are still being used at the VNA, current data indicate that 100 percent of the time the use of the catheter meets the AHCPR guidelines or the patient has been informed of the risks and refuses other interventions to manage incontinence.

CONCLUSION

The nature of UI and its complexity will increase the need for, use of, and cost of nursing care for homebound patients. This presents a unique challenge to home health agencies, which are being asked to provide cost-effective, quality nursing care. The VNA's approach to UI through the development of the QI team demonstrated that the AHCPR UI guidelines can be implemented in home care practice. The VNA had the advantage of the expertise of a continence nurse practitioner specialist as a consultant. The results of this project show improved quality of care for incontinent patients when these patients are provided safe alternatives to catheters. Future data collection may determine changes in cost of care, length of service, and visit patterns, all of which are certain to have growing importance as health care dollars are reallocated.

REFERENCES

Agency for Health Care Policy and Research, Urinary Incontinence Guideline Panel. 1992. *Urinary incontinence in adults* (Clinical Practice Guideline, AHCPR Pub. No. 92-0038). Rockville, MD: Department of Health and Human Services.

Baker, D.I., and T.W. Bice. 1995. The influence of urinary incontinence on publicly financed home care services to low-income elderly people. *Gerontologist* 35:360–369.

ConvaTec. 1996. *National home care survey.* Princeton, NJ: Bristol Myers Squibb.

Day, A.N. 1996. Characteristics of elderly home health care users: Data from the 1994 National Home and Hospice Care Survey. Atlanta: Centers for Disease Control and Prevention.

Fantl, J.A., et al. 1996. *Urinary incontinence in adults: Acute and chronic management* (Clinical Practice Guideline, No. 2, 1996 Update). Rockville, MD: Department of Health and Human Services.

Flaherty, J.H., et al. 1992. Impact on caregivers of supporting urinary function in non-institutionalized chronically ill seniors. *Gerontologist* 32:541–545.

Flynn, L., et al. 1994. Effectiveness of pelvic muscle in reducing urge incontinence among community residing elders. *Journal of Gerontological Nursing* 20:23–27.

McDowell, J., et al. 1994. Successful treatment using behavioral interventions of urinary incontinence in homebound older adults. *Geriatric Nursing* 15:303–307.

Rose, M., et al. 1990. Behavioral management of urinary incontinence in homebound older adults. *Home Healthcare Nurse* 8:10–15.

Ruther, M., and C. Helbing. 1988. Health care financing trends: Use and cost of home health services under Medicare. *Health Care Financing Review* 10:105–108.

Strahan, G.W. 1994. *An overview of home health and hospice care patients: Preliminary data from the 1993 National Home and Hospice Care Survey.* Hyattsville, MD: National Center for Health Statistics.

Thompson, R.L., et al. 1984. Catheter-associated bacteriuria. *JAMA* 251:747–751.

Warren, J.W., et al. 1988. Acute pyelonephritis associated with bacteriuria during long-term catheterization: A prospective clinicopathological study. *Journal of Infectious Diseases* 158:1341–1346.

Tools for UI Assessment and Intervention

Incontinence History

Assessment: Duration of incontinence:_____

Prior treatment (medical/surgical/behavior modification):_____

Use of self-care items (pads/diapers):_____

Exam: Abnormality of genitalia:_____

Altered sexual function:_____

Functional Evaluation of Environment: 1.   Distance to bathroom/toilet:_____

2.   Barriers to commode access:_____

Clutter_____Yes_____ No

Stairs_____

Equipment: 1.   Commode:_____

2.   Adaptive equipment for toilet:_____

3.   Other:_____

Urinalysis Results:

_____Leukocytes_____Nitrite_____pH_____Protein_____Glucose

_____Ketones____Urobilinogen_____Bilirubin_____Blood

Definitions:

61. *Stress Incontinence:* Involuntary loss of urine during coughing, sneezing, laughing, other physical activity. Confirm diagnosis by observing urine loss during activities that increase abdominal pressure.

63. *Urge Incontinence:* Involuntary loss of urine associated with an abrupt and strong desire to void. Often associated with frequency; may be massive and sudden urine loss. (Mixed incontinence: May have components of urge or stress. Use diagnostic category that predominates.)

59. *Functional Incontinence:* Involuntary loss of urine associated with altered environment and sensory, cognitive, and/or mobility deficits.

60. *Reflex Incontinence:* Involuntary loss of urine occurring at somewhat predictable times with a specific bladder volume. Often associated with neurological impairment.

62. *Total Incontinence:* Continuous unpredictable urine loss associated with neurological impairment, including neuropathy, dysfunction, or trauma.

Courtesy of Visiting Nurse Association of Eastern Montgomery County/A Department of Abington Memorial Hospital.

Incontinence Assessment: Parameters and Interventions

Goal: By discharge < 8 voids/day, 2 voids/night, and/or 50% reduction in incontinence episodes	Date	Date	Date	Date	Date
Character of continence voids/UI:					
Frequency					
Time of day					
Amount (mL/pads)					
Precipitating factors (alcohol, medications, caffeine)					
UTI: Signs and symptoms					
Intake: _____oz/day					
Bowel pattern					
Cognitive/mental status					
Examination:					
Abdominal shape					
Bowel sounds					
Palpation of suprapubic tenderness					
Perineal skin					
Rectal examination					
Instructions:					
Kegel exercises					
Bladder/bowel training					
Diet/fluid intake					
Skin care					
Reportable signs and symptoms					
Interventions:					
Evaluate effectiveness of treatment					
Coordination with UI specialist					
Note: See Incontinence History for incontinence types, history, and UA. Choose appropriate diagnosis.					

Courtesy of Visiting Nurse Association of Eastern Montgomery County/A Department of Abington Memorial Hospital.

Bladder Record

Name: _____   Date: _____

Time	Voided (X) in Toilet	Urine Leakage S M L	Activity with Leakage	Fluid Intake

Number of Pads Used Today:_____

COMMENTS:_____

Patient Education Tools—Guide for Restoring Bladder Control

Foods To Avoid

Caffeine-containing foods and fluids can act as bladder irritants and should be limited or eliminated. These include colas, coffee, tea, and dark chocolate. Some medications also contain caffeine (e.g., Midol, Anacin, Excedrin, and Dristan).

The artificial sweetener aspartame (Nutrasweet) and alcohol may also contribute to frequent urination.

Fluid Intake

Many incontinent patients limit their fluid intake to avoid accidents, but this contributes to incontinence by making concentrated, irritating urine. Try to drink 8 to 10 8-oz glasses of fluid every day.

If nighttime accidents occur, drink most fluids before 6 P.M. Also, lie down in your bed or recliner for 1 or 2 hours during the day. This helps your kidneys make more urine during the day, reducing the amount in your bladder at night.

Bowel Habits

Sometimes incontinence may be caused by rectal pressure related to constipation or impaction.

High fiber intake helps overcome this problem. Eat fiber-rich foods, including whole grain breads, cereals, nuts, raw fruits, and vegetables. You may also add whole unprocessed bran (available in health food stores) to cereals and other foods to boost fiber intake. Start slowly (1 T of bran daily) and gradually increase until bowel functions return to normal.

The following recipe can also help bowel function:

1 cup unprocessed bran

1 cup applesauce

1 cup prune juice

Mix and store mixture in refrigerator. Start with 2 T daily. Increase by 2 T a week until bowel function is normal.

Remember: Do not rush to the bathroom. Try to practice relaxation breathing until the urge to urinate lessens, then walk slowly to the bathroom.

Pelvic Floor Exercises (Kegel Exercises)

Find the Right Muscle

The pelvic floor muscle is the same one you use to purposefully stop urinating or hold back gas.

How To Exercise

Tighten the pelvic floor muscle and hold for 10 seconds. Then relax for 10 seconds. Repeat 15 times, morning, afternoon, and night. Work up to 25 repetitions.

Problems: Place your hand on your abdomen while you do your exercises; if your hand moves, you are also using these muscles. If you experience back or abdominal discomfort or headaches, you are probably holding your breath and/or using stomach or back muscles, too. Refocus on contracting just the pelvic floor.

When and Where To Exercise

Anytime. No one can see you exercise because the pelvic floor muscles are internal. Most people exercise while seated or lying down.

Steps to Intermittent Clean Catheterization—Women

1. Gather equipment and place in a convenient area. You'll need catheter, water-soluble lubricant, moist towelette or soap and water, and a small, dry towel.
2. Wash hands with soap and water and dry.

3. Position yourself comfortably with thighs spread apart on toilet or chair across from toilet.

4. With one hand, spread labia and wash from front to back with soap and water or moist towelette.

5. Lubricate catheter end that enters urethra (tip to 2 inches up catheter) with water-soluble lubricant.

6. Slowly insert catheter into urethra until urine flows. Insert about 1 inch farther, hold until urine stops flowing.

7. When urine stops, gradually withdraw catheter. Slightly rotate catheter and stop each time more urine flows.

8. Check color, odor, and clarity of urine. Report changes to your health care provider.

9. Do not reuse damaged, worn, or discolored catheters.

10. Clean the catheter with warm, soapy water, rinse well, and allow to dry in a clean towel. Store in a clean plastic bag.

Steps to Intermittent Clean Catheterization—Men

1. Gather equipment and place in a convenient area. You'll need catheter, water-soluble lubricant, moist towelette or soap and water, and a small, dry towel.

2. Wash hands with soap and water and dry.

3. Position yourself comfortably on toilet or chair across from toilet. Some men stand during procedure.

4. Hold penis up with one hand. Wash to base of glans with soap and water or moist towelette. Wash in circular motion from urethra outward.

5. Lubricate tip of catheter with water-soluble lubricant up to first 6 inches of catheter.

6. Hold penis straight up from body at 60° to 70° angle. Slowly and gently insert catheter approximately 6 to 8 inches until urine begins to flow. Insert about 1 inch farther and hold until urine flow stops.

7. When urine stops, gradually withdraw catheter. Slightly rotate catheter and stop each time more urine flows.

8. Check color, odor, and clarity of urine. Report changes to your health care provider.

9. Do not reuse damaged, worn, or discolored catheters.

10. Clean the catheter with warm, soapy water, rinse well, and allow to dry wrapped in a clean towel. Store in a clean plastic bag.

CHAPTER 32

Home Health Care Benchmarking

Michael F. Kaufman

The concept and theory of benchmarking as it specifically relates to the health care environment are relatively new. Every time we compare ourselves with some determined level of achievement, however, we have engaged in the most basic form of benchmarking. This general concept of benchmarking has become one of the most powerful methodologies to improve organizational effectiveness.

Most companies, regardless of product or service, perform various degrees of benchmarking to gauge their performance against that of a similar industry or hierarchical structure. Until recently, organizations often used a rudimentary set of factors by which to gauge themselves (e.g., productivity, costs, etc.). Lately, however, benchmarking has become a more complex methodology for an organization to determine its place or standing in the market.

The following definition, which applies to all industries, including health care, was espoused by Spendolini (1992): Benchmarking is "a continuous, systematic process for evaluating the products, services and work processes of organizations that are recognized as representing best practices for the purpose of organizational improvement" (p. 9). This generic definition can be interpreted in many different ways. This chapter examines the structure behind benchmarking and how it applies to the health care environment. To delineate the process, exam-ples from health care and non–health care settings are identified.

Health care organizations typically perform benchmarking in one or more of the following ways, which can be administered locally, nationally, or through networks such as a formal system or alliance:

- *Internal benchmarking*. Who, in our facility, does things well? This form of benchmarking occurs when an organization analyzes activities, functions, or processes within its own boundaries. Examples include comparing nursing units with similar models of care (e.g., total care) or different models (e.g., total care versus patient-focused care). Because no two departments will ever run identically, looking at different internal units or departments is an excellent way to begin the benchmarking journey.

- *Global benchmarking*. What trends are occurring in our local market or nationally? An excellent way to experience "breakthrough" thinking is to examine what others are doing throughout the country. This method is more of a "shotgun" or general approach because many issues are identified internally, national contacts are subsequently made, and the information is used to improve processes within any of the contact organizations.

Benchmarking contacts should always attempt to glean information as well. The process then becomes an optimal process of information and idea exchange.

- *Best practice benchmarking.* Who is a recognized leader in a certain area? This methodology was popularized by Xerox. Simply stated, once a process or technique is poised for improvement, who is achieving the results that we seek? The difficulty in health care is determining who is truly the best and defining exactly what the best is. This classification follows a period of internal scrutiny, so that prioritization is based on organizational need.

All these approaches can be used concurrently. Access to state or national information will certainly enhance the outcome because a universally accepted source is used as a basis for comparison. The issue rampant in health care revolves around the methodology used or definitions of the data collected and analyzed. The proactive organization accepts imperfections in the data comparison and creates a process-driven, rather than data- or target-driven, mentality. The greater the concentration on the process, the less the likelihood of a need for identical benchmarking contacts. Finding such contacts is, of course, almost impossible.

BACKGROUND

A competitive advantage is quickly becoming more of a necessity than a choice for health care organizations. The advent of diagnosis-related groups in 1983 changed the way reimbursement occurs. Health care organizations became faced with the realization that the days of receiving payment for charged services were ending. To remain profitable in the new operating environment, organizations had to seek ways to reduce costs significantly.

The need for this paradigm of cost reduction strategies has been further emphasized by the emerging presence of managed care. The existence of managed care has basically reversed the view that most of us have had about the current health care delivery system. The concept of capitation enables health care providers to make a significant profit, assuming, however, that the patients making up the payer mix utilize few, if any, services. In other words, providers attempt to ensure that their populations remain healthy. Capitation is a managed care payment methodology whereby a provider receives a set or capitated dollar amount for each covered person per month. The fewer services consumed, the greater the profit realized by the provider. Because services will probably be used, the prudent organization proactively minimizes expenses.

An interesting trend related to managed care is its varying strength in markets throughout the country. States such as California and Arizona have witnessed greater levels of managed care and capitation. In areas such as Texas and Georgia, the degree of market penetration is extremely low. This phenomenon enables later markets (those with limited managed care) to learn from early markets (those with high levels of managed care). For example, a health care organization in a late market can observe the trends and results of one in an early market, such as a potential decrease of more than 70 percent in the number of patient days per 1,000 covered lives or a precipitous drop in the average length of stay. Studying and reacting to these trends will ensure the long-term viability of an organization. Furthermore, learning from the experiences of others can help an organization avoid costly mistakes.

Providers nationwide are facing similar challenges. Common trends include a changing focus from inpatient care to a continuum of care, rapid penetration by managed care in the form of health maintenance organizations or preferred provider organizations, increasing dependence on Medicare revenues as a result of the aging population nationally, consolidations of local competitors in the form of alliances or systems, the loss of ancillary service revenues, and the increasing demand for primary care services. A typical result from these changes takes the form of stagnant or declining profit margins.

The major economic issue with the health care industry is that the delivery of care is viewed as a right, not a privilege. Because the industry is so labor intensive (50 percent to 70 percent of the expenses are related to personnel), a balance must be struck between maintaining access and quality while reducing the costs associated with delivering care. Benchmarking has becoming a formidable tool in the quest for determining this balance.

THE BENCHMARKING PROCESS

Benchmarking, like all methodologies, has a formal structure to it. The typical process or journey that an organization undertakes is based on the following steps:

1. determining benchmarking issues
2. performing internal analysis
3. searching for benchmarking candidates
4. making contact
5. planning action
6. implementing
7. maintaining

Determining Benchmarking Issues

The process must commence with the understanding and support of administration. A champion driving the process should incessantly inculcate the need for and benefits of change. He or she must develop a cogent argument to inspire administration to learn more about the benefits of benchmarking. Education of the executives will give them a basic foundation in the principles and methodologies. Furthermore, acceptance from the executives eases acceptance by the managers. The managerial buy-in builds teamwork throughout the organization, which is vital because of the complexity of the issues discovered.

Many of the findings will cross functional lines and will involve core processes of the organization. Those embarking on this journey of discovery need the ability to effect change once the need for it has been identified. The

organizationwide issues are often chosen in alignment with the long-term strategic plan of the organization. This ensures that all efforts directly benefit the goals and objectives deemed necessary by administration and the board. The issues should be specific enough to give direction yet general enough to obtain support by employees, so that the process is truly theirs.

Most employees have a strong sense of what the benchmarking issues might entail in their particular department. In a home health agency, the issues might include the following:

- the department operating statistics, such as client visits and miles logged
- staff configuration, including paid full-time equivalents and skill mix by discipline
- workload/service intensity, such as miles logged per client visit and client visits per day
- organizational characteristics

All these issues involve more than one person or even one department. Each also is related to core needs of a home health agency, such as improving profitability or quality, and each also gives the organization a base from which to begin its benchmarking journey.

A good foundation can be built into the process by following the guidelines set forth by Xerox in its benchmarking approach. The company developed 10 questions to ascertain direction from an organizational or departmental standpoint:

1. What is the most critical factor to my function's/organization's success (e.g., patient satisfaction, test turnaround time, average length of stay)?
2. What factors are causing the most trouble?
3. What products or services are provided to customers?
4. What factors account for customer satisfaction?
5. What specific problems have been identified in the organization?

6. Where are the competitive pressures being felt in the organization?
7. What are the major costs (or cost drivers) in the organization?
8. Which functions represent the highest percentage of cost?
9. Which functions have the greatest room for improvement?
10. Which functions have the greatest effect (or potential effect) on differentiating the organization from competitors in the marketplace?

Applying Xerox's 10 questions will assist the home health agency or hospice in creating the benchmarking foundation; the prioritization, once accomplished at the administrative and/or departmental level, will provide a specific framework for the process. The organization now must decide which benchmarking issues will receive priority. Usually, the processes with the greatest impact on profitability (cost or revenues), customer satisfaction, and quality are those that command attention.

Performing Internal Analysis

Once the direction has been established in the first step, a thorough analysis of the operation must ensue. The success of any benchmarking endeavor, whether organizational or departmental in nature, rests on the premise that the survey tool and methodology will be a result of a complete understanding of the current process status.

The formation of a benchmarking team precedes the analysis. This team will initially conduct the internal overview of the processes to be studied; then it will become the accountable entity charged with the improvement of the process via the benchmarking methodology.

Members of the Team

The team typically consists of a team leader, a facilitator, internal and external customers, members, and support staff. The team composition should be based on process or functional

expertise, project management skills, ability to communicate well, internal credibility, and motivation to seek improvement. Membership often will include individuals who have been skeptics, the theory being that these individuals will become the strongest drivers of the benchmarking initiative once they accept the need for it. Ad hoc members are also welcomed when their expertise is warranted.

The team leader structurally has ultimate responsibility for the success of and adherence to the initiative. He or she will also serve as liaison to a reporting body (administration, oversight committee, etc.) as well as coordinator for all benchmarking activities. He or she must ensure that the initiative is viewed as ongoing and not a project with a specific time line. Even though milestones and specific successes during the journey are vital, benchmarking is a continuous process. The leader will be wise to reinforce this to all levels of management in the organization from the outset.

The facilitator often serves in either of two ways: as an internal team facilitator or as an external team facilitator. The internal facilitator is an individual who maintains guidance and order of the team meetings, but he or she may also actively participate in the planning, contacting, and implementation phases of the initiative. The external facilitator is an individual who is a passive participant; he or she only ensures adherence to the time and agenda of the meeting. The facilitator may, in either role, assist in a supporting function to the team (e.g., report generation, graphing, etc.).

External customers, who may be more difficult members of the team to involve completely, can give external expertise and insight into the existing process. Such insight can be extremely useful in designing the future process and in assisting in the creation of the benchmarking survey tool. The customer often is involved in an ad hoc capacity.

Internal customers should be integral team members because of their desire to impart improvement. Their input can include not only specifics relating to their department or services but also the perception of how one department interacts with another. The customers with the greatest process impact must be identified immediately and included as full team members.

Finally, the members are the core of the team. They are responsible for ensuring that the expectations set forth by the leader are met. Members will conduct the internal analysis, employ the benchmarking concepts, and develop and implement the action plan that results from the initiative. Basically, they are active participants in all facets of the process.

The Analysis

The team analyzes the benchmarking issues. The priorities are mandated from the top of the organizational hierarchy. Internal analysis is one of the key success drivers of the benchmarking journey. This analysis needs to be both quantitative and qualitative in nature. Quantitative measures in a department might include productivity, expense ratios, quality indicators, and service intensity. For example, a home health agency might analyze the following indicators:

- Productivity: Hours worked per client visit.
- Expense: Regional adjusted rate per hour; or expense per client visit.
- Quality: Routinely cancel or reschedule staff.
- Service Intensity: Total client visits per day or per year.

There are many possibilities, and some home health agencies may find the process more conclusive by looking at multiple indicators for a measure. Additionally, more comprehensive analysis assists the organization and process outcome by improving acceptance.

Qualitative measures such as brainstorming, nominal group technique, and cause-and-effect diagrams are extremely useful. These measures involve many of the guidelines of total quality management (TQM). Such methods include flowcharting processes, Pareto diagrams, run

charts, and control charts. These TQM tools assist in the analysis process not only by identifying many of the underlying problems but also by creating an environment that is conducive to teamwork.

Once the data have been collected and studied, an interview outline is helpful to guide the benchmarking process toward action planning. The outline is typically either a delineation of needs and expectations or a detailed questionnaire. The outline form will be determined by the methodology chosen to obtain answers to the process problems identified. The need to identify types of benchmarking candidates will drive the outline.

Searching for Benchmarking Candidates

The next step in the benchmarking process is to find external candidates with whom to benchmark, assuming that the organization has chosen to pursue either the global or the best-practice approach to benchmarking. Often, a well-designed process does exist within the organization itself. Starting internally is a good method for some basic departmental processes, but for true breakthrough thinking candidates should exist not only in a variety of locales but also in a variety of industries.

Insular thinking at this point can become a major hindrance. Department managers, and even administrators, should not view the industry as different in all regards. Truly dynamic organizations can look beyond the minutiae and perform benchmarking on a process-by-process basis. As mentioned earlier, an acceptance of minor data discrepancies is of paramount importance to success.

The benchmarking team must decide first the appropriate method and second how to find the contacts. The method will be based on factors such as available resources (time, money, and people), organizational goals (long and short term), and competitive pressures (other hospitals, home health agencies, hospice, or managed care). Finding the contacts will be a process of significant information gathering and analysis.

Benchmarking databases are an excellent start, but they do not give complete information. State and federal data are often confusing, and statistics may not have been captured identically. The team must identify a source and agree that it is reasonably acceptable, then attempt through professional organizations, known contacts in the industry, journals, and any other sources to find the best practice candidate.

Most teams wish to look at best practices, but in many industries, including health care, this can be difficult. For example, what measure or combination of measures signifies best practice: patient satisfaction, turnaround time, or low cost? The team needs to agree on these issues if best practice benchmarking is to be attempted. Additionally, discovering a best practice can be extremely cumbersome. No lists exist as to the best practice for a process that is universally accepted across the industry.

Global benchmarking is less exact than best practice but can definitely lead to the breakthrough thinking sought by benchmarking teams. Based on the data provided by national comparative databases or system-based databases, enough information can be gleaned to discover benchmarking partners for process improvement or redesign. The main issue with this methodology is the need for an "apples-to-apples" comparison. Many home health agencies take this philosophy one step further by looking for identical matches. The inherent danger in this view is simply that no two organizations are the same, if for no other reason than the people involved. Potential sources for any type of benchmarking contacts include the following:

- government publications (federal, state, or local)
- professional organizations and networks
- publications (health care and non–health care)
- the Joint Commission on Accreditation of Healthcare Organizations
- employees, suppliers, and customers (patients)
- past benchmarking partners

- consultants
- the media

The team can determine from this list which contacts are best for the organization's particular needs and how to design the interview methodology.

After the determination of potential benchmarking candidates, the team begins to develop an interview guide. The interview guide may take a variety of formats depending upon the volume of information sought from the different contacts. The standard formats for the purposes of benchmarking include a detailed interview guide and a simple questionnaire format. The latter can be targeted to specific contacts or can be sent as a general survey via fax or electronic mail. One or both of these formats can be used concurrently when the team is seeking information.

The detailed interview guide is useful when direct contact is made (i.e., telephone interview or site visit). The questions are open ended and require clarification and, occasionally, documentation. This is the best format for major changes in processes because it will yield the most information. Questions might include:

- What is your scheduling process?
- How is your Patient-Focused Care model defined?
- What were some strategies to decrease supply costs?

The simple questionnaire will yield some benefit, but the depth of information is often limited. The questionnaire is usually based on some supporting information as well as comparative data. This tool is useful in obtaining clarification in focused areas. The questionnaire should consist of questions that are concise and unambiguous. The author should read each question and ensure that none is open to interpretation. Questions are direct and clear and ask for information about the following parameters, for example:

- the number of patients served per month
- the number of admissions per month

- geographical service area (rural, suburban, or urban)
- percentage of managed care patients or visits
- type of clinical documentation (e.g., manual or computerized)

Questions may vary by candidate, but all should focus on a limited number of identified and prioritized processes. Once the methodology and survey tool(s) are established, the benchmarking candidates become contacts.

Making Contact

The establishment of a benchmarking team has given the initiative a formal body of authority. The team has performed the introspective analysis, developed appropriate tools for obtaining information, determined the approach, and chosen multiple contacts with whom to share information. At this point, the team is prepared to engage in a benchmarking contact. Three approaches to contact are common: fax or mail survey, telephone interview, or site visit. Each, like the format of the interview tool, will yield different levels of information. Additionally, all three methods are applicable when one is attempting a full-scale redesign effort.

Sending a survey to many respondents is the quickest method to obtain some rudimentary information. A large sample size (more than 30 contacts) is essential to ensure statistically significant results. This method for gleaning benchmarking information is relatively simple and inexpensive. Unfortunately, the responses must be unambiguous because clarification of answers is not possible. Additionally, the responses will yield little information. The survey should pose yes or no, scale-rated, or numerical type questions to minimize the potential for various interpretations. A final drawback is the response rate. A rate of 20 percent to 30 percent should be considered successful, so the number of questionnaires disseminated must ensure a rate that will meet the needs of the organization.

A telephone interview is another method for contacting benchmarking partners. Often, the telephone interview can be used in conjunction with the fax or mail survey as a means to obtain greater depth in an answer or simply clarification. The interview can yield responses that minimize information collection time and can be used to develop an action plan. Like the fax or mail survey, the telephone survey is inexpensive (from a materials standpoint) and can provide useful results. A major issue with this method, however, is time. Receiving return calls or setting aside blocks of time to initiate the interviews can be cumbersome. To ensure a positive experience, the interviewer should plan the conversation and make an appointment with the interviewee. Also, direct questions with little room for ambiguity can expedite the process. The interviewer must decide the level of detail that is expected to result from the telephone survey. Extremely detailed information might best be obtained through a site visit.

The site visit is the best method for obtaining the most comprehensive information. Also, this method enables multiple individuals to experience the benchmarking journey firsthand. Additionally, the quality of the information will be the highest. Not only can clarification be accomplished verbally, but it also becomes visual when the team is on site. This fact makes the site visit the most cogent and effective contact method for initiating change; a working model of a best (or better) practice is tangible.

This method is not without problems, however. Having a benchmarking team visiting multiple sites can be both time consuming and expensive. The team must establish the interview tool to ensure that the visit time and information are maximized. The team must also be aware of the specific elements that are sought. Simply put: Know what you are seeking before you go.

The benchmarking team must follow some universal rules while making external contacts. Basically, the interview process, whether it occurs on or off site, must be legal. The team must not attempt to partake in any questioning of improvement approaches that could be deemed illegal. A simple rule of thumb to allay any confusion is: Concentrate only on process improvement or design. Any questions that appear to be essential but may cause problems should be reviewed with legal council before partners are contacted.

A second important rule, and one that is more commonly broken, is confidentiality. Often, a team will obtain proprietary information from an organization. Such information cannot be reviewed or shared with the next benchmarking contact without express consent from the source. Because benchmarking is an information sharing process, the team might be the originating source of some information about its organization at one of the contacts. The team should expect the same respect and voice its opinion on how public the information truly is.

All three methods of contact enable the benchmarking team to obtain useful information to lay the foundation for creating an action plan. Before the creation of the action plan, the information gleaned must be collated and analyzed. Depending on the method of the benchmarking contact, many useful approaches to analysis can be used. Flowcharting can delineate new processes. Matrix charting can be used to create comparative analyses between the benchmarking organization and its contacts. Check sheets can tally the raw number of certain responses for use in prioritization of process design. Finally, any type of statistical analysis (e.g., run charts, regression analysis, etc.) can be employed to dissect the interview responses. Utilizing these tools enables the benchmarking team to organize the action plan.

Planning Action

Once the contact has been made and the information collated and dissected, the team is prepared to create the action plan. An important note is that benchmarking is not a report writing endeavor. The action plan should be an internally created road map of responses to the organization's needs. It should also be viewed as an

accountability tool. Assignments with milestones should be included to ensure timely implementation of the recommendations.

The first step in an organized approach to developing an action plan is to review some of the established elements. For instance, the needs of the organization should have been declared before the benchmarking journey ever commenced. Those needs flowed into process improvement initiatives. The improvements must affect the short- and long-term needs to make benchmarking successful. Ideas for improvement should also have been generated. During the contact phase, processes targeted for change were analyzed via the interview tool and the contact approach. These ideas should be varied enough to have created a pool of potential alternatives if the prioritized changes do not meet improvement expectations. Finally, the team members should always maintain solid communication so that the action plan will be an extension of planning that has occurred throughout the process.

The team now needs to assess how to prioritize the action planning steps. Issues to evaluate include ease of implementation (time, staffpower, and expenses), risks, financial objectives, impact on quality, and the political atmosphere. Through brainstorming and/or nominal group technique, an action plan can be developed by the team.

The plan needs to encompass the organizational needs, identified core and/or departmental processes targeted for improvement, implementation steps for creating new or redesigning existing processes, associated time frames to the action steps, force field type analysis, and the resulting financial impact. Embedded within the plan, assignments of either individuals or specific teams can be noted to maintain the necessary level of accountability throughout the implementation phase. A Gantt chart is an excellent tool to delineate both the time expectations and the assignments for each milestone. Final considerations in the creation of the action plan include how changes will be monitored (and calibrated when expectations are not met) and how various individuals, departments, or others will be affected by the changes, both positively and negatively.

Monitoring the changes involves creating a set of variables that can be tracked. For example, cost per unit, productivity, and patient satisfaction are all measurable indicators that can guide a team to its improvement objective. When indicators take an adverse turn, the team can know whether the changes should be calibrated. Sources for the indicators can be the monthly budget, spreadsheets in departments undergoing process improvement or reengineering, or a productivity monitoring system whereby the tracking is modified to allow trend analysis to delineate operational alterations. The team should meet to assess the data and ascertain what, if any, action should be taken.

The final facet of the action plan is the determination of how the implementation will occur. For instance, should the organization consider small-scale pilots of the recommendations, or is the implementation plan comprehensive enough to alter all departments or services affected by the recommendations? The approach to change must be considered carefully.

The change process resulting from benchmarking may gather skeptics throughout the process (i.e., those who say "We have always done it this way"). Small successes in most organizations are the best choice. Attempting to force change throughout the organization will lead to failure if the culture is not completely open to the suggestions and findings in the action plan. The team must communicate the objectives clearly and allow an "open book" policy around the action plan so that all parties either directly or indirectly involved will know the expected outcomes and the logic behind the plan. Many organizations, particularly those in health care, have a long tradition of order. Chaos, as change is often viewed, must be slowly integrated into the mindset. Constant updates and education will ensure better results and a greater level of buy-in.

The format of the action plan can be as basic or as detailed as needed. A sample format could consist of the following sections:

- a definition or listing of organizational needs
- team members
- issues that were chosen to benchmark
- a list of contacts and how they were chosen
- survey tool(s) used
- data analysis of findings
- team recommendations
- funding assumptions (dollars, time, and staff)
- integration plan with time table and team or individual assignments

The integration plan should also include an overview of how process improvement will be prioritized, potential issues, monitoring techniques, the methodology chosen to accomplish improvements (e.g., TQM), and any narrative that may be necessary to clarify outstanding issues. The communicated plan should also be embedded within the integration area.

This format is only a guide. The needs of the organization, as well as the acceptable time limitations, will also dictate how spartan or comprehensive the action plan will be. Furthermore, the action plan is by no means the result of the benchmarking journey. This plan should be a well-defined road map of the future. The team should constantly refer to the document to ensure timely progress and delivery of milestones. As mentioned earlier, this document is an ideal way to ensure accountability.

The overseeing body has to review the document to address any obvious pitfalls before it is presented to administration. Once the amendments, if any, are complete, buy-in has to occur at the top echelon. The change agents of the benchmarking journey must have solid support from the administration of the organization. The actual improvements outlined in the action plan, however, have to be driven by the owners and users of the process. Internally, the administration has to be willing to fund the changes to ensure that the journey has not been an exercise in report generation. Top-level support will make or break the implementation of the changes.

Implementing

Everything accomplished thus far has been directed toward planning. The action planning document is the device to begin making the changes that were proposed. This step in the benchmarking process is the point at which the journey will either succeed or fail.

As recommended earlier, organizations resistant to change should implement process improvement plans slowly and directly to ensure small victories for the benchmarking team. The credibility gap that may exist will gradually close. Also, administration has to initiate this phase by creating organizational awareness of the forthcoming initiatives as well as by clearly expressing support. The tone set before actual implementation can greatly diminish the magnitude of any dissension. It will also enhance the internal atmosphere by giving the employees the knowledge and ability to be active participants.

The methodology of implementing improvements or design strategies has to correlate closely with the action plan. This is why the plan can be simple or comprehensive; the degree of the need for change will drive the complexity of the benchmarking journey. If a good road map has been developed, the implementation of the changes becomes greatly simplified.

The approaches should involve many of the tools and techniques that are employed in any change or improvement endeavor: team establishment, flowcharting, statistical analysis (before and after), brainstorming, nominal group technique, or any other TQM methodology that a team believes applies to a particular situation. The body that oversees the progress of the benchmarking journey should maintain constant communication with teams established to carry out the changes delineated by the action plan. It must also guarantee that the time lines are met adequately. Each organization has to derive a method for maintaining accountability (e.g., incentive-based pay models). This assurance is another safeguard in the process to maintain progress and achieve completion of the action plan.

Regardless of the accepted time lines outlined by the plan, the teams and the administration have to be open to deviations in the course. Often, process improvement initiatives spawn new ideas that are noteworthy and should be considered. Flexibility in the implementation can be a difficult balance, but the success level can dramatically increase when teams are free to become independent and creative. A major objective of the oversight group becomes balancing the flexibility with the creativity. Even the best laid plans will overlook something.

Finally, the benchmarking journey is truly continuous, referring to the Spendolini (1992) definition. Once process improvement has been completed according to the action plan, continuous refinement, and potentially further benchmarking, will ensure that change will remain embedded in the organizational mindset and that teams will always be active participants in the long-term viability of the organization.

Maintaining

The changes initiated by the action plan have been implemented. The benchmarking team's new objective becomes twofold: Refine what has been accomplished, and instill continuous process improvement (CPI) into the refinements. Both the refinements and CPI should be based on the information provided by the monitoring indicators developed in the action plan. For instance, assume that the benchmarking journey led to major changes in the admissions process, a process that spans many departments and service lines. What are the indicators telling the team? Has cost per 100 admissions decreased? Productivity can also show results. What are the old and new ratios for hours worked per 100 registrations? Quality has to be considered throughout this process. Are the patients more satisfied with the admissions process after the modifications? Simple quantitative indicators can direct a team's effort more effectively.

The action plan can explain the indicators, but the owner of the process must maintain and interpret what the data are saying. When the indicators are moving in an adverse direction, the team must make major refinements in a timely fashion. The owner has to track the data at least on a biweekly basis so that the retrospective analysis will still be useful.

When changes are proven to be successful through the monitored data, the CPI aspect comes into play. What was done well and poorly in the modifications has to be noted so that the pitfalls are eliminated. The benchmarking team has to look for ways to maintain the gain (i.e., ways not to revert to prebenchmarked levels of performance). CPI is certainly the best method because it creates a process in constant evolution.

A final target for the improvements can be constantly to seek better performers so that a goal is never actually attained. If the process becomes a best-in-class effort, internally set hurdles should be placed to prompt the organization perpetually to seek a higher standard.

BENCHMARKING KEYS TO SUCCESS

The benchmarking journey is one of excitement and apprehension for an organization. The outcomes are dependent on adequate planning and execution. To ensure outcomes that exceed expectations, a number of keys to success should be considered during each phase of benchmarking:

- *Communicate the plan and progress.* Communication is an aspect of the journey that is vital. Administration must clearly convey the intentions of benchmarking as well as the goals of the organization. Additionally, a primary objective of the benchmarking team is ongoing communication

throughout the organization to instill a sense of continuity, build awareness of progress, and announce and celebrate successes.

- *Accentuate the benefits.* Inculcation of the benefits of the benchmarking journey must occur from the outset. An administrative champion should leverage benchmarking methodology as a continuous process that will enable the organization to reach its long-term objectives (e.g., financial viability, process improvements, competitive advantage, etc.). Tying the benefits to the organizational direction aligns the vision of all employees with that of administration.

- *Know yourself first.* Before contacting benchmarking partners, the team must fully understand those processes that are undergoing scrutiny. The outcome of the contact is directly dependent on the quality of the team's knowledge of the present departmental or organizational situation. Internal analysis should be detailed and complete to ensure the highest-quality outcome.

- *Maintain accountability.* An individual or team must be challenged with keeping the milestones and time frames on target. Also, the team or teams should conduct frequent but concise status checks. Expectations for each milestone must be clear and realistic so that goals are reachable.

- *Be open minded.* Whether a team leader, member, or administrative champion, all individuals involved in the process must understand the objectives of the benchmarking journey so that breakthrough thinking becomes the norm rather than the exception. Maintaining the realization that current processes may change dramatically is important to ensure success.

- *Document/record changes.* The individuals involved in benchmarking should document changes that are implemented. New process flowcharts or statistical analyses can provide immediate insight into the changes. Action can thus be immediate if further alterations are necessary, or celebration can occur when implementations meet or exceed expectations.

CONCLUSION

The benchmarking team must understand that the net goal is process improvement, not target setting. Managers often find themselves studying comparative or internal information only to set productivity or cost per unit targets prematurely. The contact that ensues is either a brief set of questions or a faxed questionnaire, both of which ask little about the process. The interview focuses solely on the comparative data (e.g., volumes, allocated costs, skill mix percentages, etc.). This does nothing to improve processes; rather, it gives a manager cause to question the comparative data. In the long run, the manager and the home health agency or hospice loses because the information obtained is of little value.

The power of benchmarking as a process improvement tool should be stressed. Setting goals is useful, but targets based on unadjusted numbers can be a dangerous precedent. The journey is time consuming and continuous, but the outcomes can be significant. Any process can be benchmarked, and any team can reap the benefits of this power tool.

REFERENCE

Spendolini, M. 1992. *The benchmarking book.* New York: AMACOM.

PART V

Management Issues in Home Health Administration

CHAPTER 33

Administrative Policy and Procedure Manual

Marilyn D. Harris

A current policy manual is essential for administration and service delivery of home health care. Webster's defines a policy as "providence or wisdom in the management of affairs; a definite course or method of action selected from among alternatives in light of given conditions to guide and determine present and future decisions; a high level overall plan embracing the general goals and acceptable procedures."

Rowland and Rowland (1992) advise that there are three general areas in nursing that require policy formulation: areas in which confusion about the focus of responsibility might result in neglect or malperformance of an act necessary to a patient's welfare, areas pertaining to the protection of patients' and families' rights (e.g., right to privacy and property rights), and areas involving matters of personnel management and welfare. Barnum and Kerfoot (1995) state that a policy is a guideline that has been formalized by administrative authority and directs action to some purpose. Policies should be revised periodically for efficiency, safety, and effectiveness. There are three major components in a policy system: a purpose, a policy rule, and an action directive or procedure. A procedure details the means to be used to achieve the ends specified in the purpose and further delineated in the policy (Barnum and Kerfoot, 1995). Perrow (1979) states that policy rules are necessary in complex organizations

because of such things as variability in personnel, clients, and environment. These policies delineate an area of freedom in which a staff member knows when he or she can make a decision. The absence of written policy leaves staff in a position where any decision they make may infringe upon an unstated policy and produce a reprimand.

Before any service is provided, an approved policy must be in place, according to §484.16 of the Medicare conditions of participation (COPs; Health Care Financing Administration, 1989). This policy gives direction to staff as to what services will be provided under what conditions. It also should state what is not provided and the rationale, if appropriate.

POLICY DEVELOPMENT

Multiple levels of agency personnel should be involved in revisions or deletions of policies from an agency's manual as well as in the development of new ones. The development of a policy can take several forms. For one, staff at all levels may identify a need to provide a specific service. This could be done through systematic logging of requests for a service that is not already available through the agency. Information can be gathered from staff as to the volume of requests for the new service and also as to the rationale. A review of the literature or contact with other agencies that provide the service and their success or failure rate with this service is also beneficial. If staff initiate the request for a policy, it can be anticipated that some preliminary homework has been done to substantiate the request.

For another, physicians or other referral sources may request that personnel perform a specific service. If the request is initiated from an outside source, staff who are knowledgeable in the specific procedure under discussion should be involved in the development of the policy. For example, pediatric nurse practitioners should be allowed to give input into development of pediatric-related policies, and nurses with expertise in intravenous administration should be involved with intravenous policies.

Finally, policies can be developed as a result of the internal quality assessment/performance improvement program. Specific areas may be identified through the quarterly record or utilization review process that could benefit from a new or revised policy.

ROLE OF THE PROFESSIONAL ADVISORY COMMITTEE IN POLICY DEVELOPMENT AND REVIEW

A professional advisory committee (PAC) is important for the delivery of home health care services for several reasons. For one, the Medicare COPs require a group of professional personnel (i.e., a PAC), for another, a PAC provides an array of professionals who can contribute their expertise to the formation and updating of service-related policies and procedures. Home health care staff at all levels of the organization should be familiar with the PAC and its responsibilities, membership, and manner of operation.

Section 484.16 of the COPs states:

A group of professional personnel, which includes at least one physician and one registered nurse (preferably a public health nurse), and with appropriate representation from other professional disciplines, establishes and annually reviews the agency's policies governing scope of services offered, admission and discharge policies, medical supervision and plans of treatment, emergency care, clinical records, personnel qualifications, and program evaluation. At least one member of the group is neither an owner nor an employee of the agency.

(a)   Standard: Advisory and evaluation function. The group of professional personnel meets frequently to advise the agency on professional issues, to participate in the evaluation of the agency's program, and to assist the agency in maintaining liaison with other health care providers in the community and in its community information program. Its meetings are documented by dated minutes.

Because this committee is required to meet frequently enough to carry out its responsibilities, the number of meetings each year will vary with the agency.

At the Visiting Nurse Association of Eastern Montgomery County/Department of Abington Memorial Hospital, the PAC is an important advisory committee to the board of trustees and staff. This group of experts has a vital interest in the agency and its services. The committee meets quarterly on a volunteer basis. A subcommittee of the PAC meets on an annual basis to complete the annual program evaluation. This annual report is submitted to the hospital's Professional Affairs Committee, which includes physicians, trustees, and administration, for review, discussion, and approval. It is also shared with the full PAC at the next scheduled quarterly meeting report. The report is shared with the hospital's board of trustees by the executive vice president/chief operating officer for final approval. A cover sheet that is signed by these two executives, the chair of the PAC, and the executive director is added to the front of the policy and procedure manual each year to verify that the manual has been reviewed and updated to reflect current practice.

POLICY REVIEW PROCEDURE

Policies can be reviewed on an ongoing basis so that all are reviewed annually. Existing clinical service policies should be reviewed by representatives from each discipline to ensure that they are in keeping with current professional standards. Comments and suggestions are then shared with the PAC or board. Other policies, such as admission and discharge criteria and personnel qualifications, should also be reviewed by appropriate committees from the governing body as well as by administrative staff. Still other clinical service policies may need to be reviewed by legal counsel (e.g., do not resuscitate policy). At other times, an agency may need or want to seek expert advice from an outside consultant, such as an insurance carrier, for related policies.

To make the best use of meeting time and to facilitate approval, copies of proposed policies or changes to existing policies should be mailed to the committee with the agenda before the meeting. If there is an age- or disease-specific policy, it is helpful to have a knowledgeable staff person discuss the change and the rationale with the professional on the committee who has expertise in this area (e.g., chemotherapy policy should be discussed with an oncologist). With this prior knowledge, this individual's support can be beneficial at the time of the meeting.

One important aspect of the development of sound policies is to include professionals and lay personnel with a wide array of expertise in multiple areas of current or projected services. This expertise should be available at the staff, contract, board, and PAC levels. All individuals, whether on a paid or volunteer basis, are interested in the agency they serve and the patients to be served by the agency.

Sound policies are important for several reasons, including risk management, meeting of state and federal regulations, and fulfillment of agency and professional standards. Once these policies are in place, they must be communicated and made available to all levels of personnel in the agency so that compliance is ensured.

APPROVAL PROCESS

The approval process can take several directions depending on the type of agency and policy. Ultimately, the governing body or individual is responsible for approval. This body may not have the expertise to develop or revise specific policies (e.g., use of infusion pumps). For Medicare-certified agencies, COP 484.16 requires that an agency have a group of professional personnel, many times referred to as a PAC. As noted earlier, the PAC is charged with establishing and reviewing the agency's policies related to scope of services, admission and discharge criteria, clinical records, and other related issues. The PAC should meet frequently enough to fulfill its responsibilities.

After review of the policies by the appropriate committee, recommendations are brought to the governing body for final approval via minutes and discussion by the administrative staff. Board committees and the governing body should meet on a scheduled basis that provides for timely approval of new or revised policies.

Each policy must be dated to reflect the date on which it was initiated, initially approved, and revised. All policies should be reviewed each year. The cover page, as described above, verifies that this review process is completed on a timely basis.

CONCLUSION

Although the final approval of the agency's policies rests with the governing body or individual, the recommendation for the development of new policies is a team effort. All levels of personnel within a home care agency should share ideas that will keep the agency current and competitive with other home care providers. Finally, approved policies must be communicated to all agency personnel and followed by those to whom they apply. An agency's policy and procedure manual does not belong on the library shelf. It should be readily available to all staff and referred to on a frequent basis by all levels of personnel.

REFERENCES

Barnum, B., and K. Kerfoot. 1995. *The nurse as executive.* 4th ed. Gaithersburg, MD: Aspen.

Health Care Financing Administration. 1989. *Part II. Medicare program. Home health agencies: Conditions of participation and reduction in recordkeeping requirements: Interim final rules* (42 CFR Part 484). Washington, DC: Government Printing Office.

Perrow, C. 1979. *Complex organizations.* New York: Random House.

Rowland, S., and B. Rowland. 1992. *Nursing administration handbook.* 3d ed. Gaithersburg, MD: Aspen.

CHAPTER 34

Discharge Planning

Joann K. Erb

Discharge planning is defined as "the process of activities that involve the patient and a team of individuals from various disciplines working together to facilitate the transition of that patient from one environment to another" (McKeenan, 1981, 3). Successful discharge planning requires a thorough understanding of the concepts described in this definition and attention to all these components as a plan is developed.

Discharge planning directly affects the delivery of services by home health agencies. To provide efficient, cost-effective care, home health agencies must have accurate information about the patient's living situation, caregivers, insurance, diagnosis, and plan of care. Equipment and supplies must be available, and patients and families must have received adequate education regarding postdischarge care. Absence of any of these factors compromises continuity of care.

Discharge planning consists of a series of well-defined steps to achieve continuity of care. Use of a decision-making model in this process acknowledges the multidimensional nature of the problem and the impact of a plan on all aspects of the patient–family–provider system. It also encourages involvement of the patient/family in the development of the plan, assists in formulation of reasonable goals, and identifies appropriate outcomes. This process promotes the movement of the patient along the health care system's continuum of care.

HISTORICAL DEVELOPMENT

The health care system in this country continues to be influenced by changes in society and advances in technology. Formal discharge planning programs developed in response to changes in both provision of and payment for health care services as well as changes in illness patterns and social supports for patients.

Before World War I, the sick were traditionally treated at home by the physician and cared for by the family. As medical technology advanced, the hospital became the center of the physician's practice, and the ill were treated primarily in hospitals. The entrance of large numbers of women into the workforce during World War II and a decline in the role of the extended family resulted in decreased availability of the family to care for sick members after hospital discharge. Interest in discharge planning as a method to reduce costs, lower hospital readmissions, and provide the patient with options spurred the development of discharge planning after World War II.

One early example of the interest in discharge planning was the Montefioro Hospital Care Program, the first hospital-based program, established in 1947. This program coupled physician home visits with visiting nurse services to produce a therapeutic environment for patients in their own home. This program highlighted the need for health care professionals to consider the patient's posthospital situation and develop a plan to extend the benefits of hospitalization after discharge.

The inception of Medicare in 1966 added legislative clout to the development of discharge planning as an essential component of patient care. Hospitals were required to provide some form of discharge planning as a condition of participation.

Implementation of the prospective payment system by the Health Care Financing Administration (HCFA) in 1984 caused heightened interest in discharge planning. No longer could hospitals submit a bill to Medicare at the end of a patient's hospitalization and receive full payment. Hospitals recognized that their financial stability, even their very existence, depended on their ability to care efficiently for patients and prevent unnecessary days of hospitalization. Since implementation of the diagnosis-related group system, hospitals have focused on the need to control patients' length of stay (LOS) to remain competitive. An institution's discharge planning program became the obvious means to address LOS issues.

Other societal changes that affect discharge planning include increased life expectancy and an increase in chronic illness. The "graying of America" has resulted in an increased number of elderly patients being served by the health care community. Although individuals older than 65 years represent 11 percent of the U.S. population, at any given time they occupy 40 percent of the hospital beds. From 1981 to 1994, the average LOS for those older than 65 decreased by 2.2 days, from 10.0 to 7.8 days (National Center for Health Statistics, 1996). Because of this decreased LOS and the slower recuperative powers of the elderly, more individuals now require some sort of posthospital care. They must rely on their elderly spouses and often on aging children to provide assistance and/or care, which may prove inadequate and taxing to the family unit.

"Quicker and sicker" became a widely heard phrase during the period after prospective payment as accusations were made that, to maintain financial security, the health care system was compromising patient welfare by discharging patients too early. As concern grew, Congress responded with legislation aimed at preventing early, unsafe discharge of Medicare patients. Section 9305, Improving Quality of Care with Respect to Part A Services (P.L. 99-509, 1986), required hospitalwide discharge planning services as a condition of Medicare participation. In June 1988, HCFA published regulations concerning the implementation of this legislation. For hospitals to be in compliance with this legislation, the American Hospital Association recommends the development of policies addressing when to discharge a patient, how to discharge a patient, and how to evaluate a patient's decision-making capability. In general, the focus should be early identification of patients needing intervention by the discharge planning team, designation of the hospital professionals who are responsible for dealing with potentially difficult discharges, and the general circumstances that must be met to discharge a patient appropriately.

The Joint Commission on Accreditation of Healthcare Organizations (Joint Commission) has also increased its emphasis on discharge planning. The 1995 edition of the *Accreditation Manual for Hospitals* (Joint Commission, 1995) includes standards that require hospitalwide policies and procedures on discharge planning with emphasis on early identification and intervention for patients with potential discharge problems. In addition, the standards require that hospital policies identify the role of the discharge planner in the initiation and implementation of the discharge plan and the interaction of other health care professionals. Collaboration of disciplines across the care continuum, inclusion of the patient/family in care planning, and provision of adequate education for the patient/family to meet ongoing health care needs are areas designated by the Joint Commission as essential for hospitals to ensure. Documentation of the discharge plan, including the availability of appropriate services to meet the needs of the patient, must be present in the medical record.

The new nursing care standards of the Joint Commission also address the importance of nursing involvement in discharge planning activities. One standard stipulates that assessments, identification of the patient's needs, and discharge planning activities be documented in the medical record. Other standards provide for development of programs and policies that describe how nursing care needs are assessed, evaluated, and met. Joint Commission standards now focus attention on how nurses collaborate with other disciplines in planning postdischarge care.

The American Nurses Association's *Standards of Clinical Nursing Practice* (1991) emphasize the importance of discharge planning as an essential component of the nursing process. McKeehan (1981) notes that, when the nursing standards are applied to patient care, discharge planning is inherent in the provision of patient care.

Third-party payers such as health maintenance organizations and preferred provider organizations have recognized discharge planning as a key element in cost containment. Some companies have attempted to assume the discharge planning function for their clients in an effort to ensure that care is provided at the most appropriate and cost-effective level. One potential problem with this system is that hospitals could face liability if the discharge plan developed by the insurer is inadequate or inappropriate. Hospitals are required to ensure that the patient's needs are met, and their ability to accomplish this may be diminished if cost containment is the primary determinant of the discharge plan. In addition, fragmentation and duplication of services may result if hospital staff and insurers are both responsible for arranging follow-up services. The hospital's ability to comply with the Joint Commission requirement for monitoring quality and appropriateness of the discharge plan may be adversely affected by sharing this responsibility with other parties.

As health care delivery systems have attempted to improve patient care while simul-taneously promoting cost-effectiveness, case management has emerged as an innovative model to accomplish these goals. Case management encourages collaboration by coordinating the care provided to the patient by many disciplines across the continuum. Review of the major goals of case management—quality of care, reduced LOS, continuity of care, resource utilization, and cost control—reveals that this model incorporates discharge planning at every level of involvement because the case manager has responsibility for the patient's outcomes over time.

CONCEPTUAL FRAMEWORK FOR DISCHARGE PLANNING

Discharge planning is based on the philosophy that patients are individuals with unique health concerns and have the right to coordinated discharge planning and that hospitals have the responsibility to provide discharge planning as an essential component of patient care. Key concepts include the following:

- a holistic approach to the patient and family and their ongoing involvement in the process
- integration of discharge planning at all points on the continuum of care
- philosophy and objectives of the institution that support the concept of discharge planning
- support and involvement of a multidisciplinary team that includes the physician
- education of health care professionals about available resources and criteria for services

GOALS AND OBJECTIVES OF DISCHARGE PLANNING

The goals and objectives of discharge planning are:

- to help patients return to or improve the level of functioning they experienced before hospitalization

- to ensure continuity of care in the transition from the hospital to the posthospital environment
- to promote cost-effectiveness and appropriate use of institutional and community resources

The discharge planning process affects not only the patient but also the hospital and community. Because acute care hospitals are now viewed as only one point on the continuum of care, the discharge planning process has been recognized as an essential element in patient care that contributes to the patient's progress along that continuum.

Because discharge planning affects three systems (patient, institution, and community), each system will have its own expectations.

Patient Expectations

Discharge planning must recognize the individuality of the patient and family and promote the development of a plan of care that recognizes and utilizes the resources of the patient and family. It must accurately identify the patient's needs and develop a plan to ensure continuity of care in the transition from the hospital to the posthospital environment. Discharge planning must educate the patient and family about the options available and encourage their participation in the decision-making process. It must promote attainment of the patient's maximal potential and personal dignity, and it must assist the patient and family in resuming control of their own welfare and educate them about the resources available to assist in that process.

Institutional Expectations

Discharge planning will promote quality patient care by providing a mechanism to identify a patient's needs and developing a plan to meet them. It will provide for cost-effectiveness by promoting early identification of high-risk patients, timely discharge, and reduction of inappropriate readmissions. The discharge plan-

ning process will educate health care professionals as to the structure and function of the process, how that process promotes compliance, and how available community resources are used to meet the needs of the patient. Discharge planning will promote holistic patient care by focusing attention on the impact of illness on the patient/family, and it will promote good public relations by demonstrating the institution's responsiveness to the needs of the patient.

Community Expectations

Discharge planning will provide needed services to individuals who are vulnerable from illness on their return to the community. It will promote use of health resources at the proper level and promote cost-effectiveness. Discharge planning will promote identification and use of community resources and will identify gaps in services and community needs, and it will promote linkages between health care institutions and community agencies.

COMPONENTS OF THE DISCHARGE PLAN

Patient/Family Involvement

The involvement of the patient and family in all aspects of plan development is essential to success. Because discharge planning occurs at a point in a patient's life when he or she is vulnerable, health care professionals must be sensitive to the patient's fears and supportive of his or her needs. Including the patient and family in the planning process demonstrates concern for them and affirms the patient's rights and responsibilities for his or her own health. By presenting alternatives and assisting the patient and family in choosing the best option for their situation, discharge planning affirms the dignity of the individual and helps ensure the success of the plan.

The most effective way to do this is by meeting with the patient and family as early as possible in the hospitalization. The discharge planner not only can become aware of the patient's unique situation but also can be identified as the individual in the hospital who is aware of the patient's postdischarge needs and is committed to providing a means to meet those needs. Early involvement also helps prevent the predischarge panic that some families feel as they realize the magnitude of the task ahead.

Family involvement in the planning stage helps identify any area of confusion or conflict and allows for resolution of problems before discharge. Families need to understand what resources, such as home care services or rehabilitation centers, are available and what the family's role in the patient's care will be. Families must have a realistic expectation of the patient's abilities and prognosis, and this requires open communication between the family and health care provider.

MULTIDISCIPLINARY COLLABORATION

Another essential component of the discharge planning process involves multidisciplinary collaboration. The primary physician must take a leadership role in moving patients along the continuum of care. Just as the physician is the gatekeeper for inpatient services, the physician's referral and plan of care are required for posthospital services. Rehabilitation facilities, long-term care facilities, and home care services all require physician input. Optimally, physicians will know which discharge planner is involved with their patients. For example, many hospitals assign discharge planners to a service or general area, such as orthopedics, oncology, cardiology, or surgery. The benefits of this model are that the discharge planners are aware of facilities and services for the specialty and are well known to both the physicians and the agencies providing postdischarge care. Ongoing communication with physicians is enhanced by use of a referral form, which can be used to document the ongoing development of the discharge plan. Another efficient method of

communication is the use of a computer system with the capability of isolating notes on plan development for easy access by the physician and other involved disciplines.

The importance of involving the primary nurse in discharge planning cannot be overstated. This is the individual who assesses the patient daily, interacts with the family, evaluates the patient's response to teaching, and identifies subtle changes in both patient and family. Part of the discharge planner's role is to educate nurses about requirements for reimbursement, available resources, and the cost of outpatient care. In addition, feedback about the success of past referrals for patients helps ensure continued cooperation. Also important, although less pleasant, is information about plans that did not work—those that resulted in readmission to acute care, a poor patient outcome, or delays in service. These discussions can help pinpoint what, if anything, went wrong and how a similar situation could be handled. Tips on documentation can also help the primary nurse meet Joint Commission requirements related to patient education and discharge planning.

Because of the complexity of a patient's needs, input from disciplines such as physical therapy, occupational therapy, speech therapy, nutrition support, and other departments is often necessary to establish a comprehensive discharge plan. This requires ongoing education of hospital departments as resources and regulations change. As described earlier, computer access to the discharge plan can allow efficient input from involved disciplines.

There has been much discussion in the past as to which discipline should be responsible for discharge planning. Traditionally, this was the responsibility of the social services department. As the need for home care services grew in response to decreased LOS, more nurses became involved to assess skilled care needs and develop a plan for services to meet them. Models of discharge planning are discussed later in this chapter, but it is imperative to state here that both nursing and social services are essential for successful discharge planning. The expertise of both disciplines is required to assist patients and families in achieving their goals. In this era of cost containment, it is imperative that turf issues not be allowed to hinder the discharge planning process. Coordination, collaboration, and communication between these two disciplines are prerequisites for success.

Although multidisciplinary involvement is essential for successful plan development, it may be confusing for the patient and family unless there is a designated person in the role of discharge planner with whom they can communicate in an ongoing manner. Lack of such a designated person can lead families to feel that "no one is in charge." In addition, families as well as patients need support, and this can be provided as the discharge planner involves the family in the development of the discharge plan.

RESOURCES

The availability of key resources will have a profound influence on a patient's discharge plan. If community resources are inadequate to support a patient in his or her own home, other options, such as the patient going to the home of a family member or being transferred to a boarding home, nursing home, or extended care facility, must be considered.

One important community resource for patients returning home after hospitalization is the home health agency. There has been a dramatic increase in the number of agencies since 1980, resulting in improved access to skilled home care services. New programs, such as 24-hour on-call availability and the ability to care for patients with high-technology needs, including home intravenous therapy and ventilators, have allowed more patients the option of returning home.

Unfortunately, access to unskilled services has not kept pace. Medicare does not cover custodial care, and therefore chronically ill patients with long-term needs cannot receive homemaker services under Medicare. These are the types of services that many chronically ill, elderly individuals require to remain in their own homes. Availability of low-cost supportive services varies by locality but is generally agreed to be insufficient.

Philadelphia is typical of many cities nationwide in the deteriorating access to affordable homemaker services. The *Philadelphia Inquirer* edition of September 12, 1991, reported the findings of the Philadelphia Health Management Corporation, a nonprofit research organization that followed 60 elderly patients upon discharge from Philadelphia hospitals (Kaufman, 1991). These patients had been identified as needing more assistance than the family could provide. The survey found, however, that 31 percent of those patients referred for homemaker services had received no in-home assistance 6 to 8 weeks after discharge. Even those individuals who received services generally received 5 hours a week, less than needed.

This lack of homemaker services has a dramatic effect on a patient's ability to remain independent and a family's ability to maintain a patient at home. Mundinger (1983) noted that between 25 percent and 50 percent of nursing home patients could be maintained at home with supportive services. This lack of adequate homemaker services may require implementation of a discharge plan that is contrary to patient and family wishes, such as a change in living situation.

The availability of senior transportation services, adult day care, Meals-on-Wheels, hospice, and respite care influences the discharge plan. Transportation services provide free or low-cost transportation for eligible individuals. Elderly patients who require frequent medical follow-up or outpatient services may not be able to manage if a transportation service is unavailable. Even when senior transit is available, patients may encounter problems. For example, in Pennsylvania, senior transportation services do not cross county lines. If a patient resides in one county and needs to travel to the next county for physician visits or services, the senior transport cannot provide services. Also, not all transport services are equipped to assist physically handicapped individuals, the very group most in need of them.

Adult day care is another service that influences patients' discharge disposition. These programs provide structured, supervised activities for individuals who are unable to be left alone for long periods of time. These programs offer an alternative to institutionalization by providing care during the time when caregivers work. They may provide enough of a respite to caregivers to enable them to continue caring for the individual at home. Problems arise, however, if the patient is receiving skilled services under Medicare because attendance at day care negates the homebound status required by Medicare for service. Thus a family may be forced to choose between day care and the continuation of skilled services, including home health aide services.

Another supportive service that benefits many elderly individuals is the Meals-on-Wheels program. This program can provide an option to individuals who are unable or unwilling to do their own cooking. Programs vary in style and cost; they may be too expensive for individuals on a limited income, and they may not be able to provide special diet needs.

The ability of families to care for a terminally ill individual often hinges on the availability of a hospice or palliative care program. These programs offer skilled, Medicare-covered care and supportive services, including volunteers, chaplains, and a multidisciplinary team approach to the care of the dying. The focus is symptom control and support to the patient and family members.

Respite care is the provision of temporary relief to the caregivers of the chronically ill. Some facilities provide short-term inpatient care to allow the family temporary relief of the burden of caring for chronically ill members.

The availability of all these community services influences the development of the discharge plan. An individual who might otherwise be destined for nursing home placement may be able to be maintained at home with community services. Cost is an important consideration, however, because many elderly on fixed incomes may not be able to afford the regular supportive services that they need to stay at home. Because unskilled services are not covered by Medicare but rather are usually funded through state programs, access varies considerably from area to area. Urban areas are more likely to provide a wider range of services than rural areas. It is imperative that discharge planning professionals remain aware of community resources and educate patients, families, and health care providers of their existence.

Thus far, the discussion of resources has focused on services available to patients returning home. Other factors that must be considered during the discharge planning process include availability of rehabilitation centers, skilled nursing facilities, nursing homes, drug and alcohol treatment centers, and vocational training centers. Because acute care institutions are just one point of care on the health care continuum, access to other specialty facilities promotes optimal patient care. Access can be hindered by availability or reimbursement considerations. Discharge planning professionals must be cognizant not only of the existence of such programs but also of their financial and medical requirements and must serve as a resource to health care providers.

REGULATIONS

Another essential element that affects the discharge planning process is the regulations affecting the delivery of health care in general and discharge planning in particular. As discussed earlier, Medicare legislation has had a tremendous effect on health care delivery, and regulations initiated for the Medicare population have often been used by other third party payers. Medicare's influence has not always been positive, however, because Medicare has encouraged the use of a medical model in the care of the elderly when most of the elderly's needs are social or nursing related. To qualify for any unskilled services under Medicare, the elderly must be eligible for skilled services. It is important that professionals involved in discharge planning be active in influencing the development of future legislation and in educating society about the consequences of proposed legislation.

INTEGRATION OF DISCHARGE PLANNING ACTIVITIES

The final element affecting the discharge planning process is the integration of discharge planning activities into all aspects of health care delivery by primary providers. This requires consideration of the significance of illness for patients and families and the need to plan for postillness care. Physicians in particular, as gatekeepers of the health care system, must recognize that the health care delivery system is a continuum and that a patient's progress along that continuum requires planning and multidisciplinary cooperation that includes the patient and family. As noted earlier, increased use of case management by both hospitals and third-party payers to coordinate care and manage cost has incorporated discharge planning as an essential step in moving the patient along the continuum of care.

RESEARCH RESULTS

Recent research efforts have focused on the elderly as a population that would benefit from specific discharge planning programs, and studies have yielded results significant to all discharge planners. Dugan and Mosel (1992) described a review of medical records for 101 patients aged 75 years or older. One disturbing finding was that 43 patients had no documentation of discharge planning activities. Equally alarming was the finding that patients living alone were least likely to receive support services after discharge, whereas those living with a spouse were most likely to receive them. This finding supports the idea that, without family to advocate for them, many elders do not get information about possible postdischarge services.

Haddock (1991) also targeted the frail elderly as a population at risk for postdischarge difficulties as a result of their more complex needs and often fewer resources. This research studied the relationship between the structure of discharge planning programs and patient outcomes. Analysis of results revealed that institutions with more highly structured discharge planning programs were associated with significantly greater provision of services and greater patient satisfaction. A focused admission assessment tool and a formal postdischarge follow-up program were identified as two important factors in promoting positive patient outcomes in this study.

An innovative program aimed at the population 75 years old and older was described by Aldridge (1990). A major premise of this program is that the frail elderly require more intensive postdischarge care than younger patients but that, with a longer rehabilitation period, many patients can progress to less restrictive environments. Premature institutionalization may result if an individual's activities of daily living ability at discharge is the only factor considered in developing the long-term plan. This project, a joint effort of the Denver Regional Council of Governments, the Colorado Hospital Association, and the Colorado Association of Homes and Services for the Aging, utilized the interventions of a housing counselor specialist in planning and follow-up of the postdischarge disposition of this population. Because the counselor followed the patient for 2 months after discharge, he was able to revise the plan of care toward more independent housing as the patient's condition improved. The results of this study showed there was a 21 percent decrease in the number of discharged individuals remaining in nursing homes 8 weeks after discharge and an increase in those persons going home. The potential benefits of such a program, both financial and in terms of patient satisfaction, should prompt further attention to this type of service.

Elderly patients were also the subject of a study by Naylor and colleagues (1995) that was designed to use the expertise of a gerontologist nurse specialist in the development of a comprehensive discharge plan. The results indicated that the use of this specialist helped reduce the number of rehospitalizations and the cost of postdischarge care in the study period. Results also supported the need for intensive services in the first few weeks after discharge because of the decline in function experienced during hospitalization. These services can prevent costly rehospitalizations, promote good patient outcomes, and reduce costs for the Medicare patient.

Research has also shown that information needed by home care agencies is often not provided. A study by Anderson and Helms (1993) revealed that pertinent information about the patient and family was frequently omitted in referrals. The results also indicated that the model of discharge planning used did make a difference and that liaison nurses provided the greatest amount of data. Based on the results of a follow-up study, these same investigators (1995) proposed the adoption of a standardized referral form for all patients referred for postdischarge services that includes nursing, medical, and psychosocial information as well as demographic and financial data.

STEPS IN THE DISCHARGE PLANNING PROCESS

Assessment

This process involves identification of patients who will require assistance in planning for postdischarge disposition and evaluation of the patient's medical and nursing needs as well as psychosocial and financial resources. Because of diagnosis-related groups and the resultant decrease in LOS, this phase of the discharge planning process has grown in importance. Prompt identification of patients requiring intervention by discharge planners promotes development of a suitable plan and timely discharge.

To accomplish this step effectively, discharge planning professionals must have open access to all patients. They must be able to screen patients and begin to develop a plan without a physician's order. Screening activities include the use of patient care rounds and high-risk criteria to identify those needing intervention.

High-risk criteria have helped quickly identify patients who may need the involvement of the discharge planner. Some high-risk criteria commonly used in screening are as follows:

- age older than 65 to 70 years
- lives alone or with poor support systems
- life-threatening illness (e.g., cancer, acquired immunodeficiency syndrome)
- conditions requiring a change in lifestyle (e.g., cerebrovascular accident, amputation)
- disease conditions requiring instruction or supervision after discharge (e.g., colostomy, open wound, cardiac or respiratory disease, insulin-dependent diabetes mellitus)
- suspected abuse or neglect
- admitted from nursing home
- multiple readmissions or history of disposition problems

In an effort to refine further the screening of patients for discharge planning needs, unit-specific criteria have been developed. These include criteria for neurological, surgical, pediatric, and orthopedic units.

The purpose of using high-risk screening criteria is to identify patients quickly and reduce the possibility of patients "falling through the cracks." Even though high-risk criteria are becoming more sophisticated and sensitive, there is still the chance that patients will not be identified. All professional personnel, and nurses in particular, must be alert to identify patients who require discharge planning activities and refer them to the appropriate person in a timely manner.

Tools have also been developed to assist in the identification of patients. These include a screening tool used by primary nurses, a form filled out by the patient or family on admission, and an assessment form completed for patients in the preadmission phase. More and more health care professionals, however, are concerned about the vast amounts of time spent by various disciplines in documentation of the same data. The ideal would be a multidisciplinary assessment form that includes self-reported information from the patient and family that could be used by all disciplines, including the discharge planner, and a form that could follow the patient from one point of service to the next.

Patient care rounds are invaluable in alerting the discharge planner of patients needing intervention who may not be identified by screening alone. An ideal example is a daily meeting involving the discharge planner, social worker, and primary nurses in which every patient on the unit is discussed briefly. This may sound impossible to achieve and would require intensive education of primary nurses about the information needed, but with practice it could be accomplished in a 20-minute session and could be done in walking rounds, with those involved meeting briefly with each primary nurse. In the long run, it is much more efficient than the frantic Friday afternoon phone call concerning the fragile patient suddenly discharged to an unprepared family.

The second part of the assessment involves the evaluation of community resources available to meet the patient's needs. Availability of skilled nursing facilities, rehabilitation centers, nursing homes, and home care services, as well as the patient's eligibility for them, must be identified.

Planning

Once a thorough assessment has been completed, planning can be initiated. The goal should be to return the patient to the least restrictive environment possible to promote the most independent level of functioning. The plan should include short-term and long-term goals,

and reflect a mechanism to adapt the plan to changes in the patient's condition. As discussed earlier, family involvement results in the most successful discharge plan. This is especially true when a patient has been referred for high-technology therapy at home.

High-Technology Therapy

Advances in technology and the impetus for early discharge have combined to foster the development of an entire industry devoted to caring for patients with high-technology needs. For example, intravenous therapy, including antibiotics, pain control, and hydration, can be managed in the home via peripheral lines and central access devices. Enteral feedings are routinely delivered in the home setting via percutaneous endoscopic gastrostomy (PEG) tubes, duofeed tubes, and other types of gastrointestinal tubes. Feedings may be delivered by gravity pumps or, more commonly, by enteral feeding pumps. Recent advancements in equipment design have enabled home management of apnea monitors and home ventilators. These treatment modalities have become more common in recent years, and patients are being maintained for longer periods of time in the home setting.

Numerous companies have specialized to meet the growing need for high-technology care in the home and also to take advantage of what can be a lucrative business opportunity. Many of these companies provide not only the necessary equipment and supplies but also the personnel to train family members. Professionals from the supply company may take responsibility for the teaching provided to the patient and family before discharge as well as for providing regular in-home education and supervision. Many companies offer 24-hour coverage for troubleshooting and responding to emergencies.

High-technology therapy at home has become much more common as the cost-effectiveness of such treatment has been documented. Because of the financial benefits to insurers, many patients and families will be presented with, and even encouraged to accept, a plan of this kind. Cost should never be the sole deciding factor in the development of a plan, however. The discharge planner, as a patient advocate, has a responsibility to elicit the family's concerns and make a professional assessment of each family's ability to assume this added responsibility. Families may be pressured by health care providers and insurers to accept a plan that realistically they are incapable of carrying out. Many high-technology therapies, such as home ventilation or continuous intravenous therapy, require 24-hour supervision and a high degree of psychomotor skill. The family of any patient being evaluated for such therapies in the home setting must receive comprehensive instruction about the commitment and responsibilities involved before an informed decision can be made. The family members must also be evaluated for their ability to cope with this added stress. The availability of a primary caregiver is essential for successful management of high-technology therapy in the home setting. Finally, the environment of any patient being considered for high-technology therapy must be evaluated before the plan is instituted. The environment must have adequate space, have proper electrical equipment, and, most important, be free of substance abuse. Because many of these therapies will place equipment such as syringes and needles in an individual's home, safety must be ensured for the patient and family.

Implementation

Implementation of the discharge plan involves making the referral for follow-up care, if needed, and coordinating continuity of care in the transition. For patients who will be receiving home care services, the referral should be made before discharge. Information about the course of hospitalization, the medical and nursing plan of care, medications, and follow-up is essential to the home care agency. If a patient will require complex treatment at home, it may be necessary for the home care nurse to visit the patient in the hospital and educate him or her

before discharge. Because this may require time to arrange, a home health agency should be given ample notice of the discharge date. Continuity of care can be ensured only by thorough, timely communication.

Because home care personnel lack access to the medical record, the referral should include as much information as possible about the patient's history and treatment. It is also important to provide families with written information about follow-up services, including the names and telephone numbers of the agencies involved, the type of services and start dates, and the name of a contact in case of problems.

If a patient is to be transferred to another institution, such as a nursing home or rehabilitation center, the initial communication can take place verbally, but a written referral with pertinent information and a copy of the patient's chart should accompany the patient at the time of transfer.

Evaluation

The final stage in the process is the evaluation of the plan for appropriateness and effectiveness. This phase may be more difficult than it appears because it is easy to "forget" patients once they are discharged. For the discharge staff to evaluate the plan, adequate documentation must have occurred. Documentation should be ongoing and should include elements of the plan as they develop. Effective documentation is concise and thorough and outlines the options available and the patient's and family's response and preference. At the time of discharge, a summation note that includes disposition, agencies involved, and services to be provided will facilitate evaluation.

In evaluating the plan, some pertinent factors to consider are as follows:

- Was the plan appropriate for that patient and his or her unique situation?
- Was there adequate coordination with posthospital providers?

- Did the patient and family participate in the plan development, and were they satisfied with the outcome?
- Did the plan provide continuity of care in the transitional period?

For these questions to be answered, data must be collected. Some techniques that can be used in data collection are direct contact with the patient after discharge by means of telephone surveys and written questionnaires, feedback from the agencies providing services after discharge, and ongoing communication with patients, agencies, and physicians. The degree of sophistication utilized depends on the resources available to the discharge planning department. Even departments with limited resources can accomplish the evaluation procedure by using trained volunteers or clerical staff to collect data as long as the selection is random and the sample size is adequate.

DISCHARGE PLANNING MODELS

Numerous organizational models exist for discharge planning programs. There is no perfect model, and the best model for each particular institution depends a great deal on the institution itself. Hospitals are all unique, with different structures and power bases, and the placement of the discharge planning program should be where it will be most successful in that organization. Three of the most common sites for discharge planning departments are the social work department, the nursing department, or a separate department under administration. Wherever the placement, the process must be a multidisciplinary one.

Until recently, social work was traditionally responsible for discharge planning in acute care hospitals. Changes in health care delivery, however, have necessitated an increased understanding of sophisticated medical treatment and the skilled care needs of patients for the development of an effective plan. This requires increased involvement by nursing.

Fullan (1996) describes Abington Memorial Hospital's recent incorporation of team-centered discharge management as the most effective way to permit easy identification of and intervention for patients who require discharge planning services. Begun in July 1994, this model employs daily scheduled meetings of discharge planning nurses, social workers, and unit nurses to screen newly admitted patients and to discuss care needs of previously identified patients. At the same time that this was occurring in discharge planning, managed care insurers were making increased demands on utilization review, and reviewers were being shifted from Medicare to managed care reviews. Because the discharge planning nurses had been reviewing most of the Medicare charts because of the hospital's high-risk screening criteria, the decision was made to cross-train these nurses in utilization review. This resulted in reduced duplication; these nurses now perform utilization review and discharge planning for home care services for Medicare patients simultaneously.

The joint form used by these nurses for utilization review and discharge planning is shown in Exhibit 34–1; the form in Exhibit 34–2 is used only for a prolonged stay. When a referral is made for home care services, a copy of this form, as well as a copy of the computer generated Kardex, which is updated every shift, and the patient's demographic sheet is sent to the home care agency. Use of these forms prevents needless duplication, ensures accuracy of information, and provides the home care agency with a thorough database on which to base care.

The goals of this program are to identify patients needing discharge planning within 24 hours of admission, to assign responsibility to the discharge planning nurse or social worker based on the patient's needs, and to promote team communication related to changes in the patient's condition and discharge needs. This new model resulted in a dramatic drop in LOS for Medicare patients in the first month of the operation of team-centered discharge management.

Exhibit 34–1 Abington Memorial Hospital Case Management Review/Referral Form

Patient I.D. Label	Ins.	LCD.		D/C
	Tel. #	Date due		

Ins. Ref. # _____

Primary Diagnosis_____ Lives with: _____

Secondary Diagnosis_____ Allergies: _____

_____ P.M.H._____

Procedure/Date _____   _____

_____

ADMISSION REVIEW DATE _____ INITIALS _____ INS. REVIEWER _____

Clinical findings/Studies: _____

_____

_____

_____

_____

_____

_____

_____

_____

Treatment: _____

_____

_____

_____

_____

_____

_____

_____

_____

_____

continues

Exhibit 34–1 continued

HOME CARE REFERRAL

Address change: H.C. Consent: _____

_____   Initial Visit: _____

_____   LMD/Phone# _____

_____   Ht/Wt: _____

Home Services: Nsg ____ PT ____ MSW ____ SP ____ OT ____ HHA ____ HOSPICE _____

CR Assess _____ Med. Teaching _____ Diabetic Teaching _____ Diet Teaching _____

Please see Kardex and/or Discharge Instructions for Discharge Meds.

Specifics: Labs, Wound Care, Ostomy, Foley, etc.: _____

_____

_____

_____

_____

_____

Equipment ordered/from/phone#: _____

_____

_____

_____

_____

_____

Condition on discharge _____

_____

_____

_____

T _____ P _____ R _____ BP _____ Lungs _____

I certify this patient is essentially homebound and requires professional services related to the diagnoses stated above and/or the condition for which the patient was recently hospitalized.

CM _____ Date _____   _____
                                         Physician's Signature

Exhibit 34–2 Continuation of Case Management Review/Referral Form for Extended Stay

Patient I.D. Label	Ins.	LCD.		D/C
	Tel.#	Date due		

CONTINUED STAY REVIEW   DATE: _____ INITIALS: _____ INS. REVIEWER _____

Clinical findings/Studies with dates and results: _____

_____

_____

_____

_____

_____

_____

_____

Intensity of service/Treatments (Dates begun and ended): _____

_____

_____

_____

_____

_____

_____

_____

CONTINUED STAY REVIEW DATE: _____ INITIALS: _____ INS. REVIEWER _____

Clinical findings/Studies with dates and results: _____

_____

_____

_____

_____

_____

_____

continues

Exhibit 34–2 continued

Intensity of service/Treatments (Dates begun and ended): _____

_____

_____

_____

_____

_____

_____

CONTINUED STAY REVIEW DATE: _____ INITIALS: _____ INS. REVIEWER _____

Clinical findings/Studies with dates and results: _____

_____

_____

_____

_____

_____

_____

_____

_____

Intensity of service/Treatments (Dates begun and ended): _____

_____

_____

_____

_____

_____

_____

_____

_____

_____

_____

_____

Courtesy of Abington Memorial Hospital, Abington, Pennsylvania.

QUALITY ASSURANCE IN DISCHARGE PLANNING

Quality assurance can be defined as a process in which standards of care are identified, observed, and measured to ensure the achievement of proper standards; the goal of quality assurance is to make certain that care practices will produce satisfactory patient outcomes. Quality assurance activities can be viewed as an extension of the evaluation phase of the discharge planning process because quality assurance activities also focus on the quality and suitability of the discharge plan. Outcome criteria include:

- patient/family satisfaction and compliance with the plan
- appropriateness of the plan and adequacy of information provided by the hospital discharge planner
- quality of the services delivered to the patient by the posthospital provider

There are other outcomes of interest to the institution that should also be evaluated, such as:

- LOS and decreased discharge delays
- decreased readmissions due to inadequate discharge plans
- improved coordination and efficiency in service delivery and decreased duplication of effort

In addition, quality assurance addresses the process of discharge planning. Examples of criteria that evaluate the process include the following:

- the procedure for timely identification of patients requiring discharge planning activities
- the timeliness of response to referrals for discharge planning
- evidence of patient/family involvement in plan development
- documentation of physician involvement in discharge planning
- documentation of interdisciplinary communication and collaboration

- integration of discharge planning activities into all health care delivery by all disciplines

The objective of a quality assurance plan is to identify areas of deficiencies, make data available to aid in developing solutions to problems, and improve the quality of patient care.

ETHICAL ISSUES IN DISCHARGE PLANNING

Prospective payment for hospitals and diminished community resources have caused changes in health care delivery that can result in ethical dilemmas for discharge planning personnel. As hospitals are pressured to decrease LOS to maintain financial solvency, the frail elderly are increasingly being discharged "quicker and sicker." At the same time, more stringent interpretation of the Medicare home care benefit has resulted in reduction in eligibility for home care services. Tightening restrictions have also decreased the availability of nursing home care under Medicare. The vise is closing, and the victim is the patient.

Concepts such as the inherent dignity of individuals, the right to self-determination, and access to optimal health care may be in conflict with an environment created by prospective payment and inadequate community resources. Discharge planning professionals, whose practice has been guided by ideals that protect the rights of individuals at a vulnerable period in their lives, are being required to facilitate discharge of patients without having adequate community resources available for postdischarge care.

This is a major stressor for discharge planners as they realize that the plans they have developed are inadequate or only temporary solutions to patients' problems. One common situation is that a frail, chronically ill elderly individual will be hospitalized with an exacerbation of a chronic condition. Because the patient has been acutely ill, he or she often will qualify for short-term home care services. Because Medicare does not cover custodial care, however, once the patient is stabilized he or she must be discharged from home care services. Discharge planners may make referrals for home care services realizing that these services are short term and that there is inadequate long-term care for the majority of patients who need it.

Another example of an ethical dilemma that discharge planners face is that of a patient being discharged with complex care needs, such as pump-regulated enteral feedings, Hickman catheter, or home ventilator. These patients no longer require hospital-level care and want to return home, but they may not have the necessary support from family or community agencies.

As health maintenance organizations and preferred provider organizations become more interested in discharge planning as a means to control costs, discharge planners may be faced with attempts by providers to implement a discharge plan that is primarily motivated by financial considerations. This will require vigilance by discharge planning professionals to protect the best interest of the patient.

Because these problems are complex, multifaceted solutions must be sought. Community agencies need to be responsive to the needs of complex patients, expand services, and educate staff to care for these patients. Hospitals need to be made aware of limitations in community resources and assist in planning solutions. Families need to have sound education in the care of complex patients and the equipment used by such patients. Most important, discharge planning professionals must join forces and lobby for programs to ensure availability of care to those who need it.

INTERFACE WITH THE HOME HEALTH AGENCY

As noted at the start of this chapter, discharge planning has a strong effect on the home health agency. Lack of coordination of services can result in omission or duplication of services. An incomplete referral results in agency providers attempting to provide quality care without adequate data. Because the patient's well-being depends on the care delivered by the home health agency, it is imperative that discharge planners provide thorough, accurate information at the time of the initial referral.

Discharge planners need feedback on the quality of the plans that they develop and areas that need attention. Home health agencies that maintain close contact with referring institutions can alert discharge planners to problem areas and also to changes in the medical and social conditions of patients referred. This information assists in refining discharge plans if the patient is readmitted.

CONCLUSION

Discharge planning is a multifaceted process that seeks to promote optimal care for patients in the transition from one point on the health care continuum to another. Prospective payment for hospitals has resulted in increased attention to discharge planning as a means to reduce LOS while promoting optimal patient outcomes. Multidisciplinary cooperation, communication, and collaboration and the involvement of the patient and family in the development of the discharge plan are key elements in the discharge planning process. This process consists of four stages: assessment, planning, implementation, and evaluation. Discharge planning programs need a formal evaluation procedure to identify areas of weakness and develop strategies to improve delivery of services. Discharge planners must educate health care professionals, patients, families, and communities about the services available and the limitations and gaps in service.

REFERENCES

Aldridge, S. 1990. Counselor intervention enhances life, reduces costs. *Discharge Planning Update* 10:3–9.

American Nurses Association (ANA). 1991. *Standards of clinical nursing practice.* Kansas City, MO: ANA.

Anderson, M.A., and L. Helms. 1993. An assessment of discharge planning models. *Orthopedic Nursing* 12:41–49.

Anderson, M.A., and L. Helms. 1995. Communication between continuing care organizations. *Research in Nursing and Health* 18:49–57.

Dugan, J., and L. Mosel. 1992. Patients in acute settings: Which health-care services are provided? *Journal of Gerontological Nursing* 18:31–35.

Fullan, R. 1996. Team-centered discharge management: On a fast track to performance improvement. *Continuum* 15:1, 3–9.

Haddock, K. 1991. Characteristics of effective discharge planning programs for the frail elderly. *Journal of Gerontological Nursing* 17:10–13.

Joint Commission on Accreditation of Healthcare Organizations. 1995. *Accreditation manual for hospitals*. Chicago: Joint Commission.

Kaufman, M. 1991, September 12. After hospital care needs of elderly not being met. *Philadelphia Inquirer*, Section B, p. 9.

McKeehan, K., ed. 1981. *Continuing care: A multidisciplinary approach to discharge planning*. St. Louis: Mosby.

Mundinger, M. 1983. *Home care controversy*. Gaithersburg, MD: Aspen.

National Center for Health Statistics. 1996. *Health, United States, 1995* (DHHS Pub. No. [PHS] 96-1232). Washington, DC: Government Printing Office.

Naylor, M., et al. 1995. Comprehensive discharge planning for the hospitalized elderly. *Annuals of Internal Medicine* 120:999–1006.

SUGGESTED READING

American Hospital Association (AHA). 1974. *Discharge planning for hospitals*. Chicago: AHA.

American Hospital Association (AHA). 1984. *Guidelines for discharge planning*. Chicago: AHA.

American Hospital Association (AHA), Society for Hospital Social Work Directors. 1985. *Discharge planning statement*. Chicago: AHA.

Beck, L., et al. 1993. Use of the code of ethics for accountability in discharge planning. *Nursing Forum* 28:5–12.

Bull, M. 1994. A discharge planning questionnaire for clinical practice. *Applied Nursing Research* 7:193–207.

Bull, M. 1994. Elder's and family members' perspectives in planning for hospital discharge. *Applied Nursing Research* 7:190–192.

Congdon, J. 1994. Managing the incongruities: The hospital discharge experience for elderly patients, their families, and nurses. *Applied Nursing Research* 7:125–131.

Cooke, P., and J. Alley. 1992. Discharge planning: Whose responsibility is it? *Caring* 11:28–32.

Farren, E. 1991. Effects of early discharge planning on length of hospital stay. *Nursing Economics* 9:25–30.

Haddock, K. 1994. Collaborative discharge planning: Nursing and social service. *Clinical Nurse Specialist* 8:248–253.

Hansen, J. 1966. *Continuity of nursing care from hospital to home*. New York: National League for Nursing.

Houghton, B. 1994. Discharge planners and cost containment. *Nursing Management* 25:78–80.

Jackson, M. 1994. Discharge planning: Issues and challenges for gerontological nursing. *Journal of Advanced Nursing* 19:492–502.

Jones, S., et al. 1995. Changing behaviors: Nurse educators and clinical nurse specialists design a discharge planning program. *Journal of Nursing Staff Development* 11:291–295.

Lowenstein, A., and P. Hoff. 1994. Discharge planning: Study of staff nurse involvement. *Journal of Nursing Administration* 24:45–50.

Luken, P. 1991. Hospital-based discharge planning. *Caring* 10:18–23.

McWilliams, C., and C. Wong. 1994. Keeping it secret: The costs and benefits of nursing's hidden work in discharging patients. *Journal of Advanced Nursing* 19:152–163.

Nash, T. 1988. What's new about the new discharge planning standards? *Discharge Planning Update* 8:1, 11–13.

Naylor, M. 1990. Comprehensive discharge planning for the elderly. *Research in Nursing and Health* 13:327–347.

Naylor, M., and E. Shaid. 1991. Content analysis of pre- and post-discharge topics taught to hospitalized elderly by gerontological clinical nurse specialists. *Clinical Nurse Specialist* 5:111–115.

Pray, D., and J. Hoff. 1992. Implementing a multidisciplinary approach to discharge planning. *Nursing Management* 23:52–56.

Robinson, J., et al. 1992. Balancing quality of care and cost-effectiveness through case management. *American Nephrology Nurses Journal* 19:182–187.

Schneider, J.K. 1992. Clinical nurse specialist: Role definition as discharge planning coordinator. *Clinical Nurse Specialist* 6:36–39.

Steele, N., and Y. Sterling. 1992. Application of the case study design: Nursing interventions for discharge readiness. *Clinical Nurse Specialist* 6:79–84.

Stiller, A., and H. Brown. 1996. Case management: Implementing the vision. *Nursing Economics* 14:9–13.

Titker, M., and D. Pettit. 1995. Discharge readiness assessment. *Journal of Cardiovascular Nursing* 4:64–74.

Wilson, E., et al. 1991. Take a fresh look at discharge planning. *Geriatric Nursing* 12:23–25.

CHAPTER 35

Referral Sources in Home Health Care

Domenica M. Chromiak

Referral sources are important to the financial survival of any agency. This chapter discusses important factors in developing and keeping referral sources. The referral is the very core of the home health care industry. Without it, the business would certainly not survive. The referral is a critical component of the discharge planning process, a process that is crucial in every health care setting. Discharge planning, as defined by the American Nurses Association (ANA), is "the part of the continuity of care process that is designed to prepare the patient or client for the next phase of care and to assist in making any necessary arrangements for that phase of care, whether it be self-care, care by family members, or care by an organized healthcare provider" (ANA, 1975, 1). Discharge planning includes three components: the assessment and identification of the actual and potential physical and psychosocial needs of the client, the planning for care that is needed when change in or cessation of services by the present health care provider is indicated, and the preparation of the client for self-care when organized care is terminated or the preparation and referral of the client for transfer to another health care organization (ANA, 1975). In light of the components above, a referral may then be defined as the compilation of pertinent client-related information that is communicated to an organization for the purpose of obtaining the needed health care services. In home health care, this information would include both demographic and health-related facts about the client. The referral information may be given to or by the home health agency and may vary depending on the needed phase of care as determined by the discharge planning process.

REFERRAL SOURCES

The sources of referrals to home health agencies can be described simply and in one word: limitless. In other words, an agency can receive a referral from almost any source. The types of sources for any given agency would depend on factors such as its size, structure (free-standing, hospital related, public, nonprofit, voluntary, or proprietary), location, services offered, surrounding competition, and so on. For example, a hospital-affiliated agency would probably receive most of its referrals from the hospital. Other examples of referral sources include managed care and third-party payer arrangements, skilled nursing facilities, transitional care facilities, rehabilitation facilities, community centers,

Source: Adapted with permission from Lucas, M., and Pancoast, L.D., Referral Sources in Home Health Care, *Journal of Nursing Administration*, Vol. 22, No. 12, pp. 39–45, © 1988, J.B. Lippincott Company.

physicians, families, neighbors, and clients themselves. Each of these referral sources probably differs in its reasons for making the referral and in its expectations of the needed services. For example, a health care facility should be able to provide the agency with more complete referral information and should be more realistic in its service expectations. On the other hand, lay referral sources would probably require more intense screening and are probably limited in their understanding of the agency's role. Physician referrals generally vary in their reasons, quality of information, and service expectations, depending on the individual. The collection and maintenance of referral source data represents a wise practice for all home health agencies. Analysis of these data can be useful for internal agency evaluation as well as for agency marketing practices.

REFERRAL INFORMATION

As stated earlier, home health referrals generally include both demographic and health-related information about the client. The quantity and quality of this information vary and depend on factors such as the referral source, the needed level of care, the amount of information available, and the purpose of the referral (intake versus interagency referral). Despite variability, the agency can control some of the information received or provided by its staff via the design of its forms.

Intake Referral Form

This referral form is designed for initial intake purposes and can be thought of as a preadmission screening tool. The staff use this form for collecting or receiving information from an outside source about a prospective client. The form, usually developed by agency staff, varies according to the agency's needs. If Medicare certified, the agency is subject to federal requirements for clinical records. The record must contain "appropriate identifying information; name of physician; and drug,

dietary, treatment, and activity orders, signed and dated clinical and progress notes, copies of summary reports sent to the attending physician, and a discharge summary" (Department of Health and Human Services, 1994, §484.48). At the very least, the agency should obtain these facts when recording preliminary intake information. It is obviously beneficial for the agency to obtain as much additional information as possible when receiving a referral. If the referral source cannot provide the desired information, staff should be encouraged to pursue other possible sources. For example, if the original referral source is a family member, the staff member can confer with the appropriate physician for the desired medical information. If a physician referring a case offers only scant information, the staff member can confer with the prospective client and family for additional facts.

Interagency Referral Form

This referral form is designed for interim referral purposes and can be thought of as a transfer summary. The staff use this form to convey pertinent demographic and health-related facts about a client under their service who will be cared for by another agency. The most common reason for an interagency referral is relocation of a client to another geographic area. The *National Home Care and Hospice Directory* is an excellent reference for locating an agency in an unfamiliar area (National Association for Home Care, 1997). Like the intake form, the interagency referral is usually developed by agency staff and varies according to the philosophy of the agency. Although there are no specific content requirements for Medicare-certified agencies, there is a general requirement that, "if a patient is transferred to another health facility, a copy of the record or abstract is sent with the patient" (Department of Health and Human Services, 1989, §484.48). Thus it is wise to use a form that provides a sufficient amount of information about the care rendered, the client's status, and the services needed.

CRITERIA FOR SERVICE

The development and use of service criteria represent a wise practice for all home health agencies. Agency policies can be of immense benefit to the staff when decisions are made about whether a referred client is appropriate. Of particular benefit is the agency's policy on criteria for acceptance to service. These criteria provide parameters for the staff in determining whether the agency can safely and adequately provide the needed services. This is especially important in light of the increased demand for high-technology therapies to be provided in the home. Many agencies have developed additional policies for these requested special procedures that include admission criteria specific to each. Here, the staff would use both the general criteria and the special procedure criteria to decide whether the client is appropriate. If it is determined that any referred client cannot be appropriately cared for and therefore must be rejected for service, the reasons should be clearly documented on the referral form and the form maintained in a separate file. Agency staff may need to access these data later should a question arise about why service was not provided.

Admission or acceptance criteria may vary among home health agencies. These differences result from such factors as the size, structure, location, services offered, philosophy, and goals of the agency. In some agencies, the staff may develop the criteria. If the agency is Medicare certified, however, there must be a group of professional personnel who are responsible for advising and evaluating the agency, establishing agency policies (including admission and discharge policies), and reviewing them annually (Department of Health and Human Services, 1989, §484.16). Proposed regulations may eliminate this requirement (Department of Health and Human Services, 1997, vol. 62, p. 15). Medicare also provides a general guideline for admission policies, which states, "patients are accepted for treatment on the basis of a reasonable expectation that the patient's medical, nursing, and social needs can be met adequately by the agency in the patient's place of residence" (Department of Health and Human Services, 1989, §484.18). The agency therefore must include at least this concept when developing its admission criteria. In addition, the criteria for continuation of service (if used) and termination of service should logically flow from the criteria for acceptance to remain consistent. Exhibit 35–1 shows a sample of acceptance criteria, and Exhibit 35–2 presents some general admission policies.

REJECTION OF REFERRALS

Even if a referral is rejected because the patient is totally inappropriate for the services

---

Exhibit 35–1 Service Acceptance Criteria

- The request for service is based on a health need, not primarily a social or environmental need.
- A physician will assume responsibility for medical direction. If the source of medical care cannot be identified, a home visit may be made at the discretion of the agency management staff.
- For certain third-party payers (e.g., Medicare), the client is essentially homebound.
- Someone is available to the client to provide care between agency visits if necessary.
- The agency has the capacity to provide the kind and amount of service required or requested. Although the agency provides service to adults and maternal–child service, it does not provide service to the pediatric population.
- The home setting is safe for the patient. There is provision for shelter, food, clothing, and protection of the individual.
- The patient and/or significant other is able and willing to participate in the patient's care as necessary.
- The situation does not endanger agency staff.
- The environment is one in which service can be provided effectively.

Exhibit 35–2 Service Acceptance Policies

- Acceptance of a request for service does not ensure the continuation of further service beyond the initial visit. The decision to accept a patient for service is made after the initial visit, when it is determined that the criteria for acceptance have been met.
- The patient or patient's family will be contacted within 48 hours of receipt of referral, or sooner or later as indicated by the situation of the referral; at that time the plan for the initial home visit (if appropriate) will be established. The initial home visit is generally made within 24 hours.
- If an individual meets these requirements, he or she will be accepted for home health services regardless of age, race, creed, color, religion, sex, sexual preference, handicap, national origin, and socioeconomic status.
- If the patient does not meet admission criteria, the referring individual or organization is notified.

---

that a particular agency provides, the agency runs the risk of alienating the referral source. The dilemma is whether an agency should simply accept all referrals for evaluation and be responsible for the disposition or whether it should explain to the referral source why the patient does not qualify for services and leave the disposition to the referral source. One advantage of the former is the sense of ease that a referral source will have in expediting discharge of patients to any agency. For harried discharge planners, physicians, or others trying to arrange follow-up home care services, the referral process must be as efficient as possible. In addition, if all referrals are evaluated, some will be inappropriate. It is the responsibility of the agency to advise the patient or family member about other community resources from which needed services could be obtained. It must then be decided whether to inform the referral source of the disposition. If the referral source is a managed care company, the agency will not have this flexibility. It will be the man-

aged care entity that decides the disposition. The second approach provides an opportunity to clarify to the referral source the eligibility requirements and admission criteria of the agency.

Because of the frequently changing interpretation of eligibility for services under third party payers (and Medicare in particular), it is not possible for referral sources to keep abreast of all home care regulations. Agencies are in a position to provide the most current information to those sources as inquiries are made about referrals. An agency that refuses to evaluate a patient for admission to service should give the referral source a reason why. Such reasons may include the following: no skilled services are required, the patient is not home-bound, the agency does not provide service in that patient's home area, and services required are not available through that particular agency (e.g., high-technology therapies or pediatric care). Giving feedback to the referral source about the inability to provide requested services can, however, result in "agency shopping" by the referral source. If this shopping is successful, rapport with another agency may be established, resulting in loss of future patients from the referral source. In light of the above choices, agency managers must clearly define how an inappropriate referral is to be handled. Because confusion on the part of intake personnel will negatively affect the agency, intake policies should be established and communicated clearly to the staff.

INTAKE PERSON

The intake person is one of the most important agency persons in terms of public image. He or she is the agency's link to the outside and can be the difference between whether a referral source does or does not use the agency again. Ideally, the intake person should be a registered nurse because the majority of referrals require home nursing services. A clerical person may be able to record demographic data, but health-related information will be more accurately

Exhibit 35–3 Qualities of the Ideal Intake Person

- A pleasant and dynamic voice
- The ability to get along well with people
- Good communication skills
- Good working knowledge of the agency's policies regarding patient eligibility for service
- Ability to seek and obtain patient information
- Knowledge of community resources
- Nonjudgmental and caring attitude
- Organized approach to information collection
- Knowledge of community health principles and practices
- Sense of humor
- Good listening skills
- Ability to maintain a positive professional attitude

interpreted and transcribed by the health care professional. A referral involving only therapy services could be processed by a rehabilitation specialist, such as a physical therapist or occupational therapist, if available. Exhibit 35–3 highlights the qualities of an ideal intake person.

Intake personnel should be readily available to receive information on referrals as soon as the call comes in. The easier it is to make a referral, the more likely the referral source is to use the same agency again. This is especially true of managed care companies. The following factors can have a negative impact on a referral source: a constantly busy telephone signal, being put on hold (for more than a minute or two), constant interruptions when talking with the intake person, inefficiency of the intake person in obtaining information (writes too slowly or constantly asks the referral source to spell or repeat words), inability of the intake person to hear information being conveyed or to decide whether the referral is appropriate, and the intake person asking too many questions, being sarcastic, and displaying inappropriate, unprofessional behavior.

LIAISON

Some agencies provide the service of a liaison to major referral sources, such as hospitals and skilled nursing facilities. The liaison is an employee of the agency, usually a registered nurse, who collects information about patients referred to the agency from that institution. The nurse can also act as a resource for questions regarding home care services and appropriateness of referrals. The liaison can facilitate the transition from institution to home by meeting with referred patients and their families and discussing available, appropriate home services and the roles of the home care staff and by scheduling the first visit and arranging for necessary medical supplies and equipment before discharge. Services from the agency can be processed and initiated more promptly because the liaison is in a position to evaluate personally the patient's needs before discharge from the institution. The liaison can ascertain directly from the institution's nurses how the patient is learning and performing specific techniques, such as insulin administration, emptying drainage bags, and changing dressings.

Two major responsibilities of the liaison are to review the medical records of all patients referred and to complete the referral form, noting relevant demographic data, medical history, history of the current problem, a brief description of pertinent facts regarding this admission, rehabilitation notes, discharge medications, psychosocial information, and pertinent laboratory and radiology findings. Special instructions for the home care staff, such as specific dressing techniques, monitoring of weight, and requests for laboratory studies at home, can be obtained by the liaison as well.

The liaison position must not be confused with the discharge planner, who is an employee of the referral source. This distinction is particularly important in terms of separating the job responsibilities and the costs attributed to these positions. The discharge planner is responsible for the discharge needs of the institution's patients. This may include such planning as nursing home placement, evaluation for a rehabilitation center, and arrangement for private pay homemaker service or home-delivered meal services. The discharge planner can also initiate the referral to the home health agency through the liaison or another intake person. The liaison may not solicit patients at the institution. A referral process between the discharge planner and the liaison should be established and adhered to by all parties. Good communication between them will ensure more efficiency and smoother transition for the patient from institution to home.

SEASONAL TRENDS

Agency managers need to be aware of any trends in the referral pattern that will affect staffing. For example, the agency that employs sufficient staff to handle 50 referrals per week will experience a significant amount of downtime for its staff and resultant financial difficulties if the referral rate suddenly drops to 25 per week. One way of tracking trends is to plot agency activity, such as numbers of referrals and total visits, on graphs. These data can be analyzed to identify trends related to seasons of the year, holidays, or new legislation that will affect census. The ability to predict referral patterns allows an agency to handle overflow and staff appropriately during leaner times. The agency administrator can use trend data from the previous year to develop a realistic budget for the upcoming fiscal year. Projections for staffing can also be made based on these data. Because the home health industry is labor intensive, salaries and wages account for a major portion of the expenses. The fluctuation in caseload can be managed in a more fiscally prudent fashion through the use of part-time staff and contractors. The referral profile can assist in overall agency planning and budgeting.

MARKETING

The rapidly changing health care environment mandates that an agency market and sell its services. The increasing number of and competition among home health agencies require an active sales campaign to capture a share of the market, particularly for agencies without managed care arrangements or affiliations with health care institutions that guarantee a minimal flow of patients.

Marketing simply means selling the agency's services. This can be accomplished in many ways, but the process involves increasing the visibility of the agency. The most important aspect in a coordinated marketing campaign is repetition. Repetition is essential because it improves product recognition. The process begins with choosing an appropriate agency name that is easy to remember and relates to the services offered. Brochures and pamphlets describing the agency and its purpose should be developed and distributed in as many locations as possible, preferably where referrals are initiated. Examples include physicians' offices and waiting rooms, hospital waiting areas in various departments, senior citizen centers, community social service agencies, school nurse offices, church bulletin boards, rehabilitation centers, nursing homes, retirement communities, and so on. Brochures can be included in admission packets given to patients in hospitals and health care institutions where appropriate arrangements exist.

Each member of the staff can market the agency on a daily basis. Identification badges bearing the title of the agency as well as the individual's name and photograph should always be worn. Staff should always introduce themselves by name and give the agency name as well, such as by saying "I am Ms. Jones from the Jeanes Home Health Agency" rather than "I am Ms. Jones from the home health [or visiting nurse] agency." The latter is too generic and does not give the agency recognition. Equipment bags carried by the staff should have the agency emblem and name prominently displayed. Vehicles owned by the agency should be lettered with the agency name and phone number. For staff using their own vehicles, identification cards can be placed in the window.

Public appearances, such as speaking engagements to different community groups on a variety of health-related subjects, can also bring more visibility to the agency and its staff. Health fairs, school fairs, and shopping mall displays provide additional recognition opportunities. Giving away items with the agency's name, such as pens, pencils, refrigerator magnets, telephone stickers with emergency numbers, memo pads, and key chains, helps keep the agency's name in the public eye. Public service announcements on radio and television are also appropriate.

An agency designee should periodically visit referral sources to discuss problems or issues of mutual concern. Requests should be made for feedback from these sources and suggestions solicited on ways to improve service or add to services already being provided. Personal contact with a referral source will make a more lasting impact than a letter or evaluation card. Referral sources should be encouraged to become involved in the agency, if possible, as consultants, as members of an advisory committee, or as part of the record review process. Those who have more frequent and personal contacts with the agency will tend to use the agency more. Finally, the best way to market an agency is through satisfied clients and referral sources. Appropriate, timely, high-quality service speaks for itself.

LEGAL ISSUES

Many providers in the health care system, such as acute care facilities, have become more cognizant of liability issues and have taken steps to avoid legal problems. An example is the development of ethics committees in hospitals. Home health agencies are joining their provider colleagues in becoming more aware of potential liability concerns. Increased numbers of home health agencies and more creative business arrangements have resulted in greater competition and an increased likelihood of liability and legal problems. One of the major areas in

which agencies need to exercise caution is their referral practices.

Collection of Referral Information

It is crucial that the agency's intake staff collect as much information as possible when taking a referral. This serves two useful purposes. First, it provides agency personnel with the facts necessary to make a decision about whether the client's needs can be met adequately by the agency. Second, it results in a reduction in the amount of staff time spent in obtaining information needed to complete documentation requirements and to plan for appropriate service. As a result, the patient, who is often frustrated with the many questions asked, may feel more relaxed and may perceive the agency as being more organized and knowledgeable about his or her situation.

Maintenance of Referral Information

When as much referral information as possible is gathered, a decision is made about what types of service, if any, are indicated. If the agency plans to evaluate or admit a patient, the referral should then become part of the legal record. If, however, the patient is deemed inappropriate and will not be seen, the reasons should be documented and the referral maintained in a special file. With this practice, the agency can access the information later should a question arise about why service was not provided or should the patient be referred to the agency again in the future.

Agency Policies

In determining whether a patient is appropriate for agency services, the intake staff would benefit from having parameters by which to be guided. One way to provide such guidelines is through clearly stated agency administrative and clinical policies. A home health agency, like any other health care provider, is compared against standard practice when any legal situation arises. The agency should therefore model its policies after those of the agencies in the surrounding area. The most highly regarded agencies should be used as role models if possible. Agency policies will probably vary according to the location of the agency as well as other factors. Examples of administrative policies that can be used by the intake staff for referral-taking purposes may therefore include, but are not limited to, statements of philosophy, goals, services provided, geographical area served, service hours, patient choice, and nondiscrimination practices. Clinical policies on topics such as admission criteria and medical supervision may also be helpful. The individual policies need not be lengthy or elaborate to be of value to the staff; rather, they need to state clearly the agency's perspective so that the staff can refer to and be guided by them in making referral decisions.

ANTITRUST ISSUES

The significant changes in the home health care industry have resulted in increased competition. In particular, hospitals have sharply increased their participation in the business by either developing their own agencies or establishing arrangements with already existing agencies. Hospitals are also purchasing physician practices in increasing numbers. These trends raise concerns about potential antitrust issues related to recommending patients to the affiliated agency and about the lack of disclo-

sure of the relationship that exists. Regulations of the Health Care Financing Administration bar a physician from certifying or recertifying plans of care for an agency with which he or she has a direct or indirect financial interest of $25,000 per year or 5 percent of operating expenses.

CONCLUSION

Home health agencies are dependent on referrals for survival, and sources of referrals are limitless. It is imperative that administrators have systems in place to accept referrals, collect and maintain referral source data to use as one aspect of the agency's internal evaluation process, and target its marketing efforts. A home health agency must have approved policies and procedures available that address criteria for admission to, continuation of, and discharge from service. These must be shared with the personnel of the referral sources. The admission criteria should state the types of referrals that are not appropriate for service and how these referrals will be handled. As part of the overall management of the agency, administrators must also be aware of seasonal trends and how they may affect staffing and total budget. A positive relationship between the staff of the home health agency and the referral source is one way to generate needed referrals. The end result will benefit the patient, the agency, and the referring source.

REFERENCES

American Nurses Association (ANA). 1975. *Continuity of care and discharge planning programs in institutions and community agencies.* Kansas City, MO: ANA.

Department of Health and Human Services. 1989. Medicare program, home health agencies: Conditions of participation and reduction in record keeping requirements, interim final rule. *Federal Register*, part 2, 42 CFR, part 484, vol. 54:33354–33373.

Department of Health and Human Services. 1994. Medicare program, home health agencies: Conditions of participation and home aide supervision, final rule. *Federal Register*, part 409, 413, 418, and 484, vol. 59:65482–65498.

Department of Health and Human Services. 1997. Medicare and Medicaid programs: Conditions of participation for home health agencies, proposed rule. *Federal Register*, part 484, vol. 62:15.

National Association for Home Care (NAHC). 1997. *National home care and hospice directory.* Washington, DC: NAHC.

Administrative Priorities: Decisions and Strategies That Attract and Retain Quality Staff

Elissa DellaMonica, Marilyn D. Harris, and Joan Reynolds Yuan

PART I

Position available in home health agency for registered nurse with a wide range of clinical skills; must be familiar with countless Medicare and other third-party payer regulations, computer literate, research oriented, capable of perfect documentation.

It is also expected that the applicant will take 24-hour on-call duty on a rotating basis and make necessary home visits after stated working hours; maintain productivity standards established by management. Must also have a commitment to excellence and quality patient care.

The applicant should also be able to smile while coping with traffic problems, detours, school buses, dogs, fleas, inclement weather, and other work-related pressures such as paperwork.

Excellent, competitive salary and benefits are available in many agencies.

Only applicants who are of stout heart and courage should call for an interview.

This ad may appear exaggerated to anyone unfamiliar with home health care today. To those of us who provide and manage quality home care services, however, these job characteristics are all too familiar. Many of us can remember just a few years ago when nurses selected home care because it was a 9 to 5 position, Monday through Friday, with many weekends off. This is no longer a realistic expectation. Understandably, some nurses are deciding to seek employment in other, less stressful and restrictive settings. The question for administrators is what to do to attract and retain quality staff.

EXTERNAL FORCES THAT HAVE AN IMPACT ON HOME CARE STAFF

The home health care environment today includes multiple factors that can be viewed as negative forces affecting home care. A few of these are increased government legislation and regulations, restrictive reimbursement patterns, and a sense of decreased professional control

Source: Reprinted by permission of the National Association for Home Care, from *CARING* Magazine, Vol. II, No. 2. Not for further reproduction.

over the care provided (for example, a reviewer in a distant office determines who will receive what care and in what amount). This is the age of case management, health maintenance organizations, and other managed care options (Exhibit 36–1).

The caregiving process is further complicated by the increased age of the patient and spouse or caregiver, the increased acuity level of patients, decreased length of stays in the hospital and under home care services, and immediate family members living in distant places. Added to this is the decreased availability of some levels of human resources.

All this comes at a time of increased emphasis on quality assessment/performance improvement activities, requiring frequent monitoring and reporting; outside agency, such as peer review organization (PRO), accreditation and certification; and Medicare's proposed patient-outcome based requirements through the use of the Outcome and Assessment Information Set

Exhibit 36–1 External Forces That May Affect Home Care Staff

Demographic characteristics

- Nuclear family changes
- Aging population
- Two adults working in the household

Increased legislation/regulation
PRO reviews
Certification/accreditation requirements
Shortage of human resources (selected
  disciplines/specialties)
Documentation requirements
Restrictive reimbursement by third-party
  payers
Increased percentage of individuals enrolled in
  managed care programs
Capitated contracts
Sense of decreased professional control over
  patient care

Source: Reprinted by permission of the National Association for Home Care, from *CARING* Magazine, Vol. IX, No. 2, February 1990. Not for further reproduction.

(OASIS; Shaughnessy and Crisler, 1995). Agencies need to remain financially solvent; because home care is still reimbursed on a per visit basis in 1997, it is necessary continually to monitor productivity (Harris, 1989). Considering these factors, it is possible to be a good nurse, therapist, social worker, or homemaker–home health aide but not do well in the home health care setting.

JOB AND PERSONNEL CHARACTERISTICS IN HOME CARE

To attract and retain home care personnel, it is important that agencies accurately describe the current job characteristics. Glueck (1974) states that two general sets of factors make up any task: the technology of the task, and the working conditions. He also states that any position can be defined by nine job characteristics: degree of physical exertion, degree of environmental unpleasantness, physical location, time duration of work, degree of specialization, educational requirements, experience qualifications, human interaction, and psychological dimensions (degree of freedom, risk taking, and responsibility). Glueck states, "In general, the less pleasant the workers perceive the work to be done, the more rewards (financial or otherwise) will be necessary to attract and hold workers in good times. In bad times, workers may be unable to quit, but they may find ways to work less or less efficiently and thus indirectly increase their rewards" (p. 80).

Harris (1977) completed her first survey of home health care nurses' job characteristics in 1975 as a graduate student. The two samples included 23 home care nurses (14 staff and 9 graduate students). In 1975, the 23 home care nurses agreed on only one item: human interaction. All rated this aspect of their job as high. The graduate students agreed on two characteristics: human interaction and psychological dimension of degree of responsibility. Staff nurses did not agree on any level of responsibility.

The same form was mailed to home health agency directors in 1988. Sixty-five nurses from six agencies in various parts of the country responded. In 1988, all 65 nurses did not concur on any one of the characteristics. The two highest areas of agreement were the degree of responsibility and human interaction. These were the same two characteristics identified in 1975.

Once the external factors that affect home care services and the characteristics of the work environment are understood, it is necessary to define the personal characteristics required for professional staff to be successful in this environment. The following characteristics are just some that should be considered:

- independent
- critical thinker; ability to make decisions related to patient care
- clinical competence and assessment skills
- high-technology skills
- involvement in educational programs, both for self and in teaching others (professionals and lay persons)
- fiscal responsibility; must have some idea of the cost of providing home care services, supplies, fee for services
- knowledge of family/patient relationships and interactions
- good listener; able to assess physical and psychosocial needs
- good interviewing skills; keeps conversations on track, collects needed information
- ability to communicate; teaching, instructions
- counseling skills; asks appropriate questions, responds to patients and help them attain goals
- high energy level
- positive outlook on life

All these characteristics will be helpful in meeting the many demands placed on home care staff.

HIRING IN AN ERA OF PERSONNEL SHORTAGE

The provision of quality care by qualified staff is the best way to market home care ser-

vices. To provide such services, agencies must find ways to attract appropriate and qualified staff. Agencies must consider not only what they are looking for in staff but what potential employees are seeking. Personnel find the following characteristics of the home care environment attractive:

- close patient relationship (what the public perceives as quality often results from a positive relationship with staff)
- independence
- recognition (financial and nonfinancial)
- work environment conducive to providing quality care

When the management staff provide the visiting and support staff with encouragement and other tangible evidence of support, staff will contribute to the recruitment and retention process.

INTERVIEWING PROSPECTIVE TEAM MEMBERS

Retention begins with the selection process. The interview provides the opportunity for applicants not only to talk about their skills and experience but also to discuss their goals in relationship to the job. This is also the time for prospective employees to ask and expect honest answers to job-related questions.

In an effort to enhance retention, the Visiting Nurse Association (VNA) of Eastern Montgomery County/A Department of Abington Memorial Hospital subjects applicants to multiple interviews and provides ample opportunity for asking questions. The director of professional services (DPS), in cooperation with the hospital's Human Resource Department, does the initial screening for professional staff, often through a telephone interview. This is done to determine the applicant's work experience, level of interest in the position, and salary requirements. This initial screening eliminates those applicants who are looking for a salary or position that the agency cannot offer.

The first in-person interview is usually done by the DPS as well. At this time, the agency's programs, services, personnel policies, salary range, and weekend and 24-hour rotation schedule are presented. Productivity standards, documentation requirements, and third-party payer restrictions are also discussed. This is also the time to discuss the agency's philosophy. Applicants must hear that quality of care is a major commitment of the agency's administration. A skills checklist is also completed by the applicant.

If there is mutual interest in pursuing employment, a second interview is scheduled. The second interview is arranged to allow as many of the clinical supervisors as possible to meet with the applicant. During the interview, the supervisors present a realistic picture of home care, discussing both the pros and the cons. All staff are free to take part and share information with the applicant. When time permits, the applicant may also spend some time with a staff nurse making home visits.

It is important, during the interview process, to determine whether an applicant's philosophy, personal goals, and expectations mesh with those of the organization. For example, if the new staff nurse comes on board with previous years of home care experience and is seeking a supervisory level position in a few months, the applicant must know that there is a limited number of these positions available and that the turnover is low (or high).

The applicant should leave the interview with a favorable impression of the institution. The agency may not be able to attract an applicant with the highest salary, but the interviewer can give her or him reasons why a particular position offers what is not available in another organization. The agency must sell itself during the interview process.

A detailed interview and selection process, although time consuming, is relevant to the retention issue. New employees will not be disillusioned, and the supervisory staff will be aware of what must be addressed during the orientation period to ease the transition to home health care. This detailed process has the potential for both positive and negative impact on the outcome. One applicant to the VNA, after meeting with several supervisors, decided she did not want to work in this type of setting. Another applicant accepted our position at a lower salary than offered elsewhere, stating that she was impressed with the total interview process, the professionalism of the staff, and the honest portrayal of the pros and cons.

All available applicants who pass the initial screening process should be interviewed. Although agencies are seeking nurses with high-technology skills, qualified staff who exhibit an interest and enthusiasm to learn new skills are desirable employees. Sometimes it is the challenge and the opportunity to develop new skills that contribute to retention of staff.

Although we usually discuss retention in the context of visiting staff, we must not forget supervisory and administrative staff. It has been stated that the public health nurse supervisor must be a virtual wonder woman (or man), that she (or he) must have the enthusiasm of a college freshman, the patience of a saint, the determination of a taxi driver, and the tireless energy of a bill collector. We should take these characteristics into consideration when we hire or promote a nurse to the supervisory level.

The basic attributes desirable in an administrator are listed in *Characteristics of the Home Health Agency Administrator* (National League for Nursing, 1977). The following personal characteristics are cited: exhibits a strong commitment and abundant energy for the task, "that something extra" required to achieve goals; shows emotional stability; possesses the ability to operate under pressure; and shows initiative, enthusiasm, pragmatism, and creativity. Interviewers should look for these characteristics with administrative applicants to lessen the possibility of surprises.

RETENTION AND QUALITY CARE

Alfano (1988) stated in a professional editorial that what keeps most people in a setting over and above money and power is the bonding with coworkers. She pointed out that recruiting people into nursing will be a wasted effort unless present staff welcome new staff rather than shut them out.

The aspects of home care that attracted applicants in the past are not necessarily the drawing features in the 1990s. Autonomy, relationship with physicians, weekend and holiday rotation, working hours, and teaching opportunities may be offset today by the increased acuity level of patients, increased paperwork and documentation requirements, and the potential for decreased patient satisfaction due to decreased length of stay on service and restrictive reimbursement patterns.

For staff, supervisors, and administrators alike, job satisfaction, salary, the opportunity for participation in policy and procedure development, a sense of belonging, and recognition of personal worth, along with the opportunity to attain personal and professional goals, are important issues. At the agency level, the mission statement, philosophy, emphasis on quality care, and financial, productivity, and documentation issues are related to retaining qualified staff as well. Administrative support and encouragement are also integral to employee satisfaction and retention. All these factors work together to ensure the retention of quality staff and thus the continued provision of quality care.

REFERENCES

Alfano, G. 1988. Editorial: Welcome to our world. *Geriatric Nursing* 9:29.

Glueck, W. 1974. *Personnel: A diagnostic approach.* Dallas: Business Publications.

Harris, M. 1977. The selection process in a community health nursing agency—A look into the future. *Pennsylvania Nurse* 32:4–6.

Harris, M. 1989. The impact of one federal regulation on productivity in a home health agency. *Caring* 7:66–74.

National League for Nursing (NLN). 1977. *Characteristics of the home health agency administrator.* New York: NLN.

Shaughnessy, P., and K. Crisler. 1995. *Outcome based quality improvement.* Washington, DC: National Association for Home Care.

* * * *

PART II

It has long been recognized that job satisfaction, salary, the opportunity for participation in policy and procedure development, a sense of belonging, recognition of personal worth, and an opportunity to attain personal goals are important issues in the attraction and retention of quality staff (DellaMonica et al., 1990). As managers in this turbulent environment, the question we frequently ask ourselves is: How do we fulfill these many staff expectations?

STRUCTURAL COMPONENTS NECESSARY TO ATTRACT AND RETAIN QUALITY STAFF

A commitment to excellence is of paramount importance and must be pervasive throughout the organization. Consideration must be given to the structural components that will ensure quality. Two key structural components that are related to the attraction and retention of staff are quality assessment/performance improvement (QA/PI) activities and education. The QA/PI activities are related to the attraction and retention of quality staff. Few people would work for an organization that they did not feel was providing quality services.

There are many ways of defining quality care. The Joint Commission on Accreditation of Healthcare Organizations (Joint Commission) defined quality patient care as "The degree to which patient care services increase the probability of desired patient outcomes and reduce the probability of undesired outcomes, given the current state of knowledge" (Joint Commission, 1989, p. 7). The staff person delivering quality care is going to be a professional who is able to achieve positive patient outcomes and who has a strong knowledge base, clinical expertise, and a caring and positive attitude.

In attracting this kind of person to the organization, the area of nursing professionalism is vital. Autonomy, independence, and the ability to practice in a professional setting are important to quality staff. Guided by the American Nurses Association (ANA) Code for Nurses (1985), the quality nurse will assume responsibility and accountability for actions, participate in implementing and improving standards, and participate in establishing and maintaining conditions of employment conducive to high-quality care. The administration must have built into the structure of the organization a QA/PI program that involves staff and provides a mechanism for change and improved patient care.

The philosophy of quality must be made known during the interview process. When the nurse is choosing an organization, she or he must understand where the priorities of the organization lie. Accreditation through the Joint Commission or the Community Health Accreditation Program (CHAP) implies that an agency adheres to a set of standards that are widely accepted in the industry. This places the organization at a distinct advantage in competing for staff. Quality staff are attracted to a quality organization.

Education is also seen as a necessity to attract and retain qualified staff. Professional nurses are concerned about the kinds of educational programs available and what kinds of educational benefits they can expect to receive. This is a frequent question during the interview. Educational programs, including orientation, could be the deciding factor when an applicant is choosing a position. Education is a professional requirement. Maintaining competence is a key point within the Code for Nurses (ANA, 1985). Relevant, ongoing education is mandated by accrediting/certifying bodies such as Medicare, the CHAP, and the Joint Commission. Service–education collaboration can help build credibility in the nursing community and attract staff.

RETENTION ISSUES WITHIN ADMINISTRATIVE CONTROL

Consideration must be given to issues related to retention that are within administrative control. The administrator has direct control over his or her style of management. Frequently, staff's perception of administration is an authority figure whose only interest is productivity and its effects on the bottom line. There is no doubt that a major responsibility of the administrative staff is to manage the business of the organization. It is, however, equally important to manage and develop staff so that their experiences and skills maximize organizational effectiveness.

CHARACTERISTICS OF PARTICIPATION AND COLLABORATION

The management style of participation and collaboration is the most effective in attracting and retaining staff. The characteristics of this style of management are based on *Stogdill's Handbook of Leadership* (Bass, 1981).

- The process is directed by authority, but responsibility is shared. Managers have the authority to direct staff to comply with the standards as set by the agency and regulatory and accrediting bodies. Staff, however, must assume responsibility for compliance with the standards.

- Individual ideas and creative thoughts are actively solicited. Managers can improve the quality of their decisions by not making them in isolation, and by using the ideas and creative thoughts of staff. This also contributes to employee job satisfaction because staff feel they made a contribution to the decision-making process.
- There is an openness to negotiating individual roles, responsibilities, and goals. The use of a self-evaluation tool enables personnel to address their personal and professional goals. Criteria-based job descriptions and performance appraisals provide a mechanism to discuss roles and responsibilities. Used correctly, they encourage open dialog between staff and supervisor.
- Control is moderated by the open direction of problem solving and discussion. Solicit the input of the staff when attempting to resolve a problem. Enable the staff to confront and resolve problems through participation at team conferences, staff meetings, and support groups. Positive results will be achieved as staff assume ownership of the problem and there is a commitment to problem resolution.
- There is an assumption of a greater equality of skills with less need to teach. Recognize the skills and expertise of employees. Allow staff the freedom to make decisions regarding patient care. This demonstrates confidence in them, thus increasing their self-esteem.

The advantages of this style of management are numerous. Participation encourages a sense of ownership and involvement by the employees and leads to greater acceptance of a decision. This strengthens staff commitment to implementation of the decision.

Participation enhances communication and an understanding of the organization. The more staff know about the organization and what will result from its effort, the more they will be committed to remaining under its employ. A commitment to quality through the QA/PI process and education must be a priority of administration. A participatory, collaborative style can be effective in managing staff.

CONCLUSION

Managers in today's turbulent environment can do much to motivate employees. Such things as recognizing accomplishments, soliciting staff participation in the QA/PI and educational programs, providing employees with appropriate responsibility, establishing a climate of trust and open communication, and providing support and flexibility contribute to job satisfaction and retention of staff.

REFERENCES

American Nurses Association (ANA). 1985. *Code for nurses with interpretive statements*. Kansas City, MO: ANA.

Bass, B.M. 1981. *Stogdill's handbook of leadership*. New York: Free Press.

DellaMonica, E., et al. 1990. Administrative priorities: Decisions and strategies that attract and retain quality staff, part I. *Caring* 2:21–24.

Joint Commission on Accreditation of Healthcare Organizations. 1989. Patient care quality defined. *Joint Commission Perspectives* 9:7.

CHAPTER 37

Flextime Scheduling

Diane T. Cass and Sharon D. Martin

This chapter describes the experience of a large, private, nonprofit home health agency in developing a flextime policy. A task force was formed to examine current models utilized in business and their suitable application to home health. The task force developed definitions, measurable goals and objectives, and a policy statement and implemented a 3-month, multi-site, multidiscipline pilot study with 16 employees flexing. The pilot was evaluated from multiple perspectives. Pretesting and posttesting of all agency employees revealed that flextime was seen as a major benefit to employees by allowing them to better meet personal and family commitments. Evaluation also demonstrated that flextime did not positively or negatively affect productivity or sick time utilization and that the majority of participating employees opted for flexing to earlier work hours.

One strategy cited in the literature for recruiting and retaining valued staff and increasing morale is the use of flexible patterns for scheduling and staffing (French, 1982; Werther, 1983). Flextime, also known as flexitime, is a work schedule that allows employees some choice of when to start and stop their work day. It provides an opportunity for the person working outside the home to mesh job, family, and personal responsibilities more easily. It can assist with meeting patient needs for variations in regular caregiving hours. Best of all, in this age of clinical and corporate complexity it is a refreshingly simple concept to implement.

BACKGROUND

The 40-hour work week has been the prevalent schedule of employment for approximately four decades. The Fair Labor Standards Act of 1938, which mandated overtime pay for work over 40 hours, seemed to influence the development of the 5-day, 8-hour work week norm. It was the most obvious schedule to fit the 40-hour mandate, and it has prevailed ever since. Sometime during the 1970s, options to that norm began to be explored (Werther, 1983). At the same time, Poor (1970) spread the idea that the traditional work week was not the only option (Exhibit 37–1).

One of the major social forces encouraging the initiation of flextime is the rise of the dual-career family, in which both husband and wife work. This results in a rise in income with a resultant desire for more leisure time. Also, if children are involved, it becomes inconvenient for parents to work the traditional hours because family obligations may be difficult to satisfy with both parents being unavailable during the same hours. Single-parent families find satisfying family demands even more difficult and need even greater flexibility in the workplace to survive (Skeler, 1981; Werther, 1983).

Exhibit 37–1 Different Forms of Flextime

- *Staggered hours:* Employees are assigned a variation of regular established work hours.
- *Flextime:* Employees choose a starting and quitting time, stick with that schedule for a period, and work 8 hours a day.
- *Gliding time:* Employees may vary their starting and quitting time daily, but they must still work 8 hours, or another company-set length of time, every day.
- *Variable day:* As long as employees work the number of hours required by the end of the week or month, they can vary the number of hours they work each day.
- *Maxiflex:* Employees may vary their daily hours and do not have to be present for a "core" time on all days.

Courtesy of Sharon D. Martin, MSN, RN, CS.

Source: Data from J. M. Roscow and R. Zager (1983), "Punch out the Time Clocks," *Harvard Business Review* 61(2) (March/April, 12–29).

A second force for change lies in the labor market. Firms have been forced to find innovative ways to attract and retain the staff they need while attempting to keep labor costs down. Flextime stands out as an excellent new benefit that in most cases costs the organization little. In many cases, such as in understaffed hospitals, flextime offers a solution to attracting staff besides costly salary increases. Often, staff who otherwise would have been unable to work at all have returned to the workforce because of creative flextime schedules (Skeler, 1981; Werther, 1983).

A third force for change is demographics. The Baby Boom years have passed. The future probably will hold a decreased workforce with decreased unemployment. Competition for the available employees will be greater. Innovative techniques such as flextime may be necessary to attract and retain sufficient staff (Skeler, 1981; Werther, 1983).

TASK FORCE ON FLEXTIME

The request for flextime, originating from staff, resulted in the formation of a task force composed of administrative and first-line managers. The task force examined models utilized in other business settings to determine their suitable application to the agency and to develop a flextime policy. As mentioned earlier, the task force developed definitions, measurable goals and objectives, and a policy statement and implemented a 3-month, multisite, multidiscipline pilot study with 16 employees. The pilot was evaluated according to criteria established initially by the task force, which included the perspective of the patient, the employee, the supervisor, the team, the payroll department, and administration.

The work of the task force took place through several meetings over a period of 7 months. The task force consisted of one administrator and four first-line managers representing the central and branch offices of the agency. It was believed that the burden of implementation would be at the first-line manager level and therefore that they should have a major role in policy formulation. The task force gathered and disseminated information to staff at team meetings so that there was ongoing staff feedback.

The task force utilized the problem-solving approach in the development of the flextime policy. The first step was the identification of problems and generation of goals. Problems identified were as follows:

- Management time was spent on special requests made by staff.
- Staff desired greater freedom in managing their own time.
- Rigid hours interfered with patient needs and desires.
- Having no nurse available after 4:30 P.M., except the on-call nurse, interfered with physician communication.
- Management reorganization had left downtime in the late afternoon for some home health aides.

- With rapid growth and resulting increases in staff, there were problems in accessing telephone lines and sharing office space.

Goals established by the task force provided the direction for developing policy. Goals identified were the following:

- There will always be coverage from 8:00 A.M. to 4:30 P.M. Flextime shall not disrupt the established levels and hours of coverage.
- Productivity will meet or exceed budgeted levels.
- Patient needs and desires will be met.
- There will be decreased management time spent on special requests made by staff.
- Staff satisfaction and morale will increase.
- There will be no lateness and less absenteeism.
- There will be increased capacity to cover cases in other than the 8:00 A.M. to 4:30 P.M. time slot.

Exhibit 37–2 Flextime Policy

The manager arrives at the decision to approve individual requests for flextime. The day-to-day decisions of a short-term nature, such as alteration of staff schedule to accommodate physician appointments, also fall within the jurisdiction of the manager. This policy, however, is intended to address longer-term alternative work schedules.

Under all circumstances, the patient's and team's needs will be met. Arrangements for supervision of flextime staff are the responsibility of the manager.

Core hours will be 9:30 A.M. to 2:00 P.M., Monday through Friday. The range of visit hours will be 6:00 A.M. to 6:00 P.M.

Starting time governs quitting time each day. Once hours are chosen, they may not be changed without due notice. Anything outside the scope of this policy requires administrative approval.

Courtesy of Sharon D. Martin, MSN, RN, CS.

- There may be increased opportunity for physician and nurse conferencing to occur.

The next step of the task force was to develop definitions of flextime and core hours and a policy statement (Exhibit 37–2). The task force's definition of flextime was:

A work schedule that leaves the standard number of working hours unchanged but allows employees some choice of when to start and stop working within the limitations set by management. There is usually a flexible window at the beginning and end of each day that surrounds a core set of hours when all employees must be present.*

THE PILOT PROJECT

Planning

Initial planning involved a literature search and survey of state and out-of-state community health agencies. Information was obtained via a literature search regarding experience with flextime in the health care setting and a procedure for considering implementing a flextime program (Rosenberg, 1983). One agency surveyed had a formal policy regarding flextime.

Specific objectives for a flextime program were developed. As a result of the flextime program, there would be increased ability to meet patient needs, maintenance of productivity at current budgeted figures, increased staff morale, and decreased or no increased supervisory involvement in managing patient care or program issues as a result of flextime. These objectives were to be utilized in planning and evaluating the pilot as well.

The next step was to determine the feasibility of a flextime program in each of the offices and departments. Each of the managers was responsible for assessing whether a flextime program was feasible in that office or department. The

*Courtesy of Sharon D. Martin, MSN, RN, CS.

feasibility was based on the function of the office or department as well as on the needs of the staff and community. The flextime program was determined to be feasible by each of the managers. Eligibility criteria for employees were developed based on those of the Cambridge, Massachusetts, Visiting Nurse Association (Exhibit 37–3).

The last step of planning for the pilot project involved developing the evaluation criteria for the pilot. The criteria developed were based upon the objectives and included the perspective of the patient, manager, employee, team, payroll department, and administration.

Implementation

The flextime task force recommended that a 3-month pilot study be done utilizing employees who had indicated an interest in flextime and who met the eligibility criteria. Managers in all offices and departments selected the individuals to participate in the flextime pilot. Five nurses, five home health aides, three outreach workers, two payroll and billing clerks, and one occupational therapist represented each office participating in the pilot. Supervision was accomplished during flexed hours via telephone availability of the manager and the on-call nurse (Table 37–1).

Evaluation

At the end of the third month, an evaluation of the pilot was conducted. Evaluation efforts focused on input from the following areas: the patient, manager, employee, team, payroll department, and administration. Employees kept a log of patients whose visits had been scheduled outside the 8:00 A.M. to 4:30 P.M. workday and submitted a brief narrative statement discussing their experience participating in the pilot. A telephone survey was done by managers to assess patient satisfaction. Individual and team visit statistics were compared with budgeted projections. Increases and decreases in lateness and absenteeism among team members were assessed. Advantages and disadvantages of flextime were elicited from the managers and administration. A presurvey and postsurvey were administered to team members. Increased time spent processing payroll was measured. The task force analyzed the results based upon each of the established objectives.

Exhibit 37–3 Eligibility Criteria

- All full-time and part-time regular staff can be considered.
- Staff must have demonstrated themselves to be responsible and independent by meeting expected agency behavior via the performance evaluations.
- Paperwork must be up to date.
- Productivity statistics must meet or exceed expectations.
- Staff must have worked at the agency for at least 6 months.
- The number of individuals participating per team is at the discretion of the manager.
- Award of the flextime benefit is for a period of 6 months.
- Management reserves the right, based on performance and productivity, to require flextime participants to return to a traditional schedule after suitable notification. A 2-week time frame, whenever possible, is the maximum notice time.

Courtesy of Sharon D. Martin, MSN, RN, CS.

Table 37–1 Employees' Adjusted Work Hours, Regular Workday, 8:00 A.M. to 4:30 P.M.

Number of Staff	Flextime Hours
12	7:00–3:30
1	6:30–3:00
2	7:30–4:00
1	8:30–5:00

Courtesy of Sharon D. Martin, MSN, RN, CS.

RESULTS OF THE PILOT PROJECT

The results of the log of patient visits outside the 8:00 A.M. to 4:30 P.M. workday were that many of the staff used the early hours to do their charting rather than make patient visits. The telephone survey of patients indicated only three negative responses among 29 patients surveyed. Regarding increased opportunity for physician–nurse conferencing to occur, many staff noted the availability of the physician for consultation in the late afternoon, although most staff were flexing to earlier hours rather than later hours. Results of the pretest and posttest did not reflect an improved ability to meet patient needs. It was believed that the results were skewed, however, because work schedules had always been adjusted temporarily to meet patient needs.

Productivity was maintained at budgeted figures. Productivity and sick time were not affected positively or negatively by flextime. Employees with health problems continued to use sick time; employees with known productivity problems did not improve their performance as a result of flextime. In general, if there were problems with individuals before the pilot study, they remained. If there were no problems, flextime scheduling did not create any new ones.

Survey results reflected increased staff morale. Flextime was valued as a real benefit to pilot participants. Managers indicated difficulties in scheduling team meetings to accommodate various schedules as a disadvantage. Advantages were increased staff morale and increased flexibility to meet patient needs.

The results of the pilot study revealed that the major benefit of flextime was an improved ability of staff to meet family and personal needs and a consequent increase in staff morale. Of those flexing, most chose to flex to earlier hours. Overall, the flextime pilot was successful. The flextime task force recommended approval of the flextime policy, and the board of directors did so.

LIMITATIONS OF THE STUDY

The objectives of the program and the means for determining success or failure of the project should be identified before a flextime study is even attempted (Rosenberg, 1983). Clearly identifying these objectives before implementation allows comparison and a means to determine whether what was planned initially was actually accomplished.

Evaluation criteria established before the study rested heavily upon a prepilot and postpilot questionnaire, which was intended to gauge staff satisfaction and morale. One of the project goals was to increase these two factors among staff. It was never determined by objective measurements whether satisfaction was to be increased among all staff or just among staff utilizing flextime. The pretest and posttest were administered to all staff, however.

Some problems can be identified with this procedure. First, administering the pretest and posttest to everyone may have measured general satisfaction with work rather than response to flextime. Many of the questions reflected factors besides flextime. This was borne out when staff discussed the test. When answering the questions, frequently they were considering events in the office at times not relating to flextime. In addition, Rosenberg (1983) suggests that the pretest and posttest should be administered no sooner than 6 months apart, giving staff enough time to feel as if flextime is the usual state of affairs. Our posttest was administered at a 2-month interval to meet the deadline of a 3-month report on the pilot. This was probably too soon to test any real changes. In fact, when the tests were examined we found that there was little or no difference between the pretest and posttest answers. Because of the broadness of the questions, the fact that the test was given to all employees, and the short time between administration of the tests, the validity of the results as a means to gauge morale in relation to flextime is questionable.

Another goal of the project was that patients' needs would be better met. From patient responses via telephone or in person, it appears that patients enjoyed the flextime visits. Patients who did not enjoy the earlier visits were rescheduled for visits later in the day.

The third goal of the project, decreased management time spent on special staff requests, was not evaluated by objective criteria. Subjective reports were the sole means of evaluating this goal. A fourth objective, no tardiness and less absenteeism, was only partially measurable. Because starting and stopping times were not measured by a time clock, it was difficult to gauge tardiness. Absenteeism was measurable, however, and no change was found before and after implementation of flextime. The fifth goal, increased capacity to cover cases outside the 8:00 A.M. to 4:30 P.M. time slot, was measured only by subjective reports of staff, patients, and supervisors, all of which were positive. The sixth goal, increased opportunity for physician–nurse conferencing, was not met because the majority of staff flexed to earlier hours.

An important factor for consideration is the use of a control group to compare with the experimental group of flextime staff. This would have given us valuable comparative information.

EXPERIENCE OVER TIME

It has been 10 years since the initial flextime pilot and policy implementation described above. A recent literature review gave the surprising result that no articles describing flextime were published in major nursing journals in the 1990s. Although many articles discuss a variety of scheduling options to improve staff retention (Erickson, 1991; Goodroe, 1992; Gowell and Boverie, 1992; Stratton et al., 1992; Sullivan, 1991), none focuses on flextime. Several articles specifically discuss staffing and retention in home care and community health (Ryals, 1991; Sherry, 1994; Whitaker, 1993), but again, none discusses flextime.

Ten years after implementation at our agency, all our eligibility criteria (see Exhibit 37–3) continue to be met. Originally developed to meet staff needs, they served as a prelude to flexing hours to meet patient needs as home care changed over the past 10 years. Flextime has contributed to our ability to meet patient needs by enabling twice-daily visits, highly technical visits at unusual hours, hospice visits, and evening visits. The flextime policy remains intact with the following changes:

- Flexible scheduling has been integrated into the corporate culture. It is no longer viewed as new or different. In fact, it is viewed as peculiar that an organization would not offer something as valuable as flextime to working men and women. It has been a particular benefit in recruiting and retaining staff and in enabling staff to maintain full-time status while meeting personal obligations. Abuses of the system have been rare. A recent survey indicated that approximately 50 percent of professional staff flex in one way or another.

- The policy applies to any agency job description. As direct care staff have flexed, support staff and supervisory staff have followed suit successfully.

- A 4-day, 10-hour schedule has been implemented. This is the most popular flextime mode. Staff nurses report that it is easier to organize their work (e.g., patient visits, phone conferences with physicians, and documentation) within the longer day. This is also the mode most frequently listed by managers as causing the most scheduling difficulties for a team, however. One manager reported asking her team to abandon the 4-day, 10-hour schedule.

- Other creative schedules have been devised, such as three 9-hour days and one 4-hour day or four 9-hour days.

A recent survey of managers at our agency indicated that, although highly valued by staff, flextime is not without its drawbacks. Comments from managers suggested that it could be difficult to keep track of everyone's schedules, to schedule meetings around diverse work times, and to meet deadlines on days when people might not be available. Scheduling problems were most commonly listed as the primary drawback of the policy, occasionally affecting patient coverage and continuity of care. One manager described developing a "buddy system" to solve these problems.

CONCLUSION

Flextime has been incorporated as a permanent personnel policy. According to the literature, attempts at flextime fail only about 5 percent of the time, generally because management has not included supervisors and staff in the planning (French, 1982). For this reason, widespread participation was used. Also, flextime, as the first step in alternatives to time management, has formed the basis for future consideration of compressed work weeks, variable days, and job sharing. As one flexing staff member put it, "It's nice to come and go when it fits the rest of your life."

REFERENCES

Erickson, S. 1991. Mother's hours: "Extra" RNs balance the workload. *Nursing Management* 22:45–46, 48.

French, W. 1982. *The personnel management process.* Boston: Houghton Mifflin.

Goodroe, J. 1992. The manager's influence on retention. *Health Care Supervisor* 11:74–78.

Gowell, Y., and P. Boverie. 1992. Stress and satisfaction as a result of shift and number of hours worked. *Nursing Administration Quarterly* 16:14–19.

Poor, R. 1970. *4 Days, 40 hours, and other forms of rearranged workweek.* Cambridge, MA: Bursk & Poor.

Rosenberg, G. 1983, May 5. Issues of the workplace. Workshop sponsored by the National Council of Alternative Work Patterns, Kennebunkport, ME.

Ryals, S. 1991. Current problems confronting community health services—Part 2. *Aspen's Advisor for Nurse Executives* 6:8–9.

Sherry, D. 1994. Coping with staffing shortages. *Home Healthcare Nurse* 12:39–42.

Skeler, J.L. 1981, September 28. Flexible work hours gather momentum. *U.S. News and World Report*, pp. 76–77.

Stratton, T., et al. 1992. Recruitment and retention of registered nurses in rural hospitals and skilled nursing facilities: A comparison of strategies and barriers. *Nursing Administration Quarterly* 16:49–55.

Sullivan, P. 1991. Common-sense ethics in administrative decision making. *Journal of Nursing Administration* 21:57–61.

Werther, W.B. 1983. Nontraditional work schedules: Their use in the health care setting. *Health Care Supervisor* 1:11–20.

Whitaker, R. 1993. A home health agency's operational model utilizing per visit and hourly staff. *Journal of Home Health Care Practice* 5:38–44.

CHAPTER 38

Evaluating Productivity

Lazelle E. Benefield

This chapter discusses the definition of productivity and how productivity is analyzed in home health services. Environmental and staff factors that affect productivity are analyzed, and a procedure to follow in determining the current productivity of staff is suggested. This discussion centers only on how to determine current productivity of staff who provide direct service, i.e., make visits. Although useful for all caregivers, this information was originally written for use with professional staff. Determining current productivity is only one part of a program that measures and improves productivity. Information about how to determine the standard necessary for agency viability and a positive bottom line, and how to institute a productivity improvement program in an agency can be found in other sources (Benefield, 1988, 1996a, 1996b, 1996c; Brinkerhoff & Dressler, 1990; Levy, 1979; McAfee & Poffenberger, 1982; Olson, 1983).

WHAT IS PRODUCTIVITY?

Several assumptions are listed below and form the basis for understanding productivity.

- Productivity is an issue in every agency. It is the current buzzword, and many people incorrectly think of productivity improvement as the sole method of improving income generation in an agency. In the

past productivity issues took a back seat in health care management. The curriculum for most clinical professions focused on improving skills in the care of individual clients and families, giving little attention to any systematic review of the relationship between efficiency and the quality of services that the professional delivered. Now, growing concern over rising health care costs and the need to better evaluate and control factors that improve efficiency have prompted a surge of interest in productivity issues.

- Productivity evaluation is a greater issue for some agencies than for others, specifically agencies that use full-time (FT) and part-time (PT) staff. In the past, agency managers with contract staff usually were not concerned with increasing contract staff visitations per unit of time. Contract staff are defined as workers who are paid a flat fee per visit. Historically, managers focused on FT/PT staff who were paid a salary for the hours worked and not the visits made. This may be changing because many agencies are investigating payment of FT/PT staff on the basis of the number of visits completed.

- The word productivity is usually viewed with some discomfort by most staff. One should expect a negative response, either

469

verbally or behaviorally, when the issue is first discussed. Staff often fear an assembly-line approach, staff cutbacks, and/or unrealistic increases in workload, leading staff to believe that they must work faster and give less quality care. Again, this is not necessarily true: Are there research data to indicate that a 2-hour home visit is more effective than a 1-hour visit?

- Productivity is a management issue and not exclusively an employee issue. First-line managers and above should be involved in the process of determining, monitoring, and, if necessary, improving productivity. Other readings provide further detail (Benefield, 1996a, 1996b; Epstein, 1991).
- Quality can improve at the same time that productivity increases, although many professional staff and managers would initially disagree. The most pressing need in this area involves accurately determining when quality exists and when the client outcome has been achieved. If we have a clear and measurable method of determining when the outcome has occurred, then it is easier to determine the type of services needed to achieve the outcome.

Productivity is defined as any or all of the following:

- output per given input (Federa & Bilodeau, 1984)
- "the relationship between the use of resources and the results of that use" (Olson, 1983, p. 46)

The definitions are most accurate when measuring productivity in industry, e.g., assembly line work. It is easy to measure the number of items or products produced in a given period of time; however, it is difficult to do this in a health service industry. The Olson definition, "relationship between the use of resources and the results of that use," was developed to include those in white collar positions, and best describes productivity in professional positions

in the home health care service industry. Productivity in health care measures both the quality and quantity of work done (Sullivan, 1995).

For example, in home care the use of resources may include everything necessary to complete the home visit, known as the product. This can include the caregiver's time, supplies, agency management time, and other indirect expenses. Historically, the results or output of using these resources have been defined as the number of visits per discipline per time period. The time period may be 1 day, 1 week, or 1 month. Visits may be separated by type—maternal-child, pediatrics, or hospice—and/or by discipline—registered nurse (RN), therapist, or social worker. Examples include the following:

- 6 reimbursable visits per RN each day
- 25 pediatric visits per therapist per week
- 120 reimbursable RN visits per week (Monday through Friday, 4 RNs at 30 visits each week, each RN averaging 6 visits per day)

When staff hear the word productivity they may think only of increasing the number of visits, because the measurement of productivity is the number of visits completed. Staff infrequently assume that work can be simplified, reorganized, or delegated. Because of the negative press surrounding productivity, all agency personnel need a great deal of information and reeducation to understand exactly what productivity is and what it means to the agency.

Having defined productivity, and before we analyze how productivity is determined, this is an appropriate time to clarify why productivity is important to agency viability. First, a cost-efficient operation is a primary goal. No agency will survive without being at least being self-sustaining, and to do that personnel must be efficient. A productivity analysis program can assist in monitoring efficiency. Quality service delivery is also a primary goal, and monitoring productivity can enhance the likelihood of providing quality services. A quality service is expected and valued by clients. Providing quality services involves encouraging staff, who are the agency's most valuable resource, to work toward their potential, i.e., to use the skills they were trained to use. The premise here is that monitoring and analyzing productivity will assist staff to use their skills efficiently.

WHAT WE KNOW ABOUT PRODUCTIVITY

What is known about productivity in home health care can be summarized as follows:

- Productivity is difficult to measure in a health service industry (Linn & Karsten, 1982).
- Improving only one area/component of an agency will not affect overall production; assessment includes all areas.
- When evaluating productivity, look at the 20% of the budget that amounts to 80% of the dollars and work on these areas. This is usually the cost of personnel (Burdo, 1993).
- Professional productivity does not depend on how fast an employee works but rather on the efficient use of time (Olson, 1983).

Productivity is difficult to measure in a health service industry. It is difficult to measure because of our limited knowledge of what we are measuring. The quantity (number) of home visits can be measured, but we are less skilled in measuring and evaluating the quality of the visit. Therefore the product, the provision of a service, called the home visit, is variable. The components of a home visit, including the tasks and the staff behaviors, are complex and difficult to quantify. In addition, the recipient of the service or action, the client, is variable (Martin, Scheet, & Stegman, 1993). The client will demonstrate changing characteristics, and no two clients with the same diagnosis will ever demonstrate the exact same needs. Physical, psychosocial, and environmental needs (e.g., lack of financial resources or limited support system) make each client and each visit unique and therefore difficult to quantify and evaluate.

Linn and Karsten (1982) suggest that we have an uncertain product definition, meaning that it is unclear what the agency is trying to produce (visits or health). To take it a step further, how much of whatever health is do we wish to produce? The agency's philosophy statement, e.g. service to anyone regardless of ability to pay or service to those with the ability to pay, and administrative style begin to define what the mission of the agency is and what the agency is producing: health, visits, or both. In addition to using agency philosophy as a guide, managers at the service delivery level are assisted in defining health production by insurance companies that define the services to be reimbursed and by consumers' demands for certain states of health. In other words, agencies provide services that are reimbursable and for which consumers are willing to pay. With little agreement over what range or depth of services should be provided, it is understandable that it has been difficult to measure productivity in the health services industry.

Improving only one component of an agency will not affect overall productivity. Productivity improvement involves a systematic assessment of the entire organization rather than just a staffing review. For example, a physical therapist's job tasks may be tied to secretaries who answer the phones and screen calls, to data processing (records may not be transcribed and given back to the therapist for use during the scheduled visit), and to other disciplines. The therapist may have to wait for the home health aide to arrive to supervise the visit or to meet with an RN regarding the client. One provider group cannot improve or change productivity unless other components of the system are evaluated. Therefore, do not expect the RN staff to increase productivity unless productivity improvements occur in other components of the system in which RNs work.

Start by looking at the 20% of things that cost 80% of the dollars, and initially work on these areas. Look at a budget sheet for a home health agency; the majority of costs are attributed to staff or personnel. This includes staff who deliver the service or product, the home visit, and other personnel whose job it is to support the caregivers. Evaluate this area first, then expand to the larger organization. Remember, productivity is a people issue. Professional productivity depends not on how fast an employee works but on the efficient use of time (Olson, 1983). This is the key to beginning an analysis of productivity and is probably the most important statement in this chapter. Staff should not be encouraged to work faster, to rush through visits, or to do more with less time. Rather, staff should be encouraged to use their time efficiently by spending time performing skills they were trained to use.

Managers should assist staff to identify their professional strengths and skills, refer non-nurse activities to others, and continually focus on whether the task or action being performed is relevant to achieving client outcomes. Productivity is clearly a management issue and not solely an employee issue. Management creates the climate and sets the pace for effective productivity. An agency manager that embarks on a productivity analysis should assess the entire organization for unnecessary activities, simplification of work, and a clear definition of the product, the home visit. The goal is not to improve one subset of the organization (personnel) but to maximize the entire organization's productivity.

ANALYZE SERVICE DELIVERY: EFFICIENCY, EFFECTIVENESS, AND EQUITY

Analysis of productivity involves identifying variables that are unique to each agency, including both agencywide and personnel reviews. Before reviewing personnel productivity, determine the efficiency, effectiveness, and equity of services provided by the agency as a whole. Gather historical and baseline information, then embark on a productivity review of personnel.

Efficiency involves the production of a certain amount of output within a unit of time. An efficiency goal may be to increase the amount

of output produced by a given input or to decrease the amount of input (skilled services) required to produce a given output (home visits). A specific visit has been provided efficiently if there is little time or material waste. Consider more than just the volume of services. Include information about service intensity, e.g. the complexity level of clients and the case mix of the population served. Case mix may include the type of client, severity of illness, and the service under which clients are admitted. At this stage the degree of agency efficiency may be hard to identify, so list the methods/strategies that the agency has used in the past to maintain efficiency. Identify which ones worked and why—incentive pay for visits over a certain number, fear of job loss if visit numbers were not increased, streamlined organization of paper flow.

Effectiveness of the service, a second variable to consider in productivity analysis, is the degree to which a production process has accomplished what it was intended to do. Analysis should include an evaluation of whether the correct job was done and the quality of service provided. Use staff and management input to determine the expected outputs for the visit. What activities and tasks should be completed during the home visit? This process is useful in clarifying the standards by which one can measure the care given and received. For example, evaluate the activities that should occur during a home visit for a diabetic client. What activities should the staff complete during the home visit? Determine a range of expected client responses. As necessary, use clinical paths or care maps as templates to match nurse-specific activity to achievement of client goals. These types of data may be retrievable through the agency's quality improvement program.

The *equity* of services is defined as the distributional effects of a given productivity scheme (Linn & Karsten, 1982), or, in other words, which population receives the services and whether the services are fairly distributed. How one defines fairly distributed is based on agency philosophy and policy. Horizontal equity is how the effects of production are distributed across the population as a whole, e.g., all the types of clients who are seen by the agency from the geographic areas served. Vertical equity is how a given production function affects a specific target population, e.g., among all the clients who need intravenous (IV) therapy, have all received the service, and does the agency wish to provide service to all or only a segment of the population? Determine what the agency philosophy is regarding equity (for example, service to clients with the ability to pay or quality care to all), and use that as a framework when analyzing productivity.

Do not expect a greater level of productivity than is possible. For example, if the agency serves a large rural area, the staff productivity standard will be different from that of an agency that provides only hospice services to a population in an urban area or a maternal-child health program that serves essentially a healthy population.

EVALUATE CURRENT PRODUCTIVITY

To develop productivity standards in an agency, use the following sequence of steps:

1. Analyze environmental factors that affect productivity.

2. Analyze staff factors that affect productivity.

3. Determine the current productivity of staff.

4. Develop a standard through a management blueprint.

Exhibit 38–1 is an overview of the process detailed here. The process identifies and reviews the specific characteristics of the agency's service delivery, including both office and field work, to identify current productivity. Evaluate efficiency, effectiveness, and equity to determine what productivity standard is needed to maintain agency viability. Evaluate whether a

productivity improvement program is needed to meet the productivity standard. This section analyzes environmental and staff factors to determine and evaluate current productivity.

To determine and analyze direct caregiver productivity, evaluate the provision of direct client care and environmental factors that affect the provision of services. Analyze environmental and staff factors that contribute to the efficient use of staff expertise. Identify areas that hinder and help staff in completing their work.

Environmental Factors

Include all indirect care factors that affect the staff member's provision of direct client care.

Exhibit 38–1 How To Develop Productivity Standards

1. **Analyze environmental factors that affect productivity.**
   - geographic area
   - paperwork
   - type of program
   - amount and quality of group work
   - staff scheduling
   - percentage of unnecessary activities
   - other
2. **Analyze staff factors that affect productivity.**
   - experience
   - length of service with agency
   - morale and motivation
   - other
3. **Determine the current productivity of staff.**
   - Determine baseline data on staff.
   - Collect visit data.
     - type, diagnosis, complexity
     - reimbursement source
     - completed visits
     - travel between visits (time, distance)
     - time spent in direct service, preparation, documentation, other
   - Determine productivity (product number divided by hours of labor).
4. **Determine a standard through a management blueprint.**

Geographic Area

- Determine, if not already known, the geographic area served by the caregiver. Is it a densely populated urban area or a sparsely populated rural area?
- Is travel time great? What is the distance between clients in driving time and in miles?
- Do staff physically report in each morning or evening from the field? What is the time allotted to travel in to the office?

Paperwork

- Which programs generate the most and least paperwork?
- Determine the length of time to admit a client. Which type of client (older, complex diagnosis, particular payer source) requires additional time for the admission?
- Are charts available for charting when needed? Are computer terminals available and used, are dictaphones used, and are progress notes called in for transcription?
- Are secretaries used for completing all insurance forms, or do staff do this?
- If staff do paperwork by hand, ask them where changes can be made to reduce redundancy. Do they write the client's name on four different sheets when admitting the client? Are addresses copied on more than one form?

Type of Program

- List the programs in which the caregivers are involved—hospice, pediatrics, high technology, maternal-child health, adult care.
- Is the average visit length different for each type of program? Are there different lengths within each program based on severity of clients' needs? Which programs consume longer visit times? Review agency policies and practices to determine why particular programs have longer visit times.

- Which programs do staff consider emotionally draining? Productivity and motivation may decrease as a result of the type of clients cared for, e.g., pediatric oncology clients, stroke clients, clients without family support.
- Which programs do staff shy away from, and why? Are these programs emotionally draining because the clients are noncompliant, the environment is unsafe or staff perceive it to be so, or the travel distance within one day is taxing?

Does the financial reimbursement for the service, be it fee-for-service, prospective payment, or capitated fee, influence the visit length, staff morale, or staff hesitancy to complete the home care services? Identify the specific payer plans and their real and perceived influence on staff decisions regarding visit length.

Amount and Quality of Group Work

- List the frequency and duration of inservice and administrative meetings. Is a new program or service creating a need for more meetings? Remember that meetings cut into the number of visits possible in a day.
- Are staff returning to the office for informal support from other staff? Often, new or inexperienced staff want contact with other staff for technical or moral support. As the complexity of the work increases the need for peer consultation may also increase. Some agencies require that all staff return to the office at day's end to encourage this peer consultation and to decrease the number of team conferences.

Staff Scheduling

Supervisory skill at scheduling staff affects productivity. Yes, productivity is a management issue. Consider these areas:

- How is scheduling done? Are visits planned with geographic proximity in mind? For example, do staff meet each morning, then drive to a distant locale to complete home visits, then return to the office in the evening to check in? When staff must come to the office before beginning visits, they may drive from home, passing their first client's residence on the way to the office to check in, then retrace the drive to the first client visit of the day. Perhaps staff can phone in to document when they have begun the day at the first client's home.

- Is there a specialty program, e.g., IV therapy, that covers a wide geographic area with staff expected to cover the entire area? Although acceptable in one agency, another agency may wish to hire contract staff who reside near the client.
- Do staff live adjacent to their service area? Are caregivers purposefully assigned to areas other than where they live? Consider reevaluating this practice.
- Review the assignments that inexperienced and more qualified staff receive. Determine whether there are differences in the assignments (there should be) and what they are. Is the newer or novice staff member assigned to a complex client? Is the expert staff member working with clients whom he or she finds unchallenging?
- Assuming that there is a choice of staff in a geographic region, assess how cases are assigned, taking into account an already full caseload, vacations, and other variables specific to the agency. Are staff being used effectively?

Percentage of Unnecessary Activities

Review the caregiver's day to identify where staff are involved in nondirect care activities that may be better delegated to others. Follow a staff member for a day, and ask him or her to identify redundant activities.

- Answering phones is a major time waster for caregivers. This is an especially troublesome problem in small agencies that may not provide coverage for telephones when the secretary goes to lunch. Consider

call forwarding to another site, using an answering service (this is costly and bad for public relations during working hours and overall not the best choice), or using a part-time secretary or clerk to cover busy times, e.g., early morning or lunch.

- Do nurses and therapists stock their own bags? It may be easier to provide staff with a check-off sheet listing the needed supplies. This sheet can be turned in and supplies can be packaged by a paraprofessional or office staff member for pick up the following day.
- Are staff providing services that can be done by other professional or paraprofessional staff? For example, are therapy staff providing counseling that could and should be done by social worker staff? Are RNs completing daily care activities that aides are trained to do? Evaluate the degree to which professional staff provide tasks that, although satisfying to the staff, may limit the time they have to provide interventions that they are uniquely trained to provide and will more directly impact client outcomes. This is one of the more difficult areas to correct; however, change in this area will reap major gains in productivity.

Other

What agency-specific factors affect the manner in which staff do their jobs? Is there a seasonal workload change—are admissions highest in the winter months with slack time in the summer, or just the reverse? Track the visits done by month over the past 2 years. Determine any trends in workload volume or complexity. Review and, as needed, modify the number of FT positions that are required. If historical trends indicate periods of lower census and visit activity, consider promoting the use of employee vacation and compensation time. Many agencies use PT/contract staff for periods of peak volume.

Staff Factors

Experience

- Experienced staff should complete more visits per unit of time than do inexperienced staff. Experienced staff should be more efficient in their use of time. Assuming a similar caseload mix, are experienced staff visiting more clients than less experienced caregivers? What is the difference in average visit time between experienced and less experienced staff? If visit time is the same, does that mean that experienced staff are seeing the more complex clients?
- What defines an experienced, effective staff member? A productive staff member may have skills such as:
  1. ease in charting
  2. greater expertise in assessing client needs, prioritizing, and goal setting
  3. the ability to deal with flexibility (the new staff member often complains of having no guidelines)
  4. expertise in health assessment
  5. expertise in counseling/therapeutic conversations. The staff member is able to avoid overinvolvement in only the social or financial aspects of care and can effectively delegate roles to other professionals. Further definition and discussion of the knowledge and abilities of productive RN staff is detailed elsewhere (Benefield, 1996).
- Is there a certain tenure or time in practice that is required before a staff member is deemed *experienced*? Since each agency has different expectations, manage each staff member individually and develop caseloads that are appropriate for both new and seasoned staff members. Identify your best staff members, and determine the knowledge and abilities that define their skill level. Then, encourage these behaviors in others (Benefield, 1996a, 1996b).

Length of Service with Agency

All staff need time for orientation. What is the expected orientation time for staff to become fully functional? Are prospective staff made aware of these expectations in preemployment interviews and during orientation? Do managers assist new staff in developing expertise in efficiency as well as in the traditional aspects of providing effective home care services? Determine the point at which you expect a full contribution by staff: 2 months, 6 months, 1 year?

Morale and Motivation

Is there good, average, or poor morale among staff? Although many variables contribute to changes in morale, among them the frantic pace of change in the home care industry, consider how the agency management style influences morale. Poor management may lead to poor morale and a decrease in staff motivation, resulting in decreased productivity. Carefully analyze the changes that have occurred in the agency within the last 6 months to 1 year, then view the managers' responses to the changes and their interaction with staff. Perhaps everyone needs morale- or team-building.

Other

Miscellaneous occurrences can affect productivity, such as illness among staff, leaves of absence, and vacations. Identify and list these and any other factors within the agency that affect productivity.

Summary

For an agency to be productive we must maintain and retain qualified staff. Since staff generally take their cues for performance expectations from management, staff productivity is a management issue, not just an employee issue. Management personnel, including first-line supervisors and above, should have the responsibility and accountability to control many of the factors that affect productivity. When managers organize the work environment and encourage professional growth in staff, the efficiency and quality of services are improved and productivity is increased.

Current Productivity

What is the current productivity standard in the agency? Is there an expectation that staff complete a certain number of visits per unit of time? The productivity standard that is established should be unique to each discipline and to each program. The variables discussed earlier are unique to each agency; therefore, the productivity standard should reflect the unique characteristics (type of agency, philosophy, financial expectations) of each agency.

Assume that the agency has a productivity standard in place. Are staff members aware of the standard and involved in completing the expected standard? The staff may understand the standard of 6 visits per day, averaged at 30 visits per week; however, they may not be clear that these visits must be reimbursable, meaning that the agency can bill and receive payment for the visits. For example, staff may assume that as long as they log six visits per day they meet the productivity standard. They may not take into account that the first visit was to a client without the ability to pay, and the second was to a client who was not home. Even though six homes were visited, the staff member provided only four reimbursable visits. Thus, the established standard should delineate whether all visit types are included, i.e., reimbursable and nonreimbursable. Reimbursable visits may include those paid for by Medicare, Medicaid, third-party payers, grants, and donations.

Identify the unique agency factors, listed in the preceding section, that affect the productivity of staff. Then determine the current productivity of staff using the following guidelines. Investigate computer analysis of this information:

1. Determine baseline data (categories) to indicate what defines:

- an experienced staff member, e.g., more than 3 years of experience
- a staff member who is oriented to the agency, e.g., service for more than 3 months
- contract, PT, and FT staff

2. For a week selected at random, preferably nonvacation and without heavy admissions, determine the following for each staff discipline, e.g., speech therapy, nursing:

- basic information: name, discipline, experience level, and type of employment
- number of visits done in a specific time frame, daily and weekly. We are determining the present productivity now; analysis of the specifics of the visits can be done later.
- evaluation of the visit/travel sheet. Note:
  - whether the visit was reimbursable or nonreimbursable. Count only reimbursable visits in determining productivity unless otherwise noted by the agency.
  - whether the visit was completed or the client was not home
  - travel distance between visits. Are staff determining the most efficient travel route? Do they drive greater distances than necessary? Is client care mandating early morning or late evening visits? Could a contract staff member do these visits?
  - travel time between visits. Is inner city travel taking as much time as travel to/from a rural area? In other words, should geographic areas be reassigned, or are there extra slow/extra speedy drivers?
  - visit length, matched with the type of visit (maternal child health, adult care)
  - the type of visit: an admission, a recertification, an emergency, a discharge, or any other type that indi-

cates the expectation of a longer or a shorter visit

– time spent in other activities, such as telephone calls to physicians or clinic personnel, communication with families, return calls to clients, and gathering supplies. Staff should be completing a travel sheet documenting visits and mileage. This area can be adapted to include nonvisit time and activities. These might be turned in weekly for the initial productivity review; later, once a month reviews should suffice.

3. Use this information, tabulated over a 5-day period, to determine the productivity or output per unit of input for each staff member. Then combine these data by discipline to determine an overall figure (the number of visits divided by 5 days equals the number of visits per day). Beware of combining figures from dissimilar programs; for example, staff who do postpartum visits may achieve a higher visit rate than those working within the hospice program who may have lower productivity expectations. Use the overall productivity figure as a guide, and compare it with staff productivity in different programs, in varied geographic areas, and for various employment statuses.

4. Ask these questions when analyzing the information:
   • Are certain geographic areas more difficult to service than others? Are there fewer clients in the area, greater distance between clients, geographically isolated clients, or specific factors such as a bridge or tunnel that causes delays?
   • Which visits take the least and most time? Do additional analysis to identify specific issues. Ask the staff to assist in analysis. They can identify the complexity involved in certain types of visits and identify roadblocks to the provision of care. Managers can then determine whether support services can be used to remove barriers.
   • On the average, does the visit length differ among PT, contract, and FT staff? Are contract staff, who are paid by the visit, hurrying through the visit, or are they the most efficient of the staff? Note that many agencies pay FT, PT, and contract staff by the visit, so determine whether these data are important for the agency. Perhaps of greater significance is whether the visit length is different between experienced and new staff.
   • What special circumstances may have skewed or altered the data? Were there increases in sick leave or increases in the number of emergency visits or admissions during the sample week?
   • What do the staff make of the data? Because they provide the day-to-day service and are involved in the complexities of the provision of services, they should be able to describe why the results of the review look as they do.
   • Which staff members are productive? Evaluate the characteristics of the staff with the highest productivity. What knowledge or abilities do they possess and use on a consistent basis? Interview these staff members to determine how they describe their ability to provide both efficient and effective care. Are productive staff members ones whom managers would easily identify? What characteristics do these staff have; why are they productive? A profile of a productive employee is one who is well qualified for the job, highly motivated, has a positive job orientation, and communicates effectively.

THE NEXT STEP

The purpose of this chapter is to provide a method for evaluating the current productivity of all or a segment of the staff who provide direct service to clients. It involves analyzing the environment in which staff work, reviewing the type and quality of staff working in the agency, assessing what is included in a home visit, and having a good idea of what makes a productive staff member in the agency.

The next step is to determine, using fiscal data, the productivity standard necessary to meet expenses and/or generate revenue over expenses. Indirect costs (supplies, overhead, etc.) and direct staff costs are matched to income generated from billable visits to determine the total cost of doing a home visit. The information is analyzed further to determine (1) the number of visits necessary to cover the cost of agency operation, and (2) the number/types of visits necessary to generate a predetermined percentage of revenue over expenses. This is defined as the number of reimbursable visits per staff per unit time. This is the standard for the agency or specific program.

The standard, considered the benchmark or guide to the expected level of work, should be unique to each discipline. For example, therapy visits per day may be different from expected RN visits per day. Brinkerhoff and Dressler (1990) also provide reviews of how to determine a productivity standard for the agency.

Having determined what current productivity is and what the productivity standard is, evaluate whether there is a need for a productivity improvement program. If the current productivity does not equal or exceed the standard established for agency viability, then a produc-

tivity improvement program is essential. Likewise, if staff productivity cannot increase without a decrease in quality, a productivity improvement program is needed to assess and organize those people and things that affect caregivers' time. Perhaps the productivity standard is being met, staff morale is high, management is totally efficient, and the quality of client services and outcomes are good. Clearly, there is no need for a productivity improvement program.

A productivity improvement program includes five dimensions: systematic education of all personnel about the relationship between productivity and agency viability, an assessment of the total operation, adequate staffing and performance measurements, implementation of incentives for increasing productivity, and continual evaluation of the productivity standards.

CONCLUSION

Remember the basic assumptions when evaluating productivity. First, productivity improvement is not completed in a vacuum. Improving only one component of an agency will not increase overall productivity, so consider an agencywide program. Second, involve all staff, particularly direct caregivers, in planning and evaluating the productivity of an agency. Third, management holds the key to effective productivity through effective supervision and the ability to create environments that challenge and motivate staff.

REFERENCES

Benefield, L.E. (1988). Productivity. In L. Benefield (Ed.), *Home health care management* (pp. 164–179). Englewood Cliffs, NJ: Brady.

Benefield, L.E. (1996a). Component analysis of productivity in home care RNs. *Public Health Nursing*, 13(4), 233–243.

Benefield, L.E. (1996b). Productivity in home health care: assessing nurse effectiveness and efficiency. *Home Healthcare Nurse*, 14(9), 699–706.

Benefield, L.E. (1996c). Productivity in home health care: maintaining and improving nurse productivity. *Home Healthcare Nurse*, 14(10), 803–812.

Brinkerhoff, R., & Dressler, D. (1990). Productivity measurement. *Applied social research methods series* (Vol. 19). Newbury Park, CA: Sage.

Burdo, D. (1993). Cutting down. *Modern Healthcare*, 23(51), 49–58.

Epstein, P. (1991). Productivity analysis of professional staff and services. *Public Productivity and Management Review*, 15(2), 141–145.

Federa, R.D., & Bilodeau, T.W. (1984). The productivity quest. *Journal of Ambulatory Care Management*, 7, 5–11.

Levy, G. (1979). Productivity for home health services. *Home Health Review*, 2(2), 24–29.

Linn, N., & Karsten, S. (1982). Managing public health productivity—The art of taming conflict and chaos. *Public Productivity Review*, 6(3), 170–183.

Martin, K., Scheet, N., & Stegman, M. (1993). Home health clients: characteristics, outcomes of care, and nursing interventions. *American Journal of Public Health*, 83(12), 1730–1734.

McAfee, B., & Poffenberger, W. (1982). *Productivity strategies*. Englewood Cliffs, NJ: Prentice-Hall.

Olson, V. (1983). *White collar waste: gain the productivity edge*. Englewood Cliffs, NJ: Prentice-Hall.

Sullivan, M. (1995). *Nursing leadership and management*. Springhouse, PA: Springhouse Corp.

BIBLIOGRAPHY

Bermas, N.F. (1984). The positive side of productivity for ambulatory care management. *Journal of Ambulatory Care Management*, 7(8), 1–40.

Humphrey, C.J., & Milone-Nuzzo, P. (1996). *Orientation to home care nursing*. Gaithersburg, MD: Aspen Publishers, Inc.

Orefice, J.J., & Jennings, M.C. (1983, August). Productivity key to managing cost per case. *Healthcare Financial Management*, 20.

Ozcan, T.A., & Shukla, R.K. (1993). The effect of a competency-based targeted staff development program on nursing productivity. *Journal of Nursing Staff Development*, 9, 78–84.

CHAPTER 39

Labor–Management Relations

Jessie F. Rohner

Institutions are often thought to be the bricks and mortar of their buildings, which are easily seen. In reality, people are the institution. If they leave, the institution no longer exists. What is important for any institution, therefore, are the interactions, supports, feelings, frustrations, challenges, and hopes which come from the people who constitute it. The combination of these elements forms the institution's climate. (Lockhart & Werther 1980, p. 103)

The characteristics of the institution's climate influence the relationship between labor and management and affect the effectiveness of the health agency. This climate also influences whether staff feel the need for a union. Administration must therefore be alert to the climate and be aware of and practice ways to enhance a positive relationship with nursing staff. How management responds to employee needs, requests, and concerns will be a major determinant of the climate; a positive environment will be produced if needs are met. It is a major task for administration to find a "balance between people's needs and organizational needs" (Lockhart & Werther, 1980, p. 132), for such a balance will create and sustain an organization that is effective and vital.

CONCEPTUAL FRAMEWORK

The home health agency should be viewed from a systems theory framework in which both labor and management are seen as vital units of the system. There must be interdependency among the units if the agency is to be effective. The agency as a whole has a need for unity, and each of the units must cooperate with the other. This cooperation will build cohesion among the units, which will enhance the effectiveness of the agency. Labor and management need to view themselves as existing in a partnership in which everyone works for the patient's benefit.

FACTORS INFLUENCING THE LABOR RELATIONS CLIMATE

Many authorities have identified various factors that influence the labor relations climate of an organization and methods for enhancing the positive relationship between labor and management. Zacur (1982) has identified environmental factors, both internal and external, that influence the labor relations climate of certain organizations. Although these organizations were primarily acute care hospitals, it is possible that the same factors would be important in a home health agency. Zacur (1982) identified the following external factors:

- laws such as the 1947 Taft-Hartley Act, which guaranteed the rights of representation and collective bargaining with a nonprofit employer
- professional organizations such as the American Nurses Association (ANA), which has attempted to improve the economic status of nurses
- the state of the economy, which has put pressure on female employees to request and demand increased salaries and has focused attention on the comparable worth issue
- public sentiment regarding health care professionals.

Internal factors identified by Zacur (1982) include the organizational climate, the organization's administrators, the nurses' roles, and the nurses' views.

If the organizational climate is one that tolerates change and new ideas as opposed to being repressive, the labor–management climate may be positive and vital. If administration is parochial in its approach to managing human resources, lacks sensitivity to internal conditions encountered by staff, fails to recognize the professional issues of concern to nurses, and refuses to negotiate or discuss certain issues, the environmental climate will not be healthy and will reduce the effectiveness of the staff.

Another factor affecting the labor relations environment is how decisions are made and policies are determined. If agencies are administered through a bureaucratic organizational structure, and if processes and policies are issued from administration without any participation from caregivers, the environment may be conducive to collective action. Nursing staff cannot be viewed as functionaries at the lower end of the hierarchy without any participation in decision making if their contributions to the attainment of agency goals are to be maximized. Ginzberg (1966) suggested that, because nurses are influenced and affected by conditions in the environment, management needs to maximize opportunities for them to succeed, should care-

fully match people to jobs, and should provide maximum support to nurses in these positions.

Levitan, Mangum, and Marshall (1981) indicate that the organizational climate and administration should be secure and certain because uncertainty breeds frustration and dissatisfaction. Another important factor in determining environmental climate is the sense of fairness exhibited or practiced by administration (Gregorich & Long, 1980). Lack of this, perhaps more than any other factor, will promote a sense of collective action.

How nurses view their roles and responsibilities within the organization and how they view the nursing profession will influence the labor relations climate of the organization. These views and perceptions are influenced by factors such as length and type of education. As nurses have received increased education with a more professional orientation, they appear to have become more dissatisfied with an environment that does not acknowledge professional autonomy (Zacur, 1982). Home health nurses need to be involved in decision making regarding patient care, and this must be fostered by administration.

In a study by Meyer (1970), job security, social esteem, autonomy, self-realization, job and salary satisfaction, chance for advancement, membership in state nurses associations, beliefs about union power, and feelings toward authority were some of the variables examined in relationship to nurses' attitudes toward collective action. The following specific variables were found to be significantly related to a positive attitude toward collective action: lack of autonomy, self-realization, and security; low predisposition to submit to authority; low salary satisfaction; and lack of belief that trade union power is too great. Further analysis revealed that, when respondents in the study perceived the organizational climate as more autocratic, their need deficiency scores increased significantly, and mean collective action attitude scores were significantly higher.

Another study by Alutto and Belasco (1972) indicated that those nurses who were most militant and pro-strike were younger nurses with a low feeling of organizational commitment and strong dissatisfaction with their careers. According to Zacur (1982), the primary condition within a hospital that precipitates a nursing militancy or pro-strike attitude is administrators' use of a bureaucratic approach in dealing with human resources and failure to recognize the professional concerns and abilities of the nursing staff. Such a management approach breeds resentment and appears to initiate militant or strike behavior.

Ginzberg (1966) indicates that individuals have a value orientation and a preference system in their work. These are based on needs, goals, and values. Management, therefore, needs to be aware of preference systems and to assist nursing staff in achieving goals and meeting needs within this framework.

Four value orientation categories have been derived empirically and can be used as guidelines by management to identify employee types and their general value orientation (Ginzberg, 1966): individualistic, leadership, social, and ideological. The individualistic type wants to be free from strict direction and interference, choosing to structure his or her own activities while making optimal use of individual capacities in the work setting. The leadership type has an orientation toward building and maintaining relationships with others, having authority over others, directing and leading others, and being more involved in the organizational structure. The basic orientation of the social type is to be a member of a group or team and to be accepted by group members. Individuals of this type strive for group esteem. They have no intention or desire to become "the boss"; they derive satisfaction from the social context of their work. The greatest number of people in the workforce is of this type. The ideological worker is committed to a system of ideals or ideas and has a goal to serve a higher value than meeting personal needs. These individuals seek autonomy not for themselves but for the cause. Although these four types are not mutually exclusive, most individuals exhibit one orientation more

strongly, and management could identify this and use it to promote individual well-being and consequently organizational well-being.

Any home health agency that is attempting to promote positive labor–management relations should concentrate on identifying internal and external environmental factors that affect the organizational climate. Attempts should be made to understand the nurses' perceptions, needs, and value orientations so that both individual needs and organizational needs can be planned for and met.

COMMUNICATION AND INTERPERSONAL SKILLS

Communication and interpersonal skills, which are vital to promoting helping relationships, can aid in creating effective labor–management relationships. Scott (1962) proposed that the health of an organization depends upon successful communication, or the imparting of information to all employees. If the home health agency is viewed as a system, then communication can be viewed as a linking process, binding together the various system units (management and labor). Rothstein (1958) states:

> Organization presupposes the existence of parts, which considered in their totality, constitute the organization. The parts must interact. Were there no communication between them, there would be no organization but merely a collection of individual elements isolated from each other. (p. 34)

Communication networks should exist in the organization. These networks are decision centers interconnected by channels of communication. A feedback system is crucial for the network because it helps maintain balance among all components of the system. Change can occur, and the system can self-regulate when feedback is received.

Davis (1958) states that communication is the process of passing information and understanding from one person to another. This implies that communication does not occur unless the receiver understands the transmitted information. In organizations, the greater the degree of understanding by the receiver (worker), the more likely the receiver will be to behave and act so that organizational goals are attained (Scott, 1962). Thus communication is viewed as a manager's tool for accomplishing agency goals.

The focus of communication has shifted from being persuasion and conversation oriented to being understanding and negotiation oriented (Cushman, 1980). Talking and discussing provide both labor and management the opportunity to understand and accept diverse points of view and alternative solutions to a problem, which then allows for the successful negotiation of a solution.

For a positive relationship to occur between labor and management, both parties must practice effective sending and receiving skills. Both verbal and nonverbal channels can be used to send messages. The majority of messages are sent without words, however; messages are most often conveyed by body language, facial expressions, gestures and body movements, eye contact, tone of voice, use of silence, and other behaviors. Individuals must constantly be alert to the congruency between their verbal and nonverbal messages. Verbal messages are meant to convey ideas as well as feelings. An important component of verbal messages is asking for reactions or verbal feedback to ensure that the intent of the words is being understood by those receiving them.

Receiving skills are as critical to effective communication as sending skills. Primary skills in receiving messages are observing behavior and listening actively. An active listening response consists of a feeling component and a content component (Gerrard, Boniface, & Love, 1980); the receiver attempts to understand not only what the sender is saying but also what he or she is feeling. The sender does this by concentrating and asking reflective questions. This aspect of communication indicates interest in the speaker, conveys acceptance, builds trust, and assists the person in developing problem-solving skills. It is important that both labor and management take the time to learn, practice, and participate in actively listening to each other. Furthermore, effective sending and receiving of messages require that clarification occur. Eliciting feedback from all parties generates understanding between labor and management.

The interpersonal skills of showing respect, empathizing, and developing trust can assist in promoting a positive labor–management relationship. "Showing respect means conveying the attitude that the client has importance, dignity and respect" (Spradley, 1985, p. 273). Respect should be conveyed by both labor and management through tone of voice, recognition of valuable ideas, and the manner in which people are addressed. Empathizing is a skill that can be used by all individuals to show that they are attempting to understand feelings expressed by others. This skill also encourages the sharing of concerns.

Developing trust is critical if individuals are to work effectively with each other. Management and labor can develop trust for each other by showing acceptance of each other, treating each other as partners, and having open discussions to share feelings. Candid discussions can be part of a labor–management committee approach (discussed later).

Various reasons for communications breakdown exist, but most can be traced to the following (Scott, 1962):

- the nature and functions of human language
- purposeful misrepresentation
- the size of the organization
- lack of acceptance
- failure to understand

Distortion and filtering are severe and frequent problems in the communication process. Distortion occurs because messages sent up and down in an organization have to be interpreted by receivers. Because human language is so complex and can be interpreted differently by different individuals, messages can become distorted as they are passed among various individuals. Management can minimize distortion by asking for feedback from receivers to determine whether the content of the message is being interpreted as intended. The existence of social barriers or social distances or a difference in thinking between staff and management can also create distortion. Scott (1962) suggests that most communication breakdowns occur because subordinates do not agree with their bosses about obstacles and problems they are facing. He recommends empathy as one method by which social distances between different levels of employees can be overcome. If managers can project themselves into the framework of the employees, then any messages sent by managers will be more likely to be received and understood by the employees.

Communication breakdown can be caused by deliberate misinterpretation of a message. This occurs primarily in upward communication, when subordinates send to managers the material that they believe will be most accepted. Filtering includes errors of both commission and omission.

As an organization increases in size and complexity, management becomes buried in communication to which response is impossible. Optimum flow of material is necessary if managers are to communicate successfully with staff; thus irrelevant information should be monitored and handled by middle management personnel.

Poor timing and short-circuiting are other serious communication problems related to the size and complexity of the organization. Information needs to be released at the appropriate time and received by all employees at the same time or in sequential order. Short-circuiting occurs when someone is missed in the communication chain who should have been included. An employee's status may be lowered and angry feelings may result when the employee

does not get necessary information at the appropriate time.

Communication breakdowns also occur because staff lack acceptance and understanding of the conveyed information. Even though staff may receive the appropriate material at the right time, they may choose not to accept it for various reasons, such as incongruence in reality between sender and receiver, an ambiguous or unclear message, lack of faith in the sender (low credibility), and incongruence between the content of the message and the receiver's value system. As ambiguity of the message increases, as the credibility of the sender decreases, and as conflict between message content and value system of the receiver increases, the receiver becomes less likely to accept the information (Scott, 1962). These are all affected by the receiver's perception of reality, so that the manager should work first to understand and change the receiver's view of the reality of the situation. Teamwork has been recommended as a mechanism for effectively changing an individual employee's view of reality and thus promoting acceptance of the information.

The last cause of communication breakdown is lack of understanding by receivers who inaccurately translate the symbols used in communication. Scott (1962) suggests that a climate for understanding can be established by management by planning for communication, tailoring the information to fit the employee's frame of reference, and listening to what employees have to say. This last step can be carried out in a nondirective interview between staff and management, which will generate information about needs, complaints, and employee goals. The manager acts as a sounding board only, gathering information that will allow him or her to respond to the needs of staff.

PROBLEM SOLVING

Creative problem solving is another management tool for promoting a healthy labor–management relationship. The use of conceptual models such as an open systems model assists in improving interdepartmental communications (Golightly, 1981). Use of a model serves as a discussion point as information flows from one area to another and discussion occurs among components of the system, between the problem solvers and those who are affected by the solution. This method enhances effective communication, which then facilitates the problem-solving process.

Three levels of problem solving exist in an organization such as a home health agency: the individual process, the group process, and the organizational process, which contains several groups. The normal group approach, the Delphi problem-solving method, and brainstorming can be used by groups to solve problems creatively. Certain factors that affect group problem solving are the problem information held by the group, the extent to which the group accepts that there is a need for action, and the extent of congruence between goals of the individual members and the goals of the group (Vroom & Yetton, 1976).

Organizational problem solving is much more complex than the individual or group process because of the increased number of environmental and personal variables involved. As more individuals are involved, the potential for conflict increases. Objectives for organizational problem solving must be explicit, providing a framework for goal-directed behavior.

Many situations exist in a home health agency that are complex, with many variables interfacing and contributing to the situation. In approaching these situations, it seems appropriate to identify all the contributing factors that interface so that a reasonable problem statement and a solution can be formulated. Figure 39–1 illustrates a model in which all the information is collected, processed, and expanded (Golightly, 1981). Such a model would be useful as labor and management begin to formulate a solution to a complex problem. A systematic gathering of data is done to produce issues, facts, and givens, which are analyzed to formulate problem statements. The middle funnel is inverted to indicate that there are many problem

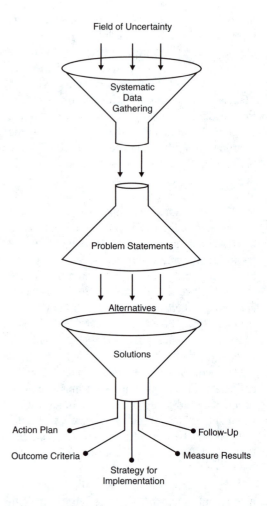

Figure 39–1 The Funnel Analogy. *Source:* Reprinted from C.K. Golightly, *Creative Problem Solving for Health Care Professionals*, p. 60, © 1981, Aspen Publishers, Inc.

statements rather than just one, and that problem statements may overlap.

As these problem statements are constructed, a people-centeredness approach is emphasized. This approach facilitates change from the manager's perspective and recognizes the contributions of the worker. Management must indicate a willingness to help and to work with the work group. Golightly (1981) indicates that, when management begins to pay attention to the work group, the out-of-balance state begins to change and improve.

After data have been collected and processed, the problem and all its parameters can be defined in small groups. A large group can be divided into smaller groups to address specific issues. Use of such a model with group involvement fosters employee involvement, promotes ownership, and accelerates group acceptance (Golightly, 1981).

After the data have been collected and analyzed and alternatives have been generated, some time should elapse before solutions are recommended. The work group, in identifying the best solution, should consider how a specific solution contributes to the agency objectives, the cost in dollars, the time needed to implement the plan, and the feasibility of the solution (Golightly, 1981).

GENERAL RECOMMENDATIONS

Various authorities have made recommendations on how to promote a positive labor–management relationship. Some of these are as follows:

- Establish a patient care committee. Such a committee should comprise all categories of caregivers and should provide a forum for discussion of general concerns regarding patients. This approach promotes a team concept, creative problem solving, and involvement in decision making.
- Establish some mechanism for recognizing nursing staff's professional contributions. A variety of positive reinforcements can be used to reward and thus motivate organizational commitment and performance. The rewards can range from monetary compensation to citations to verbal recognition only. An important criterion is that the reward be perceived as valuable by the employee, which necessitates that such programs be designed with input from the employees themselves. It seems necessary to define what nurses perceive

as professional recognition and how it can be achieved. This would indicate to management what motivational methods to use.

- Encourage a policy of informal staff meetings between nurses and supervisors. Communication can be facilitated during these meetings as input is solicited from nurses and feedback is given regarding the disposition of such suggestions. Critical components of such meetings should be a two-way communication process, the giving of much information and praise, and an emphasis on positive reinforcement and possibilities rather than constraints (Zacur, 1982).
- Use career counseling to promote professional commitment. Zacur (1982) states that "a long-term developmental approach to staff nurses and their careers can foster organizational commitment and decrease interest in militancy as a means to professional recognition" (p. 76). Administration has a responsibility to ensure that career needs of individuals are maximized, that nurses have the skills and knowledge necessary to perform their jobs, and that they have the opportunity to utilize these skills. This can be accomplished when staff and administration engage in joint planning.
- Provide orientation update sessions. These sessions provide employees with information about current developments and future plans and allow nurses to share their perceptions with management (Gregorich & Long, 1980). Problems can be presented during these sessions, but this is done in a positive, constructive atmosphere.
- Fill front-line supervisory positions with the best possible people and provide education for them to increase their effectiveness. Individuals hired for these positions should demonstrate excellent interpersonal skills, communication skills, and labor relations training. Personal attention should be given by the supervisor to all employees, especially those with great needs. The

literature indicates that an organization must meet the needs as perceived by employees, or the union will come along, meet these needs, and win approval of the group (Cangemi, Clark, & Harryman, 1980). It is suggested that the supervisor's treatment of employees is a critical factor in establishing a positive labor–management climate (Lockhart & Werther, 1980).

- Prepare an employee-oriented publication. Items concerning employees should be incorporated into the publication, along with pictures and praise. Controversial and threatening messages should not be included.
- Support athletic and recreational programs or social events sponsored by employees.
- Design an acceptable suggestion system.
- Develop a plan for rewarding loyal, dedicated employees who have demonstrated commitment to the agency.
- Develop a system to audit and identify feelings, opinions, and needs of employees. This system provides information that can be used to initiate action to meet employee needs and to facilitate movement in accordance with employee goals. Creating a more positive environment requires proactive behavior by management and allows actions to be taken before, not after, a crisis situation occurs.
- Foster a cooperative environment. "Cooperating is largely a matter of consultation between the two sides" (Werther & Lockhart, 1980, p. 156). Cooperation is sometimes difficult to achieve because both labor and management harbor fears and misconceptions based on past experiences. A cooperative relationship can begin when either side is in a desperate situation and needs help. Favors are given and reciprocation is expected. These requests form the beginning of a cooperative environment. Such an environment can also be initiated by having a formal suggestion plan in which employees can be consulted and encouraged to give suggestions. Jointly sponsored athletic, recreational, and social events provide the opportunity for each side to have a mutually satisfying interaction, to reevaluate opinions of each other, and to build teamwork. For labor–management relations to be positive, adversarial relationships must be abandoned; each side must view the relationship as a cooperative and a helping one, and each side must agree to consult the other before taking action.
- Establish an employee relations program. This program must be perceived as equitable and consistent by staff. This applies particularly to wages, which must be perceived as satisfactory. If this occurs, the employee relations program and management will have credibility. Nonunionized agencies need to act as though a third party is standing by, judging their actions for fairness and consistency. Agencies should have as part of their employee relations program a philosophy that recognizes the needs of both labor and management. Specific components of such a philosophy include the following (Werther & Lockhart, 1980):

  1. Management should recognize staff needs, and all actions should consider these needs.
  2. Staff must respect management's need for efficiency and effectiveness.
  3. Problem solving should be a joint endeavor between staff and management.
  4. Cooperation is the most viable long-term strategy for ensuring agency success.
  5. Survival of the agency is paramount.

- Establish a position of employee relations manager. The primary role of such a person would be to act as management's conscience, reminding management of its commitment to an employee relations program. The employee relations manager serves as the expert in resolving employee relations problems, designs two-way communication systems, and assists both parties in utilizing these systems to promote positive interactions and mutual understanding.

- Provide for a formal grievance procedure. "Union leaders stated publicly that the best defense against union organization is an effective grievance procedure" (Gregorich & Long, 1980, p. 109). Having a formal grievance procedure in a nonunion setting provides a mechanism for release of pressure, assurance that employee grievances will be considered, an avenue for communication, and a stimulus for discovering needs and implementing change. For the grievance procedure to be successful, members of management who have decision-making responsibility in a grievance must be credible, fair, and impartial. Second, employees must have an advocate available to assist in preparing and presenting a grievance. All employees should be encouraged to use the grievance process, without fear of reprisal or being labeled as a troublemaker.

- Establish a labor management committee. This committee is usually found in an agency that has a collective agreement for the purpose of discussing issues not covered in the collective bargaining process (Hemsworth, 1978). It also facilitates communications between management and selected members of the bargaining unit in the following ways (Centre County, 1984):

1. It allows employees to share concerns and suggestions regarding agency service.
2. It identifies employee concerns that do not qualify for the grievance procedure and are not within the scope of the supervisor.
3. It provides a mechanism for nursing staff to give input to administration on their policies and procedures.
4. It provides a sounding board for management to get input from staff.

5. It encourages a feeling of unity throughout the agency in responding to problems.
6. It facilitates a clear and consistent interpretation of the collective bargaining agreement.

Such a committee is usually composed of equal numbers of management and nursing personnel. Management can be represented by the executive director, personnel director, nursing manager, or a member of the agency's board. Members of the collective bargaining unit would represent the nurses.

One agency that instituted a labor management committee discussed the following issues as part of the monthly agendas over a period of 1 year: recruitment of nurses and supervisors; physical plant, including telephone workstations; the need for a nursing support group; charting procedures; agency finances; new services; the agreement with the local hospital; increasing referrals from special hospitals; the employee handbook; and communication patterns. Some time was spent discussing communication patterns. Staff would hear comments made by management that they perceived as derogatory and resulted in angry feelings and low morale. Discussions centered on how to prevent this from happening and how to establish open, candid communication between management and staff.

COLLECTIVE BARGAINING

Another way in which the labor–management environment is influenced is through collective bargaining. Historically, attempts at collective bargaining were met with resistance by nurses who felt it was not professional to withhold services from patients. The conflict of professionalism and unionism existed and prevented nurses from bargaining with employers. However, the trend has changed and unionization is now an acceptable way to ensure that employers recognize and discuss the economic and professional needs of nurses.

The National Labor Relations Act of 1935 was the first piece of social legislation that required employers to engage in collective bargaining with employees. Employees in nonprofit health care organizations, however, were not protected by this federal law to engage in collective bargaining. Not until 1947, when the Taft-Hartley amendment to the National Labor Relations Act was passed, could such employees organize. This legislation enabled health care workers to enter the mainstream of American labor to promote their own professionalism and unity.

The ANA, formed in 1896 as a professional organization committed to quality patient care, approved collective bargaining for nurses in 1946 to assure the public that adequate, high-quality nursing care would be available to all sick people (Kruger, 1961). Thus began an era when collective action was accepted as one way to ensure professionalism. In 1950, however, ANA members approved a policy that no strikes would occur as this would be inconsistent with nurses' professional responsibility to patients. In 1966, the ANA Commission on Economic and General Welfare determined that changes were necessary in the economic security program and rescinded the no strike policy.

During the 1970s, the ANA mounted an aggressive campaign to support the nation's nurses in collective bargaining activities. The numbers of persons covered by collective agreements increased significantly, indicating that the ANA was working to advance the economic and general welfare of nurses.

Hemsworth (1978) outlines what nurses have gained through collective bargaining:

- professional strength through unity
- the legal right to voice concerns for patient care and professional improvement
- the right to contribute to the decision-making process through negotiations
- improved benefits, including job security
- the right to challenge rules through grievance procedures

These gains have been attained primarily through presentation of a unified approach and negotiation.

Although collective bargaining can be viewed as an infringement of management prerogatives and an interference in the employer–employee relationship, nurses have continued to choose such activities as a way to affect employment conditions and to determine and control their practice.

CONCLUSION

In a home health agency, management must strive to create a healthy work environment in which labor–management relationships are positive. Management must be sensitive to perceived staff needs and to ways to meet these needs. Programs should be designed to maximize all employee contributions to the program. Both labor and management must work together, using a team approach, effective communication, and problem-solving skills and consulting with each other in an atmosphere of fairness, respect, empathy, and trust. A variety of methods can be used by management to ensure that labor–management relations are positive, that quality patient care is achieved, that employee welfare is maximized, and that organizational goals are met.

REFERENCES

Alutto, J.A., & Belasco, J.A. 1972. *Determinants of attitudinal militancy among nurses and teachers*. Bethesda, MD (ERIC Document Reproduction Service No. ED 063 635).

Cangemi, J.O., Clark, L., & Harryman, E. 1980. Differences between pro-union and pro-company employees. In C.A. Lockhart & W.B. Werther, Jr. (Eds.), *Labor relations in nursing*. Wakefield, MA: Nursing Resources.

Centre County Home Health Service Labor Management Committee. 1984, May 23. *Minutes of meeting.* Bellefonte, PA: Author.

Cushman, D. 1980. Organizing campaigns: An analysis of management's use of communication techniques, suggestions for union strategy. In R.J. Peters, H. Elkiss, & H.T. Higgins (Eds.), *Unionization and the health care industry: Hospital and nursing home employee union leaders conference report*, Nov. 29–Dec. 1, 1978 (pp. 24–31). Urbana, IL: University of IllInois.

Davis, K. 1958. *Human relations in business.* New York: McGraw-Hill.

Gerrard, B.A., Boniface, W.J., & Love, B.H. 1980. *Interpersonal skills for health professionals.* Reston, VA: Reston Hall.

Ginzberg, E. 1966. *The development of human resources.* New York: McGraw-Hill.

Golightly, C.K. 1981. *Creative problem solving for health care professionals.* Gaithersburg, MD: Aspen.

Gregorich, P., & Long, J.W. 1980. Responsive management fosters cooperative environment. In C.A. Lockhart & W.B. Werther, Jr. (Eds.), *Labor relations in nursing.* Wakefield, MA: Nursing Resources.

Hemsworth, M.J. 1978. *Nurses in collective bargaining.* Ann Arbor, MI: University Microfilms International.

Kruger, D.H. 1961. Bargaining and the nursing profession. *Monthly Labor Review* 84:699.

Levitan, S.A., Mangum, G.L., & Marshall, R. 1981. *Human resources and labor markets: Employment and training in the American economy* (3rd ed.). New York: Harper & Row.

Lockhart, C.A., & Werther, W.B., Jr. (Eds.). 1980. *Labor relations in nursing.* Wakefield, MA: Nursing Resources.

Meyer, G.D. 1970. *Determinants of collective action attitudes among hospitals nurses: An empirical test.* Unpublished doctoral dissertation, University of Iowa.

Rothstein, J. 1958. *Communication, organization and science.* Indian Hills, CO: Falcon's Wing.

Scott, W.G. 1962. *Human relations in management: A behavioral science approach.* Homewood, IL: Irwin.

Spradley, B.W. 1985. *Community health nursing: Concepts and practice* (2nd ed.). Boston: Little, Brown.

Vroom, V.H., & Yetton, P.W. 1976. Leadership and decision making: Basic consideration underlying the normative model. In W.R. Nord (Ed.), *Concepts and controversy in organizational behavior* (2nd ed.). Pacific Palisades, CA: Goodyear.

Werther, W.B., Jr., & Lockhart, C.A. 1980. Collective action and cooperation in the health professions. In C.A. Lockhart & W.B. Werther, Jr. (Eds.), *Labor relations in nursing.* Wakefield, MA: Nursing Resources.

Zacur, S. 1982. *Health care labor relations: The nursing perspective.* Ann Arbor, MI: University Microfilms International.

CHAPTER 40

Human Resource Management

Robert J. Tortorici

THE HUMAN RESOURCE DEFINED

The value of the human resource to the home health agency directly relates to the importance the agency places on its image as a provider of service to the community. Manufacturers and most service providers depend on quality, pricing, packaging, and the efficiency of their delivery systems to promote their products and services to their customers. Hospital inpatients and outpatients have perceptions based on all their observations and experiences. The home health agency, however, is dependent on the quality of the relationships that exist between caregivers and their patients. Because there is often no other frame of reference for the home care client, the aide, the nurse, the therapist, and other members of the care team assume the identity of the agency itself. The responsibility and accountability are significant and extend well beyond the caregiver's ability to provide a competent level of clinical care. Often, the caregiver is expected to satisfy all the patient's needs, whether these are communicated or not, and is held accountable by the client for doing so. The patient and members of the household may perceive the nurse in stereotypical terms, the selfless Florence Nightingale, committed to service and receiving only intrinsic rewards in return. Whether the agency and its employees are motivated by such humanitarian purposes or not, the agency's success as a service provider is somewhat dependent on the nurse's ability to transform that perception into reality.

The importance of the human resource in home care is significant. The success of the home health agency as an employer is measured by its ability to attract and retain highly skilled and talented individuals for employment. Although the notion that health care attracts altruistic humanitarians who receive their rewards from the services they provide may or may be true, the health care workers of the 1990s expect their employers to provide the same rewards received by workers in other industries. Today's employees seek and expect income commensurate with the level and scope of their responsibility and benefits that provide security for them and their families. Other priorities include a safe and comfortable working environment, fair and consistent personnel policies, equal employment opportunities, free-flowing communication, opportunities for professional growth, and the ability to participate and become involved. Proactive home health employers, and specifically individuals charged with the responsibility of managing the human resource, go farther to create a comfortable and positive employee relations climate. They understand that individuals should give their work 100 percent of their attention to ensure desired agency outcomes.

Discussion and resolution of work-related and personal problems should be encouraged and should take place in a comfortable, non-threatening setting to minimize distractions. These encounters are often convened within the personnel department, which proactive employers promote as a confidential staff resource.

Perhaps the greatest challenge of home care in the 1990s is its extraordinary growth within the largest segment of the U.S. economy: the health care industry. As the Baby Boomer generation ages, the demand for home care services will surely experience exponential growth. Yet the national labor force is declining. Health care and home health care must compete aggressively for a larger proportion of a limited human resource, and they must do so at a time when the industry is being pressured to contain costs. The staffing challenge requires a comprehensive, introspective review of the industry's personnel management practices as well as aggressive and innovative recruitment and retention strategies. The planning and implementation of such strategies fall within the scope of the personnel department's responsibility.

THE PERSONNEL DEPARTMENT AND ITS ROLE, GOAL, AND STRUCTURE

Essentially, the personnel administrator and the line manager share responsibility for managing the human resource or, more specifically, for achieving results through the efforts of others. Although the manager's focus is often limited by boundaries of departmental responsibility, the personnel administrator's view is global in scope and spans the entire organization. As a result, the personnel department is positioned appropriately as a management resource and conceptually as the initiator of consistent, proactive "people" policies and practices that enhance the recruitment and retention of staff and ultimately promote the agency as an employer of choice. Most often the personnel department reports directly to the chief executive officer and appears as a staff

(support) rather than a line (operational) function on the organizational chart. As a result, the personnel department does not exist in the chain of command of most employees. It extends its role as a resource beyond the management group to all employees and provides each individual with a safe haven for discussing concerns, issues, and interests that may affect morale. The personnel administrator may help the employee find a solution and may participate with the employee and manager to develop an appropriate action plan. The personnel department exists as a resource to encourage the personal and professional growth of staff and managers, and the personnel administrator of the 1990s will have the expertise to do so.

When each and every employment relationship between employer and employee is perceived as being mutually satisfying, or, in other terms, when each partner in the relationship believes that mutual expectations have been and will continue to be met, the personnel department may close its doors and cease to exist. Such is the goal of every personnel administrator. Is this goal achievable? The answer would clearly be yes if there existed an unlimited financial resource. The reality of the 1990s is the challenge of cost containment, however, a term of particular relevance to the health care industry. Government increases its intervention into health care in response to the public's demand for containment of health care costs, yet the health provider is expected to provide more and better care. This trend has implications for the employee relations climate of the health care employer. The prospect of developing an inventory of employer and employee expectations and a mutual commitment to satisfy such expectations may be an appropriate first step toward the goal. It is clearly necessary for both employer and employee to prioritize their mutual expectations, however, and to develop an action plan within the framework of the organizational planning process. The personnel department should contribute personnel policies and programs to the plan after receiving input from staff. To ensure progress, the approach should be comprehensive and should address the broad scope of employee and employer expectations. Typically, the personnel department and its agenda are organized according to the following professional disciplines (Figure 40–1).

Recruitment and Selection

Recruitment and selection involve reaching out into the community and beyond to ensure an adequate supply of qualified candidates for a variety of agency functions. The number of vacancies and the length of time for which positions remain open affect the agency's ability to deliver service. The selection process must ensure that all qualified candidates have an equal opportunity to be considered for employment and that the candidate who offers the best prospect for a mutually successful and satisfying employment relationship is selected. Moreover, an important consideration for personnel department staff is the realization that the impressions of all applicants may affect the agency's image in the community as an employer.

Salary Administration

Whether or not a formal plan and structure exist, the personnel department must ensure fair and equitable pay practices for all employees based on the requirements of the job performed. Therefore, standards should exist that reflect reasonable differences between jobs. Personnel department staff use objective tools for measuring the value of such jobs to the agency. Jobs are then arranged in a hierarchy according to the level and scope of responsibility assigned to each. Salary surveys are conducted to ensure that salary levels are consistent with prevailing rates in the community. In addition, salary practices include mechanisms for staff to achieve salary growth as they accumulate experience and longevity and perform at required levels.

Benefits

Often grouped with salary administration, benefits administration requires periodic marketplace studies and comparisons to enhance the agency's ability to recruit and retain. The benefit program should be designed to address the specific needs of employees with attention given to cost. Insurance plan premiums are often based on the claims filed by staff. Therefore, cost containment measures and policy provision revisions should be considered to provide the best benefit value for the employer and the employee. Staff surveys should be conducted periodically to determine benefit options that may be of interest. It is important, however, that expectations are not raised beyond the agency's ability to deliver.

Training

In the health care industry, and likewise in home health care, clinical training is often the responsibility of the professional and paraprofessional departments. The personnel department, however, shares responsibility for ensuring that all employees are adequately trained to perform their job activities. It is also appropriate to provide every employee with an opportunity to develop new skills and to keep them current. Such initiatives may include policies and programs that encourage continuing education for staff, perhaps in traditional educational settings, and financing their participation in seminars and symposia on related topics. The value of providing training programs internally should be emphasized as well because there is usually a wealth of specialized expertise among employees within each home care organization. The internal instructor is able to tailor a program with a specific agency relevance, which participants may find particularly useful. Personnel-sponsored training programs should be conducted for administrative support and management employees because specialized skills are necessary throughout the agency's opera-

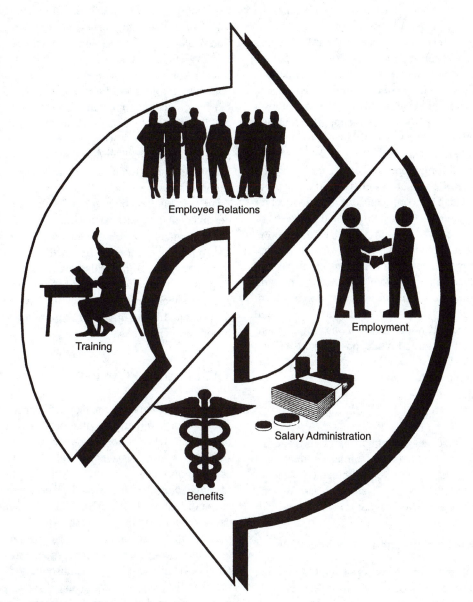

Figure 40–1 Personnel Department Services

tional department. In addition, an orientation presentation for all staff, which introduces newcomers to the agency and gives them an opportunity to meet and greet others, will enhance their ability to adjust to their new environment.

Employee Relations

The agency's ability to attract and retain highly qualified individuals is linked to the employee relations climate. Although all personnel disciplines have impact, perhaps the most significant measure of an agency's employee relations climate is the effectiveness of its communication network. Unless employee and employer needs and expectations are freely discussed, they cannot be addressed. The personnel department functions as a forum for such discussions. It also supports managers and staff by helping them find ways to create an atmosphere that supports a free and comfortable flow of information. Of course, effective and meaningful communication is a bilateral process in which the communicator and the receiver accept mutual responsibility for the quality of communication. It is important to note, however, that appropriate and timely action is often necessary after the communication of an employee relations issue. When concerns and problems are communicated but not resolved, they begin to fester, only to affect the employee's comfort level in the employment relationship. Poor morale on the part of one individual can disrupt the morale and effectiveness of the entire team.

Labor Relations

The personnel department is often responsible for the negotiation of union contracts and for the administration of the agreement while in force. Essentially, the department assumes the role of the employer's agent for such purposes.

Personnel Policies and Record Retention

An overwhelming list of federal, state, and municipal laws and regulations guides the personnel administrator, particularly in the employment, salary, and benefit administration and labor relations disciplines (Exhibit 40–1). Whether mandated or not, policies should be organized into a manual or, ideally, into an employee handbook, written in language easily understood by all staff, and distributed to ensure that every employee has access to it. It is inappropriate to hold individuals accountable for meeting organizational expectations when such expectations have not been communicated effectively. Personnel-related laws and regulations also require personnel departments to review and maintain certain documents and information for each employee. In addition, a complete employment history is maintained in the personnel department that is used for a variety of reasons to benefit both employer and employee. The employee, however, should be assured that all such information is kept absolutely confidential and that certain control procedures have been established to ensure the security of such records. It is important to note, however, that an official personnel file should not be in an employee's general correspondence file. Official personnel transactions, performance reviews, commendations, and required employment documents should be maintained, and extraneous information should be kept in department files or given to the employee for his or her own personal records.

THE PERSONNEL DEPARTMENT STAFF

As mentioned, the personnel department often reports directly to the chief executive officer, and when it does it gives staff the message that senior management places considerable importance on the agency's human resource. Normally the size of the organization, scope of responsibility, credentials, and qualifications determine the personnel administrator's place on the organization chart. The administrator is usually a generalist with responsibility for all personnel disciplines. It is absolutely essential that the administrator manage the department with sensitivity and flexibility while ensuring fairness and consistency. The individual must have the ability to motivate others, to be empathetic, to place equal value on each employee, and to appreciate the contribution that each makes to the overall mission of the agency. The role also requires exceptionally good judgment and, above all, an ability to communicate effectively. This includes, of course, exceptional listening skills as well.

Exhibit 40–1 Sections of the *Health Care Labor Manual* (Vol. 2, Chap. 12; Skoler and Abbott, 1983 (updated quarterly)) of Interest to Personnel Department Staff

Topic	Page
Labor–Management Relations Act	12:1
Hazardous Communication	12:31
Labor–Management Reporting and Disclosure Act of 1959, As Amended	12:81
The Equal Employment Opportunity Act of 1972	12:111
Fair Labor Standards Act of 1938	12:135
Age Discrimination in Employment Act	12:173
Public Law No. 72-65	12:181
Occupational Safety and Health Act of 1970	12:187
Public Law No. 73-376	12:217
Extremely Hazardous Substances List and Threshold Planning Quantities; Emergency Planning and Release Notification Requirements	12:219
Health Maintenance Organizations—Employee's Health Benefits Plans	12:230(5)
Nondiscrimination on Basis of Handicap	12:231
Final EEOC Guidelines on Affirmative Action	12:259
Questions and Answers Clarifying Uniform Guidelines on Employee Selection Procedures	12:263
Labor Department Interpretation of Effect on Employee Benefit Plans of Amendments to Age Discrimination in Employment Act	12:273
Restatement and Clarification of NLRB Rules on Election Objectives	12:281
Final EEOC Interpretations: Age Discrimination in Employment Act	12:283
Revised NLRB Procedural Rules	12:287
Final Immigration and Naturalization Reform Rules	12:291
Civil Rights Restoration Act of 1987	12:305
Employee Polygraph Protection Act of 1988	12:309
Drug-Free Workplace Act of 1988	12:315
Interim Final Rules—Drug-Free Workplace Act of 1988	12:317
Guidelines for Federal Workplace Drug Testing Programs	12:337
Americans with Disabilities Act	12:341
Older Workers Benefit Protection Act	12:385
Civil Rights Act of 1991	12:391
Family and Medical Leave Act of 1993	12:405

The personnel administrator is challenged to represent the agency's best interests and to promote its personnel policies and programs while also playing the role of advocate for employees. This dual responsibility should not present a conflict to the skilled and effective administrator. A large home health agency may also have specialists, particularly in the area of salary and benefit administration and in recruitment and selection. Support staff are normally responsible for record retention and a variety of administrative and clerical functions.

The individual who has responsibility for meeting and greeting applicants is often the only person who will have the opportunity to leave an applicant with an impression of the agency as an employer. It is obviously important that a person with superior "people" and communication skills be selected, although all members of the department should possess such skills and abilities.

Although there has been much debate about the size of the personnel department, a general rule of thumb is 1 full-time personnel employee for every 100 employees in the organization. Of course, this guideline should be modified to reflect the actual activities assumed by the department, and the talents, abilities, and interests of managers and support staff assigned.

The quality of the personnel department's outputs cannot be predicted by the number of individuals who work in the department, and the cost of the function and its impact on the budget should be a major consideration as well. The notion that the personnel department does not contribute to the bottom line is simply not true. This is especially the case in home health care, where the ability to recruit and retain staff is closely linked to the agency's ability to generate revenue.

FINDING THE RIGHT CANDIDATE FOR EMPLOYMENT

During the late 1980s, health care employers were stunned to discover that their former proportion of the national labor force was no longer available to the health care industry. A nationwide shortage of health care workers, particularly nurses, physical therapists, and home health aides, reached crisis proportions, and health care employers began to experience double-digit vacancy rates with single-digit applicant inquiries. Although the effects were devastating to employers and employees alike, the crisis was a catalyst for positive change. Perhaps the greatest change of all was the industry's realization that health care workers have many of the same needs and expectations as workers in other industries. Employee relations and salary administration practices were revised to accommodate such expectations. As a result, the status of health care workers has escalated in the past few years at a greater rate than it did in the past 25 to 30 years. Recruit-

ment strategies, once passive, were developed to compete aggressively with those of other industries for a greater share of a limited human resource. The trend is positive, but the momentum must continue because the demand for health care, and particularly home care services, will continue to rise. The proactive recruiter will therefore develop a comprehensive plan that will include initiatives specifically designed to attract candidates who meet job-specific qualifications. The plan will also include an assessment mechanism to provide information about the effectiveness of such initiatives. Of course, the most progressive recruiter will also consider future needs and will target applicants for future consideration.

Advertising

Although advertising is costly, it is often most effective for reaching large numbers of people. There is no magic formula as to the day, frequency, style, or format of the advertisement. Successes and failures, however, could be charted over a period of time and analyzed, thereby providing the recruiter with information that may be useful for future advertising decisions. The look and theme of an ad could enhance or detract from the image that the agency wants to project to the community. It is therefore advisable to consult with advertising experts, perhaps within the agency itself, to find a design that attracts applicants and promotes the agency as a service provider as well. Content should be developed after a careful review of the job description. Presumably, the requirements have been appropriately set, and if so the ad copy should specifically state required qualifications, salary range, and significant benefits. The goal is to attract as many qualified candidates as possible, but only those who would give the position serious consideration. Although the salary range provides the reader with needed information, a precise salary implies that there is no room for negotiation and should be avoided. Generally, imaginative copy sells. Standard phrases and lead-ins, such as

"Large home health agency seeks . . . ," do not project a progressive employer image, and everyone wants to work for a progressive employer.

Professional journals are also effective for certain vacancies, but they are generally used to build an applicant bank for specific programs or departments rather than to fill current vacancies. This venue is particularly appropriate when the number of jobs exceeds the availability of skilled workers. Such periodicals are published infrequently and do not provide an immediate prospect for producing large numbers of candidates quickly.

An even broader approach to advertising may include radio, television, and perhaps mass transit advertising, particularly for difficult-to-fill positions and when large numbers of staff are required. Such techniques have been used effectively for home health aide recruitment. During the nursing shortage, the broadcast media was used extensively to generate interest in the nursing profession. Nonprofit agencies are often able to obtain no-cost public service air time or low-cost local advertising council assistance in developing their advertising strategies.

Equal employment opportunity employers should draw attention to their interest in minorities and people with disabilities in their employment advertising. Tag lines appear insincere, however. A more innovative approach would be to work such commitments into the main body of the text. Also, advertisements should be placed in publications that have a significant readership among such populations, at least periodically.

Again, advertising can be expensive, and responsible recruiters will assess the results of all their advertising initiatives on an ongoing basis.

Community Outreach

There are always opportunities for presentations at schools and other community forums. Career days at the secondary school level and college career forums are effective and rela-

tively inexpensive mechanisms for cultivating short- and long-range employment and career prospects. Imaginative recruiters may develop audiovisual presentations that describe employment and career opportunities while subtly promoting the agency as an employer of choice. More important than the presentation itself, however, is the relationship between the recruiter and the school guidance counselor or placement director. These individuals will often refer promising students, recent graduates, or alumni to the agency for consideration. In fact, every recruitment outreach into the community should have as its primary goal the development of a network that will serve the agency as a megarecruitment resource. Community agencies that work with individuals returning to the workforce are excellent sources for qualified and eager candidates for employment, as is the state employment service, which is usually more than willing to assist by providing space and candidates for on-site interviewing. Agency-sponsored events, such as job and health fairs, open-house receptions, and on-site seminars, expose participants to other staff members who may be equipped to represent home health care and the agency effectively. They also serve to validate information shared by the recruiter, who is generally expected to accentuate the positives.

Permanent and Temporary Employment Agencies

Temporary employment agencies are excellent sources for satisfying temporary and supplemental staffing needs. There is a growing trend in all industries to utilize temporary agencies for permanent staffing as well. There are advantages in doing so. Although fees tend to be higher than starting salaries for most jobs, the employment agency normally provides and pays for benefits. Generally this represents a savings for the health care employer. The temporary who presumably comes to the employer with the requisite skills becomes acclimated to the health care agency's working environment while satisfying the temporary need. More important, both the employer and the temporary have the unique opportunity to assess each other before entering into a regular and binding employment relationship. Most temporary agencies have buy-out provisions, which essentially permit employers to accept temporaries for regular employment for an additional fee.

Search firms and permanent employment agencies assume advertising and recruitment costs and will produce applicants for employment who have been screened, presumably according to the employer's specifications. Fees for such services are usually a percentage of salary and are somewhat significant. The recruiter must therefore analyze the cost-effectiveness of using such a resource. For certain difficult-to-fill positions, or when a confidential search becomes necessary, search firms are often useful. The quality of the service provided by the temporary or permanent referral source, however, should be evaluated according to its track record of referring qualified and talented candidates on a timely basis.

Employee Referrals

Employees are excellent referral sources for highly qualified and talented candidates for employment, and many employers encourage staff to do so. Many individuals associate with others with similar occupational interests. This recruitment source normally offers a built-in screening mechanism because most individuals will refer people whom they know well and who offer the employer a good prospect for success. Organizations often develop referral incentive plans that reward employees who refer applicants selected for employment. Generally, there is a requirement that the new hire remain on the job for some months before the bonus is actually paid to the referring employee. Before implementing an employee referral incentive program, the employer should at least consider the possibility that it may be perceived as a bounty to induce people to work there. To be safe, the personnel department may want to solicit feedback from a representative sampling of employees.

Promotion from Within

The ultimate recruiting pool is the employer's existing staff. A meaningful training and development program, tenure and experience, and an objective performance assessment system should provide the agency with a mechanism for cultivating and identifying employees within the organization who are ready to step up to higher levels of responsibility. A succession planning process (a schematic of possible replacements for key positions in the organization), a job posting policy, and development programs such as career ladders provide opportunities for upward mobility throughout the organization. The positive impact of a successful promote-from-within policy on the employee relations climate can be enormous, and its value as a cost-effective recruitment tool is as significant. A large percentage of positions filled as promotional opportunities is an indicator of an organization that is well on its way toward becoming an employer of choice.

The goal of an agency's recruitment plan is to locate the candidate for each vacancy who will meet and preferably surpass the agency's expected results. Timeliness is important because vacancies may result in lost revenue and employee dissatisfaction. The selection standard established by the agency should never be compromised. When the applicant flow is insufficient, the recruitment initiative should be adjusted accordingly. Outreach into the community may have to be expanded, a larger geographic area may have to be considered, and multiple recruitment sources may have to be utilized, but the selection standard must remain constant.

SELECTION AND THE HIDDEN AGENDA

Everyone has a hidden agenda. There may be certain events in the past that are not appropriate for an applicant to share with an employment interviewer. Applicants who are skilled at the art of interviewing will provide as many positives as anyone would want to hear while skillfully avoiding negatives. The smart consumer learns as much information about a product as possible before making a purchase. The employer's representative, the interviewer, has the responsibility for learning as much information about the applicant's qualifications as possible before extending a job offer. Thus the object of the interview is to expose the hidden agenda. Certain preparations should be made to create the right environment for this.

First Impressions

The physical surroundings of the employment reception area and the applicant's interaction with the receptionist provide an instant impression of the organization. It is essential to the agency's community image that this impression be positive. The area should be neat and organized and, if possible, attractive. The receptionist's greeting should be pleasant and sincere with a genuine attempt to put the applicant at ease. In fact, a comfortable applicant is often a talkative applicant, which will only enhance the interviewer's ability to develop relevant information. The agency that is interested in promoting an employer-of-choice image may want to go further by providing a beverage and by having written information available in the reception area.

Although the employer should be committed to making a positive first impression, the applicant is certainly expected to do the same. Generally, the candidate does not consider the receptionist a member of the selection team and may display behavior while waiting to be interviewed that could in fact be relevant. The receptionist should therefore be observant and should pass relevant information to the interviewer before the meeting.

It is obviously important that the interview start on time. The applicant who arrives late for an interview should leave the interviewer curi-

ous and possibly concerned. It would be appropriate to explore the reason for the tardiness. An interviewer who leaves an applicant waiting beyond the scheduled time of the interview demonstrates insensitivity to the applicant. The applicant may in fact question the sincerity of his or her candidacy for the position.

Before the interview, the interviewer should review the resume and application form to note inconsistencies, overlapping employment dates, employment gaps, and omissions of fact. Such matters should be explored further during the interview.

Every interviewer should be well versed in a variety of state and federal laws and regulations that govern the preemployment process. Generally, all individuals, including persons with disabilities, who possess bona fide occupational qualifications for a position and are legally permitted to work in the United States must be afforded an equal opportunity for employment consideration. Questions must be carefully constructed to guarantee equal employment opportunity for all who apply (Exhibit 40–1).

The interviewer should develop a series of questions before meeting the applicant that probes beyond information already provided on the resume and application form. A particularly effective line of questioning places the applicant in a similar hypothetical work setting. Questions that start, "How would you handle . . . ?" produce information that can be evaluated objectively against the requirements of the actual position and work setting. Inquiries that test applicants' proficiency in dealing with difficult and stressful situations and questions that assess their comfort level with the exercise of independent judgment should be considered if, in fact, such issues may be encountered on the job. All questions should be asked in a way to encourage conversation (e.g., "Tell me about a particularly stressful situation that you encountered and how you handled it"). On the other hand, leading questions that invite a specific response or a simple yes or no should be avoided.

The interviewing area should be comfortable and arranged to encourage a free flow of information. The interviewer sitting across a desk from an applicant can be intimidating for the applicant. An arrangement that has the interviewer and applicant sitting in closer proximity, perhaps at a right angle to each other, is less formal and more congenial. The interviewer should have allotted an adequate amount of time for the meeting and should also have arranged to have telephone calls and other unannounced visitors intercepted. Of course, privacy is also necessary and the interviewing area should be free of clutter and distractions as well.

The Interview

A smile, a firm handshake, and a sincere "Welcome to the XYZ Home Health Agency" are absolutely essential first steps. A good interviewer will recall the anxiety he or she experienced during his or her last interview and will take appropriate steps to put the applicant at ease. Small talk about the weather or about the applicant's trip to the interview site may seem contrived, but extended salutary remarks and perhaps 5 minutes of light conversation about something that they have in common can reduce interview jitters. The goal at this point is to establish rapport. Ultimately, the interviewer strives for trust and confidence and tries to convince the applicant that their relationship has evolved into one where a free exchange of information would be to their mutual benefit. This, of course, is true because both the employer and applicant have a vested interest in making the right employment decision, which would not be inappropriate for the applicant to hear.

After these introductory remarks, a limited amount of information about the agency and position should be shared to confirm the applicant's continued interest in the position. Incidentally, asking about an individual's motivation for applying for a job is appropriate, and the response should be weighted heavily. The next part of the interview is fact finding. In a sense, this segment could be considered a contest, a competition, or perhaps a game. The object for the interviewer is to gain control of the dialog and to steer it to those areas of the applicant's work history that are not apparent. To do so, the interviewer should listen and observe and talk only to facilitate the discussion. The more information that the interviewer develops, the better equipped he or she will be to consider the applicant's inventory of positives and negatives and to make an educated employment decision. The applicant, on the other hand, also strives for control and in doing so tries to steer the interviewer's probe away from areas of discomfort and back to the positive attributes of the work history. When each is skilled in the art of interviewing, the interview can be an exhilarating experience for both. Certain techniques are particularly effective for developing additional discussion. Great communicators know how to use body language to solicit additional information. A pause, a gesture that implies interest, and then continued silence imply "keep talking." At the same time, the interviewer should receive messages from the applicant's body language and should follow up with questions as appropriate. The probe should continue until enough relevant information is accumulated to facilitate an objective decision.

When the interviewer is comfortable that the profile developed is sufficient, the interviewer's role should change. This part of the selection process is devoted to ensuring that the applicant will accept the position if offered and, if not, that he or she will at least speak highly of the agency to others. This is therefore an opportunity for the interviewer to provide specific information about the position and to accentuate the positive aspects of having an employment relationship with the home health agency. An enthusiastic presentation will certainly imply that the agency is certainly an employer of choice.

The Employment Decision

It should be noted that the manager with the vacancy is generally the hiring manager. The personnel department interview is primarily a screening procedure. Presumably, however, the personnel interviewer is the agency's selection expert, and his or her recommendation should be taken seriously. The personnel department is also responsible for ensuring compliance with legal employment obligations and advises the hiring manager accordingly. The hiring manager and the personnel interviewer must ensure that the decision is based on the applicant's skills and abilities as they apply to the specifications of the job. The person selected should also be the individual who offers the best prospect for success. All applicants, however, should receive periodic updates of the status of their applications. When the position is filled, applicants who were interviewed should be contacted, personally if possible, and thanked for their interest. Obviously, close runners-up should not be rejected until the applicant of choice accepts the employment offer.

MAKING A MEANINGFUL EMPLOYMENT OFFER

Regardless of the persuasive skills of the individual making the job offer, the individual in the personnel department responsible for salary administration has the greatest impact on whether the offer will be accepted. The employer, even one that hopes to be an employer of choice, does not have to pay the highest salary in the community, but it does have to set its salary levels according to the market standards that exist for positions with similar requirements and equivalent responsibility. Before developing a wage and salary program, senior management must decide just how competitive the agency's salaries should be. For example, management may decide that salaries in general or salaries for specific positions should be set in the midrange or perhaps in the top 25 percent of local labor market salaries. Management establishes the overall pay philosophy, thereby giving the salary and benefits experts in the personnel department a frame of reference.

To ensure the appeal of an employment offer, wage and salary decisions are based on a thorough and current review of salary ranges and average salaries for similar positions within the employer's recruitment pool. Periodic salary and benefit surveys are published from a variety of local, regional, and national trade and professional organizations. In home health care, state home care associations often provide annual industry surveys, as do the National Association for Home Care and the Visiting Nurse Associations of America. These surveys include data on a variety of caregiver and administrative support positions. Also, job descriptions are included to facilitate appropriate comparisons. Although the process is somewhat more complicated, the goal is to compare apples to apples and to ensure that salary levels are set to enhance the agency's ability to fill its vacancies on a timely basis.

Based on the information developed, the compensation specialist can set in-hiring salaries for specific positions and develop ranges that include midpoints and maximum values for each position. Because the base rate is normally paid to individuals with minimal qualifications, decisions are also required about an experienced person's placement on the range. This is a challenge for the salary administrator. In addition, consideration must be given to those who have been in the agency's employ for some time. Thus the job offer for the new hire must be determined precisely to ensure external equity (competitiveness in the community) and internal equity (fairness and consistency within the agency).

A structured wage and salary program also includes a job analysis methodology for arranging positions in a hierarchy according to levels of responsibility and a number of other factors. An objective process is selected from a number of possibilities and is used to determine pay grades. New positions and revised positions should be put through this process as they are created or changed.

Finally, consideration must be given to the method of assuring an employee of ongoing salary growth. Experience and longevity, and per-haps performance, should be compensated. There have been debates about the concept of pay for performance for decades, particularly across the collective bargaining table. The pro argument places a motivational value on a merit increase. The con argument is related to the premise that an objective assessment of perfor-mance is unattainable. Regardless of the deci-sion, a wage and salary program must afford staff the opportunity to be paid fairly and com-mensurate with their responsibility, and it must be perceived as such.

BENEFITS

Benefit costs are on the rise, particularly those that offer medical reimbursement. We are acutely aware of rising health care costs, but workers' compensation premiums represent a staggering expense to employers, particularly those in health care. The good news, however, is that such plans are experience rated and that claims can be controlled with appropriate edu-cational programs and proactive risk manage-ment strategies. Risk management committees should be convened to conduct studies of the causes of work-related injuries and illnesses and should be empowered to develop appropriate follow-up plans. Perhaps a staff awareness pro-gram that includes training sessions, posters, articles in agency publications, and staff discus-sion groups would be an appropriate response to a recurring occupational injury. Also, periodic inspections of the workplace to identify and report safety hazards may reduce future occur-rences and serve to increase every employee's awareness of such issues. In home care, where significant numbers of employees spend much of their working days driving, representatives of state motor vehicle departments are often will-ing to conduct on-site driving safety courses. The proactive employer realizes that cost con-tainment of insurance premiums will result in savings that could be applied to other benefit options that better meet the specific needs of the employee population.

EMPLOYEE RELATIONS FOR RETENTION

The first 6 months of employment are the most stressful. This is especially true for care-givers making the transition from acute care to the independent environment of the home health agency. Adequate training and develop-ment for all new employees are important, whether on the job or in the classroom. Equally important is the need for the employee to have a mentor, preferably someone other than the man-ager, who can assume responsibility for provid-ing support and assistance with workplace issues. The manager, however, is the key resource. The new employee's progress should be charted and discussed with the individual on an ongoing basis, and adjustments to this initial training program should be made appropriately. Above all, encouragement and support should be provided by the manager and every other member of the team. The personnel department plays a special role because the initial employ-ment relationship began there. The members of the personnel department should look for opportunities to interface with the recent hires, even simply to ask how things are going. Peri-odic progress interviews should take place in personnel, and information shared should be used to make adjustments and interventions on behalf of the newcomer. An orientation presen-tation for all new employees is an effective mechanism for introducing a group of new employees to the agency and perhaps to the var-ious operational departments as well. Participa-tion on the part of senior staff goes a long way toward placing value on the human resource.

As previously discussed, communication and staff involvement enhance the employee rela-tions environment (Figure 40–2). Programs and practices that promote such efforts serve to improve the climate within the organization. Satisfied employees are only too anxious to talk about their employer in favorable terms to friends and acquaintances, thereby enhancing the agency's community image as well. Finally, the personnel department's role as a staff and

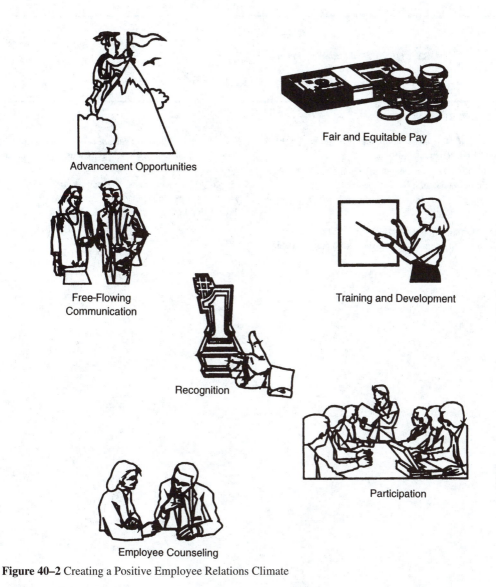

Figure 40–2 Creating a Positive Employee Relations Climate

management resource should be communicated regularly to staff. Its credibility as a resource will be tested by every employee who visits the department for help and assistance. The personnel department staff must be equipped to handle effectively every employee issue with sensitiv-

ity and expertise and every person as a client with needs and expectations that should be met.

The *Health Care Labor Manual* (Skoler & Abbott, 1983) provides a thorough overview of personnel management topics and is recommended (Exhibit 40–1).

REFERENCE

Skoler, M., & Abbott, R., Jr. (1983). *Health care labor manual* (Vol. 2). Gaithersburg, MD: Aspen, p. 12:i.

SUGGESTED READING

Belcher, D. 1974. *Compensation administration.* Englewood Cliffs, NJ: Prentice-Hall.

Cook, M. 1993. *The human resource yearbook* (1993/94 ed.). Englewood Cliffs, NJ: Prentice-Hall.

Henderson, R. 1984. *Performance appraisal* (2nd ed.). Reston, VA: Reston.

Jones, J., Murphy, W., & Belton, R. 1987. *Cases and materials on discrimination in employment* (5th ed.). St. Paul, MN: West.

Morano, R. 1989. *Managing human behavior and development in organizations.* New York: Cummings & Hathaway.

Rothstein, M., Knapp, A., & Liebman, L. 1990. *Employment law—Cases and materials* (2nd ed.). Westbury, NY: Foundation Press.

Tortorici, R. 1988. The nursing shortage . . . crisis or catalyst? *Nurses Network,* 2(4), 22–24.

Chapter 41

Staff Development in a Home Health Agency

Joan Reynolds Yuan

Nursing is a progressive art, in which to stand still is to go back. A woman who thinks to herself, "Now I am a full nurse, a skilled nurse, I have learnt all there is to be learnt." Take my word for it, she does not know what a nurse is, and never will know. She has gone back already. Progress can never end but with a nurse's life.
—*F. Nightingale* (1914)

The concept of furthering one's education is an age-old one in nursing. Traditionally, it has been an important area in community health agencies. Currently, professional development is vital to the existence of any community or home health agency. In this era of high-technology–high-touch home care, an extensive knowledge base, sharp technical skills, and appropriate attitudes are necessities for providing quality care to patients, families, and communities; preventing litigation; and remaining in business. With a view to the individual, one considers personal and professional growth, stimulation, motivation, and increasing or maintaining competence. In viewing an agency, one considers the necessity for providing quality care to clients. To accomplish this, a qualified staff must be employed. With advances in theory and technology, education is necessary to ensure understanding and competence.

Ongoing education is mandated by regulatory and accrediting bodies such as the Community Health Accreditation Program (CHAP) and the Joint Commission on Accreditation of Healthcare Organizations (Joint Commission). Staff development presents as a core standard in the CHAP program: "The organization provides for staff development through orientation, inservice education, and continuing education programs" (National League for Health Care, 1993, p. 33). A key factor in the Joint Commission accreditation process appears as standard HR.5: "The organization has established methods and practices that encourage self-development and learning for all staff" (Joint Commission, 1996, p. 394).

The Medicare conditions of participation mandate education, as evidenced in these sections:

- Section 484.14: "The administrator . . . employs qualified personnel and ensures adequate staff education and evaluations" (Department of Health and Human Services, 1991, p. 32973).
- Section 484.30: "The registered nurse participates in in-service programs" (Department of Health and Human Services, 1991, p. 32974).
- Section 484.32: "The qualified therapist participates in in-service programs" (Department of Health and Human Services, 1991, p. 32974).
- Section 484.34: "The social worker . . . participates in in-service programs"

(Department of Health and Human Services, 1991, p. 33371).

- Section 484.36: "The home health aide must receive at least twelve hours of inservice training per calendar year" (Department of Health and Human Services, 1991, p. 32975).

Staff development is a necessity for home health agencies. It plays a critical role in the recruitment and retention of personnel. Staff development refers to "learning activities designed to facilitate the nurse's job-related performance" (American Nurses Association [ANA], 1994, p. 5). It has three dimensions: orientation, inservice education, and continuing education (ANA, 1994). Nursing professional development encompasses continuing education and staff development. It builds upon educational and experiential bases to enhance nursing practice. This active participation in learning activities to enhance professional practice occurs through academic education, continuing education, staff development, and research activities (ANA, 1994).

The ANA has developed six standards for nursing professional development (ANA, 1994):

1. Administration: The mission, philosophy, purpose, and goals of the provider unit are consistent with the organization's. The organizational structure facilitates the provision of learning activities.
2. Human resources: Qualified administrative, educational, and support personnel are provided to achieve the goals of the provider unit.
3. Material resources and facilities: Material resources and facilities are adequate to achieve the goals of the provider unit.
4. Educational design: Educational offerings are designed through the use of educational principles and incorporate adult learning principles.
5. Records and reports: A record-keeping and report system is established and maintained.

6. Professional practice: The educator enhances learner's competency to provide quality health care.

ROLE AND RESPONSIBILITIES OF THE EDUCATOR

The title of the person responsible for the staff development program will vary from one organization to the next. Such titles may include director of education, nursing supervisor, staff development supervisor, and clinical educator. In this chapter, the person responsible for staff development is referred to as the educator. The role of the educator in a home health agency is complex. Responsibilities include continuing education, inservice education, and orientation of employees. Depending on the size and educational philosophy of the organization, the educator may be responsible for an agencywide program for all employees. This position requires a blend of educational, clinical, and administrative knowledge and expertise. It is commonly filled by a nurse with a Master's degree. This person typically reports to the executive director. The educator may not have line responsibilities, but power is inherent in the role. In many organizations, this person, by virtue of his or her educational background, experience, and knowledge of the organization, has the authority for decision making in the absence of the executive director and the director of professional services.

ORIENTATION

Orientation is defined in the ANA's *Standards for Continuing Education in Nursing* (1984) as

> . . . the means by which new staff are introduced to the philosophy, goals, policies, procedures, role expectations, physical facilities, and special services in a specific work setting. Orientation is provided at the time of employment and at other times when

changes in roles and responsibilities occur in a specific work setting (p. 5)

The educator has the responsibility to orient new employees to the organization as a whole. He or she orients new nursing personnel to the nursing service department. Depending on the structure of the organization, he or she may be responsible for specific orientation to other departments as well. In a general orientation, the new employee is introduced to the physical setting, specific work area, and personnel. The philosophy, purpose, and goals of the organization are addressed. The spirit of the organization is discussed (e.g., "This is a team effort; each job is important to the functioning of the organization, the attitudes of all staff members are important in a service organization, and in this highly competitive era, one must be aware of the treatment of the consumer"). A lesson can be learned by looking at the orientation process at organizations such as Disney, where attitudes toward the consumer are of paramount importance. The administrative policies and procedures are reviewed. Orientation to the specific job is provided during orientation (see Chapter 42). Competent and willing preceptors are invaluable in this process. Organizations differ in preceptor responsibilities as well as recognition. In addition to a certificate or luncheon, if the budget allows, a monetary bonus even of $100.00 is appreciated. Exhibit 41–1 shows a sample orientation form for a nursing department. Clinical policies and procedures are reviewed with the professional staff. In the nursing department, the nurse completes a skills checklist (Exhibit 41–2). This allows for individualization of the orientation program. It enables the educator to identify the learning needs of the new employee, and it enables the new employee to request a review of clinical skills that have not been fully developed. The educator or designee evaluates initial competencies.

Documentation is an area of concentration in the orientation process. Accuracy in documentation is necessary for both quality care and reimbursement purposes. It is important for the educator not only to review the orientee's documentation but to make home visits with the new nurse to assess his or her ability to function as a home health nurse and to allow for questions and discussion.

In agencies that are hospital based, downsizing may provide opportunities for transfer of experienced specialized nurses such as maternal child health or intravenous (IV) nurses. Orientation to this new position setting is required. Home care's requirements and standards are different from those of the inpatient facility. The nurse's practice is grounded in clinical knowledge and skills but within the framework of family, home, and community concepts (ANA, 1992). Case load management responsibilities and coordination with insurance case managers require orientation. Joint Commission standards are setting specific. A competent IV nurse could be knowledgeable of the Intravenous Nurses Society (INS) standards but without orientation to the home care setting would have no knowledge of home care standards.

Orientation to a new position within the home health agency is another area addressed by the educator. This becomes important as staff nurses move into supervisory positions. Management training can be done in-house or at area institutions. Many consultants are available for this purpose. This is a vulnerable time for the employee, and support in the new role is essential.

Documentation of orientation must be provided. This is necessary for both new employees and employees who have changed positions. The employees will sign the orientation forms as well as their job descriptions. These forms will remain in the personnel file.

INSERVICE EDUCATION

Inservice education has been defined in the ANA's *Standards for Continuing Education in Nursing* (1984) as "activities intended to assist the professional nurse to acquire, maintain, and/or increase competence in fulfilling the assigned responsibilities specific to the expecta-

Exhibit 41–1 Orientation Program

	DATE	SIGNATURE

Name: _____   Date of Employment:_____

Position: _____

Day One:

I.　Orientation to Agency Structure/Policies _____

　　A. Introduction to VNA-EMC _____

　　　　1. Philosophy _____

　　　　　　a. Self-Care Theory _____

　　　　　　b. Community Health Standards _____

　　　　2. Organization _____

　　　　　　a. Organization Chart _____

　　　　3. Introduction to Office Personnel and Facilities _____

　　　　4. Sources of Financial Support _____

　　　　5. Geographic Area Served _____

　　　　6. Scope of Services: Total Program and Services Provided _____

　　B. Medical Policies and Standing Orders _____

　　C. Nursing Service Policies _____

II.　Personnel Issues: Review and Discussion _____

　　A. Payroll Procedure _____

　　B. Schedule of Pay, Time, Hours of Work _____

　　C. Auto Insurance/Reimbursement _____

　　D. Dress Code _____

　　E. Insurance Benefits _____

　　F. Reporting Illness _____

　　G. Staff Inservice Meetings, Outside Activities, and Advanced
　　　　Individual Educational Opportunities _____

Day Two: Field Observation with Staff _____

Day Three:

I.　Individual Responsibilities _____

　　A. Job Description _____

　　B. Standards _____

　　C. Skilled Care vs. Nonskilled Care _____

II.　Field Assignments: Days and Type of Patient Services _____

III.　Criteria for Admission of Patients to VNA _____

IV.　Regulations Governing Home Health Aides _____

　　A. Type of Care Provided _____

　　B. Supervision of Care _____

Day Four:

I.　Relationship of Nurse to Other Members of Staff: RNs, PT, OT, ST, MSW,
　　HHAs _____

　　A. Individual Responsibilities and Relationships _____

continues

Exhibit 41–1 continued

	DATE	SIGNATURE

B. Coordination of Services

C. Role of Nurse as Case Manager

II. Explanation of the Role of Supervisor and the Methods Used for Evaluation Performance and Identifying Needs

III. Terminal Care/Hospice

IV. VNA Specialty Services

A. IV Team

B. Maternal/Child Health

C. Psychiatric

D. Enterostomal Therapy

E. Incontinence Management

V. Discussion of Referral Sources

A. Hospital: Social Worker, Discharge Planner

B. Doctor

C. Family

D. Social Agencies

E. Staff

VI. Relationship of VNA-EMC to Other Agencies and Organizations

A. Contractual Agreement with Homemaker/Home Health Agencies

B. Contractual Agreement with Other Agencies

VII. Instructions on Use of Day Sheets

Day Five:

I. Funding Sources: Discussion of the Requirements of the Following Funding Sources:

A. Medicare

B. Medicaid

C. Blue Cross

D. HMO

E. Private Insurance

F. Veterans Administration

G. Self-Pay

1. Full Pay

2. Part Pay/Fee Adjustment

3. No Charge

II. Discussion of the Role of Insurance Case Manager

III. Discussion of Paper Flow

IV. Discussion of All Other Forms Utilized in the Agency

V. Competency Review and Testing

Day Six:

I. Discussion of Professional Ethics

A. Patients'/Families' Rights

B. Confidentiality

continues

Exhibit 41–1 continued

	DATE	SIGNATURE

II. Review of Policies and Procedures

    A. Infection Control: Universal Blood and Body Precautions

    B. Safety (Patient/Staff)

    C. Equipment Management

    D. Quality Assessment/Improvement

    E. Emergency Preparedness

    F. Violence/Neglect/Abuse

    G. Advance Directives/DNR

    H. Conflict of Interest

    I. Other Relevant Policies/Procedures

III. Community Resources

IV. ATT Language Line

Day Seven:

    PC 101

Day Eight:

I. Physical Assessment

II. High-Volume Disease Entities

III. AHCPR Guidelines

    A. Pressure Ulcers

    B. Urinary Incontinence

    C. Pain

IV. KePro Standards

Day Nine:

    Field Observations with Staff/Clinical Link Daily Visits

Day Ten:

    Independent Visits Using Clinical Link

Day 11 through Day 14:

    Independent Visits Using Clinical Link

Day 15, 18, 21, 22:

    Clinical Link Openings

    I have read my job description and understand that I will be evaluated against these performance criteria.

EMPLOYEE SIGNATURE: _____

Source: Reprinted with permission of the Visiting Nurse Association of Eastern Montgomery County/Dept. of Abington Memorial Hospital, Willow Grove, Pennsylvania.

Exhibit 41–2 Competency Self-Assessment

NAME: _____ DATE: _____

   Using the scale below, please rate each skill according to your knowledge of and/or experience with the competency:

RATING SCALE

1. I have had no experience with this competency.
2. I know the basic concepts related to this competency but need review.
3. I consider myself competent with this skill.

GENERIC COMPETENCIES

		1	2	3	N/A
1.	Document in SOAP format				
2.	Perform female catherization				
3.	Perform male catheterization				
4.	Insert suprapubic tube				
5.	Care of patient with gastrostomy/jejunostomy tube				
6.	Insertion of gastrostomy tube				
7.	Care of the patient with a feeding tube				
8.	Auscultation of breath sounds				
9.	Perform oropharyngeal/nasopharyngeal suctioning				
10.	Care of the patient requiring tracheostomy tube				
11.	Insertion of tracheostomy tube				
12.	Care of the patient with an ostomy				
13.	Perform blood glucose monitoring				
14.	Care of the patient with a Jackson-Pratt drain				
15.	Perform wound care/dressing changes				
16.	IV catheter insertion				
17.	PICC line insertion				
18.	Midline catheter insertion				
19.	Postpartum assessment				
20.	Newborn/pediatric assessment				
21.	Mental status assessment				

Source: Reprinted with permission of the Visiting Nurse Association of Eastern Montgomery County/Dept. of Abington Memorial Hospital, Willow Grove, Pennsylvania.

tions of the employer" (p. 5). According to the Joint Commission Standard HR5.1, "The organization provides ongoing education, including inservices, training, and other activities, to maintain and improve staff competence" (Joint Commission, 1996, p. 396). CHAP requires that the organization have "a mechanism for providing that employees receive current professional information specific to their respective field" (National League for Health Care, 1993, p. 33).

For an inservice program to be viable, it must be backed by the administration. It is the responsibility of the educator to assess the educational needs of the employees. A regularly administered needs assessment tool is helpful. Inservice education may be required in several different areas (Barnum & Kerfoot, 1995). Preparatory education such as a physical assessment course may be required. Supplemental education such as management theory may be necessary. Maintenance education for cardiopulmonary resuscitation (CPR) certification, new product orientation, or new procedure orientation many times is indicated. Remedial education for foundational support is another area that is addressed by the educator.

Planning the inservices is the responsibility of the educator with the assistance of the interdisciplinary education committee. It is recommended that a long-range 12-month plan be made. This must be flexible, however, because new products, new procedures, and new needs will arise throughout the course of the year. In planning inservices, one must consider the cost of providing the inservice, including the cost of the instructor, the materials, and the time of the staff. It is important to remember that the time staff spend in an inservice must be deducted from the time they spend on reimbursable patient care activities. Consideration must be given to utilizing the least amount of time required to accomplish the task adequately. For example, CPR recertification may be given to two staff members in 1-hour increments rather than to four staff members in 2-hour increments. If the staff are recertified in 1-hour rather than 2-hour increments, an additional hour

becomes available for reimbursable patient activities.

The characteristics of the adult learner are another important area for consideration in planning inservices. Adult learning principles have been defined by the ANA (1984) as:

> approaches to adults as learners based on recognition of the individual's autonomy and self-direction, life experiences, readiness to learn, and problem-orientation to learning. Approaches include mutual, respectful collaboration of teachers and learners in planning, diagnosing needs, formulating objectives, designing sequences, and evaluating learning. Learning activities tend to be experiential and inquiry focused.

For example, an inservice on diabetic management would include hands-on experience with a glucose monitoring device. Creative strategies can be utilized to present mandated maintenance education material such as Occupational and Safety Health Administration (OSHA) programs. This information can be formatted into skits, bingo, or Jeopardy (Harris & Yuan, 1994) to better meet the needs of the adult learner.

Resources to consider utilizing for inservices include the agency's staff. An adult nurse practitioner may teach physical assessment. A physical therapist may teach proper body mechanics or chest physical therapy. A social worker may discuss available community resources. Staff attending conferences may have valuable information to share. Schools of nursing can be another valuable resource. State school extensions may have staff, such as nutritionists, who are available as educational resources. Community resources such as the American Cancer Society can be utilized. Manufacturers of equipment such as colostomy supplies, ventilators, and glucometers are often utilized.

Implementation should be carried out in accordance with written policy. The inservice should take place in an appropriate meeting room. If the agency does not have sufficient space, arrangements can be made with a local church, library, or school. The educator will keep attendance records of the inservices. Individual staff members will maintain educational program records, which will be collected annually and kept in the personnel file. Evaluating educational programs is not an easy task. A written content evaluation is one method. The result of education is an increase in knowledge or skill. The quality assessment/improvement program can be utilized to assess the effects of education on patient care.

CONTINUING EDUCATION

One component of staff development is continuing education. In the ANA's *Standards for Continuing Education in Nursing* (1984), continuing education is defined as "those planned educational activities intended to build upon the educational and experiential bases of the professional nurse for the enhancement of practice, education, administration, research, or theory development to the end of improving the health of the public" (p. 5).

The educator controls the budget for the continuing education program. Because funds are not endless, a determination must be made of how much money is allotted for each person. To get as much for the educational dollar as possible, other avenues should be investigated. Affiliating educational institutions may allow a free conference for an agency staff member in exchange for using the agency as a site for student experience. Participation in a planning committee and a cooperative effort with a providing institution can be other ways in which the agency can have staff attend a conference free of charge or at a discounted rate.

In some areas, many continuing education programs are available. Information regarding the continuing education programs can be posted for staff perusal. The individual staff member files a request to attend a conference. Depending on the conference, staffing, and budget, the request is granted or not granted by the educator. Although time off to attend a confer-

ence is costly (not to mention the cost of the conference itself), it is usually most helpful for the professional to meet with colleagues from other organizations and to broaden the individual's scope of experience. Attending conferences outside the institution often increases job satisfaction and ultimately may have a positive effect on patient care. It is often valuable to have the individual report the findings from the conference to his or her colleagues.

It is important that accurate records be kept. The educator will maintain records of the conferences attended by members of all disciplines. In addition, a record is kept in the personnel folder. In some areas of the country, continuing education programs are not readily available. Independent study and self-learning modules can help fill this void. Continuing education units are available through some nursing journals.

ACADEMIC EDUCATION

In this era of high-technology home care and economic restrictions, the need for highly skilled professionals with a broad knowledge base is evident. Many agencies require a Bachelor of Science in Nursing or that a registered nurse be working toward this degree for entry into the organization. The need for specialists in clinical and administrative areas is growing, hence the need for graduate education. Personnel policies should include provisions for furthering one's formal education. This can range from having time off and flexible scheduling to attend classes to taking a leave of absence or a sabbatical. This encompasses undergraduate as well as graduate education.

Among the benefits to an organization of utilizing the sabbatical are employee retention, stimulation of employees, development of employee talent, and increased commitment to the organization. The organization must cope with finding temporary replacements and reentry into the organization, however.

Many organizations will maintain a library for staff use. Often, this is the responsibility of the educator. Requests for new books and journals are submitted to the educator. He or she oversees the library budget and maintains adequate records. It is particularly helpful to have a library that includes literature related to community health and home care for staff members who are attending school and doing research. Education in a community or home health agency is viewed not just as a requirement but as a necessity and an integral part of an organization concerned about the provision of quality care.

REFERENCES

American Nurses Association (1984). *Standards for continuing education in nursing.* Kansas City, MO: Author.

American Nurses Association (1992). *A statement on the scope of home health nursing practice.* Washington, DC: Author.

American Nurses Association (1994). *Standards for nursing professional development: Continuing education and staff development.* Washington, DC: Author.

Barnum, B., & Kerfoot, K. (1995). *The nurse as executive* (4th ed.). Gaithersburg, MD: Aspen.

Department of Health and Human Services. (July 18, 1991). Medicare program: Home health agencies: Conditions of participation: Final rule. *Federal Register, 56,* 32967–32975.

Harris, M., & Yuan, J. (1994). Oh no, not another handwashing in-service! *Journal of the Society of Gastroenterology Nurse and Associates, 16*(6), 269–272.

Joint Commission on Accreditation of Healthcare Organizations. (1996). *1997–98 Comprehensive Accreditation manual for home care.* Oakbrook Terrace, IL: Author.

National League for Health Care, Inc. and Community Health Accreditation Program, Inc. (1993). *Standards for excellence for home care organizations.* New York: National League for Health Care.

Nightingale, F. (1914). *Florence Nightingale to her nurses.* London: Macmillan.

BIBLIOGRAPHY

American Nurses Association. (1992). *Role and responsibilities for nursing continuing education and staff development across all settings.* Washington, DC: Author.

Joint Commission on Accreditation of Healthcare Organizations. (1993). *Quality improvement in home care.* Oakbrook Terrace, IL: Author.

CHAPTER 42

Transitioning Hospital Nurses to Home Care

Carolyn J. Humphrey and Paula Milone-Nuzzo

With increasing numbers of patients cared for in their homes, the practice of home care nursing has grown significantly, with the trend promising to increase well into the next century. This trend to more home care services has resulted in an increased demand for home care nurses; therefore, many nurses whose educational background and practical experience are focused in acute care settings are finding themselves working in home care. What they find upon entering this new area of practice is not only an adjustment to caring for patients in a different environment, but the need to learn many new competencies. There is no doubt that home care is not just hospital care provided in the home.

The process a nurse must go through to make the move to home care has often been called transitioning to home care nursing. Just as the term *transition* is defined as "a movement, or evolution from one form, stage or style to another" (*Webster's Ninth*, 1988), so must nurses who are used to caring for patients in a structured hospital environment transition their skills to a work situation that is both different and unique. It is up to both the nurse and the agency administration to work together to see that this transition is as effective and efficient as possible.

This chapter discusses the definition of home care nursing and identifies the ways this prac-

tice is different from acute care practice. Additionally, the key content areas found in orientation that a nurse must master to become an effective practitioner are outlined. Other chapters in this book that deal with competency evaluation and staff development also should be consulted as orientation programs are developed and nurse administrators identify their roles in the important function of assisting the nurse in transitioning to home care.

DEFINITION OF HOME CARE NURSING

Home care nursing is a unique field of nursing practice that focuses on caring for an ill patient in the home while also providing anticipatory guidance and teaching the patient to be independent in his or her care to the extent possible. This unique field of nursing practice requires a synthesis of community health nursing principles with the theory and practice of medical/surgical, maternal–child, pediatric, and behavioral health nursing.

Home care nursing is provided to clients experiencing an illness outside the confines of an acute care hospital and integrates caregivers and families within the context of the community to reach the desired outcomes. Home care nurses care for acutely and chronically ill clients of all ages, those who have procedures and treatments conducted in their homes and those who wish to live out the final stages of their lives in their homes rather than in an institution.

Reflecting this philosophy, the following definition of home care nursing is offered as a framework to assist the new nurse in understanding this important new role:

> Home care nursing is the provision of nursing care to acute, chronically ill and well clients of all ages in their home while integrating community health nursing principles that focus on health promotion, environmental, psychosocial, economic, cultural and personal health factors affecting an individual's and family's health status. (Humphrey & Milone-Nuzzo, 1996, p. 2:2).

It is important that administrators understand the various ways this definition is used with clients in their agency so that ways can be found to teach this role to new nurses. Even though in the current regulatory and economic health care climate it is increasingly difficult for the home care nurse to practice this comprehensive role with clients, the nurse manager must operationalize the philosophy and style of practice the agency has agreed to provide. As managed care companies focus more on medical diagnoses and often are not supportive of what they perceive as the "extra" care a client may need, the staff nurse and the manager need to form a team to ensure that comprehensive care is provided when needed to reach desired outcomes, that long-term cost savings are realized, and that risk management issues are considered in determining length of the patient's time on the service. The foundation for this teamwork is laid during orientation.

Many home health agencies require at least one year of acute experience prior to employment. As hospitals have downsized and hospital-based home care agencies are often required to hire from within, however, orientees often do not have a strong acute care background, and this too must be assessed and covered in an orientation program. Miller and Daley (1996)

identified four domains of home care practice, each with varying levels of expertise that managers should recognize as they begin the education process with new nurses. They are as follows:

1. assessing and using physiologic data
2. initiating and monitoring therapeutic interventions
3. assessing and using family and environmental data
4. integrating data, interventions, and context

It is critical that the manager determine both the clinical practice expertise listed above and the caseload management competencies the acute care nurse brings to home care and build upon these during orientation and throughout employment. It is equally important that, if the new nurse is to make a successful transition to home care, the major differences in the two areas of practice be clarified from the first day of employment and throughout his or her orientation period.

DIFFERENCES BETWEEN HOSPITAL AND HOME CARE NURSING

Some of the specific areas that are different when hospital nurses make the transition to home care are listed below. These are the critical areas that a manager must integrate into orientation and daily practice to ensure that the new nurse understands the role transition that must be made from hospital to home care. These areas are also important to cover in competency evaluations during orientation and throughout the nurse's employment in the agency.

Assessment Skills

In the hospital, the nurse mainly focuses on physical and psychological assessment skills for the individual patient cared for in the structured institutional environment. Some acute care nurses who work in specialty areas such as

orthopaedics or oncology may have more limited assessment skills that focus on a few systems. In home care, the nurse must not only
complete physical and psychological assessments, but additionally assess social, economic,
environmental, home safety, and family issues
that affect the client's care. There is more paperwork in home care to track these assessments,
set goals, and identify outcomes. To accomplish
this, the home care nurses must learn how to
conduct these assessments efficiently and to
determine their impact on the patient's situation.

Autonomy

Even when an acute care institution has a primary nursing system for delivering patient care,
acute care nurses care for clients on only one
shift (8 to 12 hours). There is always another
shift that comes in and considers the nursing
needs of the client for those other hours of the
day. In home care, the client's 24-hour care
must be considered in the care plan that is monitored by the primary nurse. Time management
is a critical attribute of a successful home care
nurse because the nurse must plan the day efficiently, balancing travel and visit time, professional activities, and paperwork to maximize
time. If the nurse has not been called upon to
manage many roles at once, often a time management course or specific instruction in this
area should be included in the orientation.

Communication with the Physician

The patient and nurse see a physician at least
daily in the hospital, and specific physician
orders are written directly on the chart based on
the physician's direct assessments. Since the
nurse can talk with the physician in the hospital,
there are opportunities for face-to-face communication and collaborative problem solving. Clients receiving home care may not have seen
their physician for several days or weeks. The
physician relies on the nurse to make skillful
assessments and communicate them concisely
and in a timely manner regarding significant

changes in the client's condition. This means
that the home care nurse must learn how to
communicate concisely with the physician by
"painting a picture" of the client over the telephone and suggesting possible causes and interventions that might be successful. Most
interactions with a physician or the physician's
office nurse consist of less than a minute to
report the patient's condition. The new home
care nurse should practice communicating this
information within that time frame and suggesting interventions.

Determining Frequency and Duration of Care

The discharge date of a hospitalized client is
determined predominantly by the physician, the
hospital's utilization review department, and the
insurer; rarely does the acute care nurse become
involved with making this decision. In home
care, the nurse, in collaboration with the physician, uses the client's needs and the criteria of
the payment source to determine the frequency
(how many visits per week) and the duration
(how many weeks) of care. The need to communicate with the case manager, to receive
prior authorization (if applicable), and to ascertain the client's ability to learn the procedure
also factor into determining the frequency and
duration.

Direct Care

The technical skills provided to the client in
the hospital center around interpreting laboratory values, monitoring physical reactions to the
treatment regimen, overseeing the use of high-
technology equipment, and providing hands-on
care that focuses on the acutely ill. In the hospital the nurse is often in an emergency situation
and has the resources of everyone in the institution to assist, if needed. In home care, the nurse
often has to be able to improvise equipment or
suggest the lowest-cost supplies for clients with
limited resources. Additionally, an understanding of how to provide services in a home envi-

ronment and the roles of other professional and paraprofessional services is also critical for the home care nurse. Often, direct care involves teaching the client and the caregiver how to do the procedure or treatment, rather than doing it for them, as might be done in the hospital.

Documentation

The hospital nurse focuses client documentation on improvement that is being made with an eye to a quick discharge to another level of service. Many hospitals use charting by exception and therefore record only the patient behaviors that are different from what is expected. Since home care is reimbursed by using the chart as the legal guide to services that were provided, the documentation is much more complex and involved than that in the hospital. Documentation in home care must focus on the goals set and the outcomes achieved, as well as the variances experienced by specific patients. Many home health agencies are using critical paths or some kind of preprinted care plans that identify what needs to be documented and how to note what is specific for each patient. In general, the home care nurse charts negatively, with a focus on what the patient has yet to achieve based on the goals and outcomes identified. Progress toward the goals must be measured and also reflected in the patient's record.

Home Visiting

Seeing patients in their own environment involves the new competencies of planning the visit so all needed supplies and paperwork are in the home when the nurse is there. New skills of reading a map; understanding that the nurse is a guest in the patient's home and must ask to do things such as washing hands, using the phone, and turning the television off; and knowing the best way to implement universal precautions in the home setting and using proper bag technique all are new skills the home care nurse must learn before being able to conduct home visits.

Patient Teaching

No matter how competent the hospital nurse is in teaching clients, the health care system demands that clients be discharged from the hospital before adequate teaching can be completed. One of the main roles of the home care nurse is in patient teaching and the nurse most likely will need to be oriented not only in how to teach but in how teaching outcomes are monitored and recorded in the agency. Teaching is a skilled service that is Medicare reimbursable; many managed care programs stress teaching as a way to move the patient to be more independent and to identify problems early, before they require more costly interventions such as an emergency department visit or a hospital admission. The home care nurse must remember that patient teaching is just as important as technical, hands-on care.

Referral to Community Resources

While in the hospital, the social services department and the discharge planning department primarily assess and coordinate the client's need for external referrals, including home care. As the coordinator of the client's care, the home care nurse is responsible for identifying the needs and ensuring that the client and family are aware of what might be helpful. This means that the home care nurse must develop knowledge of the community resources available both locally and nationwide and must learn to work with other disciplines, especially the agency's social services staff, in referring patients to the appropriate resources.

Reimbursement

In the hospital, the admission and billing office, in conjunction with the physician, handles all the client's financial information. Although home health agencies have similar departments, the nurse validates and discusses these issues with the client and the family in the home and verifies the client's eligibility for home care services with the physician. As service progresses, the home care nurse may work with a case manager, reporting directly on the goals accomplished and the ones remaining; determine time of discharge based not only on client needs, but also on requirements of the payer source; and constantly determine whether the patient is eligible for home care services and whether the care provided meets the requirements of the payer source.

Safety

In the hospital, workplace safety issues center on institutional Occupational Safety and Health Administration (OSHA) regulations, hospital security and implementation of internal clinical safety practices such as universal precautions, and safety in the parking areas when the nurse leaves work. Home care nurses who visit clients' homes may often be faced with aggressive patients, dangerous neighborhoods, or other dangerous or violent situations. OSHA has recently released guidelines for preventing workplace violence for health care and social service workers (U.S. Dept. of Labor, OSHA, 1996), which should be integrated throughout the agency's employee policies and perhaps in a specific policy that deals with workplace violence. The nurse transitioning to home care not only must be aware of how to implement these policies in practice, but also must be able to identify situations that may be potentially violent.

Work Environment

In the hospital, the client is always there, usually in the bed or in the room. Everything is familiar and handy for the nurse, and he or she is supported with a myriad of departments such as dietary, laboratory, radiography, pharmacy, laundry, and housekeeping. If something goes wrong with the client, the nurse can call others to assist. In home care, the nurse is always a guest in the client's home and often has to adjust to variations in a client's environment.

The family and caregiver, if present, should be included in the plan of care when appropriate. If on a visit the client is found to need further assistance, the nurse must rely on her or his assessments to make clinical judgments in collaboration with others (such as with the physician via the telephone) if available.

KEY CONTENT AREAS FOUND IN ORIENTATION

Organization of the Home Care System

The nurse transitioning to home care may be unfamiliar with the home health care system and with its internal and external influences. By including a discussion on the various personnel in a home care agency; the types of home care agencies; and a description of licensure, certification, and accreditation into the orientation program, the orientee can have a foundation for understanding home care practice. Since the nurse transitioning into home care may be familiar with the accreditation process from an institutional perspective, the various roles that nurses play in accreditation must be stressed. For example, issues that would be appropriate for a surveyor to discuss with a staff nurse include a review of the process for care and service planning, the process for coordination between nursing and pharmacy, interventions used by nurses for medication administration, and the management of hazardous waste in the home.

The Specialty of Home Care Nursing

The core of an orientation program for a nurse transitioning to home care will focus on understanding the roles and functions of a home care nurse. Hospital nurses may be unfamiliar with determining financial coverage for their care, which is an essential component of home care practice. Other aspects of the home care nurse's role that may be unfamiliar to the nurse transitioning from the hospital setting include identification of and referral to community resources, supervision of paraprofessionals and unlicensed assistive personnel, assuming responsibility for the coordination of care, and ensuring continuity of care and client advocacy.

The nursing process is a framework that helps to organize and systematize the care provided to clients. Although the nursing process is used in all care settings, application of the steps varies from setting to setting. In home care, the nurse must use keen assessment skills to evaluate the client because access to laboratory values and other high-technology assessment methods may be unavailable. The intervention phase of the nursing process is heavily focused on patient and family teaching, rather than direct intervention. Since the goal of home care is to assist the client toward independence, the home care nurse must be a skilled teacher. Evaluation is the planned comparison of the client's health status with the objectives identified in the early stages of the nursing process. In home care, evaluation can help the nurse, in collaboration with the physician, determine when the client can be discharged from home care services.

The Home Visit

The home visit is the single most important tool of the home care nurse. The home care nurse must combine knowledge of the home visiting process with organizational skills and common sense. The nurse transitioning into home care should become familiar with the nursing bag and its contents. An understanding of the bag technique and of the knowledge and skills associated with use of the nursing bag is essential to providing safe and efficient care in the home. A description of the stages of the home visit—the previsit stage, the visit stage, and the postvisit stage—is an essential component of the orientation program. One of the major differences between home care nursing and hospital nursing is the environment in which the care takes place. Given that the nurse is in the client's home, the issue of the personal

safety of the nurse is important. An orientation program for a nurse transitioning into home care must include strategies for maintaining personal safety. Such strategies include having available emergency telephone numbers, having information on what to do if the nurse feels unsafe in the home, knowing how to diffuse crisis situations, and knowing policies and procedures for the use of escorts.

Infection Control

Infection control in the home is very different from that in the hospital setting. Although the underlying principles and OSHA regulations are often the same, the application of those principles is modified in the community. Compared with the hospital, the home is considered a safer environment for a client. Infection is less of a problem because of the fewer numbers and types of microbes, greater resistance of most people to their own household microbes, and exposure to fewer health care workers. Yet the home provides some unique challenges that the home care nurse must confront. For example, the primary caregiver for the client is usually a relative or friend who is untrained in aseptic technique and infection control measures. A client's environment may lack running water or may be extremely disorganized, making it difficult to minimize the risk of infection. The home setting makes it imperative that the home care nurse have the skills to develop creative solutions to infection control problems.

The familiar red biohazard bags that are seen regularly in the hospital are not used in client homes; rather, trash bags that are disposed of in the general trash are used. Responsibility for disposal of waste often rests with the home care nurse, so a full understanding of the regulations surrounding the disposal of infected waste in the home is important. Additionally, the orientation program must include agency policy and procedures for cleaning contaminated plates and eating utensils, linens, bedclothes, and medical equipment used during the home visit.

The Medicare Home Care Benefit

The hospital nurse transitioning into home care likely will be unfamiliar with the intricacies of the Medicare home care benefit. Since the nurse's judgment of the client's clinical situation is integral to Medicare reimbursement, a thorough knowledge of Medicare regulations is essential. A working knowledge of the skilled care definition (nursing, physical therapy, and speech therapy) forms the foundation for discussing Medicare. Understanding the critical elements that constitute skilled nursing (direct care, new teaching, skilled observation and assessment, and management and evaluation of the plan of care) is essential to planning care that meets criteria for reimbursement under Medicare. The coverage criteria (homebound, skilled care, plan of care signed by a physician, reasonable and necessary, and part-time and intermittent) that are so familiar to the experienced home care nurse also must be discussed for the new nurse. Since one of the many roles of the home care nurse is that of the coordinator of care, the nurse must be very familiar with the different professionals and paraprofessionals in the home and the reimbursement guidelines that govern their practice.

Home Care Documentation

Although nurses in all practice settings are accustomed to the requirement for documentation, the unique aspects of home care documentation are essential components of an orientation program for the nurse transitioning to home care. In home care, the nurse's documentation not only serves as the written account of the client's history, status, and progress toward identified goals, it serves as the basis for the justification of reimbursement for third-party payment and is the keystone to risk assessment programs. Regardless of whether the client is on managed care or in a fee-for-service insurance program, the ability to provide nursing services in the home is dependent on the home care nurse's skill in describing

what the client's needs are, justifying the skilled care needed to meet those needs, and describing how the intervention will assist the client in meeting planned goals. The home care nurse must understand and be adept at using the myriad of forms that are unique to home care (i.e., Health Care Financing Administration [HCFA] Forms 485 and 486, physician order forms, and verbal order forms).

Client Teaching

Client and family teaching is one of the most frequently used interventions of the home care nurse. With the reduction in the number of hospital days for most patients, hospital nurses have very little time to teach their patients, so the majority of teaching for self-care must occur in the home following discharge from the hospital. Just as hospital stays have shortened as services move into a managed care environment, the number of home care visits is usually reduced. This shortened number of visits requires that the home care nurse be expert in teaching clients self-care. The home care nurse must understand concepts of clients' internal and external motivation, teaching strategies, and independent learning approaches if teaching is to be conducted in the most efficient and effective manner.

Strategies for Effective Clinical Management

Nurses transitioning into home care are often unfamiliar with the process of collaborating with others for authorization to provide care to clients. The home care nurse must be an expert in collaboration with others, especially case managers. A full discussion of the case management process must be included in an orientation program for nurses transitioning to home care. This discussion should include the following:

- a definition of case management
- the role of a case manager
- where case managers are employed

- what case managers expect from a home care agency
- what case managers are concerned about
- how to develop a relationship with a case manager

A full discussion of case management and its role in home care can be found in Chapter 43.

Home Care Nursing Strategies for Success

One of the biggest differences between home care nursing and hospital nursing practice is the degree of autonomy in home care. Nurses new to home care need to be helped to develop organizational skills to manage the activities of the day in the most efficient manner. Because the nurse cannot pass duties and activities that were not accomplished to the next shift, the nurse new to home care may feel overwhelmed by the burden of the autonomy. Time management, caseload management, and stress management strategies should be included in the orientation program.

Along with the benefits of independent practice come the isolation and loneliness that nurses new to home care feel. This isolation may result in frustration in practice, with the new nurse eventually leaving the agency to return to nursing in an inpatient setting. The nurse transitioning into home care must be given the tools to be effective in the role while learning strategies to remain connected to her or his nursing colleagues. These strategies may include weekly lunch meetings with other nurses in the agency and attendance at continuing education seminars and case conferences with other professionals involved in the care of a complex client.

Legal and Ethical Aspects of Home Care

Some of the most difficult issues facing home care today are the ethical problems that arise in practice. Changes in the way health care is provided, changes in the structure of the family, limited resources for all types of care, and regu-

lations protecting the rights of the individual all serve to make home care nursing practice increasingly complex. Legal issues in home care are also beginning to become more complex. Home care agencies were often excluded from litigation because they didn't have the deep pockets of hospitals or long-term care facilities. Now that home care is growing and there are large, national chains that have significant financial resources, home care agencies are often included in lawsuits. Knowledge of risk management, fraud and abuse regulations, and the guidelines around abandonment are among the many topics that a hospital nurse transitioning to home care should have later on in an orientation program.

Specialized Home Care Programs and Services

Many nurses entering home care from the hospital setting are being recruited for their specialized skills with clients from specific populations. For example, nurses who are expert in cardiac care often will be recruited into home care to staff a cardiac rehabilitation program. Even though these nurses are specialists, home care practice requires an understanding of the basic aspects of the home care delivery system to be effective. The nurse transitioning into home care must have an understanding of other programs in the agency and community, including high-technology programs, hospice care, psychiatric home care, and early newborn discharge programs. Consider this example: The expert cardiac nurse may be seeing a patient in the home who has severe cardiomyopathy. Instead of being rehabilitated, the client seems to be on a downward progression in his or her illness. The home care nurse in collaboration with the physician determines that the client is terminal. Without a basic understanding of the criteria for enrollment in hospice care and the benefits afforded the client, the nurse will be unaware of this strategy that might be helpful to the client.

TEACHING STRATEGIES

While the key content areas are important to an effective orientation program, so too is the method by which the material is delivered. Since the relationship between the new nurse and the home care agency begins during orientation, a poorly planned experience will set a negative tone for the relationship. The teaching strategies that are incorporated into the orientation program are critical to the learning that takes place and can reduce the agency investment of time and money. Examples of teaching strategies that can be integrated into an orientation program for a nurse transitioning into home care include the following:

- Self-directed learning: This strategy calls upon the learner to read information and accomplish learning activities independently.
- Clinical simulation/documentation exercises: These activities duplicate common experiences so that the learner can practice new skills in the supportive environment of the home care agency. New nurses are given the opportunity to problem solve, question, and develop interventions with the direction of an experienced nurse.
- Role play: Using experienced home care nurses in a role-play situation, the new nurse can learn about complex processes of clinical practice, such as admitting and discharging a patient.

- Field trips: Field trips can be designed to provide a comprehensive understanding of the community and the home care agency (Humphrey & Milone-Nuzzo, 1996).

CONCLUSION

Acute care nurses can bring a great deal of expertise and experience to home health care that can be adapted to their practice. There is, however, a body of knowledge specific to the specialty of home care nursing that the acute care nurse must learn before being expected to be an efficient and effective home care practitioner. This chapter has outlined the operational definition of home care nursing that home care nurses should practice, even in the changing health care climate of today and the future. The differences between acute care and home care nursing practice as well as orientation content areas have been outlined to give the manager direction as to what should be taught to new nurses transitioning to home care. Making the transition from acute care to home care is a collaborative effort. Nurses should begin to learn basic home care nursing principles in their educational experience and build that knowledge throughout employment with a home care agency. It is up to the nurse manager to find ways to teach the new nurse this important content and constantly reinforce the learning throughout the orientation period and beyond.

REFERENCES

Humphrey, C., & Milone-Nuzzo, P. (1996). *Manual of home care nursing orientation*. Gaithersburg, MD: Aspen.

Miller, M., & Daley, B. (1996). Home health care nursing: There is a difference. *Home Health Care Management and Practice*, 8(4), 64–70.

U.S. Department of Labor, Occupational Safety and Health Administration. (1996). *Guidelines for preventing workplace violence*, Publication #3148. Washington, DC: Author.

Webster's ninth new collegiate dictionary. (1988). New York: Merriam-Webster.

CHAPTER 43

Case Management

Linda A. Billows

Case management has been a hot topic of conversation among home care providers for more than 20 years. The debate has been fueled by a number of factors: the variety of interpretations of what case management is, the concern over duplication of functions already performed by providers, and the use of case management to reduce costs by reducing services. This chapter attempts to bring some clarity to the definition of case management and raises some issues and questions for ongoing discussion.

As we prepare for the year 2000, one cannot look at case management in isolation. Health care reform has introduced an array of concepts and terms, all of which describe control of and access to health care services. Let's begin by looking at the terms under discussion:

- Managed care: the care typically provided by a health maintenance organization designed to enhance cost-effectiveness by eliminating inappropriate service.
- Managed competition: a health care theory, largely untested, based on free-market competition. Groups of providers would compete to offer services, and consumers would choose health plans based on which ones offer the best quality for the lowest price.
- Case management: as generally interpreted, a term with two contradictory aspects. The first aspect relates to fiscal management, that is, whether a person falls within certain policy limits. This has to do with whether people are eligible for a service and what level of payment will be made. The second aspect relates to clinical management, which means a determination of what kind of medical, nursing, or social service interventions are necessary and in the best interest of the client. There has been a fairly good separation of these functions until the past 10 years or so, when insurance companies, either in their private insurance role or in their role as administrator of Medicare programs, have blurred that separation to control what payers feel is overutilization (Halamandaris, 1990).

The Government Affairs Committee of the National Association for Home Care, which I chaired, prepared a White Paper on case management approved by the board of the National Association for Home Care in January 1991. The following is from that document.

CASE MANAGEMENT DEFINED

There are two fundamentally different types of case management: one performed by providers as an essential part of their caregiving activities, and one that some payers have superimposed on the provider system primarily as a mechanism to control costs. In some cases, both systems are responsible for assessing client needs, developing plans of care, coordinating the various services that clients receive, and carrying out monitoring and quality assurance activities. The committee concluded that the duplication by payer of caregiving activities is costly, that documentation reduces provider efficiency and adds to provider cost, and that there is no documentation of improvement of care or cost reduction.

COMPONENTS OF CASE MANAGEMENT

The committee's next step was to delineate payer case management functions and provider case management functions. The characteristics and functions of a financial manager are as follows:

- assessments: determining whether the client is eligible under the terms of the payer's program and applying the program's coverage limits
- planning: validating the home care agency's care plan
- coordinating benefits (where there are two or more payers)
- defining the payment system
- conducting program evaluations and provider audits

A payer financial management system should have the following characteristics:

- a proven track record as a fiscal conduit for health and social service programs
- a staff of professionals with home care experience to validate care plans
- an appeals process that is readily accessible to beneficiaries and providers
- an approved cash management plan and/or approved performance bond
- annual outside performance audits

Case management, as practiced in the clinical setting by home care providers, should consist of seven essential functions:

1. assessment: physical, environmental, psychological, socioeconomic, and eligibility under various third-party programs
2. planning: care plan development and validation
3. coordination: interdisciplinary and inter-agency/intraagency coordination
4. organization and staffing
5. staffing and resource allocation
6. implementation or care provision: implementation of care plans and delivery of service
7. evaluation: quality assurance measures to ensure that standards of care are met.

Care management is done in collaboration with the patient, family, physician, and provider.

Given the central role that the care manager plays in determining the effectiveness of the care that is provided, it is essential that the care manager be fully qualified. Care managers should meet the following criteria:

- employ the interdisciplinary team approach
- operate as an established legal entity recognized by the state
- meet all applicable local and state standards
- carry professional liability insurance
- have an established and recognized quality assurance program
- have a proven track record of providing patient care
- conduct business 24 hours a day, 7 days a week, including all holidays.

Additional recommendations include the following:

- Case management is not needed by all clients.
- Case management should be patient driven.
- Patients should choose whether they need case management.
- Case management should promote patient independence.

- Case management should be available to patients of all ages.

The committee also believed that it was important for quality assurance to be a part of any discussion of case management.

QUALITY ASSURANCE

Quality assurance programs in case management settings need to start with the development of meaningful but accessible measurements of the administrative and supervisory activities, compare program costs with benefits, and monitor progress toward objectives. The development of structural aspects of case management may include the following activities:

- a survey of the extent to which qualifications of case managers hired meet job performance expectations
- a review by supervisors of case managers, job descriptions, and requirements
- an ongoing review of recruitment activities.

Process aspects of case management provide an opportunity to look at how resources are used. The following process activities should be included:

- an evaluation of the effectiveness of preservice and inservice training provided to case managers, supervisors, billing staff, and so forth
- the development of agency norms with the objective of monitoring performance outliers to identify both ineffective case management activities and efficient activities that need to be shared to improve activity of other staff.

Outcomes are summary indicators of resource utilization and include efforts such as the following:

- costing out of care plans (by caseload or case) in the context of specific case mix factors

- development of a scale to indicate the level of diversity in care plan services and to determine whether client needs are generally met within a caseload context
- measurement of client satisfaction and client understanding of the case manager's role.

All three of the domains used in the approach by Donabedian (1978) (structure, process, and outcomes) need to be included for a quality assurance program to address all facets of a service. Additionally, this effort should be done in light of the need to identify values that are attached to the measurement within each area (Yee, 1990). Is the case manager primarily an advocate or care accountant? Does the agency respond to client crisis or only to ongoing needs after the client has stabilized? To what extent do case managers make care plan and service decisions with supervisors or other reviewers?

RESEARCH ON CASE MANAGEMENT

It is important to ask what we know about case management and to look for evidence of its accomplishments. The National Long Term Care Channeling Demonstration was the most elaborate of the demonstrations that employed case management. It was designed to demonstrate whether a home care program for older persons with chronic functional impairment would reduce spending overall by reducing nursing home and hospital expenditures. It was carried out at 10 different sites from approximately June 1982 to March 1985.

The study compared the overall home care and health care spending for a control group (a group that received no assistance from the demonstration) with that for two comparable groups of elderly disabled persons who were case managed. One of these two groups was placed under a basic case management model and the other under a financial control model. In both case management models, each client received a complete assessment, a care plan was developed, services were arranged, the plan was monitored to ensure that the care that had been ordered was being provided, and the client was periodically reassessed. The primary difference between the two case management models was that in the financial control model the case managers were authorized within prescribed limits to purchase services not otherwise available under existing programs, whereas the basic model was largely limited to the services that could be funded by other programs.

The channeling demonstration confirmed the findings of previous studies, which had concluded that case management tends to increase overall costs, not reduce them. It was estimated that it would cost the government $2,500 (under the basic system) and $3,100 (under the financial control plan) per month per client to operate a permanent channeling program. These amounts represent increases of $200 and $500, respectively, over the costs that government would have incurred in the absence of case management by the project.

The case management costs themselves accounted for much of the difference between the costs of the groups in the demonstration and the costs for those who received their care through the conventional home care delivery system. Under the basic case management method, the cost of assessment, care planning, and other preservice activities was $330 per client. The cost of ongoing case management was $92 per month per client. The figures for the financial control group were $346 and $86, respectively.

There were few real differences in the client outcomes for the two case management groups, and the differences between the case-managed groups and the control groups were not great. There were no measurable differences in mortality rates or nursing home or hospital use. Clients in the two case management models had fewer unmet needs, however, and they and their families were more confident and satisfied with their care arrangements than the group that received no assistance from the demonstration project.

A study of 48 case management systems conducted by the University of Minnesota tends to confirm the potential costliness of case management. Half the programs could report the cost of their case management activities as a percentage of the cost of services they managed. Their case management costs ranged from 7% to 50% of the cost of services (Hoyer, 1990).

TRAINING OF HOME HEALTH AGENCY STAFF

As home health agencies expand their experience in working in the managed care environment many are including case management training for their staff. The training may include such topics as costing out of care plans, case mix analysis, outcomes, development of agency norms, and so forth. Sharing these training programs with managed care companies increases their understanding of the expertise of home health agencies. Home health agencies are broadening their capabilities in outcome data, and this increased capability will be extremely useful to agency staff as well as managed care companies.

CONCLUSION

Case management and other types of management are being proposed as ways of improving the health care system, yet one has to search far and wide for reference to improved client satisfaction. Discussion is focused on cost and impact on providers and insurers, yet there is lack of clarity about exactly what outcomes we can expect from case management. One would hope that answers to the following questions about case management will soon be known:

- How will case management affect clients?
- How will it improve care?
- What outcomes are expected from a case management system?
- How much will case management cost?
- How much will case management save?
- How will it be monitored?

- Who will be the case manager?
- What are the qualifications of the case manager?
- How will duplication be reduced?

As the discussion continues on both state and federal levels regarding case management, it will be important for home care providers to continue to be active participants in the debate.

REFERENCES

Donabedian, A. (1978). The quality of medical care. In R.H. Abelson (Ed.), *Health care regulation, economics, ethics, and practice*. Washington, DC: American Association for the Advancement of Science.

Halamandaris, V. (1990). The paradox of case management. *Caring, 9*, 4–7.

Hoyer, R. (1990). Where are we and where do we go from here? *Caring, 9*, 4–12.

Yee, D. (1990). Developing a quality assurance program in case management service settings. *Caring, 9*, 30–36.

CHAPTER 44

Managed Care

Nina M. Smith

Health care services and payment systems have been developing and changing in the United States for the last century. Medical care has evolved from the simple family doctor to hospital-based technological advances. Changes in location of service have affected the method of payments. Systems of care have became more involved, and layers of specialists and alternative care providers have grown. With increasing technology has come the demand for improved and more expensive services. Lines have been drawn between the payer and the provider, each feeling the need to protect its territory. Unions, employers, social organizations, and individuals have struggled to pay for the escalating services.

The twentieth century has been an amazing time for medical and psychiatric breakthroughs. Advances have provided control and eradication of life-threatening illnesses and debilitating diseases. No longer does the average citizen have to suffer. Cutting-edge treatment is available. Unfortunately, however, the cost for some of these services is too expensive. Often, treatment can be provided only to those who have a way to pay. Health care costs have escalated in the past 30 to 40 years. In 1960 the percentage of the gross national product (GNP) spent on health care was 5.2%. In 1992 the percentage of the GNP spent on health care was 14%, approximately $840 billion dollars (Baldor, 1996). As

costs continue to spiral, payer systems are creating ways to provide necessary services and to maintain quality care, yet limit costs and create savings.

In the last 20 years several payer systems have been developed as a way to deal with the health care crisis: diagnosis-related groups (DRGs), utilization review, case management, health maintenance organizations (HMOs), and managed care are examples. Health care reform has dominated legislative discussions. Improving payment systems, reducing costs, stretching dwindling budgets and reserves for Medicare and Medicaid, and providing universal health care coverage are just a few topics under review.

As a response to the evolving and changing crisis, managed care and managed competition have shown themselves as the systems of choice best able to create the environment for change. Managed plans are growing larger, merging with other health care systems to provide an integrated delivery system. Health care providers, payers, and customers are coming together, albeit slowly, to work together toward a mutually agreeable system. Paradigms are shifting from specialists to generalists; physicians to complementary team members; inpatient to ambulatory services; and available services to necessary services. As these paradigms shift and the focus of services changes, unique ethical dilemmas and new legal issues will occur. Health care providers will be required to learn vital information early and to recognize the need for change in order to be positioned for survival.

HISTORY OF MANAGED CARE

The health care systems in the United States started changing in the early to mid-1900s. To economize time and resources, family physicians started practicing in an office environment and no longer in the home. Hospitals increased in number to accommodate physician specialists needing to utilize the technology available in the hospital setting. Payment systems were on a fee-for-service basis. The older general practitioner often was forced out of practice or into a "lodge practice" as a means to maintain business. A lodge practice was supported by union members or fraternal organizations as a way to provide prepaid health services to their constituents at a reasonable price. The American Medical Association (AMA) strongly opposed lodge practices and supported only those physicians and hospitals that worked with a fee-for-service plan. HMOs formed as a counterresponse to the AMA and emerging indemnity plans that covered fee-for-service costs.

GROWTH AND DEVELOPMENT OF MANAGED CARE*

- **1863**—Case management was defined through social work systems to coordinate public human services and conserve public funds.
- **1900**—Case management started as a part of public health nursing.
- **1929**—A rural farmer's cooperative health plan was established in Oklahoma.
- **1929**—Two California physicians entered into a prepaid contract to provide compre-

hensive health care to 2,000 water company employees.
- **1937**—The Group Health Association was founded in Washington.
- **1942**—The Kaiser-Permanente Medical Care Program was started.
- **1945**—After World War II necessary community services were extended to discharged psychiatric patients.
- **1947**—The Health Insurance Plan of Greater New York was begun.
- **1950**—The Hill-Burton Act created a number of community-based regional medical centers.
- **1950s**—Employee assistance programs (EAPs) were started as an occupational health service for alcoholics.
- **1951**—The Joint Commission on the Accreditation of Healthcare Organizations (Joint Commission) was formed.
- **1954**—One of the first Independent Physician Association (IPA) plans was started in California.
- **1963**—Community mental health centers programs were initiated.
- **1965**—Medicaid was established by the federal government to provide health care services to the poor.
- **1965**—Medicare was introduced to ensure health care access for the elderly.
- **1965**—The Older Americans Act was passed to provide federal funding support for older Americans and the development of the Administration on Aging.
- **1970s**—Workers' compensation case management was begun.
- **1973**—Congress passed the HMO Act to encourage third-party payers to increase control of medical care delivery and enable managed-care plans to increase in numbers and to expand enrollments.
- **1974**—The Nixon Administration made an attempt to control costs by freezing physician fees.
- **1974**—The Employee Retirement Income Security Act (ERISA) allowed self-funded insurance plans to avoid paying premium

*Source: List reprinted from Baldor, 1996, Department of Health and Human Services, 1994.

taxes and to avoid compliance with state-mandated benefits, even though these costs were necessary for insurance companies and managed care plans; it also required that plans and companies provide an Explanation of Benefits (EOB) statement in the event that a claim was denied and to inform the individual of his or her right for appeal.

- **1979**—Seventeen utilization review companies were operating for disability and medical-surgical cases.
- **1979**—The National Committee for Quality Assurance (NCQA) was founded by the Group Health Association of America and the American Managed Care and Review Association.
- **Early 1980s**—Telephonic utilization review for patients with psychiatric and substance abuse problems was started.
- **1981**—The Omnibus Budget Reconciliation Act (OBRA) was passed to encourage community-based alternatives to provide care to the elderly in lieu of institutional placement.
- **1982**—The Tax Equity and Fiscal Responsibility Act (TEFRA) was created to control Medicare costs.
- **1983**—DRGs were used as a means for TEFRA control of medical-surgical diagnoses.
- **Early 1980s**—Preferred provider organizations (PPOs) began to develop.
- **1985**—The Consolidated Omnibus Budget Reconciliation Act (COBRA) was passed to require employers to offer continued health insurance coverage for a certain length of time after the group health insurance had been terminated.
- **1986–1992**—Managed behavioral health care companies were carved out of traditional indemnity medical-surgical plans.
- **1989**—The Physician Payment Review Commission was created to implement legislation that introduced a resource-based fee schedule that limited the amount physicians could charge patients above the fee schedule and volume performance standards.
- **1993**—The Health Security Act (HR 3600) was enacted to provide the security of a comprehensive health benefit plan to all Americans that could never be taken away.
- **1994**—The Medicare Choice Act was passed to allow Medicare-eligible beneficiaries the choice of traditional Medicare benefit plans or enrollment in an integrated health plan.
- **1996**—Congress is considering parity for behavioral health programs by carving them back into medical-surgical plans.
- **1988 to present**—Industry consolidation of managed care companies is occurring through mergers and acquisitions to achieve economies of scale and reduce redundant costs (Baldor, 1996; Freeman & Trabin, 1994).

The growth and development of managed care shows the change from utilization management and controlling access to the future development of specific, cost-effective services in the least restrictive environments. Managed care organizations (MCOs) are moving toward constructing organized networks of providers to deliver care in a coherent, integrated, and efficient fashion (Sederer & Bennett, 1996).

STRUCTURE OF MANAGED CARE

By definition managed care is any plan, process, or mechanism that attempts to affect the price of health care, the site where health care is delivered, and the utilization of services. Further definition is difficult because managed care is an evolving concept provided by many organizations, with payers and providers continually seeking ways to provide more efficient care at a lower price. Understanding the structure, function, and history of managed care is like learning a new language and alphabet. As plans merge, separate, and grow they take on characteristics of each other. There are two major types of managed care organizations, payer-based and provider-based organizations. Payer-based organizations include insurance companies, HMOs, PPOs, self-insured employers, third-party administrators (TPAs), and workers' compensation administrators. Provider-based organizations include hospitals, medical groups, and alternate-site companies. Following is a brief description of the types of managed care organizations:

- Insurance companies are difficult to define since they may offer a wide variety of managed care plans, such as an HMO, a PPO, or a hybrid.
- HMOs can be both financiers, and providers of health care services that assume all or part of the risks of providing services.
- There are four major types of HMOs and several hybrid plans.
  1. An independent practice association (IPA) is a separate legal entity formed by physicians for the purpose of contracting with payers; physicians are contracted by the IPA to provide medical services for a negotiated fee, which is either per capita or fee for service; physicians retain their individual practices and service IPA patients; this structure comprises 60% of HMO plans.
  2. Staff model HMOs have physicians as employees of the health plan, with a broad range of specialties; the premiums and revenue compensate physicians with salary and incentive programs; this structure comprises 14% of HMO plans.
  3. Group model HMOs subcontract for services with multispecialty group practices to provide all or part of the medical services; physicians are employees of the group practice; the health plan compensates the medical group for services at a negotiated rate; captive group models recruit and form their own physicians group; indepen-

dent group models contract with existing, independent multispecialty groups; this structure comprises 14% of HMO plans.
  4. Network model HMOs contract with two or more medical practices to provide medical services that are single-specialty, independent practices, single-specialty medical groups, or multispecialty medical groups; network physicians can service their own patients as well as the HMO patients; this structure comprises 12% of HMO plans.
  5. Other HMO structures include point of service (POS) or open-ended plans (care from any willing provider with higher out-of-pocket expenses), self-insured HMO plans, and any number of other hybrid plans.
- PPOs contract with preferred providers who agree to accept discounts, comply with utilization review guidelines, and assume no financial risk for providing medical services. The incentive to the employee is to use preferred providers to lower their out-of-pocket expenses.
- An exclusive provider organization (EPO) is a type of PPO in which enrollees are covered only for services by network providers.
- Self-insured employers manage their own health care benefits. A company might be a large corporation or a number of smaller, self-insured employers enrolled in a large pool.
- TPAs are local, regional, or national companies responsible for managing health care benefits established by self-insured employers. TPAs are service management providers and do not establish benefits.
- Workers' compensation administrators work with the insurance commissioner in most states to establish workers' compensations benefits and are highly regulated.
- Managed indemnity plans impose utilization review on care delivered by any pro-

vider, and providers do not have contracts with the plan.

- Provider-based organizations include hospitals, medical groups, and alternate-site companies that provide care with financial risk (Cherney, 1995).

STAGES OF MANAGED CARE DEVELOPMENT

Managed care markets differ in terms of their stage of development. Cities and states across the United States are in various stages of managed care penetration. Understanding where a particular area is in development will assist providers in working with the level of managed care company present.

Stage I: Unstructured Markets

An unstructured market is essentially a non–managed care market and includes the following:

- independent hospitals
- independent physicians
- unsophisticated purchasers
- fee-for-service pricing
- 0% to 20% managed care market penetration, such as rural United States, Iowa, Alaska, and Wyoming

Stage II: Loose-Framework Markets

MCOs enter the market, and providers receive contact from case managers, utilization reviewers, and other personnel who are interested in reducing costs. This is characterized by the following:

- proliferation of HMOs and PPOs
- formation of provider networks
- declining hospital bed capacity
- discount and per diem pricing
- 20% to 50% managed care market penetration

Stage III: Consolidation Markets

MCOs compete heavily for patients, and this causes some MCOs to lose business or to go out of business. It is difficult for providers to distinguish the appropriate targets in this market. Stage III is characterized by the following:

- the shakeout of marginal MCO players
- the emergence of dominant MCOs
- the formation of provider/payer alliances
- per diem, per case, per episode, and capitation pricing
- 50% to 75% managed care market penetration

Stage IV: Managed Competition

The majority of alternate-site referrals are controlled by MCOs. Providers without MCO contracts have difficulty generating nongovernmental business. This is characterized by the following:

- fewer MCOs
- fully integrated systems
- direct employer/provider contracts
- high MCO penetration
- pricing strategies that are capitation, risk sharing, and outcomes based
- 75% to 100% managed care market penetration, such as Los Angeles and Minneapolis (Cherney, 1995)

PAYMENT MECHANISMS AND PRICING STRATEGIES IN MANAGED CARE

There are eight major types of pricing strategies that can be developed for managed care organizations. The degree of risk associated with each pricing structure varies from low risk to high risk. The eight strategies from low to high are as follows:

- fee for service—a specific fee for each product or service provided
- discounted fee for service—a fixed amount or percentage is subtracted from the list price fee

- per diems—a set daily rate for all of the products or services over the course of a day
- per case—a fixed dollar amount for care per case
- per episode—a fixed dollar amount per episode or occurrence
- capitation—provider receives a per member per month flat fee
- risk sharing—arrangement made with MCO to share the cost for care on a select risk population
- outcomes-based pricing—fixed dollar amount per case based on expected outcomes

IMPLICATIONS OF MANAGED CARE IN HOME CARE

Home care markets grew rapidly during the 1980s, and profit margins were at their all-time high. With the introduction of managed care into the home care arena, reimbursements and intensifying competition have affected many businesses negatively. To ensure operational success, home care companies must begin a strategic analysis of their operations and plan for the future. Agencies that adjust their marketing and operational strategies will be able to position for survival into managed care.

Strategic Planning

Developing a strategic plan is a simple yet difficult process. The steps are simple, but the honesty it takes to review organizational systems comprehensively might be difficult. Using a SWOT (strengths, weaknesses, opportunities, and threats) analysis as a method of review can be an effective tool in honestly recognizing difficulties and strengths. It is important to review current operations, financial status, mix of payer sources, quality, reputation, staff, internal and external opportunities and threats, and the impact of change on the organization. Representatives in the process should come from all

levels of the agency, and honesty should be encouraged. Administration should realistically assess all aspects of goal setting, objectives, priorities, time frames, methods of achieving results, understanding costs, and implications to agency survival (Good strategic plans, 1995).

What MCOs Want from Home Care Organizations

- effective ways to control overall cost while maintaining quality
- risk-sharing capability
- comprehensive services, networks, "one-stop shop"
- continuum of care, least restrictive level of care
- outcome measurement information, outcome-driven delivery
- clinically effective programs, specialty niche programs
- critical pathways, case management
- patient satisfaction
- consolidated billing process
- good communications
- collaborative relationships
- accreditation—Joint Commission, CARF, and Medicare (if applicable)

NETWORKS

A network is an affiliation of health care providers organized to broaden their service and geographic capabilities. Network affiliates can be bound by loose-affiliation management agreements or as owners in a new legal entity. In order for smaller agencies to work with managed care companies and maintain their position in the larger playing arena it is important to establish professional relationships. Networks are formed to provide participants a stronger position with MCOs by working together. There are three major types of network structures:

1. Management service organizations (MSOs)—participants form a separate

entity that coordinates marketing and contracts and brokers services.

2. Physician hospital organizations (PHOs)—PHOs are part of an integrated delivery system, usually with equal ownership and a separate legal entity that provides joint managed care–contracting opportunities for acute care and medical services; PHOs can add home care and other alternate site providers.

3. Foundations—foundations typically comprise hospitals, physicians, and community-based affiliates to serve the community's health care needs in a not-for-profit, tax-exempt structure.

Selecting professional affiliates for networking is a process that is determined through a criterion selection to ensure that the same standards and similar philosophies are provided. Issues to consider when selecting others for a network affiliation are as follows:

- accreditation, licensure, and certification
- geographic coverage
- community reputation
- satisfactory working relationships with physicians, patients, and payers
- similar rates and pricing structures or willingness to work on similar rates
- current professional working relationship (agency to potential affiliate)
- financial stability
- referral reliability
- scope of services provided
- on-call and after-hours systems
- history, willingness, and operational ability to work with MCOs
- case management and utilization management abilities and experience
- current contractual relationships with subcontractors and MCOs
- availability of data: financial, clinical, administrative
- clinical supervision
- verification of professional licenses
- validation of staff competency

CONTRACTING WITH MANAGED CARE COMPANIES

To contract successfully with an MCO it is necessary for the agency to ask itself basic questions before committing to any type of contract with financial, legal, or clinical obligations that contain risk. An agency must ask whether it knows what it does, how it does it, the true cost of doing business, and whether it has developed a way to capture statistics that allows it to identify trends early. Since education is critical, it must ask itself whether it has learned everything it can about the managed care marketplace and whether it has developed the management skills and tools needed to succeed. There is no guessing; the agency must know the answers and be prepared to defend the information to the MCO. The agency must know its competition and find out what others are providing and what it costs them. The agency must find its niche, discover where opportunities lie, find a gap, and learn how it can fill the need. Management must be committed to the goal, plan on constant refinement of procedures, and consider risk taking and change as creative and empowering. The agency must invest in staff, training, development, and technology to provide alternative, cost-effective, and time-efficient methods of care to position itself. Once an agency has completed its strategic plan it is time to find out about the MCO.

To learn about MCOs the agency must do its homework. It is common for an MCO to ask many questions of an agency but not be willing to provide much information in return. Asking critical questions is necessary for making an intelligent contract decision. Ask assertive and probing questions, and understand all contract terms. Ask whether the MCO is experienced, financially strong, and well established in the community. Does it provide services similar to the agency's ability? Ask what other providers are affiliated with the MCO. Is it clear what benefits are covered or what the utilization review (UR) procedures are for each plan offered? Is a clean claim identified or the payment cycle for a clean claim? Was the MCO informative about submission and payments of interval claims for patients requiring a long duration of service? Before accepting a risk-based contract, does the agency need a trial period with limited risk before a full-risk assumption is achieved? Has the agency considered which conditions will be excluded from capitation or risk-based contracts? Has the agency determined whether the contract is legal in light of changing federal and state laws? Is the agency aware of the potential for customer satisfaction and dissatisfaction and whether this will affect renegotiation at contract renewal time? Is there understanding throughout the agency about the lengthy time for negotiations and contract closure? Does it know that all the time and effort spent in negotiating can be lost in just one phone call, if the basic tenets of customer services and telephone etiquette are not maintained?

With the information obtained, it will be possible to assess the risk quotient. Most managed care contracts contain some level of risk, and this must be weighed against the financial, clinical, and administrative operations of the agency. The decision to become part of a managed care network or to enter into a managed care agreement requires careful evaluation. If it meets all criteria, then the contract may be signed. Once the contract is established, it must be maintained. Keeping communication open and responsive will ensure success.

DILEMMAS IN MANAGED CARE

Quality

Quality is no longer a critical indicator showing the worth of a provider or payer; it is now the baseline industry standard. Quality is expected, demanded, and provided by the majority. Therefore, providers and payers must show special abilities that set them apart from others, such as management and organizational development success; financial stability; strate-

gic planning and goals; contracting and negotiating skills; understanding and compliance with legal and regulatory issues; risk management plans; and creative, innovative, and flexible program services with outcome measurements.

Ethics

While ethics and managed care are not mutually exclusive, it does take a concerted effort to find a collaborative middle ground where care and cost can meet. A number of ethical issues have emerged in response to managed care's growth:

- provider-patient relationships—in which mutual trust and cost factors are at odds
- confidentiality—the more individuals who have access to medical information, the higher the potential for breach of confidentiality
- universal care—how the present system structures provide, at least, minimal care to everyone
- conflicts of interests—questions exist as to the role and ownership of services related to the payer, provider, or customer
- clinically appropriate levels of care—providers and payers at odds over patient treatment plans
- contracting—leads to questions on how to structure appropriate and necessary provision for services
- capitation—raises questions of incentives and motives for treatment or nontreatment
- rationing of care—is this done universally for all, or is it only for specific populations
- for-profit corporation—medical care is no longer a cottage industry but a large corporate structure in which medical professionalism is becoming managerial professionalism
- ethical guidelines—identification, education, and awareness are necessary to inform the leaders, providers, and public of their responsibilities and methods to

address their needs (Appleby, 1996; Baldor, 1996; Dacso & Dasco, 1996)

Teaching and Research

While the need for outcome measurements and statistics to determine the quality of health care exists, managed care has not been positioned to support the necessary research or teaching efforts needed to gain this information. Managed care has traditionally contracted with nonacademic hospitals to provide services. Teaching and research institutions generate additional overall costs for management of these programs and often cannot provide services at the reduced rates necessary. Managed care is now collaborating with some academic systems, but the funding and sample are limited. It may become necessary for the provider to create, at its own cost, the research, outcome measurements, and statistical analysis necessary to prove that its service is efficient, economical, and effective.

Evaluation of Managed Care Organizations

Hospitals, long-term care facilities, ambulatory services, home care agencies, rehabilitation facilities, and behavioral health care systems have long been aware of the accreditation and survey process. The standards that apply to these surveys often function as indicators of quality performance and assist managed care organizations in their determination of a provider with which to contract or negotiate services. MCOs are now being held to the same accreditation and survey processes by employers and providers to determine with which managed care company they will choose to contract. The National Committee for Quality Assurance (NCQA) initiated by the Group Health Association of America (GHAA) and the American Managed Care and Review Association (AMCRA) was established in 1990 to provide an evaluation process for managed care companies. MCOs were rapidly expanding in numbers, and it was becoming harder for employers

to assess the quality and efficiency of each organization. The Health Plan Employer Data and Information Set (HEDIS) was developed in response to employers. The HEDIS 2.0 system measured an MCO's quality of service based on access to care, appropriateness of care, efficiency, technical outcome, and member satisfaction.

In 1995, additional reviewing agencies came into prominence as a result of the negative press that NCQA was receiving in regard to the survey and accreditation process. Opponents to NCQA and HEDIS cited a conflict of interest in NCQA's relationship to the founding agencies (GHAA and AMCRA) and also in the fact that GHAA and AMCRA were managed care organizations and did not provide an impartial, independent audit process. As a result, the Joint Commission, the Utilization Review Accreditation Commission (URAC), the American Accreditation Program Inc. (AAPI), and the Accreditation Association for Ambulatory Health Care (AAAHC) have shown an increased presence in the survey and accreditation process for managed care organizations. Each survey agency evaluates similar standards, but no one scoring system exists to compare results. As managed care increases its presence in the health care arena, accreditation will be a basic requirement for each MCO to prove to employers its ability to provide cost-effective yet consumer friendly service (Caldwell, 1995; Dacso & Dasco, 1996; Changing landscape, 1996). The Foundation for Accountability (FAcct) is a new, nonprofit organization dedicated to providing consumers information they need to make decisions about their health care. Founded in 1995 and headquartered in Portland, Oregon, FAcct is currently composed of employers, consumer groups, and government health care purchasers. FAcct has taken the HEDIS instrument and has worked with NCQA to update HEDIS to a 3.0 version, released in late 1996. HEDIS 3.0 allows employers to compare plans directly and provides performance measurements for Medicare and Medicaid. FAcct will use the information obtained to monitor and improve the quality of health care (Caldwell, 1995; Changing landscape, 1996).

Legal and Regulatory Issues

Legal and regulatory issues are changing as fast as managed care can create new problems and stretch the already difficult to interpret laws.

Antireferrals

The Omnibus Budget Reconciliation Act of 1993 (OBRA '93) extended the prohibitions related to physician referrals to cover several additional categories of health services and to include the Medicaid program (Stark I). Stark I regulations were proposed in March 1992 and completed with final publication in August 1995. Before the final revision was published the regulation had undergone many changes, was renamed Stark II, and included 11 designated services for which a bill or claim could not be made pursuant to a prohibited referral, with the focus on services provided rather than the entity providing the services. The law also requires that entities providing designated services report ownership information and arrangements to the Department of Health and Human Services (Dacso & Dasco, 1996).

Safe Harbors

Safe harbor provisions are payment practices that would not be subject to criminal prosecution and that would not provide a basis for exclusion from the Medicare program or from the state health care program. In November 1992 the Office of Inspector General issued two safe harbor regulations governing managed care activities and they were published in 57 *Federal Register* 52724–52730, effective immediately. The regulations protect health plans that offer increased coverage or reduced costs to enrollees and protect reductions offered by health care providers to health plans so that neither would be considered illegal remuneration subject to fraud and abuse penalties under the Antikickback Statute (Tamborlane, 1993).

Antitrust Issues

Integrated delivery systems, whether horizontal, vertical, or conglomerate, are business relationships that can easily cause antitrust violations if not carefully negotiated. Horizontal integration involves similar businesses that may be direct economic competitors. Vertical integration involves businesses that may be economically related but are not direct competitors. Conglomerate integration involves businesses that produce unrelated products or services. Price fixing, division of markets, exclusive contracts, and noncompete agreements are the common violations that need to be addressed before contracting (Dacso & Dasco, 1996).

Liability Issues

Major liability exposure issues in managed care are related to malpractice and professional liability, contract liability, and bad faith claims. Managed care organizations can be held liable under independent corporate liability theory for failure to credential and monitor providers appropriately or for utilization review processes. To minimize risk the MCO should have a comprehensive risk management and quality management system with ongoing review of clinical competence for providers (Dacso & Dasco, 1996).

Reducing Risk for Antikickback and Antireferral Laws

In developing an integrated delivery system it is advisable to consider the following suggestions:

* Choose advisors carefully—use qualified health care attorneys and consulting experts.
* Recognize trouble spots in advance—ask whether there is a conflict of interest or an inducement for future referrals.
* Don't overvalue goodwill—use a reputable third-party valuation expert to document value.

- Check out the billing arrangement in advance to avoid assuming any false claims liability.
- Scrutinize intragroup referrals for medical and ancillary services—ask whether they meet necessary Stark II amendments.
- Observe caution when upcoding—upcoding can be another source of false claims by using a code that is more remunerative than necessary.
- Be aware of the safe harbors—there are no loopholes.
- Avoid anything that looks like a kickback—any financial relationship with a hospital may be suspect (Gosfield, 1994).

State Regulation of Managed Care

Each state manages the regulation of health insurance and managed care plans, even though each differs in its approach. AMCRA, in its "1995 State Managed Care Legislative Resource," has issued a state-by-state breakdown of any willing provider (AWP), UR, Medicaid, Managed Care, HMO, PPO, and TPA laws and regulations.

THE FUTURE OF MANAGED CARE

The next 10 years are being described as the era of the megaprovider. Managed care companies will continue to merge, acquire, and evolve into an even larger entity; however, futurists predict that the system as we know it today will not look the same. Because of the downward price pressures the larger organizations will benefit from economies of scale. Large insurers will move away from their origin of underwriting risk and paying claims and into the business of direct health care delivery. This strategy positions behavioral MCOs to be required to integrate into their parent company health care plan and carve back in, possibly eliminating their own structure in the process (Freeman & Trabin, 1994). The 1996 Mental Health Parity amendment has been proposed to provide mental health coverage in parity with physical health coverage; as good as this major change

could be, however, it is still being much debated and is not yet through Congress.

Somatization and medicalization of problems is one of the most costly services for managed care. The concept of medical-cost offset programs will become more involved in treatment and outcomes research. It has been noted that if treating concomitant behavioral health problems along with physical problems the cost offset in medical dollars spent will be significant (Barsky & Borus, 1995).

Community consortiums, direct employer-provider contracting, telephone counseling and treatment, and telephonic monitoring are just a few of the newest trends on the horizon (Meyer, 1996). One potential future scenario is that HMOs will evolve into organizations that control the health care system's information infrastructure, and whoever controls information technology will control care. To control care it will be necessary to coordinate elements of care, conduct population-based risk analysis, provide information for clinical decisions, and provide information for financial functions such as billing, collections, and funds distribution (Solovy, 1996). HMOs could develop the systems and then lease them back to the providers.

Hospital systems potentially could be the casualties of the managed care revolution, unless they recognize the strategy needed to survive. If hospital systems can teach employers about purchasing health care services based on the quality that hospitals can prove they provide, as opposed to MCOs' not being able to prove they can provide, then employers might be more willing to contract directly with providers. The strategic advantage will go to the hospital, as long as the public perceives that managed care companies are not able to provide quality care. If MCOs continue to implement global, restrictive utilization controls and to control costs, the consumer and the employer will consider other strategies and advantages proposed by the hospitals through direct contracting (Solovy, 1996).

Managing the future effectively will be possible by understanding some basic principles.

- Continuing the old ways will not help prepare for the future.
- It is necessary to create the future rather than defend the present.
- Change happens quickly.
- Clinical decision making must remain in the hands of properly trained and experienced clinicians.
- Effective care costs less than ineffective care.

- Liability for adverse outcomes must be shared by all levels involved in care.
- Means must be provided for research and education to ensure the future of health care.
- Professionals will need to collaborate and cooperate for health care reform and public trust (Sederer & Bennett, 1996).

REFERENCES

Appleby, C. (1996). Ethics and managed care. *Hospitals & Health Networks, 70*(13), 20–27.

Baldor, R.A. (1996). *Managed care made simple* (pp. 2–22, 30–32). Cambridge, MA: Blackwell.

Barsky, A.J., & Borus, J.F. (1995). Somatization and medicalization in the era of managed care. *Journal of the American Medical Association, 274,* 1931–1934.

Caldwell, B. (1995). Employer alliances, direct contracting, physician networks new forces in managed care. *Employee Benefit Plan Review, 49*(8), 20–22.

Changing landscape of healthcare. (1996, March/April). *PSC Healthcare Consultant III,* 1–2.

Cherney, A. (1995, Sept.). *Managed care strategies presentation.* Walnut Creek, CA: Western Medical Services.

Dacso, S.T., & Dasco, C.C. (1996). *Managed care answer book: 1996 Supplement.* Gaithersburg, MD: Aspen.

Freeman, M.A., & Trabin, T. (1994). *Managed behavioral healthcare: History, models, key issues, and future course* (pp. 9–17). Washington, DC: U.S. Dept. of Health & Human Services and U.S. Center for Mental Health Services.

Good strategic plans will guide you to success in managed care market. (1995). *Managed Home Care Report, 2*(5), 2–3.

Gosfield, A. (1994). Ignorance isn't bliss: Don't ignore these fraud and abuse dangers in integrated networks. *Physician's Management, 34*(2), 21–31.

Meyer, H. (1996). The tide of times. *Hospitals & Health Networks, 70*(8), 34–40.

Sederer, L.I., & Bennett, M.J. (1996). Managed mental health care in the United States: A status report. *Administration and Policy in Mental Health, 23*(4), 289–305.

Solovy, A. (1996, April). Backlash to the future: Is an HMO and HMO an HMO? *Hospitals & Health Networks, 70,* 42–48.

Tamborlane, T.A. (1993, June). Managed care: New legal challenges. *Caring,* 62–65.

CHAPTER 45

Working with Managed Care Networks: Strategies for Success

Marilyn D. Harris and Sharon A. Lynch

Providing home care services to clients who are enrolled with managed care health insurance companies creates unique issues and challenges for both clinical and administrative staff of home care agencies. Clinical issues are related to understanding what managed care is and how it affects the way home care staff must adapt to provide reimbursable services to clients. Improved verbal and written communication between the payer case manager (PCM) and the home care case manager (HCCM) is the key to a successful collaborative relationship.

Administrative issues deal with both cost and quality of patient care. Acceptable reimbursement methods must be negotiated. A data collection and evaluation system must be in place to track, measure, and report patient outcomes. Agency administrators must be able to sort the available data to meet the needs of the home care agency's administrative staff and to respond to requests of third-party payers for enrollee-specific outcomes.

MANAGED CARE VERSUS CASE MANAGEMENT

Although the terms are frequently used interchangeably, case management is not the same thing as managed care:

Managed care is a system of cost-containment programs; case management is a process. A global term, managed care consists of the systems and mechanisms utilized to control, direct, and approve access to the wide range of services and costs within the health care delivery system. Case management can be one of those mechanisms, one component in the managed care strategy. (Millahy, 1995, p. 5)

Managed care is designed to enhance cost-effectiveness by eliminating inappropriate service (Billows, 1994). The level of reimbursement for a client is set prospectively sometimes to the financial liability of the provider home care agency. Examples of reimbursement methods include capitation, discounted charges, per diem, and case rates. "This is what is meant by the 'provider at risk' terminology commonly associated with discussions of managed care" (Cline, 1990, p. 15).

True case management is the coordination of resources to meet the needs of the client, and it is the responsibility of health care providers to ensure that these needs are met (Faherty, 1990). To the providers of home care, case management has always been a part of the total nursing

Source: Reprinted from M. Harris and S.A. Lynch, Working with Managed Care Networks: Strategies for Success, in D.L. Flarey and S.S. Blancett, (Eds.), *Handbook of Nursing Case Management,* pp. 348–361, © 1996, Aspen Publishers, Inc.

process: assessment, planning, implementation, revising, and evaluation. With health care reform, home care is emerging as the primary site for the most cost-effective delivery system of health care. This positions the family system as the focal point for delivering health care (Sampson, 1994). Much family education will need to be done by the HCCM to make this alternate site of care a reality. Education can help clients and families change to more positive health behaviors and lifestyles.

At any given point during the client's transition through the health care system, more than one case manager (CM) might be involved, for example, the PCM and the HCCM. Each CM's different perspective can be a source for conflict. An alliance between providers of care and payers needs to evolve with the common goals of strengthening and supporting the family unit and using community resources (Wolfe, 1993).

The PCM typically wants quality patient care but with financial restraint. The role of the PCM is to assist clients in obtaining services in the most cost-effective manner. The HCCM wants quality patient care; cost is secondary. The conflict occurs as a result of each one's different perspective. Perspectives of different CMs vary, but their functions within the process are similar. The challenge is to balance client advocacy and quality with appropriate resource allocation (Sampson, 1994).

There are two different types of case management in home care: clinical (HCCM) and fiscal (PCM). To understand managed care from the vantage point of both the PCM and the HCCM, one of the authors interviewed a nurse who left her home health agency to work as a PCM in a managed care company. After a few weeks, this nurse resigned her position with the managed care company and returned to her former staff nurse position with a home health agency. The following is an excerpt from that interview:

I left my position in home care in search of another challenge. At that time, I believed that case management

in a managed care company would enable me to help patients by giving me the authority to institute care and services, assisting home care nurses in decision-making, and overseeing total patient care. As I experienced case management, I realized that I missed patient contact. I felt distant from the aspect of home care that I enjoyed the most, total patient care. I was not prepared for the attitudes that prevailed with reference to cost control. As a case manager, I dealt only with numbers. I had only basic knowledge of the patient and at times had to interrogate the client's nurses to gain more knowledge of the patient. I guess, due to my home care background, I wanted to know too much, which became time-consuming. I resented doing cost reports each week to show how much money was saved caring for the patients at home as opposed to being in the hospital. At the time, I didn't see the relevancy in this with reference to quality care. In many cases, indifference prevailed among staff of the managed care company. I missed being with the patients and the coordination of care required of the clinician. In my experience, managed care case managers dealt with numbers, not patients. Cost seemed too often more important than quality. It didn't take long to realize that I could not continue in the position of PCM.

This nurse's experience can be summarized as follows: "Managed care as used by insurance companies and increasingly by the federal government, reduced to its simplest form, is finding an excuse not to pay or to delay in making payments. What this means in simple terms is that dollars are becoming more important than people" (Halamandaris, 1990, p. 52).

ADVANTAGES AND DISADVANTAGES OF CONTRACTING WITH MANAGED CARE COMPANIES

In home health care there are advantages and disadvantages associated with contracting with managed care companies that are identified by the administrative, supervisory, business, and visiting nurse staff.

Advantages

- Payment is known in advance.
- There are service limits on clients who demand more service than is required.
- There are established contracts for servicing clients.
- Cost-efficient health care is provided.

Disadvantages

- The PCM may not authorize payment for needed services as assessed by the HCCM.
- Physicians may not order what the PCM has authorized.
- Increased staff time is required for multiple telephone calls to the PCM.
- Increased documentation is required of each PCM (no standardization of what is needed; each payer is different).
- Increased supervisory time is required to appeal denials of care when client referrals are received from hospital discharge planning nurses or social workers without pre-authorization by the PCM.
- There is duplication of PCM and HCCM duties (e.g., telephone calls to the physician).
- Increased time is needed to educate staff related to each payer's specific requirements. Some insurance payers require pre-certification and provide specific authorization numbers prior to the first visits. Other payers want a telephone call after the first visit, at which time visits are authorized for the first 2 weeks. Telephone reauthorizations every 2 weeks or once a

month are required for approval of continued service. Some payers do not require precertification authorization numbers.
- Increased time is associated with the billing process when supplemental materials such as copies of the chart must be submitted with bills.
- There are different coverages related to supplies (e.g., supplies may be billed separately, included as part of visit cost, or supplied by the managed care company).
- There are ethical issues related to balancing cost-containment versus patient advocacy.

In addition to all that the HCCM needs to remember in the care of the client, the HCCM now has to add insurance rules and related paperwork for payment to the body of knowledge. Since there are so many types of payers (state, private, preferred provider organizations [PPOs], health maintenance organizations [HMOs]) and each has its own rules, and possibly its own forms, it is almost impossible to know and remember all of this information without constant cues.

At the Visiting Nurse Association of Eastern Montgomery County, a department of Abington Memorial Hospital (VNA), there is an insurance advisor in the business office who helps clarify what the professionals need to complete in order for the VNA to be reimbursed for services provided. Staff education related to payment sources begins with the orientation of new employees and continues with ongoing staff development programs. Formal sessions as well as verbal and written memoranda are used to share current information with all staff.

ROLE OF THE HOME CARE CLINICAL CARE MANAGER VERSUS PAYER CASE MANAGER

The challenge for HCCMs is to make sure that they have a collaborative, not an adversarial, working relationship with the PCM (Wolfe, 1993). The most effective working relationship is one in which both parties focus on the health care needs of the client. This requires accurate assessments by both case managers of medical/nursing needs and the patient's personal needs and desires. The HCCM has essentially seven functions:

1. assessment
2. planning care to be provided
3. coordination: interdisciplinary and inter-agency/intraagency coordination
4. organizing and staffing
5. resource allocation
6. implementation of the plan of care
7. evaluation: quality assurance measures to ensure that standards of care are met.

The PCM has five functions that are different from those of the HCCM:

1. assess eligibility
2. validate plan of care presented
3. coordinate benefits if two or more payers
4. define payment system
5. conduct program evaluations and provider audits (Billows, 1994, p. 412).

STRATEGIES FOR CULTIVATING A SUCCESSFUL RELATIONSHIP

Negotiating for patient care is one important strategy. "Home care interests (providers) must be on the alert and demand that all home care services be delivered in conformance with the highest quality standards by licensed agencies through trained and supervised personnel" (Halamandaris, 1993, p. 6). It is difficult for case managers to be cooperative and competitive at the same time. There are two basic types of negotiation: cooperative (everybody wins) and competitive (only one wins). There are three criteria for negotiation to occur, as follows:

1. The issue must be negotiable.
2. Negotiators must be interested in both taking and giving.

3. Negotiating parties must trust each other, as both have needs to be met (Smeltzer, 1994).

The PCM and the HCCM need to be proficient in negotiation skills for the good of the patient. Following are some questions to determine the success of your negotiations (Smeltzer, 1994):

- Is the progress worthwhile for both parties?
- Do both parties feel that self-respect was maintained?
- Did both parties leave with positive feelings?
- Were both parties sensitive to the needs of the other during the process?
- Did both parties achieve the majority of their objectives?
- Would either party be willing to negotiate again with the other?

One can imagine how disastrous it would be for patient care if one of the parties did not want to talk with the other again because of negotiation problems. Home care agencies could lose a contract if their HCCMs were rude or unreasonable. Thus, skillful, professional communication is necessary, along with accurate documentation, for the ultimate benefit of both the client and agency.

Verbal communication is a second strategy for success. Administration had initial communication that resulted in your home health agency's meeting the criteria for participation in the plan. From an administrator's vantage point, this new or continuing relationship must be cultivated and nurtured on an ongoing basis. Frequent one-on-one communication with the PCM is not only required but essential. It can also be time consuming and stressful. The administrator must work with the HCCM and the PCM to develop mutually beneficial communication patterns. There are many demands on the time of both the PCM and the HCCM in providing care to the patient. In many instances, the patient's primary nurse/HCCM is the best person to have this communication.

At the VNA, the HCCMs have the primary responsibility of managing all clients' care in the assigned caseload. Administration prefers to have the HCCMs call the PCMs to give clinical reports, since the HCCMs are the nurses who have seen the patients in the home. They can give accurate clinical and home environment information that provides a clear picture and could affect the care at home. Frequently, family and a safe environment play a large role in whether a patient can be maintained at home. The HCCM who saw the patient is in the best position to answer questions posed by the PCM. The HCCM in the home is literally the "eyes and ears" for the physician and the PCM. For example, one plan has prearranged times when the PCM calls the VNA office. This schedule is known to the staff. All HCCMs who need to talk to that PCM that day inform the receptionist so that each HCCM can be paged when his or her turn comes to present patient updates. The VNA nurses do not sit and wait for numerous busy signals, nor does the PCM play telephone tag with the VNA staff. Although voice mail messages are authorized in some circumstances and do have a role in communication, there is no substitute for personal contact with the patient's PCM.

At the VNA, the HCCMs get to know the different PCMs. We make available lists of names and telephone numbers of certain PCMs, obtained from the payer companies. Supervisors distribute, or have a book of, frequently used names and numbers at each nurse's workstation. When a new PCM is responsible for clients, that information is added to the current list. Some PCMs also call when a new PCM takes over existing cases to provide for continuity of care.

The HCCM needs to be aware of the limited resources imposed by the managed care payer to plan within those boundaries. The home care supervisor gets involved only when there is a problem between the HCCM and the PCM. For example, if the HCCM and the supervisor determine that a client needs more care at home than

the PCM will approve, an appeal can be made to the medical director of the PCM, if necessary. This often requires the patient's physician to write letters of medical necessity to justify the care. The Joint Commission on Accreditation of Healthcare Organizations (Joint Commission) addresses such conflicts as follows:

> At times, indications for ongoing care may run contrary to the recommendations of an external entity performing utilization review (for example, peer review organizations, insurance companies, managed care reviewers). If such a conflict arises, care, services, or discharge (including transfer) decisions must be made in response to the care required by the patient, and not solely in response to the recommendation made by the external agency. Home health agency administrators and staff must be aware that accreditation standards require that a process exists and is implemented for resolving internal and external denial issues, when appropriate, to meet ongoing care and/or discharge (including transfer) needs of the patient. (Joint Commission, 1996, Sect. CC.6, p. 264)

Written documentation of the verbal process of informing the patient of changes in the plan of care, and obtaining the patient's consent to the plan, must be included in the clinical record.

As part of the communication network, it is important to keep the payers informed of the types of computer linkages currently available or planned for the future. In this time of instant communication and need for up-to-date patient and billing information, discussions should be ongoing to determine the compatibilities between the automated systems used by the home health agency and those used by the managed care company. Some home health agencies have installed a computer terminal in the managed care company's office that provides "view-only" access to the plan subscriber's patient care information. Current patient data and visit statistics can be retrieved at the convenience of the PCM. All home health agencies need to strive to meet the computer-age need for instant information.

Written communication is the third strategy for success. Verbal communications must be supplemented with written documentation that is readily available to the clinical and billing personnel. At the VNA, a standardized form, the Service Authorization Progress Note (Exhibit 45–1), is used to document contacts with the PCMs. This form records the patient's name, identification number, and designated PCM. Authorized services are listed with visit frequency, duration, and total visits. Space is provided for authorization codes, if needed. If there are denials of payment for bills, the supervisor can use this form to substantiate that a certain number of visits was approved, by whom, and on what date. Often, the PCM will adjust the payer's records and pay the bill if the error was on the part of the PCM. Without this type of documentation, the home health agency has no grounds to substantiate that telephone approvals were obtained.

Clinical documentation in the form of clinical notes and medical orders is contained in the patients' records. These essential written communications among the PCM, the HCCM, and the physician are readily available to meet myriad standards such as professional, legal, agency, certification, and accreditation.

QUALITY ASSESSMENT/ PERFORMANCE IMPROVEMENT ISSUES

The National Committee for Quality Assurance (NCQA), located in Washington, D.C., evaluates health plans' internal quality processes through accreditation reviews and develops measures to gauge health plan performance. Quality improvement, physician credentialing, member rights and responsibilities, utilization management, and medical records are evaluated for each plan. Plans may receive full, 1-year, or

provisional accreditation (Hospital Association of Pennsylvania, 1995). This same reference listed the status of Pennsylvania HMOs as of January 31, 1995: "Managed care plans are eager to develop comparable data because they increasingly see quality of care as a sales tool. Employers want quality data for use in choosing plans. Those that offer more than one plan also want employees to be able to compare them before choosing one" (Knox, 1995, p. 5). The value that is placed on the public release of this type of status report is evident from an article that describes a Florida HMO lawsuit to block release of a negative report (Bell, 1995).

As one aspect of attaining and maintaining an individual plan's accreditation, a plan may require a home health agency with which it contracts to submit to one or more of the relevant reviews mentioned above. It is important that a home health agency have and be able to sort its internal quality outcome data as related to patients who subscribe to a specific plan in order to report back to that plan. For example: one plan that contracts with the VNA requests that the VNA submit the results of its quality assessment (QA)/performance improvement (PI) reports for patient satisfaction for the subscribers of the plan as compared with the agency's patient satisfaction report for its total population (Figure 45–1). The plan also carries out its own patient satisfaction survey. Another plan sends a representative to the agency, where selected records of the plan's subscribers are pulled on site and reviewed to determine that standards of care are met. A written summary report is sent to the VNA director following the site visit that compares the VNA results with the standards established by the plan and the average for all other agencies.

It is imperative that the home health agency administration and staff have the written standards that the managed care company uses in reviewing utilization and quality of care. These standards need to be incorporated into the home health agency's policies, procedures, and QA/PI plan. It is not adequate, however, to be paper compliant. These standards, and expectations

Exhibit 45–1 Service Authorization Progress Note

Patient #: _____ Patient Name: _____

Telephone call to: _____ at _____

Insurance Co. Name _____

Contact Person _____

Services	Frequency and Duration	# of visits	From – Thru Dates	Authorization #	MA Alpha Modifier

Treatment Plan: _____ Initial POT _____ Interim Update _____ Recertification _____ Service Addition or Modification

Call for additional approval on: _____

Comments: _____

Signature: _____ Date: _____

White copy—Patient Chart   Pink Copy—Business Office   sapn.wk3

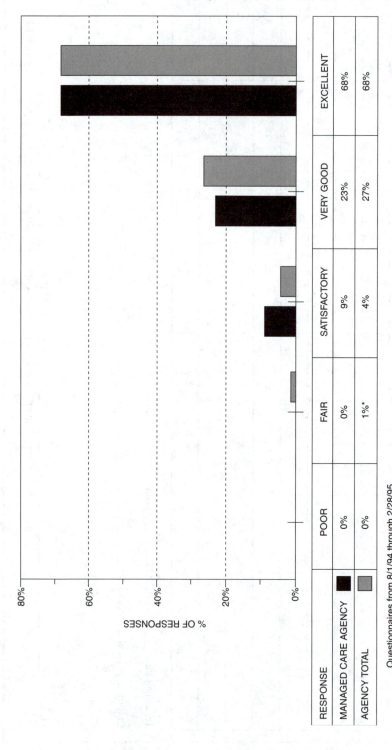

RESPONSE	POOR	FAIR	SATISFACTORY	VERY GOOD	EXCELLENT
MANAGED CARE AGENCY	0%	0%	9%	23%	68%
AGENCY TOTAL	0%	1%*	4%	27%	68%

Questionnaires from 8/1/94 through 2/28/95

* = One patient indicated that the patient wanted additional service (homemaker) not covered by third-party payer.

Figure 45–1 VNA Home Care: Discharge Patient Satisfaction Questionnaire

that they will be met, need to be communicated to the staff. Specific requirements of each plan are shared with staff by the supervisors in formal conferences and inservice programs. The sharing of new and supplemental information is accomplished through written and verbal memoranda from administration and clinical supervisors. When requirements are included that the administrative staff know are not currently met (e.g., cardiopulmonary resuscitation for all staff and contracted home health aides) or will not be met based on current practice, the administrator must communicate these concerns to the contract manager so that contract-related issues can be addressed and resolved before they become a noncompliance issue. From our experience, the representatives from the plans have been willing to discuss specific issues or requirements and make revisions when there is candid communication and rationales are expressed.

A home health agency must have systems in place to identify, collect, track, analyze, and present information on the outcomes of patient care for the patients they serve. One reason is to share this information with the managed care company. Another reason is to compare the agency's data with published national data based on studies that compare fee-for-service patient outcomes with patient outcomes for HMOs and other managed care plans (Shaughnessey & Schlenker, 1992).

Only 21% of 314 home care executives who responded to an informal poll stated they used a management information system (MIS) to calculate outcomes for either Medicare or private insurers (Rak, 1995). A manual or computerized MIS is essential for a home health agency administrator who is interested in survival in the age of managed care. This is necessary to identify patient outcomes by myriad methods, including payer source, disease categories, and costs.

Quality standards also need to address the qualifications of the home care staff. This is extremely important when new services are added to the agency. Information must be communicated to the managed care company's

PCM and the person responsible for modifications or additions to the existing contract to make them aware of new patient care programs and services and assure them that staff meet professional licensure and/or certification standards. It is important to both provision of care and payment for the services rendered. Most times, the contract, or addendum, must identify the covered disciplines prior to billing.

Accept opportunities to participate on a professional advisory committee (PAC) or clinical committees that enable the agency's representative to have input into the plan's QA/PI process. The home care administrator, although often the person to whom the invitation is extended, may not be the appropriate person to serve on these committees. Another member of the administrative team, possibly the director of professional services or director of QA/PI, may be more familiar with the clinical operations and may provide the needed input and expertise on a committee.

The role of advocate is another administrative responsibility. This includes being an advocate for quality patient care for individuals who do not know what services they are being denied. Staff also need an advocate as they seek to provide quality patient care while meeting the home care agency's expectations. Therefore, establishing smooth working relations that are efficient and effective will convey administration's commitment. Sometimes this may mean running interference by scheduling a face-to-face meeting with personnel from the managed care company.

Home care administrators also need to be aware of the many opportunities to be on the cutting edge of technology. This includes availability to monitor a patient's status via computerization, for example, daily checkups of expectant mothers with high-risk pregnancies and other electronic "visits" in the home (Joyce, 1994; Mahmud & LeSage, 1995). Administrators must also be aware of special clinical programs that are promoted by insurers (e.g., cardiac care, asthma, back pain). Your home health agency may provide the same type of service under generic names such as skilled nursing or physical therapy. The managed care company needs to be aware of this information.

Current managed care enrollment represents less than 10% of the Medicare population (Cerne, 1995; Kertesz, 1995). According to a 1995 Health Care Financing Administration (HCFA) publication, the percentage of Medicaid enrollees in managed care plans has increased from 9.5% in 1991 to 23.2% in 1994 (American Hospital Association, 1995). A survey of 547 managed care organizations showed that a little more than 18% of the population of the United States is enrolled in HMOs (American Hospital Association, 1995). As of April 1995, 21% of the VNA's discharged Medicare patients' services were paid by a managed care plan. Twenty-nine percent of the VNA's total patients are currently enrolled in some managed care plan (Figure 45–2). In Pennsylvania, all individuals who are on a medical assistance program are covered by a managed care plan, either through the department of health or a private HMO. It is anticipated that the percentage of individuals who choose to enroll in managed care plans will continue to increase.

A recent article (Friend, 1995) states that

> HMOs want your nurses and therapists to show up on time and look presentable. They want you to respond to their calls for a nurse at 5 pm on a Friday. They want you to provide specialty home care services if you claim to be a full-service provider. And if you want to contract with them, managed care companies want you to fill out their forms completely, follow their rules, and not be an administrative nuisance for them. (pp. 1 and 2)

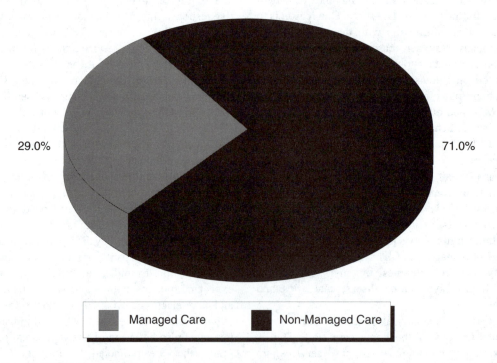

29.0%   71.0%

[ ] Managed Care   [ ] Non-Managed Care

Figure 45–2 VNA Homecare: Payer Type—April 1995

The article gives the following advice for a successful experience with a managed care company:

- Be professional.
- Be punctual.
- Be reputable.
- Be available.
- Complete the job in the fewest number of visits.
- Be your own utilization reviewer.
- Understand how HMOs work.
- Be persistent.
- Follow through on provider credentialing.
- Don't demand too much.
- Don't make waves.

In addition to these criteria, home health agency administrators and staff must be aware of the recently published home care and case management guidelines (Doyle, Pinney, & Spong, 1994). Previously published guidelines for inpatient and surgical care are widely used by case managers across the country. The new home care–oriented guidelines, published in June 1994, are for use with both commercial and Medicare populations, with straightforward cases. The issue of patients with multiple diagnoses is not addressed (Mann, 1995). These guidelines, which do not appear to be widely used as yet, could give home health agencies a preview of case managers' future expectations of home care services (Mann, 1995).

CONCLUSION

Home health care agencies are experiencing rapid changes in this era of health care and insurance reform and cost containment. Working with managed care companies brings new opportunities, challenges, and stress. The key is to be flexible, cooperative, and cost-effective while continuing to provide high-quality care to clients in their homes. Emphasis must be placed on administrative and clinical communications. Continuous QA/PI efforts must receive high priority with the goal of attaining positive outcomes for patients and families while at the same time keeping the home health agency financially viable. "How home care providers respond to the reforms and opportunities will determine the future fate of many agencies. Limited thinkers will be left behind" (Coleman & Algie, 1994, p. 36). These are the challenges of the 1990s as health care reform progresses into the twenty-first century.

POSTSCRIPT

As of January 1997, the VNA added an Insurance Liaison Nurse to the staff. This position was created to meet the requirements of several managed care companies. As of January 1997, the PCMs will not accept telephone calls from individual professionals. All communication is to be done through a contact person who will handle questions/authorizations for all patients rather than through the CHHM. The insurance liaison nurse is responsible for the insurance pre- and re-certification process for all skilled services. This nurse designs, implements, and coordinates the insurance approval process for patients of all ages.

REFERENCES

American Hospital Association. (1995). *AHA News, 32*(17), 2–8.

Bell, C. (Ed.) (1995). Florida HMO sues to block release of negative report. *Modern Healthcare, 25*(10), 56.

Billows, L.A. (1994). Case Management. In M.D. Harris (Ed.), *Handbook of Home Health Care Administration* (pp. 411–415). Gaithersburg, MD: Aspen.

Cerne, F. (1995). Rehabbing Medicare: Is managed care a cure-all or just a crutch? *Hospitals & Health Networks, 69*(8), 23–26.

Cline, B. (1990). Case management: Organizational models and administrative methods. *Caring, 9*(7), 14–18.

Coleman, J.R., & Algie, B.A. (1994). Health care reform: Reinventing health care provides new opportunities for ancillary and alternate site providers. *Remington Report, 8*(6), 36–39.

Doyle, R., Pinney, M., & Spong, F. (1994). *Healthcare management guidelines*, Vol. 4: *Home care and case management*. Radnor, PA: Milliman & Robertson.

Faherty, B. (1990). Case management: The latest buzzword: What it is, and what it isn't. *Caring, 9*(7), 20–22.

Friend, A. (1995, Febr. 13). Wake-up call for home care providers: Managed care decision-makers tell what they want and what they're willing to pay (special report). *Home Health Line.*

Halamandaris, V. (1990). Case management: Blessing or curse? *Caring, 9*(7), 50, 52.

Halamandaris, V. (1993). Cooperation in competition: E pluribus unum. *Caring, 12*(10), 4–6.

Hospital Association of Pennsylvania (1995). National accrediting agency evaluates Pennsylvania HMOs. *Pennsylvania Hospitals Nineties, 6*(8), 2.

Joint Commission on Accreditation of Health Care Organizations. (1996). *1997–1998 Accreditation manual for home care* (Sect. CC.6, p. 264) 1995. Oak Brook Terrace, IL: Author.

Joyce, M. (1994, Oct. 7–13). HMOs turn to home health firms to monitor patients. *Philadelphia Business Journal*, pp. 1, 13B.

Kertesz, L. (1995, April 3). Medicare: The final frontier for HMOs. *Modern Healthcare*, pp. 76–84.

Knox, A. (1995, Febr. 25). HMOs' quality of care reviewed. *Philadelphia Inquirer*, Sect. D, pp. 1, 5.

Mahmud, K., & LeSage, K. (1995). Telemedicine: A new idea for home care. *Caring, 14*(5), 48–50.

Mann, L. (1995). Milliman & Robertson home care management guidelines expect a lot from both nurses & patients. *Home Health Line, 20*(5), 4–7.

Millahy, C.M. (1995). *The case manager's handbook* (pp. 3–13). Gaithersburg, MD: Aspen.

Rak, K. (1995). Only 21% of home care companies track outcomes and costs electronically. *Home Health Line, 20*(5), 7.

Sampson, E. (1994). Offensive case management vs. defensive case management. *Pennington Report, 8*(6), 17–19.

Shaughnessey, P., & Schlenker, R. (1992). Medicare home health reimbursement alternatives: Access, quality and cost incentives. *Home Health Care Services Quarterly, 13*(1/2), 91–115.

Smeltzer, C.H. (1994). The art of negotiation: An everyday experience. In E. Hein & M. Nicholson (Eds.), *Contemporary leadership behavior* (pp. 351–356). Philadelphia: J.B. Lippincott.

Wolfe, G. (1993). Cooperation or competition? Collaboration between home care and case management. *Caring 12*(10), 52–60.

CHAPTER 46

Community-Based Long-Term Care: Preparing for a New Role

Emily Amerman and David M. Eisenberg

Directing health or social service organizations in an era of rampant change and heightened competition challenges managers' every waking moment. As government and private payers shift costs, tighten reimbursement, and experiment with prepayment and capitation, the truism that "form follows finance" is brought home anew. Reimbursement policy and economic incentives have a profound impact on the delivery of service by home health care providers and indeed by all providers. More than ever before, our vision of service delivery must not be limited by current regulatory parameters.

A tremendous demographic and cultural shift has been occurring, one that will have a major effect on home health care. The number and proportion of older Americans are increasing dramatically. The number of people older than age 75 years is expected to double between 1980 and the year 2010. By the year 2020, one in five people will be older than 75. People over the age of 75 are more likely than younger persons to experience chronic illnesses and other disabling conditions that interfere with their ability to function independently. They are more likely to be at risk of institutionalization in a nursing home or to be in need of ongoing health and social services. This surge in numbers of disabled older people, coupled with shortened acute care stays, means an increasing emphasis on long-term care. The demand for long-term

care services will compel policy makers and providers to respond. Ultimately, home health agencies will provide greater and greater proportions of service to patients with needs outside those currently defined as "skilled care."

The combination of increasing demand for long-term care and the interest by governments and private payers in substituting long-term home care for institutional care when clinically and economically feasible bodes well for home health agencies. The growth in demand for community-based long-term care will create both an opportunity and a challenge for home health agencies in the next decade. Since 1982, home health agencies in Philadelphia have had this opportunity. This chapter describes the Philadelphia model of community-based long-term care and the critical role home health providers play. To place the model in context, current trends in long-term care policy and program are outlined. In concluding, the chapter offers observations and recommendations that may assist home health administrators in planning and competing for involvement in community-based long-term care programs.

LONG-TERM CARE DEFINED

The original version of this chapter was first written 10 years ago, and not much about long-term care has changed since then. For decades, "long-term care" has referred to a place or a facility where chronically ill, old people are cared for until they die. The reality is that for every older person in an intermediate or skilled care facility, there are two people who look the same and who live in the community. Thus, approximately 5% of those over age 65 are in a nursing home at any one time; another 10% who need comparable levels of long-term care are at home. This is due to the fact that the largest provider of long-term care services is the American family. Studies continually demonstrate that about 80% of all long-term care is performed by family caregivers, despite myths to the contrary. Families are caring for a pool of highly impaired older people that creates ongoing, ever-increasing demand for long-term care.

More recent definitions of long-term care refer to a systematic plan of care provided over an indefinite time period to chronically ill, functionally disabled adults, most of whom are old. Since many older people have multiple health and social service needs, and since they may not remain medically stable, long-term care must cut across service delivery systems (health, mental health, aging) as well as across levels of care. Long-term care consumers may need acute care in a hospital, then restorative care, rehabilitation over an extended period, and then maintenance or custodial care. They may need institutional care or they may be cared for at home. Their *level of care* no longer automatically determines their *locus of care*. The goal of long-term care is to promote the highest level of independent functioning possible in the least restrictive setting while attending to the client's preferences and ensuring his or her safety.

CURRENT POLICY AND PROGRAM TRENDS

Despite the rapid increase in the number of persons needing long-term care and a high level of interest in community-based care, federal and state investment remains limited almost entirely to institutional care. Only a fraction of the Medicare and Medicaid budgets is spent on home care and almost none on long-term home care. At all times, there is a pool of highly impaired older people residing in the community that forms the basis of the ever-present demand for institutional care. Yet the current cost of institutional care is staggering. Some states spend as much as 10% of their entire state budget on institutional long-term care. As the very old population doubles in number, policy makers have a powerful incentive to develop a range of long-term care options that are less costly than nursing home care, or they will face doubling the current investment in institutional care.

The notion of community-based long-term care is not new. For the past 25 years, the Health Care Financing Administration (HCFA) has been experimenting with community-based long-term care for older people at risk of institutionalization. In the mid-1980s, the federal government financed a nationwide study of the viability of in-home long-term care called the National Long-term Care Channeling Demonstration. The HCFA continues to study the efficacy of health maintenance organizations (HMOs) with long-term care benefits added, called social health maintenance organizations. Several groups and at least one state are financing "continuing care without walls," in which participants receive in-home long-term care benefits to enable them to remain at home as long as possible and have access to nursing home care should such a need arise. A particularly innovative program, originally called On Lok after its San Francisco–based parent, is the Program for All-Inclusive Care for the Elderly (PACE). PACE offers the full spectrum of long-term and acute health care to nursing home–eligible elderly, operating under combined Medicaid and Medicare waivers from HCFA. Finally, Pennsylvania and other states have implemented nursing home diversion programs since the mid-1980s. In these programs, a subset of people applying for and identified as clinically eligible for nursing home care is given the option to remain at home, assisted by a case manager and provided with home health care and other services, at a cost to the state that is lower than the cost of a state-subsidized nursing home bed.

During the 1980s, half a dozen bills were introduced into the House and Senate proposing publicly financed long-term care programs encompassing in-home and nursing home care, but none was passed. In 1993 President Clinton introduced a sweeping health care reform plan that would ensure coverage for health care and, based on functional criteria, long-term care for all Americans. The plan, which failed to garner sufficient political support, proposed structural and financing changes that would make it possible for all uninsured people to receive basic health care, and it provided guidelines for long-term care reform. The model proposed by the President's Task Force was very much like the Philadelphia model of community-based long-term care. Both models suggested relying on case managers to develop and oversee individual care plans and the provision of benefits, which include personal care and other support services in addition to skilled nursing and rehabilitative care in the community.

Another significant development over the past decade is the proliferation and evolution of private long-term care insurance. There are now more then 100 policies on the market, most of which cover both institutional and in-home long-term care. As the insured come into benefit, they will need home health care and an array of other services. In the summer of 1996, the Health Insurance Reform Act, which makes long-term care expenses—including home health care—tax deductible, was passed by Congress and signed into law.

Nationwide, the majority of community-based long-term care programs rely on a model with two principal components: care management, which includes assessment, development of a plan of care, arranging for services, regular follow-up and monitoring of services, and periodic reassessment of the client's needs; and the provision of a range of concrete services that includes, among others, home health services, personal care and home management (home-

maker) services, heavy cleaning and minor home repairs, home-delivered meals, adult day care, transportation, emergency response systems, legal services, and help with daily money management. In recent years, support to caregivers in the form of caregiver assessment, education, training, peer support, and various kinds of respite is becoming an integral part of community-based long-term care programs, to bolster and preserve this silent, unpaid workforce.

Emerging from practical experience, and increasingly confirmed in the literature, is the fact that nurses and social workers are the two professional disciplines most appropriate to direct the provision of community-based long-term care. The interrelationships among medical history, current health status, functional capacity, cognitive status, emotional well-being, family relationships, and the physical environment are complex and demand the knowledge and skills of both nursing and social work. Nurses or social workers may be selected to provide care management; the best service delivery models use both.

THE AREA AGENCY ON AGING: A PARTNER IN SERVICE DELIVERY

Area Agencies on Aging (AAAs) were mandated by the Older Americans Act of 1965. Numbering more than 600, they form a nationwide network of planning and service agencies focused on the well-being of older citizens. Their major responsibilities include planning, advocacy, program development, and the prudent purchase of services. AAAs prepare an annual area plan delineating demographic trends, projected service needs, gaps in service, and priorities for program development and service delivery in their planning and service area. Each year, a fixed allocation of federal and state money, derived from several funding streams, is made to each AAA, with which the AAA is to carry out its plan. AAAs fund a wide array of services for older people, including senior center nutrition and recreation programs; health screening and promotion programs; and services to homebound people, such as home-delivered meals, homemaker services, and chore services. In their role as advocate for older people, AAAs often fund employment programs, legal services, and public education programs on issues relating to aging. AAAs also may host a nursing home ombudsman.

In their role as prudent purchaser, AAAs develop specific program standards and specifications for services. Because they are not usually direct service providers, they endeavor to create and encourage a climate of healthy competition among providers. Whenever feasible, AAAs select service providers on a competitive basis so that all potential providers in the service area have the opportunity to seek public funding to deliver services to AAA clients. Providers are selected on the basis of written proposals, price, in-person presentations, and other criteria. This process promotes a high quality of care and simultaneously keeps prices down.

With public resources both costly and scarce, states are becoming increasingly interested in the AAAs' capacity to serve as gatekeeper, conserving resources by ensuring that the most needy people are served and by using scarce and costly resources prudently. The AAA is viewed by policy makers as a logical choice for gatekeeper because of its ability to assess need and allocate resources without being affected by the economic incentives that drive the behavior of provider agencies. Provider agencies have incentives to prescribe their particular service and to prescribe it in amounts and ways that increase revenue but decrease burden and expense. AAAs, which are one step removed, are in a more objective position to determine client eligibility and to conserve public dollars. Organizations naturally view patients' needs in terms of the solutions they have most readily available, whether or not other approaches to care may be better. In the early days of the AAA network, AAAs commonly allocated blocks of funds to homemaker agencies, for example, and permitted those agencies to identify needy clients and prescribe service. AAAs found that providers tended to serve fewer clients with

larger blocks of hours of service than judged necessary. On the other hand, control of client assessment and care plan development by case managers employed by the AAA has led to an increase in the number of clients served, an increase in the choices of delivery patterns, and a reduction in average client cost.

AAAs, then, become the point of access to publicly financed service and, in the minds of some policy makers, are in a position to control that access consistent with larger policy goals. In some states, the AAA network is the basis for the expansion of publicly funded, community-based long-term care benefits. The Philadelphia model is an example of this role for AAAs.

THE PHILADELPHIA MODEL

The AAA for Philadelphia County is the Philadelphia Corporation for Aging (PCA). Since 1982, PCA has hosted a community-based long-term care program called Community Care Options (CCOs). The PCA receives state lottery funds to maintain a caseload of very frail adults in their own homes. To be eligible for CCOs, each client must be assessed by PCA's preadmission assessment program and judged to be eligible or near-eligible for nursing home care but able to be cared for at home. Care at home is feasible because of willing family caregivers and the availability of an enriched array of health and social service support through CCOs. CCOs provide care management as well as home health care, homemaker services, home-delivered meals, adult day care, chore service, mental health evaluation and treatment, transportation, respite care, and many other related services.

A PCA assessor, in consultation with other involved disciplines, does a global, multidimensional assessment of the client's medical history, current health, functioning, mental status, morale, environment, social supports, and resources (personal, social, and financial). A careful assessment of caregiving efforts by informal supports is included and reflected in the subsequently individually tailored care plan.

The case manager determines the type, amount, scope, duration, and pattern of delivery of the service to be provided. All care plans are discussed with the primary care physician. Case managers are vested with responsibility for orchestrating all services noted on the care plan and monitoring the client's overall care. Case managers periodically reassess the needs of their clients and caregivers, and monitor the performance of service providers.

Case managers purchase service on behalf of the clients on their caseload in accordance with the specific tasks and schedule in the care plan. Every day a client is on the active caseload, funds are encumbered with which to purchase services. Case managers can spend up to 45% of the daily medical assistance reimbursement rate for a nursing home bed. In 1996, this was about $40.00 daily. Funds are earned on a client-day basis but are controlled on a caseload basis. Case managers are responsible for maintaining their aggregate caseload cost at or below the 45% cap. They are permitted to shift funds between clients as long as the total caseload expenditure is below cap. This ability to treat clients differentially has a powerful effect on case manager behavior. Case managers allocate resources with caution, recognizing that preserving a cushion of dollars permits them to respond more fully if a client temporarily needs more intensive, and therefore costlier, service. Case managers have strong incentives both to serve and to conserve. They quickly become prudent purchasers of service on behalf of their clients and invariably keep their caseload expenditure level below the cap. This occurs despite the fact that some of their clients may be using resources temporarily at twice the level of the cap.

In addition to planning, authorizing, and orchestrating service delivery for clients, case managers perform functions historically associated with social casework. While they encourage and facilitate medical follow-up and compliance with health care regimens, they also counsel clients and families. They negotiate with them about caregiving tasks. They provide short-term, problem-oriented counseling. They arrange access to entitlements, housing, and protective and legal services when necessary. They serve as a general source of information and as a "one-stop shopping" resource for questions or problems facing clients and their families. Our analysis of their job responsibilities suggests strongly to us that social work is a necessary prerequisite for the job of case manager.

Care management staff of the CCOs now consist of 49 social workers organized in seven teams of seven. Given the number and complexity of health problems faced by our clients, nurses could also be an intelligent choice for case managers, but we selected the more generalist social workers for line staff, choosing to employ community health nurses at the supervisory level. Nursing expertise is critical and must be easily available. Each team of social workers has a social worker and a nursing supervisor. The nursing supervisors are responsible for adding nursing perspective to clinical decision making and to the overall program design and operation. They review assessments and make recommendations concerning individual client needs. They represent the goals and objectives of the program to providers and conduct orientation sessions for health subcontractors. They assist in development of contract specifications for health services and in monitoring the performance of health care providers. They identify training needs of case managers in the area of health care assessment and service delivery, and they provide or arrange training. The nurses essentially define the relationship between case managers and home health providers.

The provision of health and social services by multiple organizations usually involves end-to-end relationships, as when a discharging hospital refers for home health care and then home health care discharges to a social service agency, or parallel service delivery without collaboration, as when one agency provides counseling and another provides medical transportation. Interactive, collaborative relationships between different providers is atypical, but in the provision of long-term care it is a necessity.

Analysis of service utilization by clients of CCOs shows that the principal expenditure is for homemaker service. As would be expected, community-based long-term care clients need high levels of personal care (bathing, grooming, and toileting) and home support (shopping, cooking, and cleaning). At any time, about 95% of these clients are receiving homemaker service. The second most frequently used service is nursing care. Approximately three quarters of the clients are in receipt of nursing at any one time. All other directly controlled services are utilized at comparatively much lower rates. By far, the critical professional dyad is the social work case manager and the provider's home health nurse. Although all service providers must seek prior authorization from the case manager to initiate or change the delivery of service to a client, in the case of home health services, case managers exercise administrative authority over service provision while relying heavily on the clinical judgment of the nurse or other home health professional. Case managers rely on their subcontractor nurses for frequent updates on client condition and guidance on plans of care. The experience of reporting to case managers is a new one for home health nurses, but the level of conflict between staff of CCOs and home health subcontractors has been surprisingly low from the outset. Nurses sometimes find the need to get prior authorization to visit cumbersome, but case manager involvement has its benefits, too.

Several other aspects of the case manager and community health nurse collaboration should be highlighted. The capitated approach to financing care and the case manager control over spending creates cost consciousness among providers as well. In this model, home health professionals become sensitized to the economic consequences of providing service. For example, nurses who are aware of the cost of consumable medical supplies use them in a way that is different from that of their colleagues who are not attending to cost. Providers become conscious of the cost of the care they are giving and assist case managers in their efforts to be prudent, recognizing that unused resources are available for use when necessary later on. Another benefit is that when nurses identify client needs in the normal course of their duties that they or their agency are unable to meet, they can contact the case manager and immediately enlist a powerful ally in addressing those needs. Last, but no less important, providing ongoing care to long-term care clients is physically and emotionally exhausting. Home health nurses have the assurance that they are not solely responsible for the welfare of their patient; they can readily share their clinical and emotional burden with their case manager colleague. Joint home visiting, case conferencing, and peer support have strengthened service delivery in many difficult case situations.

BECOMING A LONG-TERM CARE PROVIDER: OBSERVATIONS AND RECOMMENDATIONS

Since 1977, PCA has been selecting providers, by using a competitive bidding process. The PCA has been competitively selecting home health providers since 1982, at first annually and more recently every 3 years, with annual performance audits and price negotiations. The PCA has received proposals from many home health agencies, has experienced a wide range of provider behavior, and has worked closely with a dozen different home health subcontractors. The selection process used by the PCA includes a written proposal, an oral presentation, submission of references, and a weighted list of criteria by which judgments are made that result in the selection decision. With the tightening of budgets, price has become an increasing concern. Selection decisions revolve around factors such as demonstrated experience in home health care delivery, history and reputation of the agency, current patient census (Medicare and others), past performance, conceptual understanding of the long-term care program and the special characteristics of service delivery in long-term care, the longevity and experience of nursing and rehabilitation staff, and responsiveness as a prospective subcontractor.

The differences between long-term care and skilled care are important to understand before entering into a contract. Long-term care is different from skilled care in several significant ways. Rather than a focus on diagnosis and treatment of medical problems, long-term care assumes one or more chronic conditions and a degree of permanent (if not progressive) disability. Long-term care is therefore principally concerned with functioning and the way a person lives and operates within his or her environment. Ideally, long-term care services create a prosthetic environment within which a functionally disabled person can live as independently as possible. A second difference between long-term care and skilled care is apparent when analyzing the tasks involved in the care. Eighty percent to 90% of long-term care in nursing homes, for example, is either personal care or tasks such as laundry and housekeeping, provided by paraprofessionals. The role of the physician points to a third difference. For most people receiving long-term care, daily oversight by a physician is unnecessary. What is needed is organization, coordination, and supervision of paraprofessional caregivers by health and social service professionals. *Physicians are critical to the provision of long-term care but are not central.*

A final difference between long-term care and skilled care that must be clearly understood is the nature of the clinical problems presented and the characteristics of the clients served. Although we have clients ranging in age from 18 to 103, the vast majority are older than 80. Although many need skilled care intermittently, such as expert wound care, incontinence evaluation and training, infusion therapies, or medication teaching, often the number of visits they are allowed by the insurer is very limited. About 20% of the nursing care provided is custodial; the care manager can authorize continued nursing visits to monitor skin integrity, ensure proper medication administration, support families with tube feedings and other tech-

nical caregiving tasks, and ensure that small functional gains are maintained. Some professionals, by focus or personality, prefer to tackle reversible or unambiguous problems. Most long-term care clients suffer from multiple chronic conditions or impairments. At a minimum, the professionals who serve them must be able to tolerate ambiguity, comparatively small gains, and the eventual decline of most of their patients. Professionals do best who are mature, thrive on complex problems, appreciate small signs of progress, and enjoy extended relationships with their patients. Home health agencies serving long-term care patients will need to take this into account as they select and train personnel.

Good agencies are rightfully proud of their track record, and past performance is an important ingredient in selection. To the extent that becoming a subcontractor, providing long-term care, or interacting closely with a care management entity are new experiences, past performance does not take the place of a well-informed commitment to the new program by the bidding home health agency. Prospective bidders should be sure that they understand what is being asked for and that their agency is committed to the new program requirements and whatever adjustments will need to be made. We have had contact with agencies that wish to generate additional revenue as a subcontractor but steadfastly refuse to consider different ways of operating from their tried and true traditional approaches. Such organizations may provide high-quality care but they make unsuitable partners in a new enterprise. The relationship invariably ends up conflictual and frustrating for all parties.

At the other end of the same continuum are organizations that have developed as temporary staffing agencies. Typically proprietary, they have a comparatively less developed vision of good service and agency mission as a community caregiver. They often present a posture that communicates, "We will be happy to serve you in any way you require, as long as you pay us." The motivation of these organizations is clear and their flexibility is appreciated, but their apparent lack of internal performance standards shakes our confidence.

New financing arrangements, combined with the special nature of long-term care patients' needs, are propelling home health agencies into highly interactive relationships with gatekeepers and other providers. This too requires a conscious commitment and careful orchestration of effort to achieve success. In the Philadelphia model, it is the AAA that identifies eligible clients, assesses them for service need, develops the care plan, and then arranges for the provision of home health care as part of a larger care plan, which the AAA controls. When long-term care benefits are financed by payers such as long-term care insurers or Medicare-risk HMOs with expanded care benefits, a similar gatekeeping and allocation function is likely to exist outside the home health provider. Many home health agencies are gaining experience in contracting with HMOs to serve enrollees in their Medicare risk plans. As such, participating home health agencies have two clients when before they only had one. They must serve their patients but also serve the needs of the organization that has overall care management responsibility. Thus concomitant with the development of this new long-term care market, there may be a diminishing of previously enjoyed autonomy on the part of the home health provider.

Two questions for agencies contemplating the provision of long-term care are: Will they be able to grasp the complexities of the new enterprise and perform the clinically and administratively challenging tasks required? Will they strike an adequate balance between dedication to an agency mission and performance and productivity standards and a position of flexibility and openness to new ideas and program requirements? In our experience in working with agencies of very different identities—voluntary, religious, and proprietary—that balance has been struck successfully.

PART VI

Financial Issues

CHAPTER 47

Understanding the Exposures of Home Health Care: An Insurance Primer

Brian M. Block

You have reached this chapter in one of three ways. Either you have read directly through the book to get to this point, you have read a bit and then skipped around, or you have turned directly here. It all really depends on your interest. In any event, there is an essential need for those that administer or manage home health care organizations to protect the present and future financial security of their businesses.

Those who have been in the field for any length of time know the home health care organizations that have failed. Some of the failures include organizations with poor fiscal and reimbursement planning, lack of accreditation, and poor human resource practices; organizations that are too narrowly defined in scope and wind up working with too few referral sources or are too focused on one patient type (which becomes extinct in the reimbursement community); and those that do not cooperatively work with the continuum of other services and organizations necessary for the comprehensive care of their patient cohorts. Each of these examples of failure, as well as many others, unfortunately and typically represents a slow occurrence that takes place over years of struggling to continue to provide essential clinical services.

The insurance question that must be asked is, What are the risks inherent in doing business as a home health care organization? Even if the myriad of reasons for failure that are implied above are planned for, monitored, and controlled, negligence on behalf of the professional

home health care staff can, in a very short time, create a decline in the public and professional community's opinion of the organization and can precipitate a financial disaster that will probably force the organization to close its doors.

A home health care organization must transfer and then actively control its risk of loss. Insurance provides for security from unforeseen events that cannot be controlled by other means. Insurance is necessary to protect an organization from a loss or losses that cannot be afforded. From any perspective, risk management involves a group of active techniques that evaluates and monitors an organization's exposures—the possible events, property, or behaviors that can cause a loss. These activities are integral to the home health care organization's strategic plan, which will then control the probability of a loss actually occurring.

The goal of this chapter is to introduce the reader to the basic principles of insurance and the types of coverages that are available, to describe what exposures are present in home health care, and to discuss some techniques for risk management.

TYPES OF INSURANCE

Insurance is the transfer of pure risk from one party to another for a price through a legal contract that spells out the terms, the perils covered, and the property excluded. Insurable risk is defined as the uncertainty of loss, the chance of loss, or the probability of loss.

565

Certain factors and/or conditions must be present for insurance. These include an insurable interest, the ability to predict losses, the ability to predict the monetary value of the losses, and a certainty that the losses are accidental or unplanned. In addition, to meet these criteria for home health care organizations, any insurance company or carrier must have enough experience with the home health care industry.

Insurable interest is based on the principle of indemnity, that is, placing the insured in the same financial position following a loss that existed before the loss occurred. The insurable interest is usually the financial stake in the property or casualty to be covered.

Experience with the industry would include a sufficiently large number of insured organizations so that the law of large numbers would apply. These home health care organizations should be similar in operation, exposures, and losses so that the type, scope, and monetary value of losses can be anticipated and trended by insurance industry monitors.

Losses must be unplanned or accidental; organizations must not cause losses to occur. Furthermore carriers recognize that the probability of most losses can be lowered through an active program of risk management. Home health care organizations are responsible for minimizing their exposures and for complying with the standards of local, state, and federal regulatory and accrediting bodies that define the safe operation of their business.

Home health care organizations should consider the purchase of insurance for the following exposures:

- property
- professional and general liability (including umbrella coverage)
- directors and officers of the corporation
- automobile/vehicle
- workers' compensation
- crime
- easily transportable equipment such as computers

Property

Property insurance provides security from losses related to the direct physical loss or damage to covered property. Property is defined as a building or dwelling, and includes all permanently installed indoor and outdoor fixtures, machinery and equipment, and other personal property used to maintain the building; business personal property such as furniture; and personal property of others in the care, custody, and control of the organization. Home health care organizations minimally should make sure that their policy insures against fire, lightning, internal explosion, volcanic action, vandalism, sinkhole collapse, and sprinkler leakage. Other coverages that can be purchased include loss of business income; damage from falling objects; damage due to the weight of ice, snow, and sleet; damage due to glass breakage; and damage due to collapse. Organizations in geographic areas where there is a high risk of flood or earthquake should consider these additional coverages as well. Home health care organizations should work closely with their insurance agent or broker to make sure that the proper perils are covered by insurance.

Home health care organizations may not need the entire extent of coverages available. The business office space may be within a singular building that is leased or rented or may be a suite of offices within a larger complex of offices. In either case, the property exposure would be the actual business furnishings owned by the organization; any personal property of others in the care, custody, and control of the organization; and other building and property exposures agreed to by the organization and spelled out in the rental agreement.

Property exposures for home health care organizations are managed through good basic business practices because the actual building within which business is conducted usually performs secretarial, accounting, or business management functions. If the organization stores medical supplies (including pharmaceuticals), however, the organization's exposure increases.

The agent or broker securing insurance for the organization should be aware of this risk when placing coverage.

Liability

Liability is defined as the failure of an individual or organization to exercise the proper degree of care required of a sensible person. The guideline driving this definition is that of negligence. Negligence is a wrong committed by one person or organization on another. It is an improper action that causes bodily injury or property damage and is usually in the control of the negligent party. A home health care organization's liability exposure, however, may also be present because of an accidental occurrence. All employees, contracted professional staff, and the organization itself may be held legally responsible for any action that leads to the bodily injury or property damage of others. Liability insurance covers both the financial obligations resultant to the injured person's claim and the cost of legal defense.

Liability insurance is available in two forms: occurrence and claims made. Both forms provide a home health care organization liability insurance for bodily injury or property damage to others. The occurrence form of liability insurance furnishes coverage during the policy period regardless of when a claim is reported and filed with the carrier by the insured. The claims made form of liability insurance furnishes coverage only for claims that are reported or filed during the policy period or within 60 days of the policy's expiration, and only when the date of alleged negligence occurred after a retroactive date. The retroactive date defines the specific date when the policy actually begins.

Home health care organizations have a vicarious liability as well. This means that the organization itself may be held liable for any negligent act committed in the performance of assigned duties or on behalf of the organization by employees or contracted professional staff.

Liability of Directors and Officers

Directors and officers of any corporation are defined by the organization's bylaws and usually include the board of directors and administrative/senior management employees such as (but not limited to) the chief executive officer, the chief operations officer, and the chief financial officer. These individuals can be held liable, or have an exposure, for any and all activities of the home health care organization. Liability insurance for directors and officers provides coverage for the identified individuals who commit wrongful acts such as error, neglect, or breach of duty. Examples of wrongful acts include fiduciary malfeasance and misfeasance, failure to adequately supervise professional activities, improper hiring, and wrongful termination. It is the responsibility of the board of directors and officers of a home health care organization to ensure that recognized standards of care are followed, that staff have earned appropriate academic degrees and hold proper licensure to do their job, and that the environment within which business is conducted is free from defects that might cause bodily injury or physical damage to others. These basic principles apply whether professional staff are employees of the organization or are performing duties for the organization on a contractual basis.

General Liability

General liability coverage provides insurance for bodily injury or property damage to clients, their families, vendors, or others not employed by the home health care organization caused by perils within the organization's premises or resulting from its business operations. General liability coverage also includes protection from a claim that is the result of an accusation of libel, slander, or invasion of privacy, as well as medical payments for bodily injury.

General liability exposures faced by home health care organizations are centered primarily on the premises from which the operation is directed. Examples are failure to remove ice from the entryway to the building, failure to post notice of a wet floor, failure to repair expediently or to remove dangerous physical plant problems (for example, wet ceiling tile).

Fire legal liability is also a possible exposure. It is essential for the home health care organization to check its lease or business complex agreement about this liability and to enforce strictly its necessary policies about smoking and emergency procedures regarding smoke and/or fire.

Professional Liability

Professional liability insurance protects professionals or an organization's professional staff who fail to meet the standards of skill and care generally accepted for that profession or occupation. The protection afforded by this coverage includes both direct injury or harm and indirect injury or harm (emotional trauma, pain, and suffering). A claim may be filed by an individual, the legal guardian of an individual, or an individual's estate. Professional liability also includes the failure of any professional with regard to "duty to report" or "duty to warn."

Home health care organizations are faced with exceptional professional liability exposures. Two essential questions should be asked:

1. Are the professional staff credentialed and trained, and supervised properly for the performance of all aspects of their duties?
2. Are the duties performed under the direct order of a professional legally and medically authorized to order such duties?

Even if the home health care organization contracts for the services of any or all professionals, the organization itself is liable for the professional activities performed. Contractual professional staff may be included in professional liability coverage as contingent employees.

Umbrella Liability

An umbrella policy provides insurance for liability claims when an award for damages is in excess of the limits of the general and/or professional liability policy. There are multiple limits of insurance that apply to liability coverages; however, the two major limits to consider are the per occurrence and the aggregate limit amounts. The occurrence limit is the dollar amount the carrier will pay for a single, individual claim. The aggregate limit is the maximum amount an insurer will pay for all covered losses during the policy period. When limits are reached, additional coverage is provided by an umbrella policy.

Home health care organizations might consider the purchase of umbrella liability coverage to provide coverage in the event of a catastrophic loss, such as a wrongful death.

Automobile/Vehicle

There are two different forms of insurance that compose an automobile policy. Both include property and casualty coverages.

The property section of the package policy protects an insured from loss due to comprehensive or collision damage and is specific to an insured's vehicle(s). The vehicles that are covered must be scheduled (i.e., listed specifically). Comprehensive coverage is defined as the direct and/or accidental damage to an insured's vehicle from anything other than collision. Collision is defined as a direct and/or accidental loss that results when two vehicles collide, when the vehicle collides with another object, or when the vehicle is upset (overturned).

Protection from economic loss due to negligent ownership (failure to repair bad brakes), poor maintenance, or negligent use of an insured vehicle is provided in the liability section of an automobile policy. As with all liability coverages, this protection is designed to cover damages that an insured is legally obliged to pay as a result of bodily injury or property damage to others as a result of a vehicular accident.

A business auto coverage form may be necessary for home health care organizations. For example, if the organization owns a fleet of vehicles, coverage would be essential in order to conduct business. If the organization requires that professional staff drive their own vehicles in order to conduct business, however, the business auto coverage form would specify coverage for nonowned autos only. Nonowned autos may, depending on the carrier, be added as an endorsement to the general liability section of an organization's commercial policy. This is also true for hired autos (i.e., any vehicles hired, leased, rented, or borrowed and used for business purposes).

The use of nonowned autos raises an additional exposure for home health care organizations. Whenever a vehicle is used on behalf of a home health care organization in the course of business, the organization has a responsibility to ensure that the vehicle is properly registered (and, if applicable, inspected) and that the driver of the vehicle is licensed and insured. It is best to make sure that the organization's policies and procedures incorporate the aforementioned points and that all staff are properly educated.

Workers' Compensation

Most states have promulgated compulsory laws that require employers to provide coverage for employee work-related injuries and for employer protection against common lawsuits that may be brought by employees (or their survivors) to recover damages from job-related injuries. All injuries sustained by an employee arising out of and in the course of employment are covered. Additionally, occupational diseases specific to a particular trade or occupation are covered. Workers' compensation insurance provides cash (a portion of wages), medical benefits, and rehabilitation for injured employees. It doesn't matter who, why, or what caused the injury to occur and as such is considered a no-fault type of coverage.

Workers' compensation insurance implies that employers should provide as safe a work environment as can be maintained, given the scope of the organization, and that employees should be integral to the maintenance of the

worksite. Furthermore, employers must consider their return-to-work and modified-duty policies. Also, employees must be informed of their workers' compensation rights and their duties should an injury occur.

It is strongly suggested that organizations establish a safety committee, contract for the assistance of a workers' compensation loss control expert to assess an organization's exposures (and to make recommendations), and educate their employees regarding safe work practices. Although carriers recognize that a zero employee injury policy is impossible, all organizations can improve their safety record continually.

Home health care organizations have distinct workers' compensation exposures. The nature of the work may demand lifting, entering buildings and dwellings that may not be in the best repair, physical activities with clients, and performing duties with individuals who may be less than cooperative. For organizations that provide injections, there is always the risk of needle sticks and exposure to communicable diseases. For this reason, as well as others, a strong education program related to safety procedures and potential risks is necessary; even the basics (e.g., universal precautions, proper lifting techniques) need to be reviewed at least yearly with the most experienced employees. Organizations that contract for professional staff through another organization or agency also hold a responsibility to ensure that the employing organization or agency has workers' compensation insurance.

Crime

Very simply, crime insurance protects an insured from burglary, robbery, theft, forgery, mysterious disappearance, extortion, and computer fraud. Although crime insurance does not cover dishonest acts committed by the insured (see Liability of Directors and Officers), coverage is extended to all employees, a custodian of the insured's property, a messenger transporting an insured's property (including money and securities) from one location to another, and individuals watching over or guarding an insured's property.

There may be a loss due to typical crime exposures (robbery, burglary, etc.); however, the primary exposures for home health care organizations are employee dishonesty, forgery, or alteration (particularly of client records) and mysterious disappearances of equipment, supplies, or medicines. The single best method for controlling these exposures is focused on the organization's record-keeping procedures, including the location of client records (and the method of checking them in and out) and the supplies allocated. An occasional field check of activities is strongly recommended.

Transportable Equipment

Inland marine coverage is insurance to protect a home health care organization's easily transportable property (e.g., computers). The home health care organization needs to consider that an investment made in electronic data processing, including computer hardware and software, is an insurable interest and can be covered by an inland marine policy form called an electronic data processing floater.

RISK MANAGEMENT

The exposures of home health care organizations have been touched upon in each section of this chapter. As the field continues to mature there will be additional exposures not already mentioned; however, there are some good basic principles of risk management to consider. Risk management is loss control or the strategies applied by management that minimize an organization's exposure to potential claims. Risk management activities focus on the corporate culture necessary to develop, carry out, and coordinate activities; it involves all levels of the organization, centers on employee behavior, and is an essential ingredient in an organization's quality improvement plan.

A good risk management program includes the following components:

- a mission statement developed and understood by the directors and officers and staff at all levels in the organization
- routine organizationwide strategic planning, with an ongoing analysis of goal attainment that drives the organization forward
- a quality improvement or quality assurance plan that is developed and monitored by all levels of the organization
- solid employee practices, including screening and hiring, orientation, annual performance evaluations, and staff development
- consumer satisfaction analyses, including an evaluation of the organization's primary customers, referral sources, and the community within which the organization does business
- a safety committee that monitors the mechanical and physical plant and infection control, and holds regularly planned disaster drills
- a mechanism to ensure inventory control and minimize employee theft
- a system minimally to oversee transportation issues and to review annually all policies and procedures
- a workers' compensation review, including return-to-work/modified-duty policy and loss analysis
- an active training program that focuses on risk management issues
- a plan to have all facets of the risk management program linked to administrative planning and decision making

PURCHASING INSURANCE

Home health care organizations should evaluate carefully their exposures, develop and actively pursue loss control/risk management activities, and assess carefully their insurance needs. It is important that home health care organizations earnestly consider working with an insurance agent or broker who can understand the unique aspects of their business.

Home health care organizations should purchase insurance coverages to match their risks. The types of insurance described here can be put together into one commercial package policy when only one insurance company writes all coverages. Some carriers will have a better form (coverages within the policy itself) for a particular type of coverage, however, and then the home health care organization could purchase their policies from several companies. This too

is an issue to discuss with the organization's broker or agent. Remember, the single goal in purchasing insurance is to provide proper coverages for the organization's unique needs.

CONCLUSION

This chapter has purposefully outlined the possible exposures of home health care organizations through a delineation of the various types of insurance coverages available and provided descriptions of how those might apply to home health care organizations.

BIBILOGRAPHY

Bickelhaupt, D. (1983). *General insurance.* Homewood, IL: Richard D. Irwin.

Head, G, & Horn, S., II. (1991). *Essentials of risk management (2nd ed.).* Malvern, PA: Insurance Institute of America.

Levick, D., & Grzincic, N. (1994). *Workers compensation: Exposures, coverage, and claims.* Boston: Standard Publishing.

Mehr, R., & Cammack, E. (1972). *Principles of insurance.* Homewood, IL: Richard D. Irwin.

Mehr, R., et al. (1983). *Fundamentals of insurance.* Homewood, IL: Richard D. Irwin.

CHAPTER 48

Budgeting for Home Health Services

Gregory J. Brown

The budgetary process obligates management to make an early study of its current and projected operating problems. It instills in the organization the habit of making a thorough and careful study of information before making decisions. When all programs have been evaluated through a well-thought-out budget process, the budget becomes management's written plan for the future. The budget should enlist the aid of the entire management organization so that final decisions represent the combined judgment of the entire organization and not merely that of an individual or small group of individuals. The budget promotes increased coordination of limited financial resources for use by all agency programs. The budget allows current operations to be measured against a financial and statistical model that incorporates management's projections of anticipated operational activity. The budgetary process has three fundamental phases: program planning and evaluation, statistical and operational budget development, and analytical budget controls.

PROGRAM PLANNING AND EVALUATION

To gain a broader base of information about each program, the agency may choose to establish a program review team as part of the budgetary process. The program review team should involve only as many administrative personnel and/or agency board members as considered practical. While each review team member should represent an area of expertise, the team's composition must be balanced to maintain subjectivity between clinical and financial program issues. The higher the degree of scrutiny that each program receives during the review process, the more reliable will be the data on which the upcoming budget will be based. The greater the involvement of the board and administrative staff in the budget review process, the greater their commitment to operate those programs within the approved budget parameters.

One of the most important tasks that the home health agency must accomplish during the program review and evaluation process is to evaluate the effectiveness of all existing programs and to ensure that the programs continue to meet the established organizational goals and objectives.

The continued viability of each program should be determined from answers to questions that the agency considers important, such as the following:

- Has each program met its established goals?
- Are any changes necessary for the program to be more effective?
- If the program is to be continued, are there any changes in the demand for that program?

- Are there sufficient controls established to monitor the program's progress?
- Can the program generate sufficient revenues to cover expenses, or must it rely on alternate sources of funding?
- If funding cutbacks dictate program cuts, what is the program's rank of importance in relationship to other programs?
- What other risks are there associated with maintaining this program?

STATISTICAL AND OPERATIONAL BUDGET DEVELOPMENT

The primary focus of the budget development section is identifying the various steps and components utilized in the preparation of the statistical and operating budgets. During this phase of the budgetary process, the agency will establish specific parameters within which it will prepare the budget. The agency will also establish the time frame for accomplishing the budgetary process. A list of all budget procedures and required items is identified and prioritized in the order of date required. Budgetary assignments are delegated to appropriate administrative personnel or board committees with due dates for completion.

Cyclical versus Noncyclical Operating Year

Budget information is usually based on the time period covered by the operating or fiscal year. The budget comprises 12 monthly periods from which comparisons can be made against the actual monthly and year-to-date levels of activity. If the organization operates in a noncyclical environment, with flat or nominal growth projections, the operating budget can be prepared as 12 individual monthly budgets, all presenting identical levels of activity. If the organization operates in a cyclical environment (i.e., seasonally or with specific growth projections), the annual budget can attempt to reflect these projections by presenting the 12 monthly budget periods in a manner that would coincide with the cyclical or projected levels of actual activity. Presumably, most organizations will plan for a favorable rate of growth. As we all are aware, however, organizations may at times need to project a downward growth pattern. In either case, if this information is known at the time of the budget preparation, it should be incorporated into the annual budget projections.

My experience has shown that unanticipated fluctuations in visit volume will occur during any given period of time. When comparing several years of our agency's historical visit data, I observed a definite pattern as to when the high and low visit cycles occur during each year. Upon analysis of the statistical data (visits, referrals, discharges, and staffing activity), it was possible to identify several recurring relationships. For example, the effects of a severe winter season will tend to produce an increase in the number of referrals for patients with muscular-skeletal injuries, influenza, and respiratory problems. A winter with high levels of snowfall also tends to decrease staff productivity because of hazardous road conditions, safety issues, and school closings. Conversely, these seasonal problems do not occur during the warmer spring and summer months. The warmer months generate as many referrals, but vacations by agency staff tend to decrease the availability of personnel to perform visits. If per diem help is unavailable to make up for the shortage of visiting staff, patient admissions may have to be delayed or visit frequency for other patients may have to be decreased.

Immediately prior to weekends and during major holidays, many home health agencies receive an above-average number of referrals for patients being discharged from hospitals. This may be attributed to hospitals' discharging patients to reduce their staffing costs during these time periods and patients' scheduling elective surgery with a planned recovery at home during the weekend and holidays.

Although these visit and staffing patterns recur with regularity, I have not encountered a model that will reliably forecast the timing and magnitude of each recurrence. Because of the absence of cyclical staffing data, our agency budgets for a static core visiting staff supplemented with an adequate number of employee and contract per-diem staff to absorb the visit volume fluctuations. On an annual aggregate basis, utilization of the noncyclical budget has been adequate for our purposes.

Case Mix Analysis

After having evaluated the services and programs the agency chooses to provide, the agency must develop the cross-section (case mix) projection of individuals who would actually utilize the agency's services. The agency can make this projection from historical data or from a demographic market survey studying population and medical care requirement characteristics of potential consumers. From these data, the agency must make a projection of when and how many units of service will need to be provided to meet the demands of the consumers. Consumers may be state and county agencies, individual patients, other home health agencies, hospital home care departments, managed care entities, health maintenance organizations, preferred provider organizations, insurance companies, and even private industries. Although a significant amount of data can be collected on prospective consumers, only a limited amount is required for preparing a basic case-mix analysis.

As the case mix data are being collected, they should be classified as units of service in each of three categories: types of services required, reimbursement resources available, and time frame for services required. Types of services required would comprise all of the services the agency chooses to provide (e.g., skilled nursing, physical therapy, home health aide, hospice, and maternal–child health programs). Reimbursement resources would comprise all the reimbursement types and sources the agency would utilize for payment of services (e.g., Medicare, Medicaid, managed care, patient pay, and uncompensated care). Time frame would comprise the number of monthly operating periods

during which the service would be provided (e.g., throughout the year, summer only, from the date a new contract starts, and, if applicable, cyclical visit data).

Once sufficient case mix visit data have been collected, the data are recorded on a table format worksheet to observe the units of service required for each category of service offered and the units of service to be paid for by the reimbursement resources available. At this time, it is not important to classify the information by time frame; however, the time frame information is important for planning staffing level changes. (See Exhibit 48–1 for an example of the case mix analysis worksheet.)

The visit data on the initial case mix worksheet represent only potential clients. Agency administration must further review these data to identify the exact case mix of clients for which it intends to provide services. For example, if the administration chooses not to provide homemaker service to clients who have no reimbursement resources, then the corresponding units of service should be removed from the worksheet. The worksheet should continue to be reworked until it represents what administration considers to be a realistic representation of the types and units of service to be provided under each program and reimbursement resource.

Additional data collection and analysis will be required if the agency becomes involved with programs that are reimbursed by other than the traditional fee for service (e.g., per diem, per case, per member per month capitation, etc.). To succeed under these types of reimbursement, the agency must have access to excellent historical data that can be analyzed to determine the service requirements for patients under each reimbursement arrangement. Upon completion of the data collection these data can be processed as a subset of the agency case mix data.

Because the case mix analysis is the foundation for all subsequent budget analysis, it is important to take the time to validate your assumptions before proceeding further in the budgeting process.

Exhibit 48–1 Example of Table Format Worksheet

Budget Worksheet # ____

Service Type   Reimbursement Resources

	Medicare	Medical Assistance	Private Insurance	Self-Pay	Hospital Home Care	Home Health Agencies	Total
Nursing							
Physical Therapy							
Speech Therapy							
Occupational Therapy							
Medical Social Service							
Home Health Aide							
Homemaker							
Total							

Productivity and Staffing Requirements

Although the case mix analysis indicates the annual projection of the units of service to be provided, a separate analysis must be made to calculate the number of full-time equivalent (FTE) staff required to service those projections adequately. Several calculations must be performed when analyzing how many staffing hours of each profession it would take to provide the units of service projected in the case mix analysis. These are the employment factor and average visits per day calculations.

Employment Factor

The employment factor is a calculation to project the actual annual productive work hours that are available from staffing a full-time position. The available productive work hours are determined by taking the annual payroll hours paid to staff, regular hours (skilled visit time, skilled nonvisit time, and all nonskilled service time), overtime hours if significant, and any types of paid leave time (vacation, holiday, and sick time). From these annual payroll hours paid, deduct all leave time and non–service-related hours paid, and divide the results into the total annual hours paid. An analysis of the

agency's historical time records will provide data on the average annual leave time taken. The basic concept for calculating the employment factor is shown in Exhibit 48–2.

If the nonservice time and leave benefit levels provided to an agency's employees are significantly dissimilar, an agency may need to calculate separate employment factors for each service provided. The employment factor calculation provides two pieces of information: It indicates the amount of time that can be utilized for revenue-generating activity, and it provides a factor from which one can calculate FTE staff-

Exhibit 48–2 Nursing Employment Factor

Total annual paid hours		1,950.00
Less paid leave hours		
Average annual vacation	(112.50)	
Average sick time usage	(52.50)	
Holidays	(67.50)	
Personal days	(15.00)	
Less nonservice hours paid		
Administrative functions	(20.00)	
		(267.50)
Available work hours		1,682.50
Employment factor (1,950.00/1,682.50)		1.16

ing requirements. For example, in Exhibit 48–3, if the services being provided are to be sold by the hour (e.g., home health aides), you would multiply the total projected case mix hours of service to be provided by the employment factor for that service to determine the FTE staffing requirements.

Although historical data are typically the most valid source of information available for this analysis, you also need to consider what impact a proposed procedural change would have on staffs' utilization of time. For instance, as part of our hospital's plan to cut operating expenses, the annual payment for the unused sick time program was eliminated. Although the payout ratio was modest, many hospital workers looked upon this payment as a reward for prudent use of sick leave. During the following year we observed a 100% increase in the amount of sick time taken by our hourly home health aide staff. This specific circumstance increased the home health aide employment factor by just 6%, but a combination of unanticipated events can have a significant impact on an agency's operations.

Average Visits per Day

If the services provided are made on an encounter basis and without regard to length of time spent on the visit, then the staffing requirement calculation must take into account the productivity capacity of the employees. This requires that the agency calculate the average visits per day productivity statistic for each group of service providers (see Exhibit 48–4).

The agency's historical time study data are the best source of data to use when making the average visits per day calculations. If historical data do not exist, an agency may wish to survey other home health agencies to obtain average visits per day productivity statistics. Exhibit 48–5 is an example of how the employment factor and the average visits per day statistic can be utilized to calculate FTE staffing requirements when services are provided on an encounter basis.

When the FTE calculation for each service is completed, a comparison should be made between the existing staffing levels and the new staffing requirements. If the new staffing requirements exceed the existing level of staff, at least four options exist: Add new employee positions to the budget; attempt to increase productivity of the existing staff; begin or increase utilization of contract personnel; or implement a cost-effective and practical combination of all three options.

If projected staffing requirements are less than the existing level, a reduction in staff is warranted. Reductions in staff should be accomplished in a manner that would not jeopardize the provision or integrity of services being provided. Reductions could be accomplished via layoffs, natural attrition, or reducing workweek hours for all or specific staff of the program in question. Whichever scenario occurs and whichever option is chosen, consideration must also be made for the effects that service expansion or reduction will have on the administrative and supervisory capacities of the organization.

Expense Classifications and Departmental Expenditure Budgets

Expense Classifications

Once administration has identified its staffing requirements, it will begin identifying expense categories and preparing departmental expenditure budgets. The goal of expense budgeting is to identify, on an accrual accounting basis,

---

Exhibit 48–3 Home Health Aide (HHA) Staffing Requirements

Projected HHA hours to be sold	25,000
HHA employment factor	× 1.06
Total payroll hours budgeted	26,500
Payroll hours budgeted/ 1,950.00 = FTE staffing requirement	13.59

Exhibit 48–4 National League for Nursing Productivity Calculation: Home Visits per Day per Employee

$$\text{Average visits per day} = \frac{\text{Number of visits during period}}{\text{Number of days available for visiting}}$$

To count visits:

- include all completed visits by discipline (maternal–child health, health promotion, and care of sick, whether billable or not)
- exclude not home, not found, supervisory, and observation visits (two persons in home) and office visits

To calculate available days:

1. from attendance records, enter total hours on duty for each discipline on staff level (exclusive of holidays, vacation, time off, and sick time; include weekend time if on duty)
2. subtract nonvisiting service time (in clinics, schools, etc.); time spent in supervision, orientation, and the like; inservice time; and office visit time
3. add time spent in home visiting by agency personnel above staff level replacing staff
4. divide resultant hours by working hours per day in agency to calculate equivalent full days available for visiting

Source: Reprinted with permission from *Productivity Home Visits Per Day Per Employee* ©1979, National League for Nursing.

expenses that will be incurred during the provision of services to patients. Every expense category listed in the agency's chart of accounts will need to be classified as either a direct or an indirect expense. Expenses that can be directly identified with a service or department are known as direct expenses (e.g., salaries, benefits, conferences, and automobile allowances). Expenses that cannot be directly identified with a service or department are known as indirect expenses. Indirect expenses, also known as overhead expenses, will need to be allocated equitably to each service program to determine the true cost of providing that program. Examples of indirect expenses are plant operation expenses, administrative services, general and professional liability insurance coverages, marketing, and legal and accounting services.

Departmental Expenditure Budgets

The departmental expenditure budget comprises at least three components: direct compensation and benefits analysis, direct contract services analysis, and other direct departmental expenditures analysis.

Because one aspect of the budgetary process is the need to identify the total direct operating cost of each service offered, a departmental expenditure budget would be the basis for this analysis. Typically, for every general ledger

Exhibit 48–5 Employment Factor Calculation

Projected skilled nursing visits	35,000
Divide by average visits per day	5.20
Service days required	6,730
Multiply by 7.50 daily work hours	7.50
Service hours required	50,481
Multiply by nursing employment factor	1.16
Total payroll hours budgeted	58,558
Divide by annual work hours	1,950
FTE staffing requirement	30.03

expense account that the agency uses, a corresponding budget projection would be made. In the event an agency has designated one general ledger account to record a specific multidepartmental expense (e.g., health insurance expense), the general ledger chart of accounts should be revised so that each department has the same set of direct expense categories. For example, the health insurance expense category would be listed for each service as nursing health insurance, physical therapy health insurance, homemaker health insurance, and finance health insurance. An advantage to using such a detailed classification process is that it will specifically identify each direct cost incurred by the department and, conversely, no department receives a cost allocation of a direct expense that it did not legitimately incur.

Direct compensation and benefits analysis. A detailed compensation and benefit analysis will allow administration to evaluate the direct cost associated with every position within the agency. This information is helpful when doing a cost-benefit analysis evaluating staffing versus contracting for services. The compensation and benefit analysis will list each position required by that department, projected annual working hours, proposed hourly wage, projected annual salary, projected annual cost of mandatory payroll taxes and insurance, and annual cost of each optional health and welfare benefit provided. Mandatory payroll-related costs include social security wage tax, Medicare wage tax, state unemployment tax, federal unemployment tax, and workers' compensation. Optional health and welfare benefits include pension plan, life insurance, health insurance, disability insurance, and tuition reimbursement.

Direct contract services analysis. If an agency has done a cost–benefit analysis and has determined that it is to its advantage to utilize contracted services in lieu of hiring additional employees, the cost for the contracted services is considered a direct expense of the department for which the services are provided. Projecting the cost of contracted services for a direct ser-

vice contractor is usually a matter of multiplying the projected units of service the contractor will perform by the contractor's negotiated charge per unit of service.

Projecting the cost of contracted administrative services can be accomplished by obtaining fixed bids for the contractor's services, reviewing historical cost data, or a combination of both.

Other direct departmental expenditures analysis. The other direct departmental expenditures analysis will list the remaining expenditure categories that can be directly associated with a department (e.g., conferences, seminars and education, uniforms, books and periodicals, automobile allowance, direct supply purchases, and any other expense item that can be directly associated with a department's operation). Other agency expense categories not directly incurred by a service department are the indirect cost associated with plant operations and maintenance and the administrative and general categories. Within these two expense classification categories, an agency may wish to establish several functional departments. As stated previously, these categories of expenses are considered overhead and will need to be allocated to each service being offered to arrive at the true cost of providing that service.

Typical plant operation and maintenance expenses include the following:

- heat, light, and power
- building repairs and maintenance
- janitorial and groundskeeping service
- real estate taxes
- depreciation of buildings
- depreciation of furniture and equipment

Typical administrative and general expenses include the following:

- administrative services
- financial services
- data processing services
- medical records and transcription services
- contracted professional services (legal, accounting, marketing)

- general and professional liability insurance coverages

Estimating the expenditure level for these expense categories can be accomplished in several ways:

- **Incremental:** The projected percentage of change (increase or decrease) in the annual visits, or growth rate, could be added to an across-the-board rate of inflation to increase expenses incrementally. This method is fast and uniform but will overstate those expense categories that do not increase proportionally with volume increases (e.g., depreciation, real estate taxes).
- **Zero base:** Justify every dollar of expenditure based on known occurrences or consumption levels. For example, for data processing expenses multiply total projected visits by the quoted per visit processing fee. This method provides very specific results but can be very time consuming and does not account for unforeseen occurrences.
- **Combination:** Utilizing a combination of zero-base and incremental budgeting can provide an agency with optimum levels of expenditure projections.

Allocating indirect cost. If an agency is going to provide care to Medicare patients, there are specific guidelines established for allocating indirect expenses to existing departmental expenses. This allocation procedure is known as the Medicare step-down method of cost allocation. Agencies may want to review Part II of the *Medicare Provider Reimbursement Manual*, on provider cost reporting forms and instructions, to determine the exact parameters that they must follow. While some agencies may have a reason to use an alternative to the Medicare step-down methodology during the budgetary process, most agencies will find it practical to allocate indirect cost according to the Medicare guidelines.

Plant operations and maintenance costs are allocated on a square footage basis. This requires that a floor plan for all leased or owned space occupied by agency personnel be prepared, allocating the square footage to a service or department by actual square footage occupied by each employee or, if the employee participates in several activities, by division of the employee's square footage by time spent in each activity. The actual cost attributed to each service is calculated by multiplying the square footage for each service by the projected cost per square foot.

Cost per square foot

$$= \frac{\text{Total projected plant operation cost}}{\text{Total square footage occupied}}$$

Administrative and general costs are allocated on an accumulated cost basis. If one were to total all direct costs that have been identified with a service (e.g., salaries and benefits, direct departmental expenses, direct contract services, direct costs associated with adjustments, and allocations from other departments), this total would be referred to as the department's total direct accumulated costs. When total accumulative costs have been calculated for each service, it is possible to allocate administrative and general costs that have not previously been assigned to a service or cost center as a percentage of the total accumulated costs of all services.

When all agency expenses have been allocated to a service program, the agency can determine a per unit cost for each service it intends to provide. This is done by dividing each program's total accumulated cost by the units of service (visits and/or hours) to be provided by that program as indicated in the case mix analysis. Once the agency knows what the projected cost of providing each unit of service will be, it can construct a charge structure and begin making revenue projections and profitability analysis of each service provided.

Revenue Projections

Revenue, like expenses, should be recorded on an accrual accounting basis and by the corresponding service or revenue center established during the preparation of the expense budget. Revenue for home health agencies falls into two major categories: revenue from patient care services, and nonoperating sources of revenue.

Revenue from Patient Care Services

An accurate projection of patient care services revenue must take into account the sources of gross revenue and any deductions from gross revenue that would represent a less than full-charge reimbursement for provided services. Revenue from patient care services represents gross revenues, measured in terms of the agency's full established rates earned from all services rendered to patients by the various revenue-producing centers in the agency. Deductions from patient service revenues represent reductions in gross revenues arising from charity service, contractual adjustments, policy discounts, administrative adjustments, and bad debts (Serluco, 1984).

Several worksheets will need to be prepared to assist in the cost and profitability analysis. These worksheets will be prepared in the same format as the case mix analysis: by service by reimbursement source. By completing the worksheets in the indicated order, an individual reviewing the worksheets will immediately be able to observe trends or variances occurring for any program and payer source combination. The following worksheets will be required:

- cost per unit of service: gross service cost divided by case mix units of service provided by each service provided
- gross cost of services: cost per unit of service times case mix units of service
- charge per unit of service: projected gross charge for each type of service being offered

- gross charges for service: charge per unit of service times projected case mix units of service to be offered
- expected net revenue per unit of service: gross charge per unit of service adjusted for deductions from patient care services
- net revenue from services: net revenue from service times case mix units of service
- gross allowances on services: gross charges less net revenue
- gain or loss on service: net revenue from services less gross cost of services

Many home health agencies are faced with a reimbursement environment where revenue from fees for service fall far short of the actual cost of providing the services that the agency has stated it will provide. For example, unexpected clinical needs of patients may force program costs to exceed the revenue-generating capacity of the established charge structure. Revising the charge structure to cover the increase in cost may only complicate matters if the new charge structure sets the price for service higher than what consumers are willing to pay. Because this scenario has become a routine occurrence, it has become a commonplace practice for agencies to institute cutbacks to reduce program expenditures, to limit the quantity of care being provided to patients, to pool any unrestricted program surpluses to offset losses incurred by other programs, or to secure other sources of nonoperating income to supplement program losses.

Nonoperating Sources of Income

Nonoperating sources of income are often acknowledged as a reason why many nonprofit home health agencies have been able to continue surviving in today's health care environment. Home health agencies have come to rely heavily on the funds made available by United Way, fraternal organizations, public and private contributors, interest income, and the allocations that state and local governments have earmarked for the provision of public health services.

When one is preparing a nonoperating sources of income budget worksheet, two pieces of information can be obtained: total anticipated nonoperating income, and monthly cash flows from receipt of the nonoperating income. The financial data required for preparation of the nonoperating sources of income analysis typically are obtained from the agency's current and prior year deferred income analysis. All anticipated sources of nonoperating income should be listed on a worksheet indicating source of funds, the period the funds cover, and the amount expected.

Expense and Revenue Summary Analysis

The completion of the worksheets and procedures outlined in the budget development stage will give the agency an idea of how much it will cost to provide services, how much revenue is expected to be received, and how much money the agency expects to gain or lose on the services provided. The expense and revenue summary analysis worksheet (Exhibit 48–6) will summarize the gains and losses of the service programs and the sources and distribution of nonoperating income. Observation of this analysis will indicate those service areas that require additional review and revision. By following any service program backward through each series of worksheets, unacceptable variances can be identified and the budget review team can concentrate its efforts on reviewing the circumstances of that specific area, modifying budget parameters as appropriate until the profitability results are within the limits established during the program planning and evaluation process.

Other Budgets

Two additional components required of the budget development process are the cash budget and the capital acquisitions budget.

Cash Budget

A cash budget involves detailed estimates of anticipated cash receipts and disbursement requirements coinciding with the 12 monthly periods of the projected budget. The cash budget is an important management tool for monitoring the operating condition of the organization.

Specifically, the cash budget will indicate the effect on the agency's cash position for changes in service utilization patterns, routine and unusual cash receipt or expenditure items, and inefficient accounts receivable collections; the cash requirements for capital acquisitions; when cash shortfalls may make it necessary to borrow or utilize credit lines; and when excess cash balances will be available for investment purposes.

Most cash budgets are prepared from cash receipt and disbursement data. Items to be considered when preparing the cash receipt portion of the cash budget would be all anticipated incoming cash from the provision of patient care services, state and local government allocations, United Way allocations, fund-raising revenues, restricted and unrestricted contributions, grant and trust moneys received, interest income, proceeds from sales of assets, and rental and lease income. Projecting the actual period of time during which the cash receipts are going to be received is difficult because of problems with accounts receivable collections, the unpredictability of planning contribution receipts, and the uncertainty of knowing when private and public allocation funds are going to be made available to the agency.

Expenditure items of the cash budget would be payroll, payroll-related taxes, employee health and welfare benefits, the cost of operating supplies and operating expenses, capital expenditures, income taxes, and dividends paid to owners.

Expenditure items are easier to project because the majority of a home health agency's costs are payroll related and would occur in a predictable pattern.

Exhibit 48–6 Sample Expense and Revenue Summary Analysis Worksheet

AGENCY NAME SUMMARY OF REVENUE AND EXPENSES FY 19___	FY 19___ BUDGET PROJECTIONS			DISTRIBUTION OF DONOR RESTRICTED INCOME			
	Program Revenue ($)	Program Cost ($)	Gain/Loss ($)	United Way Allocation ($)	Municipal Allocation ($)	Foundation Grant ($)	TOTAL ($)
Nursing	1250000	1263200	–13200				–13200
Physical Therapy	350000	343000	7000				7000
Speech Therapy	125000	119000	6000				6000
Occupational Therapy	175000	160000	15000				15000
Medical Social Service	85000	123000	–38000				–38000
Home Health Aide	650000	655000	–5000				–5000
							0
Special Program 1	10874	16418	–5544	5544			0
Special Program 2	0	12000	–12000	0			–12000
Special Program 3	4374	13889	–9516	9516			0
Special Program 4	10812	26254	–15443	15443			0
Special Program 5	46871	226350	–179479	79498	28915	30074	–40992
Special Program 6	0	17860	–17860			10389	–7471
Special Program 7	0	6254	–6254			14217	7963
General Contributions	7500	0	7500				7500
Municipal Contributions	28915	0	28915		–28915		0
Misc. Income	3500	0	3500				3500
Interest Income—All Sources	76500	0	76500				76500
Foundation & Trust	54680	0	54680			–54680	0
United Way Individuals	5000	0	5000				5000
United Way Allocation	110000	0	110000	–110000			0
	0	0	0				0
	0	0	0				0
Total	2994026	2982226	11800	0	0	0	11800

Capital Expenditure Analysis Budget

The capital expenditure budget will contain several analyses that would indicate the impact of leasing versus owning an asset, the impact of financing versus utilization of cash reserves to purchase the asset, annual costs associated with depreciation and maintenance of the new capital equipment, and additional cash expenditure requirements for the upcoming year under any of the above-mentioned options. When agencies have many requests for new equipment, a capital equipment requisition form can assist with the evaluation process. The capital equipment requisition form should indicate the purchase priority of the item (new, replacement, and date required), a brief description of the item and why it is needed, potential vendors, the item's cost, and its expected useful life. Cost association with the installation, delivery, and annual maintenance of the equipment also should be indicated.

ANALYTICAL BUDGET CONTROLS

The budget control phase of the budgetary process is intended to give management the ability to monitor, alter, or limit the degree to which actual agency activity deviates from budgeted activity. Monitoring can be achieved by having the agency's internal financial statements prepared in a manner that presents actual activity against budgeted activity on a monthly and year-to-date basis. It is also helpful if the agency has the ability to compare current year activity against prior year activity. The monitoring of the agency's financial activity must be done in a manner that is as accurate and timely as possible because the significance of the data representing the agency's current financial activity loses its importance as time passes. If management is to make sound decisions regarding the future of the agency, it must have timely information measuring the results of decisions it has made previously. This can be accomplished by having the financial statements prepared and presented to the agency's governing body on no less than a monthly basis. The financial statements should be accompanied by analytical reports that indicate variances between the actual and budgeted monthly and year-to-date levels of activity.

Suggested variance reports include the following:

- employee productivity (total visits, mileage, visit and nonvisit time, average visits per day)
- payroll hours (regular, overtime, on-call, etc.)
- visits by discipline/payer
- free care, allowances, and bad debts
- accounts receivable turnover (aged by date/payer source)
- inventory withdrawals (patient and administrative)
- sources of referrals

These reports, in conjunction with any other variance reports an agency determines to be appropriate for management and supervisory staff to monitor their areas of responsibility, are essential to good budgetary control.

REFERENCE

Department of Health and Human Services. (1966). *Medicare home health agency manual* (5:71). Washington, DC: U.S. Government Printing Office.

BIBLIOGRAPHY

Frank, Barry H. (1989, December). Independent contractor vs. employee: Guidelines for the practitioner. *Practical Accountant.*

National League for Nursing and Council of Home Health Agencies and Community Services. (1979). *Productivity (home visits per day per employee).* New York: Author.

Rasmussen, B. (1992). Contracts and fees: Parts 1, 2, and 3. *Clinical Management, 12*, No. 2; No. 3; No. 4.

Serluco, R.J., & Institute of Public and Private Service, Trenton State College. (1984). *Innovative financial management and reimbursement strategies for the home care agency.* Trenton, NJ: Trenton State College.

CHAPTER 49

Reimbursement

Charlotte L. Kohler

Home care expenditures for the federal government have grown by $10 billion since 1993. Home care costs in 1987 were a small portion of total health care costs, estimated at $4.1 billion, but were projected by the U.S. Department of Commerce to be $26.5 billion in 1995, or 3% of the national health care spending. This 60.6% increase is one reason why Medicare (and Congress) is very much interested in home care as an industry. Although this continual increase was spurred, in part, by the federal government (i.e., Medicare) and other insurance carriers seeking alternative ways to hold costs down, perhaps the biggest push in the growth of home care came from managed care and hospitals/hospital systems seeking more cost-effective ways to provide care. For example, many managed care organizations (MCOs) and hospitals have mandated home care as a component of postpartum care for the new mother and baby as the hospital length of stay has been shortened. Overall, home care providers have also been increasing the types and sophistication of services provided.

A survey by SMG Marketing of Chicago identified up to 14 types of services offered by home care providers directly by agency personnel or by a contractor. These included intravenous (IV) infusion care, new birth services, pharmaceuticals, durable medical equipment (DME), and day care/personal service care,

among others. In many cases, a "primary" agency, under contract or agreement, will be responsible for coordinating or triaging all home care services to other home care providers because of geographic coverage or specialty requirements or limitations. Technology continues to play a part in the growth of home care. Services requiring sophisticated and stationary equipment can now be provided in the home care setting with miniaturized versions. Applications, such as new methods of treating severe wounds (e.g., decubitus ulcers), allow this care to be home based. Increased use of home care is often cost/benefit based, given the increased cost of hospital or other inpatient facility daily care.

Over the years, the ownership of the home health agency (HHA) has changed. HHAs started out as independent or visiting nurse associations (VNAs), but there has been a progressive change from these independent (often nurse-driven) agencies to those owned by larger business entities and hospitals. Between 1980 and 1990 the number of community hospital home health programs increased from 610 to 1,801, according to the American Hospital Association. The Health Care Financing Administration (HCFA) has reported growth in Medicare-certified agencies from 1989 to 1995 to be over 200%, or 9,147 agencies at the end of 1995. Some of these programs were developed by the acquisition of local agencies, and a few were developed from within the hospitals. Many individual agencies became part of a regional chain, with smaller chains merging into large industry leaders, and hospital-based agencies (or VNAs) consolidating into a component of an integrated delivery system (IDS) or a unit of the MCO. Consolidation has been forced over the last several years by competition and a focus on cost reduction. Hospitals first entered the market with expectations of engaging in a money-making venture, but now that dream has been replaced by the need to "position" the agency in a way that will allow it to secure MCO contracts and/or be part of an IDS that needs to minimize the leakage of patients out of the system and that was established to provide the continuum of care with less expensive alternatives. Over the years, hospitals and managed care programs have learned to move patients through a system with more physician/clinical overview of treatment and utilization; this has proved the strength of the affiliated or owned agencies in surviving Medicare restrictions on payment.

In a recent article in *Modern Healthcare*, Greene (1996) discusses the significant growth in home care as a key to the IDS strategy. Others have attributed this growth of the required coordination of care after hospitalization to the movement of patients more quickly out of the hospital, in part as a result of the prospective payment system (PPS) of the hospitals. In a more recent article in *Outreach*, Schaffer (1996) explains the trend in hospitals to use home care as a means of securing managed care contracts by using lower-cost home care to offset costly acute hospital care (and reduce the number of days of stay) in a continuum of care approach. Based on a multiunit provider survey in 1995, hospital-based agencies grew 156.5% between 1993 and 1994, and profits in the last quarter of 1995 increased by 12% over those of 1994 (Lutz, 1996).

This chapter covers current reimbursement trends for home health care services with a concentration on Medicare because Medicare still

pays for a substantial portion of home care provided (Shaw, 1985; Stewart, 1979). The chapter concentrates on the basic aspects of current Medicare reimbursement and addresses changes that are being proposed by HCFA and the major home care industry organizations. Medicare has been the most restrictive agency in determining eligibility for coverage, and it is a good starting point in a discussion of reimbursement. Already we have seen that the major changes for home care have not been HCFA reimbursement driven, but have been responsive to the initiatives of MCOs. Nevertheless, HCFA has tried to jump-start a movement to a PPS for home care. Early efforts in the 1980s were dropped, and demonstration projects were started again in 1995. Congressional activity regarding home care has increased as a result of pilot projects in Texas and New York that found improper billing in 40% of the cases reviewed (Weissenstein, 1996). Operation Restore Trust is the Department of Health and Human Services (DHHS) program initiated in 1996 to stamp out fraud and unnecessary costs in home care paid for by Medicare. The White House estimates that $3.5 billion could be saved over a 6-year period.

Cost containment parallels the continuity of care focus of Medicare and other payers. Managed care and other insurers or approvers of care are less restrictive in coverage, but being part of the payer's panel has become more restrictive in the marketplace because of its exclusive contracting goals. Consequently, the home care administrator's knowledge level must be increased regarding contracting and knowing the cost to provide specific services for which the organization is contracting. The contract is often offered at reduced rates or for differentiated services, unlike those provided to Medicare patients.

CURRENT MEDICARE REIMBURSEMENT TRENDS

The federal government provides home health care or funding for such care under a variety of programs created by the Social Security Act, including Medicare (Social Security Act Title XVIII), Medicaid (Social Security Act Title XIX), and the Older Americans Act (P.L. 89-73, 1965; P.L. 98-459, 1984), to name a few. These programs provide specific approaches and funding for specific aspects of home care. Medicare was enacted July 30, 1965, and became effective on what has since become known as M Day, July 1, 1966. Medicare is a two-part program commonly referred to as Part A Medicare and Part B Medicare. Under Part A Medicare, beneficiaries receive certain insurance coverage for hospitalization, specifically defined medical care provided in a skilled nursing facility, and specifically defined home health care. In addition to Part A coverage, Medicare beneficiaries may purchase, for a small monthly premium, supplemental insurance for Part B coverage. The 1996 monthly premium paid by the patient for Part B Medicare was $42.50. The monthly premium is determined by a formula that sets the rate at 25% of the aggregate amount needed to cover program costs. Physician services provided on an outpatient (physician's office) basis, pathology services, outpatient hospital services, and others are covered by Part B. On July 1, 1981, Part A began to pay for home health services to beneficiaries who are covered by both Part A and Part B. There are currently no deductibles or coinsurance amounts charged to the patient for home health services (with the exception of DME); however, a PPS for home care may include one.

Medicare is an entitlement program with benefits offered to persons who are at least 65 years of age and eligible for Social Security retirement benefits, who are younger than 65 but have been eligible for at least 2 years for Social Security benefits as a result of a disability, or who have end-stage renal disease. There are six types of services for which Medicare provides reimbursement under its home care schedule of benefits: skilled nursing, home health aide service, physical therapy, occupational therapy, speech therapy, and medical social work.

Skilled nursing is care rendered by a licensed nurse or care provided under direct supervision. Observation and assessment, care of wounds, administration of injections, and patient teaching are some of the many services provided as part of skilled nursing. For HHAs to be reimbursed, patients must require skilled care on a part-time (less than 1 hour per visit with the exception of home health aides) or intermittent basis. To be considered intermittent, care must be for a medically predictable, recurring need for which the patient requires skilled nursing at least once every 60 days. Currently, intermittent skilled nursing visits are allowed on a daily basis for up to 8 hours a day for up to 3 weeks. The interpretation of intermittent care has been the subject of much debate and confusion between HCFA and HHAs and often centers on the definition of *homebound*. Additional confusion exists when a minimum number of skilled nursing visits per week are mandated (e.g., three per week) to warrant the medical necessity aspect of home care nursing.

Complementing skilled nursing is home health aide service. A home health aide performs many necessary, although nonmedical, tasks such as helping patients with personal hygiene, retraining the patient in self-help skills, and performing certain household services such as changing the bed. However, household services are limited to the medical needs of the patient and not to general cleaning services. The services provided by the home health aide must be determined by a registered nurse and not by the home health aide. Like skilled nursing, home health aide services may be provided only in the patient's home and should conform with the guidelines for intermittent care. Any care provided in a skilled nursing or hospital facility is part of that facility's costs and will not come under the home care reimbursement provisions (and the facility should pay for the care provided by the HHA, if it had requested the service).

Additional types of home health care provided for under Medicare Part A are physical therapy and speech therapy. Occupational therapy helps beneficiaries gain the necessary skills to resume the activities of daily living, and physical therapy helps patients regain physical functional skills such as increased mobility. Speech therapy is provided to help patients overcome speech problems, and for these services to be covered by Medicare, there must generally be a restorative potential demonstrated in the treatment of the patient. Medicare will allow several visits to teach a patient how to maintain function if there is no restorative potential. Although physical therapy and speech therapy are services that can be rendered either at the patient's home or in a hospital outpatient department, skilled nursing facility, or rehabilitation center, only when the services are actually rendered at a patient's home will they be reimbursed under Medicare's home care provision. Social work services such as counseling and referral to appropriate community agencies are covered by Medicare if they are considered necessary to further a patient's medical progress. Recently, this was interpreted to include the spouse when he or she becomes emotionally unable to care for the Medicare beneficiary who has Alzheimer's disease. To receive any of these home health services, Medicare beneficiaries must meet program requirements. The beneficiary must be *homebound*.

To be considered homebound, the patient must have physical impairments that make access to outside care difficult. The patient need not be bedridden. Lack of readily available transportation, however, does not constitute homebound status. The program also requires that the beneficiary must be under the care of a physician (including doctors of medicine, osteopathy, and podiatry) and that the physician place the order for care prior to the initial visit. In addition, the physician must submit a plan of treatment (POT) in writing to the appropriate fiscal intermediary (FI). The POT is reported on HCFA Forms 485 and 486 may be requested with the initial claim.

The FI is the third party designated by HCFA to process claims and payment contractually to Medicare providers. The POT must be reviewed and signed by the attending physician and an agent of the HHA at least every 2 months. If a recertification has not been made and home health services have not been provided in 60 days, the home health plan is considered terminated by Medicare.

BASIC TENETS OF MEDICARE REIMBURSEMENT

Methods of Reimbursement

Under the Medicare program there are three methods of determining reimbursement to providers: reasonable cost, lower of amount charged or fee schedule, and prospective payment. Currently, HHAs are reimbursed under the reasonable cost method, that is, on the basis of the cost deemed necessary to deliver services efficiently to beneficiaries subject to a mandated limit. This method takes into consideration both direct and indirect costs. To determine reimbursable costs, HCFA carries out a process called cost finding by a standardized reporting of data. This is accomplished by having the HHAs complete the Cost Report (HCFA Form 1728); the methodology used in the cost report is discussed below.

Cost-based reimbursement must be distinguished from charged-based reimbursement and prospective payment. Charge-based reimbursement is generally used under the Part B portion of the Medicare program. Under this process, Medicare uses the amount billed (charges) as one measurement for the basis of payment. Providers that fall under this methodology are reimbursed at the amount of current charges or the current Medicare Fee Schedule (effective after December 31, 1991), whichever is lower. Physicians, DME suppliers, and hospital outpatient services are reimbursed under this methodology. The PPS, as the term implies, is the methodology that reimburses hospitals for inpatient services at a predetermined rate. The hospital PPS was enacted as part of the Tax Equity and Fiscal Responsibility Act of 1982 (TEFRA). A fixed amount is paid to hospitals according to each patient's admitting and/or discharge diagnosis, which is categorized into a diagnosis-related group (DRG). The hospital receives a fixed per DRG payment regardless of service intensity (except for certain outliers), which may vary as a result of intragroup differences in severity of illness. The general concept is that the hospital must manage its use of resources to provide the required care within the average amounts paid. To the extent that the hospital is able to provide care for less, the difference can be kept. This provides the incentive for reduction of costs.

The amount paid under the Medicare hospice provisions is a type of prospective payment methodology. Efficient use of resources is rewarded. Generally speaking, under the Medicare PPS, if the hospital (or hospice) incurs less than the payment under that specific DRG-based (or set payment) PPS payment, the difference (or profit) is kept. If either the hospital or hospice incurs more than the PPS payment, no more is received unless the patient falls within an outlier status. In both cases, the hospital and the hospice have the opportunity to offset profits and losses for each case because the limit is calculated on an aggregate basis.

The last area that may be of interest to the HHA in terms of reimbursement is the various ways in which the HHA can be paid for medical supplies. Medical supplies must be broken down between routine and nonroutine supplies. Nonroutine supplies, requiring specific orders from the physician, include IV supplies, ostomy supplies, catheter supplies, syringes and needles, and home testing equipment (such as home glucose monitor strips). For DME, the HHA must use the cost of the DME (nonroutine supplies) on the cost report, since other costs must be allocated to it, but it must obtain a Part B provider number and bill (and collect) based on the DME fee schedule and limitations. There is a 20% copayment. In addition, corporate reorganization is generally needed to maintain appropriate reimbursement for DME from those

of the home care services without falling into the necessary allocation of costs from Medicare.

Cost Finding through the Cost Report

Because of the implications of cost-based reimbursement, a working knowledge of the cost-finding process and a knowledge of cost accounting are basic management skills. Cost finding is the process of identifying those costs that are to be reimbursed as defined by the Medicare regulations. This is a regulatory process that can have little to do with the actual cost of providing services, but rather is the methodology prescribed (required) by the Medicare program. Cost accounting, on the other hand, measures the resources (expenses) required for each service based on the actual use of the resource, and allocates overhead (or non–directly related expenses) based on its use of the overhead. The methodology is internally developed based on accounting principles and studies of the specific agency's approach to patient care and business.

Because of the unique Medicare regulation requirements, the mechanics of cost finding must be understood because it has an impact on all costs to other payers as well—even if only for its absence of cost-accounting common sense. Nevertheless, in discussing the overall intent of the Medicare rules of cost finding, two major goals of the principles of reimbursement as stated in 42 CFR 405.402 have been noted (Booth, 1985):

1. There is a division of the allowable costs between the beneficiaries of this program and the other payers' patients of the agency that takes account of actual use of services by the beneficiaries of the program.
2. There should be a recognition of the need for hospitals and other providers to keep pace with growing needs and to make improvements.

To identify appropriate costs, the HCFA requires HHAs and other home health providers

Exhibit 49–1 Cost Report Form

Worksheet S & S-1	HHA cost report—identification and certification This first page of the report shows the identification name and provider number as well as details of visits, statistics, and the composition of full-time equivalent employees. This cover page is also where the report is signed and certified by the responsible officer of the HHA.
Worksheet A	Reclassification and adjustment of trial balance of expenses Worksheet A shows the total expenses per the general ledger trial balance and the impact of adjustments and reclassification, leading to total costs available for cost allocation on Worksheet B.
Worksheet A-1	Compensation analysis, salaries, and wages Worksheet A-1 provides details of total employee compensation.
Worksheet A-2	Compensation analysis, employee benefits (payroll related) Worksheet A-2 provides details of employee fringe benefits.
Worksheet A-3	Compensation analysis, contracted services/purchased services Worksheet A-3 provides details of amounts paid for personal services of independent contractors.
Worksheet A-4	Reclassification Worksheet A-4 is used to detail reclassification between cost centers as shown in column 7 of Worksheet A.
Worksheet A-5	Adjustments to expenses Worksheet A-5 is used to furnish details of adjustments to general ledger trial balance expenses as shown in column 9 of Worksheet A.
Worksheet A-6	Statement of costs of services from related organizations Where Worksheet A includes costs of goods or services purchased from related organizations, the identity of the related parties and the overall cost amounts are detailed in Worksheet A-6.
Worksheet A-7	Depreciation Details as to any depreciation expense included on Worksheet A are provided on Worksheet A-7.
Worksheet A-8	Reasonable cost determination for physical therapy services furnished by outside suppliers Where independent physical therapists are used to provide patient services, Worksheet A-8 is used to compute the salary and travel Medicare limitations for comparison against actual expenses.
Worksheet B	Cost allocation—general service cost The general service cost centers are allocated among the specific service cost centers on Worksheet B.
Worksheet B-1	Cost allocation—statistical basis The statistical data supporting the allocation of general service cost centers as reflected on Worksheet B are detailed on Worksheet B-1.
Worksheet C	Apportionment of patient service costs Worksheet C shows the computations of actual costs per visit and the cost limitations applicable to each discipline and to DME sold or rented as well as cost of medical supplies.

continues

Exhibit 49–1 continued

Worksheet D	Calculation of reimbursement settlement
	Worksheet D furnishes the bottom line of the cost report, comparing net total allowable costs against interim payments and yielding the net overpayment or underpayment of the Medicare program for the HHA.
Worksheet D-1	Analysis of payments to providers
	The details of interim payments to the provider during the cost report are furnished on Worksheet D-1.
Worksheet D-2	Calculations of reimbursable bad debts
	Where total allowable costs include Medicare bad debts (deductibles and copayment only), the summary details are provided on Worksheet D-2.
Worksheet D-3	Recovery of unreimbursed cost
	The carryover of unreimbursed cost under the lesser of cost or charges is shown on Worksheet D-3.
Worksheet F	Balance sheet
	The balance sheet of the provider, by fund type, is furnished on Worksheet F.
Worksheet F-1	Statement of revenue and expenses
	The income statement of the provider is provided on Worksheet F-1.
Worksheet F-2	Statement of changes in fund balances
	Changes in the fund balance accounts of the provider, by fund type, are detailed in Worksheet F-2.
Worksheet F-3	Return on equity capital of proprietary providers
	This schedule, applicable to proprietary providers, details the computation of allowable return on equity capital includable in allowable costs.
Worksheet K	Cost and data report
	This schedule furnishes information of a general nature regarding the hospice.
Worksheet K-1	Patient care service utilization analysis
	Worksheet K-1 provides for reporting of visiting service data applicable to the four levels of hospice care.
Worksheet K-2	Analysis of direct costs
	This schedule shows the expenses account trial balance for the hospice.
Worksheet K-3	General service cost allocation statistics
	Worksheet K-3 furnishes the statistical data necessary to compute the allocation of HHA general service cost centers to hospice cost centers.
Worksheet K-4	Hospice general service cost allocation statistics
	Worksheet K-4 provides the statistical data necessary to alleviate the general service costs of the hospice that are included in the hospice cost center.
Worksheet K-5	Analysis of shared services
	This schedule provides for the identification of shared service data for the HHA and the hospice.

Source: Reprinted from HCFA, Form 1728.

to complete a predefined cost report form (Form 1728). The cost report is a financial summary that must be submitted at the end of the provider's fiscal year (FY). It contains a number of schedules that are designed to identify Medicare home health costs (Exhibit 49–1). It is important to realize that, through the use of adjustments required by regulations and nonallowable expenses, Medicare regulations will reduce the expenses of HHAs to Medicare-allowable costs.

Cost reporting involves a three-step process: allocation, cost finding, and cost settlement (Figure 49–1). The first step in the process is to allocate expenses by Medicare-defined cost centers. A cost center is an administrative unit or subunit defined by Medicare that in theory provides a specified service. Cost centers are divided into three different areas: reimbursable services, nonreimbursable services, and general services. Those services included under reimbursable costs are skilled nursing, home health aide services, physical therapy, and the other Medicare-covered services. Nonreimbursable services include non–Medicare-covered services such as home dialysis, homemaker service, private-duty nursing, meal services, and health promotion activities. General services include administration, plant operation and maintenance, and depreciation on buildings and fixed equipment. This breakdown is accomplished on Worksheet A on the cost report.

Both direct and indirect costs are allocated by cost center. Direct costs are any costs incurred for the benefit of and traceable to a specific cost center. Salaries of employees, such as registered nurses and physical therapists, are direct costs that may be allocated to the specific reimbursable cost center. Indirect costs are those incurred for the benefit of the organization as a whole. The costs of administration, depreciation, and accounting are indirect because they benefit the entire HHA. Moreover, all other costs under the general service cost center are indirect.

At this point, adjustments are made on Worksheet A. Certain adjustments are required, such as adjustments for insurance and interest. Other adjustments for nonallowable costs must be

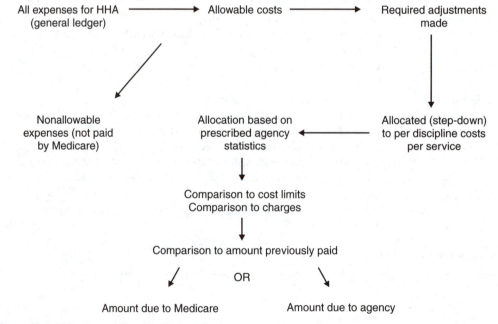

Figure 49–1 Flowchart of Cost Finding and Settlement

Exhibit 49–2 Nonallowable Medicare Costs for HHAs

Generally, costs will be allowable for Medicare purposes where they are related to patient care and conform to the prudent buyer concept. Under this concept, costs will be minimized by arm's-length bargaining for the best available prices and terms.

Following is a partial listing of costs that have been found to be unallowable for Medicare purposes:

- Federal income and excise taxes
- Net operating losses
- Advertising (for the purpose of increasing patient utilization or for fund-raising purposes)
- Research
- Uninsured theft and casualty losses (where insurance was available)
- Life insurance premiums (where the provider is a direct or indirect beneficiary of a policy on the life of an owner, key employee, provider-based physician, or officer)
- Bad debts (unless specifically attributable to unpaid Medicare deductibles or coinsurance)
- Charity and courtesy allowances (these are reductions of revenue)
- Compensation of owners in excess of a reasonable allowance
- Accelerated depreciation
- Interest expense (to the extent of interest income; any excess over interest income is allowable, however)
- Legal fees (incurred in the defense of criminal charges)
- Costs of meals sold to visitors

- Costs of drugs sold to persons other than patients, including employees
- Costs of the operation of a gift shop
- Alcoholic beverages for medical staff meetings
- Meals-on-Wheels
- Political contributions
- Nonvisiting costs (including school visit programs and well baby programs)
- Contracted services where the contract term exceeds 5 years
- Costs of drugs in excess of the maximum allowable cost limitation
- Fines and penalties
- Taxes that could have been avoided by a legally available exemption
- Reorganization costs
- Membership dues and costs in social and fraternal organizations
- Malpractice and general liability losses and related expenses where the provider is uninsured
- Costs of influencing employees in respect to proposed unionization
- Possibly, 800 number costs
- Possibly, cellular telephone costs

Following are costs that are not allowable in full in the year in which they were incurred but are allocable as amortized over a period of years:

- Special water and sewage assessments (these should be capitalized and depreciated)
- Start-up costs (amortizable over 60 months)
- Issue costs for stocks or bonds (amortizable)

Source: From HCFA.

made before cost finding is started (Exhibit 49–2). The regulations identify the entries to be made. Specific reference is made to those costs that Medicare may find excessive, such as excessive compensation of the executive director or administrator.

Once costs have been allocated on Worksheet A, the second step in the process is to separate Medicare and non-Medicare costs. In assigning costs as either Medicare or non-Medicare, providers must carry out a process known as cost finding, which consists of allocating indirect costs to reimbursable and nonreimbursable services. This is accomplished on Worksheet B (and B-1). This method recognizes that services are rendered by certain non–revenue-producing centers as well as by revenue-producing centers. The stepping down (allocation) of costs is performed on a statistical basis. The statistics are developed on Worksheet B-1 using the requirements and guidelines as set forth in the regulations. Specifically, an HHA must allocate general service cost centers in the order prescribed by regulation, using the required statistical allocation basis. If permission is obtained from the FI, as discussed under Discrete Costing later in this chapter, the allocation may be done in a different order or with the use of some other statistical basis; otherwise the order and the statistical basis as listed below must be used.

- *Depreciation—Building and Fixtures*: This cost center includes not only depreciation but also other expenses pertaining thereto, including insurance, interest, rent, and real property taxes. Costs should be allocated to each cost center based upon the proportion of square feet occupied by that cost center to total square feet.
- *Depreciation—Movable Equipment*: This cost center includes expenses closely related to movable equipment such as interest and personal property taxes, in addition to depreciation on such equipment. Costs should be allocated according to square feet, similar to the allocation done for building and fixtures.
- *Transportation*: The transportation cost center includes the cost of vehicles owned or rented. Costs should generally be allocated on the basis of miles per cost center. As an alternative to this statistical allocation basis, weighted trips may be elected upon request.
- *Administrative and General*: Administrative and general expenses should be allocated on the basis of net costs per cost center after reclassification, adjustments,

and the allocation of other general service cost centers.

Where a given cost center has a negative balance immediately prior to the allocation of administrative and general expenses, such cost center should not be included in the allocation base. Total indirect costs, such as those for administration, are divided by a unit multiplier set by the provider. Transportation costs, for example, are distributed on the basis of mileage; depreciation of buildings and fixtures and plant operation and maintenance are allocated by square foot usage by the various cost centers. Depreciation costs for movable equipment are distributed by dollar value; administrative and general costs are allocated by accumulated costs.

Cost finding calls for the distribution of these indirect costs on a per discipline basis. That is, indirect costs are distributed to skilled nursing, speech therapy, medical social work, and the other types of covered and noncovered services. The allocated, indirect costs for each of these areas are added to the expense derived from the original direct cost allocation (general ledger distribution) of expenses by cost center. The sum represents the total costs by Medicare-defined reimbursable and nonreimbursable cost centers. The next step in the cost-finding process is identifying the per visit cost by discipline. This is done on Worksheet C. This is simply the total per discipline costs divided by the number of visits. For example, if the results of the allocation and step-down indicate that the cost for skilled nursing is $528,398.00 for 10,125 visits, then the cost per visit is $52.19. Medicare reimburses providers on the basis of per discipline visit costs subject to certain aggregated upper limits (current reasonable *cost limit* provisions are discussed below). Therefore, the last step in this process is to determine whether the agency is below the aggregate cost limit and therefore can be reimbursed for all its costs. There are some specific exemption of limit filings that can be done to allow an HHA higher reimbursement, but these must be handled carefully and by experienced reimbursement advisors.

The final step in the cost-reporting process is the calculation of the reimbursement settlement. On Worksheet D the provider's reimbursable costs are applied against a variety of payment adjustments, including payments already made under the periodic interim payment (PIP) program (see section on PIP) and lower of cost or charges limitation. If there has been an excess of reimbursement to the provider, the provider must remit the amount due to Medicare with the cost report. If there has been an underpayment to the provider, the provider will be reimbursed the deficit after a desk review of the cost report by FI. The cost report is due 5 months after the end of the agency's FY.

The remainder of the cost report consists of financial statements, including a balance sheet and statement of revenue and expenses, and certain other required disclosures, including the Provider Cost Report Reimbursement Questionnaire (HCFA Form 339) and the Summary of Medicare Uncollectibles. Exhibit 49–3 explains Form 339 in more detail.

Changes in the statistical basis can have a dramatic effect on the Medicare reimbursement received. That is why careful planning by means of a pro forma cost report is necessary to avoid an unfavorable effect on Medicare reimbursement: one can actually see the financial impact of any proposed change. This is of specific concern when managed care contracting is done within a Medicare HHA.

The Summary of Medicare: Uncollectibles provides a unique opportunity to recover any Medicare copayments or deductibles (should there be any established by Congress). The important point to remember is that there are strict documentation standards and the required adherence to claim the recovery.

Cost Limits

Cost limits are the predetermined maximums placed on per visit reimbursable costs by discipline to ensure the efficient delivery of care.

Section 223 of the Social Security Amendments of 1972 granted the authority for limits to be set on the costs that Medicare would recognize as reasonable for the overall efficient delivery of health services. Cost limits are developed using labor and nonlabor costs as separate costs. Before July 1, 1985, and after the Omnibus Reconciliation Act of 1986 (P.L. 99-509), the limits were based on the aggregate: the per discipline limits were established by type of service and compared with the per discipline costs in the aggregate based on the number of visits for each type of service. The aggregate was used to determined whether the HHA was above the limit. In the short period in between, the limit was issued and its impact calculated by the individual disciplines without the offset of gain of one discipline's offsetting the loss of another discipline.

Each year the *Federal Register* sets forth a new schedule of limits on HHA costs for cost-reporting periods as developed by HCFA. However, there had been a freeze on the cost limits. For cost reporting periods starting after October 1, 1996, HCFA imposed an across-the-board 1.078 budget neutrality adjustment on the wage index component of the cost limit. This revision was made in November 1996. As the cost limit concept is discussed below, understand that budget neutrality is a concept of ensuring that no more is paid than prior to any increase. Table 49–1 illustrates what impact the new (1996–1997) limits, including the budget neutrality adjustment, can have on a large HHA. Although the goal is to establish cost limits based on the actual costs in the industry, there has been a problem in obtaining reliable information on a current basis. The wage index used has often been questioned. In setting limits, HCFA first pulls information about costs per visit from the filed and audited cost reports. Consequently, there can be a significant lag between the cost-reporting periods and the time when limits are set, requiring adjustments by HCFA to reflect the best guess of what the current year's costs should be. In recent years, HCFA has updated cost information on a more timely basis and has

Exhibit 49–3 HCFA Form 339

Provider Cost Report Reimbursement Questionnaire Form (Required Attachment on the Medicare Cost Report)

Medicare continues its efforts to identify the payments made to owners and other employees who have significant authority within a home care agency. The HCFA Form 339 always provided some information, but now the level and detail of information requested have paled previous reporting requirements. Effective for cost reports filed for fiscal years ended November 30, 1995, and later, an expanded HCFA Form 339 is required. The most significant changes to this questionnaire are as follows:

Exhibit 6: Owners/Management Personnel Compensation

"Management personnel" are defined as persons "in positions that have influence or control of your operations and/or your ability to prepare an adequate cost report." At a minimum, HCFA lists the following as examples: executive director, medical director, nursing director, controller/financial officer, billing director. Beyond the specific employment title, HCFA requires the top 10 compensated "management personnel" to be included in Exhibit 6 filings.

In addition to completing Exhibit 6 itself, the job description and copy of the W-2 must be attached for each position.

A second group of individuals fall within the reporting requirements of HCFA 339: "Immediate relatives" are defined as spouse, parent, child, sibling, adopted child (or parent, stepparent, child, or sibling), all in-laws one generation up or down and their spouses or siblings. This second group is also required to file a completed Exhibit 6 with the related-job description and copy of the W-2.

Exhibit 7: Wage Related Cost Care

The datum required for this filing is a required resummarization of expenses from the way in which costs are normally allocated within the general ledger of the HHA. *At this point,* Exhibit 7 is *not required* for HHAs. However, it does include the following:

Retirement costs:
1. 401K employer contributions
2. Tax sheltered annuity (TSA) employer contribution
3. Qualified and nonqualified pension plan cost
4. Prior year pension service cost

Plan admin. costs (paid to external org.):
5. 401K/TSA plan administration fees
6. Legal/accounting/management fees—pension plan
7. Employee managed care program administration fees

Health and insurance costs:
8. Health insurance (purchased or self-funded)
9. Prescription drug plan
10. Dental, hearing and vision plans
11. Life insurance[*]
12. Accident insurance[*]
13. Disability insurance[*]
14. Long-term care insurance[*]
15. Workers' compensation insurance
16. Retiree health care cost (current year portion only—not the extraordinary accrual required by FASB 106)

Taxes:
17. FICA—employer's portion only
18. Medicare taxes—employer's portion only
19. Unemployment insurance
20. State or federal unemployment taxes

Other:
21. Executive deferred compensation
22. Day care cost and allowances
23. Tuition reimbursement
   [*]If employee is owner or beneficiary.

Source: From HCFA, Form 339.

Table 49–1 Impact of New Cost Limits on Baltimore Area HHAs

	Skilled Nursing	PT	ST	OT	MSW	HHA	Total
Labor portion	$76.57	$83.84	$84.11	$83.41	$110.59	$37.14	
Wage index—MSA adjustment	0.9865	0.9865	0.9865	0.9865	0.9865	0.9865	
Budget neutrality	1.078	1.078	1.078	1.078	1.078	1.078	
Adjusted labor portion	$81.43	$89.16	$89.45	$88.70	$117.61	$39.50	
Nonlabor portion	21.62	23.59	23.88	23.84	31.46	10.56	
Cost limit FYE 6/30/97	$103.05	$112.75	$113.33	$112.54	$149.07	$50.06	
FY adjustment factor	1.01524	1.01524	1.01524	1.01524	1.01524	1.01524	
Cost limit FYE 12/31/97	$104.62	$114.47	$115.05	$114.26	$151.34	$50.82	
Current cost limits	99.55	100.25	101.75	100.17	141.53	50.20	
Net change	5.07	14.22	13.30	14.09	9.81	0.62	
Number of visits by discipline	× 21,630	8,640	4,320	3,800	6,870	17,280	
Impact	$109,664	$122,860	$57,456	$53,542	$67,383	$10,714	$421,576

Source: Reprinted from *Federal Register* 61(127) July 1, 1996, and November 1996 HCFA Program Memorandum A-96-11.

worked to develop price indices that are more truly HHA related, which is a marketbasket of the goods and services used by the home health industry. The current cost limits are based primarily on 1995 wage index effective July 1, 1996. The HHA price index is monitored by the HCFA in an effort to minimize the difference between the estimated marketbasket rate and the actual rate which is why the positive budget neutrality factor was warranted.

The second step used by Medicare in setting per visit limits is to divide each cost limit into the labor and nonlabor components of costs so that an adjustment may be made to the labor portion of costs based on the location of the HHA. Referring to the price index, labor costs include employees' wages and benefits and a share of the contract services and are 79.25% of the limit (down slightly from 79.301% in the 1993 cost limit). The wage portion of costs is adjusted by multiplying it by the appropriate metropolitan statistical area (MSA) index based on the location of the HHA. This specific area adjustment is illustrated in Table 49–2. This wage component would be added to the nonwage component to equal the limit for that discipline within that region. Each HHA should receive a notice from the FI indicating the appropriate limits to use for Worksheet C of the Medicare cost report.

As a result of the increased limits, all agencies will have an easier time maintaining profitability until a prospective reimbursement system is implemented.

To explain further the mechanics used by HCFA, before HCFA establishes the wage portion of costs, the cost data are screened for outliers. These are costs that are either above or below the mean (arithmetic average) cost by a predetermined range. To screen for outliers, the cost data are transformed into their natural logarithms to determine the mean cost and standard deviation for each group. All costs not within two standard deviations of the mean are excluded from the calculation of the mean. A per service limit is then determined. Currently, the basic service limit is 112% of the mean labor and nonlabor portions of the cost per visit.

Table 49–2 The Limits for 1996 Are Compared with Limits for 1993

| | Per Visit Visit Limit | | | |
| | Urban | | Rural | |
TYPE OF SERVICE	1993	1996	1993	1996
Skilled Nursing	96.17	104.16	105.52	116.60
Physical Therapy	96.79	113.97	111.57	127.26
Speech Pathology	98.29	114.55	116.73	138.90
Occupational Therapy	96.77	113.76	113.09	137.49
Medical Social Worker	136.72	150.68	173.95	195.72
Home Health Aide	48.50	50.60	48.94	50.63

Source: Reprinted from *Federal Register* 61(127), July 1, 1996, p. 34353 and November 1996 HCFA Program Memorandum A-96-11.

To account for a variety of circumstances, adjustments are made to the service limits. These include an adjustment for hospital-based HHAs and an adjustment for the fiscal reporting year that is different from the years that coincide with the limit's effective date. The first adjustment was designed to account for the higher administrative and general costs related to the Medicare cost allocation requirement for hospitals. The *Federal Register* of January 6, 1994, published regulations for the elimination of the additional payment for administrative and general costs of hospital-based HHAs effective for cost-reporting periods on or after October 1, 1993 (Medicare Program, 1994). The adjustment for the cost-reporting year helps account for the higher prices that HHAs will be expected to pay after the limits have become effective; in terms of inflation, these adjust for increases relating to inflationary pressures.

"Before the limits are applied at cost settlement, the provider's actual costs will be reduced by the amount of individual items of cost (for example, administrative compensation or contract services) that are found to be excessive under Medicare principles of provider reimbursement" (*Federal Register*, 1996, p. 104). In this way, Medicare reduces costs during the cost-finding process before the question of cost limitation is to be addressed.

Under certain circumstances, a new provider can request an exception from the cost report for discipline limits. To qualify, the agency must demonstrate that the limits were exceeded as a result of the initial setup to comply with Medicare regulations of participation. HCFA strictly enforces the new agency requirements and will not consider a newly certified Medicare agency that preexisted as a non-Medicare agency a new Medicare agency (Department of Health and Human Services, 1985).

In addition to limits based on per discipline costs, there is also a limit based on the lower of costs or charges. This is the only case where charges have a basis for determining the reimbursement under Part A. The theory behind this limitation is that the provider must charge an amount at least equal to (or greater than) cost. Should the provider charge an amount (in the aggregate) less than cost, the amount charged will be the maximum that the provider can receive from Medicare. This is true even if the provider is under the per discipline limits. Amounts not received as a result of this limitation can be carried forward until the difference between cost and charges is enough to absorb the carry forward.

PIP

HHAs are reimbursed on the basis of the lower of reasonable costs or customary charges.

Reasonable costs are developed through the Medicare cost report and cost-finding process. *Customary charges* are the aggregate amount billed by the HHA. There are other limits, as previously discussed, based on an aggregated per discipline amount.

There are three different methods by which payments are made to HHAs on an interim basis, that is, during the course of the year as services are provided. In practice, most FIs use all three and use the first two to validate the amount to be paid via the third. Of course, as with any cost-based reimbursement procedure, the annual cost report will determine the final allowable costs of the provider; hence, any overpayment or underpayment for the period will be settled.

Of the three Medicare payment methods, the per visit method is the most basic. Under the per visit method, estimated total Medicare costs of the provider based on the prior year cost report are divided by total estimated Medicare visits to yield a cost per visit amount. Because Medicare visits are then billed to the FI, reimbursement will be made at the predetermined cost per visit amount.

Another method used by Medicare FIs to pay providers is based on a percentage of charges. Under this method, an estimate is made of expected total Medicare costs and total Medicare charges for the period. By dividing the charges by the costs, a rate is determined for the reimbursement of the provider. As an example, imagine a provider with anticipated total Medicare costs of $800,000 and anticipated total Medicare charges of $1,000,000; the costs expressed as a percentage of charges would be 80%. For each Medicare visit billed by this provider to the FI, the provider would be reimbursed for 80% of the charges billed. Medicare found that the providers could manipulate reimbursement by increasing charges. Although notification by the provider to the FI is required for any changes in charges, the FIs were not always adjusting the percentage to compensate. To establish better reporting and payment control and to provide an even, expectable payment

from Medicare to health care providers, the PIP method was developed. The PIP method is the third and most popular method of Medicare payment. Under this method, total estimated Medicare costs are reimbursed to the provider evenly at regular intervals. The interval is usually every 2 weeks but can be from weekly to monthly based on the agreement of the provider and the intermediary. The interval is generally established to coincide with HHA payroll requirements. Reimbursement under PIP is available to qualified providers upon election of that provider in a formal written request to the FI. The request for PIP reimbursement is reviewed by the FI, which results in a recommendation to HCFA to allow or disallow the election.

To be eligible for PIP reimbursement, a provider must meet certain qualifications. The HHA must have a total Medicare reimbursement of at least $25,000 for the year or an estimated Medicare reimbursement equal to at least 50% of total allowable costs. In addition, the agency must have already filed at least one acceptable cost report, thus providing the FI with a basis for making an accurate estimation of payments to be made. This requirement generally restricts use of the PIP reimbursement method to providers who have been in operation for at least 1 year. Most important, the provider must possess the capability to maintain accurate and timely data regarding costs, charges, and statistics to monitor properly the status of PIP payments against actual costs. As an additional requirement, a provider that commences PIP reimbursement must first make arrangements to repay any overpayment due to the intermediary under the reimbursement in effect before the conversion to PIP.

Once a PIP reimbursement amount is determined, it will be paid to the provider on a regular basis until modified. Modifications to the PIP reimbursement amount result from any of several different factors. HCFA requires the FI to monitor the PIP status on at least a quarterly basis. The provider is required to furnish a quarterly report of such items as total costs, adjustments to costs, the number of total visits, the number of Medicare visits, total charges for the quarter, and whatever other information the intermediary may need to perform the review and adjustment function. Upon review of the quarterly report, the intermediary may adjust the PIP reimbursement amount accordingly to approximate a break-even position in the final settlement. In some cases, the results of the review of the quarterly report will show that the provider is in an underpayment situation. In these cases, the provider may receive a lump sum adjustment (payment) simultaneous with the adjustment of future PIP payments to compensate for the underpayments. The intermediary is also required to review the PIP reimbursement amount and to adjust as necessary upon its completion of the desk review of the annual Medicare cost report.

On its own, the provider may act to adjust PIP reimbursement amounts whenever it has reason to believe that costs of the provider have decreased (or increased) significantly. Similarly, the FI has the responsibility to act to protect the financial interest of Medicare whenever a provider is found to be in a situation of impending bankruptcy or insolvency. Here, as in all cases, the fundamental objective of the FI is to attempt to ensure that periodic payments made to the provider exactly match the allowable costs, thus avoiding underpayment and overpayment situations.

The FI may terminate the PIP status of a provider based upon the provider's failure to comply with certain standards. Such termination is generally not automatic, and the standards are used more as general guidelines. If the provider's cost reports show an overpayment situation on a consistent basis (within prescribed parameters), the FI may terminate PIP status on the basis of abuse. Other potential reasons for termination include failure to file accurate cost and quarterly reports in a timely manner, failure to notify the FI of a significant decrease of Medicare service levels (volume), and failure to notify the FI in cases of significant overpay-

ments where the provider either knew of the overpayment or should have known.

In the case of a new provider that is not eligible for PIP, as discussed above, reimbursement for Medicare visits is made under special conditions and results in a percentage of charges payment or a cost per discipline payment method. Because there are no actual historical cost data to rely on, the FI will first attempt to base the reimbursement upon payments made to a similar provider, using the budget of the new provider. In cases where the FI can find no similar provider on which to base the comparison, the budgeted costs of the new provider will be used as a reimbursement basis. After the first quarterly report is reviewed, the FI will adjust the reimbursement rate as appropriate to take into account the actual cost experience of the new provider. The HCFA has continued the effort to eliminate the use of PIP for HHAs, but it still exists, and will probably not be phased out until a prospective payment methodology is in place for home care. At this point, only demonstration projects on prospective payment are in process.

To remain on PIP, the HHA must have an error rate of less than 2.5%, and be billing timely (monthly) for at least 90% of all services. Additionally, the PIP must be based on a realistic budget. Agencies found to have budget-reporting problems can be denied the use of PIP because they cannot project an estimate of their Medicare allowable costs.

Denials and Waiver of Liability

The term *technical denial* was created by the HCFA to label a denial of a visit when the FI believed that the HHA should have known that the patient's condition would not qualify for Medicare reimbursement. In the use of technical denials, the HCFA is distinguishing between a situation where a particular visit to a patient is determined to be unskilled care and a situation where all visits are denied because the patient's condition does not warrant medical coverage. These include denials for patients who are too sick for intermittent care, those who are not sick enough, and those determined not to be homebound. Currently, technical denials are not subject to waiver of liability (as defined below) and are appealable by the beneficiary with assistance from the HHA provider. Technical denials do not become part of this calculation. The impact of these denied or rejected claims is significant on the Medicare cost report and the fiscal viability of the HHA. This stems from the following:

- Services rendered that are deemed to be technical denials are not paid by Medicare and are considered due from the patient. The patient generally does not understand why Medicare will not pay, however, and therefore the patient will not pay, causing a loss to HHA.
- Because services were rendered, they are counted in the total visits by discipline for the HHA. When the Medicare cost report is prepared, costs are allocated to the denied visits and away from the Medicare program. This reduces the total Medicare costs and reimbursement. Through this analysis, the HHA may never be paid for the services determined to be technical denials.

The waiver of liability principle was created by Section 213 (a) of the Social Security Amendments of 1972. The purpose of the waiver principle is to hold harmless a beneficiary or provider that acted in good faith in accepting or providing services later determined to be noncovered because they were either not reasonable or necessary or custodial in nature. Specifically, the program will make payments in those instances where "the provider and beneficiary did not know, and could not reasonably have been expected to know" that payment would not be made for such items or services. Because of the many claims that providers submit to Medicare, a system of presumptions was devised to avoid case-by-case review of liability waivers for providers. Under this system, if a

provider's denied claims for a year fell below certain preestablished percentages, the provider would be presumed to be capable of making accurate Medicare coverage decisions (this is called a favorable waiver presumption), and therefore would be entitled to a waiver of liability for the few cases where a wrong coverage decision was made.

A favorable waiver presumption is granted to HHAs with claim denial rates of less than 2.5%. The denial rate is calculated by dividing the number of visits for which the intermediary denies coverage by the number of covered visits billed by the HHA. Under a presumptive favorable waiver, payments are made and then the paperwork supporting the visit is reviewed. If an HHA loses its presumptive waiver status, all billings and supporting paperwork (UB-92, Forms 485 and 486) is reviewed by the FI before payment is processed (there is no PIP payment allowed).

Early in 1996, it seemed that HCFA was eliminating the use of waiver of liability for HHAs and skilled nursing facilities. However, in May 1996, HCFA agreed to continue its use. Previously, regulations enacted in February 1986 had eliminated the favorable presumption waiver, thus requiring review of denied claims on a case-by-case basis. HCFA estimated in the *Federal Register* (February 12, 1985) that elimination of the favorable presumption waiver would save Medicare $93 million in FY 1987, $22 million of which would have been reimbursed to HHAs. The Consolidated Omnibus Budget Reconciliation Act, however, which was passed on April 7, 1986, restored the favorable presumption waiver (except for denial on custodial care grounds) at the 2.5% rate.

Appeals on Medicare Cost Reports and Services

There are certain appeal rights granted to HHAs through Section 1878 of the Social Security Act and the implementation of Medicare regulation (DHHS, 1985). The procedures for appeals are specifically stated in the regulations, including the time limit in which such an appeal must be made.

Provider representation is allowed for the beneficiary for both Part A and Part B claims. Only the cost of successful appeals is an allowed (reasonable) cost for cost reporting, however. The HHA cannot charge the beneficiary (patient) for the service. Under Part B, an administrative law judge (ALJ) is provided for amounts of $500 to $999, and a judicial review is provided for amounts greater than $1,000. In general, the amount of reimbursement in dispute (as a result of the Medicare cost report) must be $10,000 or more to qualify for review by the Provider Reimbursement Review Board (PRRB). For amounts greater than $1,000 but less than $10,000, a Medicare ALJ will review the dispute at the request of the provider. This is called an intermediary hearing. Although the route is generally not taken, the provider has the right to seek judicial review (in a district court) of a final decision by the PRRB or any action by the ALJ involving a question of law. Civil action must be commenced within 60 days after notification of determination is received.

The PRRB is composed of five members who are knowledgeable in the field of health care reimbursement; these individuals are appointed by the Secretary of DHHS. At least one member of the board must be a certified public accountant. As required under Section 1878(h) of the Social Security Act, the Secretary selects two members from qualified and acceptable nominees of the providers. The PRRB is authorized to make rules and to establish procedures necessary to its operation in accordance with regulations established by the Secretary. The general requirement for a PRRB appeal is as follows:

- The provider must have filed a timely cost report.
- The adverse final decision of the FI must result in a disputed amount of reimbursement of $10,000 or more. (*Note*: Any cost to be disputed must have been originally filed in a cost report or in an acceptable

supplemental filing to come under these regulations.)

- The appeal must be filed within 100 days after the FI renders its final determination.
- Group appeal must be filed by providers under common ownership, and the amount at issue must aggregate to $50,000 or more.

The HHA has rights as to notice (of time and place) of the hearing, representation by counsel, and introduction of reasonable and pertinent evidence to supplement or contradict the evidence considered by the FI. All decisions by the PRRB must be made based on the record from this hearing, which can include evidence submitted by the Secretary.

The positions of the PRRB and ALJ are unusual in the American judicial system. Both come under the jurisdiction (and are employees) of the government unit upon which they are ruling and can be reversed, affirmed, or modified (Social Security Act, Section 1878(f)(1)) by the Secretary or Assistant Secretary (on behalf of the Secretary). In other words, they are reviewing the work of their boss.

GENERAL DISCUSSION OF INCREASING REIMBURSEMENT

Discrete Costing

The HHA cost report reflects the three different types of cost centers found within an HHA. General service cost centers are those for divisions or departments operated for the benefit of the provider as a whole. Reimbursable cost centers are those for which Medicare will reimburse the provider on a reasonable cost basis. Nonreimbursable cost centers are those relating to services not covered by the Medicare program. The nonreimbursable and reimbursable cost centers are also known as specific service cost centers, in contrast to the general service cost centers, which represent overhead costs. The objective of cost finding in the context of preparing the cost report is to allocate the general service costs among the various reimbursable and nonreimbursable cost centers.

Until the mid-1980s, HHAs were required by regulations to allocate general service costs using the step-down method of cost finding. Under this method, the general service cost center costs were allocated among the other cost centers (both reimbursable and nonreimbursable) on a prescribed statistical basis. For example, depreciation expense is allocated to the specific service cost centers on the basis of square footage. Accordingly, a specific service cost center occupying 10% of the total provider floor space would be allocated 10% of the depreciation expense.

A similar allocation is made for administrative and general costs. This is a sort of catch-all cost center, which tends to accumulate all those costs that cannot be specifically assigned elsewhere. In the case of administrative and general costs, allocation is made to the specific service cost centers based upon total accumulated costs. This includes not only those costs specifically attributable but also those costs allocated from the other general service cost centers, all of which are allocated before the administrative and general cost center. This means that previous allocations increase further allocations, a sort of snowball effect to the allocation of expenses.

The step-down method of cost finding was not considered satisfactory by many HHAs, which felt that the prescribed statistical allocation basis did not fairly allocate general service overhead costs between the reimbursable and nonreimbursable cost centers. A specific example of the impact of cost finding on non–Medicare-reimbursable centers is found in HHAs that contract with health maintenance organizations (HMOs), provide IV therapy, or provide DME. The accounting and administrative costs are allocated based on the accumulated costs in this cost center even though, in the case of the HMO contract, little accounting and administrative time is required. The portion of these expenses that is allocated to the HMO contracts would share a direct percentage with

the Medicare cost centers even though it is not reflective of actual costs incurred. In response, many providers initiated corporate reorganization designed legally to segregate the reimbursable and nonreimbursable activities and the related general and administrative costs.

In response to the trend toward reorganization, the HCFA prepared a position memorandum on discrete costing by HHAs (Booth, 1985), which resulted in the revision of Chapter 23 of the *Medicare Provider Reimbursements Manual* (HCFA Publication 15-1) in early 1986.

Discrete costing involves the direct assignment of general service costs to specific service cost centers based on measurements of actual usage instead of the prescribed statistical allocation basis per the step-down method. The advantage of discrete costing is that overhead costs can now be assigned to specific service cost centers before the step-down process, resulting in what is presumably a more equitable cost finding.

Although the cost-finding methodology allows the provider relative flexibility in establishing cost centers within what was previously the administrative and general catch-all category, there are other specific requirements that must be met. To take advantage of discrete costing, the entities within the provider must be kept physically distinct. In addition, they must be operated and supervised separately and must maintain separate records and accounting data contemporaneously: separate personnel, space, records, phone number—at a minimum. Also, the provider must request permission from the FI to use discrete cost finding in advance of the start of the FY in which it is to be adopted. To obtain this, the provider must convince the FI that the cost-finding changes proposed by the HHA represent an improvement to the step-down method and will result in greater accuracy in cost finding. This approach to cost finding is, of course, subject to audit verification. Cost reports prepared and filed using the discrete cost-finding methodology must be accompanied by supporting schedules detailing the cost allocations reflected in the report. Shared overhead cost centers must be directly costed between the reimbursable and nonreimbursable cost centers; the total portion attributable to reimbursable cost centers will then be allocated to specific reimbursable cost centers using the step-down method.

There are two critical factors to be considered in the decision to use discrete cost-finding in lieu of the traditional step-down method. The first is the need to establish and maintain wholly separate records and accounting. Where this is not or cannot be done, the step-down method remains mandatory. The second is that, although the HCFA has published revisions to the *Medicare Provider Reimbursement Manual*, specific instructions were not given to the FI; only guidelines allowing a certain level of discretion in the application of these regulations were supplied.

Impact of the Restructured Agency on Medicare Reimbursement

After one reviews the methodology behind Medicare cost reporting and cost finding, it is often fiscally and physically possible to separate noncovered Medicare activities from the Medicare-covered services. Even if fiscally and physically possible, the effort and cost associated with discrete costing can be overwhelming. Consequently, a more effective choice can be corporation reorganization. Medicare will review such reorganization carefully, but as long as the organizational structure and operations actually conform to the new corporate organization, these attacks can be mitigated. The use of the corporate structure that includes a parent foundation and subsidiaries for the different services requires the use of a home office cost report, but it does provide for the most defensible structure (Figure 49–2).

The reimbursement impact of providing non-Medicare services in a traditional Medicare agency is that the costs will be allocated to all cost centers (Medicare and non-Medicare) based on the allocated costs (and other statistics). This generally results in the higher costs of Medicare billing and compliance (plan of treatment, documentation, audit, etc.) being shared by non-Medicare cost centers and payers, and thereby not being paid by Medicare. Because non-Medicare services are generally lower-cost services, there is not enough gross margin in these services to cover their own direct and indirect costs plus the shifted costs from Medicare caused by the cost-finding and allocation methodology of the Medicare cost report. With the increased purchase of HHAs by publicly traded companies and also the development of integrated delivery systems (multiple hospitals and other providers under the same corporate parent), there is a potential to separate further traditional (Medicare) and nontraditional home service agencies. In addition, by removing the nontraditional agency from the hospital or HHA, licensed vocational or licensed practical nurses can be used to provide care. Other costs, such as Joint Commission on Accreditation of Healthcare Organizations (Joint Commission) or other certification surveys, can be eliminated.

Although hospital-based HHAs are reimbursed the same as free-standing HHAs, costs can be allocated downward. In addition, if a free-standing HHA is part of an IDS, there may be many opportunities to improve the overall reimbursement of the HHA in certain ways as well as have a very positive impact on the IDS. For example, HHAs are often faced with the physical therapy limitation when using outside contractors. There are special provisions, however, when the source of the physical therapists is other cost-based providers. This means that a hospital or other rehabilitation entity that is Medicare cost-based can provide the therapists, and the amount paid is cost settled. This eliminates the problem with the limitation and also allows for other members of the IDS to utilize their staff more fully. (Of course, the downside is that the management within each of these entities must be able to utilize staff and to coordinate their needs effectively.)

Experienced legal and accounting counsel should be obtained to determine the impact on the agency (reimbursement, legal, functional)

TWO TRADITIONAL APPROACHES:

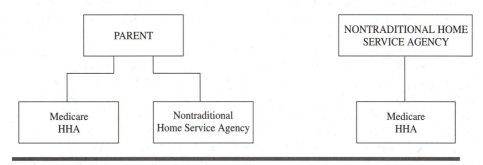

INTEGRATED DELIVERY SERVICE OR PUBLIC CORPORATION APPROACH:

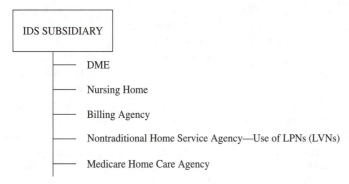

Figure 49–2 New Wave of Corporate Reorganization within the IDS

and the many options available to meet the objectives of restructuring.

SOME THOUGHTS ABOUT THE FUTURE

The National Association of Home Care (NAHC) has led the industry in recommending and evaluating the current proposals for a PPS for home care, which NAHC has called the unified plan. Although there have been nuances to the model being discussed, the general attributes include payment based on an episode of home care, provided over a defined period of time, with valuations in payment based on a case mix adjustor (similar to a DRG methodology), with outliers defined and paid on a separate payment schedule, and finally a mechanism to reward overall savings. Savings are measured in terms of both cost per service and volume of services provided and are measured based on geographic/census tract medians rather than based only on the specific HHA itself.

Other types of PPS payment plans have discussed the use of payment by enrollee or by outcome base. Regardless of the approach, defining and measuring both the base in development of the payment and the results of the PPS implementation are major ongoing concerns.

NAHC has estimated the average number of visits per patient to be 66 in 1995. This is up from the General Accounting Office (GAO) March 1996 study (GAO/HEHS 96-16), which found the 1993 mean visit per patient to be 56.71, and the median to be 24. It is the average number of visits per patient that has concerned both Congress and HCFA. Consequently, PPS for HHAs needs to address the volume issue as well.

Some proposed features of the PPS system have been rigorously opposed, such as a copay, which was recommended by ProPac (*Federal Register*, 1996).[*] Other features of the PPS are of concern, such as the use of the current case mix adjustor, which HCFA admits may explain only 10% of the differences between cases (*Home Health Line*, June 10, 1996). Currently, there are 18 categories for case mix adjustors that look to whether the patient had been hospitalized prior to home care, whether there are other medical conditions that contribute to the intensity of care, age, and the support at home (including factors relating to activities of daily living). Another concern is the base year to be used. The base year is the starting point to measure any savings.

To alleviate some of these concerns, a phase-in of PPS is being recommended, generally over at least 3 years, which has several components to the calculation for the final PPS payment and settlement. Nevertheless, HCFA chief Bruce Vladeck informed members of House Ways and Means Health Subcommittee in late July 1996 that HCFA "is certain that it would take two to three years to develop the systems and gather the data necessary to implement the [prospective] payment system" (*Home Health Line*, July 29, 1996). He also addressed the case mix

---

[*]ProPac is the Prospective Payment Assessment Commission, which reports to Congress with recommendations on prospective systems and rates. This report is published generally in March of each year. It can be ordered by calling 202-401-8986.

adjustor and the definition of an episode of care or significant concerns.

The GAO, from its standpoint, wants to target Medicare's high-cost, high-utilization area for running demonstrations with specific focus on particular high home health costs per beneficiary. Demonstration projects for home care are not new—the first were started in 1987, 1988, and 1989.

Even without PPS, the new (1996) cost limits will challenge the smaller HHAs to find additional volumes to spread the fixed costs of the agency in order to survive. When managed care is seen as a solution to increase volumes, it is often at a payment rate lower than Medicare, which may cause other problems and reduced payments from the Medicare component of the HHA. To deal effectively with managed care, the HHA must have good cost accounting.

The ultimate solution will focus on necessary care at the most cost-effective approach, ultimately using outcome determination as the measurement. The challenge to the HHAs will be to manage themselves in a business manner, realizing the reduction of financial resources and the loss of the cost report mentality safety net. In the interim, having an adequate means of measuring cost and payer mix change and being effective in the negotiation and provision of home care within the managed care environment will provide valuable experience to test the agency's ability to survive.

REFERENCES

Booth, C. (1985). Cost finding for home health. *Caring,* 4(7), 72–73.

Department of Health and Human Services. (1985). *Code of federal regulations (Title 42): Section 405.1801 et seq.* Washington, DC: U.S. Government Printing Office.

Federal Register. (1996, May 31).

Greene, J. (1996, January 29). Home health a key factor in systems' integration efforts. *Modern Healthcare.*

Home Health Line. (1996, June 10):7.

Home Health Line. (1996, July 29):2.

Lutz, S. (1996, March 19). Double-digit growth continues. *Modern Healthcare.*

Medicare Program. (1994). Eliminating additional payment for administrative and general cost of hospital-based home health agencies. *Federal Register, 59,* 760–762.

Schaffer, C.L. (1996, March/April). Hospital–home care integration: Society of Ambulatory Care Professionals. *Outreach, 17,* 2.

Shaw, S. (1985). Market and program changes for the traditional intermittent provider. *Caring,* 4(7), 8–9.

Stewart, J.E. (1979). *Home health care.* St. Louis, MO: Mosby.

Weissenstein, E. (1996, May 20). HCFA to respond to home-care fraud. *Modern Healthcare.*

CHAPTER 50

How To Read, Interpret, and Understand Financial Statements

D. Scott Detar

Financial statements used by administrators of home health organizations vary from organization to organization. Home health organizations may be nonprofit or commercial enterprises operating for profit. Depending on the organization, financial reports may be on a cash or accrual basis. This chapter approaches the reading and understanding of a home health organization's financial statement from the perspective of a nonprofit organization. Many of the interpretations, ratios, and conclusions are the same regardless of the type of enterprise (nonprofit or for profit). Where there are differences, they are noted and explained. This chapter assumes that accrual basis financial statements are prepared.

CASH BASIS OR ACCRUAL BASIS

Cash basis accounting simply means recording only those transactions when cash is received and disbursed. There is no attempt to record receivables for service rendered or payables for amounts owed by the organization. Many small nonprofit organizations use the cash basis of accounting during the year, principally because it is the most simple method of record keeping. The cash basis method of accounting is merely the recording of the activity in the organization's checkbook.

As organizations grow in size, however, there is a need to see not only a more accurate, but a more complete, picture of their financial results on a regular basis (i.e., monthly, quarterly, or annually). Organizations will use the accrual basis of accounting to record transactions during the accounting period. The accrual basis requires organizations to record transactions resulting from the receipt and disbursement of cash as well as amounts owed them for services rendered and the amounts they owe for goods and services. The underlying accounting principle used in recording accrual basis transactions is to match revenue earned during the accounting period to expenses incurred to generate that revenue for the same accounting period.

Many administrators or executives of organizations, whether nonprofit or commercial enterprises, operate using the cash basis theory. They understand what is going into the bank and what is coming out of the bank. These same administrators or executives many times mistakenly believe that the accrual basis is more complicated. In fact, accrual basis statements can be quite easy to read. A thorough understanding of the financial statements will assist the administrator in his or her ability to make informed day-to-day operational decisions. The informed administrator each month should be reviewing four financial statements and at least one schedule of statistics.

The first statement is the income statement, or, for nonprofit organizations, the statement of revenue and expenses for the period under review. The second statement is the balance sheet, listing all assets and liabilities at the end of the period. The third statement, the statement of functional expenses, allocates expenses by program. The fourth statement, the statement of cash flows, is a meaningful and integral part of the financial picture relating the accrual basis to the cash basis. The schedules of statistics needs to be available and reviewed in conjunction with the above four financial statements for the administrator to be properly informed. This chapter discusses how to read and interpret each of the four financial statements.

SCHEDULE OF STATISTICS

A thorough understanding of home health agency financial statements involves a careful review and understanding of the basic statistics or data used to generate the financial statements. Three basic statistical essentials are described below.

Visits

For all accounting periods shown, visits are the number of visits performed for each period. Visits should be detailed by fee source (the payer) and also by discipline (the type of service, e.g., nursing, therapies, etc.). Many home health agencies also provide hours in addition to or in lieu of visit data.

Personnel

Employee statistics for the period reported on are the number of employees (full- and part-time) in each service area calculated in terms of a full-time equivalent (FTE). FTE equates all full- and part-time employees into a common denominator for employment. This statistic should be available for service areas (nursing, therapies, etc.) as well as administrative departments.

Accounts Receivable Aging Percentages

Accounts receivable aging percentages by pay source must always be presented when reviewing balance sheets and income statements. The aging columns should be labeled as current (0 to 30 days), 30 to 60 days, 60 to 90 days, 90 to 120 days, and more than 120 days. Aging is usually based on the month in which services were performed.

Analyzing statistics along with financial statements is likely to have an immediate impact on the administrator's understanding of an agency's operations, but their longer-term benefits may have even greater value. As third-party payers move toward capitation as a method of reimbursing health care service providers, the pressure on those providers to control costs per capita is sure to increase. That's when an even closer look at the numbers—revenue per visit, personnel cost per visit, and the like—will make a critical difference in an agency's financial success.

INCOME STATEMENT

The income statement details revenue and expenses during the accounting period reported. In Exhibit 50–1, the accounting periods shown are 1995 and 1996. Revenue, or the fees billed for the home health visits and services provided to patients, is reflected in the period the services were provided by agency personnel. Revenue is generally reported net of any contractual allowances or reserves for uncollectibles. Revenue is the dollar equivalent of service agency individuals (nurses, therapists, etc.) provided patients during the period.

In the example, the administrator should ask the question, "Why did revenue increase by $528,000?" This can be answered by reviewing the visit activity for each of the two accounting periods included in the schedule of statistics. Normally, published financial statements do not present visit activity for the accounting period. As an administrator, however, you should request visit activity as an integral part of the

Exhibit 50–1 Home Health Agency Statement of Revenue, Expenses, and Changes in Fund Balances: Years Ended December 31, 1996, and December 31, 1995

	1996	*1995*
REVENUE		
Nursing and related service fees	$1,823,146	$1,294,811
Investment and other income	10,207	10,590
TOTAL REVENUE	1,833,353	1,305,401
EXPENSES		
Program services	1,459,188	990,221
Administrative	511,123	417,562
TOTAL EXPENSES	1,970,311	1,407,783
LOSS FROM OPERATIONS	(136,958)	(102,382)
NONOPERATING INCOME		
United Way appropriation	78,290	76,000
Municipal appropriations	57,250	59,330
Grant	17,588	—
Contributions and bequests	33,434	45,350
Total Nonoperating Income	186,562	180,680
Revenue and Income in Excess of Expenses	49,604	78,298
Fund Balances at Beginning of Year	452,039	373,741
Fund Balances at End of Year	$501,643	$452,039

financial statements your controller provides you on a monthly and year-to-date basis. Increases in service fee revenue should be consistent with increases in service volume measured in visits or hours. If the change in revenue is not proportional to the change in service volume, then other factors, such as rate increases or a large bad debt reserve adjustment, should be investigated.

Expenses are reflected, as noted, in terms of program services and administrative expenses. Program service expense represents the direct cost of providing visits and services to patients during the accounting period. Program service expenses generally include salaries and contract services for personnel, payroll taxes, benefits, transportation, and other related direct costs of providing service. These expenses, over time, should remain fairly constant as a percentage of revenue. As with service volume, there is a general expectation that program service expenses change in the same relationship as revenue changes from accounting period to period. Pro-

gram service expenses that increase faster than revenue may be an indication of inefficiency in productivity (simply stated, people doing fewer visits for the same or more dollars) or general overspending in nonpersonnel areas. In addition, it may also be an indication that the agency needs to increase its revenue rates to keep up with the inflationary cost of providing service. Increasing individual rates for visits may not be easy with managed care fixed-price contracts becoming the norm for an agency.

Administrative expenses typically are the fixed expenses necessary to handle the agency's day-to-day operations. This category generally includes administrative and clerical personnel salaries and related payroll taxes and benefits, occupancy expenses, office operation, legal and professional expenses, professional dues, publications, public relations, and any other related expenses. These expenses do not increase significantly from year to year unless there are changes in the fixed operations, such as a new facility, more people, or a significant change in visit volume. When one compares the expenses on a month-to-month basis, there should be small or insignificant variations each month. When making long-term comparisons, increases in the level of administrative expenses that are in excess of the local inflation rate and are not accompanied by significant increases in the level of administrative services may indicate a lack of control over spending and should be addressed immediately.

The term *operating income (loss)* indicates whether the organization is charging enough fees for the services provided to cover the cost of delivering services and managing the operation. Income is a positive number and mathematically indicates that fees are greater than costs. (Loss) is a negative and indicates that fees are less than costs. Typically a nonprofit organization reports an operating (loss). Generally, the operating (loss) is planned, and the planned loss is covered by other items of income or support included under the title "nonoperating income." The for-profit service provider does not usually report an operating loss. If the organization is reporting several successive periods of losses, the cash flow statement (explained later) must be reviewed fully to determine how the organization is paying for the losses.

Nonoperating income generally reflects the results of fund-raising activities conducted by the nonprofit organization during the accounting period. Typically in this category, you may expect support from individual or corporate contributions, federated fund-raising organizations (e.g., the United Way), or local municipal governments supporting general purpose services or objectives. A review of this category for several years offers a basic understanding about the level of independent (board) fundraising activity compared with that of the administrative staff. Administrative fund-raising typically results in United Way or municipal support and grants for specific programs.

In reviewing the income statement, the administrator will learn how much revenue was generated for the accounting period, how much it cost to generate the revenue, whether the agency made a surplus, and whether it received any contributions during the period. However, for an accurate understanding of the organization, the administrator should not look at the income statement alone. This is only one part, and reading and understanding it must be interrelated with the other financial statements.

BALANCE SHEET

The income statement provides the administrator an indication of what happened during the accounting period. The balance sheet provides the administrator with a picture of the financial health of the agency at a point in time. The financial health is gauged by the relationship of total cash and receivables to the amount of liabilities and debt. A large amount of cash with a low amount of receivables indicates that the organization is collecting its receivables on a regular and frequent basis. A small cash balance with a large amount of receivables and a large amount of liabilities may indicate that the organization is unable to collect its receivables in a timely manner. The administrator should review the aging of accounts receivable in conjunction with the review of cash, accounts receivable, and liabilities.

The balance sheet is a financial statement that must balance. The amount of the assets owned by the organization must equal the amount of liabilities owed by the organization plus the equity. In comparison, the income statement does not balance but provides the results of operations.

In analyzing a balance sheet (see Exhibit 50–2), there are several key ratios of which the administrator should be aware in order to understand the organization. First is the current ratio. The current ratio equals the total current assets divided by total liabilities. Current assets consist of cash, accounts receivable, and inventory. Current liabilities consist of accounts payable, accrued expenses, and the amount of debt the organization must repay in the 12 months after the close of the accounting period. This ratio

Exhibit 50–2 Home Health Agency, Balance Sheet: December 31, 1996, and December 31, 1995

	1996	1995
ASSETS		
Cash	$170,768	$251,398
Accounts receivable, net of allowance for doubtful accounts of $66,300 (1990) and $43,000 (1989)	252,254	136,501
Interfund receivable	—	341
Prepaid expenses	9,319	6,365
TOTAL CURRENT ASSETS	432,341	394,605
Land, building, and equipment, at cost, less accumulated depreciation	262,718	139,899
TOTAL ASSETS	$695,059	$534,504
LIABILITIES AND FUND BALANCES		
LIABILITIES		
Notes payable	$ 9,007	$ 13,384
Deferred grant	75,892	5,260
Interfund payable	—	341
Accounts payable and accrued expenses	108,517	63,480
Total Current Liabilities	193,416	82,465
Fund Balances	501,643	452,039
Total Liabilities	$695,059	$534,504

provides the administrator with a benchmark of the amount of assets readily available to liquidate the liabilities. In the example in Exhibit 50–2, current assets divided by current liabilities equals a current ratio for this organization of 2.24. Usually any ratio above 1.5 to 1.0 indicates better than average financial health. The larger the ratio the better the health of the organization.

A second basic ratio is working capital. Working capital quantifies available liquidity. Working capital is the excess of current assets over current liabilities, theoretically an amount that can be turned readily into cash. In Exhibit 50–2, working capital is current assets minus the current liabilities, which equals a working capital of $238,925.

Our particular example indicates a significant amount of working capital and a high current ratio. A closer look at the components, however, may yield slightly different results. Both the above indicators measure liquidity, the amount of liquid assets available to cover current liabilities. The example organization has a deferred grant. The deferred grant represents a cash grant provided to cover certain designated expenses for a particular program. It is deferred because the grant funds were not spent in the reporting accounting period and will be spent or refunded in a succeeding accounting period. If one reduces both current assets and current liabilities by the amount of the deferred grant, the current ratio and amount of working capital are 3.04 and $238,925, respectively. These amounts are still high for a home health agency.

Another area to analyze is the change in and the level of accounts receivable. Accounts receivable should be analyzed in conjunction with service fee revenue, the change in units of service or visits, and the accounts receivable aging listed on the schedule of statistics. First, how does the amount of accounts receivable at the balance sheet date compare with total service fee revenue for the accounting period? Or, how much of the revenue billed during the accounting period has not been collected as of the balance sheet date? In the example agency, 13.8% of the period's revenue is receivable. Is 13.8% meaningful? The 13.8% may be more meaningful if reflected in terms of days accounts receivable are outstanding. How many days does this represent? Is this an improvement over last year, or are collections slower? These are among the questions to be asked.

To determine the number of days of service revenue in accounts receivable, a simple equation is used:

$$\frac{\text{Total amount of accounts receivable}}{\text{Total revenue} \div \text{the number of days in the accounting period}}$$

where accounts receivable represents the total amount as of the balance sheet date, total revenue is the total billed for services for the accounting period, and number of days represents the number of days in the accounting period. In the example agency, this number is 50. For the prior year, it is 38. Now one year can be compared with the previous year. We know the period-end receivables represent more days of revenue than the previous period. We do not know the cause. The administrator must investigate reasons, such as above-average billing in the last 2 months of the year or a general slowdown in collections, or a combination.

Another common financial ratio used to analyze accounts receivable is turnover. Turnover is the number of times accounts receivable are collected during the accounting period. A high turnover number indicates quick collections, and a low turnover number indicates slow collections. To calculate turnover, simply divide the days in the accounting period as calculated above by the number of days in accounts receivables. In our example, 365/50 equals 7.3 times. This compares with 9.6 times the previous year. If the turnover ratio is decreasing from period to period, this is a strong indication of a deterioration in collections. The reasons need to be investigated further and corrective action put into place immediately.

Generally, the type of pay source will determine the number of days and the turnover. Insurance companies, Medicare, and other third-party payers often pay no more quickly than 60 days after billing, which may be 90 days after service. This payment time frame will cause the days in accounts receivable and turnover to be closer to 90 and 4 times, respectively. Typically, home health organizations have turnover ratios in a range of 3.0 to 4.0. Any turnover number lower than 3.0 indicates serious cash flow problems and the inability of the agency to regularly pay current expenses in a timely manner.

The last major ratio on the balance sheet is fund balance or equity. This category indicates the amount of investment in the organization. Equity is usually compared with total debt to determine a relationship between the amount of investment by the owner and the amount of investment by creditors. In a nonprofit organization, the owner is replaced by the board or the community benefiting from the services provided. Generally, a financially sound organization maintains a ratio of debt to equity no worse than 1:1. In a labor-intensive service business, debt compared with equity should not be lower than 1:1. If not, the organization may experience shortages of cash from time to time.

In conclusion, the balance sheet is a snapshot. Look at its details. Compare it with prior years. What are the trends? Often, trends provide an indication of what is around the corner in the next accounting period.

FUNCTIONAL EXPENSES

The statement of functional expenses (see Exhibit 50–3) details expenses for the accounting period by type of expense (i.e., salaries, benefits, taxes, etc.) in the program service and administrative areas. The statement should be reviewed and analyzed in conjunction with the income statement, and the visits and FTEs in the schedule of statistics for each accounting period presented. The statement of functional expenses will provide information to answer questions concerning a fluctuation between accounting periods (e.g., Why are salaries higher? Why did transportation expense more than double?). The

Exhibit 50–3 Home Health Agency Statement of Functional Expenses: Years Ended December 31, 1996, and December 31, 1995

	Program Services	Administrative	Total Expenses 1996	Total Expenses 1995
Salaries	$959,804	$314,293	$1,274,097	$883,684
Employee benefits	153,167	59,894	213,061	137,941
Payroll taxes	76,138	28,186	104,324	72,135
Total Employee Compensation	1,189,109	402,373	1,591,482	1,093,760
Professional fees and contract service payments	177,398	35,112	212,510	187,964
Clinic expenses	2,074	—	2,074	2,273
Supplies	19,130	10,429	29,559	24,041
Telephone	—	10,510	10,510	8,912
Postage and shipping	—	7,700	7,700	5,862
Occupancy	9,457	14,563	24,020	22,176
Local transportation	52,636	2,110	54,746	32,674
Conferences, conventions, and meetings	1,437	5,144	6,581	4,965
Printing and publications	—	6,276	6,276	4,863
Membership dues	—	5,930	5,930	4,843
Interest expense	—	1,529	1,529	1,411
Total Expenses before Depreciation	1,451,241	501,676	1,952,917	1,393,744
Depreciation of land, building, and equipment	7,947	9,447	17,394	14,039
Total Expenses	$1,459,188	$511,123	$1,970,311	$1,407,783

schedule of visits for each accounting period will assist in this review and in answering those questions.

Additionally, there are certain basic relationships that should be consistent from period to period. Payroll taxes and employee benefits are expense categories that should remain consistent when expressed as a percentage of salaries. Transportation expense generally changes in direct proportion to any changes in visits provided. Occupancy expense (e.g., building costs, maintenance, and insurance other than health and workers' compensation) is usually predictable and generally does not vary from accounting period to accounting period, except in cases of major repairs.

The functional expense statement also will provide the administrator with information on a program basis. The administrator will note the direct cost of each program. Administrative cost also may be allocated to each program to reflect the real cost of the program or service. The programs should be compared with the same programs in prior accounting periods for variances.

An interesting and informative analysis pertaining to the functional expense statement is to review the direct expense categories (salaries, payroll taxes, benefits, contract services, transportation) in relationship to visits. This analysis can be performed on both a total agency basis and an individual program basis. In addition to reviewing direct expenses in relation to visits, the direct expenses should be reviewed in relation to FTEs.

Experience shows that administrative expenses generally are consistent from period to period. If visits are increasing over time, program service costs should increase, but the administrative or indirect costs should remain fairly flat. There is a visit volume level in every organization at which another administrative function or person may be required. When additional administrative personnel are hired, administrative costs could change by a percentage usually greater than the percentage change in visit volume.

In summary, the functional expense statement is used to review consistent spending patterns from accounting period to accounting period, to verify that spending bears some consistent relationship to the level of service provided, and to review expenses on a program basis, all in conjunction with the schedule of statistics.

CASH FLOWS

The statement of cash flows provides a reconciliation of net income reported on the accrual basis to the change in cash for the accounting period. The statement reports cash flow from operations, cash flow from the purchase of fixed assets, and cash flow from financing activities. The statement answers the question, "Where did the profit go?" or "What did the organization do with the profit?"

In the example agency statement in Exhibit 50–4, the reader will note that net income for the year of $49,604 resulted in cash provided by operating activities totaling $63,960. In examining the components resulting in positive operational cash flow, note that three items changed significantly: accounts receivable, deferred grant, and accounts payable. These are line items on the balance sheet with significant variance from the prior year. The positive operational cash flow is a result, however, of the agency receiving a grant and not spending the entire amount in the accounting period.

What did the organization do with the $63,960 of cash provided by operations? The statement tells us the organization made its regular debt service payments on a note payable and purchased fixed assets. In this example, the cost of the fixed assets purchased exceeded the

---

Exhibit 50–4 Home Health Agency Statement of Cash Flows: Years Ended December 31, 1996, and December 31, 1995

	1996	1995
Cash Flows from Operating Activities		
Revenue and income in excess of expenses	$ 49,604	$ 78,298
Adjustments to reconcile revenue and income in excess of expenses to net cash provided by operating activities		
Depreciation	17,394	14,039
(Increase) decrease in:		
Accounts receivable	(115,412)	(17,873)
Prepaid expenses	(2,954)	(1,559)
Increase (decrease) in:		
Deferred grant	70,632	(432)
Accounts payable and accrued expenses	44,696	4,949
Net Cash Provided by Operating Activities	63,960	77,422
Cash Flows from Investing Activities		
Purchase of fixed assets	(140,213)	(11,281)
Cash Flows from Financing Activities		
Principal payments on note payable	(4,377)	(3,651)
Net Increase (Decrease) in Cash	(80,630)	62,490
Cash Beginning of Year	251,398	188,908
Cash End of Year	$170,768	$251,398

cash flow from operations, and beginning year cash was required to purchase the assets. Therefore, the informed analyst may conclude that fixed assets were purchased by $63,000 of deferred grant funds and $77,000 of the organization's cash reserves.

This statement completes the link between the balance sheet and the income statement. Some financial analysts choose to review this statement first when analyzing operations. Regardless of the order of review, the statement of cash flows is a necessity to give a full understanding of the agency during the reporting period.

CONCLUSION

To fully understand a financial statement, notes should accompany the statement. The notes should be read and analyzed in conjunction with statistics and ratios. Many times the notes provide information that may answer questions or explain hidden liabilities and obligations or one-time transactions significantly affecting relationships.

This chapter only scratches the surface of financial statement interpretation. It gives administrators a basis for understanding the financial statements provided by their financial departments. Many administrators receive more information and detail than is explained here. You should sit down and review with your controller certain basics and attempt to build from there. Look at the information supplied with a skeptical eye. Ask questions. Look at relationships. This will provide the basis for informed, educated decisions.

CHAPTER 51

Management Information Systems

Charlotte L. Kohler

THE EXPANSIVENESS OF A MANAGEMENT INFORMATION SYSTEM

Methods of data acquisition and use continue to broaden at a speed that can be disabling to the administrator who wants to make the best decision for the home health agency (HHA). However, by looking at the term *management information system* (MIS), it is easy to see that the word *computer* is not a limiting component in the concept. MIS has been defined as any systematic information-gathering and recordkeeping method that makes accurate, timely, and useful information available to the management of a business. In a guideline provided by the Society of Management Accountants of Canada, MIS has been broadened into a concept called *information resource management* (IRM), which includes the creation, use, management, and delivery of relevant data with the goal of helping the business enterprise capitalize on its base of information. IRM focuses on designing, implementing, and maintaining a balanced, enterprisewide system of information, processes, and technology. In the IRM environment, technology is viewed as a means to assist the business to do things faster, better, and cheaper—not as an end in itself. An effective IRM program provides for continuously scanning the environment for opportunities that could enhance an organization's business.

In the 1980s, the term *MIS* became closely aligned with the concepts and theories of computerization. The term *data processing* implied the need to process a large volume of data elements to provide needed information to management. Data were fed (by paper) to one central entry point. Having a computer, however, does not mean that MIS provides necessary management information. Consequently, today most agencies are computerized because of the need for analyzed information from the data entered. Agencies are reviewing their need to upgrade systems to provide even more information beyond that which is gathered from the billing process, including direct entry of more extensive clinical data by the caregivers at the home of the patient.

Agencies that are not computerized or are computerized with a system that is incapable of using available data are disadvantaged. Successful managed care contracting requires high use of data, and knowledge of services and related costs. Trying to capture the necessary data from the care provided, as well as billing the time and personnel requirements without an integrated computer system, is beyond burdensome. As a result, in agencies without adequate computer systems, the amount of analytical data is reduced to levels justified by the cost and the time available. Competitive disadvantage extends to those agencies with a highly sophisticated and flexible MIS if they have not yet learned how to use the system to assess the agency outcomes and attributes. Management requires data to be effective. The HHA needs the data to remain profitable and viable.

WHY COMPUTERIZE WITH A SYSTEM THAT ALLOWS DATA ANALYSIS?

The overall benefit of computerization is that, after data are entered from various sources and the billing is prepared, the data can be summarized, analyzed, and reported. Where a database software package is used, the reports available to management are generally unlimited. A true database system treats each element of information as unique and provides the user with a means, often a "report writer," that allows the agency to select the data and how it is to be analyzed. Data may be compared to other current information, to prior months or years, or to other data elements that are important in the management of the HHA. In highly sophisticated systems, benchmark standards or care plans can be set up to monitor, report, and compare agency (or patient) results. Data can be manipulated after selection to produce reports upon which sound business decisions can be made.

Data elements may change in their relative importance to an HHA well after the initial analysis of the data has been performed. For example, consider the analysis performed to determine the financial implications to an HHA that is considering prospective payment based on episodes of illness. Since this methodology may also include additional payment for outliers, it is necessary to determine the HHA's experience regarding care plans that fit the new criteria. Prior to this, the HHA had no reason to analyze and compare these data elements. Although this information has not yet been analyzed, it is available as a byproduct of patient registration, daily charge input, and care provided (medical record) data entered by the caregiver. By selecting and analyzing the data from previous admissions and substituting the pay-

ment proposed by the prospective payment alternative, managers of these agencies can develop a clear understanding of the impact of prospective payment and appropriately respond to the proposal to switch to this method. The current movement toward some prospective payment mechanism, or specific managed care contract payment provisions, for both traditional and extended home care reinforce the need for MIS and for managers to be able to effectively use the information available to them.

The new concept in MIS for home care introduced by J.H. Muellin (1986) in response to changes in prospective payment systems for hospital reimbursements has moved HHAs toward the gathering of clinical as well as financial data. The integration of clinical (or medical record) information is necessary to provide both administrative (business) and care effectiveness (clinical) information. The availability of these data will assist HHAs in becoming strong providers of those services not found in the traditional HHA. Portable data acquisition devices can obtain clinical data such as electrocardiogram (ECG) rhythm strips and can transfer this information electronically, either by radio wave unit or modem, to the computer system for clinical analysis.

Technology is catching up with the HHA, through the use of more sophisticated MIS, which has effectively leveraged its primary assets: "cost-effective and timely access to patients at home" (Muellin, 1986, p. 36). Small hand-held or palm-sized computers, allowing nurses and aides to enter data about their patients while in the patients' homes, have been developed. The data entered into these devices can be transferred via phone lines by a modem and used by employees once they return to the agency. This improves productivity and reduces clerical time, while improving the quality and accuracy of data obtained.

CURRENT COMPUTER TECHNOLOGY

Selecting and evaluating a computer system for the HHA can be difficult, especially since there is no perfect system, and because systems are continually upgraded and made more sophisticated. Nevertheless, prospective micro-computer purchasers can fall into two categories (Knauer, 1984):

1. *Extinct by instinct:* This is the impulsive decision maker who is easily persuaded by the flashy demonstration and dazzling display of a computer show.
2. *Paralysis by analysis:* The mystery of computers causes these managers to ponder all avenues while waiting for better prices, technology, or products. No decision is ever made.

Add to these two polar positions the intensity of change and the increasing level of sophistication in both hardware and software, and computer selection can become a daunting task. The solution to such dilemmas is to establish a framework of needs and decisive deadlines. One must stop and proceed slowly but diligently. The selection of an appropriate computer system is one of the most important financial decisions an HHA must make—not just the amount paid to the vendor who sold the HHA the system, but more important, the internal costs for development, setup, training, and data entry. Although reduction of personnel was often used as a sales pitch in the 1980s, the current selection criteria for the appropriate MIS is one of minimizing the number of administrative people in a time of growth or when data analysis or summarization is needed. At a fall 1996 National Association for Home Care (NAHC) conference, there was a general agreement between the speakers that the consolidation of the managed care and insurance companies will have a positive impact on the data processing (for billing) requirements for the HHAs—as the mergers continue, these merged companies will standardize the claims submission requirements.

As difficult as this decision may be in this period of continuous upgrading of both hardware and software, the goal is to computerize with the most flexible and upgradable system available. The increased complexity in home health care billing and reporting increases the need for management to have a sophisticated computer and MIS. The selection of an automated system must be made systematically to obtain the desired results. Otherwise, the HHA may find out what the first theorem of computerization really is: GIGO (garbage in—garbage out), while the last theorem is "don't convert bad or incomplete data."

The decision of whether to use consultants in selecting a computer system must first be examined in terms of what the system is to do. Outside consultants can help or hinder the process. Presently there is no certification process identifying a consultant with bona fide training and experience in computer applications related to home health care organizations. The contract between the HHA and the consultant is established on an hourly fee basis with specific limits on fees and timing of deliverables. In any case, it is important to have your attorney review the consultant's contract to ensure its completeness. Although it may seem cheaper and easier to have one of the vendors perform this function, the vendor is not in a position to provide you with an *independent* analysis of which system would be best for your HHA. The consultant's role is to facilitate the process of selection within the time frame established, to assist in the development of the selection committee, to ensure that MIS selection committee members are able to fulfill requirements, to ensure that all important needs are met (requirements are included in the request for proposal [RFP]), and in general to ensure that the selection decision is made. Because of this, the consultant's people skills are as important as his or her computer and agency industry knowledge.

APPROACH TO SELECTING AUTOMATION AND MIS

Computerization or automation is available to the HHA on several levels. Although some HHAs may still opt for a pre-1990 approach to data accumulation and bill processing (ranging from batch processing to HHA terminal entry whether batch processing or on-line), most will select an in-house microcomputer-based system. Few mainframe HHA software applications are cost-effective or available, and in recent years, they have extended to integrated linked systems with hospital or managed care payer computers (Table 51–1). The choice of processing type depends on the internal application needed by the HHA, the available staffing and capabilities, and the initial and ongoing costs. These costs are measured by including the costs of software, hardware, on-line processing, personnel, office space needs, paper, insurance, and any other directly related costs associated with each option. There is a significant, and generally underestimated, cost of setup, training, and conversion of data.

When one is making the decision to computerize, software should be selected first, and then the compatible hardware should be selected. The most common mistake for the first-time buyer is selecting hardware first, or when upgrading, limiting the selection process because of the desire to reuse as much of the existing hardware as possible. Only if the HHA is part of an integrated delivery system (IDS) that has a "deemed" (preselected by the IDS) platform selected for all MIS use, should hardware be one of the initial parameters of the selection. An excellent, top-of-the-line machine may be easy to select but becomes a large paperweight if the software selected to run on it does not meet the agency's current and future needs. This is why the MIS selection committee is so important (Exhibit 51–1). With this committee, the following steps must be taken:

1. A chair should be selected and a specific timetable established. It is also helpful to establish a standard format to be used by each committee member for the next three steps.
2. For each area within the agency, each committee member solicits ideas and concerns from colleagues.
3. For those agencies that have some form of automation (Exhibit 51–2), each committee member solicits ideas and comments regarding the current system.
4. Each committee member summarizes these comments in two lists: needs (requirements) and wants (would be nice to have).
5. With these lists, the committee constructs an agreed-upon system needs/requirements list.
6. This will be attached to an RFP that is sent to potential vendors. As part of the RFP process, committee members should try to project future volumes and needs as well as any constraints—pricing, platform, integration.
7. The responses from the vendors are received and evaluated (by number grading) based on the system needs/requirements list. The list of system needs/requirements should have each element ranked according to its relative importance in the selection. (The relative ranking of each system attribute should be agreed to before receipt of vendor responses.)
8. From this review, two or three vendors are selected for an in-house demonstration.
9. Further evaluation by the committee members is done after the demonstration, and one or more vendors are selected for an on-site visit.
10. The committee performs site visits and ranks vendors.
11. The committee selects a negotiator.
12. An attorney is selected to review the contracts.
13. The selection is made and the final points to the contract and pricing are resolved.

As part of this process, the proposed software programs should be seen in a functioning setting, so that committee members can be assured that the program is complete, available, and free of problems.

TYPES OF SYSTEMS AND FEATURES

As shown in Table 51–1, there are various approaches to the types of system used in the

Table 51–1 Comparison of Data Processing Levels

Type	Consideration
Batch Processing	Low front-end dollar commitment Monthly processing costs directly related to volume Little control over processing time Balancing with service bureau may be difficult Little management reporting above basic (standard) level Reporting to management at specific time (monthly) Little customizing
Batch processing with HHA terminal input	Monthly processing costs increase over batch processing but are generally directly related to volume; include data transmission costs More control over processing Balancing done by HHA staff at time of entry Generally, reports have the same level of sophistication as those from batch processing
On-line processing (service bureau)	Front-end dollar commitment covers terminals and printers Monthly costs are a combination of volume-related processing costs and fixed payments relating to equipment Balancing and processing performed at HHA (some service bureaus may perform certain tasks such as mailing bills or statements from the service bureau location) More control over processing Reporting may be more responsive and flexible by allowing the HHA to run its own specialized reports
In-house system	Front-end costs can be significant in both hardware and conversion Monthly costs tend to be at a fixed level regardless of volume All processing performed internally with schedule established by HHA based on its need May include customizing of software for the HHA Responsibility for data backups left to HHA
Electronic interface	Can be costly to set up Good sharing of data Best use in IDS where data needs to be shared

Exhibit 51–1 The MIS Selection Committee

- Administrator
- Financial manager
- Billing representative
- Home care nurse
- Home health aide
- Consultant on computer (internal or external)

agency. The modules, or application programs, commonly available are as follows:

- billing, statistical reporting, and accounts receivable
- general ledger
- accounts payable
- payroll
- sick and vacation time (accrued and taken)

Exhibit 51–2 Issues To Be Handled by the MIS
Selection Committee

Internal staff/administrative time
Lost income from providers while in
committee meetings
Consultant review
Attorney review of contracts
Software
Hardware
Internal facility construction/reconstruction
for system use
Conversion data
Training (outside services and lost time by
staff)
New forms/filing system
Maintenance agreements
If upgrade, loss on old system

- fixed asset reporting
- inventory/durable medical equipment (DME) control
- plan of treatment (and Health Care Financing Administration Forms 485 to 488)
- word processing
- report/spreadsheet program (for modeling, end-of-year planning, etc.)
- cost reporting
- electronic bill transmission
- scheduling
- outcome analysis and costs

Other modules that are becoming increasingly available are: electronic receipts, collection follow-up, third-party contracting, and managed care cost analysis.

The terms *bundled, unbundled*, and *turnkey* are often used in the sales presentation of in-house systems (see Appendix 51–A for a glossary of terms). Bundled or turnkey systems are substantially the same in concept: The vendor combines hardware and software into a package to be sold as one unit. Unbundled software allows you the choice of several hardware vendors with which the software is compatible. If a turnkey or bundled system is chosen, the vendor is responsible for any problem with both soft-

ware and hardware. If an unbundled computer package is chosen, the HHA must coordinate activities and problems between the software vendor and the hardware vendor. In some cases, the unbundled system is the better choice if:

- the software vendor's location is far from you and faster service could be provided from a local hardware vendor (downtime is caused more often by hardware problems than by software problems)
- you can negotiate a better price for hardware from local vendors (this savings, however, must be offset by the future coordination time between hardware and software vendors)
- you already have compatible hardware in your HHA and want to use it with the new system

With the use of modems, the software company generally has the capability to analyze computer problems from a distance (by looking inside your system), which could require the cooperation by several vendors when the HHA includes existing (compatible) hardware within their contracts. Consequently, the risk that there may be unresolved issues between the hardware and the software vendors may result in more down time and personnel frustration.

Further, the HHA must decide whether to choose multiuser (at multiple branch locations) or multitasking systems. Multiuser systems can accept and process information from several terminals at a time. Multitasking permits several users, all doing different things, to be on the system. For example, the accounting department could process general ledger and payroll at the same time that new patients are being entered and scheduling is being revised by someone else within the HHA. If care providers are also using the system to enter care plan and care results from the field, the capacity of the system must be increased significantly.

In the last few years, with the growth of larger agencies and IDSs, the use of linking programs with managed care companies, hospitals, and other providers as well as automated medical records is becoming more important. This is due to the rising cost of personnel and the need to collect the data for outcome studies. After the software is selected, the hardware needs should be determined. The pertinent areas to be considered are:

- *processor size:* this equates to the speed required for the number of unique data elements and the volume of visits (or data elements) to be processed
- *memory size:* this is a result of determining the storage capacity needs based on the size of the HHA, the software file structure, and the level of multiuser, multitasking sophistication
- *monitors and printers:* the number of each must be determined based on function, staff, and layout of the office (or branches)
- *communication lines:* these are used for electronic billing and also for communication between different locations; in considering modem communications, the cost/benefit of this method of data transfer must be investigated.

An experienced systems analyst from the selected software vendor can take the HHA's written list of needs/requirements and assist in many of these decisions. It is prudent to have a guarantee by the vendor for upgrade requirements above those recommended for the first year. The goal of the vendor guarantee is to prevent the agency from incurring substantial additional costs if the hardware or software requirements have been underestimated by the vendor in an effort to make the sale. To do this, however, the vendor will require volume projections from the HHA to estimate the input/output specifications, and base the guarantee on that level of volume. In other words, the vendor will guarantee functionality of the system to the maximum level.

An attorney experienced in computer contracting should review every contract. There are many concerns often overlooked in computerizing: freight, supplies, sales tax, installation, training (cost and location), conversion (costs and timing), hardware and software support, computer consulting, legal review of contracts, adequacy of air conditioning, special carpeting, and costs of laying cables. Considering these factors is important in order for the agency to obtain the desired result.

WHY SHOULD AN HHA COMPUTERIZE?

Few, if any, agencies are not automated in some form. Generally the decision faced by HHAs is to what level the sophistication should be increased and at what cost. The decision to change systems is often caused by some painful experience by the agency. Sometimes the feeling starts as an uncomfortable choking experience: mounds of paper swell and management and staff are overwhelmed until it becomes impossible to make decisions required in managed care contracting or other business opportunities that must be based on data, trends, or projections.

Although reasons to move to more sophisticated MIS may be more subtle, the basis for automation should be evaluated by considering the current and future needs of the HHA. Small or rural agencies must weigh the cost against the need for good management information with limited resources. On the other hand, large agencies must be concerned with finding a system large enough to handle multiple locations and able to report data from each office as well as to summarize data selectively. Add to this the need found in IDSs to share data on patients.

For hospital-based agencies, the concern is often whether the hospital system can handle the needs of the HHA. Baker (1986) was concerned about the transition from having the hospital perform the billings and statistical reporting to having a computer system that the HHA could use itself to perform these functions. He also believed that increased and more sophisticated reporting from the home health MIS system was required for productive management. This industry-specific data gathering and analysis is still not normally available from a hospital system even now, 10 years later.

Although home health agency directors define the needs of their agencies based on differences in growth, size, and corporate structure, the concerns are similar and their analysis very similar. General concerns developing into a "why should we upgrade our computer system?" question are:

- *more efficient managing*: The type and details of reports that can be generated weekly, daily, or immediately, allowing HHA management to make better decisions based on analyzing historical business and patient care patterns and trends, which can be developed into realistic projections and forecast techniques.
- *reduced costs*: This is a "maybe." The system can reduce costs by collapsing the effort for necessary paperwork and clerical activity, but the cost of sophistication may eliminate any initial savings.
- *increased profit potential*: The system should minimize increased costs for generating all insurance and third-party invoices quickly (including the follow-up on overdue accounts), but the greatest potential is in managing patient care and the business.
- *increased competitiveness in the marketplace*: Increasing productivity, improving efficiency, and raising the level of patient service enable an HHA to become more competitive. The financial impact of a capitated or prospective payment system can be evaluated, and the HHA can become one of the leaders in home health care. Before choosing to computerize, each HHA must analyze what is needed and whether a specific system meets its specific needs.

"Keeping up with the Joneses" by selecting the computer system they use, is not a good approach unless the Jones HHA has the same needs as your HHA, and Jones is becoming stronger as a result of better management, better

marketing, and better fiscal planning resulting from their selected MIS.

WHEN SHOULD AN HHA COMPUTERIZE? THE ANSWER IS: "YESTERDAY."

It would be simple if there were an HHA industry standard based on the number of patients or visits that said, "An HHA should always automate when it reaches 12,000 visits per year." However, there is no simple and fixed rule. However, advisors often use the following indicators to gauge the need to evaluate the current level of computerization:

- *disappointing revenue growth:* Because of the past, the economy, the competition, or Medicare reduction in coverage, business growth is not matching predictions and management is not sure why.
- *disturbing profit trends:* Compared with previous performance in the industry, profits are down.
- *various financial and statistical indications of suboptimal operation:* These include factors such as lengthening of the average age of receivables, increases in bad debt losses, excessive employee overtime, reduction in the ratio of reimbursement to revenue-generated equity or other assets, and reduced revenue dollars per patient.
- *a chaotic work environment:* Employees rush frantically from problem to problem.
- *lack of information:* Knowing too little about what is happening reduces productivity and reimbursement.
- *lack of uniformity:* Records are not updated with any degree of standardization, procedures are not followed in every situation, and decisions are not always made on a uniform basis.

After one determines that it is time to computerize, there will be some normal hesitation as to what the change may bring. Additional hesitation is a natural response to realizing the high level of effort required to computerize. If the agency is still in doubt about whether now is the time to purchase the computer system, three additional points should be considered:

1. If a small business computer would save money or make money for the HHA now, then the HHA is losing money by not having it.
2. Peripherals (e.g., printers, hard disks, etc.) and software will be useful even if the computer becomes obsolete. The computer itself is usually the least expensive component of all and can be used for other, noncritical processing.
3. By owning a computer now, an HHA can obtain the benefits of automation while learning to use the system. If the need arises to upgrade to a larger, more powerful system, it will be easier to do so.

Additionally, even though Medicare's reimbursement under cost finding requires depreciation of the computer system, many of these costs for computer conversion will be covered by Medicare in the year of the conversion, if the cost of the conversion is separately stated. A prospective payment methodology will not generally provide additional payments to the HHA to automate. *Consequently, it is important to improve the level and sophistication now of the computer system while it's a covered expense.* Finally, the cost to computerize has dramatically reduced even as the sophistication has increased.

The DME industry set some standards in the mid-1980s for computerization: when a DME company reached 75 to 100 patients per month (Liska, 1986) it was at the optimal point for automation. DME companies are generally more aggressive about automation and are outspoken about the consequences of not automating: "After the dust settles I think you will find out the strong [DME] dealers will survive, the weak will not. The strong ones will appreciate the value of a computer to keep them managed and expand their business and to pinpoint mar-

keting effort" (Liska, 1986, p. 138). In 1996, this has proven to be true for the DME companies. These comments are appropriate for HHAs as well. The HHA that has strong data processing and management reporting systems early in its development will manage its growth with effectiveness and efficiency.

DEVELOPING YOUR OWN SOFTWARE

By using existing software products that meet its specifications, the HHA saves time and money. One disadvantage often cited in using standard, or "canned," packages is that the HHA often has to make some compromises in its specifications or in the way it has traditionally processed its paperwork or coding. This need for compromise generally is mitigated when a database system is selected.

Even when the compromises are made in the system selected, the vendor will ensure that it works and does most of what the HHA wants (and needs). The desire for a "perfect system" is generally what compels an HHA to develop its own, although this goal is rarely achieved. Consider the lost opportunity costs and the overall drain on the management and staff of the HHA: after an experienced systems analyst (with home health care experience) is hired, the development of a new home health care billing, statistical reporting, and accounts receivable package can require 18 months for programming and testing, development of documentation and the user manual, and creation of support services; add to this time factor several hundreds of thousands of dollars.

It is important to determine whether the cost to create a system is really worth it: it takes the time of people at the agency to work with the programmer, time that should be spent running the business of the agency and pursuing opportunities in the marketplace. One of the prime risks of using customized software is that it can contain bugs or errors that, surprisingly, can exist undetected for months or even years before making a sudden and unwelcome appearance—often after the programmer has left and the documentation is not adequate to make a fast fix.

Existing software packages, on the other hand, allow users to examine their performance. Even if a package has been on the market for only a few months, it probably has the equivalent of many years of usage. This extensive usage tends to minimize the risk of bugs or errors. In an industry that must adapt quickly to new Medicare requirements, the vendors with existing software are ready to make these changes. The HHA needs software that is specifically developed for home care, that can accommodate changes quickly, and that is at the forefront of improving management and the medical information system.

ARE THERE ANY GUARANTEES?

No. Even though warranties may be given, they are a source of continuing and troublesome questions. Generally, existing software is provided "as is" without any warranties. Unlike many other products, software is subject to so many variables in use, and its evaluation is so subjective, that vendors, as a practical matter, could not charge enough for mass-marketed software to cover their exposure to warranty problems. This means that the HHA assumes all risk for the operation and suitability of the selected package. Thus the HHA must be aware of the strengths and weaknesses of a given package before selecting it. This starts at the selection process: even with significant diligence it is possible to purchase "smokeware"—software that doesn't exist as described or promised.

An HHA that contracts for custom software may be able to obtain a warranty that the product will substantially conform to the agreed specifications for some period of time and will be covered (as long as the vendor is in business) for any determination that the warranty has been breached. Even these guarantees, however, will not protect you from missing requirements in your specifications. For existing or canned

packages, use the following steps to test the software package:

1. Use the package itself for testing, not the demonstration model. Try a section of the program yourself.
2. Determine whether the software is user-friendly by determining how the help screens, menus, and on-line tutorials assist you.
3. Test your requirements against the features included in the package.
4. Review the documentation (instruction manual) to determine that it is clearly written, understandable, and helpful.

Even though a contract disclaims all warranties, vendors will generally attempt to limit their liability for damages, usually to the cost of the package, if they are found liable for breach of contract. Consequently, the best "insurance" is to purchase from a known vendor and hold back a portion of the purchase price until you test and accept the product.

There are two other ways to improve your chances for success: the first is to develop a high level of expertise within the HHA. In some cases, it may mean that a few people will receive a more comprehensive level of training; this is often called the "train the trainer" approach to implementation and support. These people become the internal resource, which is more cost-effective in larger organizations. This approach has been successful at several VNAs. The second method is to standardize throughout the HHA: the same information services (IS) support, the same hardware and software/communication vendors, the same machine layout (capacity and program set-up), and the same implementation (or roll-out) plan that eliminates multiple steps to reach the same result or end.

ACCEPTANCE TESTING FOR SOFTWARE

Because software is intangible, there is always the question of whether a package (written or modified to the HHA's specifications) is performing in accordance with specifications. Consequently, an acceptance test should be incorporated into either a software development contract (for custom software) or in purchased software to provide an objective measure of whether the software corresponds to the specifications using data supplied by the HHA. This test should be performed on the vendor's premises to the satisfaction of the user before the software is installed in the HHA's place of business and before any final payment is made.

FINAL THOUGHTS ABOUT CUSTOMIZED AND PURCHASED SOFTWARE

Custom software is the most expensive option in software selection. It will require the greatest expenditure as well as the greatest effort from agency staff. The HHA will generally need to hire an experienced systems analyst or developer to assist in negotiating with the software development house. During the time of development, the HHA must have another system to handle the ongoing billing and reporting. It is a decision to be made with a great deal of forethought. In contract negotiations, be sure that software is written in a platform or language that is generally used in the industry, and that the source code and all documentation will be property of the HHA. In this way, if the HHA and the software development company eventually choose not to work with each other, the HHA is safeguarded by owning all its programs, which can be maintained and modified by some other software house.

For "canned" or purchased software, the source code should be maintained by some third party (a banker, lawyer, or trade association) so that the HHA will be protected if the software vendor goes out of business. To the extent possible, the agency should learn of other HHAs who are using the products and go to user group meetings.

In the software and hardware maintenance agreement, be sure that the response time is stated and that there is a clear description of costs of software upgrades. In all cases, have an attorney write or review the contract. A performance bond or some other note to ensure program completion should also be seriously considered. The sad story is that software often turns out to be unsuitable or unworkable. A great deal of time and money can be devoted to entering data and learning software that does not perform as expected. The ultimate costs of poorly performing software can far exceed the direct costs paid for the package. To minimize risk in the software purchase, unexpected problems should be avoided. To avoid these problems, the following five major reasons why users encounter software problems and the appropriate response to each should be understood:

1. Software cannot be examined. Only the results of using it can be examined. The HHA staff will purchase the software but may fail to test all functions of a given piece of software. As a result, inadequate capabilities, such as insufficient report-generation capacity or inability to retain month-to-month data for comparison or update purposes, may go unnoticed.

2. There are no objective HHA industry standards for comparing the capabilities of various software packages (each package is, to a great extent, unique). To a certain degree, this difficulty can be surmounted by the use of standardized tests, called benchmarks. Although these are time-consuming and expensive to develop, the HHA is often left to develop them on its own based on what may be limited exposure to software selection requirements.

3. Many users, surprisingly, do not really understand their business operations. This problem is often compounded by the unrealistic assumption that a few hours of discussion will allow a software vendor to understand both the HHA's business operations and the HHA's data processing needs.

4. Many prospective computer users do not have a clear understanding of the capabilities and inherent limitations of computerization.

5. Users and vendors have substantially different expectations of the transaction. Users (HHAs) expect to obtain a program that will make a continuing contribution to their business operations, whereas vendors are interested in concluding the sale and moving on to the next one. Before the HHA can evaluate software, it must define its needs. This is not only a time-consuming process but also one of the biggest stumbling blocks for first-time users. A critical, multifaceted review of current and future operations will affect selection, implementation, and results.

REFERENCES

Baker, D. (1986, March). Managing a hospital based home health information system. *Computers in Healthcare,* 7(3).

Knauer, C. (1984, August). The microcomputer in hardware purchaser decision from the user's viewpoint. *Healthcare Financial Management.*

Liska, J. (1986, April 28). *Home Health Line, xi,* 138.

Muellin, J.H. (1986). Strategic importance of MIS for home healthcare. *Computers in Healthcare,* 7(6).

Tolos, P.C., and D. Moody. (1986). *Choosing and using the right medical office computer.* Oradell, NJ: Medical Economics Books.

Glossary

Application program—Program written to accomplish a specific purpose.

Applications software—A computer program that carries out a specific task or tasks, such as verifying patient eligibility, scheduling appointments, generating bills, or recording laboratory test results.

Architecture—The general technical layout of a computer system, usually including the hardware, operating system, and applications software. Common choices for architecture are mainframe and distributed client/server computing. See also **Open architecture.**

Artificial intelligence (AI)—An application capable of mimicking human thought or generating new knowledge, such as a program that suggests treatment protocols based on a patient's condition.

ASCII—Pronounced "AS-KEY." American Standard Code for Information Interchange character code; used for representing information by most non-IBM equipment.

Audit trail—Records of every transaction with a record of the source of the entry; a means of tracing errors.

Back-up—Duplicate of a file made to protect information.

Batch processing—Method by which data are handled by an outside organization and the results sent to the submitting office; see **Offline**.

Baud—Speed of communications between devices (300 baud is 30 characters per second).

Billing and statements

- **Contract billing**—Bills sent out for a set amount per month as agreed to under a contract and not for services as they are rendered (such as health maintenance organization).
- **Cycle billing**—Statements sent out at specific times for part of the accounts (A to L on the 15th and M to Z on the 30th).
- **Monthly statements**—Sent to all patients when a balance is owed.
- **Statement**—Notification of the status of an account, even though the balance may be zero.
- **Third-party billing**—Bills sent to insurance companies or other guarantors, such as UB-92, the billing form for home care.

Bit—Contraction of binary digit; operating unit of a computer (essentially an on/off switch).

Board—Thin, flat component that serves as the base for one or more layers of electronic circuits.

Boot—Starting up a computer.

Bridge—A simple, limited-function device for connecting a series of two or more segments of a local area network (LAN). A bridge has a physical interface or port for each LAN to which it is connected.

Broadband network—A network capable of transporting voice and interactive full-motion video and data services.

Buffer—Memory that holds data before transactions are performed on it, to speed up processing.

Bug—Error or anomaly in a software program.

Byte—Usually eight bits; the unit of symbolic transfer (i.e., every character, alphabetic or numeric, is one byte).

Cartridge disk—Removable disk (five megabytes or more) in a convenient cartridge form.

Central processing unit (CPU)—Part of a computer where data are processed and manipulated; contains the main memory, operating system chip, RAM and ROM, and the controller for the entire system.

Chip—Integrated circuit; the building block of a computer.

Circuit board—Systematic arrangement of circuits that can be easily inserted or removed; electronic building blocks of a computer.

Clinical decision support—The capability of a system to provide key data to clinicians in response to certain rule-based triggers.

COBOL—Common Business-Oriented Language.

Community health information networks (CHINs)—Networks that are forming to exchange data electronically among computer systems of various health care financing and delivery organizations serving a defined geographic region. CHINs would facilitate seamless care and community-wide analysis of information on resource utilization, patient outcomes, and health status.

Compatibility—The ability of one computer system to accept data and commands from another computer. The technical characteristics of the hardware, operating system, and applications software determine compatibility.

Configure—To design the components of a computer to perform assigned functions in a particular manner.

Console—Terminal that has the most control in the system; sometimes used to refer to any terminal or monitor.

Continuous form—Fan-folded, pin-fed paper.

Controller—Device to control peripherals.

Conversion—Entry of manual records into a computer.

Coprocessor—A second CPU in a single device.

Core or core memory—Central or main memory.

Custom program—Software written especially for an individual application that has limited use outside that application.

Data—All information processed by the computer.

Database—Organized information available for access by a computer (e.g., names and addresses, diseases and their symptoms, a bibliography, etc.).

Data dictionary—A list that describes the specifications and locations of all data contained in a given system.

Data element—A specific piece of information or required content, such as a subscriber's name or identification number; when arranged in a specific grouping or order, data elements constitute a format.

Data repository (Clinical repository)—A place or system that maintains information electronically. Examples include a hospital's clinical data repository, a claims administrator's claims history database, or a community health information network's distributed database.

DBMS—Database Management System.

Debug—To identify and eliminate errors and anomalies in a software program.

Disk crash—Destruction of information on a disk by a mechanical malfunction in the disk drive.

Diskette—Another term for a floppy disk.

Disk file—File residing on a disk.

Distributed client/server computing—A type of architecture in which many computer terminals are distributed throughout an organization and are connected to one or more servers and to each other through a network. The operating system, applications software, and data are stored on various servers but are accessible throughout the network.

Documentation—Written instructions for operating hardware or software.

DOS—Disk Operating System.

Downloading—Sending information or programs from one system (generally larger) to another (generally smaller) through the modem.

Down time—Time when a computer is not operational.

Dumb terminal—A computing unit that has a keyboard and a screen but no internal memory; it functions as an input/display unit only. A dumb terminal can function only because it is attached to another unit that serves its processor.

DBCDIC—Like ASCII, a means of assigning binary codes to character sets on IBM computers.

E-mail—Electronic mail; it allows users to send notes and other types of textual information—such as a physician's referral instructions to a consultant and the consultant's report back to the referring physician—from one computer to another. Newer e-mail systems allow the exchange of voice and digital information, as well.

Edit—To correct and maintain text.

Electronic billing—To submit insurance claims electronically via the computer and modem instead of manually via the mail.

Electronic data interchange (EDI)—The electronic transmission of data in a standard syntax or format by means of computer-to-computer exchange—either real time or batch—via a standard on-line transmission method between sites not on the same computer network.

Electronic medical record (EMR)—Although the exact nature of what constitutes an EMR is still a topic of debate, it generally is considered to be progress notes, test results, consultant's reports, medication records, and other aspects of patient care stored in electronic form, allowing immediate exchange of information across the network. EMRs also facilitate data analysis, such as the impact of a particular anesthetic on time spent in the recovery room. An EMR is part of a managed care information system.

Executive information system—A software application that allows senior leaders to make straightforward inquiries on their computer and receive information from a mainframe or server immediately in easily understood formats, such as graphs showing monthly admission trends or a list of frequently ordered medications categorized by subspecialty.

Field—A database reserved for specific information.

File—Collection of records in the same type and in the same format, such as patient demographic information.

Fixed disk—Hard disk that is permanently attached in a computer.

Flag—Indicator associated with a special condition (an insurance flag would indicate that a patient has insurance).

Flow chart—Symbolic representation of a program sequence.

Gateway tools—Tools that permit entering and exiting a communications network.

GIGO—Garbage In—Garbage Out.

Graphical user interface (GUI)—Applications that display icons and buttons that a user can point to or press to carry out various functions. GUI programs allow "intuitive" computer use.

Hard copy—Printed copy or microform output.

Hard disk—Peripheral memory storage unit in a rigid format.

Hardware—The computer onto which the operating systems and applications software are loaded.

Head crash—Head failure that damages the disk.

Hospital information system—Computer system used by a hospital primarily to register patients, record services performed, and generate bills and other financial information. In recent years, these systems have expanded to include clinical as well as financial information.

Index—Shortcut means of locating specific data on a file; a key for accessing data.

Infrastructure—The basic facilities and installations needed for the functioning of an information system. It includes cable links among providers and existing data centers, computer hardware and electronics, personnel, and financing.

Interactive—Equipment that responds directly to the user's input.

Interface—*1*, Boundary, meeting, or connection between components; *2*, Ability of components to work synergistically; *3*, Human/machine interaction.

Interface engine—The software that permits communication between various components of an information system.

Internal memory—Memory of the central processing unit.

Internet—An international computer network known as the "network of networks."

IS—An acronym for information systems.

IT—An acronym for information technology, which broadly refers to knowledge about and knowledge generated from information systems.

Legacy systems—Computer applications that have been "inherited" through previous information system acquisitions and installations. Legacy systems run business applications that generally are not integrated with each other. Open and distributed systems are enabling organizations to make the transition from maintaining older legacy systems toward taking an enterprisewide network approach to systems development.

Line surge—Sharp change in voltage that can cause equipment damage.

Linking—To connect two software packages or applications to transfer and share data.

Load—Transfer of data or a program to execute a set of commands.

Local area networks (LANs). See **Network.**

Longitudinal patient record—An electronic or paper record detailing a patient's lifetime medical history, showing diagnoses, treatments, pharmacological interventions, and other health care efforts.

LPs—Lines per second (speed of a line printer).

Mainframe computing—An architecture in which the operating system, applications software, and data all are stored in a single, large computer and accessed by terminals.

Main memory—High-speed, readily addressable memory.

Managed care information system—An information system designed to automate the major functions of an organization engaged in managed care. Components may include patient eligibility and benefits, registration, electronic medical records, authorization and referral tracking, capitation and billing, scheduling, and utilization management.

Master patient index or Master person index—A single patient identification number or code that is recognized by every individual IS within a network.

Medical workstation—See **Terminal.**

Memory—Data held in storage.

Menu—Listing of options in functions or programs.

Merge—To combine two or more records or files into one.

Microcomputer—Small computer system usually costing less than $40,000.

Microprocessor—The CPU of a microcomputer.

Modem—A device that connects a computer to a telephone line, allowing data to be transmitted and retrieved via phone lines.

Module—Pertaining to software, any part of a software program that performs a specific function (e.g., billing, patient/staff scheduling, recertification, and so on).

Monitor—Computer readout terminal (CRT) for displaying computer information.

Motherboard—Essential electronic board in a computer to which daughter boards may be connected to extend functions.

MS-DOS—Microsoft Disk Operating System; IBM personal computer operating language.

Multiplexon—Device to tie in several modems.

Multitasking—Performs more than one task simultaneously.

Multiuser—System that allows multiple terminals to be used simultaneously.

Network—The interconnection of computers by cables, telephone lines, or wireless communication. Networks allow data transmission among computers. Local area networks (LANs) generally reside in one location. Wide area networks (WANs) span geographical boundaries, linking, for example, hospitals and physicians' offices.

Object code—Output code readable by the computer.

Off-line—*1*, A processing operation completed separate from the mainframe (e.g., batch); *2*, Storing mass memory in a removable disk format.

On-line—*1*, Direct processing between satellite or peripheral equipment and the host computer; *2*, Having data or information available to call immediately into use.

Open architecture—A computer network that allows integration of various types of components.

Operating system—Computer software that controls the allocation and use of hardware resources and the execution of application programs. Common operating systems are Unix and Microsoft Windows™ NT.

Optical disk archiving—A process that stores large amounts of information on optical disks and allows rapid retrieval of specific information, such as medical records or radiological images.

Output—Information delivered by the system after processing.

Overhead—Amount of disk space or main memory consumed by system requirements, including keys, indexes, programs, and instructions.

Parallel—Simultaneous performing of tasks.

Parameters—Descriptions of limitations or control levels.

Password—User identification to allow access.

Peripherals—Devices attached to the computer, adding to its value and the functions it can perform.

Power surge—Current exceeding 110 to 120 V that may damage the data set, programs, or computer.

Platform—Word used to describe an operating system for a new generation of software.

Program—Logical sequence of instructions.

Protocols—Standardized formats that allow file exchange between computers.

Purge—To clean or eliminate data.

RAM—Random access memory; a portion of the core memory dedicated to the storage and manipulation of data.

Random—Not sequential; accessible at any point.

Record—Data arranged in sequence to make up a file.

Record length—Limit to the amount of information in a file.

Relational database—A database model in which information is stored in two-dimensional tables consisting of rows and columns. The rows represent records and the columns represent data fields—the pieces that form the entire record.

Report writer—Program enabling the user to prepare an analysis or report from the data in the system and to define the information, the order, and the presentation format.

Response time—The method of timing different computer operations; a measure of speed and efficiency.

RFP—Request for proposal; formal document used to gather consistent information from a vendor for making a decision.

Save—Reading information from temporary storage into permanent storage.

Server—The main computer on a network, which holds the network's applications software and, sometimes, its data.

Smart card—Memory cards the size of a credit card that can be carried by the patient, some holding more than 2,000 pages of medical and personal information.

Software—The instructions written to tell the hardware what to do.

Sort—To sequence data according to specified parameters.

Source code—Original program code that is translated to object code for the computer to use.

Spool—Allows an action, such as printing, to occur while the computer can still be used for other work.

Standalone—Hardware and software combined, making a complete system.

Standards—Clearly defined and agreed-upon conventions for the operation and behavior of specific computing functions, formats, and processes.

Streaming tape—Quick back-up system for a hard disk.

Surge protector—A device used to prevent line surges from damaging data or equipment.

Systems analysis—Determination of the detailed components that make up a system and the development of specifications.

Systems design—Plans drawn up to achieve the specifications, tasks, and objectives of a system.

Systems integrator—Vendor that puts together hardware and software from different manufacturers and sells it as a system (also called a value-added resaler).

Telemedicine—The practice of using two-way audio and video communications (via telephone lines or satellite) to link patients and caregivers or allow caregivers access to medical and technological resources.

Terminal—A workstation hooked up to a mainframe or network server. A dumb terminal cannot perform computer functions by itself. Smart or intelligent terminals contain their own operating system and applications software, allowing users to perform tasks on and off the network.

Throughput—Speed at which processes occur.

Time sharing—Multiple users on one system.

Turnkey system—Computer system completely assembled, installed, and ready to use.

Unbundled—When software, hardware, and other components are sold and priced separately.

Upgrade—To improve a system by trading up.

UPS—Uninterruptible power supply; a device to maintain a constant current preventing power surges or brownouts.

User-friendly—System that is designed to be easy to learn and use.

Utilities—Programs used to accomplish normal data processing tasks (e.g., sort).

Volatile storage—Storage device, such as RAM, that loses data when the current is turned off.

Virtual integrated delivery system—A term applied to companies that buy group practices in a market and tie them together with information technology that enables the exchange of clinical and financial information. It is expected that a group practice owner will enter into contracts with other providers to offer the full continuum of care to capitated managed care plans, then electronically link all of the sites in a region.

Voice recognition—The ability of some programs to understand the user's voice and translate that voice into action or into dictation by digitizing speech.

Winchester disk—Sealed high-density hard disk.

Windows—Ability to look at and process information in a second file or record while the screen continues to show the original record.

Write—Process of entering or changing data.

Write-protect—Process or code preventing overwriting of data or programs.

Xenix—Platform/operating system allowing for multiusers and multiactions (sometimes referred to as UNIX).

CHAPTER 52

An Overview of One Home Health Agency Management Information System

Charles G. Farber

Computer software designed explicitly for use in home health agencies has been available for more than 20 years. During those years, an astounding rate of change has been maintained in the computer sciences, the application systems available, the computer industry in general, and the home health industry as a whole. Some architectures such as batch processing by service bureaus have come and gone only to return in more modern form. The batch processing of yesteryear has been expanded to include more features and user access and is now marketed as outsourcing. This is based on a theory that any entity should focus on what it does best. Home health agencies deliver care; data processors deal with computing. This makes a great deal of sense and may gain popularity. Currently a great many home health agencies opt to install a computer system in their offices. There are a variety of vendors with adequate systems, each unique in scope and approach. These systems may be installed in a variety of configurations that are chosen to best suit the needs of an individual agency. The complexity of these will vary from a "shrink wrap" product for use at small sites, to self-contained standalone systems and complex hybrid systems utilizing processing power at the agency as well as at a remote service provider.

GENERALIZED SYSTEM ARCHITECTURES

One recognized name in the home health software industry is Delta Health Systems of Altoona, Pennsylvania. The software marketed by Delta has evolved over more than 20 years from a small service bureau package to a complex application containing a number of modules, each designed to address specific needs. Flexibility has been maintained, which allows a single product to address multiple configurations. Batch processing services are still provided, as are standalone systems and the hybrids that combine local processing capabilities with the remote mainframe power maintained at the vendor location. The batch and hybrid systems are available on multiple host-based computing platforms using the open architecture of AT&T's UNIX SVR5, SCO UNIX, and IBM's AIX. Earlier systems tied to a vendor-specific, proprietary operating system are still supported, as are two of the more prevalent network protocols: Novell *NetWare* and TCP/IP. These are supported on a variety of topologies. An important aspect worthy of consideration is the number of product variants needed for one to make use of such an array of computers. In this case, only one system has been developed and is maintained with no special platform-dependent code. A single product removes the need for large numbers of slightly different product releases, allows for more rapid response to changes, and frees support personnel from being overly concerned about the specific pieces of hardware in use at a given site. Another benefit of this technique is seen in the ease of movement between platforms brought on by an inherent forward compatibility. All this has been referring to the primary data processing system, whose purpose is seen as managerial in nature. This type of system is used to collect and use demographic data, caregiver activity data, charge and payment data, and statistical data. In a business setting, this might be described as a back office system.

A new class of product that would have been inconceivable just a few short years ago has come to market and is now offered by several vendors. These are the field automation systems used at the point of care to collect and process data needed to run the primary back office system as well as to provide a repository of clinical data. These systems utilize portable computing devices in the hands of the caregiver as well as some type of central processor that serves as a global data store. Although some experimentation is being done with hand-held as well as pen-based computing devices, the *Clinical-Link* system has been based on more conventional notebook computers with the familiar keyboard user interface. The more sophisticated products of this class will provide each caregiver with a copy of assigned patient charts and will resolve data conflicts that arise when multiple caregivers make redundant data changes. The data gathered in these clinical systems ought to be accessible to the main processor and, as such, will eliminate redundant data collection and entry. In other words, if a caregiver sees a patient and records clinical data, the systems ought to have sufficient integration to avoid the need for a separate data entry operation informing other modules or systems of such an occurrence.

Field automation is also useful in establishing a more uniform standard of care. Certain key elements may be authored into such an application that guides caregivers through a common data set of questions and possible responses. An example of this can be seen in the automation of care plan generation. In a system based on either nursing or medical diagnosis, a decision tree can be established to isolate possible and probable responses. More comprehensive software will allow a user more or less flexibility in certain areas of the care plan. Computer-generated data are not really computer generated; they are merely selected from a database using the parameters supplied during an interview session. A desire to tailor this database to the preferences of each agency might be expressed, and a more flexible software module will provide for this. Even if the main database is not modified, it will be desirable in some situations to allow the caregiver to tailor the resulting data. Some data from the database will probably require some tailoring because many suggested interventions are frameworks needing additional data, such as number of times per day, anticipated schedule, and the like.

DATA COLLECTION

Assuming the absence of a field automation system, an examination may be made of the fundamental management of data within any of the three aforementioned categories of systems: batch, standalone, and hybrid. In any of these, data are captured at some point in space and time (not necessarily during a data entry session). The norm for this data collection uses simple paper forms. Data relevant to any particular process are captured as written notes or completed preprinted forms containing either summary or detailed data. Detailed data specific to a single patient will begin to be recorded during the admission process. Subsequent data will be provided as they become available during assessments or other functions. Summarized data might be presented in the form of a day sheet or daily report, which records data about each visit, encounter, or activity. This form will be completed for an individual caregiver on a daily or other interval basis. The data from these sheets will be input to the computer and used for billing, statistical, and payroll functions. It makes little difference whether a system is batched or standalone when data originate on paper. The recipients are different, the timings may vary, and some additional paper management may or may not be required, but the end result is still a person seated at a data entry device transcribing data from paper to electronic media.

MASTER FILE MAINTENANCE

A great deal of data are required to operate a computing system. It would be unwise to portray a picture of a system driven by only patient and activity data because, although this is certainly crucial, it is by no means all the data required to support the applications in question. A significant number of data types are required to configure and support the use of this system. Configuration issues such as options to be enabled are vital but usually are visited infrequently. Supporting files or data tables must be in place and kept current to reflect accurately the physician population, the specific pricing structure to be applied, employees and their levels of functions or authorizations, and so forth. Separate tables whose use will vary are needed to assign passwords and other more generalized system functionality. Because this is not intended to be an exhaustive list, only the patient master file is detailed further. It is also assumed and not mentioned again; any system ought to provide a means by which hard copies of the master file contents can be produced.

PATIENT MASTER UPDATE FORMS

Patient update forms (Exhibit 52–1) are used for each new patient to be added and for all subsequent changes. A number may be assigned and placed on this form, or the system may optionally generate the next available number.

This number will become the permanent key to a particular patient. Because the system will not allow the entry of a patient with essential data missing, this form must be completed before it is passed for data entry. Significant amounts of related data will be accumulated in the patient master file during an episode, but this is not required for initial entry and is not included on the paper form. All demographic data for a patient are stored in this file. Some of the accumulated data will be used for a variety of statistical reports, including service statistics and some hospice reporting. Some of the key data elements on this form are substation, payers, Social Security number, primary physician, and International Classification of Diseases (ICD-9) codes. Because these are simply paper forms meant to collect some subset of the patient master data, a great deal of flexibility may be exercised in their design, and the forms in use at one agency might be quite different from those at another. A generic form set is supplied with a system; images of these are shown in this chapter.

A substation is a vendor-specific implementation and allows an agency to define various offices or programs within the agency structure. Other fields, such as team and county, are available and can be used as reporting criteria later. For instance, an agency might use a substation to define a program, a geographic office location, or both. That agency might also provide service in a number of counties. Certain reports will allow grouping of data by substation(s) or county codes. With this parameterization, the same report is used to present data in the same format, but with distinct sorting and totaling. Patient billing data are also present in this master file, and subsequent processing functions will make use of it. For example, a change to the primary pay source can be entered with an effective date.

Another vendor-specific function known as the automatic payer change will examine the monthly visit file and adjust each record found to be out of conformance with the pay source and effective date contained in the patient mas-

Exhibit 52–1 Patient Master Update Sample

DATE COMPLETED _____

PATIENT NUMBER ☐☐☐☐☐☐☐☐☐   ACTION CODE   3 ☐ NEW PATIENT   5 ☐ CHANGE

SUBSTATION ☐ ☐

☐ A. NAME _____ _____ ___   READMIT ☐ Y

   LAST   FIRST   M.I.

☐ B. ADDRESS _____ _____ _____

   STREET   CITY   STATE   ZIP   ☐☐–☐☐–☐☐

☐ C. STATUS   DISCHARGE REASON   DISCHARGE DATE

   3 ☐ SAVE OLD PLAN   1 ☐ EXPIRED   5 ☐ MOVED
   3 ☐ ACTIVE   2 ☐ SERVICES REFUSED   6 ☐ OTHER
   4 ☐ DISCHARGED   3 ☐ INDEPENDENT   7 ☐ NURSING HOME   ☐☐–☐☐–☐☐–☐☐
   4 ☐ HOSPITAL   SERVICE CODES

☐ D. BILLING   PRIMARY   SECONDARY   ☐☐☐☐☐☐☐☐☐☐

   10 ☐ MEDICARE A   43 ☐ PRIVATE INS.   A ☐ SELF   MEDICARE NUMBER
   20 ☐ MEDICARE B   44 ☐ CMAAA - WAIVER   B ☐ PRIVATE INS.
   29 ☐ MEDICAID   45 ☐ CMAAA - HBCA   C ☐ BC & BS   ☐☐☐☐☐☐☐☐☐
   30 ☐ MEDICAID LTC   47 ☐ MEDICARE OUTPATIENT   D ☐ EMPLOYER
   38 ☐ BLUE CROSS   48 ☐ ADULT PROTECT CARE   E ☐ MEDICAID   MEDICAID CASE NUMBER
   39 ☐ COORD. HHC (HOSPICE)   49 ☐ OTHER   F ☐ OTHER
   41 ☐ SELF-PAY   ☐☐–☐☐–☐☐
   42 ☐ V.A.   PAYER CHANGE EFFECTIVE DATE

   PAY STATUS   1 ☐ NO FEE   INSURANCE DESCRIPTION ☐☐☐☐☐☐☐☐☐☐☐☐
     2 ☐ PART FEE
     3 ☐ FULL FEE   CHORE PAY ☐☐   EFFECTIVE DATE ☐☐–☐☐–☐☐

   HOMEMAKER PAY ☐☐   EFFECTIVE DATE ☐☐–☐☐–☐☐

   BC GROUP ☐☐☐☐☐☐☐   CERTIFICATE ☐☐☐☐☐☐☐☐☐

☐ E. DOCTOR _____ NO. ☐☐☐   START CARE ☐☐–☐☐–☐☐   PLAN ☐☐–☐☐–☐☐

   HOSPITAL _____ NO. ☐☐☐   STAY FROM ☐☐–☐☐–☐☐   TO ☐☐–☐☐–☐☐

   HOSPITAL _____ NO. ☐☐☐   STAY FROM ☐☐–☐☐–☐☐   TO ☐☐–☐☐–☐☐

   RE-CERTIFIED DATE ☐☐–☐☐–☐☐

☐ F. ILLNESS ☐☐☐,☐☐   DIAGNOSIS ☐☐☐☐☐☐☐☐☐☐☐☐☐☐   EMPLOYMENT RELATED

   ☐☐☐,☐☐   DIAGNOSIS ☐☐☐☐☐☐☐☐☐☐☐☐☐☐   Y ☐ N ☐

   ☐☐☐,☐☐   ☐☐☐,☐☐   ☐☐☐,☐☐

☐ G. PATIENT INFORMATION   REFERRAL   1 ☐ HOSPITAL   5 ☐ STAFF   RACE _____   SEX
     2 ☐ DOCTOR   6 ☐ SOCIAL AGENCIES   M ☐
     3 ☐ FAMILY/FRIEND   7 ☐ NURSING HOME   F ☐
     4 ☐ OTHER

   LOCALITY ☐☐☐ _____   DATE OF BIRTH ☐☐☐☐☐☐☐   PHONE ☐2☐0☐7 ☐☐☐☐☐☐☐
      MO.   DAY   YEAR   AREA   NUMBER

   LIVES ALONE   0 ☐   MARITAL STATUS   VISITS AT LEAST EVERY ☐0☐3☐0 DAYS
     1 ☐ SINGLE
   LIVES WITH OTHERS   1 ☐   2 ☐ MARRIED
     3 ☐ WIDOWED   EMPLOYEE ☐☐☐☐☐
     4 ☐ OTHER

☐ H. SELF-PAY AMTS.

   A-SKILLED NURSING ☐☐–☐☐   F-HOME HEALTH AIDE ☐☐–☐☐   K-RN PRIV DUTY ☐☐–☐☐
   B-PHYSICAL THERAPY ☐☐–☐☐   G-CHORE ☐☐–☐☐   L-LPN PRIV DUTY ☐☐–☐☐
   C-SPEECH THERAPY ☐☐–☐☐   I-CNA ☐☐–☐☐   O-OFFICE VISIT ☐☐–☐☐
   D-OCCUPATIONAL THERAPY ☐☐–☐☐   J-PCA ☐☐–☐☐   S-HOMEMAKER ☐☐–☐☐
   E-MEDICAL SOCIAL WORKER ☐☐–☐☐

Courtesy of Delta Health Systems, Inc., Altoona, Pennsylvania.

ter file. Use of this function provides a measure of confidence that all charges submitted to a pay source are truly intended for that pay source. Other fields such as physician and hospital are referenced by number. Use of numeric codes reduces the storage requirements within the system. Special studies requiring unique classifications not found in the standard file can be accommodated through the use of service codes, which are nothing more than free form codes available for agency definition. Selected reports may then accept service codes as parameters to produce detailed analyses as needed. ICD-9 codes are utilized in later reporting and are also referenced and carried into the visit files. Again, detailed reporting may be invoked to incorporate illness codes into certain sorting and totaling algorithms.

Throughout the data entry process, a series of cross-checks and validations is performed. When the system allows the operator to complete a patient entry/edit activity, there is assurance that no required data are missing and that no known inconsistencies exist. Two illustrations are the requirement that an effective date be entered along with a change to a pay source and the cross-validation involved in verifying a health insurance beneficiary number against a variety of tables, Social Security number, and/or patient sex.

DAILY REPORT FORM

Every caregiver is assigned the task of recording on paper the activities of his or her day. These data are batched according to agency desires or entry into the system. This form (Exhibit 52–2) will be used to record the employee completing it, the patient seen, supplies used, actual time used, miles driven, and the visit reason code. Visit reason codes are agency-defined codes used to classify any particular encounter between patient and caregiver. These codes might be used for a simple definition of discipline involved, or they can be used to define the primary purpose or nature of a specific visit (e.g., skilled nursing or IV change).

For brevity, these are treated as alphanumeric codes and do not need to be explicitly written out. The concept of nonvisit time is implemented on this form; time spent charting, attending inservice presentations, or participating in other related activities not involving patient contact can be captured here through the use of nonvisit codes and time fields.

Other fields are available for use on this form as well. Treatment codes can be agency-defined and will act as parameters on later reports for use in identifying high-technology visits or hospice services. Override fields are provided for pay source and charge information. These fields might be filled in by the caregiver or by some person doing subsequent reviews and adjustments. Since their use is agency-specific, they might be meaningful only at data entry time.

Once a number of forms are in the hands of data entry personnel, batching methods are applied. The forms may first be sorted by employee or date. Then a number of forms will be selected for inclusion in one batch. Batch totals will be calculated on key elements such as number of lines and charge overrides. For ease of action, should a batch be out of balance after data entry, the number of lines entered in any particular batch is recommended not to exceed 200. Because a variety of data files are updated with information from these daily forms, it is also recommended that batches be posted at least daily. These data are not available to all reporting functions before posting; frequent posts will allow all reports to reflect the most up-to-date information to be had. Frequent posts also distribute the processing over a wide time span; this is appreciated at month closing time, when there is no need to run a single process to post every visit made during the month. Also, unposted visits are considered only tentative until posting and will not appear on a bill. This has an effect if bills are produced more than once per month.

The data entry function used will do a number of cross-checks and validations to ensure accurate data. The optional requirement of entering some number of characters from the

Exhibit 52–2 Daily Report Override Charges

Courtesy of Delta Health Systems, Inc., Altoona, Pennsylvania.

patient's last name as well as the patient number works to guarantee that data are applied to the proper patient. Messages will be generated during entry if a visit is being made after the patient has been discharged from a discipline or from the agency. Checks will be made to verify that the employee discipline code allows visit reasons of the type entered. Specific billing data might also be presented as a trigger, telling the entry person to adjust the pay source or rate for one or more lines of data. An optional payroll interface may be added that will request additional verification of data. These data will ultimately be passed on to the available payroll module.

At the end of entry, batch totals are calculated and verified against the manual totals, which are also entered as part of the batch. Discrepancies must be resolved before a batch is permitted to move from a status of entered to a status allowing printing and posting. Batch balance lists are available and present data in a format much like the format in which they were entered. These are quite useful for balancing and as audit trails. Visit registers show the data in a much different format with a variety of sort and total parameters.

YEAR-TO-DATE VISITS

A file is maintained for long-term storage of visits. This file is generally required by stand-alone systems because there is no other long-term repository of details concerning individual visits. Many of the statistical reports use this file as a data source. The year-to-date visit file is maintained on the vendor mainframe for hybrid system users. An option to maintain a redundant copy at the agency is useful for inquiries and reporting. Full editing capability is provided, and activity will be transmitted to the vendor mainframe system, ensuring data integrity. A year-to-date visit correction form (Exhibit 52–3) is normally used to record changes before data entry. Other functions are also available linking accounts receivable records to the source visit in the year-to-date file. With this system function, alterations of the

two related data sets are kept in sync. A simple question at the end of this activity allows a user to specify whether a rebilling is to be done.

ACCOUNTS RECEIVABLE FILE

Posting visits or other charge-generating items will create accounts receivable records that are stored separately. Bills are generated from this file, and individual items are stamped with a billing date. A separate data field is reserved for the payment date. Because bills are prepared according to an astounding collection of rules that vary wildly among agencies and payers, some additional flexibility has been created. A system function is configurable to merge billed accounts receivable detail records into a single receivable file in a condition matching the expected cash receipts. In this scenario, the application of cash to a specific item is made clear. Some pay sources are now providing electronic cash remittance through the use of magnetic tape or processor-to-processor transmission. Use of this option reduces or eliminates the task of cash application and adjustment. Should cash be applied manually, it will first be recorded on the cash and accounts receivable adjustment transmittal form (Exhibit 52–4). For auditing and balancing purposes, these data need to be batched into workable groups. The cash entry process calculates batch totals and compares them with the totals entered at the start of a batch. Individual cash transactions may involve complex adjustments and are verified by the system to be in balance. Appropriate debit and credit indicators are shown on the form to assist in the preparation of cash transactions and batches. During cash entry, transfers of full or partial amounts may be entered to move dollars to or from bad debt accounts or allowance accounts or between pay sources.

AD HOC REPORTING

Several optional report-generating modules are available. Although the design of this sys-

Exhibit 52–3 Year-to-Date Visit Corrections

AGENCY NAME _____ DATE / /

ACTION				KEY					
ADD 1	CHG 2	DEL 3	PATIENT NUMBER	VISIT DATE	VISIT TYPE	BATCH	SEQUENCE NUMBER		

SUB	PAYER	VISIT CHARGE	ALLOW	SUPPLY CHARGE	SUPPLY CODE	SUPPLY QUAN	TOTAL CHARGE	VISIT HOURS	ILLNESS CODE	R/X	EMPLOYEE NUMBER	NON-VISIT TIME CODE	NON-VISIT TIME HOURS	MILES	P/C	REF	HOSP	CITY CODE	LOCALITY	DOCTOR #

Courtesy of Delta Health Systems, Inc., Altoona, Pennsylvania.

Exhibit 52–4 Cash and Accounts Receivable Transmittal Form

MONTH OF _____ 19 _____ AGENCY NAME _____ PAGE ____ OF ____

BATCH NUMBER _____

CASH & A/R ADJUSTMENT TRANSMITTAL

PAYER	PATIENT NUMBER	PATIENT NAME	SERVICE AMOUNT	SERVICE DATE	AMOUNT PAID +	CREDIT REMOVAL +	PAYMENT ON ACCT. –	DATE PAID	AMOUNT	TRANSFER			SERVICE DATE	SUB
										TYPE	TO	HOURS		
PAGE TOTALS														

Courtesy of Delta Health Systems, Inc., Altoona, Pennsylvania.

tem allows a single product to be portable across a number of platforms, the lower levels of functionality must use distinct data storage techniques. Because a report generator is closely tied to the data storage model, report writing software is not always portable. For this reason, the choice of report writer may be driven by the hardware and operating system upon which a particular site has chosen to run. Two report writers are used with the home care system. One of these is called *Just Ask*, and the other is marketed as *Bbase*. The *Just Ask* product will run on host-based platforms utilizing the proprietary CADOL environment. *Bbase* is used on DOS-based platforms. These report writers are rather limited in scope and do not eliminate the need for custom programming, but they provide economical data access and are fine for use in list making based on easily expressed parameters. Advanced users have created some impressive applications using an included screen builder and forms printer. With the introduction of relational database technology in the recent *Clinical-Link* product, a new natural language-based technology can be installed. This product is structured query language–based and through training emulates an expert system of sorts. A great deal of logical power is easily accessible to the end users of this class of product.

FINANCIAL MANAGEMENT REPORTS

An extensive array of reporting options is included in the various versions of this system. These reports have been developed over many years and with the input of hundreds of customers. There should be few reporting needs that cannot be met with the standard software, but regulations and business methodologies change. As new needs arise, additional reports or variations are added. Audit trails are produced throughout the system. Functions such as the automatic payer change will print every altered piece of data. General ledger entries are built at various locations depending on the system version chosen. These may optionally be directly interfaced to an available group of financial modules. A variety of sort and total options offer a method of further tailoring reporting to specific needs. Many reports can be produced for individual or groups of substations, pay sources, and/or visit reasons. Totals of gross charges, allowances, supply charges, and net charges are produced for various selection criteria. Detail listings can be generated to support these totals. Bills or statements can be produced according to various cycles, and thereafter these amounts can be tracked through the receivables system through the generation of aging analysis and receivables schedules. An optional collections module can be added to facilitate further action as required. Users of this system have seen a significant reduction in the average age of outstanding receivables.

ACTIVITY REPORTS

Employee productivity and activity may be tracked and analyzed through several specialized reports. The caseload summary can be used to group employees by a substring of the employee numbers. Totals for these groups are then presented. This report will provide data on the number of visits by type, hours of service provided, average visit duration, number of visits made per day by an individual, nonvisit time, and miles driven. These same elements are also shown for the group as well as for the overall agency. From this, a good analysis can be made and standards established and monitored. For isolating the visit patterns of an individual, a couple of optionally sequenced employee registers may be printed. A similar report can be produced from the data in the year-to-date visit file. This is quite useful in assessing both patterns and revenue generation of a particular employee.

STATISTICAL REPORTS

Using the same source of data as the financial and other system reports, the statistical reports present a different view of the database. As with most reports in the system, a substation is typically used as a primary sort and selection parameter. Monthly and yearly versions are available for most reports. The service statistics report is a single report showing a variety of summaries in a format of one page per substation. Each page will have a collection of data boxes listing visits and hours of service by discipline, pay source, category of illness, locality, and patient age. A separate area of the page lists the number of patients served, admitted, and discharged. Yearly visits within localities can be shown on a similar report summarizing visits and hours in a specific locality with one locality per page and data boxes as previously discussed. Patient analysis reporting can be generated to show patients served, admitted, and discharged according to various criteria, such as referral source, age, race, sex, illness category, pay source, and the like. A unique method of defining ranges of illness codes provides a reasonable way of dealing with the number of ICD-9 codes in use. The number of patients, visits made, hours of service, and average time per patient and visit can be detailed for a specific ICD-9 code or group of codes. By providing data for the current month as well as year to date, trends or variances in personnel utilization might be spotted. This same report may be produced for specific pay sources, and interesting variances worth investigation might be noticed. In many cases, these variances will be due to patient age differences among pay sources.

A discharge summary report is also available and uses an agency-defined set of parameters. This report shows lengths of stay within discipline in each diagnosis. Patient and visit data are used to show averages and revenue figures. By using this report as a historical document, a projection regarding resources required by any specific illness can be made.

QUALITY ASSURANCE REPORTS

Several reports are available for use in a quality assurance program. A visit pattern alert report provides extensive evaluation of visits and conditions regarding a particular patient. Messages alerting staff to items that are likely to cause concern are shown along with pertinent data regarding that patient. By using a maximum expected visit interval stored for each patient, one of several simple lists can be produced. If a patient has not been seen in that period of time, a simple report can trigger personnel to initiate an appropriate check and response. Another report shows patients about to turn 65 years of age. This report should trigger a pay source review and possible adjustment. For agencies that wish to select patients for quality review, a quality assurance report will sample the patient database and suggest 3.33% of the total patients for review. Because some preference is applied within the software to filter out patients reviewed in the last six months, this is not a true random selection, but it serves a useful purpose.

CLINICAL-LINK FIELD AUTOMATION

Using DOS-based notebook computers and a central host, the *Clinical-Link* product offers caregivers access to a current collection of clinical data. Caregivers in the field will have a complete patient electronic chart, to which they may add progress notes and other required clinical data. The system also supports an electronic mail capability, through which other caregivers as well as office personnel may be contacted. The basic architecture builds a system around the concept of forms that are completed as part of an activity. The forms are tailorable to present and record data in a format modeled after existing agency paper forms. Exhibits 52–5 through 52–7 show paper copies of three related patient forms. These forms are larger than a normal 24-line computer screen and will scroll up or down as a user progresses through them. Activities are collections of various forms used in the course of any particular function performed by a caregiver, such as an assessment, a recertification, a daily visit, and so forth. The forms required within an activity are determined by the agency. The contents of each form are also determined by the agency. Various levels of validation are

Exhibit 52–5 Referral Demographics Form

```
┌─────────────────────────── GENERAL INFORMATION ───────────────────────────┐
```

Referral Information

    Referral Date: _____   Referral Time: _____

    Referred By: _____   Phone Number: (_____)_____

    Referral Source:_____

Patient Information

    Last Name: _____   First Name:_____ M.I.: _____

    Address: _____

    City: _____   State:_____ ZIP:_____- _____

    County: _____   Phone: (_____)_____

    Medical Record Number: _____

    Comments/Directions: _____

    SSN:_____   Date of Birth:_____Sex:____Race:_____

    Marital Status:_____ Lives Alone (Y/N): ____   Special Case: _____

    Employment Code 1: _____   _____

    Employment Code 2: _____   _____

    Locator Code: _____   _____

    Locality Code: _____   _____

    Miles to Residence: _____ Duplicate Patient:_____   Possible Disability: _____

    Emergency Contact:_____   Phone: (_____)_____

    Caretaker: _____   Phone: (_____)_____

Case Information:

    I.D. Number: _____

    Last Name: _____   First Name:_____ M.I.: _____

```
┌────────────────────────── PHYSICIAN INFORMATION ──────────────────────────┐
```

Physician Signing Initial Orders:_____

    Name:_____

    Address: _____   _____

    City: _____   State:_____ ZIP:_____- _____

    State License #: _____   Phone: (_____)_____

    Return to Clinic Date: _____

Second Physician: _____

    Name:_____

    Address: _____   _____

    City: _____   State:_____ ZIP:_____- _____

    State License #: _____   Phone: (_____)_____

Third Physician:_____

    Name:_____

    Address: _____   _____

    City: _____   State:_____ ZIP:_____- _____

    State License #: _____   Phone: (_____)_____

    Specialty: _____

    Comments: _____

```
┌────────────────────────── INPATIENT INFORMATION ──────────────────────────┐
```

Most Recent Inpatient Stay

    Facility: _____   Type of Facility:_____

    Admission Date: _____   Discharge Date: _____

    Facility Floor: _____   Phone: (_____)_____

Courtesy of Delta Health Systems, Inc., Altoona, Pennsylvania.

Exhibit 52–6 Referral Clinical Form

MEDICAL DIAGNOSES

	Code	Description	O/E	Date	Patient Aware?
1st Dx:	_____	_____	_____	_____	_____
2nd Dx:	_____	_____	_____	_____	_____
3rd Dx:	_____	_____	_____	_____	_____
4th Dx:	_____	_____	_____	_____	_____
5th Dx:	_____	_____	_____	_____	_____
6th Dx:	_____	_____	_____	_____	_____
7th Dx:	_____	_____	_____	_____	_____

SURGICAL PROCEDURES

Code	Description	Date
_____	_____	_____
_____	_____	_____
_____	_____	_____

Prognosis: _____ Patient Aware of Prognosis? (Y/N): _____

Patient Aware of Referral? (Y/N):_____ Purpose Code: _____

Communicable Disease? (Y/N): _____ Priority Code: _____

Goal Code: _____ UR Code:_____

Determination Date: _____

Vital Signs: _____

INTRAVENOUS INFORMATION

IV? (Y/N): _____

BLOOD WORK TO BE ORDERED AND FREQUENCY

CBS:_____ Blood Sugar: _____ Electrolytes:_____

BUN: _____ Magnesium: _____ Others: _____

IV EQUIPMENT TO BE SENT HOME WITH PATIENT

Equipment: _____ Type: _____

Company Supplying Equipment: _____ Phone: (_____) _____

Completed Orders To Be Obtained by High-Tech Department? (Y/N):_____

DIET

_____

_____

FUNCTIONAL LIMITATIONS

_____ _____

_____ _____

_____ _____

ACTIVITIES PERMITTED

_____ _____

_____ _____

_____ _____

continues

Exhibit 52–6 continued

EQUIPMENT

Equipment? (Y/N): _____

Code	Description	Needs or Has? (N/H)	Supplier	Ordered by Intake?	Purchase Order Number
_____	_____	_____	_____	_____	_____
_____	_____	_____	_____	_____	_____
_____	_____	_____	_____	_____	_____
_____	_____	_____	_____	_____	_____
_____	_____	_____	_____	_____	_____

Comments:
_____
_____
_____

INTAKE LAB WORK ORDERS

Lab Work Orders? (Y/N): _____
A6. RN to Draw Lab Work:
    Orders (Include Freq./Duration) _____
_____
_____
_____

A145. RN to Arrange Lab Work:
    Orders (Include Freq./Duration) _____
_____
_____

Lab: _____   Lab Phone: (_____) _____
Lab Work Ordered in Intake? (Y/N): _____   P.O. Number: _____
Comments:
_____
_____
_____
_____
_____

Courtesy of Delta Health Systems, Inc., Altoona, Pennsylvania.

---

performed based on the combination of form and activity. For instance, a pay source may not be known during the referral activity and will not be required on the patient master form. A certification cannot be completed without a pay source having been specified; therefore, this is required even though the certification activity is dealing with the same patient master form used during the referral.

Data are transmitted automatically each evening from each notebook to the central office system. This may or may not be the same machine upon which the home care system is running. Once all the notebooks have called in or a preset time has been passed, the server will prepare newly updated data for retransmission to each notebook. Again using a predefined schedule, each notebook makes a second call and is presented with current data for each assigned case. These data will now include all entries made by other users of the system regarding any individual patient. Should a user

Exhibit 52–7 Patient Status Form

PATIENT STATUS

Region:_____District: _____   Tract:_____Team: _____
Sub-Effective Date: _____
Referral Priority Code: _____   Evaluation Date: _____
Intake Evaluation Code: _____
Service Codes:
    1. Service Code 1: _____
    2. Service Code 2: _____
    3. Service Code 3: _____
    4. Service Code 4: _____
Goal Code:_____
Start of Care Date:_____   Agency Discharge Date: _____
Certification Period From:_____   To: _____
Plan Established Date:_____
Case Manager #: _____   Name: _____
SN Supervisor #: _____   Name: _____

REFERRAL TO DISCIPLINE

Discipline: Status:

_____   _____   _____
_____   _____   _____
_____   _____   _____
_____   _____   _____

Discipline: _____   _____
Referral Date: _____   Referral Source Code: _____
Referring Physician: _____
Referring Hospital: _____
Referring Employee: _____
Other:_____
Anticipated D/C Date: _____
Admitted or NTUC? (A/N): _____   NTUC Code: _____

              Date   Employee
Assessed By: _____   _____
Admitted/NTUC:_____   _____
Discharge: _____   _____
_____ Frequency and Duration: _____
Orders: _____
_____
_____
_____
_____
_____
_____
_____
_____

Courtesy of Delta Health Systems, Inc., Altoona, Pennsylvania.

need to access data currently on the host or another notebook, a demand communication mode is supported. Using this feature, data entered into one notebook in the morning could be immediately transferred to the host and subsequently transferred to another notebook. This feature is especially valuable for on-call personnel, who may be assigned a case only for the weekend or some other short time.

The *Clinical-Link* product is based on the UNIX or AIX operating system and makes use of a commercial relational database engine. Bidirectional interfaces are provided to achieve system integration with the standard home care software. An included print manager detects newly completed forms and produces printed outputs suitable for signatures or paper medical record archiving. A range of reporting options provides supervisory reports showing activities required, in process, or needing attention for some reason. Other reporting allows complete referral tracking and general management lists. Much of this system's repetitive processing is carried out at night or during other off-hour periods and does not require an operator.

OTHER MODULES

Two other modules have not yet been discussed: the scheduling system and the Health Care Financing Administration (HCFA) system. Both have been designed for complete integration with the base system and have interfaces built in such a way as to eliminate redundant entry of data. They have also been built to allow their use as standalone packages if desired. Scheduling, although frequently used in aide programs, has use in the nursing arena as well. Benefits include a more organized and documented schedule with reporting and partial automation of the scheduling process. Criteria matching may be used to make sure patients with special needs are seen by appropriate personnel. Scheduling may be done by allowing the system to suggest the person who is best suited and has the most available time within a district or by simply telling the system which

person to utilize. Users have often seen greatly reduced travel time and effort, which is due in large part to this simple matching. Automatic transfers may be made to shift some or all of a caseload from a sick or vacationing caregiver to other employees. With the same feature, a caseload may be transferred to a temporary holding area on holidays or during emergencies. Another key feature is found in the use of the visit interface. As part of the verification process, numbers of changes and missed visits are recorded and can be shown on a score card report. This might give a clear indication of missed visits or unexpected visits and can allow managers to be proactive in cases where revenue will be lost. Completing the visit interface eliminates the need for a separate data entry function to record visits from daily activity sheets.

The HCFA system is internally tied to care plan software as well as to the billing subsystem. The HCFA system in itself is based on data entry from code-driven forms completed by caregivers. The use of simple codes for common responses minimizes the need for extensive handwriting. Tracking of these worksheets begins at the time of a recertification need in the base system and continues through receipt of a signed copy from the physician. If the *Clinical-Link* product is in use, the data needed for production of HCFA forms 485 and 486 are gathered directly from it and require only review and approval without redundant data entry. The care plan system, available in a base system implementation as well as in a *Clinical-Link* version, is based on a nursing diagnosis methodology. This system uses a response tree mechanism to automate the production of a care plan. The care plans are interfaced with the HCFA system and also serve to limit redundant data entry. Billing, including electronic bills, is tied directly to the HCFA system and will run a variety of data checks, as would be found with certain intermediaries. A bill and HCFA set failing any of the edits will not be generated for submission because it would probably be rejected. Instead, audit trails and error listings guide a user through a process of revision until a bill may be reliably produced.

CONCLUSION

Software systems have become much more complex and comprehensive, as have the needs of most agencies. Failure to match vendor, product, and agency properly will result in unmet expectations and unmet needs. Cost is always a factor, and the correct system ought to demonstrate a payback expectation in the form of reduced personnel costs, increased productivity, higher levels of care, greater consistency of care, revenue maximization, or any number of other attractive reasons. As the home care industry grows, matures, and reacts to changing situations, the need for flexible and reliable computing systems is compounded. The proper system not only will meet the requirements of doing business but also will provide a window into how the business runs, its health, and its future needs. A data processing system should not get in the way of patient care. As information becomes available at all levels of an organization, the key is not the data but the use of that data in the most beneficial manner.

PART VII

Legal/Ethical/Political Issues

CHAPTER 53

Legal Issues of Concern to Home Care Providers

Ann P. Sherwin

INTRODUCTION

Home care providers come in a variety of forms and types. Providers may include the various business forms of sole proprietorships, partnerships, limited partnerships, corporations, and limited liability companies. Home care providers hold a variety of tax statuses that may be for profit, not for profit, or charitable.

The types of home care providers include but are not necessarily limited to home health agencies, visiting nurse associations, durable medical equipment companies, infusion care or high-technology companies, diagnostic testing companies, medical supply companies, hospices, specialized service agencies, private duty nursing services, homemaker–home health aide services, and companion services.

The laws of an individual state govern and may limit the organizational forms, tax status, and types of home care providers who are authorized to operate within that particular state. The state may require that the home care provider qualify to provide services through the state's registration, certificate of need, licensure, certification, and/or accreditation laws.

Failure to meet these minimum threshold legal requirements of the individual state law may prevent a home care provider from lawfully operating within that particular state.

Even after the home care provider has met the state's legal requirements for operation within a state, a number of evolving legal issues are likely to continue to affect the practices of the home care provider.

This chapter on legal matters in home care highlights a number of legal issues affecting home care providers in their business dealings and in the provision of health care and health-related services.

ANTITRUST

Antitrust is activity that restricts trade and discourages free competition in the marketplace.

The general purpose of both state and federal antitrust laws is to promote and maintain free and fair competition in the marketplace. The federal antitrust statutes are the Sherman Act, the Clayton Act, the Federal Trade Commission Act, and the Robinson Patman Act. The provisions of these laws prohibit certain artificial business manipulations such as the unfair competitive practices of group boycotts, dividing up the marketplace, exerting undue monopolistic practices, illegally tying products, and price fixing. The antitrust provisions basically bar an agency from agreeing with or conspiring with its competitors not to compete and from competing unfairly. The business practices of health care providers have come under increased scrutiny by the Federal Trade Commission for activities that may have an anticompetitive effect in the healthcare marketplace. Mergers, joint venture activities, and other combinations engaged in by a wide variety of health care providers have exposed the health care industry to examination for possible antitrust violations.

This increased scrutiny should be of great concern to the health care community. A judgment or finding of a violation of the antitrust laws against a home care provider poses great risk. In addition to a court order halting the illegal antitrust activity cited as the violation, the violator is exposed to high penalties. Moreover, private parties who successfully prosecute an antitrust violation against a business may recover triple monetary damages and attorneys' fees in amounts that can be staggering and fatal to that business's viability. In a recent Florida case, the court determined that the intent of a joint venture between a hospital and a durable medical equipment company and the manner in which it was implemented were anticompetitive. A $2.3 million dollar jury verdict in the case was recently upheld on appeal to the Eleventh Circuit Court of Appeals.[1]

CORPORATE LIABILITY OF PROVIDERS

There are a number of legal theories of liability under which a health care company may be found liable to other parties. These legal theories are breach of contract, agency, respondent superior, ostensible agency, and the evolving theory of corporate negligence.

A breach of contract requires that a contract exist between the parties whereby an offer is made, acceptance is given, and some form of consideration is given to bind the contract. This may involve an activity between the patient and a home care agency whereby the home care provider offers certain services to the patient, the patient agrees to accept the services, and the consideration to the contract is the agreement of payment for the services. A patient may have a cause of action for breach of contract against the home care provider if services were not pro-

vided as agreed to, such as if the program's marketing materials promised certain high-quality services and the provider did not deliver the quality or scope of services promised in its agreement.

The principle of respondent superior is that employers are liable for the acts of their employees when employees act within the scope of their employment. It is also known as the master and servant rule in that the master is deemed to be responsible for the acts of his or her servants.

Theories of vicarious liability hold a health care company/provider indirectly liable for the action and omissions of its employees, agents, and ostensible agents. Ostensible agents are those persons who act with the apparent authority of the health care provider, in that the health care provider holds out these agents and/or persons as employees, and the public would have no reason not to consider these persons as agents or employees of the health care provider. This theory of negligence requires that the patient look to the health care provider rather than the individual health care practitioner for care, and that the health care provider hold out the practitioner as its own employee. This holding out or appearance occurs when a health care provider acts or omits to act in some way that leads the patient to a reasonable belief that she/he is being treated by the health care provider and/or one of its employees.

A number of courts have created a direct legal duty owed to the patient by the health care provider as an additional duty to the already established legal duty held by each individual health care practitioner to his or her patients. This new theory of liability is a departure from the notion that a corporation could not be directly liable for the negligence of health care practition-ers because corporations are prohibited from practicing medicine and from practicing under any individual health care practitioner's individual professional license. This prohibition, also known as a prohibition against the corporate practice of medicine, has now evolved into a direct duty to patients under a new theory of corporate negligence.

This direct duty and/or theory of corporate negligence reflects a growing appreciation on the part of the courts and of consumers that health care providers play an increasing role in the selection of health care practitioners on behalf of the consumer. Evidence of this increased role of the health care provider is found in the selection of health care practitioners as employees and independent contractors for the patient. Of special note are health maintenance organizations and preferred provider organizations and their duties in their selection of health care service providers and health care practitioners made available to the consumer. The duty owed to the patient under this theory of corporate negligence is measured in activities such as the selection of the health care practitioner, the credentialing and recredentialing of staff, the supervision of the quality of care rendered, and the verification of skills, training, and retraining required to maintain optimal levels and reasonable standards in the provision of health care services as promised to the consumer by the health care company/provider.

TORTS AND CIVIL LIABILITY

A home health care provider can be liable for damages if it is found to have committed a tort. A tort is a wrongful act or injury committed by one person against another. The types of torts are defined and governed by the laws of each particular state.

Intentional torts require the intent to commit harm, that is, an actual, conscious desire on the part of one person to harm the other. Examples of intentional torts include an intentional act to commit harm, battery, the intentional infliction of emotional distress, fraud or willful concealment, and misrepresentation or deceit.

A battery is an intentional touching without permission or consent. No harm need occur to the patient for a finding of battery to be lodged against a health care provider. Patients have successfully sued health care providers for bat-

tery where treatments to their person were provided without their consent.

Fraud is defined as a concealment or misrepresentation of a material fact that induces a patient's reliance. When a patient reasonably relies on a home care provider's misrepresentations and then suffers damages as a result of that reliance, the patient has a cause of action in negligence against the provider.

Intentional infliction of emotional distress is usually defined as outrageous conduct that results in physical and emotional harm to an injured party. Its finding by the court involves activities by a party that are in themselves sufficiently outrageous to warrant a separate tort of intending to cause the other party emotional distress.

Negligence is behavior that falls below the legal standards defined to protect people from harm or the lack of due care that a reasonable person would be expected to exercise in given circumstances. To determine negligence, a court examines whether the wrongdoer knew or should have known how to act in the circumstances, and whether the wrongdoer did not take reasonable precautions or did not act in a way to avoid or prevent harm and injury to the patient. In other words the home care provider is held to a standard of care, defined as the reasonable standard under which home care providers generally operate in order to provide safe, reasonable care that protects patients. If the home care provider's actions or inactions fall below this reasonable standard of care and harm to the patient results, the provider is guilty of negligence.

In any tort, the injured party must show a causal relationship between the wrongdoer's conduct and the resulting damage to the injured party. As such, the injured party or patient must show that the home care provider engaged in conduct that involved a foreseeable risk of harm to the patient, and the injury resulted from this action or omission on the part of the home care provider.

Damages in such circumstances may be either compensatory or punitive. Compensatory damages are those that compensate the injured party for loss of earnings, diminution of earning capacity, medical and other expenses, and pain and suffering. Punitive damages are punishment damages. Punitive damages may be awarded where the wrongdoer's conduct is sufficiently outrageous to warrant punishment beyond the simple compensation of the injured party for actual damages. Punitive awards are often made in cases of willful and negligent behavior where the wrongdoer knew of the danger and willfully acted to harm the injured party or willfully failed to act, knowing that likelihood of harm was great.

Criminal liability covers prosecution by a state or by the federal government against a home care provider who commits an act that is specifically punishable under the law.

FRAUD AND ABUSE

The federal laws under the Social Security Act and its amendments established the health insurance programs that we know as Medicare and Medicaid.[2] Medicare is a federal program that provides health insurance for the benefit of the elderly and disabled as well as other programs for dialysis patients. Medicaid is a state-administered program designed to help needy citizens pay for medical expenses. Medicaid is funded jointly by the federal government and by each state, and serves impoverished individuals who are aged, blind, or disabled, or members of families with dependent children. States are responsible for setting standards for reimbursement and claims processing through the adoption of regulations and the development of policy within federal guidelines according to an individual state plan.

The Medicare Statute authorizes the Secretary of Health and Human Services (HHS) to administer the Medicare program to pay for health benefits for the elderly and disabled. This responsibility has been delegated by the Secretary to the Administrator of the Health Care Financing Administration (HCFA). The HCFA promulgates rules, regulations, and guidelines for the Medicare program and enters into contracts with private organizations to assist in program administration. These organizations are known as fiscal intermediaries under Medicare Part A and as carriers under Medicare Part B.

Additions to the Medicare law under the Social Security Act, known as the fraud and abuse amendments at 42 U.S.C. Section 1395nn, provide for prohibitions and penalties with respect to certain abusive and fraudulent activities in the Medicare and Medicaid programs.[3] The most basic prohibitions under the fraud and abuse amendments are those making it a crime for a provider to knowingly or willfully make false or fraudulent claims; concealing or failing to disclose certain information; soliciting, receiving, or offering to pay a remuneration in return for referring an individual to another for the furnishing of any item or services; or knowingly and willfully making a false statement of material facts with respect to the conditions of operation in a hospital, skilled nursing facility, or home health agency.

The HCFA has delegated the responsibility for investigating fraud and abuse in the federal health insurance program to the Office of the Inspector General (OIG). The OIG has independent authority to sanction providers who have violated the fraud and abuse laws. Additionally the OIG works with the U.S. Department of Justice, the Federal Bureau of Investigation (FBI), the state Medicaid Fraud Control Units (MFCUs), and the intermediaries to combat abusive and fraudulent activities within the Medicare and Medicaid health insurance programs.

The Social Security law provides that fraud and abuse of the Medicare and Medicaid programs or their beneficiaries may result in criminal, civil, or administrative actions against the perpetrators. The civil money penalty provisions of the fraud and abuse amendments authorize the OIG to assess fines and penalties in thousands of dollars for each false item claimed against the Medicare and Medicaid program. The OIG may also impose civil and administrative sanctions in the form of program exclusions or monetary penalties on individuals and entities for engaging in fraud and abuse of the Medicare and Medicaid programs and/or their beneficiaries.

In addition, the Medicare and Medicaid Patient and Program Protection Act, Public Law 1900–93, provides for a wide range of authorities to exclude individuals and entities from Medicare and Medicaid programs. Exclusions are typically made for conviction of fraud against a private health insurer, obstruction of an investigation, controlled substance abuse, and the revocation or surrender of a health license. Program exclusion is mandatory and lasts for a minimum period of five years for those convicted of program-related crimes or patient abuse.

The OIG typically refers cases for criminal prosecution to the U.S. Department of Justice, which may enlist the services of the FBI in its prosecution and investigation of the matter.

MFCUs are responsible for investigating fraud in the Medicaid program. MFCUs receive funds from the OIG. The MFCUs prosecute persons charged with defrauding the Medicaid programs and those charged with patient abuse and neglect.

Many activities may trigger an investigation of a provider by the OIG including but not limited to special areas of focused review for all providers; variation in numbers of visits or number of denials; inaccurate, inadequate, or missing documentation; complaints; and news publications.

Investigators may contact the provider directly or circumvent the provider and attempt to question employees, contractors, or suppliers, all without notice to the provider. The investigators' demeanor may vary from friendliness to hostility. They may act in a manner that causes division and dissension in your company. In any event, unless you are under arrest, an investigator has no duty to be completely up front with you, nor to inform you of your basic legal rights. You as an individual are expected to know your rights under the U.S. Constitution and the Bill of Rights.

Under all circumstances, any investigation of your company is serious business. Even the threat of an investigation can have a chilling effect on your business and employees. As such, you must take any and all inquiries and investigations about your home care business seriously. If you have any indication that you or your company may be the focus of an investigation or that your employees may have been contacted by an investigator, you should always consult with your attorney. If you do not have an attorney, you should seek counsel immediately.

In the event that your company is served with a search warrant or is informed that it is the target of a criminal investigation, you must contact an attorney to preserve and protect your rights, even if you insist that you are not guilty of any wrongdoing. Failure to protect your rights during an investigation can be evidence of a waiver of those rights for the duration of the investigation and proceedings. Therefore, it is imperative that you act quickly to protect and preserve your rights and the rights of your company.

If you are required to provide certain documents and business records as the result of a valid subpoena or official court order for such documents, then you should keep copies of, and a record of, all documents supplied to the authorities. Keep a record of all contacts with investigators whether formal or informal of which you have knowledge, including a listing of the persons who were present and the content of the contact or meeting. There is no such thing as an informal meeting during an investigation. Do not be lulled into a feeling of false security. Investigators are typically required to set forth a description of their meeting and contact in a written report to their superiors. As such, the formal report of investigation is made and written in the words of the investigators, which may vary with what you consider to be an accurate transcript of the events and commentary made during the meeting or contact.

Keep your attorney involved in all phases of your contacts. Beware of meeting informally with investigators in a way in which you may unintentionally waive your rights. You should resist feeling pressured to answer before you are prepared to discuss the issues. It is important to think out a plan of action for your home care business and your staff. Your plan might include education of your staff to defuse confusion and allay employee fears and concerns, identification of a central contact person to handle all questions and inquiries about your home care business, creation of a central distribution person for all documents released or provided to authorities, and development of a plan for dealing with the press.

A part of this process that you eventually must confront is the business decision whether to litigate the matter or whether to attempt to reach a settlement of the alleged violation. The downside risks of damage to your business, reputation, and the expense of litigation should be examined carefully by you in counsel with your attorney. Issues of collateral enforcement activities and reporting by investigators to other federal agencies, state certification, licensure and private accreditation bodies and the resultant effect on your business must be considered in your decision on how to best proceed in the matter. If a settlement agreement is reached and litigation is avoided, certain provisions such as releases and confidentiality agreements should be included in the settlement agreement as a continued protection for your health care business.

DECISION MAKING, PRIVACY, AND INFORMED CONSENT

Every individual has the right to consent to treatment and the right to refuse treatment. The legal basis for consent and refusals of consent originates from the Constitutional right to privacy and the common law right to be free from bodily intrusion. The right to privacy is not an absolute right, however, as each state holds countervailing interests that must be taken into consideration when individuals make decisions to withhold or refuse to consent to treatment for others or for themselves.

Generally speaking, consent can be express or implied. Expressed consent is by either written or spoken direct words. Written consent is evidenced by a signed consent form. Internal agency policy, state law, and licensure, certification and/or accreditation standards determine which procedures require a person's written consent. Implied consent is consent evidenced by the person's conduct. For example, a patient holding out his/her arm for a nurse to take a blood pressure is a form of implied consent. Consent may also be implied by the law in emergency situations when the patient is unconscious and relatives cannot be reached and immediate treatment is required to prevent serious bodily damage or to save the person's life. Public policy favors the preservation of life and recognizes that in emergency situations, requiring health care workers to wait would do more harm to the patient and that in such situations health care workers should take immediate actions to save and preserve a life.

For a consent to be valid, it must be informed. The doctrine of informed consent arises from each individual's right to self-determination. The law provides that each patient has the right to be free from bodily intrusion, and to decide what will or will not be done to his or her own body. The law of informed consent requires that a physician must disclose information about a medical procedure or treatment to the patient so that the patient can weigh and consider the information prior to making a decision. Generally, the courts have found that the physician's duty to inform the patient is non-delegable to other health care providers, and that the physician has the duty to disclose information about medical procedures to the patient and obtain the patient's informed consent. For a consent to be valid, the patient must be of sound mind and consent voluntarily. Ideally, disclosure of information about a treatment or procedure should be given in advance of the treatment, so that the patient has time to reach a considered decision and so that allegations of coercion are avoided.

A failure to obtain the informed consent of a patient is a form of negligence, also known as malpractice. A legally valid informed consent is one given by the patient after information about the treatment or procedure is given to the patient. The information disclosed to the patient for a valid consent includes the diagnosis and condition of the patient, the purpose and nature of the proposed treatment, material risks and adverse reactions to treatment, the probability of success of the treatment, alternative treatments, and the prognosis if treatment is not given. Courts usually hold physicians to a reasonable patient standard of disclosure. The reasonable patient standard of disclosure requires that the physician disclose those risks that are material to the patient's decision making process. For example, the risk of a hysterectomy would be material to a woman of childbearing age in her decision whether to consent to or refuse a particular course of treatment or procedure.

Just as every person has the right to consent to treatment, every person has a similar right to refuse treatment. The right to be free from bodily intrusion and the right to self-determination derived from the Constitutional right to privacy are essential rights owned by each individual. Competing with these individual rights, however, are the countervailing interests of the state. These countervailing state interests are the preservation of life, the prevention of suicide, the protection of third parties, and the safeguarding of the integrity of the medical profession. When a court determines that a patient's right to privacy outweighs the countervailing state's interest in a specific patient's circumstance, then the court will probably uphold the patient's decision to refuse treatment.

Individuals enjoy privacy rights in their health care and treatment. Persons with certain diagnoses, such as patients with a diagnosis of Acquired Immune Deficiency Syndrome (AIDS), may own an increased measure of protection in a number of states where statutory-specific protections to safeguard the patient's privacy have been put into law. Federal law protects the disclosure of the name, diagnosis, and treatment of patients undergoing treatment in federally assisted drug rehabilitation programs. The intent of these laws is usually twofold: to encourage treatment and to protect the privacy and confidentiality of the persons seeking treatment.

Privacy in the contents of medical records is deemed to be a right owned by the individual person unless proper authorization for the release of information is given by the individual. The patient's privilege and privacy rights in his or her communications and the relationship between the physician–patient has been a privilege long recognized by the courts. The patient may also own other legally recognized privileges in his or her relationship with health care providers, and these privileges are usually determined under a state's own laws and statutes.

ADVANCE DIRECTIVES

Advance directives are documents within which patients direct the kind of health care they would or would not want and/or appoint someone to make health care decisions on their behalf if they are unable to make the decisions for themselves. Advance directives are typically called living wills or health care powers of attorney. The Patient Self Determination Act (PSDA) was passed by Congress in 1990 and focused on an adult's right to refuse life-sustaining treatment and gave force to patients' rights to accept or refuse medical treatment and to state laws regarding these rights.[4]

The PSDA is an effort to allow each person an opportunity to control his or her future in the event of incapacity and the acknowledgment and response to the less often discussed issue that the past practices of life "at any cost" and even against a person's own wishes is partly responsible for the exorbitant cost of aggressive care and treatment during the last weeks of life, that such care is generally futile and not expected to improve the quality or length of a patient's life, and that many patients, if capable to decide, would refuse such care or not choose it for themselves.

State laws within which these rights are described include, but may not be limited to, durable powers of attorney, living will acts, health care powers of attorney, and surrogate decision maker laws. The PSDA applies to all health care institutions receiving Medicare or Medicaid funds, and compliance with the PSDA is incorporated into Medicare and Medicaid provider agreements as a requirement for reimbursement.[5] The PSDA requires the care provider agency to:

- Provide written information to each adult patient on admission (inpatient facilities), enrollment (HMOs), and at first receipt of care (hospices and home health or personal care agencies). The information provided must describe the individual's legal rights under state law to accept or refuse medical care and to write advance directives for incorporation into his or her medical record;
- Maintain written policies and procedures regarding advance directives and provide written information to the patients about those policies;
- Document in the patient's medical record whether the individual has executed an advance directive;
- Ensure compliance with state law requirements regarding advance directives; and
- Provide, either independently or with other like institutions, for education for the staff and community on issues concerning advance directives.[6]

Information provided to the patients should include a description of how the individual state's law handles continuation or withdrawal of treatment from incompetent patients who have not executed advance directives.

Patients are presented with advance directive information on the first visit. Due to the numerous documents signed and the limitation on time for staff to explain the directives and the capacity of patients to understand the directives, some patients do not appreciate the importance of the advance directive. Educational efforts directed toward patients should help to correct these deficiencies. Written information or brochures explaining the meaning of the advance directive and its purpose for the individual can be given to the patient so that it may be reviewed and reflected upon within the individual patient's time frame. Materials should be written in plain language, easily understood by the patient. Materials should be available in the language of the patient or via interpreters, and personnel should be available to disseminate information via appropriate means to the disabled and impaired.

A follow-up telephone call or provision of an address to write to for additional information/guidance would be helpful to some patients and families. Agency staff should be educated about advance directives so that they may easily explain the directives to a patient and answer basic questions about directives. An individual in the organization should be designated as the resource person for staff and patients for further information on advance directives.

Patients requiring specialized or further assistance should be referred to appropriate resources such as their own attorney or the local bar association.

Any patient or family member or caregiver presenting a purported valid legal paper that authorizes a health care power of attorney, durable power of attorney, guardianship, surrogacy, or similar document should be referred to the agency's designated advance directives person, so that the authenticity and legal effect of the documents may be verified and included in the medical record. Any conflicts, discrepancies, or questionable validity in the existence of or content of an advance directive document, whether it is originated by staff, patient, family, or outside parties, should be referred to the designated advance directive person for investigation and resolution. In cases of unresolved problems or questions with directives that will affect your staff and the care rendered, you need to consult your company's attorney for specific advice in the individual case.

It is important that all staff be aware that, as with any medical directive, an advance directive may be changed or withdrawn by the competent patient at any time and by any means, and that a patient may refuse to execute an advance directive. Additionally, staff should be reassured that generally states and courts protect health care providers who act *in good faith* in reliance on a valid advance directive.

State law governs the effect and interpretation of advance directives. Since these state laws are ever-evolving on the subject of advance directives, and a multiplicity of legal documents that have the effect of an advance directive may be present for a patient, your staff and company should have access to a designated advance directives resource person/contact in order to resolve questions and educate staff on the effect of an advance directive document in the care and treatment of a particular patient.

LABOR AND EMPLOYMENT ISSUES

Recent areas of concern for home care providers in labor matters are the wrongful termination of employees, negligent hiring and supervision of staff, and characterizations of workers in an employee versus independent contractor status.

The wrongful termination of employment is a matter of increased litigation in employment law. The common law recognizes that most employers and employees enjoy a relationship defined as employment-at-will, meaning essentially that either party may terminate the relationship for any reason, at any time. Due to certain federal regulatory and state law requirements, employers have increasingly utilized employee handbooks to define and describe the expectations of the employment relationship with employees. Courts in many states are increasingly taking the view that employee handbooks are evidence of, and may constitute proof that, the employment-at-will relationship

is ended or modified and that a contract of employment exists between the employee and employer.

Employment contracts confer certain duties, rights, and privileges upon employees and duties upon an employer that were not necessarily contemplated in the employment relationship, and that are not required in an employment-at-will relationship. An example of this may be a formal, written disciplinary procedure agreed to be followed prior to any termination of employment status.

Employees are increasingly invoking the existence of an employment contract when an employee handbook is utilized in a company. Home care providers should be especially diligent in reviewing their employee handbooks to include certain provisions such as a disclaimer or language indicating that the handbook is not a contract and that the handbook does not intend to alter the employment-at-will relationship between the parties. Employers should be cautious about provisions that may infer that employees hold greater rights than were intended in the employment relationship.

Negligent hiring and supervision practices should be an area of great concern to home care providers. The increase in the number of home care personnel assisting a patient in the less controlled environment of the patient's home, and an increased examination of the home care industry in its self-monitoring of home care activities, will probably cause a heightened scrutiny as to which factors constitute reasonable hiring practices in the home care industry. Medical equipment drivers and delivery persons, health care professionals, home health aides, companions, infusion care company personnel, medical diagnostic testing personnel and a variety of health care–related workers are entering into the privacy of the patient's home.

With this reality in mind, a number of states currently require pre-employment criminal records checks for all employees who provide patient care services in the home. Certain states may limit the criminal record check to home care personnel who provide patient care services to children, the elderly, or persons defined as at special risk for harm from mistreatment or abuse. A current proposal by federal regulators would require all home care agencies receiving Medicare funds to conduct criminal background checks before hiring home care workers.

Courts have recognized that health care providers and facilities that provide health care services hold a duty to protect the patients for whom they care and to whom they render health care services. This minimum protection on hiring employees comes into play in the activities of screening applicants for patient care positions; verification of valid, current, and appropriate licensure or certification for the position sought; and diligent verification of employment and personnel references as to the appropriate character and demeanor of the applicant in patient care service activities.

Negligent supervision of staff is another factor and risk in employment litigation. Current federal regulations requiring supervision of home health aides should assist to minimize findings of negligence in matters involving this category of employee. A number of states have implemented similar protective laws to require supervision of nonlicensed professionals providing health care and health care–related services to patients at home.

A continuing issue for home care providers in many states is the characterization of workers performing work for the home care providers in the status of independent contractors versus employees.

Such characterizations may carry serious tax and labor policy implications for your business. Employees are workers whose wages are subject to withholding taxes at federal, state, and, in some cases, local levels. Employee status causes the employer to both withhold and contribute to federal taxes, Social Security, state workers' compensation funds, state unemployment, and similar programs enacted for the security and benefit of employees. These programs are additional costs to all employers for their employees. Employers are exempt from

providing such benefits and treatment to independent contractors.

The home care industry has typically utilized the services of certain workers such as physical therapists, speech therapists, and occupational therapists on a per-visit basis under contract. A controversy continues as to whether these categories of workers may be classified as independent contractors rather than employees. The main issue is that employer and employee status is usually defined by control and direction by the employer over the employee. Conflicts in interpretation occur, because for many home care providers, the provider is required to have a measure of control over such workers, and yet in industry practice and according to this worker group's own professional licensure statutes, these workers have traditionally acted and been treated as independent contractors.

While it may seem advantageous to your agency to classify a worker as an independent contractor and avoid certain employer responsibilities, such a misclassification may result in major costs, penalties, fines, and liabilities to your company.

Labor matters of these types will continue to confront the home care industry as new types of workers and responsibilities to those workers and to consumers evolve in the health and home care service industry.

AMERICANS WITH DISABILITIES ACT

The Americans with Disabilities Act (ADA) gives rights and protections to individuals with disabilities to the same extent that they are presently provided to individuals on the basis of race, sex, national origin, and religion.[7] It prohibits discrimination against workers with disabilities in all aspects of employment and requires access of disabled persons to public transportation and public accommodations.[8]

In developing the ADA, Congress made note that approximately 43 million Americans have one or more physical or mental disabilities and that such persons are routinely discriminated against solely because of their disabilities.[9] An increased and more favorable integration of individuals with disabilities into society is a major goal of the ADA.

Under Title I of the ADA, employers with 15 or more employees may not discriminate against a qualified individual with a disability because of the disability of such individual, in regard to job application procedures; the hiring, job assignment, advancement, or discharge of employees; employee compensation or fringe benefits; job training; and other terms, conditions, and privileges of employment.[10] An employer must provide reasonable accommodations for disabled workers, unless that would impose an undue hardship on the employer.[11] Only employees and applicants who are qualified individuals with disabilities are protected.[12] The term disability means 1) a physical or mental impairment that substantially limits one or more of the major life activities of an individual; or 2) having a record of such impairment; or 3) being regarded as having a substantially limiting impairment.[13] In determining whether a condition is a disability one must consider the unique characteristics of each applicant or employee on a case-by-case basis.

The term qualified person with a disability means an individual with a disability who meets the skill, experience, education, and other job-related requirements of a position held or desired, and who, with or without reasonable accommodation, can perform the essential functions of such positions.[14] The identification of the essential function of each job is the key to ensuring compliance with the ADA, because the duty to employ individuals and provide reasonable accommodations, job standards, and medical examinations each relate to the essential function of the job. Essential functions are primary job duties that are intrinsic to the employment position, rather than marginal or peripheral functions that are incidental to the performance of primary job functions.[15]

A major standard of the ADA is the requirement for employers to provide reasonable accommodations that do not involve an undue hardship on the employer so that qualified persons with disabilities can perform the essential functions of jobs.[16] Reasonable accommodations also demand that the employer make equally available all services and programs provided in connection with employment, such as wellness programs, cafeterias, counseling services, and transportation. Reasonable accommodations may include, but are not limited to making existing facilities used by employees readily accessible to and usable by persons with disabilities; job restructuring; modifying work schedules; reassignment to a vacant position; acquiring or modifying equipment or devices; adjusting or modifying examination, training materials, or work policies; providing qualified readers or interpreters; and other similar accommodations.[17] Tax credits and deductions are available for some of these costs.

Employers are required to make a good faith effort to find a reasonable means of accommodation. Consultation with federal, state, or local rehabilitation and disability organizations familiar with the needs of disabled workers may provide useful input into the determination of a reasonable accommodation. Employers should prepare a written record to document the efforts taken, sources consulted, options considered, potential costs of available accommodations, and the resulting decision.

The most significant element of Title I of the ADA concerns the employment application process and determination of final hiring, promotion, or termination decisions. Employers are prohibited from utilizing any procedure or taking any action, in the process of screening applicants and during the hiring process, that could have a discriminatory effect against a qualified individual with a disability.[18] Many job applications have historically included questions regarding applicant disabilities, hospitalizations, or illnesses. It is recommended that employers review all job application forms and eliminate questions about physical or mental disabilities.

In order to establish that the disabled status of an applicant or employee was not a factor in the employment-related decision, employers should base all employment decisions on clearly articulated job criteria. In addition, the specific reasons for all adverse decisions, including all medical evidence, accommodations considered, and the reasons for rejecting such accommodations should be clearly documented in writing in the employer's personnel files.

The ADA has established prohibitions against discrimination in application and hiring that encompass a general prohibition as to the use of medical examinations and inquiries into whether a person has a disability. However, in certain circumstances medical examinations are permitted, such as when job related and consistent with business necessity or when required by federal, state, or local law.[19] In all situations strict confidentiality of the medical examination results is required and the information regarding such exams should be kept in a separate file from the personnel file.[20] When medical exams are performed as a condition of employment, the company should ensure that all of the ADA conditions are met, such as that the exam is a post-offer exam, that the physician performing the exam has been provided a written job description for each position sought, and that such physician has specified if there are essential tasks that the individual cannot safely perform without undue risk of harm to him- or herself or others.

Individuals with contagious diseases such as hepatitis, tuberculosis, AIDS, or HIV infection are considered disabled under the ADA.[21] An employer is permitted to limit the job opportunities of individuals with an infectious disease only if it can demonstrate that the infectious disease constitutes a significant risk to the health or safety of others, that is, a direct threat that cannot be eliminated by reasonable accommodation.[22] If an individual poses a direct threat as the result of a disability, the employer must determine whether a reasonable accommodation would either eliminate the risk or reduce it to an acceptable level. Actions taken against individuals because of a belief that they may communicate an infectious disease to others cannot be based on fears, stereotypes, or gener-

alizations. The Centers for Disease Control (CDC) guidelines state that HIV-infected health care workers who adhere to universal precautions and who do not perform invasive exposure-prone procedures pose no threat of HIV transmission to their patients.[23]

An employee or applicant currently engaging in the illegal use of drugs is not entitled to ADA, protection because such individuals are not included in the definition of qualified individual with a disability.[24] Alcoholism is considered a disability under the ADA, and alcoholics are protected from discrimination unless the alcoholism interferes with the individual's ability to work or poses a threat to the property or safety of others. Reasonable accommodation requires health care providers to employ former drug addicts or alcoholics for most health care positions. Nevertheless, employers are permitted under the ADA to:

- prohibit the use of alcohol or illegal drugs at the workplace by all employees
- prohibit employees from being under the influence of illegal drugs at the workplace
- require employees to follow the requirements of the Drug-Free Workplace Act of 1988
- require employees to meet the job-related requirements established by federal regulatory agencies regarding drugs and alcohol
- hold a drug user or alcoholic to the same qualification standards for employment or job performance and behavior to which they hold other individuals, even if any unsatisfactory performance or behavior is related to the drug use or alcoholism of such individual.[25]

Reasonable accommodation of the alcoholic employee and former drug-addicted employee qualified for the position may include access to substance abuse rehabilitation programs and leaves of absence for treatment.[26]

The ADA neither requires nor prohibits drug testing by employers to determine illegal drug use.[27] The ADA permits employers to adopt or administer reasonable policies or procedures, including but not limited to drug testing, to ensure that employees or applicants are not currently using illegal drugs. Drug testing is not considered a medical examination subject to the limitation of the ADA, and the ADA permits employers to conduct drug testing of job applicants and employees and make employment decisions from the results of those tests.[28] However, employers must be careful that drug testing does not violate state or local laws or patient confidentiality laws.

Your company must post notices issued by the Equal Employment Opportunity Commission (EEOC) that inform applicants and employees of the provisions of the ADA.[29] Such notices should be posted conspicuously on the employer's premises, including personnel offices and other places where applicants and employees are likely to see them, such as the cafeteria, staff meeting room, etc. Such notices must be made available in various formats so that persons with impaired vision and other disabilities are notified of the ADA requirements. Your company might also include information about ADA obligations in job application forms, job vacancy notices, and personnel manuals. Employers must retain employment records and job applications for at least one year for ADA purposes and for longer periods under certain state laws and for other federal regulatory purposes.[30]

Title III of the ADA prohibits discrimination based on disability in the full and equal enjoyment of the goods, services, facilities, privileges, advantages, or accommodations of any place of accommodation by any person who owns, leases (or leases to), or operates a place of public accommodation.[31]

A public accommodation is described as a privately owned establishment that makes its services, goods, or programs available to the public.[32] The public accommodation requirements apply to all types of health care facilities including home health agencies and to all areas in such companies such as lobbies, restrooms, parking areas, etc. In order to assist a disabled person to experience full and equal enjoyment of a facility, places of public accommodation may be required to:

- modify eligibility criteria policies or practices that have the effect of discriminating against or excluding people with disabilities
- remove architectural barriers that restrict accessibility and communications
- supply auxiliary aids and services
- provide transportation services on an equal basis.[33]

Health care providers and insurers may need to increase office accessibility by installing ramps, establishing accessible parking spaces, enlarging the office's physical entrance, rearranging furniture, and widening doors or modifying other spaces to facilitate wheelchair access or movement.[34] Bathrooms must also be accessible to disabled persons, and modifications may include installation of grab bars, rearrangement of partitions, mirrors, and towel dispensers, and raised toilet seats.[35] If your company has limited funds, the rules prioritize the order in which existing barriers should be removed:

- measures that will enable individuals with disabilities to physically enter a place of public accommodation
- measures that provide access to those areas of a place of accommodation where goods and services are made available to the public
- measures to provide access to restroom facilities
- any other changes necessary to remove barriers.[36]

The ADA does not require that alterations be made to existing facilities. It does require that if alterations are undertaken that could affect the facility's usability, those alterations must, to the maximum extent feasible, make the altered portions of the facility readily accessible to and usable by persons with disabilities.[37] New facility construction must be designed and constructed so the facilities are readily accessible to and usable by persons with disabilities, unless it is structurally impracticable to do so.[38]

Public accommodations are required to provide auxiliary aids and services to enable a person with a disability to use the available goods and services, unless to do so would fundamentally alter the program or would constitute an undue burden.[39] The term auxiliary aids and services includes methods of making aurally or visually delivered materials available to individuals with visual or hearing impairment, and the acquisition or modification of equipment or devices for disabled persons.[40] Auxiliary aids and services include:

1. qualified interpreters or other effective methods of making aurally delivered materials available to individuals with hearing impairments
2. qualified readers, taped texts, or other effective methods of making visually delivered materials available to individuals with visual impairments
3. acquisition or modification of equipment or devices
4. other similar services and actions.[41]

The ADA specifically provides in regulations that landlords and tenants are jointly responsible for public accommodation requirements; however, the responsibility for and the cost of compliance with the ADA may be allocated in the leases.[42] As such, your company should review its facility leases and amend them to include necessary changes where appropriate. Your company may claim certain tax deductions for removing architectural, transportation, or communication barriers in your physical plant and company property.[43] In addition, eligible small businesses may take a tax credit for accommodations made to comply with the ADA.[44]

The ADA, and many state and local laws, require health care providers to treat all disabled persons, including those with AIDS or HIV infection. Since AIDS and HIV infection and other infectious diseases are considered disabil-ities under the ADA, health care providers are prohibited from denying treatment to any patient because he or she has AIDS, HIV infection, or some other infectious disease.[45]

In *Glanz v. Vernick*, a patient was refused treatment due to his HIV infection.[46] The patient sued under Section 504 of the Rehabilitation Act, and the health care facility was found liable for the health care worker's discrimination under the theory of respondent superior. The court based its decision on the fact that although the treatment of AIDS- or HIV-infected persons posed a minimal risk of infection, that risk was so small that a refusal to treat was legally insupportable.

The ADA gives the health care provider a duty to communicate with all patients who have impaired hearing, vision, or speech.[47] It is very important that all patients understand the nature and risks attendant to medical treatment. Appropriate auxiliary aids must be furnished where needed to ensure effective communication. The examples provided in the ADA regulations note that an interpreter, rather than a written summary, may be necessary to communicate in an effective manner to persons with hearing, vision, or speech disabilities.[48] The ADA also requires that interpreters be qualified to provide interpretive services and be able to interpret effectively, accurately, and impartially both receptively and expressively, using any necessary specialized vocabulary.[49]

As a limitation on the public accommodation requirements, your company is not required to provide services to individuals who pose a direct threat to the health or safety of others.[50] If your company concludes that a disabled person poses a direct threat, such that he or she is violent or acts in a threatening manner, that person may be denied the services of the public accommodation.[51] Additionally, your company may deny access of accommodation to current illegal drug users.[52]

Many questions remain as to the effect and extent of rights and responsibilities under the ADA. The federal courts and the EEOC hear discrimination complaints and lawsuits under the law, and questions will likely be answered on a case-by-case basis. However, this does not mean you should wait to comply with the law. It is imperative that you seek counsel when a question arises as to compliance with the ADA that you are unable to resolve easily on review of the regulations and your own internal procedures. Due to the substantial legal remedies afforded injured persons under the ADA, it is in your company's best interest to carefully document your attempts to comply with the ADA and to seek counsel when further advice is needed. The ADA provides harmed persons with substantial legal remedies and so imposes new and increased liability risks on health care providers, employers, and public accommodations. A plethora of questions remain on the extent of a disabled worker's rights and the limitations of an employer's or public accommodation's responsibilities under the ADA.

Your company should develop its own policies and procedures to comply with the ADA and state and local laws. Legal counsel should be sought for advice in particular circumstances and to assist in developing undue hardship and business necessity defenses where a reasonable accommodation cannot readily be provided. Relevant federal, state, and local laws should be reviewed, and administrative and supervisory staff and all personnel should be educated as to their responsibilities and rights under the various nondiscrimination laws in their multiple roles as employer, employee, and care provider.

TAX MATTERS

Increasingly, the tax-exempt status of health care providers is being challenged by a variety of sources. These sources of challenge are at the municipal, city, county, state, and federal levels. Pressure on governments to secure revenues through tax funding has caused the authorities to closely examine the tax-exempt status of both nonprofit and tax-exempt 501(c)(3) charitable health care providers. In addition, the taxing authorities are taking a closer look at health care providers due to reasons such as the diversifica-

tion of health care providers into lines of business and business ventures viewed as unrelated and/or in contradiction with the provider's articles of incorporation, charter and/or mission, and the fact that a number of health care providers are earning surplus revenues and/or are operating in ways that are divergent and inconsistent with their original charitable purposes.

Tax matters of concern to home care providers may also arise in the accounting methods on which the tax treatment of certain transactions are predicated on Medicare cost accounting and allocation principles. The Internal Revenue Service (IRS) has cautioned health care providers that the IRS' method of accounting and definitions of certain transactions for tax purposes vary from those utilized in the federal health insurance program known as Medicare. These differences in tax interpretation and characterization must be carefully considered by home care providers in managing the business affairs of their home care companies.

ENVIRONMENTAL ISSUES

Environmental issues are of great legal concern for all health care providers. The increased complexity of treatment modalities, pharmaceuticals, supplies, and equipment utilized in the home environment equates with ever-increasing issues of how to deal with the waste and environmental results associated with such treatments and materials.

The Occupational Safety and Health Administration (OSHA), under the authority of the Department of Labor, is the federal agency vested with the responsibility of developing and enforcing regulations and developing guidelines that encourage and cause employers to create and maintain safe workplace environments for employees.

OSHA has become increasingly active in the monitoring of the activities of health care providers in their actions for protecting health care workers. For example, OSHA issued instructional guidelines from its Office of Occupational Medicine, Directorate of Technical Support, entitled *Work Practice Guidelines for*

Personnel Dealing with Cytotoxic (Antineoplastic) Drugs.[53] This instructional publication outlines practical precautions recommended for health care providers involved in the handling, preparation, administration, and disposal of antineoplastic agents. The main thrust of the publication is the protection of the health care worker and the environment from the unknown long-term effects and hazards of new drugs and technologies that health care providers may utilize in their everyday work. Similarly, in February 1990 OSHA issued a revised instruction CPL 2-2.44B from its Office of Health Compliance Assistance, *Enforcement Procedures for Occupational Exposure to Hepatitis B Virus (HBV) and Human Immunodeficiency Virus (HIV).*[54] This instruction provides standards for the management and treatment of health care workers potentially exposed to HBV and HIV. Essentially, the standards require that employees at substantial risk of contacting body fluids must be offered hepatitis B vaccinations free of charge by employers and that employers must report any needlestick requiring medical treatment. OSHA acts to protect health care workers by the enforcement of such standards through site inspection, citations, and fines.

Noncompliance with OSHA standards may also result in collateral enforcement activities adverse to a home care provider by the licensure, certification, and accreditation bodies whose approval is a basic legal requirement for the continued operation of the home care provider.

Other worker protection laws, such as the federal and state employee right to know laws requiring posted notices to employees of workplace exposures to known hazardous chemicals and agents, govern all employers, including home health care providers.

The U.S. Environmental Protection Agency (EPA) is also concerned with the risks that new technologies may present in the uncontrolled disposal of medical waste, infectious waste, hazardous waste, and contaminated supplies such as needles and sharps from a patient's home.

In an effort to educate home care personnel and patients about such hazards, in January 1990 the EPA issued a pamphlet entitled *Disposal Tips for Home Health Care—Educating Your Patients*, as an instruction to home care personnel in their disposal practices of medical waste from the home.[55] Similar efforts and legislation are occurring at the state level in an effort to regulate waste created in the care and treatment of patients in their homes. In a number of states, past laws that excluded home health agencies and various home care providers as generators or producers of medical, infectious, or hazardous waste are now including home care providers in their state's legal definition of a producer of these wastes. This new designation is likely to subject home care providers to a plethora of regulatory and reporting requirements. Such trends are likely to continue in the future and shall subject home care providers to even greater scrutiny and requirements under state environmental protection and waste management laws.

These issues should be of great concern to home care providers in that these environmental and worker protection requirements expose the provider to greater accountability and increased exposure for liability if it fails to comply with the regulatory standards. Environmental claims are typical exclusions in most policies of insurance, and as such, the liability exposure for home care providers is one that cannot be easily protected against by a policy of insurance. Moreover, many state environmental laws are strict liability laws that provide that if the home care company is found to have violated the environmental law, then it must pay the mandated fines and costs of cleanup or correction. Under strict liability laws, it is usually irrelevant whether the violator knew of or intended to cause the violation. All that is necessary is a finding that the violation occurred and that the home care company/provider was the violator. Environmental damage claims and fines and the costs of cleanup can be astronomical. As such, it is crucial that home care providers pay serious attention to the development of environmental laws in their communities and at both state and federal levels of government.

WHAT TO CONSIDER IN SELECTING AN ATTORNEY

"One cool judgment is worth a thousand hasty counsels. The thing to be supplied is light, not heat."[56] Perhaps we should best look to the words of President Woodrow Wilson in his address on preparedness given in Pittsburgh, Pennsylvania on January 29, 1916, for words of inspiration in your considerations of what to look for in selecting an attorney to assist you with legal matters and matters of concern to you in your home care business.

It has been evident that employer/employee disputes, conflicts with government agencies and regulators, consumer concerns, and litigation are beginning to confront, and are of increasing concern to, home care providers. In these and similar matters, your health care business may require the services of an attorney.

The key to a productive relationship with an attorney is personal compatibility. You must be able to speak openly, freely, and candidly with this individual. As a general business counselor, you should look for an attorney who offers guidance, suggests alternatives to proposed actions, and anticipates, thereby preventing, legal problems.

Legal expertise and judgment are key attributes to seek in an attorney. A lawyer should have a working knowledge of the laws and regulations that affect your business.

Legal expertise in the matters in which an attorney will likely be involved is of increasing importance for health care providers in the ever more regulated service industry of home care. However, home care providers are similar to all companies in that they face a growing complexity of business and legal issues that demand technical knowledge. Certain areas of your business that may require special attention include pension planning, complex tax matters, securities issues, labor matters, and patent and trade secret protection.

With this perspective in mind, a health care organization should seek out an attorney who concentrates his or her practice in the health care industry, and in particular in the representation of home care service and product providers. Securing the services of an attorney who concentrates his or her legal practice in health care matters may assist you to avoid the recurring time delay and frustration of educating your attorney about what that thing is that you and your company do.

Alternately, you may seek references from your accountant and banker or from other companies in the home care industry. Your trade associations may be helpful in assisting you to secure appropriate counsel. In any event, you should feel free to ask the attorney for a number of client references and check them out. The American Bar Association, the lawyer referral service of the local Bar Association, the National Health Lawyer's Association, the American Association of Nurse Attorneys, and the American Academy of Hospital Attorneys are just a few of the many organizations that may be able to direct you to attorney members who concentrate their legal practice in health care matters or in a related area of concern to your company.

Due to both the litigious and the regulatory nature of health care services, for specific matters it may be in your company's best interests to seek out experienced attorneys in special matters (e.g., malpractice defense litigators in negligence matters and criminal defense attorneys in fraud and abuse matters).

If your current general counsel is an attorney experienced in health care matters, your counsel will probably seek out these attorney specialists when it is in your company's best interests to do so. Many policies of insurance for liability require that your company utilize the insurance company's counsel in matters of defense under the policy of insurance or risk the possibility of no insurance coverage of the matter and nonpayment of attorney fees under the policy of insurance.

In any event, your company's general counsel should be experienced in home care provider matters related to your specific home care business. An experienced health care attorney is able to recognize when it is imperative for you to retain an attorney with experience in specialized matters. For example, as mentioned above, due to the legal criminal procedural issues that may occur at a certain juncture in a fraud and abuse investigation, your health care attorney may suggest the retention of the additional legal services of an experienced criminal defense attorney in order to best proceed in protecting your rights and those of your home care company. Protecting your company's legal position and putting you and your company in the best possible legal position should be the goal for you and your attorney in such matters.

REFERENCES

1. *Key Enterprises of Delaware, Inc. v. Venice Hosp.* 919 F.2d 1550 (11th Cir. 1990), vacated and reh'g en banc granted 979, F 2d 806 (11th Cir. 1992).

2. U.S.C.A. 42 § 1395 et seq.

3. 42 U.S.C. § 1395nn.

4. The Patient Self Determination Act of 1990, Pub. L. No. 101-508, 105 Stat. 1388–44–115, 42 C.F.R. § 489.100–104.

5. 42 CFR § 489.100–104.

6. 42 CFR § 489.102.

7. 42 U.S.C.A. §§ 12101–12117.

8. 42 U.S.C.A. §§ 12111–12117, 12141–12189.

9. 42 U.S.C.A. § 12101(a).

10. 42 U.S.C.A. § 12112(a).

11. 42 U.S.C.A. § 12112(b)(5)(A).

12. 42 U.S.C.A. § 12112(a).

13. 42 U.S.C.A. § 12102(2).

14. 29 CFR § 1630.2(m).

15. 29 CFR § 1630.29(n)(1).

16. 29 CFR § 1630.2(o).

17. 29 CFR § 1630.2(o)(2).

18. 29 CFR § 1630.10.

19. 42 U.S.C.A. § 12112(d)(4)(B).

20. 29 CFR § 1630.14(d)(1).

21. 28 CFR § 36.104.

22. 28 CFR § 36.208.

23. Centers for Disease Control. (July 12, 1991). *Recommendations for Preventing Transmission of Human Immunodeficiency Virus and Hepatitis B Virus to Patients During Exposure-Prone Invasive Procedures,* 40 MMWR1, 3.

24. 29 CFR § 1630.3(a).

25. 29 CFR § 1630.16(b).

26. *Rogers v. Lehman*, 869 F.2d 253(4th Cir. 1989).

27. 42 U.S.C.A. § 12114(d)(2).

28. 42 U.S.C.A. § 12114(d)(1)-(2), 29 C.F.R. § 1630, App.

29. 42 U.S.C.A. § 12115.

30. 29 CFR § 1602.

31. 28 CFR § 36.201(a).

32. 28 CFR § 36.104.

33. 28 CFR §§ 36.302–310.

34. 28 CFR § 36.304(b).

35. 28 CFR § 36.304(b).

36. 28 CFR § 36.304(c).

37. 28 CFR § 36.402(a).

38. 28 CFR§ 36.401–407.

39. 28 CFR § 36.303(a).

40. 28 CFR § 36.303(a).

41. 28 CFR § 36.303(b).

42. 28 CFR § 36.201(b).

43. I.R.C., 26 U.S.C.S. § 190.

44. I.R.C. § 44 (1992), *Disabled Access Credit*, 1992 U.S. Master Tax Guide, CCH, 1338, 1991.

45. 28 CFR § 36.104.

46. 756 F.Supp. 632 (D. Mass. 1991).

47. 28 CFR § 36.309.

48. 28 CFR § 36.309.

49. 28 CFR § 36.303, 28 C.F.R. §36.309.

50. 28 CFR § 36.208(a).

51. 28 CFR § 36.208(b),(c).

52. 28 CFR § 36.209.

53. Occupational Safety and Health Administration. (1986). *Work Practice Guidelines for Personnel Dealing with Cytotoxic (Antineoplastic) Drugs* (OSHA Publication No. 8–11). Washington, DC: OSHA.

54. Occupational Safety and Health Administration. (1990). *Enforcement Procedures for Occupational Exposure to Hepatitis B Virus (HBV) and Human Immunodeficiency Virus (HIV).* Washington, DC: OSHA.

55. Environmental Protection Agency. (1990). *Disposal Tips for Home Health Care—Educating Your Patients* (EPA Publication No. EPA/530-SW-90-014A). Washington, DC: EPA.

56. Wilson, W. (1981). *The Papers of Woodrow Wilson* (A.S. Link, ed.). Washington, DC: Library of Congress.

CHAPTER 54

Ethical Issues

Charmaine M. Fitzig

According to Bandman and Bandman (1990, p. 3):

> Ethics . . . is concerned with doing good and avoiding harm . . . possibilities of good or harm depend partly on knowledge and partly on values. Both must be consciously and critically evaluated for their potential of good or harm to human beings, well or sick.

The practice of nursing is concerned with doing good, and in attempting to define what is good one could begin with a review of several different pledges or codes that have defined the practice of nursing over time. The following is one of the statements in the Florence Nightingale Pledge, written in 1893 by Lystra Gretter (Kalisch & Kalisch, 1978, pp. 141–142): "I will abstain from whatever is deleterious and mischievous and will not take or knowingly administer any harmful drug. . . ." The International Council of Nurses code of ethics begins with the statement, "The fundamental responsibility of the nurse is fourfold: to promote health, to prevent illness, to restore health and to alleviate suffering . . ." (Kelly, 1991, p. 214). The code that is probably best known and cited most often, because of the seeming increase in ethical dilemmas due to several court cases that have had extensive media coverage (*Doe v. Bolton*

410 U.S. 179; *Roe v. Wade* 410 U.S. 113), is the American Nurses Association (ANA) code for nurses (only 2 of 11 provisions are cited here): "The nurse provides services with respect for human dignity and the uniqueness of the client unrestricted by considerations of social or economic status, personal attributes, or the nature of the health problem" (ANA, 1985, pp. 2–4) and "The nurse assumes responsibility and accountability for individual nursing judgments and actions" (ANA, 1985, pp. 7–9).

The early philosophers, such as Socrates, Plato, and Aristotle, attempted to define the meaning of good and the role of the individual and the state in achieving it. Today, however, after centuries of debates and hundreds of treatises, we are no closer to deciding absolutely what good is or what an individual or state should do to achieve it. The final decisions must be based on several factors, including time, knowledge, technological advances, the culture and values of a people, available resources, and, ultimately, cost. Given the uncertainty of the decision-making process, however, several positions or theories have been developed over the years that could serve as guidelines for action in the health care delivery system. Bandman and Bandman (1990) have developed a graphic representation of what they call traditional models of morality (Figure 54–1). They state:

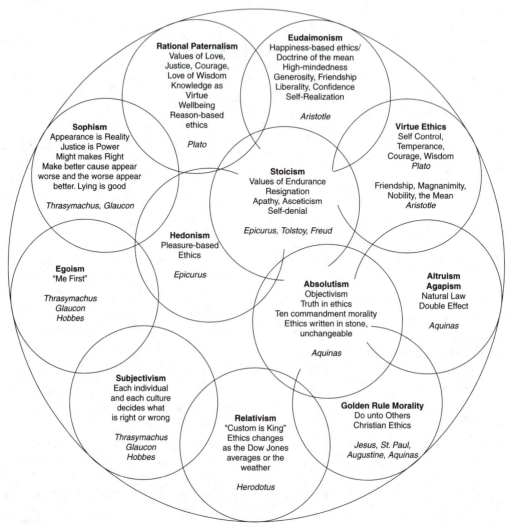

Figure 54–1 Traditional theories of ethics. *Source:* Reprinted with permission from E.L. Bandman and B. Bandman, *Nursing Ethics through the Life Span*, p. 44, © 1995, Appleton & Lange.

As one studies ethics, one finds no single science of moral values. One, instead, finds alterative theories of ethics and dialogue between these. Alterative theories of morality orient the role of nursing in the care of patients. These models of moral values are like overlapping circles. Each theory sets out its values along with an attempted justification to some decision-making aspect of nursing. (Bandman & Bandman, 1995, p. 44)

Ethics, also called moral philosophy, is generally divided into three major subdisciplines: metaethics, normative ethics, and applied ethics or bioethics. Metaethics deals with questions related to the nature of moral concepts and judgments. Normative ethics is concerned with establishing standards or norms for conduct and is commonly associated with general theories about how one ought to live. Applied ethics or bioethics is the application of normative theories to practical moral problems such as human rights, the quality of life, and the ethical implications of various developments in medicine and the biological sciences, such as *in vitro* fertilization, the operation and use of sperm banks, gene manipulation, and so forth.

ANCIENT BEGINNINGS

It has been postulated that ethics began with the introduction of the first moral codes, and examples of ancient codes or laws would certainly include the Ten Commandments and the Code of Hammurabi. Socrates (470–399 B.C.), considered one of the seminal thinkers of Greek philosophy, operated under two assumptions: the principle never to do wrong or to participate, even indirectly, in any wrongdoing; and the conviction that nobody who really knows what is good and right could act against it.

Plato (428–347 B.C.), the most important disciple of Socrates, is best known for his theory of ideas, one of which was the ideal of good, which he described as beyond being and knowledge. Aristotle (384–322 B.C.), a younger contemporary of Plato, believed in the doctrine of purposiveness. He felt that all human activities are directed toward the end of a good and satisfactory life.

The later period of Greek and Roman ethics included the Stoics and Epicureans, who presented different positions as to how one ought to live. The Stoics felt that all human beings share the capacity to reason and that what is important is the pursuit of wisdom and virtue. They rejected passion as a basis for deciding what is good or bad. Suicide, as a means of avoiding inescapable pain, was acceptable to the Stoics. The Epicureans regarded pleasure as the sole ultimate good and pain as the sole evil. Epicurus, the founder of this philosophy, taught that the greatest pleasure obtainable was the pleasure of tranquility, which is to be obtained by the removal of unsatisfied wants.

SELECTED ETHICAL THEORIES

Egoism

From the Latin *ego*, "I," egoism is an ethical theory holding that the good is based on the pursuit of self-interest. The egoist seeks perfection through the furthering of his or her own welfare and profit.

Utilitarianism

The fundamental principle of utilitarianism, a tradition in ethics stemming from the 18th and 19th century English philosophers and economists Jeremy Bentham and John Stuart Mill, is that an action is right if it tends to promote happiness and wrong if it tends to provide the reverse of happiness, not just the happiness of the performer of the action but that of everyone affected by it. This theory is in opposition to egoism.

Altruism

Altruism is an ethical system governed more by one's social aspects. It stresses the importance of the community rather than the individual.

Deontology

Deontology is a theory that judges actions by their conformance to some formal rule or principle. An example is the ethical system of the German philosopher Immanuel Kant, who felt that our actions possess moral worth only when we do our duty for its own sake.

Theory of Justice

Put forth by John Rawls, the theory of justice was a welcome alternative to utilitarianism. His theory had two principles. The first stated that each person should have the maximum amount of liberty. The second principle required that wealth be distributed so as to equalize resources and afford the greatest benefit to the least advantaged (Rawls, 1971).

Theory of Obligation

William Frankena, a modern philosopher, in 1973 published his work *Ethics*, in which he described his theory of obligation, which contains two basic principles. The first principle of beneficence includes four "oughts": ought not to inflict harm or evil, ought to prevent harm, ought to remove evil, and ought to do or promote good. The second principle was one of justice as equal treatment: the equal or comparative treatment of individuals, or dealing with people according to their merits (Frankena, 1973).

Other Theories

Two other modern philosophers have written on the rights of individuals and the role of the state. Robert Noziak (a deontologist), in his 1974 book *Anarchy, State and Utopia*, presented the ideal that life, liberty, and legitimately acquired property are absolute rights and that no act can be justified if it violates them. He further indicated that no one, not even the state, has a right to assist people in the preservation of their rights (Noziak, 1974).

Although Ronald Dworkin agreed with Noziak's theory of individual rights, his ideas were much broader. In his work *Taking Rights Seriously*, he indicated that respect for others might require us to assist them and not leave them to fend for themselves. In addition, Dworkin felt that the state had an obligation to intervene in areas where it was necessary to ensure the preservation of individual rights (Dworkin, 1977).

CHARACTERISTICS OF ETHICAL ISSUES

The five criteria proposed by Rawls (1971) for looking at the rightness of any ethical princi-

ple can serve as a guide in the identification and analysis of all ethical issues or dilemmas:

1. *Universality*: the same principles must hold for everyone
2. *Generality*: reference must not be made to specific people or situations
3. *Publicity*: the situation or issue must be known and recognized by all involved
4. *Ordering*: conflicting claims must be ordered without resorting to force
5. *Finality*: the issue may override the demands of law and custom

The health care delivery system is replete with instances where ethical dilemmas have had to be resolved through the convening of ethics committees or through the courts. In the early days of kidney dialysis (before 1972, when Public Law 92-603 was enacted and made dialysis procedures financially available to all), many hospitals initiated interdisciplinary teams to define the criteria for deciding who was to be put on the machine. Many of these teams were later called ethics committees and were involved in decisions regarding more than the kidney machines. Also, a practice that is fairly common within many hospitals and known to few outsiders is writing in pencil the abbreviation *DNR* (do not resuscitate) on selected patients' charts. This custom was discussed at length by Korein, who testified in the Karen Ann Quinlan case about the unwritten and unspoken standards of medical practice (*In the Matter of Karen Quinlan*, 1976, p. 647):

> . . . cancer, metastatic cancer, involving the lungs, the liver, the brain, multiple involvements, the physician may or may not write DNR . . . it could be said to the nurse: if this man stops breathing don't resuscitate him. . . . No physician that I know personally is going to resuscitate a man riddled with cancer and in agony and he stops breathing. They are not

going to put him on a respirator. . . . I think that would be the height of misuse of technology.

Several other important issues have been tried in the courts. Among them are the following interesting cases that have implications for public health nursing practice.

In *Roe v. Wade* (410 U.S. 113 (1973)) and *Doe v. Bolton* (410 U.S. 179 (1973)), the right of every woman to have a legal abortion was established.

Quality of life and the right to die were issues addressed in the Karen Ann Quinlan case. Quinlan's father, as her guardian, won the right to obtain a physician who would agree that the respirator should not be used based on the medical decision that there could be no reasonable possibility of Karen's returning to a cognitive state (*In the Matter of Karen Quinlan*, 1976).

The right to life issue resulted in a national debate after a 6-day-old infant, Baby Doe, born with Down syndrome and an incomplete esophagus, died from lack of food and water. The courts in Illinois supported the parents' decision to refuse surgical intervention ("The Prosecutor Closes Case," 1982). In response to the public outcry, the U.S. Department of Health and Human Services Office of Civil Rights issued the now-famous "Notice to Health Care Providers," which directed anyone with knowledge of the denial of food or customary medical care to contact immediately the department's handicapped infant hotline or the state's child protection services. These notices were to be placed in conspicuous places. This directive was later found to be invalid by a U.S. district court judge.

Many nurses and hospital administrators failed to take advantage of the furor caused by the Baby Doe case to initiate permanent ethics committees. In addition, few hospitals have realized the need for ongoing continuing education or training programs on decision making relative to clinical issues dealing with ethical dilemmas.

ETHICAL ISSUES IN THE ADMINISTRATIVE AND CLINICAL AREAS OF HOME HEALTH CARE

In general, although the types of ethical issues and dilemmas encountered in home health care are, by and large, no different from those encountered within the whole spectrum of the health care delivery system, there are several issues that are unique to home health care. The following issues are addressed:

- case finding
- documentation for reimbursement
- compatibility of public health nursing and complex care in the community
- quality of life
- role of the nurse in ethical dilemmas in a changing health care system

Case Finding

Many years ago, when I was a student and later a staff nurse in a public health nursing agency, one of the criteria used to evaluate my effectiveness was my case finding ability. In those days, we had the luxury of actively seeking out individuals and families who were potential users of health services. They were the other family members or neighbors who were present when actual home visits were made (the pregnant teenager, the elderly diabetic, etc.). These new patients were contacted and cared for without reimbursement limitations. Today, even though theoretically case finding is still considered a good public health practice, it is not pursued as vigorously as it was in the 1950s and 1960s. The general feeling is, "Why look for cases to increase your caseload when the majority may not be reimbursed?" Of course, there are some public health nurses and supervisors within the public health agencies (voluntary and public) who still do some case finding and who have budgeted a small percentage of their funds for case finding. Many, however, have developed strict criteria in deciding which types of cases to go after.

Documentation for Reimbursement

The importance of recording accurate data is stressed in nursing schools; nurses' notes have figured prominently in several malpractice suits. Many examples of court cases lost or won have been reviewed in classrooms during discussions of the legal aspects of documentation. Hospitals and home health agencies have recognized the importance of accurate recording not only to serve as evidence of good patient care but as safeguards in future malpractice suits. Many hospitals have also hired individuals, known as risk managers, to evaluate, monitor, and modify practices that can have deleterious effects on patient care and safety.

Continuation programs stressing the legal aspects of nursing, and especially the issue of documentation, have been popular among nursing audiences. In a 1974 survey on ethics done by *Nursing '74*, 4 questions of 73 dealt with recording information ("Nursing Ethics," 1974). The survey results were interesting and confirmed the fact that almost all nurses (96%), at least among those who responded, would not record inaccurate data. Some of the questions and their responses are presented in Exhibit 54–1.

Contrary to the findings presented in Exhibit 54–1, Mundinger (1983), in her book *Home Care Controversy: Too Little, Too Late, Too Costly*, found several instances where nurses omitted or adjusted data to maintain nursing services that the clients needed. The nurses ignored the Medicare restrictions and recorded whatever data were necessary to conform to the rules. To comply with these rules, three important criteria had to be met:

1. The patient must require skilled care.
2. The patient must have a physician's plan of care.
3. The patient must be homebound.

Mundinger's (1983) study involved 50 home visits in which she compared the care given with the Medicare eligibility criteria noted earlier. At the time of the visits, 16 (32%) of the clients did not meet the requirements for skilled care, only 25 (50%) of the physician's plans of care were judged to be adequate, and only 15 (30%) of the patients were actually homebound. She notes, "Nurses learn how to document cases to assure reimbursement. Fabrication is rare but adjustment of the data probably is frequent" (Mundinger, 1983, p. 66). She does not indicate how many nurses she observed in her study of 50 home visits.

Although the *Nursing '74* survey did not include the place of work of the nurses who responded, one can safely assume that the majority worked in hospitals, and there were no indications that public health nurses responded. It would be interesting to conduct a similar study among public health nurses. Invariably, the question of recording to meet the reimbursement criteria would be an important issue. It would be enlightening to know how common this practice is in public health nursing.

Hoeman (1984), in her unpublished doctoral dissertation, describes how nurses record data to ensure the maximum benefits for clients. She notes that the restrictions of the reimbursement procedures make it difficult for nurses to give care in a curing system. Aroskar (1977) describes a survey that was based on question-

---

Exhibit 54–1 Excerpts from *Nursing '74* Ethics Survey

In making notes have you ever done the following? ($n = 11, 681$)	
Question 50: Added information by writing between lines?	48%
Question 51: Erased or altered information?	11%
Question 52: Purposely omitted information because it might make you look bad?	9%
Question 53: Recorded inaccurate information because of a delicate situation?	4%

naires sent to the deans or curriculum coordinators of some 209 accredited baccalaureate nursing programs in the United States. Eighty-six schools responded. Two thirds of the respondents said that ethical aspects were integrated throughout the nursing courses.

Compatibility of Public Health Nursing and Complex Care within the Community

Many nurses working in public health or community health nursing agencies are graduates of baccalaureate nursing programs. Many of them forgo experience in the hospital and go directly into community nursing. The community agencies usually welcome these new graduates because many of them would have completed their clinical experiences at the agencies involved. Many agencies required 1 or 2 years of hospital experience for the nonbaccalaureate-prepared nurse. As a result of many cost containment strategies, hospitals have responded by discharging patients sooner and sicker. The needs of these patients are complex and include administration of peripheral and central IV therapy, passage of nasogastric tubes for feeding, ventilators, chemotherapy, and the like. To respond adequately to the increasing referrals of patients in need of complex care, many of the voluntary community home health nursing agencies have modified their services to offer 24-hour nursing and support services (Bowyer, 1986; Griffith, 1984). In addition, these agencies have identified the learning needs of their staff nurses and have, in cooperation with many hospitals and equipment companies, developed in-depth inservice education programs for their nurses and support staff.

Many proprietary home health nursing agencies and equipment manufacturers have recognized the financial rewards of establishing specialized clinical nursing teams that make home visits and care for clients in need of high-technology nursing services. Many of these nurses are recruited from the intensive care and medical-surgical units of hospitals. The majority are registered nurses without public health

preparation, experience, or orientation. Consequently, they are unable to function as public health nurses. Their purpose in the home is to complete a special task. The functions of public health nursing, which include health education, health promotion, and risk reduction, are usually not addressed. We have these mini-medical-surgical teams operating in the home, and the practice of public health nursing is non-existent.

A few of these commercial agencies employ supervisors or staff nurses who are public health practitioners and who recognize the importance of obtaining individual and family assessment data on each referral. These nurses become the coordinators and work closely with the high-technology, specialized nurse in the development of appropriate comprehensive care plans.

Quality of Life

Webster's defines quality as a "peculiar and essential character" and as a "special or distinguishing attribute." Obviously, each person who is capable of reasoning will determine what constitutes quality of life for himself or herself. The final decision as to what the individual is willing to accept will, to a large extent, be influenced by several factors, among them state of health, ability to function independently (financially and personally), adequate housing or living conditions, meaningful family or significant other relationships, changes in lifestyle, and the like.

Quality of life issues have gained importance with the increase of technological advancements. Although no age group has escaped quality of life considerations, for certain groups of people the qualify of life issue is a daily experience in decisions and choices. These groups or populations at risk include the handicapped or disabled, the poor, minorities, the chronically ill, and the elderly. There have been several situations dealing with quality of life issues among the chronically ill that have had extensive media coverage. The following court cases all have implications for public health nursing.

Elizabeth Bouvia, a 25-year-old quadriplegic cerebral palsy patient, in 1983 filed suit against the hospital because she wanted to starve to death. At the time she contended that her pain-ridden body was useless and that her physical disabilities prevented her from taking her own life. The judge refused her request ("Woman Who Sought To Starve," 1986). In January 1986, she filed suit against a second hospital where she was hospitalized because, against her wishes, the physicians had inserted a feeding tube through her nose and she was fed by force. Bouvia later stated, "I didn't want to ever depend on others in an institution. I'm caught in a legal bind because other people can't realize I'm not living, I'm existing . . ." ("Patient Finds," 1986). In April 1986, a state appeals court panel declared that the right to refuse medical treatment is basic and fundamental and ruled that Bouvia had the right to refuse to be force fed (Chambers, 1986).

Another equally dramatic case involved a 30-year-old woman. In March 1980, Nancy Jobes, who was 4.5 months pregnant, was injured in a car crash, and the fetus was killed. During surgery to remove the fetus, she had a cardiac arrest from an anesthesia accident. This resulted in severe brain damage and coma. Several months later she was transferred from the hospital to a nursing home. Nearly 5 years later, her husband and family petitioned the courts to allow her to die by removing the artificial feeding tube because she had been in an irreversible vegetative state since the cardiac arrest. The state superior court judge ruled that the artificial feeding tube could be removed (Sullivan, 1986b).

The third case deals with an individual who was maintained at home on a respirator. Ms. Farrell was 37 years old and had amyotrophic lateral sclerosis. She was paralyzed except for the muscles controlling her eyes and lips. Farrell and her husband petitioned the court to allow the respirator to be disconnected because she did not wish to live. The judge approved, saying, "it would be cruel to sustain a life so wracked with pain" (Sullivan, 1986a, p. 6). The decision by Judge Wiley of the Superior Court in Toms River was the first in New Jersey to allow the withdrawal of life support from a person who was being cared for at home (Sullivan, 1986a).

It is interesting to note that the majority of the cases involving quality of life issues were initiated by or on behalf of patients who were in either hospitals or other institutions at the time the suits were initiated. One might speculate that, for the patient receiving nursing services at home, the public health nurse would have obtained vital information (through an adequate initial and periodic assessment of the patient) before any need for emergency treatments. This would then necessitate a plan of care, with the patient's involvement, that would allow the patient's wishes to be followed. Many terminally ill patients and nurses working in oncology units have enthusiastically welcomed the expanding hospice movement.

The proportion of the population 65 years and older is growing at a faster rate than that of other age groups, and the group 85 years and older is growing rapidly. Recent data indicate that, although 60% of the 2 million users of home health services are younger than 65 years of age, the most intensive users are the elderly, who average 22.3 home health visits annually. The data show that 78% of all home health visits are received by Americans older than 65 years of age even though they account for only 43% of the user population (National Center for Health Services Research, 1985).

That the elderly are at risk for institutionalization was confirmed by a National Center for Health Statistics survey, which indicated that almost half of the elderly report some degree of limitation of activity resulting from chronic disease or impairment (Department of Health and Human Services [DHHS], 1983). These same data indicated that an estimated 4.7 million adults in the civilian noninstitutionalized population need functional assistance from another person for selected personal care or home management activities. More than half (2.7 million) are 65 years of age and older, 1.3 million are 44 to 64 years of age, and fewer than 1 million are between 18 and 44 years of age. The percentage of the noninstitutionalized population needing another person's help increases with age. Functional assistance is needed by only 1% of young adults but by 12% of the elderly. As expected, the proportion of the population needing help continues to increase with age among those 65 years of age and older. Those needing help represent 7% of those 65 to 74 years, 16% of those 75 to 84 years, and 39% of those 85 years and older (DHHS, 1983).

The ability to maintain independent living is dependent on a number of factors, including the following: extent of disability and functional impairment, sociodemographic characteristics of the individual (sex, age, and living arrangements), availability of another person to provide needed assistance, and availability of community services and their accessibility to people who need them (DHHS, 1983).

For the elderly person receiving public health nursing services at home, the countdown begins when he or she begins to have difficulty in personal care and home management skills. As his or her abilities decrease, decisions about living arrangements have to be made. As living arrangements change, whether by moving to a relative's home or to an institution or by staying at home with the assistance of a home health aide, the quality of life is compromised.

The Role of the Nurse in Ethical Dilemmas in a Changing Health Care System

The 1990s ushered in many changes as the cost of health care skyrocketed. During this time both providers of care and individuals have become more concerned about choices and quality of life issues. This heightened sensitivity has been expressed in various ways: through living wills, advance medical directives, informed consent, and so forth. Many hospitals and nursing homes have developed elaborate systems to increase the individual's ability to

make choices that will invariably affect his or her quality of life. There is inconsistency and ambivalence within the health care delivery system, however, because there are no rules or guidelines and because decisions are made individually without consideration of the impact on society or the common good. Concurrently, health care providers are being forced to contain the cost of care through managed competition. The idea of competition is based on the assumption that informed choices must be made because health care is not an unlimited resource.

In a well-documented and publicized case, Armando, 24 years of age, was admitted to a hospital in Houston, Texas (Belkin, 1993). He had been shot during a dispute, and the bullet had penetrated his spine. He was not expected to live, and initially the health team considered him a good organ donor. He was given the best of high-technology care, and he survived but was paralyzed from the jaw down. He was a ventilator-dependent quadriplegic. Later, members of the health team who had worked laboriously to keep him alive questioned him about his decision regarding the DNR order. They were sure that he would not want to live and were puzzled and surprised that he resisted their pressure to have him accept the DNR order. Where were the nurses? Did they understand the patient's choice?

A more recent case (Toufexis, 1993) involved the decision by a hospital to separate Siamese twins. The parents' own physician had put the likelihood of one twin surviving at no more than 20% and had advised them to seek an abortion. Although the parents initially agreed to the abortion, the mother changed her mind after the clinic postponed the procedure. At the hospital where the twins were delivered (Children's Hospital in Philadelphia), the surgeons indicated that the surviving twin would have only the slimmest chance (less than 1%) to survive for more than a few weeks (the twins were joined breast to belly with a fused liver and shared heart). The surgical team responded to the parents' wishes and not the medical outlook.

Nurses were not mentioned as part of the health care team.

In another highly publicized decision (Greenhouse, 1993), a hospital in suburban Virginia appealed a federal district court's ruling that it must continue to provide life-sustaining treatment for an infant born there 11 months earlier with most of her brain missing. The American Academy of Pediatrics filed a brief supporting the hospital on grounds that life-sustaining treatment for an anencephalic infant was medically inappropriate. The mother had rejected the physician's recommendation to have an abortion when the anencephaly was diagnosed before the infant was born. The pediatrician who headed the program on medical ethics at the Boston University School of Medicine and Public Health stated that sustaining the life of an anencephalic infant was the ultimate inappropriate use of health care resources. Again, decisions were made by the medical team. Should nursing have been involved?

Finances played a small role in these three cases. Armando, the 24-year-old quadriplegic, was finally discharged home after the hospital realized that he had no health insurance and that his case would cost the hospital thousands of dollars a month for the rest of his life. He had spent 4.5 years in the hospital at a cost of $727,008 dollars. He probably could have been discharged much earlier with a reduction in the total cost if nursing and discharge planning had been part of the decision. In the case of the Siamese twins, the total cost of the care of the twins up to and including surgery was estimated at about $300,000 and was expected to increase. The cost for the care for the anencephalic infant described in the third case was estimated to be about $1,464 per day in the nursing home where she had been placed. Where was the nursing input? These cases raise issues of health policy, ethics, and the role of nursing.

Alan Fleischman, director of neonatology at Montefiore Medical Center in New York City, stated, "Americans are a society of rescue rather than prevention, we are not people who really believe in community; we are a society that believes in the individual" (Toufexis, 1993).

STRATEGIES

Case Finding

Agency administrators need to decide whether case finding and preventive care are important functions and, if so, if they should include these services with the necessary criteria for eligibility. The policy should be clear and shared openly with agency staff. One way to determine the importance of case finding through the seeking out of at-risk population groups would be to compare the agency's caseload with the community's mortality and morbidity database obtained through complete and current population and community assessments.

Documentation

Accurate and timely recording can facilitate change. Policy decisions need hard data to support the need. Agency personnel and administrators need to discuss problems openly. Nurses have to accept the responsibility of recording data even if it means that a service visit will not be reimbursed. The agency then will have to assume a larger deficit until the reimbursement regulations are changed. If all the agencies coordinated their efforts and lobbied for changes based on the data that are recorded and not omitted, that would be, in the long run, a more professional and ethical posture to take.

Quality of Life

A problem that is virtually ignored is the increasing number of elderly persons committing suicide. Statistics indicate that, more than any other age group, the elderly are prone to commit suicide. According to Nancy Osgood, an assistant professor of gerontology and sociology at Virginia Commonwealth University in Richmond, 7 of 10 elderly persons who attempt suicide succeed. In addition, she indicated that 25% of the country's elderly population commits suicide. The population at risk for suicide includes the isolated lower class, elderly men in urban areas, and widowed men, who may have experienced multiple losses (physical, mental, financial, and social). According to Osgood, all these factors increase the likelihood of depression and, ultimately for many, suicide (Bugman, 1985).

Public health nurses can increase the quality of life for each patient by consistently obtaining and recording assessment data on individuals and their families. By analyzing the data, the nurse identifies those individuals at risk and develops appropriate short-term and long-term goals with the individual's and the family's participation. Within the first visit, the nurse should be aware of the patient's preference to die at home, for example, and should, with the patient's permission, engage significant others in the plan of action for the time when the patient's condition would necessitate decisions being made.

It is disheartening that, at this point in time, we do not have recreational or occupational programs geared to the homebound in any systematic fashion. Even though the Meals-on-Wheels programs are limited in their scope, at least a fair number of elderly people can get one meal per day for 5 days per week. How many "Crafts-on-Wheels" programs are there? We keep our elderly alive only to let them die of boredom or commit suicide.

Many industries have begun to implement preretirement programs to help their employees adjust to retirement. Many senior citizen centers have outreach and friendly visitors programs, but they are not organized and not widespread enough. Recreational programs should be an essential home health service. These programs would certainly add to the quality of life among our elderly population.

Questions regarding appropriateness of decisions are beginning to surface as medical costs approach a trillion dollars a year figure. Should we be content to continue the dramatic media-reported miracles such as transplants, resuscitations, and bionic type surgeries as they are being done more frequently when we are so behind in basic preventive health services such as childhood immunizations, prenatal care, screenings for high blood pressure and diabetes, and the like? What is nursing's role at this phase?

The Role of the Nurse

Nurses at all levels and types of institutions need to reacquaint themselves with the ANA code for nurses. Plank XI states that the nurse should collaborate with members of the health professions and other citizens in promoting community and national efforts to meet the health needs of the public (ANA, 1985). Nurses need to obtain information to use the legislative, regulatory, and political process to effect change in our society, specifically to strengthen the health care system and the practice of nursing (DeVries & Vanderbilt, 1992). Nurses need to know how their hospitals or other health care facilities function regarding ethics committees, informed consent, living wills, advance directives, and so forth. They need to get on ethics committees if they exist in their agencies or to develop them if not. They need to be active in their professional organizations. They need to lobby policy makers about their concerns through letter writing or personal visits to hearings, political rallies, and the like. They need to identify a system by which they can receive, on a regular basis, information about health legislation. They need to network.

CONCLUSION

All nurses need to recognize the implications of their care and the need to be actively involved in health care decisions that affect their patients' care. Nurses in community health are involved in many decisions, and increasingly these decisions deal with patients' choices. Moreover, the community nurse needs to develop an awareness of the ethical and legal principles that are involved in or have implications for practice. Community nurses need to begin thinking of, and acting on behalf of, the community and society at large even as they care for individuals and families.

REFERENCES

American Nurses Association. (1985). *Code for nurses with interpretive statements* (rev. ed.). Washington, DC: Author.

Aroskar, M. (1977). Ethics in the nursing curriculum. *Nursing Outlook, 25,* 260–264.

Bandman, E.L., & Bandman, B. (1995). *Nursing ethics through the life span* (3rd ed.). Norwalk, CT: Appleton & Lange.

Belkin, L. (1993, January 31). The high cost of living. *New York Times Magazine,* pp. 30–33, 44, 46, 56, 58.

Bowyer, C. (1986). The complex care team: Meeting the needs of high-technology nursing. *Home Health Care Nurse, 4,* 24–29.

Bugman, C. (1985, October 27). Suicide among elderly virtually ignored despite highest rate of any age group. *Star Ledger,* p. 91.

Chambers, M. (1986, April 17). Appeals panel says quadriplegic has right to end forced feeding. *New York Times,* p. A28.

Department of Health and Human Services, Public Health Service, National Center for Health Statistics. (1983). *Health United States.* Washington, DC: Government Printing Office.

DeVries, C., & Vanderbilt, M.W. (1992). The *grassroots lobbying handbook.* Washington, DC: American Nurses Association.

Dworkin, R. (1977). *Taking rights seriously.* Cambridge, MA: Harvard University Press.

Frankena, W. (1973). *Ethics* (2nd ed.). Englewood Cliffs, NJ: Prentice-Hall.

Greenhouse, L. (1993, September 24). Hospital appeals decision ordering treatment for baby missing a brain. *New York Times,* p. A10.

Griffith, E. (1984). Home care today. (Interview by E.M. Morris and J.D. Fonseca). *American Journal of Nursing, 84*(3), 340–342.

Hoeman, S. (1984). Counting whatever counts—An ethnography of a hospital-based home health agency. New Brunswick, NJ: Rutgers, the State University (unpublished dissertation).

In the matter of Karen Quinlan. (1976). 355 A2d, p. 647.

Kalisch, P., & Kalisch, B. (1978). *The advance of American nursing.* Boston: Little, Brown.

Kelly, L.Y. (1991). *Dimensions of professional nursing* (6th ed.). New York: McGraw-Hill.

Mundinger, M. (1983). *Home care controversy: Too little, too late, too costly.* Gaithersburg, MD: Aspen.

National Center for Health Services Research and Health Care Technology Assessment. (1985, October). Who uses home health care? *Research Activities 78,* 1.

Noziak, R. (1974). *Anarchy, state and utopia.* New York: Basic.

Nursing ethics: The admirable professional standards of nurses: a survey report. Part 3. (1974). *Nursing, 74* (10), 56–66.

Patient finds just existing is not living. (1986, February 13). *New York Times,* p. B3.

Rawls, J. (1971). *A theory of justice.* Cambridge, MA: Harvard University Press.

Sullivan, R. (1986a, April 24). Dying woman wins Jersey ruling to end life-sustaining care. *New York Times,* p. B1.

Sullivan, R. (1986b, April 24). Judge sanctions end of feeding in a coma case. *New York Times,* p. B3.

The prosecutor closes case in death of Indiana baby. (1982, April 20). *New York Times,* p. A18.

Toufexis, A. (1993, August 30). The ultimate choice. *Time,* pp. 43–44.

Woman who sought to starve sues hospital. (1986, January 22). *New York Times,* p. A12.

CHAPTER 55

Understanding the Political Process

Kathleen Carlson Mebus and Elizabeth Z. Cathcart

Many federal, state, and local laws and regulations have a direct impact on the ability of a home health agency to provide care. It is important that home health administrators develop an awareness of the many statutory and regulatory issues that affect their agencies. It is also important to develop positive relationships with political leaders at all levels of government and to be familiar with the legislative and regulatory processes. This chapter provides information about how to develop relationships with political leaders and an overview of the legislative and regulatory processes.

BUILDING RELATIONSHIPS

Health care delivery and the regulation of health care are changing rapidly and have become increasingly complex. Thus when a legislative crisis at local, state, or federal levels is imminent, action must be taken immediately to protect the ability of the health care providers to deliver services. There is no time to search out political allies when legislative or regulatory actions are pressing. Home health administrators therefore should develop active networks of support before crisis situations can evolve.

One of your first tasks as a newcomer to the state or to your agency's service area is to register to vote. If your state has mail registration, applications can be found in post offices and state agency buildings. If, however, you must register at the courthouse, take advantage of the opportunity to gather as much data as possible about your elected officials and the demographics of your voting district and the agency's service delivery area.

By networking with other community agencies, the administrator can ascertain whether a community is politically conservative or liberal in its posture toward health and social issues. This can be accomplished by meeting with local health and welfare councils or the Chamber of Commerce. Most chambers have regular meetings with local elected officials that vary from informal gatherings to formal meetings. Both groups have deep community roots and an astute awareness of the political and business climate.

Local politics form the base from which state and federal politics evolve. In some areas, you will find friendly political rivalries; in others, members of opposing parties will seldom be seen together at the same functions. At any function where elected officials are present, make every effort to be introduced by someone who is known to the elected official. This contact becomes a bridge for later communications with the officials.

The home health administrator should strive to develop a good relationship with at least one or two key political figures in the community. It is important to communicate with other officials periodically, however, because at some time you may need their help as well. Agency board members are an asset in identifying these key political players. They have usually been associated with many of these individuals through past community activities.

A representative of your agency should be present at major political fund raisers to create an awareness of the agency's interest in the community's political process. It is important that the agency be represented. If possible, find an individual who knows the candidate to represent you. At times, the person who represents the agency carries more weight. At the same time that the administrator is developing a working relationship with elected officials, liaisons should be forged with other agencies sharing similar concerns.

Local coordinating groups synthesize information from multiple sources. This coordination broadens the approach to resolving a problem affecting the delivery of services. Group information gathering is valuable in developing strategies and in coordinating materials to be shared with elected officials. Through memberships in national and state associations, the administrators can keep on top of issues affecting home health care at all levels.

As an administrator, you should be involved only with those legislative issues relevant to your organization. It is not effective to support or oppose every health care issue. Although legislative proposals frequently receive the most attention, changing regulations may have a greater impact on the day-to-day operation of your agency and should not be ignored.

LOCAL GOVERNMENT

The second step in the development of political and legislative awareness is to assess your county and local forms of government. By now you know their general political posture, but you also need to evaluate their positions regarding your primary interest: health care. For

example, when an agency serves more than one county, you might find a county with its own health department being reluctant to provide financial support to an outside visiting nurse association. On the other hand, another county may find it less costly to support community agencies delivering health care services and as a result may provide funding for specific programs.

Political subdivisions such as townships or wards are concerned about accessibility of public buildings by the handicapped, low-income housing, or transportation of the elderly. Whatever the subject, involvement with groups studying broader issues identifies the home health administrator as a citizen concerned for the total health of the community. All these issues bear a direct relationship to the problems faced by the clientele served by home health agencies.

Although health systems agencies are still intact in many communities, their degree of influence on health care delivery systems varies. Involvement with any local planning group, however, gives the agency director visibility in the health care community as well as an opportunity to be on the forefront of evolving changes within the health care delivery system. Some health care agencies have been leaders in identifying gaps in health care delivery as well as in providing leadership in solving the problem. At meetings such as these, the administrator collaborates not only with politically appointed individuals but also with influential citizens in the community. The major goal is to maximize your visibility as an agency administrator whose interest includes not only your own organization but also the general health of the community.

Increasingly, county officials are responsible for the direct provision of health care. Therefore, attendance at county commissioner meetings concerning special health care issues provides an opportunity for the administrator to present public testimony. A well-developed presentation with emphasis on the problem from the home health administrator's perspective has impact. You need to focus on the benefits or deficiencies of the plan under consideration rather than highlight the implications for your organization.

Another approach to increasing your visibility is to host or sponsor joint luncheons or affairs for county commissioners and state legislators. Although the emphasis may be national issues or state issues, the local impact of such meetings is of great importance. County officials frequently take advantage of this type of forum to raise pertinent questions on your behalf. Additionally, this is a good opportunity to provide legislators who sponsor health care proposals the opportunity to update the group. This reinforces the legislators' involvement in and support of health care issues. The legislator not only provides the public with information but also is viewed by colleagues as a knowledgeable resource on health care.

It should be apparent, however, after interacting with elected officials for a short time that your issues and their issues are seldom the same. The home health administrator needs to investigate an elected official's special concerns to develop a creative approach to gain attention. For example, if an elected official is concerned about a segment of the population, place emphasis on how proposed legislation will affect that group. By arranging to have your elected official accompany you on a home visit, you create a graphic impression of the legislation's impact.

How often your agency is asked to participate in county-appointed task forces or study groups is a gauge for evaluating your effectiveness in your community's political process. You will be one of the first invited if you have been accepted as a knowledgeable and politically astute individual in your field.

LEGISLATIVE PROCESS

All 50 states have an established process for creating laws. In Pennsylvania, the constitution of the state outlines the specific steps required to introduce, consider, and pass legislation. Each state has its own distinct system of checks and balances to protect the individual rights of its citizens. You can usually obtain pamphlets outlining your state's system from your elected state officials. Although it is not necessary to learn all the intricate maneuvers, it is important to understand the varying time elements involved in passing legislation.

In any given legislative session, more proposals are developed than any one person or special interest group can follow. Several thousand bills are introduced in the House of Representatives and Senate each year. These bills address many subject areas such as taxes, appropriations, licensing laws, access to health care, sunset of government agencies, insurance changes, and health care reform. When issues arise that affect your special interest, you should take time to communicate your views to your legislators. The background information you need about a particular piece of legislation can usually be obtained from a professional or trade association.

Your role in the legislative process as a member of a trade or professional organization is to follow through with association directives for legislative action. Your role as the director of an agency is to seek ways to protect or further your agency's interests. Occasionally, an association position does not exactly meet your agency's needs. When this situation occurs, contact your professional or trade association to make sure you understand its position. Associations frequently evaluate legislation based on the broadest application of a proposal to its entire membership. If, in your judgment, you cannot support the association's position, do not take any action unless the position specifically jeopardizes your agency. It is imperative that you work through your association, not your legislator, to resolve any differences.

It is helpful in communicating with your legislator to include the following: the bill number, the committee or subcommittee to which the bill has been assigned, your position, a rationale or supporting example, and a specific request for support or opposition.

The following is a list of essential items to include when you are writing a letter to a legislator:

- the proper address (frequently letters never reach their intended destination because of incorrect addresses)
- the proper salutation (although "The Honorable" is appropriate for the address, it is not appropriate within the letter. "Dear Senator/Representative/Assembly Representative" is correct)
- the bill numbers when referring to legislation
- a summary of what the bill proposes
- your position
- your rationale
- specific examples of how the legislation, regulations, or policies affect you and the delivery of client services in the legislator's district
- the action you wish the legislators to take
- clear, concise, and credible facts
- your address within the letter itself, not just on the envelope

Public hearings may be part of your state's process to give proposed legislation as much exposure as possible. Differences can be aired, and, as a result of the hearing, negotiated compromises may be achieved. Input at this stage is critical. If you have never testified before a legislative committee, it is advisable to learn the committee members' positions on the issue before the hearing. Legislators on opposing sides of an issue can become aggressive in their questioning, particularly when an audience is present. It is important to remember that the hearing's purpose is to address the issue, not the position of an individual legislator.

Even though your legislator may not serve on the committee considering the bill, his or her influence in caucus may strengthen your position. Thus, although initially communications should be with the legislators serving on the committee reviewing the bill, you should keep your own legislator apprised of your action. Personal visits to your legislator lend emphasis to a critical issue.

Once a bill has progressed to final passage and a vote is imminent, there is usually insufficient time for the U.S. Postal Service to deliver a letter. Facsimiles are appropriate for actions occurring during the next 48 hours. If an action is to occur within 24 hours, telephone contacts are of greater value.

It is appropriate to follow through after an action has occurred. A thank-you to officials who supported your position is always appreciated. If the legislator votes in opposition to your position, you have several options in your communication: Ask for the legislator's rationale, or agree to disagree, restating your position. This follow-up correspondence keeps the lines of communication open between you and the legislator. The goal is to maintain a working relationship with the official. Remember, all legislation is a compromise.

REGULATORY PROCESS

Most laws, once enacted, have implementation and enforcement provisions vested in a state authority. Rules and regulations are subsequently promulgated to outline how the government will implement the laws. State governments have various methods for proposing these rules. Some follow an orderly process; others have no specific requirements. In a few states regulations are merely guidelines, but in others they carry legal implications. You must determine what legal standing regulations have in your state. This determination could affect your next course of action. Whether you take further action or not, you need to understand the process required. Regulations may affect the delivery of home health services to a greater extent than the original law.

Frequently, the regulatory process provides for public input. If so, this is an excellent opportunity for you as a provider to influence the regulation of the health care delivery system. Once again, start with statewide organizations if you are affiliated with one that regularly follows legislative and regulatory activities. Significant groundwork and legal opinions may have already been obtained. If, on the other hand, you find that little or no work has been accomplished, volunteer to serve on a committee to address the regulatory issue, or offer to serve as a resource with expertise in the area being regulated. If public comments are requested, respond and send copies to your legislators. Also send copies of all correspondence to your national or state organizations to assist the associations in monitoring how much membership activity is taking place.

Perhaps you are not affiliated with an organization or your issue is not a priority for that organization. By networking with other organizations that share your concerns, a quality document can be produced in response to requests for public input. Although it is usually beneficial for each administrator to respond as an individual, there are also times when a group effort has greater impact.

The same strategy used by national and state associations can be applied by you as an individual. By contacting the government agency or the individual within the agency who is responsible for developing the regulations, you can express your interest in the development of the regulations, and you may be able to affect the early draft of the regulations. Some government agencies, however, prefer no outside involvement until an initial draft has been prepared, although written recommendations with a rationale may be appreciated. You should request a copy of the draft document if it is to be disseminated to special interest groups. When public input is sought, you should respond with documentation supporting your position.

POLITICAL ACTION

For educational purposes, it helps to consider political action separate from the legislative process. Political action is people oriented rather than issue oriented. Political action deals with the direct efforts of an individual or group to affect the outcome of an election to public office. Most often, political action efforts are translated into raising and expending financial contributions to run political campaigns. In addition to dollars, anything of value, such as personal services, a loan of property, or gifts of stationery, can be considered efforts to affect the outcome of an election. State laws vary concerning the amount of control they impose on campaign financing.

Because the purpose of political action is to affect the outcome of an election, before you make personal financial contributions you must carefully evaluate the potential consequences for you and your agency. As an agency administrator, you must be clear on both state and federal laws before becoming directly involved in any political activities, particularly because these activities are under close scrutiny for abuse and excessive influence. You as an individual are probably not restricted from engaging in political action, including making financial contributions to a candidate's campaign. Federal employees are regulated by the Hatch Act, and state employees may be restricted by specific state laws. At the federal level and in most states, campaign records are open to public scrutiny. As an administrator, you need to weigh carefully the value of having your name appear in these records.

The neophyte is advised to work through organized groups, such as political action committees (PACs) of state and national organizations. If you have worked with a legislator for longer than 6 months, you are in a position to evaluate how well that legislator responds to you and the issues affecting your agency. Your input can assist these PACs in their evaluations of candidates because PACs use information from many sources to determine who receives financial support or endorsement.

Involvement with a state or national PAC does not negate your opportunity to work with a specific legislator or elected official. If you are clearly identified in the community as an agency director and are personally active in party politics, however, then you should consider ways to identify yourself as a private citizen to offset any potential community backlash for your agency.

As a rule of thumb, PACs consider seniority, committee chairships, party position, committee membership, and financial need in determining whom to support. It follows, then, that the majority of financial contributions are given to incumbent candidates. Frequently, legislators who do not serve on health care committees or who do not hold party seniority are overlooked by small health-related PACs. Nevertheless, you can usually request a review of a particular legislator or candidate with accompanying documentation of how the individual supports your issues.

As a private citizen, you may also make an assessment of a candidate's commitment and make a personal contribution to the campaign fund. Agency donations are frequently restricted by state or federal campaign laws. In particular, a nonprofit agency's tax status would be jeopardized by direct political contributions.

General fund raisers for political parties provide an opportunity for the administrator to participate in political action without endorsing specific individuals. When attending political functions, make certain that the candidates know you are there. A follow-up letter commenting on the success of the event gives you yet another opportunity to point out your participation.

The objective of political action is to gain access to people rather than access to information as it is moving through the legislative and regulatory processes. There is, however, a natural flow between the processes.

CONCLUSION

Many federal, state, and local laws and regulations have a direct impact on the ability of a home health agency to provide care. Changes in any program that decrease the availability of state and local funding may be obscured by larger issues, but they can create serious service

delivery problems. An agency therefore needs many information resources to keep abreast of the constant changes.

Sometimes issues being considered are so crucial that the staff and board members of an agency should take the initiative to contact their legislators. To assist these individuals, who are not involved in government issues on a day-to-day basis, it might be necessary to circulate a legislative fact sheet stating the problem, the alternative, and the expected outcomes. Agency directors should understand lobbying restrictions placed on tax-exempt organizations before they embark on any assertive campaign.

Although it should be obvious that there are many nuances in dealing with the players in the legislative-regulatory arena, the final impact is related to your ability to communicate. Individual letters are far more effective in influencing lawmakers than petitions or form letters. At key times, telephone contacts are even more effective. Whatever the mode of communication, it should be clear, concise, and credible. There should be no doubt about your position on the issue. When it is necessary to communicate with federal legislators, the same communication techniques are appropriate; you should send a copy to your state officials, however. This creates the potential to generate a chain of support for your position. As you get more involved in the process, information sharing between you and your elected official should be mutual.

The best communication tool for all citizens and yet the most frequently ignored one is the power of the individual vote. Voting is your final evaluation of the overall effectiveness of an elected official in responding to you as a concerned citizen with a special interest. Although you cannot expect an elected official to support your position 100% of the time, nevertheless you have the right to expect a knowledgeable response to your inquiries as well as the official's rationale for his or her vote.

Home health administrators have known for years how to generate community support. Because communications and networking are common activities for any agency director, it is not difficult to expand this activity to include the politicians and key elected officials in your community. Be aware that they, too, have a role to play in the future of your organization.

PART VIII

Strategic Planning/Marketing/Survival Issues

CHAPTER 56

Strategic Planning

Edward R. Balotsky and David B. Smith

INTRODUCTION

Strategic planning is difficult, rewarding, and essential for organizations. It shapes the way an organization changes so that it can better accomplish its goals and more effectively adapt to environmental pressures. Organizational change is inevitable, but even the most effective strategic planning may not always control the way an organization changes. Successful home health agencies, so dependent on third-party payment regulations and referrals from potential competitors, are like the champion downhill skier, a little out of control.

> The Men's Downhill races in the 1976 Winter Olympics changed the strategies of racers. Franz Klammer seemed "out of control" for the entire run. Yet, he won the Olympic Gold Medal. Up until Klammer's run the prevailing thinking among downhill racers was that the winner of a race would be the one who was in the best condition, had the best technique, and skied just this side of the edge of losing control. The thinking changed. To win one now had to ski on the other side of the edge of losing control. In 1976 Klammer was the only one (of truly world class skiers) who skied out of control. Since every

other top skier was trying to ski just short of losing control and since Klammer was lucky, he won easily. Now all the top skiers, perhaps fifteen or twenty, are skiing out of control and on any given day it is largely natural selection stemming from factors beyond the skiers' control which determines who wins. During any run there are many blind variations in the form of ruts, bumps, mistakes and so forth, which are beyond the control of the skiers at the speed they are now going. The skier who skis most out of control and is luckiest in avoiding falling will win. Since there are so many good skiers skiing out of control the odds are excellent that one of them will always take enough risks and manage enough miraculous recoveries to beat the under-control skier (McKelvey, 1982, p. 447–448).

The top skiers made a strategic choice: They chose to go for the gold rather than the less risky strategy of good, average performance. Organizations can make risky strategic choices that aim for market dominance or more conservative ones that aim for average performance. The rapid technological, regulatory, and competitive changes in the home health care market, however, make almost any strategy a risky one.

Strategic planning helps make those choices and controls their implementation.

No matter what choices are made, successful strategic planning must move at the speed of the winning downhill skier. Such planning is not a special set of procedures, a committee structure, a set of statistical projection techniques, or a document that can be produced by a consultant for the right price. It involves an understanding of how organizations change and the use of that knowledge to shape changes in an organization that will, as much as possible, ensure its success. The first section describes how organizations change; the second, how strategic planning can help shape those changes; the third, how to develop strategic planning capacity; and the final section, pitfalls to avoid in the strategic planning process.

HOW ORGANIZATIONS CHANGE

Organizations resist change. It is stressful and disruptive. Figure 56–1 summarizes the process by which changes take place in organizations. An organization must adapt effectively to its environment to succeed. When it fails to achieve at least the minimum performance needed for survival, it looks for ways to turn things around. Change involves risk. The larger the change, the greater the cost and disruption and, consequently, the greater the risk. As a result, most organizations attempt to turn things around by making modest adjustments that involve incremental change for the organization. If modest changes fail, an organization searches for more drastic solutions. That search will progress through four distinct phases.

Phase I—Manipulation of the Environment

Organizations invest effort in getting others to change rather than changing themselves. One tries to change the reimbursement policies, influence the granting of certificates of need to restrict competition or change consumer patterns of utilization. If such efforts are successful, the organization does not have to change at all. Home health agencies and the associations that represent them fight such battles.

The proliferation of health care marketing reflects this concern with reshaping the environment. Many organizations equate a marketing focus with an advertising campaign designed to increase market share; their scarce resources would be better spent in changing their organizational structure or tailoring the mix of services provided to rapidly respond to market demands. As suggested in Chapter 57, successful marketing is not an isolated activity; rather, it is an integral part of the more extensive process of strategic planning and organizational change.

Most providers of health services have recognized the limits of environmental manipulation. The acute care hospital experience with the shift from retrospective to prospective payment is well documented, particularly the drastic reduction in average length of stay (ALOS) and total admissions, and the increase in case mix index. In dealing with these changes, hospitals have resorted to drastic solutions that have directly affected the character and structure of their own organizations.

The result of environmental manipulation need not be negative, however. Home health care is uniquely positioned to be a "winner" in the prospective payment wars. The growth of managed care has reversed home care's traditional role as a residual set of services provided only after other institutional interventions to one that is in the forefront of market-driven reform (Benjamin, 1993). The result has been a dramatic increase in the utilization of home care programs as providers reacted to reduced revenues by shuffling patients through less intensive treatment regimes. Between 1980 and 1993, Medicare home care visits increased from 22,428 to 184,397 and expenditures climbed by 175%. Between 1993 and 2000, total home care spending is predicted to rise by 400% (Lumsdon, 1994a). The environment for home care providers is expected to be far from tranquil, however, as consolidation among providers, regulatory changes, the continued evolution of

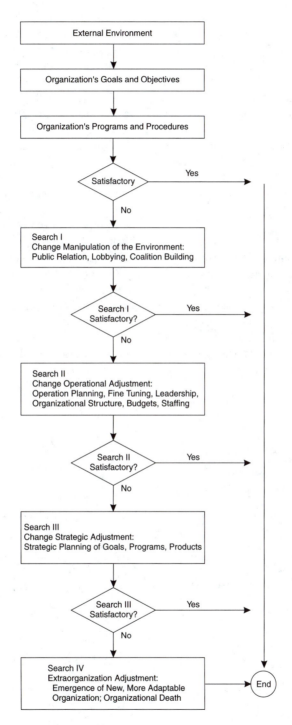

Figure 56–1 Organizational Response to Problems in the Environment. *Source*: Used with permission from *The White Labyrinth: A Guide to the Health Care System, Second Edition*, by David Barton Smith and Arnold D. Kaluzny. (Chicago: Health Administration Press, 1986).

managed care toward true capitation, the development of outcomes-based performance standards, and the rise of disease management programs will challenge industry participants (Leavenworth, 1995; Shriver, 1996). Some experts predict a health care system that is organized around home health and primary care instead of acute inpatient care (Shortell et al., 1996). The home health care "winners" will be those organizations that proactively influence these key environmental stakeholders and trends.

Phase II—Operational Adjustment

If environmental manipulation fails to ensure adequate performance, then an organization will attempt to address the immediate operational issues. Revenue shortfalls produce staff and budget reductions. The administrator may be fired and new leadership brought in to help turn things around. In some cases, this is a poor substitute for more fundamental changes that are needed. Operational adjustments can improve efficiency and quality of services. Such efforts absorb most of the time of management. Yet, no matter how well performed, these activities alone will not ensure success, or even survival.

The home health care sector is not static. As indicated in Figure 56–2, products or services have a life cycle. It is perhaps most useful to think of home care as a market rather than as a discrete product. That market existed long before the emergence of the modern hospital around 1920 (Starr, 1982) and will continue regardless of hospital structural changes. Home care products and services, however, have changed dramatically. Some, such as the remote monitoring of vital signs, are in the early embryonic and growth stages. Others, such as managed care systems (capitation case management, preferred provider organizations, and health maintenance organizations [HMOs]), have entered the more competitive growth and shake out stages of the life cycle. Other products, such as the more familiar packaged array

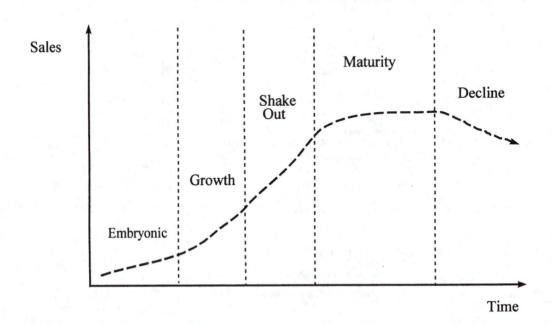

Figure 56–2 The Product Life Cycle

of fee-for-service home health services, have reached maturity, where growth in net income is restrained both by competition and restriction of third-party payment. Home care organizations must continually scan the environment, as major change in an environmental variable can decrease, accelerate, or reverse a product's position on the life cycle. The more traditional private duty nursing services that were in the decline stage of the life cycle, for example, have gained a significant life extension through the shift in Medicare payment toward subacute care. Third-party payment, technological and regulatory changes, and access to capital will continue to affect both the actual home health care products delivered and the organizations that provide them.

Fragmentation has been a characteristic of the approximately 15,000 home care agencies and hospices that deliver services across a range of free-standing and facility-based structures, but consolidation activities have begun (Lumsdon, 1994a). Hospital-based home care programs, for example, grew from 610 in 1980 to 1,801 in 1990, an increase of 200% (Cerne, 1993). Presently, 35% of U.S. hospitals offer a home care product, but the growth curve of hospital-based programs has flattened as regulation, limited reimbursement, and alternative providers have entered the market (Burns, 1994). Not surprisingly, managed care organizations are shaping the structure of home care delivery. Case management groups, such as the National Preferred Provider Network (NPPN), are developing home care networks in response to increases in home care costs (Marshall, 1996). Size is now a crucial barometer of home care success. These networks are contracting with home care providers capable of servicing large, defined geographic markets with a broad line of product diversification. The selected providers are expected to offer the benefits of economy of scale and clout in negotiating with suppliers, as well as the willingness to share any cost reductions with their clients (Burns, 1995; McNamee & Schiller, 1994; Snyder, 1995). In response, free-standing home care agencies are

using horizontal and vertical networking of all types, including home care HMOs, in an attempt to provide what has become "one-stop shopping" for everything outside the acute care setting (Lumsdon, 1994b). Revenues for home care chains, once the smallest component of the industry, grew 47% to $5.1 billion dollars in 1993 (Scott, 1994). Sixty-three mergers of home care providers occurred in 1995, a 14.5% increase from the 55 mergers in 1994 (Lutz, 1995). Insurance companies are pursuing similar strategies, including the development of internal case management, as a method to control home care expenditures (Koco, 1994). Concentrating on efficiency and quality alone, then, may not stave off the erosion of the traditional home health agency's share of health care expenditures in the face of these emerging vertically integrated hospital systems of community care, or HMOs and other emerging permutations of insurance and service organizations.

Phase III—Strategic Adjustment

A strategic adjustment involves changing goals, programs, and products to better respond to regulatory or market pressures and to adopt new products in the introduction and growth phase of their life cycle. This is not an easy thing for organizations, particularly when staff have strong professional identities. Yet the capacity to engage effectively in such adjustments will determine the ability of an organization to survive. Working effectively at this level and changing products and services to adapt to shifts in regulatory or market pressures is the acid test of effective strategic management.

It is often useful to think of products as separate and distinct from the medical specialty or allied health occupational group services that form the traditional building blocks of health services organizations. The product line management approach attempts to identify a single center of accountability for financial and quality of care issues. This is a logical extension of the matrix-type organizational structure illustrated in Figure 56–3. The traditional approach is to

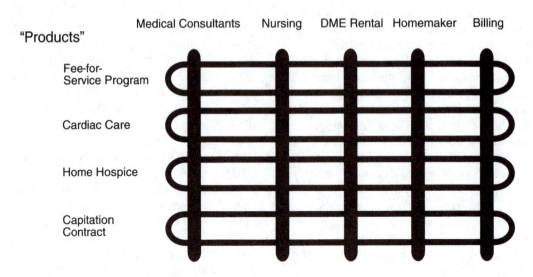

Figure 56–3 Examples of Home Care Product Management

divide an organization into major specialty areas. In Figure 56–3, these areas are the vertical columns (nursing, billing, etc.). The products are the horizontal rows. This particular hypothetical home care agency or company has defined four products: a home hospice service, a conventional fee-for-service program, a highly specialized posthospitalization cardiac care program, and a special capitation subcontract with an HMO. While there is a good deal of overlap in the kinds of services offered by each of these products (medical consultants, nursing, durable medical equipment rental, etc.), it is often advantageous, particularly in a competitive environment, to manage them separately. That is, organize the home care agency by rows (products) rather than columns. This may lead to better cost and quality control as well as more responsiveness to the needs and demands of a special segment of the market.

Defining the products of a home care program may seem like belaboring the obvious. Sometimes, however, it's not that obvious. Products may be defined by geographical boundaries, third-party markets, or medical spe-

cialty. There are also three basic additional ways health care products or services can be redefined, as illustrated in Figure 56–4. First, the time commitment during an illness episode can be either narrowed or widened. One can focus on a narrow time during posthospitalization or view the service or product as one involving a more extensive time commitment. The latter would imply a commitment to serving the chronically ill and providing long-term maintenance and rehabilitative services. Sec-

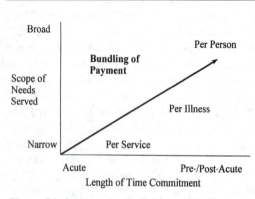

Figure 56–4 Alternative Definitions of Product

ond, the nature of the services can either be restricted to more narrow technical services or expanded to include broader social-psychological support services. The broader definition of the product, for example, might involve the development of social and recreational services. Conversely, the more narrow definition might simply include rental of specific pieces of durable medical equipment.

The relative attractiveness of these alternatives, however, depends on how specific services are bundled for payment. Arrangements for payment can be negotiated with third parties or the client for each specific service rendered, either by illness episode or admission (a DRG-type payment system) or by the person covered (HMO). The bundling of services for payment, of course, defines the time commitment and breadth of services that will be provided. The movement from a fee-for-service payment system to ones where third parties shift risk onto providers has required a fundamental change in orientation. A strong financial position for a provider is facilitated under such payment arrangements not by providing a high volume of relatively costly and complex services, but by reducing the volume of costly services and substituting less costly treatments. Health care providers are scrambling to adjust to the shift in bundling of acute care services into payments for illness episodes and bundling based on capitation arrangements. The ripple effect of these shifts in financing has forced fundamental redefinitions of most health services products as well as the organizational structures and relationships in which services are delivered. A positive outcome for home care providers has been the recognition of home care services as a competitive necessity in the prospective payment environment (O'Donnell, 1993) because the home setting is attractive to managed care payers as a less costly alternative to institutionalized care. Many home care organizations are meeting this challenge/opportunity by restructuring to offer a full line of home care products rather than single service offerings such as

home infusion or nursing care services (Lumsdon, 1994a).

Phase IV—Extraorganizational Adjustment

If none of these searches is effective, an organization either dies or is transformed into a completely different entity. The hospital industry is a prime example of both outcomes. Between 1983, the inaugural year of the Medicare prospective payment system (PPS), and 1991, 505 U.S. acute care hospitals closed (Burda, 1992). Many others have merged or been absorbed into organizations that can more effectively control external pressures. In 1993, the American Hospital Association identified 18 mergers (Lutz, 1994). In the two following years, 20% of the nation's community hospitals changed ownership, with mergers escalating to 674 in 1994 and 735 in 1995 (Lutz, 1995). This merger frenzy is expected to continue (Greene, 1996). The latter part of the 1990s is witnessing the beginning of a variety of hybrid multi-institutional, multiservice, community-based health care structures that are acquiring providers at an accelerating rate in order to develop regional integrated delivery systems (IDS) (Coile, 1995).

From Vertical to Virtual Integration

Most IDSs construct their systems through horizontal and vertical integration. This is the traditional strategy that equates the accumulation and ownership of capital, labor, and equipment with competitive advantage. However, with the emergence of global competition, and the resultant downsizing, reengineering, and reduced organizational slack, many organizations do not have sufficient capital to invest in new technology, products, or markets (Welles, 1995). At the same time, knowledge has become more important than labor and is more accessible via information technology. In this environment, few assets remain such for long. Businesses have responded by outsourcing functions previously performed in-house. In the process, vertical integration is rapidly being supplemented by a new paradigm, "virtual integration."

Virtual integration is a temporary network of independent organizations linked by information technology to share knowledge, skills, costs, and access to each other's markets (Byrne, Brandt, & Port, 1993). Participants contribute their core competencies in a combination of talents that allows the rapid exploitation of a specific opportunity. A virtually integrated structure is a strategic collaboration in which common ownership of assets is replaced by contractual arrangements (Goldsmith, 1995). The main advantage of this approach is the ability to efficiently harness separately existing resources without the capital requirements associated with in-house production of all services. The major drawback of virtual integration is the loss of control that occurs without a central entity that can force compliance among multiple organizational structures (Clark, 1995). Thus, the decision facing managers is the trade-off between the financial incentives for virtual integration versus the control possible in the vertically integrated organization. The result has been a continuum of integration in which few organizations outsource all functions. Rather, a middle ground is taken in which functions essential to unique competencies are produced internally, while less essential needs are acquired from the marketplace (Chesbrough &Teece, 1996).

Health care ventures have been no exception to this overall pattern. The newest health care organizations involve institutional providers, physicians, and payers that have linked in various organizational structures in response to managed care pressures. For example, the terms "virtual hospital" and "hospital without walls" have been used to describe coordinated health care services provided outside their traditional structures (Pallarito, 1996). The appeal of these virtual structures is simple: vertical integration in health care has proven to be expensive and very cumbersome to manage. Some describe health care's experience with vertical integra-

tion as a "costly mistake" (Goldsmith, 1994), citing the obsolescence of assets acquired by such integration as not creating the best value for health care buyers.

The virtual network model of the future may already be operating. In California, individual physicians are creating linkages through membership in giant medical groups and independent practice associations (IPAs). These evolving structures control access to extremely large blocks of patients, giving these groups real market power in negotiating capitation rates with managed care organizations. There is IDS or hospital ownership in some cases, but the majority of the medical groups and IPAs remain independent, using short-term contracts as the dominant method of maintaining an optimal provider network. As a result, hospitals and other health providers have been forced into the role of "price-taking subcontractors in the managed care food chain" (Robinson & Casalino, 1996, p. 16).

The California experience bodes well for the home health care organization. The de-emphasis of hospital-based care under full-risk capitation is well documented, as is the positive impact on home health utilization. Managed care has matured into a product line that has shifted from a hospital to a home-based focus point (Goldsmith, Goran, & Nackel, 1995). For the home care provider, the value-added argument for contracting with dominant managed care groups is compelling: these groups provide access to larger patient blocks than is possible for the unaffiliated home health agency, and providers can do so in an efficient, economical manner while maintaining the autonomy of the agency (Robinson, 1996). Given this environment, home health care organizations have become attractive partners for these emerging virtually integrated networks of providers. Home health agencies, however, must create virtual organizations of their own that can provide unified packages of cost-effective services across broad geographic areas that include the entire market areas of managed care plans.

HOW STRATEGIC PLANNING SHAPES CHANGE IN ORGANIZATIONS

Effective strategic planning radically alters the natural process of organizational change. Its focus is on change rather than the maintenance of the status quo, viewing the stages of organizational change not as places to go only in desperation, but as inevitable steps in an ongoing process of organizational development. Strategic planning transforms what is essentially a passive, often unconscious, reactive mechanism of organizational change into a self-conscious, proactive, future-oriented process. At each stage in the process of organizational change outlined in Figure 56–1, effective strategic planning anticipates the questions, develops answers, and makes choices. Those choices are based on an assessment of the external environment, a refined sense of the mission and goals of the organization, and a knowledge of the key issues in each of the four phases of organizational development.

Assessment of the External Environment

The strategic process is the search for the optimal fit between the internal strengths of an organization and external opportunities, while solving external threats and internal weaknesses. Intelligence is critical to the strategy process. What do we know and what do we need to know to position ourselves strategically? What trends in payment and regulation of the health care industry will affect home health care services? What changes in the population and economics will shape demand for home health services? The population of those over 75 is growing rapidly, and the relative wealth of this population segment appears to be growing. Household size is decreasing as well. Also, the popularity of mass-market, homogeneous products appears to be waning, as consumers are seeking more alternative product choices. For home health services, these trends represent distinct opportunities for attracting new market share.

Everyone remotely involved in the health sector is engaged in environmental assessment. Porter (1991) believes that intensity of rivalry within an industry must be an organization's first priority and lists five key factors that environmental assessments should consider:

1. The potential of an attractive and growing market invites greater competition.
2. One needs to know what new entrants to the market are likely, and what position existing competitors are likely to take.
3. There is also the threat of potential substitute products or services that will affect the competitive environment; for example, the growth and development of hospice programs, subacute care units in hospitals, life care communities, HMOs, and the return of the physician or nonphysician practitioner home visit can all affect home health care service demand.
4. Greater competition will in turn increase the bargaining power of customers.
5. Greater competition will also increase bargaining power of suppliers, who in the home health market are largely composed of the staffing resources necessary for the actual provision of care.

Wheelen and Hunger (1995) add a sixth issue to the mix: the level of stakeholder power in a market. The market share of managed care organizations, the state-level regulatory climate, and business coalition activity will all affect the strategic choices that a home care organization can consider. The importance of the environmental assessment cannot be overstated, as the future viability of the home care provider will depend upon the accuracy of this analysis.

Clarifying Goals and Objectives

Goals and objectives have to represent a good deal more than financial ratios and utilization and budget projections. There is a fine line between organizational autism, which ignores the environment, and organizational emptiness, which ignores any internal vision and is preoccupied with short-run market demand. Either extreme will destroy the organization. Strategic planning involves a wide scope of vision and a long-term perspective. One needs to articulate the special vision of the organization that helps to impose order upon the chaotic signals of the environment. It also helps to give a sense of cohesiveness and common purpose to those involved in ensuring the success of the organization.

Identifying Strategy in Each Phase of Organizational Change

At each phase of organizational change the question becomes not what action can alleviate the immediate problem, but what can be done to ensure the overall effectiveness of the organization's strategy in achieving its vision. Questions such as the following need to be asked and answered.

> **Phase I,** Environmental Manipulation: How can the market be shaped and the regulatory climate influenced to better assure organizational success?

> **Phase II,** Operational Adjustment: What changes to current activities can be made to improve the organization's strategic position?

> **Phase III,** Strategic Adjustment: What choices are available in new goals, products? On the basis of internal experience, what are the organization's core competencies, and are these competencies being utilized to the best competitive advantage of the organization?

> **Phase IV,** Extraorganizational Adjustment: What new organizational forms are possible? Which forms should be pursued? Should the organization compete with others or form coalitions?

Answers to such questions form the framework for the strategic plans of an organization,

linking immediate operational issues to efforts for the active creation of a future for the organization. The ultimate consideration for the home care organization is the development of a structure that will build and maintain the distinctive competencies of the organization.

STEPS IN DEVELOPING STRATEGIC PLANNING CAPACITY

There are many detailed outlines of the specific actions and steps involved in an overall strategic planning process (Ackoff, 1981; Day, 1986; Lorange, 1993; Nutt, 1984; Perry, Stott, & Smallwood, 1993; Weber & Peters, 1983; Wheelen & Hunger, 1995). Others have concentrated on health care as an unique industry (Duncan, Ginter, & Swayne, 1992; Harris, 1994; Hay, 1990; Koeppen, Mess, & Trott, 1995; Moldof, 1994; Shortell, Morrison, & Friedman, 1990; Stevens, 1991) or have supplied case studies of strategic planning in health care that help put flesh on the abstractions (Johnson, 1991; McKnight et al., 1991; Reeves, 1983; Shortell, Gillies, Anderson, Erickson, & Mitchel, 1996; Suver, Kahn, & Clement, 1984). In simplest terms, however, the strategic planning process can be reduced to four critical steps.

Commit the Resources To Do It Right

Strategic planning is least likely to be done by those who need it the most. Administrators faced with rapid change in their environment as well as increasing competition have difficulty stepping back from the immediate day-to-day crises they face. The result has been the use of in-house planning staffs or consultants external to the organization to dictate strategic direction to those individuals most responsible for the success or failure of the planning process. Although these groups can play a key role in facilitating the planning process, the most critical resource that has to be committed is the time of key decision makers within an organization. Initially, several full days may be needed to clarify and reach agreement on the process, as well as follow-up sessions necessary to help reinforce and further clarify the process. If effective, this strategic planning format becomes embedded in the decision-making routines of the organization and is no longer perceived by executives as "something else I have to find time for." There is also a need either to build the internal staff support or to contract out for the development of the information base to "feed" the strategic planning process. The level of effort and cost of these information-gathering activities will depend on the size and complexity of the organization, the size and complexity of the market and regulatory environment with which the organization must deal, and the level of detail and degree of certainty that the managers involved determine are necessary to make strategic decisions. Just as with the time commitments of top managers, the initial cost will be relatively high; however, as such information gathering gets built into the daily operations of the organization, these maintenance costs will decline.

Pick the Right Participants

Strategic planning must be done by the key decision makers in an organization. It is not something, such as a certificate of need application or a required long-range planning document, that can be delegated to either a staff person or a consultant. The top managers in an organization are responsible not only for strategy formulation but also for making the strategy work. It is thus the responsibility of the chief executive officer to pick the individuals that will be involved in the strategic planning process. These individuals need to have a working knowledge of the organization and the intellectual ability to think strategically, rather than parochially or defensively, about their own special concerns. The basic work group should include no fewer than 3 and no more than 12 individuals. It need not include all those that hold the key formal organization positions on the

board, medical staff, and administration, but should be designed to ensure, as much as possible, the support of all those groups needed to implement whatever strategic plans are developed.

Provide an Effective Link between Operational and Strategic Planning

Strategic planning operates in the gray area between the broad ends espoused in the organization's mission statement and the overall direction and the specific means incorporated in the operational plans of department heads and middle managers. Those operational plans include operating budgets, staffing, construction and capital equipment, and program and marketing plans. The strategic document needs to be translated into operational plans. This conversion requires the bottom-up participation of those responsible for these operational areas in the creation, implementation, and evaluation of strategy efforts.

Strategic plans that emerge insulated from any understanding of operational difficulties are doomed to failure. The strategic planning process for several for-profit hospital chains in the 1980s, for example, developed the concept of incorporating an in-house HMO into the product mix. Strategically, it was brilliant. Operationally, it almost proved disastrous because of the failure to consider the potential competitive impact upon the existing base of admitting physicians. Eventually, these chains were forced to divest their HMO products in order to maintain the good graces of their physician stakeholders. Similar anecdotes of the gaps between strategy and operations abound, illustrating the need for a regular dialogue between operational and strategic planning.

An effective dialogue between strategic and operational planning can take place through well-designed joint operational and strategic planning sessions. These sessions can also be built into the day-to-day review and consultation process between top and operational managers. The goal is to provide the opportunity for operational managers to shape strategies as well as their implementation.

Develop an Orderly Process for Accomplishing the Tasks

There are many ways that the essential tasks of strategic planning can be accomplished. The method used is not critical; what is important is that the process is well understood by and acceptable to the key participants and proceeds in an orderly manner. The opportunity for more open-ended, chaotic brainstorming and free association should not be excluded but must take place within a formal structure so that the ideas can be subjected to critical appraisal and put to work. Regardless of the method employed, the following steps should be included in the strategic planning process:

Step 1: Assess current situation. Collect information and evaluate the organization's present strategic position. Assess potential future opportunities and threats.

Step 2: Revise objectives. Set new objectives based upon the assessment in Step 1.

Step 3: Generate and evaluate strategy alternatives. Explore alternatives in all four phases of organizational change in light of their potential to achieve the desired objectives.

Step 4: Select the best strategies. Within the four phases of organizational change, make choices. The choices should have the benefit of review by operational managers as well as the support of the governing body.

Step 5: Develop detailed plans for the selected strategies. Provide opportunities for input from operational managers or, if this is a new venture for the organization, from outside consultants.

Step 6: Implement the plans. Delegate responsibility to a manager and those involved in each plan's operation.

Step 7: Monitor performance. Timing is important. Regularly review to determine whether the strategies are accomplishing their intended objectives. Make midcourse corrections as necessary.

Step 8: Update the organization's situation, using this information as input for the next regularly scheduled strategic planning cycle.

PITFALLS TO AVOID IN THE STRATEGIC PLANNING PROCESS

The strategic planning process requires no small investment of an organization's scarce material, time, and human resources. The end product, the planning document, represents a competitive advantage that can be an invaluable blueprint for guiding an organization toward the accomplishment of its goals. Yet, many well-developed, appropriate strategic plans are never implemented. The reasons why the planning process fails have been thoroughly discussed in the literature (Birnbaum, 1990; Clark & Boissoneau, 1995; Robert, 1991; Whelan & Sisson, 1993) but can be summarized as four pitfalls that, if not avoided, virtually doom any planning activities.

The Strategy Rests in the Mind of the CEO

The best strategic plan is worthless if it exists primarily in the mind of the CEO. Successful planning must be characterized by frequent, bilateral communication among the key organizational members charged with the implementation of the plan. Too many CEOs fail to take their vision from the implicit to the explicit level or develop strategy without input from other important players. Equally important, strategy must be viewed as an internally generated product, not just the recommendations of an outside consultant. A strategic plan developed in isolation will result in an underutilized and misunderstood document that may hinder rather than support the organizational mission.

The Strategic Plan Is Not Complete

Sound strategic planning must consider all pertinent issues affecting an organization's outcomes. The value of including all personnel involved with plan implementation now becomes more obvious; a broad set of opinions should facilitate the identification and consideration of potential results that may occur after strategies are operational. Information-gathering efforts should provide supporting documentation in this evaluation process. It is impossible to anticipate every contingency, but the validity of any planning activity is directly linked to the thoroughness of the endeavor.

The Planning Process Is Biased

Many strategic plans are predisposed to failure because of an organization's internal environment. Strategic potential may never be realized due to premature budgeting that establishes operating budgets prior to strategy decisions. The political climate within the organization must be controlled so that power struggles, the ability to take risks, and the tendency for people to avoid change do not circumvent the implementation effort. Employee reward systems, either financial or personal, should be linked to the process. In short, an internal environment not geared toward meaningful strategic planning will hinder a successful outcome.

Strategic Plans Are Not Monitored

Follow-up is crucial to the strategic planning process. Too many strategies are initiated but never evaluated until the next formal planning period. As a result, planning becomes meaningless to organizational members because there is no feedback or concern shown regarding the value or success of the plan, nor are modifications made to bring unsuccessful activities into line. To maximize the impact of the planning process, strategies must be monitored regularly during the lifetime of each planning period.

CONCLUSION

This brief summary may suggest that the process of strategic planning is easy and obvious. It is neither. Some readers may conclude that they are already doing it. That is probably correct. The key question is not whether organizations should do strategic planning, but how well it is done and whether the process can be improved. Many tools and techniques can be applied to strategic planning. There is no end to the information that could be collected, analyzed, and utilized in such a process. What improves the process in one setting may be ineffective in another. Strategic planning is a process for bringing about organizational change and growth. Like the process of individual change and growth, it is very personal and individualized: you learn by doing it. Organizations that have the most successful strategic planning are motivated to engage in it not so much by grim survival pressures but by the uniquely human drive to grow, and to become all that they are capable of becoming. This motivation is particularly evident in health care organizations, which have social responsibilities that may be stronger than mere survival goals (Liedtka, 1992). To paraphrase Rene Dubois's conclusion in his classic work *Mirage of Health*,

> The earth has never been a Garden of Eden but a Valley of Decision where resilience is essential to survival . . . To grow in the midst of dangers is the fate of the human race, because it is the law of the spirit. (Dubois, 1959, 281–282).

BIBLIOGRAPHY

Ackoff, R. (1981). *Creating the corporate future.* New York: J. Wiley and Sons.

Anderson, H. (1992). Hospital-based home care poised for growth in 1990s. *Hospitals, 66:* 60–62.

Benjamin, A. (1993). An historical perspective on home care policy. *The Milbank Quarterly, 71*, 129–166.

Birnbaum, W. (1990). *If your strategy is so terrific, how come it doesn't work?* New York: American Management Association.

Bommer, M., & DeLaPorte, R. (1992). A context for envisioning the future. *National Productivity Review, 11*, 549–552.

Burda, D. (1992). Hospital closings drop for third straight year. *Modern Healthcare, 22*, 2.

Burns, J. (1994). Homeward bound. *Modern Healthcare, 24*, 35–38.

Burns, J. (1995). More consolidation on the home front. *Modern Healthcare, 25*, 86–90.

Byrne, J., Brandt, R., & Port, O. (1993). The virtual corporation. *Business Week, 3304*, 98–102.

Cerne, F. (1993). Homeward bound: hospitals see solid future for home health care. *Hospitals, 67*, 52–54.

Chesbrough, H., & Teece, D. (1996). When is virtual virtuous? Organizing for innovation. *Harvard Business Review, 74*, 65–73.

Chesney, J. (1990). Utilization trends before and after PPS. *Inquiry, 27*, 376–381.

Chesney, J., & Long, M. (1986, June). *Medicare case-mix complexity and product change: what has happened since prospective payment.* Paper presented at the meeting of the Association for Health Services Research. Boston.

Clark, B., & Boissoneau, R. (1995). Strategic planning and the health care supervisor. *Health Care Supervisor, 14*, 1–10.

Clark, C. (1995). Planning along the continuum of care. *Healthcare Financial Management, 49*, 20–24.

Cleverley, W. (1991). Large urban hospitals increasingly on closed list. *Healthcare Financial Management, 45*, 77–78.

Coile, R. (1995). Assessing healthcare market trends and capital needs: 1996–2000. *Healthcare Financial Management, 49*, 60–65.

Das, T. (1991). Time: The hidden dimension in strategic planning. *Long Range Planning, 24*, 49–57.

Day, G. (1986). *Analysis of strategic market decisions.* New York: West Publishing Company.

Dubois, R. (1959). *Mirage of health.* New York: Harper and Row.

Duncan, W., Ginter, P., & Swayne, L. (1992). *Strategic management of health care organizations.* Boston: PWS-Kent Publishing Company.

Farley, D., & Rosekamp, J. (1986, June). *Changing patterns of occupancy, length of stay and admissions.* Paper presented at the meeting of the Association for Health Services Research. Boston.

Frieden, J. (1992). Growing home health care market is a boon for employers. *Business & Health, 10*, 29–35.

Gilbert, R., & Coyne, J. (1987). Should hospitals rush to diversify? *Healthcare Financial Management, 41*, 91–92.

Goldsmith, J. (1994). The illusive logic of integration. *Healthcare Forum, 37*, 26–31.

Goldsmith, J. (1995). It's time for virtual integration. *Hospitals & Health Networks, 69*, 11.

Goldsmith, J., Goran, M., & Nackel, J. (1995). Managed care comes of age. *Healthcare Forum, 38*, 14–24.

Greene, J. (1996). System size, breadth will continue to grow. *Modern Healthcare, 26*, 39.

Harris, J. (1994). *Strategic Health Management.* San Francisco: Jossey-Bass.

Hax, A., & Majluf, N. (1991). *The strategy concept & process: A pragmatic approach.* Englewood Cliffs, NJ: Prentice Hall.

Hay, R. (1990). *Strategic management in non-profit organizations.* New York: Quorum Books.

Hospital prognosis deteriorates. (1992, 20 August). *Standard & Poor's Industry Surveys: Health Care:* H15–H36.

Hospital Statistics. (1984). Chicago: American Hospital Association.

Hospital Statistics. (1992). Chicago: American Hospital Association.

Johnson, D. (1991). Planning high on agenda. *Health Care Strategic Management, 9*, 9–13.

Koco, L. (1994). AMEX brings managed care to LTC. *National Underwriter, Life & Health, 98*, 37, 50.

Koeppen, L., Mess, M., & Trott, K. (1995). Effective planning for managed care. *Healthcare Financial Management, 49*, 44–47.

Leavenworth, G. (1995). Trends in home health care. *Business & Health, 13*, 55.

Liedtka, J. (1992). Formulating hospital strategy: Moving beyond a market mentality. *Health Care Management Review, 17*, 21–26.

Lorange, P. (1993). *Strategic planning and control: Issues in the strategy process.* Cambridge, MA: Blackwell Publishers.

Lumsdon, K. (1994a). No place like home. *Hospitals & Health Networks, 68*, 44–52.

Lumsdon, K. (1994b). Home care prepares to catch wave of managed care networking. *Hospitals & Health Networks, 68*, 58.

Lutz, S. (1990). Hospitals reassess home-care ventures. *Modern Healthcare, 20*, 23–30.

Lutz, S. (1994). Let's make a deal. *Modern Healthcare, 24*, 46–52.

Lutz, S. (1995). 1995: A record year for hospital deals. *Modern Healthcare, 25*, 43–52.

Marshall, J. (1996). EPO network. *Managed Healthcare, 26*, 31–32.

McKelvey, B. (1982). *Organizational systematics, taxonomy, evolution and classification.* Berkeley, CA: University of California Press.

McKnight, J., Edwards, N., Pickard, L., Underwood, J., Voorberg, N., & Woodcox, V. (1991). The delphi approach to strategic planning. *Nursing Management, 22*, 55–57.

McNamee, M., & Schiller, Z. (1994). Prepping for radical surgery. *Business Week, 3353*, 97.

Moldof, E. (1994). Do-it yourself strategic planning provides map to the future. *Healthcare Financial Management, 48*, 26–31.

Mulner, R. (1986, June). *Hospital closures, mergers and consolidations.* Paper presented at the meeting of the Association for Health Services Research. Boston.

Nemes, J. (1990). For-profit chains look beyond the bottom line. *Modern Healthcare, 20*, 27–36.

Nutt, P. (1984). *Planning methods for health related organizations.* New York: John Wiley & Sons.

O'Donnell, K. (1993). Home care shaping up as competitive necessity. *Modern Healthcare, 23*, 34–36.

Pallarito, K. (1996). Virtual healthcare. *Modern Healthcare, 26*, 42–47.

Perry, L., Stott, R., & Smallwood, W. (1993). *Real-time strategy: Improvising team-based planning for a fast-changing world.* New York: John Wiley & Sons.

Porter, M. (1991). Towards a dynamic theory of strategy. *Strategic Management Journal, 12*, 95–117.

Reeves, P. (1983). *Strategic planning for hospitals.* Chicago: Foundation of the American College of Hospital Administrators.

Robert, M. (1991). Why CEOs have difficulty implementing their strategies. *The Journal of Business Strategy, 12*, 58–59.

Robinson, J. (1996). The dynamics and limits of corporate growth in health care. *Health Affairs, 15*, 155–169.

Robinson, J., & Casalino, L. (1996). Vertical integration and organizational networks in health care. *Health Affairs, 15*, 7–22.

Scott, L. (1994). Home care revenues soar to $5.1 billion via mergers. *Modern Healthcare, 24*, 85–90.

Shortell, S., Gillies, R., Anderson, D., Erickson, K., & Mitchel, J. (1996). *Remaking Health Care in America.* San Francisco: Jossey-Bass.

Shortell, S., Morrison, E., & Friedman, B. (1990). *Strategic choice for America's hospitals: Managing change in turbulent times.* San Francisco: Jossey-Bass.

Shriver, K. (1996). Bumpy road ahead for post-acute providers. *Modern Healthcare, 26*, 44.

Smith, D., & Kaluzny, A. (1986). *The white labyrinth.* Ann Arbor, MI: Health Administration Press.

Snyder, K. (1995). Home care marriages. *Drug Topics, 139*, 44–46.

Starr, P. (1982). *The Social Transformation of American Medicine.* New York: Basic.

Stevens, G. (1991). *The Strategic Health Care Manager.* San Francisco: Jossey-Bass.

Suver, J., Kahn, C., & Clement, J. (1984). *Cases in health care financial management.* Ann Arbor: AUPHA Press.

Wasson, C. (1974). *Dynamic competitive strategy & product life cycles.* St. Charles, FL: Challenge Books.

Weber, J., & Peters, J. (1983). *Strategic thinking: New frontiers in hospital management.* Chicago: American Hospital Publishing, Inc.

Weiner, J., & Hanley, R. (1992). Caring for the disabled elderly: There's no place like home. In Shortell, S. & Reinhardt, U. (Eds.), *Improving health policy and management*: Nine critical research issues for the 1990s (pp. 75–110). Ann Arbor, MI: Health Administration Press.

Welles, E. (1995). The awakening. *Inc, 17*, 23–24.

Wheelen, T., & Hunger, J. (1995). *Strategic Management and Business Policy, 5th ed.* Reading, MA: Addison-Wesley.

Whelan, J., & Sisson, J. (1993). How to realize the promise of strategic planning. *The Journal of Business Strategy, 14*, 31–36.

CHAPTER 57

Marketing: An Overview

Karen L. Carney

Marketing is a journey. It is the path an organization takes to move toward its strategic business objectives. It encourages an organization to understand how it relates to its environment and to identify what relationships it needs to make the trip. As in any journey, there are several steps that contribute to its success: analysis of the environment, preparation and planning, implementation, evaluation of progress, and adaptation to remain on course.

This chapter will explore marketing and how home care providers can harness the power of marketing to move their agencies along the path toward their marketing goals.

WHAT MARKETING IS AND ISN'T

Marketing is not a discrete function. It is a way of doing business that cannot be separated from the organization's overall journey. Each individual within a home care agency has a marketing role, though it is not always a consciously accepted role. Internal operations and all the functions that constitute the agency's capabilities combine to create the agency's product, which is an integral component of the agency's marketing. That means every staff member affects the product and thereby the marketing. Expensive marketing materials and promotional promises are worthless if they are not backed by the day-to-day actions that create

the agency's true product. Home care providers must foster a marketing mindset among all staff, helping them understand how they contribute to the agency's success at meeting customers' needs.

Some home care providers believe they have achieved continued growth without investing in "marketing." The truth is that they have been involved in marketing all along, any time they reached out to potential or existing customers to understand the customers' needs and helped customers understand the benefits of their agency's capabilities. For years, many agencies have relied on this informal marketing. They had a good product that satisfied customers' needs and therefore was in demand. But without a structured environmental analysis and concerted effort to regularly assess and satisfy customers' needs, this informal marketing cannot sustain any home care provider as the market changes.

To be successful, marketing demands an organized approach. The home care organization's goals must be clearly delineated and its marketplace surveyed to determine the best actions for reaching those goals. To take a trip, one first must know the destination. What are the options for traveling there? By car, by plane, by ship? What obstacles or barriers must be overcome to arrive there—immunizations, up-to-date passports, etc.? What is the climate like?

Does the terrain consist of rugged mountains or urban pavement? What clothes and how much money should be brought as resources? Is there a better time of year to visit? What types of facilities such as hotels and restaurants exist? All these questions make a difference, as there is always more than one option for reaching a specific destination. Marketing for home care works in a similar manner.

Agencies must have a good sense of their own marketplace and what is happening in their environment. Is the market growing with managed care or already saturated? Is it dominated by a few health care systems or fairly fragmented with a high level of competition? Who dominates the home care market and what services do they provide? The choices one makes for a marketing plan depend on the answers gained from this early analysis.

Based on the goals that have been set and the terrain that must be covered, the home care provider then maps a route for arriving at its goals. What marketing steps are necessary? How can the agency solve problems for its various customers and make itself indispensable? Supplies, equipment, and resources must match the terrain to be covered, and be used on a consistent and continual basis to repeatedly present the agency's capabilities to its various customers in a manner that appeals to them.

A primary tool for any marketing effort is the marketing plan, which serves as the road map. It focuses a home care organization's limited resources in a structured effort to reach specific milestones. An effective marketing plan creates an integrated array of outreach activities that build on previous efforts to move an agency ever closer to its goals. As every home care organization is different, each one's marketing plan will be different as well.

Marketing relies heavily on the principles of communication that foster the exchange of information and ideas as well as products and services. A critical component of marketing is the understanding of the customer. With that knowledge, home care providers can shape their products and marketing messages and efforts to appeal to the customer's needs and goals. The marketing process is cyclical, repeating itself as the home care provider continually seeks information to understand the customer and adjusts its products and marketing efforts.

Unfortunately, marketing is a concept that has had a troubled history in health care. Often perceived as sales, marketing has been denigrated as somehow robbing the compassion from health care and elevating concerns for money over the concerns for the patient.

In reality, marketing is the sum of any activities that help a home care organization align its goals, needs, and interests with its customers' goals, needs, and interests. By doing this, home care organizations position themselves as partners to their customers, providing services and resources that help the customers achieve their goals. Marketing is a long-term process that must continually repeat itself. Even home care providers that achieve success must reinvent that success the next year, and so on.

THE ROLE OF MARKETING IN HOME CARE

Traditionally, organized marketing has been avoided by home care providers for several reasons. Even just 20 years ago, there was little competition in home care. Most agencies served distinct territories with little overlap. As the Medicare program grew as a payer source, more agencies, especially proprietary home care providers, appeared in many markets. When the Health Care Financing Administration (HCFA) initiated the Medicare diagnosis-related groups (DRGs) for inpatient acute care in the early 1980s, home care utilization boomed. The DRGs created an incentive for hospitals to decrease hospital lengths of stays. Home care became the natural next step for hospital patients who were sent home earlier in their recuperation. Areas without certificate of need requirements experienced tremendous expansion in the number of home care providers, while existing agencies experienced double-digit growth throughout the late 1980s into the early 1990s.

At the same time, managed care became a more dominant force in the health care industry. Managed care focused on the price and value of health care services, causing many providers to rethink their approach to positioning their agencies in the marketplace. Managed care also brought a greater emphasis on accountability— what exactly is a home care agency providing when it accepts a new patient? How many visits will be provided and for how long? What outcomes will be achieved and efficiencies gained? Home care agencies needed to answer those questions, providing data and information such as critical pathways that outlined more definitively the parameters of the service they provide.

These market occurrences—increasing competition and managed care—have increasingly encouraged home care providers to adopt a more structured approach to marketing.

Yet in the midst of these changes, Medicare, the primary payer source for most home care providers, has maintained a cost-reimbursed system for financing its Home Health Benefit. Under that system, marketing is considered a nonreimbursable cost, which has created a disincentive to invest in marketing. Some agencies have interpreted the nonallowable cost issue as a mandate to avoid marketing. Others have surreptitiously invested in marketing, engaging in only those activities that fit within the ever-narrowing interpretations of allowable costs. Much of the restrictions regarding marketing should change with the advent of a Medicare prospective payment system. Regardless, home care providers should check the Medicare regulations as well as with their accountants to determine what impact marketing activities will have on their cost report and financial viability.

Marketing has also been a taboo subject for many agencies due to staff resistance. Clinical staff typically balk at marketing and its sales connotations. In practice, however, marketing is similar to the clinical assessments home care staff perform. When staff visit new patients,

they don't try to "sell" them an intravenous the patients don't need. Instead, the staff asks a series of questions, assessing the patients' conditions as well as their situations. Based on that assessment, staff develop a treatment plan that is adjusted as the patients progress toward their goals. Marketing works in the same way.

Despite home care's reluctance to embrace it, marketing remains an essential element for home care providers that want to build their business success. Marketing takes the organization's mission and strategic business goals and translates them into the marketing steps needed to realize those goals. A structured marketing effort brings a home care agency numerous benefits:

- **Focused effort:** A marketing plan captures the energy of the organization and focuses it on achieving its goals. Decisions can be made as to where to invest time and energy because the goals have been established. With a clear marketing plan, everyone in the organization can work toward the same goal. Resources can be interwoven and applied toward a common goal, multiplying the impact of the resources.
- **Consistency and cohesiveness:** A marketing plan unites the organization in striving for the same goals, ensuring that all actions and messages are geared toward those endpoints. Marketing messages presented to customers are consistent and therefore complement one another.
- **Strategic growth:** A structured marketing effort helps steer the organization in the directions of its goals, attaining growth in specific areas and product line capabilities. As opportunities arise, an agency can quickly determine if the opportunities are consistent with its goals, and based on that, whether it should pursue the opportunities.
- **Advantageous use of resources:** Every organization has limited resources. A structured marketing effort helps a home care provider use its resources efficiently

in the areas that will help it achieve its goals.

- **Ongoing customer feedback:** A key element in every organized marketing effort is the gathering of feedback, data, and information from customers. While the mechanisms for attaining that feedback may vary, the purposes don't. Feedback enables an agency to adapt and evolve its marketing efforts, responding to the inevitable changes in the marketplace.

How then can home care providers harness this power of marketing to craft a road map that will lead them to their business goals?

THE MARKET ANALYSIS

All marketing planning starts with analysis. Few home care providers can afford to stand still in the current health care marketplace. There is a constant stream of decisions to be made, from whom to partner with to which contracts to pursue. A market analysis pulls together market intelligence in a cohesive, organized format to narrow an agency's options and identify the most advantageous paths to follow. It helps an agency determine where it currently stands and identifies landmarks and milestones that will help the agency travel to its future destination.

A good market analysis does not have to be expensive, though it is usually time-consuming. Questions form the most basic level of analysis. Good questions generate good information, but few home care providers have practiced the art of asking questions. Consider how many times home care staff interact with customers, potential customers, vendors, and other market sources on any typical day. If those staff were armed with questions, they could help their agency fill in the gaps of its market intelligence. For example, if an agency is considering launching a new pediatric asthma program, it can encourage staff to ask questions such as How are children with asthma currently cared for? What other home care providers have a

special pediatric asthma program? What sets those asthma programs apart? What kinds of problems occur in managing the care of children with asthma? The answers can be jotted down and returned to the agency for inclusion in the overall market analysis that will help shape the agency's final development of its pediatric asthma program.

The goal is to ask questions that can't be answered with a yes or no. However, the most critical step in the questioning approach is to capture the answers in black and white, whether in a database or on paper or index card system. Too often the information remains in a staff member's head where it cannot be combined with feedback from other sources and cannot be retained if that individual changes jobs or moves to a new home care provider.

The market analysis can be directed toward the development of a specific program such as the example of a pediatric asthma program, or it can provide a market overview for the agency's entire operations. In the past, comprehensive market analyses were done every two to three years. In today's rapidly changing health care market, it is better to perform one at least annually and to continuously monitor the market during the year for any significant alterations that might occur in the meantime.

Competitive analysis. A competitive analysis identifies competitors, surveying their strengths and weaknesses. Gather feedback from customers and potential customers to evaluate how the agency compares. Some factors about competitors to assess include annual patient volume, referral sources, payer mix, competitive advantages, market share, market relationships, market position, weaknesses, financial viability, service record, and profile of capabilities.

A competitive analysis also should review more than just other home care providers. Competition for home care patients can stem from subacute or transitional care units, outpatient clinics, rehabilitation facilities, skilled nursing facilities, and physician offices. What are these providers offering and how does it compare to what the home care agency can provide? The same types of information gathered for competing agencies should be collected for these providers as well as to help the home care organization understand more fully how it fits into the overall health care market.

Internal analysis. An internal analysis should assess the agency's strengths, weaknesses, opportunities, and threats (a SWOT analysis). Information should be included on the agency's payer mix and its patients' demographics, including diagnoses, patient volume, and visit utilization. The home care provider needs to assess its agency's identity, financial viability, and relationships with other providers and organizations. The analysis also should answer: Where do current referrals come from and where is there potential for more referrals? Once a list of current and potential referral sources is compiled, rank the referral sources by priority based on their referral potential, revenue generated by each referral, patient demographics, and openness to new or expanded home care resources. The ranking creates a tier of customer priorities, highlighting their potential for generating business. The ranking is an

individualized decision that is determined by each agency. In one agency, a new multigroup practice of physicians that has an alliance with the hospital where the home care agency is based may be a top priority. For another agency in the same market, that physician practice may be a lower priority precisely because it has an established relationship with a home care provider that may be difficult to penetrate.

Customer analysis. Agencies need to identify their customers, who can range from consumers and patients to payers, physicians, legislators, and other local community organizations (see Exhibit 57–1). The ability to understand customers individually and to respond to their specific needs will substantially affect the agency's marketing success. For example, consumers are not physicians and do not require, or desire, the same types of marketing messages. Individual customers are seeking different assurances and information about how the home care provider solves their problems or serves their needs. The home care provider's job is to help each customer understand "What does home care mean to me? How does it help me?" At the same time, the home care agency needs to gather informa-

---

Exhibit 57–1 Key Customer Audiences for Home Care

- Assisted living facilities: administrators, social workers, clinical staff
- Community organizations: administrators
- Consumers
- Continuing care retirement communities: administrators, social workers, clinical staff
- Donors
- Hospital administrators
- Hospital discharge planners/case managers
- Industry associations
- Investors
- Legislators, local government officials
- Local businesses: owners, human resource directors
- Media representatives

- Patients and families
- Payers/managed care organizations: case managers, contract managers, provider relations directors
- Physicians
- Regulatory officials
- Senior centers and elder groups
- Skilled nursing facilities: administrators, social workers
- Specialty clinic/program managers, e.g., cancer center, etc.
- Subacutes/transitional care units: administrators, social workers
- Volunteers

tion on how the customers perceive home care and the agency. It should collect information on their needs, issues, goals, and life stages (i.e., retiring, starting families, etc.) as well as their demographics and disease incidence rates.

In addition to customer information, the analysis should provide information on a variety of factors (see Exhibit 57–2) that will help paint a picture of the current marketplace.

Agencies can gather this market analysis information in several ways. The first step should be to tap existing knowledge among staff members. Staff encounter a broad array of market intelligence daily but often aren't aware that management wants it. At the same time, staff can be encouraged to make every encounter more valuable through the use of effective questioning techniques. By asking a series of focused questions over time, staff can uncover qualitative information that can help shape the agency's marketing strategy.

There are numerous other sources of market intelligence: competitors' Medicare cost reports, research studies, Medicare program statistics, national health care statistics from various companies as well as the National Center for Health Statistics, the U.S. Census, literature searches via on-line databases, local newspapers and magazines (including help wanted ads), trade publications, division of health and human services for each state, division of insurance for each state, national associations and self-help groups (e.g., American Heart Association, etc.).

The central focus of the market assessment phase should be to identify problems and uncover unmet needs. These problems become opportunities for savvy home care providers. Take a situation where the assessment uncovers a high incidence of pediatric asthma that is causing repeated emergency hospitalizations. A home care provider could partner with a local

---

Exhibit 57–2 Elements of a Home Care Market Analysis

Identify and gather the following information to develop a home care market analysis.

Internal

- Current referral patterns, e.g., volume from specific referral sources, patient diagnoses, revenue per referral source, revenue per patient diagnosis, costs per patient, etc.
- Current referral sources
- Existing patient demographics
- Customer relationships and satisfaction rates
- Payer mix
- Agency strengths and weaknesses
- Profile of agency capabilities and services

External

- Decision makers for home care referrals
- Potential referral sources

- Relationships among referral sources as well as among competitors, e.g., networks, affiliations, integrated delivery systems, etc.
- Profile of patient demographics for each referral source
- Level of consumer choice
- Service area demographics
- Disease incidences within service area
- Health care market trends, e.g., shorter lengths of stay for inpatients, decreasing inpatient volume for hospitals, etc.
- Regulatory issues and developments
- Competitor analysis
- Customers' unmet needs and/or problems
- Managed care penetration
- Top hospital DRGs
- Number of patient discharges to home care
- Home care utilization for service area
- Community and industry leaders

hospital and area pediatricians to develop a clinical pathway that transcends various health care settings to more effectively manage the care of children with asthma, reducing the need for unplanned hospitalizations, decreasing the incidence of complications, improving the patients' quality of life, and reducing the cost of caring for those children. The pediatric asthma program would be attractive to managed care organizations and other payers who are struggling to reduce the costs of caring for that specific population. Other options would be to hire staff with special training in respiratory care or partner with a home medical equipment provider to offer a package of specialized asthma capabilities. It could be that the home care provider already has specialized pediatric asthma capabilities. The assessment then may help uncover why those services haven't been fully utilized.

The analysis will also give the provider a base of information on which to forecast demand for specific sets of services.

MARKET TRENDS AND FORCES

The health care marketplace is dynamic. There are constant changes. New roads and relationships are built. New developments occur. Construction and maintenance along familiar routes might force some rerouting. Customers may move or close their businesses, and new customers may take their places.

To complete a market analysis, home care providers have to understand that the home care industry has became increasingly complex. Multiple customers with diverse needs and goals must be satisfied simultaneously. A side issue for many home care providers during the last decade has been managing enormous growth. While that growth may level off for many agencies during the next decade, they must still grapple with a rapidly changing environment being reshaped by nine major trends and forces:

Competition. According to the National Association for Home Care, the number of home care agencies in the U.S. has more than doubled since 1975. With roughly 15,000 home care providers across the country, competition is a central force in all but the most rural markets. Competition will be a factor in reducing the overall number of home care providers by causing weaker, less resourceful agencies to close or merge.

Managed care. Managed care brings a cost consciousness about the utilization of resources and a demand for accountability. For home care providers, the increasing presence of managed care not only realigns relationships and decision makers but also requires data and measurements that demonstrate the performance of one provider over another. More important, the guiding principles of managed care have begun to spill over into other payer sources, including Medicare, Medicaid, and indemnity insurers that will increasingly demand similar cost-consciousness and outcomes measurement.

Consolidation. A side effect of competition and managed care, consolidation has become a major trend in home care as agencies pursue mergers, acquisitions, and affiliations to strengthen market positions, streamline operations, and achieve economies of scale.

New decision makers. With the onset of managed care, payers have begun wielding more power as decision makers. While hospital continuing care staff may have had significant influence in directing referrals to specific home care providers, now those decisions are determined before the patients are even admitted to the hospital. Managed care organizations establish contracts with providers, creating panels of accepted home care providers from which patients and their caregivers must choose. The redistribution of decision making is even creeping into Medicare and Medicaid programs as some states allow managed care organizations to participate in those programs. The shift in decision makers means home care providers must shift their marketing efforts to focus on these new power brokers.

Technology. Advances in technology have been a significant boon to home care, enabling ever more sophisticated capabilities to be delivered in the home setting. Technology has also changed the way information is captured, stored, and communicated. A decade ago facsimile machines dramatically altered communication between referral sources and home care providers. Now the Internet, e-mail, cellular phones, telemedicine, and laptop computers promise to do the same. Technology can be a competitive advantage, reducing costs, eliminating redundant procedures, and streamlining administration.

Aging population. The fastest growing segment of the U.S. population is the age 85 and over group. The irony of this public health success story is that, as elders live longer, they are often living longer with chronic health conditions that may limit their ability to care for themselves independently in the community. For home care providers, the aging population ensures that demand for home care services will continue. However, the flip side of that equation is that often these individuals have complex conditions that may not fit within narrow boundaries for insurance coverage or may be more costly to treat.

Integrated delivery systems. As managed care has introduced risk-sharing and capitated payment methodologies, health care providers are looking for ways to streamline operations and more completely manage patients' care as they move from one care setting to the next. The result has been the rise in integrated delivery systems (IDS)—vertical arrangements of different types of providers through contract or formal affiliation. The creation of an IDS can either suddenly constrict the referral stream or expand it for home care providers, depending on whether the agencies are on the outside or the inside of the new system.

Acceleration. The pace of health care delivery today is faster, faster, faster. Patients who are admitted to inpatient facilities find they are discharged much sooner in their recuperation. The turnaround time from admission to discharge is dramatically shorter, leaving less time for inpatient staff to provide patient education, establish a discharge plan, or even identify that a patient may need home care services. For home care providers, the result has been that patients sometimes fall through the cracks and others go home "sicker and quicker." At the same time, patients are discharged whenever they receive their physicians' approvals—evenings, weekends, and holidays as well as normal business hours. Gone are the days of keeping a patient an extra day to avoid a weekend discharge. To respond, home care providers have extended their office hours and added regular evening and weekend staff to handle the off-hour referrals and admissions.

Educated consumers. Changes in the health care system have created an impetus for consumers to become better advocates for themselves. They ask more questions, demand more information, may challenge a health care professional's guidance, command greater knowledge of health care issues and options, and are asserting their rights more adamantly.

MARKET PREPARATION AND PLANNING

Once the marketplace has been analyzed, the next step is to create a marketing plan. It takes the market analysis and weaves it with the organization's self-assessment to create a snapshot of the agency's current market position. It outlines the agency's strengths and weaknesses as well as its opportunities and threats. It should detail the primary and secondary customers, ranking them by priority and identifying the agency's marketing goals for each.

The market analysis also gives the home care provider the opportunity to assess whether its marketing goals are on track or need some adjustment. For example, if one of the agency's goals is to increase referrals from a specific hospital by 20%, it may find the goal is no longer realistic given that the hospital has merged with another hospital that has its own home care department. Or it may find that the hospital's inpatient census has dramatically decreased so an increase of 20% may be unrealistic. More important, the home care agency will want to rededicate its resources to goals that will have a better return on investment.

The process of developing the marketing plan can be as important as the finished plan. By involving various frontline staff members along with the marketing coordinator and other appropriate managers, the agency can gain different perspectives while establishing consensus on where the agency is headed and the steps required to get there. The process can foster staff participation and buy-in with the marketing effort. Based on the snapshot created by the market and organizational analysis, the home care staff select the marketing tactics that will move the agency toward its goals. Those tactics are chosen based on the resources available, the potential return on investment, the customers involved, and the marketing goals. For example, a home care agency may decide that while a newsletter published four times a year is a great public awareness tool, it has become a costly endeavor in a market where there is little consumer choice. Instead, the agency may want to invest the resources usually spent on developing and distributing a quarterly newsletter toward building stronger relationships with specific physicians and case managers.

The marketing plan becomes a road map, outlining the obstacles and opportunities as well as the steps to circumvent the pitfalls and grab the opportunities (see Exhibit 57–3).

This is the stage where an agency must determine where to focus its effort. With limited time and resources, it will have to make some difficult decisions about where to channel its resources. Ideally, it wants to build on its strengths. It can be very expensive and time-consuming to challenge a market leader or established home care provider without having a major competitive advantage or added-value capability.

Exhibit 57–3 Elements of a Marketing Plan

- **Marketing plan overview/summary**
- **External market analysis**
  - major referral sources
  - decision makers
  - market relationships
  - payer sources
  - service area demographics
  - disease incidence statistics
  - market trends
  - threats
  - opportunities
  - competitor analysis
- **Internal market analysis**
  - mission and business goals
  - existing referral sources and referral patterns
  - revenue per patient by diagnosis
  - patient profiles and demographics
  - strengths
  - weaknesses
  - customer feedback
- **Priority customers**
- **Key marketing messages**
- **Marketing goals and marketing activities for each goal**
- **Action plan**

THE MARKETING MIX

Marketing involves developing the right **product**, offering it in the right **place** at the right **price** with the right mix of **promotional** activities. Examining each of these four Ps of marketing more closely helps reveal their interrelationship.

Product. What products and capabilities will the agency offer and what competitive advantage do those capabilities hold? How will services be packaged and presented? How will the agency position itself in the market? What identity will it project? Demand for various products and capabilities varies over time. Different home care providers may serve different segments of the market. The environment changes and market forces fluctuate, creating shifts in what customers seek. A home care provider needs to continually assess its market to determine how those changes affect its products and packaging.

The product is much more than just the services a home care provider supplies. It is the sum of all the parts within the home care agency—how the phone is answered, how accurate the billing is, and how easy it is to get questions answered. The product also involves the segment of the market that the home care agency strives to serve—children, elders, people with specific diagnoses, and so on. The product is a critical decision point in marketing. It determines what the organization is "selling" and who will potentially buy it. Ideally, the agency will build on its strengths and minimize its weaknesses to maximize customer satisfaction. But the decision about the product needs to take into account the organization's mission, culture, organizational leadership, resources, and capabilities.

Packaging is how the product is presented to the customer. Is it simply skilled nursing or specialized certification in diabetic nursing? Is it the array of standard home care services (i.e., skilled nursing, home health aide, etc.), or is it a clinical pathway that more clearly defines what set of services a patient with a particular diagnosis will receive? Packaging is also an aspect of assigning specific home care nurses as liaisons to specific doctors. The doctor's liaison nurse builds a stronger relationship with the doctor and serves as the doctor's home care resource. That package of personal attention to the physicians adds value to the home care provider's product and makes it more attractive to the customer.

One of the most common marketing pitfalls for home care providers is the failure to establish a competitive advantage. To many customers—patients, families, physicians, payers, and so on—most home care providers look alike. In their eyes, home care has become a commodity product. Quality is not a competitive advantage in the current health care market. It is a baseline expectation. How an agency defines and demonstrates quality, though, can be a competitive advantage. The competitive advantage is what sets a home care agency apart from its competitors. What added value does it bring to its customers? How does it help its customers achieve their goals? What special strengths does the agency have and how do those strengths benefit the customers?

Competitive advantages come in many shapes and sizes. Special clinical skills or programs, rapid response time, streamlined paperwork, electronic medical records, laptop computers in the field, superior clinical outcomes, cross-training of staff, service guarantees, discount prices, vast service areas, disease management programs or clinical pathways for high-cost complex diagnoses, one-stop shopping, and follow-up phone calls are all examples of different competitive advantages. The competitive advantage depends on the customers involved and how they perceive the advantage.

Place (distribution). Place represents where and how the home care services are offered, which can be another differentiating factor. Many home care providers are forming networks and alliances to give managed care organizations and IDSs, a larger service area for contracts. The alliances may also provide one-stop shopping, offering an array of services through a single access point. The location of an agency's main office can give it increased community visibility, as can the location of its satellite or branch offices. Place can also relate to the relationships a home care provider has. For example, a hospital-based provider has a distinct advantage in its market because of its relationship with the hospital, a relationship that places the agency in the path for referrals from the hospital. A home care provider that assigns a liaison nurse to specific physicians' offices has multiplied its distribution network by creating an extension of its office within the physician practices.

Price. Pricing is a new arena for most home care agencies. Until managed care burst on the scene, the major issue related to fees was fine tuning the cost report for the best reimbursement rate. There were no negotiations and no real pricing strategies involved. Pricing, though, has moved to center stage in many health care markets as home care providers struggle to offset price concessions with added-value capabilities that may allow them to secure higher prices. Price is the combination of costs and value. Traditionally, home care providers have not had a good understanding of either, which has left them vulnerable to the new pricing methodologies such as risk sharing and capitation.

Pricing methodologies in home care currently range from discounted fee-for-service arrangements, per diem payments, and episodic case rates to risk sharing, performance-based compensation, and capitation. As home care providers try to negotiate higher prices from managed care organizations, they learn that price is often the only factor that differentiates home care providers from one another. Until recently, there has been little available data about home care and few benchmarks that enabled managed care organizations to compare apples to apples among home care providers. To move beyond price as a differentiating factor, home care agen-

cies need to offer other capabilities that are perceived as having value by the customers.

Promotion. The mix of marketing activities an agency selects to engage its various customers and move toward its marketing goals is called the promotional mix. Below is a sampling of promotional activities that a home care provider may select.

Media relations. News releases, television and radio public service announcements (PSAs), and feature stories have been standard elements in home care marketing outreach. A relatively low-cost promotional method, media relations have been effective in creating and maintaining the company's identity but are perhaps less effective in influencing which agencies end up on a managed care organization's provider panel. Some of the newest media avenues—the Internet and on-line forums—are low cost and offer ample opportunity for one-to-one contact with customers. Use of the media can be effective in reaching out to consumers, influencing patient choice, providing consumer education, and fostering the agency's identity.

Advertising. Advertising has become more prevalent in home care as some providers try to differentiate themselves from an increasing field of competitors and establish a market advantage. Interestingly, several managed care organizations have used home care success stories in their own advertising to consumers. A capital-intensive medium, advertising relies on frequency of the ad placement and the ad size (or duration in broadcast media).

Community relations. The general public remains a pivotal audience for every home care provider even though the public's ability to choose a specific provider may be eroded through managed care contracts. Community education programs, screenings, and immunization clinics help position an agency as a community resource. Speakers' bureaus enable the agency to present a variety of topics related to home care and general health. For those providers affiliated with an integrated delivery system, the home care agency can provide the infrastructure for the system's community outreach efforts. For free-standing agencies, the community represents a major marketing audience.

Professional relations. As decision makers have become more diverse, home care providers have placed more emphasis on professional education and networking. Health care professionals often misunderstand home care. Hospital staff and physicians who must refer patients to home care may hold outdated notions of home care and its capabilities. Education efforts must bridge this gap while engaging professionals who may feel they already know all there is to know about home care. The relationship-building process fosters an exchange of information that will help the home care provider more fully understand the health care professional's needs and concerns, thereby enabling the agency to translate its home care services into appropriate benefits based on those needs and concerns.

Special events. While often labor intensive, special events can generate substantial public and professional awareness of home care. They can help publicize a specific service or capability and help with fund-raising.

Marketing communications. Print communication has long been the mainstay of health care marketing—brochures, annual reports, newsletters, and marketing collaterals. Print communication remains a strong component in home care marketing but is taking more of a supportive role to interpersonal marketing strategies such as sales and one-to-one education efforts. At the same time, the forums for marketing communications have expanded with the advent of videos, e-mail, Web sites, and interactive software.

Contract negotiations and management. One of the newest dimensions of home care marketing, contract negotiations enable a home care provider to more fully represent itself and its capabilities with payers and other providers during the contract development. In addition, once a contract is in place, the complexities of a contract extend beyond the legal nuances and into the areas of service definition and compliance. The ability to understand, interpret, and comply with a contract can give a home care provider an advantage over competitors.

Sales. Structured sales efforts have become a familiar factor in home care marketing as many agencies have discovered that relationship building demands one-to-one interactions. The downfall of many home care sales efforts, though, is that interactions are not focused on achieving a particular goal or eliciting specific information. By asking questions and proposing case examples, sales representatives can lead health care professionals and other referral sources to a greater understanding of how home care can solve problems they face. The questions help the sales representatives to better understand the customer's role and perspective, enabling the sales representatives to then tailor their home care messages and examples to the customers' specific situations.

Fund-raising. For not-for-profit home care providers, fund-raising efforts form the cornerstone of much of their marketing outreach. Fund development can be exercised at various levels of sophistication from special events to finely timed annual appeals. For fund-raising to be successful, the target public must know and have some type of vested interest in making a donation. As a result, fund-raising efforts should be closely coordinated with the rest of the organization's marketing outreach, to provide consistent messages and leverage the potential of other marketing efforts.

Investor relations. Investors are a critical source of support for privately held and publicly traded home care providers. The ongoing communication with these key audiences often takes the form of marketing communications and relationship building.

IMPLEMENTATION

Focus. Once the marketing plan is complete, one of the toughest marketing challenges for home care providers is to maintain their marketing focus. Too often they try to be all things to all customers. The result: resources are spread too thin and the impact of their marketing investment is diluted. More important, by narrowing their targets, home care providers reduce the likelihood that they'll be overwhelmed by their marketing responsibilities, which often causes marketing tasks to be placed on the back burner. Instead of targeting 50 doctors, it may be more realistic for a home care agency to target 5. They can launch a more comprehensive campaign with the five doctors, focus a greater proportion of resources on building solid relations with those five physicians, and working with five physicians can seem much more "doable" for home care providers already saddled with other responsibilities.

Local markets demand local strategies. What works in one geographic area may not work in the neighboring service area. Each health care community has its own distinct needs and issues. Home care providers that operate several offices or regional networks know that each market demands its own version of the agency's overall marketing plan. The goals may remain the same, but the strategies and tactics may vary. In some markets, though, the goals may vary as well. Certain markets may have no need for a pediatric asthma program while other markets may find those programs flourishing.

A living document. The marketing plan should change over time, just as the market does. It is meant to be a living, breathing document. While the overall strategies should remain sound as long as the market doesn't undergo dramatic upheaval, the tactics should be adjusted to match the changing environment. Consider a situation where one marketing goal is to develop specialty programs, and the marketing plan originally recommended developing

a pediatric asthma program. Then soon after the marketing plan is complete, the major referral source develops its own pediatric asthma program. The agency must adapt its marketing plan. It can either discontinue the pediatric asthma effort, investigate how it may be able to align with or augment the referral source's program, or develop new sources of referrals by expanding its service area.

One way to keep the marketing plan from sitting on a shelf is to transform the finished plan into an action plan that lists activities that need to be accomplished month by month with the names of the individuals responsible for accomplishing those tasks (see Exhibit 57–4).

Marketing structure. The structure of a home care provider's marketing effort will affect its ability to implement its marketing tactics and achieve its goals. The structure should match the marketplace and the goals. For example, if there is a growing presence of managed care, the home care provider needs to send staff on marketing visits to build relationships with the increasing array of decision makers such as physicians, case managers, managed care contract managers, and subacute care managers.

Some agencies have decentralized the marketing effort by assigning marketing responsibilities to several staff members who also shoulder other agency responsibilities. Other agencies have designated a single individual as the marketing coordinator. Even in agencies with more extensive marketing departments, it can still make sense to decentralize some of the marketing responsibilities because this encourages staff participation in and understanding of the agency's marketing efforts.

MEASUREMENT AND ADAPTATION

Once a structured marketing effort is implemented, the evaluation begins. Evaluation and feedback enable the agency to determine not only whether its marketing efforts are working but also whether its marketing goals are on track with any changes in the marketplace. Evaluation can occur through customer satisfac-

Exhibit 57–4 Marketing Action Plan

January		February		March	
Action	**Responsible**	**Action**	**Responsible**	**Action**	**Responsible**
Meet with the three doctors in the new multigroup practice	Liaison nurse and clinical supervisor	Begin developing new agency capabilities sheet for physicians	Community relations director	Meet with three doctors in the new multigroup practice to explain new physician liaison program	Liaison nurse and clinical supervisor
Hold first meeting to develop physician liaison program	Liaison nurse, clinica supervisor, community relations director, and executive director	Compile list of physicians to be sent new capabilities sheet	Community relations director and administrative assistant	Mail new capabilities sheet to physicians	Administrative assistant

Exhibit 57–5 Key Performance Indicators

- Referral volume per referral source
- Revenue per patient
- Revenue per patient per diagnosis
- Revenue by payer/referral source
- Costs per patient
- Costs per patient by diagnosis
- Costs per patient by payer/referral source
- Agency revenue
- Patient volume
- Patient volume by diagnosis
- Customer satisfaction rates
- Visit utilization per patient
- Visit utilization per patient by diagnosis

tion surveys, data collection of key performance indicators, informal feedback from customers, market intelligence gathered through the media and other reports, and structured market research. Exhibit 57–5 offers a list of key indicators that can help measure marketing efforts.

Marketing in some respects is experimental, making it more an art than a science. Different products and promotional activities work in different situations. That's one reason why measurement is so important. Home care providers need to check whether their marketing efforts are working.

CONCLUSION

Marketing is a natural aspect of business, whether or not a home care provider consciously structures a marketing effort. However, by structuring a marketing effort that begins with analysis and continues through measurement and adaptation, the home care organization will move along the steps towards its marketing goals. The marketing plan becomes the road map, helping the agency navigate its changing health care landscape, understand and satisfy its customers' needs, and achieve its marketing goals.

BIBLIOGRAPHY

Bowen, D., & Schneider, B. (1995). *Winning the service game.* Boston: Harvard Business School Press.

Clampitt Douglas, L., Edwards, P. & S. (1991). *Getting business to come to you.* Los Angeles: Jeremy P. Tarcher.

Conrad Levinson, J. (1993). *Guerrilla marketing excellence: fifty golden rules for small-business success.* Boston: Houghton Mifflin.

Drucker, P. (1964, 1986). *Managing for results.* New York: Harper & Row.

Drucker, P. (1990). *Managing the non-profit organization: principles and practices.* New York: HarperCollins.

Fuld, L. (1995). *The new competitor intelligence.* New York: John Wiley & Sons.

Gumpert, D. (1992). *How to really create a successful marketing plan.* Boston: Inc. Publishing.

Hawken, P. (1987). *Growing a business.* New York: Simon & Schuster.

Kawasaki, G. (1991). *Selling the dream.* New York: Harper-Business.

Kotler, P. (1996). *Marketing management: Analysis, planning, implementation and control.* 9th ed. Englewood Cliffs, NJ: Prentice-Hall.

McKenna, R. (1991). *Relationship marketing: Successful strategies for the age of the customer.* Reading, MA: Addison-Wesley.

Newsom, D., & Scott, A. (1976). *This is PR: The realities of public relations.* Belmont, CA: Wadsworth Publishing.

Peppers, D., & Rogers, M. (1993). *The one to one future: Building relationships one customer at a time.* New York: Currency Doubleday.

Reilly, R. (1987). *Public relations in action.* 2nd ed. Englewood Cliffs, NJ: Prentice-Hall.

Ries, A., & Trout, J. (1993). *The 22 immutable laws of marketing.* New York: HarperBusiness.

Sewell, C., & Brown, P. (1990). *Customers for life.* New York: Pocket Books.

Tracy, B. (1995). *Advanced selling strategies.* New York: Simon & Schuster.

Whitely, R. (1991). *The customer driven company: Moving from talk to action.* Reading, MA: Addison-Wesley.

CHAPTER 58

Corporate Reorganization

Bernard R. Lorenz

Corporate reorganization is becoming increasingly more attractive to many home health agencies as they strive to expand services, meet new competition, and operate more efficiently. In many instances, Medicare cost reimbursement can be made more accurate and supportable, to the advantage of the agency.

This chapter discusses how agencies should structure themselves in a cost-based system of reimbursement. The implementation of any prospective payment system will almost certainly change how Medicare affects corporate structures. The specific incentives and disincentives that would come with prospective pay system cannot be adequately addressed until legislation is enacted. Home health agencies, however, should weigh the possibility of prospective payment when considering a corporate reorganization.

Reorganization also offers the potential to provide a number of in-home services that are not reimbursed by Medicare but for which there appears to be an increasing need. These include, but are not necessarily limited to, the following:

- infusion therapy
- medical equipment
- private duty nursing
- homemakers
- personal care
- home management
- companion services
- chore services
- medical day care
- child care

Integration and segregation of a home health agency's goals and objectives are vital in establishing and prospering in an integrated health care environment. Home health agencies are expanding into new lines of business for the purpose of being able to provide an integrated system of patient care. As populations grow and demographics change, the organizations that are able to offer a full range of health care services will be most likely to prosper and survive in the industry. As a result, it should be every home health agency's goal to provide a diverse mix of services to meet the demands of this growing and changing population.

The costs of reorganizing the corporate structure are not allowable costs, according to Medicare rules. These types of costs are allowable when starting up an agency and include legal fees incurred in establishing the corporation or other organization (such as drafting the corporate charter and by-laws, legal agreements, minutes of organizational meeting, terms of original stock certificates), necessary accounting fees, expenses of temporary directors and organizational meetings of directors and stockholders, and fees paid to states for incorporation. (Section 2134, Provider Reimbursement Manual, Part I.) However, the Provider Reimbursement

Manual states that Medicare considers the same type of costs incurred in a reorganization to be nonallowable because "they duplicate an entity's original organization costs." (Section 2134.10, Provider Reimbursement Manual, Part I.)

Being able to establish such an organization is a long-term process. All home health agencies need to create new and expand existing types of health care services. Home care has been the fastest-growing part of the health care industry for the past 20 years. All projections for the future point to an increased growth in the home health industry, and it is projected to be the fastest-growing part of the health care industry in the future.

There are many benefits agencies may realize by expanding their existing home care services. These areas are as follows:

1. **Maintaining Flexibility.** A home health agency should always have the flexibility to meet the demands of the growing and changing population. Providers that have the foresight and flexibility to meet the demands of the elderly population will be the most likely to prosper. Health care and home health care are becoming market-driven industries. Patients are now becoming much more active in the decision-making process of choosing a health care provider. By expanding their home care services, agencies will be able to provide high quality of care at a low cost to these patients.

   In order to provide the highest level of care to patients, health care organizations are being required to stay with patients over a longer period of time. During this time, the patient's needs and required services change. The patient may need a diverse range of services, including home health, mental health, therapy, and social services. An integrated health system should be able to provide all types of services that a patient demands. These services are not only the acute care that a hospital provides, but also home health care, the ability to provide durable medical equipment in the home, and other high-technology care. Expanding home care services will improve an agency's relationship with its physicians and patients in a long-term relationship that is rewarding for the physicians, patients, and agency.

2. **Advances in Technology.** The industry has also seen tremendous advances in technology over the past several years. As technology improves, the provider is able to render a higher-quality product. Other providers are now looking into enhancing the quality of life and care to patients by using this improved technology. Agencies will be required to use this technology in home care and their integrated system to maintain a competitive edge.

   Many providers of integrated services are being influenced by physicians to provide a very high quality of care. The providers realize that in order to accomplish this, they must increase the types of services and use new technology in their integrated system. The fragmentation of the various levels of services such as mental health, social services, and health care prohibits many providers from producing the level of care that physicians require. Also, the fragmentation of these services results in cost inefficiencies and duplication of administration and overhead costs and efforts.

   Many agencies are becoming increasingly involved in higher-technology care. These technologies involve chemotherapy, dialysis, antibiotic therapy, etc. The patient in such high-technology home care programs benefits by having a hospital involved. This enables the patient to remain in touch with the hospital in case more sophisticated medical technology is needed.

   Many patients are choosing integrated health care systems that offer hospice care because it not only enables them to have the availability of more sophisticated technology as a backup, but it also enables them to control the quality of their lives. Expansion of these home care programs to include these services has enabled many providers to maintain better relationships with patients, physicians, and managed care networks as well as to enhance patient care.

3. **Financial Benefits.** Providing care within an integrated health system has enabled agencies to increase their revenue. Not only are they increasing their revenue, but by emphasizing home care, they are getting more involved in another rapidly growing revenue stream. Home care has been the fastest-growing revenue stream for many delivery systems for the past 20 years.

This revenue stream will also be accompanied by additional expense. But by being able to provide an integrated system, many of the administrative expenses that are incurred by fragmented health care services are saved (i.e., they are not duplicated in an integrated environment). Hospitals can realize gains or reduce losses by moving patients within the integrated system. For instance, the patient can move out of a higher-cost inpatient service level of care to a less expensive level of care in the delivery system.

Hospitals realize greater control over patient flow. The more services that are provided within an integrated system, the greater the opportunity for the organization to maximize the use of administrative and overhead expenses for other revenue streams. The emphasis on increasing home health volume provides a tremendous opportunity for hospitals in that the hospital may allocate overhead expenses by reallocating costs to the cost-reimbursed services.

Another financial benefit is that an integrated system can benefit by economies of scale. Usually, the administrative expense of larger organizations is allocated to larger revenue streams. Also, the risk of having these administrative expenses in one health care service provider presents a greater risk of loss. This risk is spread when an integrated environment exists.

4. **Increased Market Share.** There is a tremendous amount of competition occurring in the health care industry. By becoming part of an integrated delivery system, agencies increase patient flow and keep patients within the integrated system, thereby increasing market share. Many patients will enter into the integrated system because they are attracted by the full level of care provided in the system.

Home health agencies become more attractive to managed care or HMOs by being able to provide a full level of care. A hospital, for example, that cannot provide a wide range of services may have to refer a patient to another external integrated organization. This integrated organization may provide a comprehensive level of service that the patient may like. This patient may decide to stay with the integrated system because the hospital was unable to provide a full level of care.

Many physicians expect health care organizations to be able to provide a wide range of services in an efficient manner. Physicians look very favorably upon a provider that is able to provide cost-effective services. Physicians are also attracted to organizations that are financially stable.

The decision to reorganize or restructure a home health agency must be based on careful study and strategic planning, which includes an analysis of community demographics, the agency's competition, and its goals and objectives; the last of these should be projected for at least five years. The agency's analysis must consist of projections for every service the market will support, anticipated market share, anticipated levels of changes, and expected costs. An operation budget must then be prepared to determine the potential profitability of each service and the cash flow that can be realized from it. Projections must be constructed for different volumes of services and changes in costs and charges to determine what effect they will have on profitability.

An ideal organization would meet the needs of long-range goals while providing sufficient flexibility to respond to new opportunities and to meet the competition as it arises. The variety of corporate structures available to approach the ideal is almost unlimited. Most, however, fall into two categories: the single corporate organization and the multicorporate organization.

SINGLE CORPORATE ORGANIZATIONS

Single corporate organizations, as their name implies, are the simplest type of organizational arrangement. They are a single legal entity, usually a corporation.

Single corporate organizations have several advantages. They are the least expensive to establish; they require only one corporation, one management group, and one accounting system; and lines of authority are clear. In addition, issues and problems relate to only one corporation, and additions and deletions of services can be made without creating too many problems.

There also are several disadvantages to single corporate organizations. Those that are Medicare certified find that all their operations are affected by government control through Medicare and Medicaid regulations. Hence lines of business that are not covered by government programs cannot be separated from those that are. Consequently, allocations of costs, especially administrative and general costs, using federally prescribed methods may be disadvantageous, and assignment of costs to various activities may not be as clear or defensible as they would be with a more definitive separation of program entities. Although it is true that Medicare does have some provisions for discrete cost finding, it is usually easier to justify the allocation of costs among different corporations than among different departments within one corporation.

MULTICORPORATE ORGANIZATIONS

The most common and simplistic form of a multicorporate organization consists of a parent corporation with two or more subsidiaries, depending on the size and complexity of the agency. The parent company provides overall management and some centralized administrative services such as human resources, accounting, billing and collections, management information systems, and so forth. The subsidiary companies provide the different medical and other services. For example, one subsidiary could provide the traditional home health services for Medicare, Medicaid, private insurance, and self-payers, and another could provide services not covered by federal programs. Another possible division of services would be cost-reimbursed versus non–cost reimbursed payers, which include private duty nursing, homemaker services, personal services, chore services, and the like.

There are several advantages to the multicorporate organization. First, it provides greater flexibility in operations because each corporation has its own separate legal entity, its own board of directors, its own accounting system, its own assets and liabilities, and its own financial statements. As more services are provided by the group of entities, more corporations can be added without disturbing the others. Costs can be more accurately charged against the services for which they were incurred, and allocations can be better recognized and defended. Where services are provided by related organizations, charges can be assessed between or among them. Although Medicare will substitute costs for charges for reimbursement purposes, charges are still important. Furthermore, the allocation of general and administrative costs will be clearer and more accurate because usually only the costs of the parent corporation need to be allocated. The administrative costs of each subsidiary remain within it. Finally, costs in the parent corporation that are directly allocated to the subsidiary can be directly allocated before cost finding.

Multicorporate organizations are not without their disadvantages. These begin with the costs of organizing the multiple corporations, which are much greater because everything that must be done for one must be done for all of them. In relating to one another, the entities must always remember that they are separate as well as related, and accounting and information systems must adhere to that fact.

In the event that a provider becomes a different entity in the reorganization, a change of ownership occurs. This requires that all things related to change of ownership be done (this is not usually recommended). Another problem is that staff, clients, and providers of service to the agency can become confused by the diversification. The accounting for transactions among corporations, for transfers of assets, and for the services provided can become complex and confusing. This can be reduced, however, by decentralizing management to the maximum feasible extent.

If any of the corporations is not-for-profit, great care must be taken to ensure that there are no violations of the inurement of benefit requirements for maintaining that status, especially with grants and contracts. Violations could result in loss of the tax-exempt status. Care also must be taken to account for any unrelated business income earned by the tax-exempt organizations.

CONCLUSION

There is no easy answer for any organization concerning corporate diversification. It is important for the agency to research all the possibilities of corporate reorganization but not to copy the ideas of any other organization. The agency must start with its goals and objectives and the best way of achieving them. There are no easy answers, and the agency should review this carefully from a financial viewpoint as well as from many others. The financial, management, and other benefits of diversification must be clearly seen before the agency embarks on such a large project. Also, the projections generated in the decision process can be used as a management tool in monitoring the progress of the diversified entities.

CHAPTER 59

An Experience in Diversification

Mary Ann Keirans

INTRODUCTION

In this era of managed care and changes in Medicare and Medical Assistance, many home health providers are looking for new ways to maximize payment from their cost-reimbursed product lines while responding to the demands for lower prices by insurance companies and business coalitions. Diversification can provide home health agencies with new opportunities as they cope with these challenges. However, some agencies are considering diversification without really evaluating what they want to accomplish or studying the methods of fulfilling these goals without diversifying. This chapter relates the experiences of a voluntary, nonprofit home health agency and its decision to diversify. A brief review of the agency's history is necessary to convey why the diversification route was chosen.

WHY WE DECIDED TO DIVERSIFY

The Visiting Nurse Association/Home-Health Services (formerly known as Home-Health Services of Luzerne County) is located in the northeastern part of Pennsylvania. The agency was started in 1908 by a group of local citizens who were concerned about the health and sanitary conditions of the community, especially among the families who had immigrated to the Wyoming Valley area of Pennsylvania to work in the local coal mines. The Visiting Nurse Association developed a reputation for excellent services and quickly became a primary caregiver in the health and social services delivery system.

Over the decades, the agency changed in response to community needs. These changes were spontaneous rather than planned occurrences. The board of directors was composed of numerous volunteers from the community who, according to ancient board minutes, had as their primary responsibility the financial stability of the organization. The board of directors was involved in continuous fund-raising campaigns, and the professional staff concentrated their efforts on the care of patients under the direction of the superintendent of nurses.

The primary sources of funding for the Visiting Nurse Association in the early days were the fees collected from patients for services rendered and funds raised by the board of directors or allocated to the agency through the Community Chest, which later became the United Way. The blessing of program flexibility was constantly thwarted by limited financial resources. Despite this difficulty, the Visiting Nurse Association continued to flourish and to respond to the changing health care needs of the people in the community it served.

In the early 1950s the first major changes occurred in the Visiting Nurse Association. The original agency merged with another Visiting Nurse Association from a nearby town to strengthen and coordinate the work of both agencies. A third Visiting Nurse Association joined the other two in the late 1950s, and men began serving on the agency's board of directors for the first time in its history.

When the Medicare program was introduced in Congress in the early 1960s, the board of directors actively supported passage of the legislation because Medicare was expected to take care of paying for services for all the needs of the elderly. If government money could be used for that purpose, the board of directors would be able to concentrate its fund-raising efforts on the needs of the nonelderly population and would be assured of a degree of financial stability for their organization.

The Visiting Nurse Association had had limited experiences with third-party reimbursement. Funding from insurance companies such as the Metropolitan Life or John Hancock programs had existed but was limited in scope and had few regulations about service delivery. After the Visiting Nurse Association became a Medicare provider, the board of directors became interested in expanding the scope of the agency's programs from just nursing and physical therapy to the full gamut of Medicare-allowable services. It was decided that a home health aide program, speech therapy, social work, and eventually occupational therapy would become parts of the Visiting Nurse Association's menu of services. At the same time the local Welfare Planning Council was encouraging mergers of organizations that had similar purposes.

The Visiting Nurse Association and the local Homemaker Services began to talk about a merger. The agency was also encouraged to merge with the two remaining small Visiting Nurse Associations in the county. In 1971 the first of a series of mergers took place, creating the new agency, which was known as Home-Health Services of Luzerne County. This new name was chosen to reflect the broad array of services available and to remind the community

that the focus of the agency had changed from nursing care to the total health care needs of the homebound population in the area. Expansion was rapid, with new programs being added on a regular basis. Geographical territory was increased until a countywide service covering approximately 1,300 square miles was achieved.

With the new structure, most of the professional services were reimbursable under the Medicare program, but it quickly became evident that the homemaker program, which primarily provided care to the chronically ill, would not be sustained through Medicare funding. The Wyoming Valley area experienced flooding after Hurricane Agnes in 1972 and had resources made available to it for service delivery programs that were unique in nature. Unfortunately, these funds were also temporary in nature. As flood recovery dollars were expended, the organization found itself in the unique position of having developed a large chronic care delivery system as a part of its Medicare-certified home health agency. The program was extremely popular among the elderly of the community, but it lacked an adequate funding source to support it.

The skilled services section of the organization had grown in size and complexity, causing the cost of the homemaker program also to increase to a point where chronic care services could not be offered on a private-pay basis at a price that was affordable by the average citizen in need of the services. Therefore, with great reluctance and a significant deficit, the agency discontinued its homemaker program and experienced the first layoffs in its history.

From the mid-1970s until the early 1980s, the Visiting Nurse Association concentrated on perfecting its professional health care services to the community. The agency had grown from a staff of fewer than 20 employees to more than 100 employees in a decade. Funding that had once been more than 80% United Way allocations reversed to being more than 80% Medicare reimbursement. The caseload changed in composition from maternal and child health care and care of patients with communicable diseases to an emphasis on service for the acutely ill, homebound, geriatric patient. Even the procedures performed by the nursing staff had changed in intensity, requiring the development of more sophisticated continuing education programs. The direction of the agency was no longer provided by a superintendent of nurses but rather by a team of specialists under the direction of an administrator. The qualification for the administrative function was no longer "an experienced nurse of fine repute" but rather a master's-prepared individual with extensive experience in home health administration.

The composition of the board of directors and its responsibilities also changed. The role of fund-raiser was traded for the role of policy maker. Accountability, compliance with regulations, cost analysis, personnel policies, patient rights, professional liability insurance, and other business topics became the focus of the board's agenda.

In the late 1970s the board of directors and administrative staff looked at the agency's history and realized that growth and program development had occurred through spontaneous reactions to community needs rather than through a process of business planning. Therefore, a long-range planning committee was created to help guide the organization's future development. One of the first documents reviewed by the committee, after a demographic analysis had been completed, was the agency's mission statement. The committee realized that the agency was not fulfilling its commitment to the chronically ill as stated in the agency's purpose. The members recommended to the board of directors that the organization either should change its mission statement or should find a way of serving this unmet need in the community. In response to this recommendation, an ad hoc committee was established to study the issue. An extensive survey of community resources revealed that programs existed for care of the chronically ill who were of a low income level and that resources existed for the

wealthy who could afford to pay the going rate for services from private agencies but that nothing existed in the community for the population between these two extremes.

CHOOSING A MODEL

After the need was determined, the board of directors and administrative staff had many lengthy discussions regarding the agency's responsibility to fulfill this need. The past experiences with a homemaker program under the auspices of the home health agency and the deficits that resulted from the care of the chronically ill caused the board of directors to be extremely cautious when considering the reestablishment of such a program. It was finally decided that the agency did have an obligation to fill the unmet community need if a way could be found to do it in a financially viable fashion.

At this stage in the decision-making process, the board of directors hired a consulting firm to advise the board on its various options. The board had previously decided that an in-depth marketing study performed by consultants would be too expensive to absorb. Therefore, administrative staff were assigned to perform a marketing survey on the feasibility of starting a homemaker program for the chronically ill using the caseload of the Visiting Nurse component of the agency as the population to be studied. The role of the consultants hired by the board of directors was limited to the legal structures available for consideration and the reimbursement impact of each of these structures on both the existing acute care program and the projected chronic care program.

Four corporate structures were studied in depth with the consultants. The first was the foundation model, which was rejected by the board of directors because it did not desire to commit itself to a specific volume of fund-raising annually. The second model studied was the holding company model. This model was also rejected by the board of directors because it had decided that each of the corporations involved in the restructuring would be nonprofit 501(C)(3) agencies, so that there would be no stock to be held by a holding company. The third model presented was a management corporation. This model satisfied the desires of the board of directors in the sense that it provided a logical structure for having two subsidiary corporations controlled by one management company.

The last structure studied was creating a chronic care component within the existing home health agency. This model was also rejected by the board of directors because of concern that the history of the organization could be repeated and that a chronic care program that was not financially viable could have adverse effects on the future of the home health agency. Before this concept was rejected, however, the methods of discrete cost analysis were carefully explored. The administrative staff were confident that they could avoid many of the previously encountered financial pitfalls through the use of the sophisticated accounting methods currently available. In the past, the agency had neither the knowledge nor the staff to utilize these tools. The administrative staff also recommended, however, that the acute care and chronic care programs be separately organized because the service philosophies of the two programs were different. The Visiting Nurse Association services were medically necessary and, therefore, were provided to all in need regardless of ability to pay for the services. A homemaker program was socially necessary and, in some cases, a luxury service. People might be less comfortable or less independent without the service, but they could survive without it. Implementing these different philosophies required different management techniques that were easier to accomplish in separate corporations. In addition, types of employees, training programs, personnel policies, and salary levels could be developed to suit the market of each corporation when separate organizations existed.

FUNDING CONSIDERATIONS

Now that the agency knew what it wanted to do and how it wanted to set up the structure, the remaining piece of the plan—how to fund the chronic care portion of the total program—remained to be solved. Because the home health agency was serving a large population of patients, it was felt that surveying current recipients and recently discharged patients or their families would provide the agency with sufficient data to determine whether a homemaker program could be financially viable in the community. The administrative staff developed a brief but concise survey instrument and taught the professional staff how to use it for interviewing current service recipients. The same tool was also mailed to patients or families of individuals discharged from the home health agency during the past 6 months. A total of 827 surveys were returned and tabulated for presentation to the board of directors. Included in this survey tool were questions regarding the need for services to supplement the skilled services provided by the home health agency, including its home health aide program; questions regarding the need for personal care assistance and homemaking help after discharge from the agency's skilled service component; and questions regarding the volume of services desired on a weekly basis and the fee that the individual would be willing to pay for such a program.

The results confirmed the fact that the population surveyed was highly interested in having homemaker services available as a supplement to the other services provided by the home health agency and that the clients wanted bathing as well as homemaker services to continue after the Medicare-certified agency discharged the patient. The survey also confirmed, however, that most patients desired to pay a fee lower than the one established by a budget projection as necessary to cover the cost of the program.

The survey results were logical and had been anticipated because northeast Pennsylvania has a large percentage of elderly who need help; most of the elderly in this segment of the state, however, are living on fixed incomes and are not wealthy. Because the Visiting Nurse Association was a United Way Member Agency, it received an allocation for supporting those skilled services that were not reimbursable under third-party payment. It used a sliding fee scale based on ability to pay to determine the patient's financial obligation for services whenever United Way funds were needed to supplement the patient's payment.

The United Way was asked for support for the homemaker program. A small portion of the Visiting Nurse Association's allocation was being used for care of the chronically ill. The cost of providing this service through the Medicare-certified agency's aide component was considerably higher than that projected for services under the homemaker agency. The United Way therefore agreed to shift this portion of the Visiting Nurse Association's allocation to the new program and to help the agency with the start-up expenses. It was decided that the target population would be the individual in the community who was unable to afford private pay rates and who was not eligible for services through other state-sponsored programs. As a nonprofit agency, the financial goal was to cover costs and to generate cash reserves to sustain the agency for the normal turnover period between billing and receipt of payment. It was estimated that it would take two years for volume to build up to the point where break-even occurred.

The financial consultants made numerous recommendations to the board of directors' committee regarding the structure of the organization, billing practices to be followed, documentation requirements, and the importance of good customer relations. It was recognized from the start that the philosophy of service delivery in the homemaker agency had to be considerably different from that of the Visiting Nurse Association, where all patients were served regardless of ability to pay. The homemaker agency would need to limit its free and partial-pay services to the size of the annual United Way allocation. In addition, bad debt situations could not be tolerated.

THE LEGAL ASPECTS

The ad hoc committee of the board of directors presented its findings to the full board approximately two years after the study was initiated. A number of board meetings were devoted to reviewing the committee's findings and recommendations. Finally, the board of directors voted in favor of diversification using the management corporation model. The legal work then began. It was decided that the ad hoc committee would become the incorporators for the two new organizations: the management company and the homemaker services.

It was decided that the management corporation would be called Home-Care Management of Luzerne County, with the two subsidiary organizations being called Homemaker Services of Luzerne County and Home-Health Services of Luzerne County. The home health program had as its mission statement the provision of skilled services and home health aide services to the acutely ill, homebound members of the community, a responsibility for health education and health screening, and the provision of professional services to other segments of the community. The homemaker agency, on the other hand, was clearly identified in its mission statement to be responsible for provision of homemaker, personal care, and companion services to the chronically ill segment of the community. The management corporation had as its sole purpose the provision of management services, including financial, marketing, and public relations services, to its two subsidiary corporations and to any of the corporations that the board of directors might determine to be appropriate to add in the future.

Articles of incorporation for the management corporation and the homemaker agency were filed in the Commonwealth of Pennsylvania. Bylaws were drafted and adopted by the incorporators. The incorporators also decided how the board of directors was to be divided. The original board of directors consisted of 30 individuals; therefore, it was decided that 10 individuals would serve on each of the three corporations, with the officers of the two subsidiary corporations also serving on the management corporation board. Therefore, the subsidiary corporations each had boards comprising 10 people, with the management corporation board comprising 18 people. A singular nominating committee for all three corporations now exists at the management corporation level, budgets for the subsidiary corporations must be approved by the management corporation's board of directors, and the bylaws of the subsidiary organizations cannot be changed without the approval of the management corporation. Because of the structure desired by the board of directors, it was decided that the subsidiary corporations would be related parties and that any services sold by Homemaker Services of Luzerne County to the Medicare-certified home health agency would be done at cost. Filings were made with the Internal Revenue Service for all three corporations requesting a continuation of the 501(C)(3) status of the home health agency and establishment of a 501(C)(3) status for the two new corporations. These requests were approved approximately seven months after filing.

CONCLUSION

On February 1, 1984, the management corporation became functional. Four individuals from the Visiting Nurse Association were terminated in that agency and were hired by Home-Care Management of Luzerne County. These four individuals were the administrator, the director of financial affairs, the director of marketing and public relations, and the executive secretary. It was decided that the salary and benefits of these individuals would be the same as they were in the home health agency and that the personnel policies of the home health agency would be adopted for the management corporation. Separate groups needed to be established in the home health agency's pension and health plans to accommodate the employees of the management corporation.

The following month, Homemaker Services of Luzerne County started. A nurse from the home health agency was hired as the manager of the homemaker corporation. She developed a training plan for the homemaker/personal attendants and interviewed, hired, and trained the first group of part-time workers. The title homemaker/personal attendant was chosen to distinguish these employees from the home health aides employed by the home health agency because of salary differences. Consideration was given to developing contracts between the two subsidiaries for home health aide services, but it was decided not to take that action in the homemaker corporation's formative stage. Because the subsidiaries were related parties, Homemaker Services of Luzerne County would only be able to charge its cost for aides to Home-Health Services of Luzerne County on a contract basis. This did not offer an economic advantage to either party because the home health agency was well below the Medicare cost cap for aide services and had no need to reduce its aide costs. The homemaker corporation would require more administrative staff if its initial volume was too great; therefore, it would not have a lower cost for its private-pay clients by contracting to provide aide services to the home health agency. In addition, it was felt that the homemaker corporation needed time to develop expertise in its management functions before extensive growth occurred.

Because of these decisions, the initial caseload for the homemaker program consisted of 15 patients transferred from the home health agency to the homemaker agency. All these individuals had completed their need for skilled services but still required assistance in personal care. They had been taken off the Medicare program and were personally responsible for paying for their nonskilled care.

Homemaker Services of Luzerne County offered three programs: personal care, help with household chores, and companion services. The fee for these services was set at $6.50/hour. Because this fee was considerably less than that charged by the home health agency for private-pay clients, the patients were able either to save money by being transferred to the homemaker program or to purchase additional hours of services. A sliding fee scale based upon income is used to ensure proper utilization of United Way resources and to provide equitable guidelines for adjusting client charges when necessary. Home-Care Management of Luzerne County generates its income by charging the two subsidiary corporations for its services. This means that each employee of the management corporation must maintain an elaborate time record on a daily basis. In the beginning it was difficult for the management corporation employees to get used to continuous timekeeping, but after a few months the task became routine. Funding for the home health agency did not change with the diversification.

The cost of accomplishing the diversification, excluding administrative staff and board time, was approximately $15,000. To provide cash flow for the homemaker corporation from the time of start-up until the point at which break-even volume was developed, a line of credit of $25,000 was established at a local bank using the home health agency's resources as collateral. The total of $40,000 was considered a reasonable amount to risk on the new venture.

It is almost 13 years since diversification took place. Frequently, we are asked whether the effort was worth it. Our response is always a resounding "Yes!" We feel strongly that diversification was the answer for our agency. We knew what we wanted to do, and we knew why we wanted to do it. Diversification was the only way in which our company could accomplish its objectives. The home health agency, now known as the Visiting Nurse Association (VNA)/Health Services, was not changed by the diversification. Our United Way resources and contributions are being used for more people and for more hours of client care.

The greatest advantage from diversification, however, is that a previously unmet community need is being filled. Homemaker Services of Luzerne County, now known as VNA/Personal Care of Luzerne County, provided 11,536 hours of help during the first nine months of its operations; 30,402 hours of care were provided in the following calendar year, and last fiscal year it broke the 110,000-hour mark. Most important, thousands of people have received help from the homemaker program over the past 13 years, and the agency has developed a reputation for its caring and its quality services.

The management corporation model is a comfortable one for our structure and provides us with a parent corporation that has a functional purpose that can be expanded as needed. This structure also enabled the VNA to maintain maximum autonomy in its service delivery companies after the VNA became an affiliate of the Wyoming Valley Health Care System on January 1, 1994. In addition, we are in a position to add additional subsidiary corporations with minimal cost and effort if we desire to take advantage of new opportunities to expand our service line. Late in 1994, it was decided that the Wyoming Valley Health Care System needed a hospice program to round out its service offerings. Since most hospice services are provided in the home setting, the VNA was given the opportunity to develop the program. Because of our diversified structure, another company, Hospice Care of the VNA of Luzerne County, was started and is a wholly owned subsidiary of VNA/Management Services. An experienced Director was hired and the first patients were admitted to the program just three months after the corporate paperwork was completed. Ten months into its history, this subsidiary added a nine-bed inpatient unit to its care options. One of the reasons why so much was able to be accomplished in such a short period of time, in addition to hiring the right personnel, was that the new company had the resources of the diversified structure to help support it through its start-up period.

The health care delivery system of the future will include an emphasis on the long-term care needs of the county's growing elderly population. The unknown is how those services will be paid for. It is also obvious that prospective pay and managed care will change the reimbursement method for acute home health care services. The traditional methods of caring for the sick and elderly in a home setting are changing. The simple fact that an agency is flexible and able to respond to change quickly will be of great value as we learn to work with the case managers and eldercare brokers of the future.

At our VNA we believe that we are positioned to respond to these challenges with our diversified structure until the time comes when cost reimbursement is nothing more than a memory and it is time to once again evaluate our options.

CHAPTER 60

The Process of Visiting Nurse Association Affiliation with a Major Teaching Hospital

Marilyn D. Harris

Affiliation among agencies with differing staff, resources, organizational structures, policies, and programs is never easy. This chapter discusses major components of an affiliation between a Visiting Nurse Association (VNA) and its former competitor: a major teaching hospital.

The VNA of Eastern Montgomery County was no stranger to corporate restructures. It had successfully completed five restructures since it was founded in 1919. Although I focus on the hospital affiliation in 1988, some comments apply to the three restructures that occurred since I became the director of the agency.

In 1988, the VNA was a voluntary, certified accredited home health agency and hospice that provided in-home and community health services. The VNA received referrals from physicians, hospitals, community agencies, and individuals.

Abington Memorial Hospital (AMH), a 500-bed teaching hospital, opened its doors in 1913. It established a home care department in 1979. Home care services were made available through contracts with certified agencies for all disciplines. Occupational and physical therapy services were also offered through the hospital's rehabilitation department. In 1988, the hospital had a home care director, five home care coordinators, and support staff. Although informal discussions had taken place for several years and the VNA was the hospital's contractor for home care service, formal discussions regarding affiliation did not begin until 1985.

During June 1985, when affiliation discussions began, the VNA provided services to patients referred by multiple hospitals and physicians. Staff made 4,685 visits to 646 individuals. Referrals from AMH resulted in 1,765 visits (37% of total) to 236 individuals (36% of total). The VNA had 76.6 full-time equivalent employees and made 59,294 home visits during the fiscal year.

Although the VNA was a financially sound organization when discussions began in 1985, 1988 was a deficit year. This was due in part to the large percentage of fixed-rate, rather than cost-based, reimbursement from the VNA's contract with the hospital while the negotiations were taking place.

THE NEGOTIATION PROCESS

The VNA board received a formal letter from AMH's administrators in July 1985 outlining a proposal for merger. The board met to discuss the letter, and several VNA board members and the administrative staff scheduled a meeting

Source: Reprinted with permission from M.D. Harris, The Process of Visiting Nurse Associaton Affiliation with a Major Teaching Hospital, *Journal of Nursing Administration*, Vol. 22, No. 7-8, pp. 51–60, © 1992, J.B. Lippincott Company.

with the hospital's executive vice president (EVP) and vice president for nursing to discuss the proposal. The hospital's president, EVP, and comptroller were invited to meet with the VNA board. After this meeting, an ad hoc committee including legal counsel was formed with representatives from the VNA and AMH. Regularly scheduled meetings were held with established agendas.

One of the first tasks was discussing the options available to the hospital and the VNA. There were at least four options for the VNA: to remain as is (i.e., the hospital would expand its own program and compete with the VNA); merger (dissolution of its present entity and a merger into one agency with the hospital); a joint venture with the hospital, where each organization would keep its own identity; or affiliation with a division of services. The options for AMH were to expand its existing home care department separate from the VNA or to consider an affiliation with the VNA. The advantages and disadvantages of each option had to be identified.

From the start, both organizations felt that the VNA should continue to provide service to those patients who were referred by others in the community, including hospitals and physicians. There was concern that other facilities and referral sources might be reluctant to refer to the VNA if skilled service were offered through AMH (i.e., fear of loss of control of patients). Therefore, this issue was one of the topics for discussion. As of 1997, the VNA continues to receive one third of its referrals from other agencies/facilities.

The VNA also addressed the financial impact that any decision would have on its funding sources. The executive director (ED) contacted the United Way, Office on Aging, and municipal managers to determine what effect, if any, the various corporate structures would have on current and future funding. Certifying and accrediting agencies were also contacted to discuss the impact of restructuring. The VNA management staff determined that the least adverse

effects were associated with the affiliation option.

Meanwhile, in 1986, while discussions were taking place with AMH, the VNA completed a planned internal corporate restructure. A parent company, VNA-Health Management Services (VNA-HMS), was formed with two subsidiaries, the VNA (the Medicare-certified home health agency) and VNA-Community Services, Inc. (VNA-CS), to provide the support and health promotion services. The three VNAs had separate boards of directors but shared the same administrative staff through a management agreement. A lease was established for rental space between the corporations that were housed in the same office buildings. This fact is mentioned because this internal corporate restructure with the resulting division of health care services was important in light of the decision made to affiliate the VNA with the hospital in 1988.

THE DECISION-MAKING PROCESS

The VNA and AMH mutually agreed to use a health care consulting firm to assist with data collection and analysis. The anticipated benefits of a cooperative effort were as follows:

- combined effort of two well-respected organizations
- continuation of needed patient services in a coordinated manner
- ability of the VNA again to realize costs for services by discipline rather than a fixed rate
- ability of AMH to maximize reimbursement
- opportunities for expansion of in-home and community services

The ad hoc committee met again after receipt of the consultant's report. Although the consultant recommended a community-based agency, the hospital administration determined that it would retain a hospital-based agency. Hospital administrators believed that a hospital-based agency would be financially beneficial because home care is reimbursed on a cost basis. A time frame was established for the VNA board to share its decision with hospital administration. The VNA board, in cooperation with the administrative staff, made the decision to affiliate the VNA services and personnel with the hospital. VNA-CS would remain a free-standing community-based agency with its own board of directors.

The VNA administrative staff developed a list of operational issues that were to be included in the affiliation agreement. These included use of the VNA's organizational chart, computer system, fiscal intermediary (FI), professional advisory committee, policy and procedure manual, and name. After legal counsel for both organizations finalized the agreement, the boards of the three VNAs approved the agreement on February 16, 1988. The hospital's board of trustees approved the agreement the following week.

THE TRANSITION PROCESS

The transition period between February 25 and May 31, 1988, was very busy. In addition to the day-to-day operations of the three VNAs, the administrative staff had 30 meetings with hospital staff to facilitate the smooth transfer as of June 1, 1988. The reasons for meeting with the various departments are summarized below.

Nursing Administration

In 1988, the hospital's home care department director reported to the nursing department's business manager. As of June 1, 1988, the director would report to the hospital's EVP and chief operating officer. Many meetings were held to make sure that all the necessary details were completed. There was a good working relationship with the nursing department as we addressed personnel, clinical records, physical space, and the need for a smooth transition of patient care from one to another. Much time was devoted to the placement of existing home care personnel within the new home care department.

One major project was combining two policy and procedure manuals and obtaining approval of the professional advisory committee. The professional advisory committees of both organizations had overlapping membership. The existing VNA professional advisory committee membership was expanded to include the hospital's members.

Social Service Department

Before the affiliation, two discharge planning nurses reported to the director of the social service department. One of the terms of the affiliation was that these two nurses plus three additional nurses responsible for the nursing aspect of discharge planning would report to the VNA. Numerous meetings were held with the director of social services and the director of professional service (DPS) at the VNA to develop mutually acceptable policies and procedures that identified areas of responsibilities. The entire discharge planning process at the hospital has experienced several changes over the past few years and the nurses have not reported to the VNA for several years.

It is imperative that administrative level personnel be aware of the sensitive nature of positions that overlap or have similar areas of responsibilities.

Therapy Department

The VNA provided all therapy services through contracts. The hospital's home care department had, in addition to purchasing services from the VNA, purchased service from the hospital's occupational and physical therapy departments. The therapists were assigned to the home care department on a rotating basis. The VNA agreed to continue with this arrangement, although most services would still be provided through contract service because of the shortage of staff therapists.

Medical Record Committee

All clinical record forms must be approved by the hospital's medical record committee.

This meant that all the VNA forms had to be reviewed by this committee. Forms were sent to the committee chair, who circulated them to members. The ED, DPS, and supervisor for quality assessment (QA) attended the meeting to explain the forms and answer questions.

The administrative staff also met with the director of the hospital's medical record department to review the current record system and format, the storage of closed records, and the requirements to meet Joint Commission on Accreditation of Healthcare Organizations (Joint Commission) standards. The VNA record format remained the same. The closed records are stored off site, in keeping with policy.

The VNA addressed the issue of custodian of the records as of May 31, 1988. The affiliation agreement included reference to clinical records. The hospital's medical record department agreed to accept, and the VNA board agreed to transfer, all active records with the effective date of the affiliation. All closed records were made available to the hospital.

The VNA also transferred active hospital home care patients to the VNA fiscal intermediary as of June 1, 1988. The hospital agreed to request an early transfer to the identified regional FI. This provided for continuity of clinical and billing aspects of care because the VNA was currently served by this FI. All these transactions were accomplished without major problems.

Pastoral Care

A meeting was scheduled with the ED, the DPS, and the assistant chaplain of the hospital to discuss how the VNA's certified hospice program would interface with the hospital's in-house program for terminally ill patients. We determined that the hospital's chaplains would not make home visits on a regular basis. Neither would the VNA's hospice chaplain follow patients when they were hospitalized. Continuity of care is provided through the hospice coordinator, who attends both the in-house palliative care team meetings and the VNA's hospice

interdisciplinary team meetings. In specific situations, the chaplain's visits may be interchangeable. The hospital's chaplain would continue to assist with the hospice's bereavement group meetings.

QA and Utilization Review

The VNA's QA program was extensive but had to be revised to meet Joint Commission and hospital standards. The ED, DPS, and QA supervisor attended several formal presentations on the Joint Commission standards and QA and met with the hospital's director of QA and the staff. The administrative and supervisory staff rewrote the QA policy and procedures, identified specific aspects of care to be monitored, identified indicators and thresholds, and revised our yearly calendar for reporting outcomes. The VNA's QA report is presented to the hospital's board of trustees quarterly through established committees. The VNA's DPS and discharge planner (DP) nurse supervisor participate in regularly scheduled, hospital-wide, multidisciplinary meetings to address the DP process and current utilization of hospital days.

The VNA has been accredited by the National League for Nursing (NLN), now the Community Health Accreditation Program (CHAP) since 1967. Although the agency was accustomed to the three-day site visits, we were apprehensive about the next visit because so much change had occurred. I am confident that we did an excellent job because the Joint Commission site visitor stated that the department was doing "too much" QA. At the exit conference, the hospital's EVP said he had never heard of any department doing "too much" QA.

Volunteers

The hospital had an active volunteer program. The VNA's hospice volunteer program is directed by our own volunteer director. Meetings were held several years ago to formalize policy and procedures to enable VNA volunteers to visit hospice patients who are admitted to the hospital. Arrangements were also in place to allow a hospice volunteer to begin visits while the patient is still in the hospital, if this is indicated (Harris & Groshens, 1985).

Additional meetings were held to update these procedures. Mutually agreeable procedures were implemented. To date, hospice volunteers have visited with patients at home and in the hospital. The VNA also had a friendly visitor program that was expanded to serve more patients. In 1996, a six-bed designated hospice unit was identified in the hospital. Hospice trained volunteers are available to be on the unit during the morning, afternoon, and evening hours.

Communications

Numerous meetings were held with the director of communications to discuss multiple issues. The VNA would continue to occupy two offices off the hospital campus. One office was located two blocks from the hospital. The second office was seven miles away from campus. The physical location of the DP nurses' office within the hospital was moved. Arrangements had to be made to increase the number of telephones and to change the location. The hospital's telephone directory was being updated, and the timing enabled the new numbers for all the DP nurses to be included. Arrangements were discussed for a future hook-up between the VNA's computers and the hospital computer system. Discussions were held to arrange for dedicated telephone lines when the hospital expanded its system.

Additional pocket pagers were ordered and air time was coordinated because the hospital and the VNA used different systems. It was cost-effective to purchase new beepers and to purchase air time from the hospital's system.

The hospital also initiated a voice mailbox system. The VNA was able to obtain voice mailboxes for most of its administrative staff, clinical supervisors, and all DP nurses. Staff nurses were added in November 1991. In 1997, this communication device has made it easy to accept and leave messages while decreasing telephone tag for staff and contractors.

Internal communications are an important part of the VNA operation. For several years, weekly announcements have been held at a specific time. The two VNA offices were equipped with speaker telephones so that the entire staff could hear. These weekly staff announcements are taped and transcribed and are made available on the bulletin boards for everyone to read. This method of communication continues even though all personnel are located in the same building, but in two separate offices since 1991.

Public Relations

The ED met with the director of public relations to discuss the current public relations activities and the procedures to be followed in the future. Discussions included public relations budget, news releases, articles, pictures, brochures, and handouts. Parameters were established for those activities that could be accomplished in-house and those that had to be done through freelance writers. Time frames were established for preparing new brochures and other promotional materials.

Fund-Raising

The VNA's ED and finance director met with the hospital's director of fund development to discuss the establishment of designated restricted funds specifically for the hospice program. The VNA's current fund-raising activities were also shared with the fund development director.

Personnel

The establishment of a good working relationship with the personnel department at the hospital was important before, during, and after the affiliation. Before a decision was made on the affiliation, it was important to meet with the vice president of human resources to share information about benefits available from both organizations and to make comparisons. It was important to bring the VNA benefits in line with the hospital's while seeking to preserve existing benefits (e.g., grandparenting employees at current levels). The hospital and the VNA made a comparative chart for review by the hospital's administration and the VNA's board. There was a genuine interest and concern from both organizations to preserve the best of both policies. This was accomplished to the satisfaction of both parties and the staff.

Once the decision had been made to affiliate and the VNA board had agreed to the benefits package, administrators communicated this decision to staff. The hospital's vice president of human resources and his staff met with VNA staff to review the details and answer questions. Before the meeting, information packets were distributed to all staff including information about the available hospitalization, dental plans, and other benefits. This meeting was beneficial because it enabled the VNA staff to meet with the personnel department staff and get direct answers to their questions.

Payroll

The hospital was changing from a weekly to an every other week payroll schedule to coincide with the planned affiliation. The VNA was already on a two-week pay schedule with a different service bureau. Therefore, the VNA continued to prepare its own payroll for approximately three months. The delay in the transfer to the hospital's system allowed time for the hospital to transfer its 2,500 employees to a new system without disrupting the VNA payroll. The VNA payroll transfer occurred as planned. There were some problems encountered, most of which were related to accrual of time benefits and deductions. These problems were resolved after several pay periods.

The VNA staff lost the benefit of direct deposit for several months because the hospital did not have this program in place. It was instituted by the hospital about six months later.

Hiring

As the director of a community-based agency, I had the authority to hire staff to fill budgeted positions. This process changed with the affiliation. The employment process is now the responsibility of the personnel department. Vacant positions must be posted in the hospital for five days. Internal applicants are given the opportunity to interview for a position. A classified ad is placed if no internal transfers are received.

At times, applicants apply at the VNA office. When this occurs, the applicant is given general information and asked to contact the hospital's personnel department to complete forms and discuss salary and benefits. Interviewing is done at the VNA by the DPS and supervisors. The VNA staff have the final decision on which of the applicants will be offered employment. Also, all new positions must be approved through the budgeting process.

Staff Orientation

All VNA employees must attend selected sections of the hospital's orientation program in addition to job-specific orientation. Joint Commission standards state that specific items must be included in orientation, such as safety and infection control. To orient all VNA staff in 1988, a special orientation inservice was planned at the VNA office in cooperation with the personnel department. Representatives from AMH administration were also available. New employees attend the monthly orientation scheduled at AMH, which consists of two days of general orientation. Additional orientation is then done at the VNA. Other personnel issues included the development of criteria-based job descriptions for all positions and understanding of the performance appraisal system for hourly and salaried personnel. We also had to determine how to assimilate the VNA staff into the hospital's wage and bonus system the first year. We decided that the VNA board would provide an increase as of May 31, 1988. The VNA staff would not be eligible for an increase in September 1988 that first year, although hourly rates would be adjusted at such time that overall increases were granted or the base was increased.

Finance Department Billing Activities

Continuity of business activities had to be maintained with the effective date of the affiliation. On June 1, 1988, there were two sets of bills that one VNA staff was responsible for processing. The VNA had to bill its May 1988 visits with one FI. It also had to bill the hospital's visits with a second FI. The non-Medicare billing also had to be done.

For many months, the administrative, business, and clinical supervisory staff had to deal with two FIs to answer questions on previous bills, denials, and requests for information on 485 forms. We also had two postpayment compliance audits within a short period of time from two different FIs. We also received requests from Keystone Peer Review Organization for charts for quality of care reviews for both hospital and VNA patients.

Check Requisition

Checks are issued once per week (except in an emergency). Based on internal operations, the requests must go to the VNA finance director on Tuesday. Then they are processed and sent to the hospital finance department on Wednesday, which enables processing of the checks on Thursdays. Checks can be issued and available Friday morning. This requires advanced planning, such as for last-minute registration fees, which was a change for the staff. This timing also changed the way contractor checks were processed.

Budget/Reports

The VNA prepares its own budget, which is submitted as part of the total hospital budget. Departments are expected to live within these approved budgets unless additional personnel will generate additional revenues. Reports based on budget versus actual expenses and staffing hours on a monthly and year-to-date basis are available to administrative staff. The VNA handles its own billing and posting of accounts receivable and submits monthly reports to the hospital. Cost reports are prepared by the hospital's finance department.

Contract/Policy Approval

As the director of a community-based agency, I was accustomed to receiving or gathering information, seeking staff opinions, obtaining legal advice, and presenting findings to the board for approval. I had the authority to carry out the board's action.

In a larger bureaucratic system, more departments are involved in the process, and thus it moves more slowly. Also, specific contracts may have impact on the larger organization. Therefore, all aspects must be explored, not just those of the home care agency. Administrative approval is obtained at stated meetings that the director has with the EVP every two weeks or more frequently if needed.

Other Departments

Meetings were held with the nutrition department to discuss arrangements for the hospice program. An interdepartmental agreement was arranged for a registered dietitian to be available for the hospice program. Meetings were held with pharmacy personnel to discuss services available to the hospital's home care and hospice patients and to make billing arrangements. We made arrangements to obtain the daily census sheets of admissions and current patients for the DP nurses.

I, as well as the administrative team, met with the hospital administration, including the EVP and the directors of finance, personnel, and nursing, regularly to make sure that everyone was aware of all the transition activities.

The hospital's educational department offers many excellent inservice programs each month at no cost to the departments. Programs are available for the nurses as well as clerical and business office staff. I met with the director to determine how the VNA staff would access these programs. I also met with the director of media services to become familiar with the services available to the VNA, such as videotaping, in-house television programs, and preparation of slides.

The VNA would be ordering patient and office supplies through the hospital's purchasing department. We had to prepare policy and procedures and become familiar with time frames (e.g., length of time between placing an order and receiving it).

External Contacts

In addition to the meetings with AMH staff, it was essential to determine that the hospital and the VNA continued to meet all federal and state requirements during the transition process. This required early notification of the state licensing/certifying agency and the FIs.

State Certifying Agency

The hospital and VNA home care directors contacted the Pennsylvania Department of Health/Division of Home Health. The hospital had to continue to provide those services for which it was certified during the transition phase. The VNA had to advise the state agency that it planned voluntarily to terminate its participation in the Medicare program as of May 31, 1988. Because the hospital did not have a Medicare-certified hospice, the VNA's Medicare hospice was transferred to the hospital by completing change in ownership forms. These changes were forwarded by the Pennsylvania Department of Health to the federal agency. The action required a completion of the civil rights compliance forms.

State Medical Assistance Office

The VNA's existing medical assistance (MA) number had to be relinquished when it went out of existence on May 31, 1988. Although the hospital had an MA number for the home care department, it could not be used as of June 1, 1988 because MA numbers are issued in Pennsylvania by address codes. The VNA/AMH home care department was no longer going to be located in the hospital. Therefore, the VNA had to apply for a new number for services provided as of June 1, 1988. MA billing had to be held for several weeks until the new number was issued.

FI

The hospital had its own FI. The VNA had Blue Cross of Greater Philadelphia, now Independence Blue Cross (IBC), as its FI. The affiliation agreement provided that the hospital would request an early transfer to IBC, one of the 10 regional FIs. The VNA had been with IBC since 1967. The hospital and VNA administrators wrote the necessary letters to both FIs. The hospital received permission to transfer to IBC. The transfer was easy to accomplish. All active hospital patients were transferred to IBC with a new form 485 as of June 1, 1988. All the VNA's patients continued on service. The transfer to the hospital's home care identification number was facilitated through a cooperative effort among the VNA, IBC, and Delta Computer System (Altoona, PA). The VNA's agency identification number was changed on the electronic billing that was completed as of June 1, 1988. Needless to say, there was some confusion until everyone became aware of the affiliation.

Accrediting Organizations

The VNA had been accredited by the National League for Nursing (NLN) since 1967. The hospital's home care department is accredited by the Joint Commission. The VNA submitted its annual report to the NLN spring board of review. Because the VNA would no longer exist as of May 1988, it would have to apply for NLN CHAP status as a new agency in the future.

Meanwhile, the hospital was scheduled for a Joint Commission survey in July 1988. The home care site visit was delayed until December 1988. At that time, the VNA had a successful three-day site visit. In 1991 and 1994, the VNA and AMH were accredited with commendation.

State/National Associations

Letters were sent to the Pennsylvania Association of Home Health Agencies and the National Association for Home Care informing them that the VNA would become a hospital-based agency effective June 1, 1988.

United Way

The VNA had frequent, informative meetings with the staff at the local United Way organization. As noted earlier, the VNA completed a corporate restructure in 1986. Before 1986, the VNA was the United Way Member Agency. Funding was received for its health promotion and support services. These services were assumed by VNA-CS in 1986, when the three VNAs were formed. In 1986, VNA-CS became the United Way Member Agency because this agency provided the supported services. Therefore, in 1988 there was no change in the United Way relationship because VNA-CS remained a free-standing community-based agency.

Contracting Agencies

The VNA director wrote letters informing all individual and group contractors of the change process. Letters of renewal sent to all contractors indicated that the hospital would be the new contracting entity. There was a slight change in the payment schedule to coincide with the hospital's weekly check processing system. There was no change in the clinical aspect of service.

Identification Numbers

It must be noted that many of the third-party payers and regulatory agencies required new agency/department identification numbers. It was important to notify all staff of the impending changes and new numbers. This was especially important in the instance of patient identification numbers. All care providers, nurses, aides, therapists, and medical record department personnel had to be aware of the change in VNA patient numbers so that clinical records and billing were correct. This took a few weeks, and some corrections or combinations of bills had to be made until all the patients were on the VNA's system.

"FEELINGS": THE IMPACT ON BOARD AND STAFF

At the board level, there was at least one resignation during the negotiating process. The plan of the VNA-CS board members was to enable interested members from the VNA and VNA-HMS boards to join the VNA-CS board as of June 1988. Although a few members chose not to continue, the board's size was increased from 15 to 22 members.

The VNA administrative staff were cognizant that the greatest impact of the affiliation would be felt at this level. The ED, Director of Finance (DF), and DPS felt that they had lost control in several areas. In the financial area, administrative personnel were accustomed to an internally generated monthly financial report showing income and expenses, profits and loss. Now, although we have control of the budget vs. actual expenses, we do not have control of the bottom line (e.g., hospital add-ons).

In relationship to operating within a larger, more bureaucratic system, the administrative staff had to learn the process. For a while, I felt totally inadequate; I had to learn what forms to use to requisition the forms I needed to requisition the clerical and clinical supplies and checks! Timing and planning ahead was critical. I went to inservices for new managers to become familiar with all the details of hospital expectations in addition to the one-to-one meetings discussed earlier.

The VNA staff involved with clinical services and related issues (computer input, billing, and medical record) felt the impact with a change in volume of Medicare business from 30% in May 1988 to 70% in June 1988. This change resulted from the loss of the hospital's home care contract services, which represented about 50% of the VNA's business before June 1988.

There was a significant increase in the paperwork that had to be done by the VNA staff. As noted earlier, we also had to deal with two FIs for clinical and reimbursement purposes for many months. There were also some changes that were initiated to meet Joint Commission requirements. The DPS and ED met with the hospital's chief of staff to review the existing procedure to make referrals for home care services and to verify physician credentials to meet Joint Commission requirements.

Once the decision to affiliate was announced, there were some resignations within the home care department. This occurred even though all employees of the VNA and the hospital's home care department were offered positions in the new home care department. Some employees chose to interview for the new position of DP nurse within the home care department. All these nurses were hired. Some took other positions in the hospital.

ADJUSTMENTS FOR STAFF

I asked the VNA staff to share written comments with me concerning the impact of the change from a community to a hospital-based agency. Exhibit 60–1 shows these selected observations and comments from staff at all levels in the organization. Personally and professionally, this was one of my most challenging experiences. Although I knew I was not personally responsible for the current health care climate, in which affiliations are common, I felt responsible for the agency's future direction

because the board depended on the administrative staff and me for direction. The process could not have been accomplished without the support and expertise of the VNA's DPS and DF.

CHANGE IN PROFESSIONAL RELATIONSHIP WITH PEERS

Ongoing professional relationships are often organized under an agency's auspices. This occurs at the local, state, and national levels. A business decision is based on facts and is made after the pros and cons have been identified and discussed. Because the staff, more than the board, are usually involved with their peers on an ongoing basis, administrative staff must be prepared for changes in professional relationships. This change occurred at the VNA when I informed organizations of the agency's planned change and requested a decision concerning future membership based on interpretation of the bylaws. Based on these interpretations, some organizational relationships were terminated as a result of our restructure.

By the time the affiliation decision was made, I felt comfortable with the terms of the affiliation and the impact it would have on our daily operations. We were prepared for our new responsibilities and the change this might require in current relationships. The reactions of administrative colleagues ranged from "You sold out" to "I envy you. You know in what direction you're headed."

One relationship that did not change in 1998 was the one with the VNA-CS board. Before the affiliation, the administrative staff were accustomed to managing both in-home and community services through a management agreement. As of June 1, 1988, a management agreement was continued. VNA-CS has a management agreement with AMH for the administrative staff's time to manage its programs and services. The workload greatly increased, however, because there were now both hospital and community agency budgets, personnel policies, meetings, QA programs, accreditation stan-

Exhibit 60–1 Selected Observations and Comments from Staff

Emotional Aspects

- Coming to grips with our feelings, specifically anger. It took the 3 years from 1985 to 1988 to move through the stages to acceptance.
- I had to look at the environment and deal with reality.

Organizational Considerations

- Excellent educational opportunities.
- Increase in income commensurate with hospital salaries is a plus!
- Less autonomy.
- It's nice to say you are truly connected to the hospital and are included in the activities.
- Involved in hospital politics.
- Trust in VNA administration to have the best interest of employees at heart.
- Confidence that concerns about the history and philosophy of the agency and the focus on quality of care have been addressed.

Operational Issues

- Identify the costs/benefits to the organization and individuals.
- Attend inservices and conferences to become familiar with new external organizations, such as the Joint Commission, and new reporting requirements.
- Stockpile supplies to allow time to fit into new time frame.
- Create position for QA supervisor or new personnel before change.
- Get to know new players (e.g., department directors).
- Prepare for increased number of meetings.
- More departments to deal with.
- Increased need to justify requests for additional positions.
- Decreased overall control.
- Biggest frustration is waiting for answers.
- The autonomy of day-to-day decision making in the provision of patient care has remained intact, dispelling fears that the hospital system would alter this autonomy.
- Difficulty adapting to new payroll regulations, benefits, and especially leaving the flexibility of a small office to join a large, more inflexible organization. Yet, the hospital administration has seemed to strive to make the changes as easy as possible and has been accessible to staff when questions arise.
- Suddenly you are working for a whole new organization and management team. It's like starting a new job when you really haven't. The adjustments required can be formidable.

---

dards, and public relations. The VNA administrative staff continued to interact with the United Way, Office on Aging, county/municipal of-fices, and the hospital administrator. The role of the ED was, and continues to be, a busy but enjoyable one to fill. The management agreement was not renewed by the hospital in 1993.

My communications with, and access to, the hospital's EVP are excellent. Meetings are scheduled approximately every two weeks. The EVP is readily available by telephone or by voice mailbox. He sends pertinent written materials and articles related to home care and the hospice to me. I am included in selected committees and asked to share my ideas on issues within the hospital. I share pertinent information with him and other staff members. I also meet every two weeks with all department directors.

CONCLUSION

I believe that the VNA's decision to affiliate its skilled home care services with AMH was the result of a sound strategic planning process. The mission and purpose of the new entity are consistent with those of the two organizations involved. The affiliation met the needs of the staff, responded to market realities, and was accomplished in projected time frames. The budget projections and visit volumes have exceeded initial projections. The VNA has grown both in volume of patients served and visits and in full-time equivalents (FTEs) since the 1986 restructure and after the affiliation with AMH in 1988. The management team is committed to meeting the challenges that con-tinue to present themselves each day. The honest discussion and compromises from both the VNA and AMH made it possible to achieve a workable and balanced approach to some difficult economic and sensitive organizational issues. I share this experience with you to assure you that there is life after affiliation with a major hospital.

REFERENCE

Harris, M., & Groshens, M. (1985). A cooperative volunteer training program. *Home Healthcare Nurse*, *3*, 37–40.

Chapter 61

Integrated Delivery Systems

Warren Lyons

INTRODUCTION

The near term movement of health care delivery toward a consolidated delivery system certainly affects home care agencies in a manner not dissimilar from the impact of national banking mergers upon local, smaller banks. The demise of branch banking, however, has been countered by the emergence of new, local bankers seeking a niche position and by unexpected competition from nonfinancial market sectors such as Internet service organizations. This chapter spotlights the impact of integrated health care delivery systems (IDSs) on your home care agency strategic planning.

As with contemporary action movies, by the time you read this chapter, the plot and actors may have changed, but the automated, digital projector continues to display new story lines against a constant screen size and color. For home health care, the constants of market consolidation, defragmentation of clinical care delivery, and cost reductions will continue to be applicable.

The definition of an IDS is an organization that has economically and clinically linked various professional health care services through ownership or intercorporate contract. This IDS definition could include these provider elements: insurance, hospital care, skilled nursing facility care, home care, physician practice, and various ambulatory care services.

The home care agency owner or CEO might ask the following questions:

- Will I continue to provide home health care as a cost to the purchaser or will I provide additional value through shared cost-risk contracts with that purchaser?
- How will my clinical care services interface with the patient's physician or payer who seeks an integrated care plan across the continuum of treatment locations over an extended time period?
- What is my plan to access capital funds for information systems and other technology and can I obtain funds during a period of intensifying price competition?
- How do I compete in the labor market with other health care providers who may offer superior employee benefits and career paths?
- What is my competitive plan to address integrated long-term care providers who have diversified into subacute care, home health care, physician practice ownership, and capitated contracts with health maintenance organizations (HMOs), both Medicare and commercial, as well as long-term care managed care insurers?

INTEGRATED DELIVERY SYSTEMS—DEFINITION AND ASSESSMENT

The development of IDSs suggests by its very name that prior models of health care have featured less integration or, indeed, disintegration. The movement toward integration has both economic and clinical dimensions affecting your strategic plans for home health care.

Economic integration, primarily driven by the growth of managed health care, has shifted the right to define covered health care benefits and to pay for medical treatment from the patient and physician to the payer who is usually a health care insurance company operating as an HMO. This shift of power has produced powerful data repositories that HMOs use to better understand the cost of care over a long period of time for individuals and population cohorts with common characteristics.

This economic integration from the payer viewpoint has reduced health care expenses through unit cost reductions by discounted provider fees, unit volume reduction through utilization review, and selective contracting with providers as a reward for achieving cost and utilization targets. The sum of these medical care costs compared to premium revenue is known as the medical loss ratio. This ratio is a key indicator for the financial performance of HMOs and often will affect stock price and credit ratings of HMOs.

The impact of economic integration on home health care agencies has been to affect the traditional sources of patient referrals, such as patients, physicians, and hospital discharge planning staff, by shifting referral power to the HMO. As employer and governmental pressure continues on HMOs to further reduce the medical loss ratio, HMOs have moved, in certain markets, to shift some of the financial risk to care for HMOs members *from* the HMO *to* the health care providers that have organized into an IDS.

When the health care provider has an economic risk to reduce the medical loss ratio, there is an opportunity to integrate physicians, hospitals, and home care agencies into an IDS that can accept limited delegation from the HMOs of the traditional insurance plan powers of provider credentialing, contracting, and referral management. If the IDS can reduce the medical loss ratio for the HMO, then the HMO can reduce premiums and maintain a competitive advantage over other HMOs.

DESCRIPTION OF "AT-RISK" IDS CONTRACTS

An HMO usually segments the expected medical expenses into several risk pool categories:

- institutional facility expenses including hospitals and skilled nursing facilities
- primary care physician expenses
- specialty care physician expenses
- pharmacy expenses

Each of these provider groups may be paid on a fee schedule, on an all-inclusive per-case rate such as all care for pregnancy through delivery, or on some form of capitation. The capitation payment based upon an assigned number of patients to the specific provider carries an assurance of "referral volume" because the provider, typically a primary care physician, has a firm revenue flow to use for all of the care required from a primary care physician. Because traditional HMO plans have asked only that HMO members select out their primary care physician, other contracted providers have had no assurance of referrals. In some cases, the HMO plan design permits the primary care physician to designate a capitated specialty provider, such as radiology, and the HMO members understand that this restriction on referral panels is part of the HMO benefit plan.

Recently, HMOs have undertaken global risk contracts with IDSs, in which the IDS is effectively capitated for all care needed by the patient in each of the risk pool categories noted earlier. The payment formula can be as simple as payment to the IDS of a percent of the premium paid by the HMO member or member's employer allocated to the medical loss ratio. The IDS can incur a positive or negative earning on these payments if the medical loss expenses meet or fail to meet the targeted medical loss ratio through use of unit cost controls, utilization controls, and effective preventive care and disease state management.

When the IDS has this type of at-risk contract with the HMO, the IDS is motivated to negotiate subcontracts with other providers, including home health agencies, so that the medical loss ratio target of the IDS is achieved. Some of these subcontracts can be at-risk relationships in which the subcontracted provider is capitated or given some other assurance of referral volumes in return for a fixed expense for the assigned or capitated HMO members. These forms of risk sharing must of course be consistent with the HMO's insurance plans as approved by insurance regulators.

The home health agency in a managed care market should prepare itself to bid for these types of IDS at-risk contracts. While the agencies failing to obtain such contracts usually will continue as non-risk contracted providers to the HMO, the market shift towards a select group of agencies will likely offer declining profitability to the non-risk contracted agency.

DISEASE STATE MANAGEMENT ISSUES

The economic integration of HMOs has produced clinical data repositories as well. The more advanced state HMOs have developed special review programs for high-risk disease states such as congestive heart failure, diabetes, and asthma. The use of disease state medical management programs by the HMOs has then led to selective contracting with designated centers of excellence, such as solid tissue transplant centers. For home health care agencies, HMOs have also targeted specialized home care providers for patients with chronic conditions or special needs such as high-risk newborns.

Home health agencies can add value to disease state management programs by offering case management programs that first help screen and identify high-risk patients *before* they are even seen by the primary care physician, then enroll that high-risk patient in the appropriate care management protocols and, finally, demonstrate quality and cost-effective outcomes for these high-risk patients.

Unless the HMO also operates its own health care delivery system, there is a limit to disease state management programs when the provider cannot enjoy the economic benefits from medical loss ratio reductions through integrated disease state management. Using an HMO at-risk contract, the IDS can economically benefit from reductions in the medical loss ratio through effective implementation of programs targeting the small population of insured patients who represent a disproportionately higher medical loss ratio per patient. The IDS can then accept delegated authority from the HMO to select preferred home health agencies capable of meeting the performance expectations of the IDS in the management of specific HMO disease cohorts.

In summary, an IDS that shares medical loss ratio risk with a managed care company can select or influence the selection of a home care agency, or, it can "recapture" the home care agency portion of the medical loss ratio by operating its own agency. As IDS risk-bearing entities become regional, statewide, or national in scope, the home care agency must find a way to share in this risk or face the unpleasant result of becoming a deeply discounted provider with no assurance of referral volume.

INTEGRATED DELIVERY SYSTEMS STRATEGIES

Recent IDS strategies seem to have several repeating themes:

- Through ownership or partnership with others, IDSs seek to obtain managed care contracts for a defined population through the assumption of risk-based contracts in which the IDS is responsible, as the "broker," to either directly provide a health care service, or to subcontract for that service.

- The decision to take economic risk has led to consolidation of physician practices into larger private or public group entities—some of which directly seek a prime role as an IDS.
- As the IDS contracted population reaches a threshold size, the IDS seeks either to share risk with a subcontractor, such as a home care agency, or to "recapture" the service by direct provision.
- To induce an IDS to accept economic risk with a much lower medical loss ratio target, the HMOs may offer to employers and enrolled members plan options that provide greater or lesser freedom to use certain panels of providers. For a lower premium or out-of-pocket copayment or deductible, the member may purchase an HMO product that has a "private label" feature. That is, the insurance product is restricted to use of an IDS whose name is applied to the product name.
- The marketing of these "private label products" explicitly removes the home care agency from marketing or referral access to the patient and physician unless the agency has either contracted with the IDS or has shared medical loss ratio risk to ensure referral volumes of sufficient size to justify the risk.
- An IDS with a risk-sharing HMO contract will need to develop quality of care measurements to demonstrate competency as the HMO's reported performance moves towards the center of the "bell curve" *and* as that curve moves upward on the quality/cost axis, the home care agency will need access to skill sets and infrastructure to maintain a competitive quality/cost index.

IMPLICATIONS FOR HOME HEALTH CARE AGENCIES

1. The traditional source of referrals and purchasing power has been redirected from patient and physician to intermediary providers whose economic risk relationship with the ultimate payer delegates legitimate authority to select or de-select home health care agencies.
2. Medicare HMOs' plans will experience significant growth as the federal government seeks to maintain solvency of the Medicare trust funds. These HMOs will offer risk-sharing arrangements to IDS and home health agencies for the Medicare product lines.
3. Long-term care companies will seek to obtain at-risk contracts from Medicare and commercial HMOs, and from long-term care insurance plans, so that they can act as an at-risk IDS. Long-term providers will then either recapture home care revenues through ownership or subcontract with non-owned home health agencies.
4. Self-pay patient demand for home health care will be influenced by the emergence of regional and national branded "marquee" home care agency providers.
5. The conversion of not-for-profit hospitals and insurers into for-profit private or public companies will also apply to not-for-profit home care agencies facing a decision to convert or to be acquired.
6. Utilization reductions throughout the provider system will cause traditional allies of home care agency to become direct competitors.
7. Assumption of risk contracts will require a minimum home care agency size, unit cost structure, and information infrastructure.

RECOMMENDATIONS FOR HOME HEALTH AGENCY SURVIVAL AND SUCCESS

1. Grow through merger or acquisition to a size that can manage a risk-sharing HMO contract and can meet the purchasing needs of emerging provider-owned IDSs.
2. Develop an automated financial and clinical information system that can track patient care and cost by payer, disease

state, or IDS and can document quality and cost outcomes.

3. Enter into a strategic alliance with more than one IDS, including physician-owned IDSs, to ensure referral volumes and market share.

4. Acquire disease state management competencies that position the home health agency for risk-sharing contracts with the HMOs or the IDSs.

5. Diversify into home medical equipment, infusion care, home chore care, health risk appraisal, and health education. Internal competency or subcontracted relationships for these services will help qualify the agency as a full-service, credentialed HMO provider that can take economic risk for patients across a broad continuum of services.

6. If the agency is a not-for-profit, consider conversion to for-profit status so that effective equity partnership can be established with for-profit IDSs such as physician-owned entities, long-term care systems, or for-profit hospital networks.

PART IX

Other Types of Relationships

CHAPTER 62

Resource Development for Home Health Care Providers

Barbara Klaczynska

INTRODUCTION

Resource development is a critical component of a home health care organization's ability to offer services that are responsive to community needs. Additional resources are often required as an agency considers developing new programs, expanding services to new populations, training staff with updated skills, and working collaboratively with other community agencies. Many home health care providers gain support for their work from individuals, foundations, corporations, and government agencies to supplement their operating income.

PRELIMINARY PREPARATION FOR SUCCESSFUL FUND-RAISING

Before an organization can approach funders, some preliminary steps need to be taken. It is important that an agency's board of directors and staff members understand that the organization will be seeking new funds and that the purpose of these funds will be to supplement, not replace, fees for service. Board members should be ready to take leadership roles in cultivating and soliciting community organizations and individuals for support.

A comprehensive planning process needs to take place so that an agency can prioritize its needs and have a clear vision of what steps it will be taking to accomplish its goals. The projects for which funds are sought need to carry out the mission of the agency and a commitment needs to be made to continue the project once outside funding is no longer available.

In addition to careful planning, an organized public relations effort is a critical component of a successful development program. A home health care agency should be publicizing the agency's accomplishments and documenting the services provided. Efforts should be made to work with community and regional newspapers, television and radio stations as well as participating in health fairs and other informational and community service opportunities. Attractive and informative brochures, newsletters, and updates can be created for public information.

Background materials must be assembled to meet the funder's need to know about the organization requesting funding. These materials include a well-written, succinct history of the agency, the agency's current budget, an audited financial statement from the previous year, a list of current income sources, documentation of tax-free status, a list of current board members including their titles and affiliations, agency brochures, and other materials that can help introduce the agency to the funder. Once these materials are in place, a home health care organization is then able to move forward with a fund-raising program.

IMPROVING THE PROBABILITY OF RECEIVING FUNDS

One of the most important steps an agency can take to submit a successful application is to know as much as possible about the organization it hopes to approach with a request. Susan Sherman, President of the Independence Foundation, a private foundation that is a major supporter of health care and community services in Philadelphia, emphasizes the critical role that information about a foundation can play in approaching a foundation:

> It is important that an organization seeking funds knows about the stated interests, guidelines, restrictions and giving history of the foundation it is approaching. Once a potential applicant has undertaken some preliminary research, and believes there is a fit between its organization and a foundation's goals, many foundations have staff members who are willing to discuss in detail the applicant's organization and the project for which funding is sought. (Personal communication, 1996)

Such discussions can help the organization shape its written proposal in such a way that it fits a foundation's purpose. Additionally, funders frequently know of projects developed by other organizations that can be examined to enhance a proposal design.

Foundation staff often network with other funders and are able to suggest other possible sources of support for an initiative. Whenever possible, it is valuable to learn about potential funding sources through library research and review of guidelines and annual reports, which are often available directly from foundations.

FUND-RAISING SOURCES

A majority of philanthropic support is provided through individuals. Never underestimate the ability of people in the community, in partic-

ular grateful recipients of an agency's services and their families and friends, to support good works. Corporations and local businesses are also important contributors to health and welfare in communities. Federal, state, county, and municipal government grants are continuing sources of support for health programs. However, nonprofit organizations new to fundraising often begin with foundations as a first place to request funds.

Foundations are legal entities established to offer families, individuals, and sometimes corporations a method of providing charitable gifts. National foundations, such as the Robert Wood Johnson Foundation, Kellogg Foundation, and The Pew Charitable Trusts provide support for health care programs with the potential to have national impact. It is more likely that a local foundation already committed to a community and knowledgeable about its needs and services would consider funding an organization providing services for a particular area.

RESEARCHING FOUNDATIONS AND CORPORATIONS AS POTENTIAL FUNDING SOURCES

Information on foundations and corporations with appreciable contribution programs is available through published directories that list each organization's address, staff, assets, giving history, interests, and deadlines. National directories of foundations and corporations are published by the Foundation Center, Taft Group, and many other publishers. In addition to national directories, many states have directories that list detailed information about foundations that provide support in that particular state.

Larger foundations have professional staff members who are willing to discuss projects and review letters of inquiry. Although it is always advisable to speak with foundation officers and corporate giving staff about their guidelines and interest in particular types of projects, some funders request that initial approaches be made through a short letter presenting background on the applicant organization and the project for which funding is requested.

The Foundation Center is an independent national organization established by foundations to provide an authoritative source of information on foundation and corporate giving. The Foundation Center has reference collections in New York City, Washington, D.C., Atlanta, Cleveland, and San Francisco. In addition, the Foundation Center's Cooperating Collections are available in libraries, community foundations, and nonprofit organizations that provide Foundation Center materials throughout the United States. These foundation libraries contain corporate and foundation directories, how-to fund-raising books, annual reports of local nonprofit organizations, publications with sample proposals, and specialized guides on topics including services for youth, the aging, women, and minority groups. The foundation libraries also provide Internal Revenue Service files on microfiche listing foundations' assets and distribution patterns. In addition, the foundation libraries have helpful staff who are able to provide guidance and resources for persons new to fund-raising research. A listing of regional foundation centers can be obtained from The Foundation Center, 79 Fifth Avenue, Eighth Floor, New York, NY 10003, 212-620-4320.

Many large foundations and corporations now provide information on the Internet. This is often a cost-effective way of learning quickly about funders' interests and giving patterns without infringing on their resources. For the most part, foundations and corporations have specific geographic locations for which they provide support.

RESEARCHING GOVERNMENT SOURCES

There are many avenues available to research government funding sources including commercially published directories and newsletters. The *Federal Register*, which lists available grants and is published every business day, can be obtained by subscription or in government document departments of university and large public libraries. Also, many government agencies have web pages on the Internet and post information about their funding interests as well as deadlines and guidelines. Individual states also publish announcements of funds that will become available. The best way to obtain information on local funding sources is to contact local municipalities. It is possible to call government funding sources and be placed on mailing lists to receive future information on new government funds as they become available.

TYPES OF FUND-RAISING PROJECTS

There are several different types of projects that can be supported through fund-raising activities including:

Capital Support: This type of support is to acquire equipment or obtain or improve a facility for use by an agency. Usually a capital campaign is undertaken after an agency has developed a successful track record of fundraising from individuals, foundations, and corporations in the community.

Programmatic Support: This type of funding is probably the most common funding that is provided by foundations and corporations. In programmatic support, specific activities are proposed in a definable time frame. Program funding allows health care organizations to launch new service initiatives and reach new populations.

"Seed Money" Support: Many funding sources are interested in providing funds that can help an organization launch a new program or move into an expanded area of service. Such grants, known as "seed money," can provide for hiring new staff, training for existing staff, creating promotional materials for new projects, and evaluating successful components of new efforts, as well as determining where additional support is needed.

Operating Funds Support: Often the funding needed most is support for the general operating budget. Most foundations and corporations are interested in funding a specific project or program rather than providing unspecified support. Once a relationship is in place with a foundation, an agency might be able to obtain operating support for its activities.

Emergency Funds Support: This funding is sometimes difficult to obtain, but there are occasions when a case can be made for emergency support to assist an agency with a particular crisis. Funders sometimes look favorably upon "bridge" grants that help a service to continue during a period when one source of support is discontinued and other funding seems likely in the foreseeable future.

ELEMENTS OF A SUCCESSFUL PROPOSAL

Many funders, particularly larger foundations and corporations, have specific guidelines to follow for organizing a proposal. If a funding source does not have a published format, applicants should provide a proposal that presents organizational information, goals and objectives, methodology, staffing, evaluation, and plans for the continuation and dissemination of the proposed project.

Developing a Written Proposal to Funders

The applicant requesting funds in most cases needs to present a well-written proposal to a funding source. Again, Susan Sherman, president of the Independence Foundation, provides guidance in this area. She states that organizations often do not clearly articulate the impact of the activities for which they are requesting support. Ms. Sherman recommends that agencies seeking funds present measurable outcomes, that is, specific, quantifiable results that will occur as a result of the support requested. The process of developing measurable outcomes moves many proposal writers from global to specific thinking and allows potential funders to understand clearly why the project should be supported.

Organizational Capability

A successful proposal needs to be introduced with a brief history of the organization to establish credibility in working with its community and providing services. The organizational capability statement should be brief and specifically emphasize the agency's experience in developing projects related to the funding received. For example, if funds are requested to deliver services to a specific group of people in the community, such as the elderly, children, or a new immigrant group, an agency's specific experience serving these populations should be included.

Since funders are interested in an organization's financial stability and management capacity, reference to past financial history and present fiscal organization is critical. The past experience of obtaining and responsibly managing grant funding is also an important component of an organization's history.

Problem/Need To Be Addressed

The problem/need statement section offers an opportunity to describe the community and the problems that will be addressed by the project for which funding is requested. The problems should be defined clearly and precisely with emphasis on the urgency of the need for a solution proposed in the project. For example, if a home health care agency plans a project that would improve services to families caring for children with disabilities, documentation of the number of children with disabilities living with their families in the community, the types of disabilities the children have, the kinds of services provided, and the need for additional assistance should be chronicled.

Goals/Outcomes

The goals section provides a global direction for the proposal, and the outcomes offer measurable purposes that will be accomplished by the project. The goals and outcomes are the basis for developing an effective description of activities, evaluation, and budget for the program. It is critical that the objectives demonstrate that the outcomes are "stretching" in new directions but at the same time the tasks are reasonable and can be accomplished during the period of time that funding will be provided.

Project Activities

In this section, the author of the grant proposal should create a scenario of how the project will operate. The project should be described to illustrate what will happen, who will be served, who will implement the project, where it will take place, and the timetable for the operation of the project. The more details that can be provided in this section the better.

Staffing

The staff who will be involved in the project should be described with attention to supervisory relationships, the role of volunteers, and relationships with other agencies/organizations. All people working on the project should be presented with detailed descriptions of their responsibilities related to the project as well as how their education and experience have prepared them for this work. If new staff members will be hired for the project, the proposal should outline the qualifications sought and the job responsibility of new staff members as well.

Evaluation

Evaluation is critical to a comprehensive proposal. Proposals should detail specific plans for evaluating the ongoing program (formative evaluation) as well as how the entire project will be assessed and analyzed. It is important that the evaluation describe how the project has been able to respond to the proposed goals and honestly assess what outcomes have not been met and the reasons for this. For the most part, a successful project achieves its stated goals, but circumstances do change and it is not always possible to carry out the project as originally described. The evaluation should discuss why the project staff was not able to meet some goals as well as areas in which outcomes were surpassed and how new outcomes were accom-

plished. Recommendations for future efforts are an important part of evaluation and in some cases can serve as the basis for developing future funding proposals.

Evaluation can be conducted internally or an outside consultant could be brought in to assist in planning or implementing the evaluation. Some tools that can be utilized in the evaluation include surveys, interviews, group interviews, sometimes called focus groups, and analysis of records for the quality and quantity of contacts. These evaluation techniques need to be described in the proposal. Project staff, clients, families, and staff in other community organizations that interact with the process are all important sources for learning the strengths and weaknesses of the project.

Continuation

Funders are reluctant to become "permanent" sources of support because of the widely held view that grant money should not replace operational money in the provision of services. It is important to plan how the project will continue beyond the grant period. For example, a foundation would be more interested in a project that would train the existing staff of an agency to provide culturally sensitive materials to underserved populations or to translate and print materials in languages for use by groups than a project that would fund a position that would be responsible for the provision of services on an ongoing basis.

Dissemination

Funders like to know that a project will have an impact beyond the immediate agency and community where the original program was developed. Programs that are models that can be adapted by other agencies and communities are desirable. The organization seeking funds should consider how the results of this project might be presented to other health care organizations through journals, newsletters, publications, and presentations at professional meetings.

Budget

The budget should realistically reflect how much the project will cost. Expenses that need to be taken into consideration are staffing (including fringe benefits), equipment, travel, printing, and supplies needed. Often organizations also include indirect costs, such as space rental, utilities, telephones, accounting work, and other support needed by the agency to operate such a project.

Funding Sources

This section should describe in detail funds in hand for the project and other funding that has been committed to the project. In most cases, funding sources are impressed by the involvement of other funders in the project. However, if no other funds are available at the time of proposal submission, a detailed description of plans to obtain these funds should be included. Letters of commitment from other funders can strengthen the case of an agency, confirming the importance of the project and the specific role support will play in enhancing the development of this project.

Supportive Materials

Often applicants provide additional materials with proposals including general background about their agencies, information about the service area, letters of support from cooperating agencies, staff or consultants who will be involved in the project, and other agencies in the community endorsing the agency and project. Selected testimonials from clients and families and newspaper clippings about the agency's track record are also helpful. If these materials enhance the application and the proposal guidelines do not restrict such materials, they can be included. However, it is important that such materials are relevant to the project and directly reinforce the ability of the agency to implement the program. It is better to have no letter of support than one that is vague or unenthusiastic about the organization or the proposed initiative.

SUBMITTING PROPOSALS/FOLLOW-UP

Once a proposal is submitted to a funding source, it is appropriate to follow up with a telephone call to ensure that it has been received, to see if there are any questions, and to determine the timetable for decision making about the project. Often if a project is to be considered by a foundation, the foundation staff contacts the agency to ask questions and obtain additional material. In some cases, foundations welcome a visit from applicants before a proposal is submitted or during the decision-making process, or might make site visits to the applicant organization. Usually applicants learn of a decision concerning their application from one month to six months after submission. If funding is not received, some foundation and corporate funders are willing to provide information on the reason for their negative decision while others make it a policy to not provide this type of information.

STEWARDSHIP OF FUNDS

If funding is received, the agency is responsible for appropriate management. Any announcement of funding needs to be made in accordance with the funder's guidelines and approval. In the course of the funding period, it is important to document the accomplishments of the grant through careful record keeping. Frequent reports are advisable to foundations by conversations and written reports as well as press clippings, publications, and other printed materials generated by the project. Meticulous financial records and reports are also required and in some cases an audit showing how the funds were spent. When appropriate, staff from the funding organization should be invited to events related to the project or to observe how services are delivered.

Although funders are reluctant to become permanent contributors to any one project or agency, once a foundation or corporation supports a successful program for an organization, they are willing to consider applications for future funding activities. Also, funders are sometimes able to introduce applicant agencies to other funders in the community and alert applicants to new opportunities for support.

CONCLUSION

A home health care agency that is interested in outside support must develop a comprehensive planning process, specific projects, and manageable activities, along with a reputation for providing caring, efficient, and responsive services in the community. Once these are in place, grants received from foundations, corporations, and government sources can become a valuable resource for the delivery and expansion of home health care services.

CHAPTER 63

Home Care Volunteer Program

Carol-Rae Green Sodano

THE NOTION OF VOLUNTEERISM

Old sailors know never to volunteer for anything. The implication is that volunteering places one at risk. Volunteering makes one vulnerable to the experience of injustice, a risk that is prevalent enough in all human interaction but is intensified by the intrinsic nature of volunteering. Volunteering means to offer one's services out of one's own volition with no guarantee of reciprocity, let alone a guarantee of equal reciprocity. The risk of experiencing injustice is high.

To volunteer means to generate a proactive statement of commitment based on faith, belief, and individually felt principle. It is a projection of personal quality, which normally can remain hidden and safe from public perusal, into a concrete act that becomes visible and subject to public judgment. To volunteer is to make an open statement of principle. It makes the individual visible and accountable and consequently binds him or her by honor to the fulfillment of a promise. Here again is the potential for felt injustice. The volunteer risks visibility and public judgment by his or her own volition; he or she stands alone. The volunteer risks exposure and judgment from those who can shout their condemnation from the anonymous safety of the crowd. The volunteer is always vulnerable to the statement, "You offered."

Most of us volunteer with the hope, perhaps even the belief, that we will feel the balance of our risk in received appreciation. Sometimes this payback comes through, but often it falls short. The self-perception of one as a volunteer can easily slip to a self-perception of one as a victim.

It is precisely this issue, keeping the volunteer a volunteer and not a felt victim, that is the key to a successful volunteer program. The object is to attract qualified, committed individuals who will risk the public statement of volunteering, to stimulate and support these individuals into working at maximum levels of investment and productivity, and finally to maintain their involvement over an extended period of time. Recruiting quality volunteers, stimulating them into maintained production, and retaining them demand a recognition of the risks incurred by the volunteer and responding to those risks by working toward a reciprocity of justice. A fundamental goal for any successful volunteer program must be mutuality: a mutuality of acted-out commitment by both volunteer and agency, a shared justice and fairness that precludes victimization.

Volunteerism is an American cultural trait and a well-established American tradition. The cultural demand to volunteer one's time, energy, and talent seems to be rooted in the American interpretation of the Protestant work ethic. In

America, not only are you expected to work hard with every anticipation of financial and spiritual reward but, once your rewards have been recognized, you are expected to share the wealth, both material and moral. In America, once the individual is in a position of relative financial stability, he or she is expected to give over time and talent for the general social good and for the good of individuals who are less fortunate. There is considerable social pressure to share the wealth; individuals who, because of the time restrictions created by their success, cannot give directly of their skills are expected to surrogate this donation with money. Government supports this practice by making contributions of this sort tax deductible and in so doing concretely acts out the social sanction of this unique value.

Money is fine, but time is better. Direct action volunteerism has always held cultural esteem in our society. Interestingly, although it has usually been a predominantly female prerogative, volunteerism has consistently been encouraged of men as well. Often men volunteer for positions that hold significant social status (e.g., volunteer heads of foundations, social and cultural committees, or political and economic organizations), whereas women often volunteer for direct service functions (e.g., the Gray Ladies, institutional fund-raising committees, and volunteer services in schools and welfare agencies). All individuals are expected to participate, and if there are inequities in the volunteer system in America, they are inequities reflective of the general social system rather than those specific to volunteerism. The culture is consistent.

In summary, volunteerism in America is a well-established cultural trait rooted in moral sanction and perpetuated through significant social pressure. Volunteerism is a collective charge, a cultural norm propounded to all members of the society with every expectation that the individual will meet every challenge to the best of his or her ability.

HEALTH CARE VOLUNTEERISM

During the 20th century, the health care institution in America gained tremendous esteem. The post–World War II period saw a dramatic rise in social and political power for the health care community, a rise that seemed to reach its peak in the mid-1970s. This rise in power and esteem appears to be rooted in the notion, perpetuated in the latter half of the 20th century, that medical personnel can do more than mitigate pain, they can in fact defeat death. With the "magic" powder of antibiotics tightly in hand, medicine in the post–World War II era came close to gaining religious prestige. Before this period, the power of life and death was pretty much in God's hands; now God seemed to have the assistance of a physician.

The public has done a great deal to increase the prestige of the health care community. It makes sense that, if you stand just under God's right hand or if the public believes that this is your designated position, you acquire a considerable amount of respect and a considerable amount of power. Add to this set of perceptions the popular American image of the life saver as a romantic hero, and you are well on your way toward sanctification.

The whole notion of a collective cultural fantasy spinning around a hero who exercises power over death is an intriguing cultural phenomenon. This fantasy allows the individual to bask in the warm light of public acclaim, of public recognition and esteem, and of direct ego gratification at the highest level through the perform-ance of an act that by its nature is the ultimate in moral behavior. Give back to an individual that which is most morally valued, most ethically weighed—his or her life—and you earn the right to direct ego gratification. It is a point of curiosity that, for many of us in America, to free ourselves, even in our fantasy, to claim recognition on our own behalf we must pay the cost of performing an act that comes conceptually close to divine.

It should therefore not be surprising that volunteerism in health care settings has been consistently popular in America. Volunteering for service in a hospital or geriatric facility, for example, fulfills the requirement to give back to the society and at the same time allows the individual to gain permitted self-gratification by engaging in good work. Whether one agrees with the ethical system or not, there is a system operative, and its reality must be recognized and worked within. Furthermore, an ethical system that manifests through altruism certainly is far better than a system that is nonaltruistic or anti-altruistic in its expression. Perhaps our motives are a bit bent, but better bent than crooked.

HOME CARE VOLUNTEERISM

Outpatient care is a growing movement in the current health care spectrum. In-home care has always been present, to a greater or lesser degree, in the general health care scene in America. Today, however, because of DRGs and the payment policies they impose, more and more individuals find themselves at home at stages of more and more acute caretaking need. In addition, the growth of the hospice movement, which in America is predominantly of the in-home care variety, has vastly contributed to the need for trained volunteers for in-home care service.

Home care volunteerism makes good sense. If properly administrated, it is cost-efficient and delivers a quality of care that can be acquired in no other way. The patient who is clinically appropriate for in-home care has the advantage of being in the security of familiar surroundings, in an environment in which he or she can usually exercise a fair degree of individual control and can remain among those who are most significant, most trusted, and most nurturing in every sense. Well-trained and well-supervised volunteers, through their facilitation, can maximize the quality of the in-home care experience, and in many cases they do more than facilitate the process: They are essential to its very existence.

In-home care volunteers come in several varieties: individuals who volunteer their time

to provide companionship for the at-home patient, and individuals who volunteer their professional services and skills, among others. Without these donations of personal resources by volunteers, many patients and their families would not be able to function effectively in the in-home setting; responsibilities would be too demanding, and costs would be too consuming.

In-house care that incorporates the efficient use of volunteers has every potential to increase the possibility and quality of good patient care and at the same time to stabilize or lower cost. There are some risks, however, that cannot be ignored.

The first issue is the possibility of legal liability. When the volunteer is sent into the patient's home, institutional environmental control is given up, and this creates a degree of risk. In addition, in-home volunteers, unlike most volunteers working in institutional settings, usually hold an extraordinary degree of personal responsibility for the patient's well-being. Often the in-home volunteer is the only individual present and responsible for the patient. This singularity of responsibility demands that the degree of trust and confidence placed in in-home volunteers be extraordinary, and in the extraordinary is risk. The second issue is the problem of burnout. In-home volunteers are giving a great deal of themselves in relatively intense doses; there is a risk of losing them or their quality if they are not treated with some degree of reciprocity and nurturing.

When the effect is balanced against the risk, most in-home care agencies choose in favor of volunteer involvement in patient care plans. Volunteers do not need to be present in every case handled by an agency to be perceived as earning their salt. They need to be present when their presence is critical and/or appropriate. In addition, they can provide peripheral services such as bookkeeping, secretarial, or library tasks, which usually translate into all-around increased quality of service. The bottom line is that volunteers enhance service at every level with a minimal cost in terms of both money and overhead.

THE PHILOSOPHICAL BASIS FOR A SUCCESSFUL VOLUNTEER PROGRAM

Program Goals

A well-organized volunteer program is designed to meet four basic program goals. These goals are internal and aimed at the creation and preservation of a productive, stable volunteer corps that in turn will provide quality service both to the service agency and, more important, to the public. Well-managed volunteer programs focus on meeting the demands of quality in (1) recruitment, (2) service, (3) retention, and (4) cost-effectiveness.

Quality in recruitment demands that the agency knows what it wants and expects from its volunteer corps and then aims its recruitment campaigns at populations best able to meet these expectations. Targeted recruitment, although demanding a greater effort and time investment up front, pays back with volunteers who bring in skills and who are more likely to remain in the program because they are wanted. They come to understand that they are wanted, and they value this recognition.

Another advantage of targeted recruitment is that only individuals appropriate to the function of the agency are approached, thus eliminating the problems that surface when large numbers of individuals who have nonspecific skills are recruited and the agency must find a use for all of them. Often it is discovered that there are too many individuals who are able to fulfill one task and not enough to fill another; consequently, more volunteers need to be recruited while volunteers already trained must remain idle. This policy is both monetarily inefficient and corrosive to morale.

Quality in service demands that volunteers be well trained and well supervised. Individuals recruited into a volunteer corps must be taught, and taught clearly, what is expected of them and how they are to meet these expectations. Little if anything should be left to chance. It is unfair to assume that the volunteer knows precisely what you want and how you want it done, even if he or she has a professional handle on a given skill. The volunteer must be helped to integrate this skill into the personality and function of the agency. Training is as much a function of integration as it is the communication of information. Similarly, the function of supervision is more guidance and development than discipline and judgment. Supervision policy and process must encourage the volunteers in the performance of their tasks and assist their growth in both skills and self-assurance.

Quality in retention suggests that skilled and well-functioning volunteers remain in a program not by accident but by design and effort. Because the economic investment in volunteers is primarily in their training and only secondarily in their supervision, it makes good fiscal sense to work consciously to maintain the fruits of the initial investment. The longer a volunteer remains productively a part of the corps, the lower the cost to train that volunteer and the lower the cost of the services provided by the volunteer. More important, the longer the volunteer remains in the corps, the greater his or her skill and adaptability to work within the process of the agency become as he or she develops into an incorporated member of the team. It takes time and effort to train new people continually; it takes time, effort, and loss of service to integrate new individuals into a team continually.

The quality of a volunteer program is often measured by its cost-effectiveness. Although cost considerations need not be the only rationale for a volunteer program, they are certainly important. Any quality program will be designed to achieve the best service for the least amount of money. Volunteer programs have their cost in the staff necessary to train and supervise them. Effective programs that result in a volunteer corps characterized by skill, adaptability, variability, and creativity will be quite cost-efficient. The measure of the cost-effectiveness of a volunteer program is not so much what it costs to create and maintain the corps but how much the corps can provide in both quality and variability of service, or what the corps allows you to offer to the public that could not be offered without it.

Basic Premises Necessary To Attain Goals

The successful attainment of these goals through a system that does not rely on monetary incentive falls just short of being an art form. Volunteerism depends virtually exclusively on an affirmative relational process to attain its specified goals. This process is a skill under any circumstance, but in the context of volunteerism, unbolstered by economic support, it becomes critical.

The relational process necessary to create and maintain a successful volunteer program must flow from a clear, committed philosophical basis. This basis consists of two concomitant sets of premises: the ethical and the relational. The ethical premises, those of integrity, justice, and humanism, are the philosophical foundation for the process. The relational premises, those of trust, fairness, mutuality, reciprocity, and dialog, are the actuating behavior of the process. The ethical premises form the essence of the process, and the relational premises form its actuality.

The Ethical Premises

The ethical premises form the value system that directs the process of interpersonal relationship. It is the commitment to these values that determines the criteria against which behavior is judged and decisions of policy and procedure are made. Successful volunteer programs are based on policies and procedures that remain committed and faithful to integrity, justice, and humanism.

Integrity is a commitment to reality, consistency, and truthfulness. Integrity demands that individuals and the systems they create recognize the nature of reality and, having recognized that nature, work compatibly and affirmatively with that reality. Integrity demands that reality not be denied, mutilated, or distorted but rather honored and credited for its existence and its

essence. Integrity demands consistency, that actions match spoken words and understood agreements and that policy mirrors principles. Integrity demands that truth be honored and continuously respected in thought and deed.

Specific to a volunteer program, integrity demands that administration have a realistic understanding about what is needed and what will be required to meet the need; that these requirements be clearly stated to both the client and the volunteer so that communication is kept open, clear, and appropriate; that what is asked of the volunteer is what is wanted and possible with no hidden messages, motives, or circumstances; and that feedback given to the volunteer is inclusive, direct, and always truthful.

Justice is a commitment to fairness, to making a return on what is received, to giving credit when credit is due, and to critiquing when critiquing is deserved. Justice flows from integrity, and although the two are separate in essence, they are experienced simultaneously. Justice in a volunteer program demands that all sides are heard and credited, that treatment of the volunteer is fair and equitable in every circumstance, and that there is a recognition of earned trust and reliability as well as open, clear statements of complaints.

Humanism is the capacity to see and respect others for the honor and dignity they hold by virtue of their status as human. Humanism demands respect, honor, empathy, and judgment that is recognized as individual and subjective, not authoritarian and absolute. Humanism in a volunteer program demands that each individual in the corps be continuously seen, perceived, and responded to with consideration and conscious recognition of his or her human dignity and needs. Humanism demands that administration relate through constructive processes with the volunteer; by doing so, administration earns the right to similar consideration from the volunteer.

Relational Premises

The relational premises are the modes of behavior that concertize and make experiential the abstract principles of ethics. They are the particulars of the processes that form and maintain relationship; they are the actions and exchanges that engender union and encourage its continuity.

To maintain itself and to create a constructive history, a relationship must be founded on trust. Trust building consequently becomes a critical dynamic in the relational process. Trust is earned over time and with experience. Trust generates out of mutual, constructive interaction that binds individuals in a common history. Trust cannot be rushed; neither can it be given away and remain in character. Trust demands mutual disclosure of individual truths; it demands that the individual speak and act with integrity, justice, and humanism. Trust demands appropriate self-disclosure and a corresponding willingness to be held accountable. Trust demands the courage to know one's truth, to say and act one's truth, to hear the other's response to one's truth, and to credit the legitimacy of the other's side.

The creation and maintenance of trust are essential to a successful volunteer program. The trust building must be mutually engaged in by volunteer and agency as well as mutually earned and mutually felt. The building of trust demands a mutually created history of integrity, of honest statements openly given and carefully adhered to over time.

Fairness encourages trust. Crediting others' positions recognizes their presence and honors their intrinsic value. Fairness encourages reciprocal behavior and works to ensure a future in the relationship.

The volunteer must be treated with fairness based on a commitment to justice. Fairness to volunteers includes working with them to help make their experience personally enriching, openly recognizing their accomplishments and their contributions, clearly communicating direction, delivering honest critiques with sensitivity and encouragement, and recognizing that they are entitled to something back for what they give.

Reciprocity is the give and take necessary to maintain the momentum of the relationship. Reciprocity is the interchange within which fairness is experienced and trust evolves. The balance that creates reciprocity actuates in the willingness to give and to receive information and assistance and to encompass attitudes and events. Reciprocity must have the perceived experience of equality, but it does not need to be tit for tat. It is the recognition of entitlement both in the other and in oneself and the capacity to act on that entitlement.

Reciprocity in the volunteer corps requires that the volunteers be encouraged to share their side and that, when they share, they be legitimately heard and considered. In turn, the agency also has its right to have its side stated, heard, and worked through to mutual understanding. Reciprocity demands again that volunteers receive from their experience as well as give and that the agency appreciate and credit what it receives from the volunteers.

Reciprocity requires mutuality. Mutuality is a recognition of relational reality and a willingness to work cooperatively with that reality. Mutuality demands that all parties affected by a given process or decision be consciously and actively included in the evolution of that process or decision. Mutuality precludes authoritarianism and the dictatorial imposition of one's wants on another. Mutuality demands that all parties involved be given an opportunity to contribute to the processes that will directly affect them, thereby encouraging their sense of inclusion, cooperation, and adaptation. Mutuality forestalls resentment, resistance, and noncooperative reaction; it assists in creating a smooth administrative process.

Mutuality with the volunteer corp requires stated recognition of the volunteers' existence and contribution to the process of the organization. It requires that volunteers be included in the development of policy that will directly affect them as individuals or the nature and manner of their work. Throughout the evolution of this process, they must be given legitimate attention and consideration, spoken to with honest, direct statements, and heard with openness and sincerity. This willingness to engage in an authentic, mutual process does not preclude the legitimate power of the agency to make final policy decisions; in fact, mutuality demands that the volunteer recognize and respect the rights of the agency to exercise its administrative function. The volunteer must credit the administration's side as honorably as the administration credits the volunteer's position.

Trust, fairness, reciprocity, and mutuality are clearly interdependent, each being interlocked and supportive of the others in a productive process of human relationship. Key to the actuality of this process is the additional premise of commitment to dialog. Dialog, the concrete, mutual, reciprocal, and fair exchange of each individual's "I" truths, may not guarantee universal positive resolution, but it will generate trust and consequently lay the foundations for a process that is most often constructive, most often progressive, and most often highly productive.

Dialog not only encourages cooperation and integration but generates creativity. It is out of dialog that new perceptions, new insights, and new approaches find their way into consideration and, often, productive implementation. Dialog engenders the productiveness of a team model. Dialog is the essential dynamic of team process, and an attempt to create and maintain a team approach without dialog is doomed to failure.

Dialog, the clear, direct sharing of "I" statements, must be encouraged with and from the volunteer corps. Volunteers must be given, in understandable vocabulary, the position of the agency, particularly on issues that directly affect them. In turn, their "I" statements must be given a time and place in which to be voiced and the credit they warrant. Volunteers must be known, they must be spoken with, and they must be credited. In turn, the agency must also be known, heard, and credited. This requires a system of practices that consciously and deliberately encourages dialog, including support groups, inservice programs, retreats, one-on-one interviews, and reasonable access to volunteer supervisors and agency personnel. The time commitment this requires is balanced with a relatively smooth and productive process. It is much easier, and much less costly in terms of time and money, to forestall personnel problems proactively than to attempt to counter and correct problems reactively.

PROGRAM DESIGN

What has been discussed so far is a consideration of desires and premises, wants and beliefs that form the abstract foundations for a successful volunteer program. How to make these principles concrete in both design and execution needs to be addressed next. With concreteness and effectiveness in mind, we now turn our attention to the specifics of program design.

Director of Volunteers

Any program, no matter how well designed, is only as effective as the individuals involved in its execution. With this postulate in mind, it seems appropriate to begin a discussion of program design with a description of expectations and responsibilities associated with the creation of the position of director of volunteers and a description and recommendations about the nature and capability of the individual hired to serve in this function. Both these points warrant careful consideration because, realistically, the function given to the position of volunteer director and how that function is executed greatly determine the success of a volunteer program.

Job Description

The director of volunteers is usually responsible for recruitment, selection, placement, supervision, and evaluation. In addition, many programs are designed so that training is included as the director's responsibility, although this can be contracted out. The advantage of facilitating new members' entry and bonding into an established corps is obviously hampered to some degree, however, when training is done by an outside individual.

The director of volunteers should hold equal status to other divisional directors in an agency and should be directly responsible to the administrative director. It must be remembered that the volunteer director will be responsible for the administration of a division that houses a significant number of people; in fact, in many home care agencies the volunteer corps represents, in gross number of personnel, the largest division in the agency. The degree of responsibility held by the director is measured by the number of functions he or she is accountable to perform, the number of personnel under his or her supervision, and the fact that personnel in this division usually have the greatest amount of contact hours with the public and consequently represent significant risk if mismanaged.

The director of volunteers is usually responsible to the executive or managing director of the agency. Occasionally the position of director of volunteers is combined with or responsible to the social services division or, in a few instances, to the pastoral unit. In still other instances, the position of director of volunteers is filled by a volunteer, an arrangement that works well provided that nothing major occurs for which the director needs to be held accountable. When this position is held on a volunteer basis, it limits the power of the executive administration to hold the division accountable; this is a subtle point but warrants careful consideration before one institutes a totally volunteer division.

In addition to administrative and educational responsibilities, the director of volunteers ideally should perform a counseling function. The capacity to defuse psychodynamic problems as they begin to evolve is invaluable in the administration of a problem-limited agency. The director of volunteers, like any director of any division, needs to be able to keep problems from developing, and must be aggressively proactive in philosophy and policy so that there is need for only a limited amount of reactive administrative decisions. This helps keep the

general balance of administrative power in place and helps the executive director maintain an effective and assertive leadership role.

In most home care agencies, teamwork is essential. First, it is the volunteer director's responsibility to inculcate and nurture a cooperative team interaction within the corps itself. Second, the director must function as the chief catalyst to assist in the integration of the corps into the general agency team. The director's responsibility is to help the corps remain cognitively, emotionally, and functionally integrated with the agency as a whole. Finally, it is the obligation of the volunteer director to ensure that the corps function meets and matches the service needs of the agency in general and of other divisions in specifics; the director is responsible for seeing that the corps delivers, and delivers with some skill, the services requested by the various divisions of the agency.

Special Skills Required

Ideally, the individual who functions as volunteer director should have administrative (particularly in health care or social areas), educational, and psychotherapeutic (counseling) skills. It is difficult to find one individual who has talent, experience, and training in all three of these areas, so compromises must often be made. It must be remembered, however, that the more compromises agreed to, the weaker the structure and the greater the potential for problems. With this in mind, a good rule of thumb is that any individual hired to act as director of volunteers should be skilled in performing at least two of the three ideal functions of the job. In addition, no compromise should be made on administrative capability. Individuals who are skilled in administration and education would be suitable; the psychotherapeutic function could be addressed by the social service division. Alternatively, individuals who are skilled in administration and psychotherapy could forfeit the educational function to an outside contract. It is risky, however, to have as director an individual who has only administrative skills;

this creates too weak a structure by dividing responsibility and thereby accountability. It is difficult, if not impossible, to administer an integrated division if the majority of responsibilities are farmed out, along with their accountability and control.

The individual should be empathetic, perceptive, and capable of being supportive to others; should have well-developed listening and communication skills; and should be relatively charismatic or at least capable of stimulating bonding, cohesion, and commitment in a group. In addition, the individual should be skilled in evaluation and decision making, should be capable of exercising his or her responsibility with decisiveness, and should have the strength and the courage to accept responsibility and be held accountable.

Ideally, the individual should hold at least a Master's degree in psychology, sociology, human services, administration, or related fields and should have a minimum of three years of experience in working with groups and/or the public. The credentials are important, but the bottom line is the effectiveness of the individual in the job; consequently, exceptions to specific credentials are always possible.

Structure of the Corps

The structure of the corps must be logically and thoughtfully developed. This structuring begins with a careful evaluation of what is expected in performance from the corps, or what the volunteers will be doing. Their various functions should be conceptualized in terms that are concrete and specific (e.g., cataloging books for a library, cooking, or filling in for personnel shortages in other divisions, such as social service or nursing). Once it is determined what the corps is expected to do, then an educated guess about how many individuals will be needed to fulfill the functions listed must be made. What should be avoided is having too many volunteers who can serve a function for which there is limited use and not enough volunteers to fill functions where there is demand.

Home care volunteer corps should contain individuals who are proficient in general social skills, homemaking, child care, fine arts, and fund-raising. In addition, a percentage of the corps should have professional skills in nursing, social work, geriatric care, business, law, library science, or virtually any area in which the agency sees itself potentially involved. The greater the versatility of the corps, the greater the agency's potential for service and for lowering the costs of service. A volunteer corps should be envisioned as a pool of resources in terms of both the skills of the individuals themselves and the potential that these individuals offer through the networking of their contacts. These individuals bring not only themselves and their skills into the corps but also their world.

All volunteers enlisted into the corps should be required to attend a training program designed by the agency to orient the individuals to the expectations and procedures of the organization. The training program should be structured so that the focus includes orientation and group integration in addition to factual data. The skills and talents brought into the corps by the volunteers must be recognized and credited, and training programs must be flexible enough to enhance and facilitate a variety of volunteer offerings; they must never suffocate, mutilate, denigrate, or disregard what the volunteer offers as his or her own. Training programs must come from a position of respect, reinforcement, and facilitation rather than from a position of haughty authoritarianism and unilateral righteousness.

PROGRAM STRUCTURE

Recruitment

Appropriate time and consideration given to a recruitment campaign can save a great deal of time, effort, and money later on in the management of the volunteer corps. As described before, targeted recruitment is well worth the time and effort it involves because it guarantees an appropriately populated resource pool and aids morale by ensuring that those recruited will be appreciated and used.

In-home care agencies should begin their recruitment programs with a careful examination of the services they offer and those that can legitimately be expected from a volunteer corps: what the corps can be expected to do for the agency, and what it can be trained to do for the public served by the agency. The outline in Table 63–1 is generally adaptable and serves as a base for virtually any in-home care volunteer corps. An attempt should be made to recruit individuals who have specialties within areas that are concurrent with the specialties of the agency. For example, if a particular agency specializes in the care of terminally ill children, then individuals who are familiar with nursing, psychotherapy, and physical therapy specific to children should be sought.

Obviously, familiarity with the structure and service function of the agency is important when one is choosing a recruitment target, but equally important is a familiarity with the demographic nature of the population served by the agency. A concerted effort must be made to recruit a complementary, representative sample of the service population. Here the issues relevant to the client population that must be considered include the following:

- number of males and females in the client population
- age factors
- racial and ethnic factors
- educational factors
- socioeconomic factors
- religious factors
- neighborhood ethnocentric factors

Every attempt should be made to recruit volunteers from each demographic group perceived as essential and representative of the client population. Good recruitment policy should result in a corps that has flexibility, adaptability, and enough variety in resources to meet creatively virtually any challenge of service offered by the population. In short, the corps should match in demographic make-up the make-up of the population served and should match in resources the wants and needs of the agency's clients.

Recruits can be gathered from a variety of sources. Individuals with professional and semi-professional skills can be acquired by tapping into business and industry volunteer programs, professional service organizations and clubs, and professional schools, particularly for combined volunteer/internship programs. Contact with these sources should be personal and ongoing, and the director of volunteers must be responsible for the cultivation of a wide-ranging, solidly woven network of personal contacts in each of these recruitment areas. In addition, volunteers from the existing corps can be trained to speak to church groups, women's organizations, general social service clubs, and special interest groups that might have an interest in the function and services offered by the agency. The development of a speaker's bureau within the corps is an excellent technique. This involves the development of a brochure listing a variety of topics on which members of the corps are willing and capable to talk, circulating these pamphlets in appropriate places (many groups are looking for speakers), and following up with

Table 63–1 Volunteers Who Have Skills Most Appropriate for the Agency and the Public

For the Agency	For the Public
Librarians	Nurses
Accountants	Physician assistants
Lawyers	Physical therapists
Bookkeepers	Educators
Grant writers	Social workers
Fund-raisers	Clergy
Secretaries	Psychotherapists
Computer operators	Homemakers
Publicity personnel	

phone calls and personal arrangements for bookings.

Publicity is an important factor in the recruitment plan. It is a good idea to begin by seeking out for recruitment an individual who has some degree of skill in creating, developing, and executing publicity campaigns. This individual might be someone who is actually in public relations but may also be someone familiar with newspaper writing, advertising, and the like. Once this individual is in place, then he or she can carry the ball in designing public relation programs aimed at general recruitment. In addition, remember that every constructively used and credited volunteer in the corps will recruit for the corps through his or her spoken enthusiasms.

Good recruitment demands that you know what you are doing as an agency and that you have a good idea where you are going and how you are going to get there. How you are going to get there should include the creation of a corps that has as its goal not only service but the capacity to be self-generating. When you begin by recruiting individuals who are skilled in recruitment, you are well on your way; simply credit their skill, maintain basic guidance and cohesiveness, and allow your original recruits to do what they do best: recruit.

Evaluation

Evaluation is one of the more difficult functions of the volunteer director. Bad decisions can be costly in many ways; consequently, it is essential that the volunteer director have some basic familiarity with standard evaluation instruments and techniques and also have well-developed and well-tested visceral reactions.

Every candidate should be required to have a private initial interview with the director. At this point, the candidate should be evaluated for basic social skills, generally appropriate behavior and expression, and the identification of any gross problems that would make the candidate inappropriate for recruitment. A conversational interview of about 30 to 45 minutes is usually enough to give you a general sense of the individual's personality. If there is a desire to be more clinical, any one of the standard personality tests could be administered at the end of the interview, and the individual could then be told that he or she will hear from the agency about the decision as to his or her status.

The guideline for this evaluation must be appropriateness for the program, not whether the director likes the individual. Evaluations must be kept as fair as possible, and that requires looking at what is needed to do the job and how much the individual being interviewed fits the need.

Once past the initial interview, the candidates should be informed that they will be under ongoing evaluation during the training period. This is one of the reasons why it is a good idea to have training periods that extend over time (4 to 6 weeks); it gives the extended opportunity necessary for a fair and accurate evaluation.

During the training period, candidates should be evaluated in terms of their creativity, insightfulness, perception, cooperativeness, emphatic capacity, adaptability, and capability to integrate relatively easily into the group. In addition, attention should be given to identification of leadership potential in general and of particular talent areas. It is an excellent idea to include a practicum period at the conclusion of the training course. This practicum should include at least 6 hours of on-site observation and supervised participation by the candidate in activities appropriate for the volunteer corps. Candidates should be evaluated by their practicum supervisor, and this evaluation should be handed in and reviewed by the volunteer director before the closing interview.

The closing interview must be perceived and conducted as a mutual dialog between the candidate and the volunteer director. Both parties must present their side with reasonably open disclosure. If a candidate has proved less than appropriate for a particular volunteer program, the individual should be credited for skills that he or she does hold, an explanation given for why this particular program is not a particularly good context for his or her offerings, and constructive suggestions given for situations that might prove more fulfilling. Candidates who do appear to be appropriate need to be credited, and clear statements must be made about how their skills will be incorporated into the program and what their rights and responsibilities are as members of the corps. Time must be given in all cases to hear and process candidates' concerns, questions, and opinions. In addition, candidates should be reminded of the fact that they are subject to continuous evaluation and that there is a mutual right to terminate the relationship at any point if either volunteer or agency finds that necessary. Finally, a contract stipulating the rights, responsibilities, and terms of the relationship should be jointly signed, and each participating party should receive a copy.

Training Program

The goals of a well-developed and well-delivered training program must be the integration of the recruit into the system and structure of the agency, the inculcation of necessary skills and pertinent information, and the encouragement and direction of preexisting skills and information brought into the program by the recruit. Training programs should be aimed at enhancement and integration rather than reformation and visionary indoctrination, at development and adaptability rather than reconstruction and remodeling. A syllabus that has proved successful with a variety of training classes is presented in Exhibit 63–1.

The case review is a method of engendering thematic cohesiveness throughout the lectures. In addition, it is an excellent method of integrating new members into the ongoing work experience of the agency. A current case seen as didactically appropriate should be chosen and introduced with initial relevant data at the second session, and then in each session thereafter the material being presented that day should be applied to the ongoing case study. The result should be clarity, concreteness, and a growing

familiarity with agency process; in addition, there should be a distinct evolution of identification, inclusiveness, and integration and a feeling of developing familiarity and confidence within the volunteer candidates.

The practicum, as discussed above, gives the agency a unique opportunity for on-site evaluation. In addition, it offers the volunteer candidates a chance to experience concretely what they might have only imagined. Experiencing the reality allows the candidates to discover whether they really want to do this work; it is one thing to imagine a role, another to live it.

There are two formats that the practicum can follow: accompanying as an observer an in-home care nurse as he or she makes rounds, or assisting a working volunteer. Ideally, both formats can be included with the nursing observation as the formal practicum experience and the volunteer assistance a primary step in actual volunteer function. It is important for the volunteer director to do a debriefing with each candidate as he or she completes the nursing observation; this gives the candidate a chance to work through any surfaced concerns or anxieties and at the same time allows the volunteer director to acquire necessary firsthand feedback from the experience.

It is important that clear recognition and crediting be given to the volunteers who successfully complete the training program. This is a factor of both incorporation and morale. Successful candidates should be formally issued certificates of completion at a graduation ceremony. It is not at all inappropriate to schedule an evening event, off site at a town hall or a church auditorium, with a guest keynote speaker, the distribution of certificates to each graduate, and a reception. Graduation should be seen as a rite of passage or initiation marking a distinct shift of status based on the recognition of skill. It is a formal recognition of the incorporation of the candidates as fully functioning members of the corps; it is a statement of welcome, trust, and inclusion.

Exhibit 63–1 Syllabus for Volunteer Training Program

Structure: Twenty-four hours of class time divided into 2-hour sessions for 6 weeks and 6 hours of practicum experience for a total of 30 instructional hours.

Delivery: Appropriate team members with one core instructor to provide continuity and integration as well as group cohesion. Methods should include lecture and discussion, demonstration and guided hands-on experience, and group process.

Content Breakdown:

- *Session 1*—general introduction (focus primarily on structure, function, and general process of agency, including introduction of personnel and demonstration of procedures)
- *Session 2*—context presentations (what they will do, where they will do it and with whom, and how the current program integrates with work they have already done in other areas), group process session, case review and process session, case review and process demonstration
- *Session 3*—history of the movement in which they are involved (e.g., if hospice groups, a full explanation and differentiation of types, forms, and methods of hospice care), discussion of philosophical roots of program, notion and practice of confidentiality and professional responsibility; group process; case review
- *Session 4*—presentation of materials by the social service division, including policy, practice, and issues of integration and cohesiveness; group process; case review
- *Session 5*—presentation by the medical division, including material on pain control, psy-

chiatry, and other relevant medical issues; group process; case review
- *Session 6*—presentation and demonstration of material from the nursing division, including basic information about lifting the patient, making a bed, etc.; group process; case review
- *Session 7*—consideration of basic sociological issues surrounding in-home care, general information and significant demographics in the catchment area served by the agency, discussion of social and legal issues, group process, case review
- *Session 8*—communication skills, including nonverbal communication; listening skills and basic evaluation methods (fact, cognitive, and affect levels of evaluation); group process and practice; case review
- *Session 9*—communication skills, including demonstration and practice in content and affect responses; application of methods to various psychological situations (e.g., responding to an agency patient); group process and practice; case review
- *Session 10*—presentation and consideration of issues on family dynamics; variability in family structure and function; what might they find, how must they adjust, and when they need to refer; group process; case review
- *Session 11*—consideration of religious dynamics and their function and influence on patient and family, presentation by chaplain, group process, case review
- *Session 12*—ethical issues (suicide, euthanasia, confidentiality, integrity, responsibility), general review, closure

Retention

The capacity to retain individuals who do their jobs with skill and dedication is always a goal for volunteer programs. Retention is usually important in any personnel program because it should guarantee a maintenance of

quality in service or product. Consistency, commitment, personal identification, and consequent responsibility, loyalty, and increased skill that comes from experience are all excellent reasons for encouraging retention. In a volunteer program, the economic factor makes retention programs essential. The cost of volunteer labor is primarily in recruiting and training. Once the initial investment has been made, the cost of supervision should be significantly lower. Because the largest cost invested in an individual volunteer comes up front, and because maintenance costs are significantly lower, it stands to reason that the longer the individual remains in active and productive service, the greater the return on the initial cost. The expense of training an individual is clearly and significantly diminished by the length of his or her service.

The key to a strong retention program is a commitment by the agency to a policy of equability, mutuality, and fairness. It is essential to remember that, although volunteers are not paid, they do need paybacks. It is essential that individuals get something back for what they give. If this balance of giving and receiving is not maintained, it will not be long before corps members will begin to feel victimized. Volunteers want to feel useful, not used.

Payback is given in recognition, reward, and authenticity of respect. Recognition demands that volunteers, both collectively and individually, be credited for the nature and quality of what they do. Individuals need to have communicated to them that their immediate supervisor and the agency see and understand what they are actually producing. The volunteer needs to know, by being told, that the director is aware and appreciative of the difficulties involved in the volunteer's performance of responsibilities. Recognition demands that the director be familiar with the person and performance of the volunteer and that this understanding be communicated to the volunteer as acknowledged praise and/or direction at regular intervals.

Rituals of reward are part of the paycheck in volunteerism. Open, formal, public rewards for quality of service are necessary for morale and to help maintain retention. Rewards, whatever specific form they take, should always involve some degree of public recognition for the individual and the corps and for the quality of their work.

Authenticity of respect can only be communicated if the director truly does know the volunteer and his or her work and takes the time and effort to communicate that familiarity. Authenticity of respect demands that the director perform his or her job responsibilities with a high degree of commitment and involvement. It is the director's responsibility to develop appropriate relationships with each volunteer and, within the context of this relationship, to understand perceptively the capacity and character of each corps member. Authenticity communicates when it exists; if the goal is to communicate authentic respect, then the director must be committed to behavior that engenders an honest and appropriate knowledge of and appreciation for each individual member of the corps. Basically, the issue here is integrity of behavior, an integrity that is quickly recognized by the volunteer and is responded to with appreciation, trust, and mutuality.

The question still remains as to how specifically the director can apply recognition, reward, and authenticity of respect toward a goal of retention. Basically, this goal can be accomplished through structures of interchange, which fall into two broad categories: those activities that are the specific personal efforts of the director, and those activities that involve the participation of the agency and the corps.

Under the first category, it is essential that the director know the members of the corps. A file should be kept on each member containing as much relevant data as can be acquired. Information that is standard to a résumé obviously should be present in this file, but the profile should be broadened to include details of life events, personal traits, unique characteristics and relationships, and anything and everything that will help the director know and understand the individual with whom he or she is working; obviously, all information should be kept confidential. A complete medical and psychological history should be acquired if possible, enhanced by an appropriate social history. Updates as to addresses, phone numbers, changes in name, marital status, and jobs are essential. The record should include basic information about the volunteer's mate and family so that a sense of the volunteer's social context and needs is continuously and accurately maintained.

The director must make every effort to keep the dialog open with members of the corps. The maintenance of dialog involves time, relational skill, and commitment to the process.

Approximately 25% of the director's time should be dedicated to the "cultivation of the garden." This cultivation involves time spent in direct interchange with the volunteers as individuals and as a group. Individual time can be created in a variety of ways. It is a good idea periodically to schedule lunch with individual members of the corps at the initiative of the director. The lunches should be informal and conducive to open dialog. They should occur at least once a year and more frequently if the calendar permits. Individual lunches offer time and opportunity for personal disclosure, for needed recognition, for mutual evaluation, and for defusing and affirmation. In addition, they serve to enhance and maintain the bonding and integration of the volunteer with the program and as such are a major tool in retention.

It is important that the director advocate on behalf of volunteers, as individuals and as a group, to the agency. The corps needs someone to speak on its behalf, to exhibit concern for its interests, and to act as a peer representative within the management level of the agency. This can be a delicate balance for the director who is obligated to meet the needs of the agency as well as those of the corps. Every attempt must be made to keep the corps bonded and integrated with the agency so that goals become reciprocal and mutual. The director must be open and truthful in all communications, both to the corps and to the agency; this includes making statements of the inability to disclose when permission to discuss an issue has not been received from involved parties. Basically, it must be recognized that it is the responsibility of the director to safeguard the fair treatment of corps members and to work to maintain trust, equability, and mutuality.

In the same vein, it is the responsibility of the director to maintain clear communication between the agency's administration and the corps. Weekly meetings with the executives are quite appropriate when possible. These discussions should center on a mutual exchange of information, interest, and concern in which management is kept informed as to the function and character of the corps and the director can in turn be informed as to management's attitude and insights concerning the corps.

In addition, it is the responsibility of the director to meet with the corps, ideally on a weekly basis. These meetings should function as an open exchange of information and attitudes. They should be conducted as open dialogs directed toward goals of understanding and cohesion. These discussions are clearly an essential tool in maintaining good communication, but in addition they serve to identify and defuse problems of anxiety, insecurity, rumor, and discontent before they fester into major administrative difficulties.

Mentioned above was the director's responsibility for the organization and facilitation of collective methods to assist retention. These collective tools include operating a weekly support group, conducting recognition events, offering periodic inservice programs, and awarding certification and credentials when possible.

Support groups are essential in maintaining an effective volunteer program. Ideally, the support group should meet once a week and be open to all volunteers. The group should not exceed 20 participants; if it does, a second group should be formed. The group must have a professional facilitator; if the director is not qualified to act in this capacity, someone who is credentialed should be brought in. The presence of a professional is required because the basic function and nature of the group are therapeutic rather than self-help. The issues that surface from in-home care volunteerism are often heavily psychologically laden and warrant therapeutic response. A well-conducted support group can forestall numerous problems, some of a serious nature, before they have a chance to begin. The group should function therapeutically (defusing emotional or conceptual issues before they evolve into a crisis), educationally (with continued instruction included that is relevant to the volunteers' current experiences), and cohesively (as members begin to identify with and support each other as a group).

Groups should be 1.5 hours in length. This gives enough time for all members to participate if they so choose. It is helpful to have a therapeutic theme for each session. For example, the issue of the volunteers' self-confidence might be chosen. The facilitator then introduces the theme, and as the group progresses with discussion around the individual volunteer's experiences and concerns, the facilitator clarifies, interprets, and interconnects individual contributions along thematic lines. This process serves to educate, affect therapeutically, and encourage the group in terms of identification and cohesion. Alternatively, the thematic line can be extracted by the facilitator from the group process. In this case, the group begins its process immediately, and the facilitator, having paid close and perceptive attention, extracts whatever thematic thread begins to surface, mirrors it back to the group, clarifies, elaborates, and again reinforces the theme as the group process continues. Here again, the same positive effect of education, therapy, and cohesion can be achieved with a final result of minimal crisis and burnout within the corps.

We all need to feel a sense of accomplishment and competency, regardless of what it is we have chosen to do; this is especially true for volunteers. For this reason, recognition events are essential to maintain individual involvement in the volunteer corps. Recognition events should include graduation, an awards lunch, a Christmas or other holiday event, a mates dinner, and a summer picnic hosted by the agency.

Graduation, as discussed above, should be a specific event, held off site in the evening, with a guest speaker and the distribution of certificates of completion. A reception after the ceremony always is well received and serves to enhance group identity and belonging.

An awards lunch, given by the director usually in the early spring or fall, serves to affirm publicly the director's recognition and appreciation for the corps and its members. The lunch is for the corps, and outside individuals should be invited only at the initiative of the volunteers; this includes invitations extended to other members of the agency. The lunch provides an excellent opportunity for a review of in-house corps business and the highlights of the preceding year of service. In addition, specific awards for contributions and performance can be given, with care being taken that presentations are always given in fairness and justice. The main theme, however, should be the affirmation of the corps as a unit, and an open statement of appreciation for the quality of the corps' performance and commitment should be the central focus of the luncheon.

A mates dinner is essential for any assertive retention program. In-home care volunteers have a degree of involvement in their work that is rivaled by few paid employees. The work tends to hold the volunteers emotionally and intellectually. It is as though a piece of them were put aside especially for this work, and those who are close to them are acutely aware of this surrender. Mates may become uneasy, competitive, and in some case jealous of the volunteers' time and vested concern. Often the mate may experience the volunteer's new commitment as a personal loss and may subtly or aggressively agitate for the volunteer to resign from the corps. This agitation can be eased by giving recognition and credit to the mate's position. A dinner, sponsored by the agency and hosted by the corps, given in February or March, again off campus, usually works exceptionally well. February and March tend to be depressed periods, times when issues that are grains of sand during the rest of the year become pebbles or perhaps rocks to stumble over. It is quite appropriate for all agency administrators to be invited, and the executive administrator as well as the director of volunteers should be asked to address the group. Regardless of the general theme chosen for the evening, it is essential that direct recognition of the mates' position and difficulties be expressed. Statements must be open and discussion direct, not subtle or alluding.

The mates' side must be clearly credited, and it is essential that the agency thank these individuals for their support and recognize them as nonrostered members of the team. Again, the goal is cohesion and dissipation of dissatisfaction before it blossoms into crisis; in addition, the dinner serves an advocacy function for the volunteers and consequently directly bolsters their adhesion to the program by increasing their trust in the agency as a concerned personal resource.

Christmas parties and summer picnics are events best sponsored by the agency. The Christmas party may include only agency personnel; the summer picnic may include family members, mates, and children. Again, the purpose is cohesion, affirmation, recognition, and nurturing of group identification. In these two events the emphasis is cohesion and identification with the agency as well as with the corps.

Inservice programs provide continuing education for the corps in addition to a psychodynamic function. A full-day inservice program in the fall, planned and prepared by the volunteers, works well. A central theme, a guest speaker, and appropriate representation from the agency are the basic ingredients. The day can be broken into a morning and afternoon session with a luncheon in between; it is a good idea to leave plenty of time for group process and participation. What is important here is that the volunteers get something, learn something, from whatever is offered and that the corps be involved in every aspect of the planning and presentation, that they own the day as their own. The goal, here again, is to reinforce involvement and commitment and to stimulate the enthusiasm and spirit of the corps with new learning, new insights, and new possibilities.

A feeling of belonging, of being an integral, appreciated part of the team, is an essential dynamic in retention. Consequently, it is important that a conscious and consistent effort be

made by the agency as a whole continuously to integrate the volunteers into the spirit and function of the agency. This is as much an attitude as it is a mode of behavior, an attitude that must pervade policy and be actively present in the day-to-day operation of the agency. The bottom line is that volunteers remain present and active if they feel useful, appreciated, and rewarded and perceive themselves as active, necessary parts of the team.

Volunteers who remain with the corps need to feel competent and successful. With this need in mind, the director of volunteers should make every effort, when placing the individual volunteer on an assignment, to place the volunteer for success. Placing a volunteer for success demands that the director know each volunteer, know the particulars of each case, and carefully match the volunteer and his or her skills and personality to the needs of the placement case. It is helpful to envision each case as a context in which the volunteer must function. The object is to choose an individual who, when placed in the case context, will connect and engage in a positive, productive process that will culminate in positive resolutions for everyone, or at least almost everyone.

Placement must begin with an evaluation visit to the family by the director of volunteers. Evaluation data to be considered should include a consideration of the following:

- the patient's physical and psychosocial needs
- the family's physical and psychosocial needs
- the family structure and basic dynamics
- relevant demographic data, such as socioeconomic level of the family, education, ethnicity, religion, race, and the like

Once this material has been gathered, a general profile of family needs and functions can be created and a volunteer chosen who is perceived as compatible with the case dynamics. A great deal of this process is procedural, but there must be, present and active on the part of the director, an intuitive capacity for matchmaking. No matter how many data are collected, and no matter how documented and procedural the evaluation is, success often rests on the intuitive, perceptual capacity of the director to match precisely the right volunteer with the right case context. If the match is fundamentally compatible, the success of the case, in terms of resultant positive resolutions, is close to guaranteed barring introduced or unforeseen circumstances.

Once placement has been made, a schedule for supervision contact must be followed. Ideally, it is good for the director to accompany the volunteer on an introductory visit to the family. This gives the director an on-site opportunity to make sure that there is in fact basic compatibility between the volunteer and the context. On the day when the volunteer actually begins his or her assignment, a brief visit or phone call to the volunteer while he or she is working on the case is both affirming and supportive. Thereafter, periodic on-site visits for evaluation and morale are appropriate. The frequency of these visits depends on the complexity of the case and its length. Cases that are complicated demand more attention, and cases that extend over lengthy durations demand periodic visits to sustain volunteer morale. In addition, periodic brief meetings in the office for review and suggestions are appropriate.

The volunteer should be present at team meetings and encouraged to participate in the case report. Here again, it is the director's responsibility to facilitate this participation and to evaluate its content and process for accuracy, compatibility, and effectiveness. The director then needs to feed back appropriate critiques or affirmation privately to the volunteer about his or her contribution, remembering always that the main objects of supervision include education and development of the volunteer as well as quality service to the client.

There are times when cases do not work out as anticipated, no matter how carefully the preparatory work has been done. It is the director's responsibility to initiate and facilitate the exit of a volunteer in these cases. Circumstances that warrant this intervention include situations where the health and safety of the volunteer are at risk, situations where gross incompatibility of personalities develop, and situations where the family dynamic is fundamentally dysfunctional and threatens the general procedure of the case.

It is the responsibility of the director to advocate on behalf of the volunteer to the family and to the agency in these circumstances and in any situation where it is critical that the volunteer's side be heard. In this regard, the director is answerable for the creation and maintenance of an open, constructive dialog. This demands a degree of diplomatic skill and courage. In the end, however, it takes less courage to deal directly with each crisis as it arrives than to let discontent and antagonism grow to proportions of a major incident and then attempt to deal with it. Again, the object is to keep problems from ever developing rather than to figure out how to cope with them after the fact. The object is to be consistently proactive and consistently in control and thereby to minimize the necessity to respond reactively, subjugated to control by the situation.

CONCLUSION

A successful volunteer program demands that the agency in general, and the director in particular, have a clear, mutual understanding of a relational ethic that is conscientiously and consistently concretized in program design and process. There must be an active commitment to the ethical values of integrity, justice, and humanism. These values must influence policy and decision making at every level, acting as an integrating thread of uniformity and consistency. In addition, there must be an active commitment by all involved parties to the relational premises of trust, fairness, mutuality, reciprocity, and dialog, premises that must be experienced in and through the daily process of the program. The bottom line is that quality recruits who are appropriately and skillfully trained and supervised are retained and remain productive, thereby increasing the quality of service and the cost-efficiency of a good volunteer program.

Fair treatment and experienced justice for all parties involved pay dividends on every level in every way, regardless of the currency used, whether monetary or relational, to ensure the magnitude of the result.

BIBLIOGRAPHY

Benton, R. (1978). *Death and dying: Principles and practices in patient care*. New York: Van Nostrand Reinhold.

Boszoimenyi-Nagy, I., & Krasner, B. (1986). *Between give and take*. New York: Brunner/Mazel.

Chapman, J., & Chapman, H. (1975). *Behavior and health care: A humanistic helping process*. St. Louis, MO: Mosby.

Danish, S.J., & Haner, A.C. (1976). *Helping skills: A basic training program*. New York: Human Services Press.

Logan, M., & Hunt, E. (1978). *Death and the human condition*. North Scituate, MA: Duxbury.

Mann, R. (1967). *Interpersonal styles and group development: An analysis of the member-leader relationship*. New York: John Wiley & Sons.

Schein, E., & Bennis, W. (1965). *Personal and organizational change through group methods*. New York: John Wiley & Sons.

Schmolling, P., Youkeles, M., & Burger, W. (1989). *Human services in contemporary America*, 2nd ed. Pacific Grove, CA: Brooks/Cole.

CHAPTER 64

The Peer Review Organization

Marilyn D. Harris and Maryanne McDonald

The Peer Review Improvement Act of 1982 established the utilization and quality control peer review organization (PRO) program. Initially, the PRO reviewed care provided to Medicare patients in acute care settings. Section 9353(c) of the Omnibus Budget Reconciliation Act of 1986 amended Section 1154(a)(14) to require PROs to respond to all written Medicare beneficiary complaints on or after August 1, 1987, concerning the quality of care provided by skilled nursing facilities (SNFs), home health agencies (HHAs), and hospital outpatient departments (HOPDs). Federal Regulation 42 CFR Section 476.131 authorized the PRO to obtain the patient's medical record to perform this required review activity. There are other criteria that can trigger a request for a patient record.

OVERVIEW OF PROCESS

The PRO review process is contracted to agencies that carry out the myriad procedures. All aspects of the review process are important. These details are included in the manual prepared by some PROs. The manual contains the PRO's responsibilities, generic quality screens (GQSs), weighted scores for severity levels, interventions required to correct identified problems, methods of chart selection, sample forms used to request documentation from agencies for medical review and letters that are issued, notice of determination, and time frame for review. Each HHA should have (or request) a copy of this manual from the PRO responsible for the agency's review process.

One criterion that may initiate a review of an HHA's clinical record is a patient's readmission to a hospital within 31 days of discharge from a hospital. The clinical record for a percentage of patients who have had intervening care, including home care, will be selected for review. The agency receives a written request from the PRO for a copy of the clinical record. The reviewer uses the GQSs (Appendix 64–A) specific to home care agencies that were developed by the Health Care Financing Administration (HCFA) to determine whether a quality of care issue exists. These GQSs address multiple aspects of care. The HCFA has recommended that the GQSs be updated by PROs to reflect current standards of medical practice.

The purpose of this chapter is to encourage HHAs to incorporate the current PRO criteria and GQSs into the agency's Quality Assessment/Performance Improvement (QA/PI) pro-

Source: Adapted with permission from M.D. Harris and M. McDonald, The Peer Review License, *Home Health Care Nurse*, Vol. 9, No. 1, pp. 37–42, ©1991, J.B. Lippincott Company, and M.D. Harris, The Peer Review Organization Process Revisited, *Home Health Care Nurse*, Vol. 11, No. 5, pp. 67–68, © 1993, J.B. Lippincott Company.

gram. Selected criteria and screens can be evaluated as one aspect of the ongoing reviews done to meet certification and accreditation standards. Data collection is beneficial to document specific patients' outcomes. Also, agencies can determine whether a quality of care issue is present within the agency.

AGENCY-SPECIFIC FINDINGS

The first request for a clinical record from the Visiting Nurse Association of Eastern Montgomery County/Department of Abington Memorial Hospital (VNA) was received in July 1988. As of August 1990, the VNA had received requests for 16 clinical records. Once additional information was requested, this was followed by a letter stating that there was no question of a quality of care issue. The VNA included the PRO criteria in its QA/PI program. Selected GQSs are reviewed as one aspect of quarterly record reviews. We have also completed two in-depth studies that used the 31-day readmission criterion as a basis for record review.

At the VNA we use our computer system to identify specific charts for review. By using Just Ask (Delta Health Systems, Inc., Altoona, PA), we are able to request our computer to sort data from the patient master file. The computer can generate a list of all patients who have been admitted to the VNA upon hospital discharge and have been discharged from VNA services because they have been rehospitalized within 31 days of discharge from the hospital.

From a clinical perspective, we are interested in answers to several questions as a result of these reviews:

- What was the patient's condition on admission to home care (medical and nursing diagnosis)?
- Was the referral appropriate in our opinion?
- Why was the patient readmitted to the hospital? Was this related to admission diagnosis at the start of home care?

- Were there factors within the agency's and nurses' control that could have prevented the rehospitalization?

The purpose of the studies in 1988 and in May 1990 was to identify areas of inappropriate assessment, planning, intervention, and evaluation during the patient's stay with the agency.

In January 1988, 207 patients were admitted and 114 discharged from service. Ten patients were readmitted to the hospital during the month. Seven patients had diagnoses that included neoplasms; other diagnoses: congestive heart failure (CHF), chronic obstructive pulmonary disease, and pneumonia.

Eight different primary nurses were involved in the care of the clients. Billing sources included Medicare and private insurance such as Blue Cross, health maintenance organizations (HMOs), and hospital home care departments. Referrals came from three hospitals.

The GQSs were used to review the records of these 10 patients. It was determined that all 10 patients were hospitalized with complications beyond the control of the nurse or the HHA. There was no evidence of inappropriate planning or administration of care.

A similar study was completed for the 17 patients who were readmitted to the hospital within 31 days of hospital discharge in May 1990 (total of 249 admissions to and 243 discharges from service). These 17 patients had 9 different nursing diagnoses. The two most frequently identified were ineffective breathing patterns (8) and self-care deficit (7). There were 11 different medical diagnoses, of which neoplasm (4) and CHF (3) were the most frequently noted.

The payer sources included Medicare, Blue Cross, and other insurers. The majority of patients were older than 70 years of age. The one difference noted was that the majority (13) were men, whereas the agency's total caseload is usually one third men. Only one of the patients did not have some type of support network available. Referrals came from three different hospitals. There were 15 primary nurses involved with the 17 patients. A majority of patients had care by multiple disciplines.

One finding that showed a change over time was the increased number of prescribed medications. Nine of the patients had an average of 8 to 11 medications, and one of the patients had more than 12.

We also correlated the admitting medical diagnoses with the reason for readmission and the nursing diagnoses. Patients readmitted to the hospital with the same diagnosis were a result of the severity of the patients' physical condition, which needed to be managed in the hospital.

In general, it was determined that home care services and the frequency of visits were appropriate in all cases. The patients' support system did not affect the outcome. Patients with poor support systems, however, were more difficult and time-consuming to manage.

The levels of care (patient classification system) of the patients reflected the general breakdown by level of all VNA patients. The majority of patients had multiple chronic illnesses. Eight of the patients had more than two nurses involved with their care within a 31-day period. There was no evidence to support the literature that multiple health providers decrease compliance (Becker & Janz, 1985; Kazis & Friedman, 1988; Matthew & Hingson, 1977; Neal, 1989).

Ten of the patients had more than eight prescribed medications. There was no evidence to support the literature that multiple medications decrease the likelihood of compliance (Spanoli, Ostino, & Borga, 1989). In 1996, Harris & Dugan described the results of a six-month study to evaluate the reasons why, and the characteristics of, VNA patients who were rehospitalized during the time that they were receiving home health care following a previous hospitalization. The findings showed that the VNA patients who experienced repeat hospitalizations were older and sicker than the average VNA patients. There was no evidence that the patients were treated ineffectively by either the hospital or the VNA. The advanced age, multi-

ple diagnoses, and increased mortality rate of these patients suggested the same conclusions. The patients were experiencing overall body system breakdown, which is consistent for patients in the last months of life. Each progressive level of deterioration required a coinciding therapeutic response, resulting in increased hospital encounters.

NATIONAL FINDINGS

The August 4, 1989, issue of the NAHC Report carried a status report on the 2,055 cases of postacute care review that were equally divided among SNFs, HHAs, and HOPD services. Quality problems appeared in 6% to 8% of SNF cases and in 3% to 4% of the home health cases.

Interventions resulting from the review of the cases have primarily been limited to letters and educational activities, although one SNF was placed on intensive review, two SNFs (as of August 4, 1989) were being considered for intensive review, and one physician had been sanctioned. No HHAs were placed on additional reviews.

CONCLUSION

The PRO process is just one of the many reviews that HHAs are subjected to at any given time. On a practical level, HHAs should incorporate current PRO criteria and GQSs into their QA program. At present, there is no mechanism in place for denial of payment for substandard care, although proposed regulations were published in the January 18, 1989 *Federal Register* (vol. 54, no. 11, p. 1956). Medicare certification, and therefore payment, could be lost if the facility or HHA is sanctioned.

The Medicare law requires PROs to coordinate their activities with other review organizations. The HCFA, however, has not established procedures for providing reports from fiscal intermediaries and PROs to the state survey agencies or for coordinating state surveys with

PRO reviews (U.S. General Accounting Office, 1989).

HHAs should have structure and process criteria (either manual or computerized) in place to identify selected records for review. This enables the agency to monitor its internal QA activities so that it has confidence that the GQSs will be met when reviewed by external agencies, including the PRO. This internal monitoring will also enable the agency to document patient outcomes. This is an important aspect of the evaluation process because the emphasis of certification and accreditation programs and site visits in the 1990s will be patient outcomes.

POSTSCRIPT

In Pennsylvania, the Keystone Peer Review Organization, Inc. (KePRO) is the designated Medicare PRO. KePRO's 1992 annual report included a description of the fourth scope of work that began April 1, 1993, and a report of the results of the record reviews completed during the year. During 1992, KePRO completed a total of 732 intervening care reviews. A total of 15 confirmed quality problems were identified for SNFs, HHAs, and HOPDs. There were five Severity Level I and two Severity Level II confirmed problems in HHAs. In comparison, the 1991 annual report stated that there were 43 total problems for HHAs, 24 Severity Level I cases, 17 Severity Level II cases, and 2 Severity Level III cases. A majority of the problems were attributable to communication/documentation issues.

The records of 28 patients who were admitted to VNA services during June 1993 and were discharged within 31 days because they were hospitalized were reviewed. The hospitalizations were planned (a patient with carcinoma who was readmitted for chemotherapy and an expectant mother who had received prenatal home care service and delivered her child) or unrelated to the care provided by the VNA staff. There were multiple payer sources, staff, and medical and nursing diagnoses associated with these 28 patients.

The number of patients at the VNA who meet the criterion discussed above has increased over the years. As noted, there were 10 patients in 1988 (9% of discharges), 17 in 1990 (7%), and 28 in 1993 (10%). To date, at the VNA no quality of care issues have been identified on final determination by the PRO for those records that have been requisitioned for review.

Effective April 1, 1996, KePRO implemented its fifth consecutive contract with the HCFA. This new contract places increased emphasis on health care quality improvement, requiring that numerous cooperative improvement projects be conducted with providers, Medicare HMOs, physicians, and Medicare beneficiaries. One of the changes in the new KePRO procedures is the cessation of the 5% beneficiary sample review. SNF and HHA individual case review will occur only when a beneficiary or other agent acting in the interest of the patient requests a KePRO review. SNFs and HHAs may be asked to participate in cooperative projects, or may suggest projects to KePRO (KEPRO Provider Bulletin, 1996).

The PRO process is just one of the many review processes that HHAs are subjected to at any given time. The complete and accurate documentation of the quality of care rendered to patients is of the utmost importance and contributes to the minimal number of confirmed quality of care problems that have been identified in HHAs.

REFERENCES

Becker, M.H., & Janz, N.K. (1985). The health belief model applied to understanding diabetes regimen compliance. *Diabetes Educator, 2,* 41–47.

Crescent County Foundation for Medical Care. (1990). *Reference manual: HHA Medicare quality review conference.* Naperville, IL: Author.

Harris, M., & Dugan, M. (1996). Evaluating the quality of home care services using patient outcome data. *Home Healthcare Nurse, 14*(6), 463–468.

Kazis, L.E., & Friedman, R.H. (1988). Improving medication compliance in the elderly. *Journal of the American Geriatric Society, 36,* 1161–1162.

KePRO (Keystone Peer Review Organization) Provider Bulletin, 96–1; April 26, 1996. Harrisburg, PA: Author.

KePRO (Keystone Peer Review Organization) 1991–1992 Annual Report. Harrisburg, PA: Author.

Matthew, D., & Hingson, R. (1977). Improving patient compliance. *Medical Clinics of North America, 61,* 879–889.

National Association for Home Care. (1989). *NAHC reports: Post acute care is focus of American Medical Peer Review Association meeting* (Vol. 324). Washington, DC: NAHC.

Neal, W.W. (1989). Reducing costs and improving compliance. *American Journal of Cardiology, 63,* 17–20.

Spanoli, A., Ostino, G., & Borga, A.D. (1989). Drug compliance and unreported drugs in the elderly. *Journal of the American Geriatric Society, 37,* 619–624.

U.S. General Accounting Office. (1989). *Report to the Ranking Minority Member, Special Committee on Aging, U.S. Senate: Medicare assuring the quality of home health services.* Washington, DC: GAO.

Keystone Peer Review Organization HCFA Generic Quality Screens for Home Health Agency Review

GENERIC QUALITY SCREENS—HOME HEALTH AGENCY (HHA)

1. **ADEQUACY OF INTAKE EVALUATION**

   a. Adequate assessment of HHA's capacity to provide the services required for recovery or maximum restoration of function. Assessment to include:
      1. History
      2. Physical assessment/functional limits/impairment
      3. Activities of daily living (ADL)
      4. Psychosocial (cognitive and affective)
      5. Caregiver
      6. Review of medications
      7. Nutritional needs
      8. Environmental risks

   b. Adequate assessment of physical environment and capability of caregiver to provide care in the home.

   c. Adequate assessment of patient before or at time of admission, and source of referral to HHA.

2. **APPROPRIATE AND TIMELY INTERVENTIONS**

   a. Presence of temperature elevation of 100°F oral (101°F rectal) or >, or presence of hypothermia without physician notification within 4 hours from the time detected

   b. Presence of B.P. reading of <85 or >180 systolic, or <50 or >110 diastolic without physician notification within 4 hours from the time detected

   c. Presence of pulse <50 (or 45 if the patient is on a beta blocker) or >120 without physician notification within 4 hours from the time detected

   d. Presence of other significant changes in signs and symptoms without physician notification within 4 hours from time detected. Examples:
      1. Mental status (re: changes in cognitive function or behavior)
      2. Loss of function
      3. Signs and symptoms of congestive heart failure (CHF), etc.

   e. Appropriate diagnostic services provided on physician's orders

   f. Abnormal results of diagnostic services addressed and resolved, or the record explains why they are unresolved

   g. Appropriate intervention if significant change in social support system, including environment

Source: Reprinted from HCFA.

h. Appropriate reporting of abuse/neglect

i. Timely reporting to physician of lack of family and/or patient compliance

3. ADEQUACY OF RESTORATIVE CARE

a. Specialty therapies

1. Restorative need identified and addressed through assessment, plan implementation, and evaluation

2. Presence of therapy plan of care and documentation of therapist's compliance with plan

3. Presence of patient education

b. Nursing instructions

1. Presence of patient education plan and documentation of nursing compliance with the plan

2. Documentation in the nursing care plan of coordination of services (interdisciplinary follow-up and reinforcement)

3. Continual reassessment of patient's needs with referrals to other disciplines as necessary

4. DEATHS

Deaths within 48 hours of transfer to hospital as ascertained from the hospital record

5. POSSIBLE INDICATIONS OF SECONDARY INFECTIONS

a. Temperature elevation >2 degrees after 72 hours of start of care

b. Any indication of an infection following an invasive procedure

6. ISSUES RELATED TO PATIENT CARE AFTER THE HOME HEALTH START OF CARE

a. Presence of incident with resultant injury or untoward effect

b. Presence of decubitus ulcer

c. Presence of life-threatening complications

d. Adverse drug reaction or medication error

e. Evidence of inappropriate planning and administration of patient care

f. Responsibility for termination of care only when services are no longer required

7. DISCHARGE PLAN AND FOLLOW-UP

Documented plan for appropriate follow-up care and discharge summary to physician(s) of record

8. ADEQUACY OF CARE

In the judgment of the professional reviewer, are there any other events/patterns of care that resulted in adverse outcomes that should be evaluated?

No __ Yes __ Explain _____

Effective for all 4SOW reviews initiated on and after 4-15-93

HOME HEALTH AGENCY GENERIC QUALITY SCREENS GUIDELINES

ELEMENTS	EXCLUSIONS	DATA SOURCES	EXPLANATORY NOTES
1. Adequacy of Intake Evaluation			
a. Adequate assessment of HHA's capacity to provide the services required for recovery or maximum restoration of function	None	HHA admission assessment form/intake evaluation, nurses' notes, physician's orders, plan of care, hospital or SNF transfer information, social service notes	Review for appropriateness of level of care (i.e., is the HHA capable of providing the care required for this patient? Did he/she require a higher level of care?)
b. Adequate assessment of physical environment and capability of caregiver to provide care in the home	None	HHA admission assessment form, nurses' notes, intake evaluation	Review home environment to determine if any changes were required (examples: open stairway, exposed electrical cords). Were solutions to the problems identified and discussed and appropriate resolutions agreed upon?
c. Adequate assessment of patient before or at time of admission, and source of referral to HHA	None	HHA admission assessment form, nurses' notes, intake evaluation, hospital or SNF discharge record, physician's orders, plan of care	Was an adequate assessment of the patient done so that the HHA was aware of all the patient's needs? The assessment should include mental status (e.g., depression, orientation). Did the patient have to be referred by a family member as opposed to the medical community?
2. Appropriate and Timely Interventions			
a. Presence of temperature elevation of 100°F oral (rectal 101°F) or >, or presence of hypothermia, without physician notification within 4 hours from the time detected	None	Nurses' notes, vital sign flow sheet, physician contact report, aide notes	Latitude is permitted for the nurse reviewer to use his or her judgment when there is a physician's order that covers the situation identified by the element.

continues

Element		Sources	Guidelines
			If the HHA identifies a temperature elevation, "physician notification" is satisfied by the agency's attempt to notify the physician within 4 hours. Note: Hypothermia as well as hyperthermia may be a problem. Therefore, −2°F from patient's normal temperature requires intervention.
b. Presence of B.P. reading < 85 or >180 systolic, or < 50 or > 100 diastolic without physician notification within 4 hours from the time detected	None	Nurses' notes, vital sign flow sheet, physician contact report, hospital or SNF discharge record, aide notes	Any patient being treated for hypertension would fail the screen if BPs were not recorded.
c. Presence of pulse < 50 (45 if the patient is on a beta blocker) or > 120 without physician notification within 4 hours from time detected	None	Nurses' notes, vital sign flow sheet, physician contact report, aide notes	Any patient receiving digoxin or an anti-arrhythmic drug would fail the screen if pulse was not recorded. If the patient has a pacemaker, physician contact is expected if the pulse is less than the ordered parameter.
d. Presence of other significant changes in signs and symptoms without physician notification within 4 hours from time detected	None	Nurses' notes, physician contact report, physician's orders	Look at visits where significant adverse changes occurred in signs or symptoms in any body systems or function without physician notification.
e. Appropriate diagnostic services provided on physician's orders	None	Physician's orders, nurses' notes	This element applies to elements 2.a thru 2.d.
f. Abnormal results of diagnostic services addressed and resolved, or the record explains why they are unresolved	None	Nurses' notes, physician's orders, laboratory reports, X-ray reports.	

continues

Home Health Agency Generic Quality Screens Guidelines continued

ELEMENTS	EXCLUSIONS	DATA SOURCES	EXPLANATORY NOTES
g. Appropriate intervention if significant change in social support system, including environment	None	Nurses' notes, social service notes, physician contact report, aide notes	
h. Appropriate reporting of abuse/ neglect	None	Nurses' notes, social service notes, physician contact report, aide notes	
i. Timely reporting to physician of lack of family and/or patient compliance	None	Nurses' notes, social service notes, physician contact report, aide notes, physical therapist notes	A benchmark of three consecutive, professional visits where noncompliance is noted without physician contact is sufficient to fail this screen. Noncompliance is defined as a refusal rather than an inability to comply.
3. **Adequacy of Restorative Care**			
a. Specialty therapies	Those not requiring specialty therapy		"Restorative care" is intended in the broadest sense here as opposed to a more narrow sense. The specialty therapies include physical, speech, and occupational.
1. Restorative need identified and addressed through assessment, plan implementation, and evaluation	As in 3.a	Nurses' notes, physician's orders, therapy notes, specialty evaluation(s), plan of care	Look at the interaction/coordinated effort of care as well as the documented evidence that the plan has been reviewed periodically and that there was adherence to it. Documentation must be present that addresses the unique needs, circumstances, and plan for each patient individually, with modification of plan as conditions indicate.

continues

2. Presence of therapy plan of care and documentation of therapist's compliance with plan	As in 3.a	Nurses' notes, physician's orders, therapy notes, specialty evaluation(s), plan of care	
3. Presence of patient education	As in 3.a	Therapy notes, aide notes, nurses' notes	Patient education involves teaching the patient how to do the required exercises. It also involves supervision and return demonstration.
b. Nursing instructions	Those not receiving nursing services		
1. Presence of patient education plan and documentation of nursing compliance with the plan	As in 3.b	Nurses' notes, physician's orders, aide notes, treatment plan, plan of care	Review for documentation that patient was taught, and patient's response to taking his or her own pulse, diabetic therapy, or exercises as his or her condition warrants.
2. Documentation in the nursing care plan of coordination of services (interdisciplinary follow-up and reinforcement)	As in 3.b	Nurses' notes, physician contact report, plan of care, therapy notes, aide notes	This screen looks at the coordination of all disciplines required to carry out the care plan for this patient.
3. Continual reassessment of patient's needs with referrals to other disciplines as necessary	As in 3.b	Nurses' notes, physician contact report, therapy notes, aide notes, plan of care	
4. Deaths Deaths within 48 hours of transfer to hospital as ascertained from the hospital record	None	Entire Home Health record	The purpose of this screen is to identify those cases where an untimely transfer to a higher level of care resulted in death.

continues

Home Health Agency Generic Quality Screens Guidelines continued

ELEMENTS	EXCLUSIONS	DATA SOURCES	EXPLANATORY NOTES
5. Possible Indications of Secondary Infections			[It is assumed that when a patient is discharged from the hospital that the patient is stable and any existing infection is under control. "Secondary" infection is defined as a new infection or a flare-up of an infection previously under control.]
a. Temperature elevation > 2 degrees after 72 hours of start of care	None	Nurses' notes, vital sign flow chart, aide notes	
b. Any indication of an infection following an invasive procedure	None	Nurses' notes, vital sign flow chart, laboratory reports, culture reports	Look for the linkage between the procedure and the infection. Examples of invasive procedures are catheterization; suctioning; tube feeding; intravenous feeding; hyperalimentation.
6. Issues Related to Patient Care after the Home Health Start of Care			
a. Presence of incident with resultant injury or untoward effect	None	Nurses' notes, physician contact report, therapy notes, aide notes	Injury or untoward effect includes, but is not limited to fracture, dislocation, concussion, or laceration. An incident that takes place when the HHA is not present in the home would cause a screen failure only if the HHA was remiss in providing education that could have prevented the incident.

continues

b. Presence of decubitus ulcer	None	Nurses' notes, therapy records, initial nursing assessment, physician orders, aide notes	Decubitus ulcer is defined as a break in the skin not present on admission, regardless of the size and depth. If an ulcer develops or a previous decubitus ulcer becomes worse while the patient is under the care of the HHA, it would also result in failure of this screen.
c. Presence of life-threatening complications	None	Nurses' notes, physician contact report, therapy notes, aide notes	Use professional judgment on a case-by-case basis in determining whether an action or lack of action resulted in the life-threatening complication.
d. Adverse drug reaction or medication error	None	Nurses' notes, physician contact report, therapy notes	An error or reaction that takes place when HHA is not present in the home would cause a screen failure only if the HHA was remiss in providing education that could have prevented the incident. Review for physician error in prescribing drugs.
e. Evidence of inappropriate planning and administration of patient care	None	Nurses' notes, physician contact report, treatment plan, plan of care	This screen looks at the planning for the delivery of services. Examples would be scheduling a physical therapy, speech therapy, skilled nursing, and aide visit all on the same day; planning one visit per week at the start of care for a patient who needs intensive teaching (diabetic care, colostomy care).
f. Responsibility for termination of care only when services are no longer required	None	Entire Home Health record	The purpose of this screen is to identify premature discharge from the HHA.

ELEMENTS	EXCLUSIONS	DATA SOURCES	EXPLANATORY NOTES
7. Discharge Plan and Follow-Up Documented plan for appropriate follow-up care and discharge summary to physician(s) of record	Death	Nurses' notes, discharge summary, treatment plan	Discharge planning is appropriate for all patients. Documentation must be present that addresses the unique needs, circumstances, and plan for each patient individually.
8. Adequacy of Care In the judgment of the professional reviewer, are there any other events/patterns of care that resulted in adverse outcomes that should be evaluated? No____ Yes____ Explain	None	Entire Home Health record	Look for mismanagement of the case, actions that should have been ordered and/or taken, but were not, and any issue that is not covered by a specific element, but may represent a quality concern.

Effective for all 4SOW reviews initiated on and after 4-15-93

CHAPTER 65

The Manager As Published Author: Tips on Writing for Publication

Suzanne Smith Blancett

Writing for publication is a process: it can be learned and it can be mastered. Although understanding the writing and publishing process can increase your chances of being a published author, it cannot replace experience.

Think of the processes, skills, and techniques mastered during your nursing education, for example giving injections. Knowledge of physiology, pharmacology, anatomy, biology, and psychology gave you needed conceptual skills. Knowing how and actually doing, however, were two different things. To develop proficiency, you actually had to administer drugs and observe client reactions.

Likewise, writing for publication has a conceptual and an experiential component. Although resources related to writing, such as this chapter, will give you information you need to write for publication, it is practice that leads to success.

BLOCKS TO WRITING

When I ask nurse administrators and managers why they do not write for publication, I get answers such as I can't seem to get started; I'm not motivated; I can't write at work; I'm not creative; I can't write at home; Other things seem more important each day; I have nothing unique to share; I don't write well; My first paper was rejected; and I'm too busy.

These reasons for not writing fall into three main categories. The first is lack of motivation stemming from inexperience, past rejection of a manuscript, and negative feedback on your writing. The second hindrance is your workload and how you choose to prioritize. The third reason is procrastination. Here are some suggestions to overcome these personal blocks to getting started.

Inexperience

If lack of motivation is due to inexperience or poor writing, take a writing or journalism course at a local college or attend seminars on writing for publication. A source of motivation and support is colleagues who have already published. Many neophyte authors attribute their success in publishing to being mentored by a nationally known and well-published nurse. This relationship is most often initiated by the neophyte author, asking the expert for advice. Do not be hesitant about establishing contact with published experts in your content area. They most often appreciate the opportunity to share their knowledge with and help develop others.

Another source of motivation can be a writers' support group. Find colleagues who are interested in writing but, like you, can't seem to get started. Form a group and meet on a regular basis. Share resources, critique small writing projects (such as an abstract or an interoffice memo), develop interesting and innovative topics, write query letters to editors about your ideas, and co-author manuscripts. For assistance in structuring a writers' support group, read Flarey's article on journal clubs (Flarey, 1991).

Workload

Overcoming the second block, setting workload priorities, involves deciding what activities you want in your life. You have to be honest about the value of writing for publication to you, your life, and your career. Do you really want to make writing a priority over reading a good novel, a trip to the gym, or a long bath? Time is always found to do what we want and value. Once you take writing into your life, when and where is it going to be done? How will you set your priorities and manage your time?

Procrastination

Overcoming the third block, procrastination, is the same as overcoming procrastination in your daily life. You have to know what motivates you, and what works to get you started on projects.

Here are some techniques to overcome blocks to getting started; all can work if you use them consistently, in a disciplined way:

- Set aside a specific period of time to write, preferably a time when you are at your peak. Write in a place that is conducive to work and where you will not be interrupted by family, colleagues, or telephone calls.
- Break your writing into reasonable time blocks. Trying to find eight hours of uninterrupted time in a busy schedule is impossible and demotivating. Instead, for example, set aside 30 minutes every other day. Work exactly 30 minutes and stop, even if you are in the middle of a thought.

This will motivate you to return to the work the next time.
- Use a tape recorder to dictate your first draft. Transcribe, cut, paste, and edit that material. This approach avoids the blank piece of paper and the "where should I start?" syndrome.
- For those who cannot work until the first sentence is perfect, start in the middle of your paper. The introduction and conclusion of a paper are often the hardest to do. Leave them until the end.
- Start in a small way by writing a query letter about your topic to the editors of several journals. A positive response from an editor can be the motivation to write the whole paper.

Another less intimidating way to overcome writing inertia is to write short, concise letters to the editor. To be timely, the letter should be written soon after the journal publishes the article you wish to critique. An effective letter will contain information that sheds additional light on the topic rather than just praises the article.

Most journals have specific departments, such as executive development, education for administration, innovations from the field, and news, notes, and tips, that accept brief manuscripts in the one- to five-page length range. Peruse journals to assess the fit of an idea you have with the department's purpose.

Use behavior modification to establish a reward system for every so many pages you write. Rosenberg and Lah (1985), using this approach, lead the reader through an analysis of tasks and overt and covert reinforcements and distractions. With this analysis, the would-be author develops a self-modification timetable and a reinforcement and evaluation schedule.

Finally, if lack of spontaneity and creativity seems to be the problem, Rico's (1983) book is a must. A well-known nurse editor referred this book to me after I asked her how she managed to write consistently interesting editorials. Rico presents a creative, developmental, step-by-step process for making writing easier. The book is interactive: as you read, you are asked to do brief writing exercises. The book's approach can be used for any type of writing.

REJECTION

Manuscript rejection can be a major block to continued writing. Too many first-time authors who have their first manuscript rejected by an editor never try again. Rather than seeing rejection as a chance to learn from mistakes, improve ideas through the use of feedback, and master a process, authors are personally crushed by their perceived failure.

Rejection of any kind sets up a grieving process. Symbolically, rejected manuscripts are seen as an attack on one's ideas and perhaps even on one's life's work. Even though it was the paper, not you, that was rejected, you still have to deal with an emotional reaction.

If your manuscript is rejected, avoid the urge to destroy it immediately. Instead, give yourself time to deal with the shock, hurt, and anger. After your disappointment has subsided to a manageable level, analyze why the paper was rejected. Ask a trusted colleague to critique the manuscript in light of the reasons given for rejection. The perspective of a person more distant from your work can be helpful as well as supportive.

If you want more feedback from the editor as to why your paper was not acceptable, call or write the editor. A large part of an editor's role is as a teacher. Ask for guidance. If you have enough feedback and your idea is still timely, revise the paper, improving your ideas and their presentation. If the editor expressed interest in your idea, resubmit the revised and improved version of your manuscript to the same journal. If the journal's editor did not indicate an interest in seeing the revised paper, submit your paper to another journal. Revise the paper based on the first journal's feedback or submit the original paper. Using either approach, you will continue to receive feedback so that you can perfect your idea and its presentation.

If your paper is rejected by several journals, you must seriously reconsider the approach, validity, and importance of your topic. At some point, cut your losses, move on to another interest, and start the process again. You will be wiser and the process will become easier. Do not quit, no matter how you are feeling.

Reasons for Rejection

Although it is important to be mentally prepared to deal with rejection, it is equally important to know and avoid the major reasons why manuscripts are rejected. Manuscripts are sometimes rejected because a journal has recently published or is soon to publish an article on a similar topic. A query letter to the editor helps avoid this reason for rejection.

Manuscripts are also rejected because the content is outdated, not important, not appropriate (e.g., a clinical topic for a management journal), too technical or too basic for the journal's readers, inaccurate, undocumented or poorly documented, or fabricated. A research paper is most often rejected because of poor research design. Finally, a poorly organized and poorly written paper is almost always rejected.

These reasons for rejection imply some obvious solutions. Know what the journal has published in the last several years related to your topic, know who the primary audience of the journal is, know the types of positions held by and the average educational preparation of the readers, and do not write a research paper for a national journal if your sample is small and geographically isolated or your methodology is flawed. If grammar, spelling, and composition are not your strengths, get editorial assistance.

MANUSCRIPT CRITIQUE

Before you complete the final version of a manuscript, have it critiqued for content, style, and relevance to the reader. Although one person might be able to evaluate all these areas of your manuscript, I recommend three different people; the task is more manageable for each, and you will receive more and better criticism than if one person does all.

First, have a content expert read your paper for the information's accuracy and completeness. The content expert should be concerned only with the paper's technical content. For example, if your topic is using financial spreadsheets, your agency's financial officer might be the reviewer.

Second, have a style reviewer read the paper for clarity, flow, organization, and grammar. This person might be a teacher or student of journalism or English, or perhaps just a friend who has good writing and organizational skills.

Third, a colleague who represents the journal's primary reader should review the paper for appropriateness and relevance of focus. If you are not the journal's primary reader, your content might be too dogmatic, might be above or below the readers' knowledge level, or might attack "sacred cows." For example, imagine that as a graduate student, a faculty member, or clinical nurse specialist, you write a manuscript on budgeting for *The Journal of Nursing Administration* (JONA). Because JONA is edited for top-level administrators and you are not in that position, find an agency administrator to check the content's level for sophistication and appropriateness for the reader.

GETTING STARTED

There are many excellent sources (Barnum, 1995; Blancett, 1988; Camilleri, 1987; Fondiller, 1992; Knox, 1989; Mateo & Meeker, 1992; Sheridan & Dowdney, 1986; Tornquist, 1986) that discuss critical elements in the writing and publishing process. The following highlights a few areas.

Generating Ideas

How many times have you read an article and said, "I've been doing that for years," or "I could have written that article"? The difference between you and published authors is that they actually did it. Too often, we feel that our ideas

are commonplace. A better thought to have is, "If I have a problem, other people around the country probably have it too. If I have a solution that's working in my institution, other people would probably be interested in hearing about it." A few telephone calls to colleagues will confirm the validity and timeliness of your idea.

If you do not have an idea, become a critical reader and observer. As you read professional and nonprofessional literature, ask what the implications of the information are to you, your institution, other nurses, and the profession. What problems are common at work and how are they being addressed? What trends are emerging that will affect how nursing is practiced and how can we be proactive now? What have you learned through your work with community and professional groups? How could that knowledge be applied to the profession or your work situation? Answering these questions can be the basis of a publishable idea.

The often maligned technique of brainstorming is always a good way to generate ideas alone or in groups. Brainstorming works when care is taken to avoid premature criticism of ideas. Productivity is increased by brainstorming answers to a specific question. For example, what is the most difficult job-related problem you expect to face in the next three years? Answers to questions such as this can lead to interesting, innovative, and visionary manuscripts.

Selecting an Idea

Before committing to an idea, assess it for timeliness, focus, interest to readers, and interest to you. You need to know why your idea is important (perhaps because of recent advances in technology or new legislation or because it is a new way to do an old thing). To pinpoint hot topics, go to the literature. You probably have a hot topic if there is little to nothing in the professional literature.

The best articles also have a specific slant. Article titles and abstracts often reveal an article's focus. Know the particular point your article will make before you start writing. For example, a manuscript on developing a capital budget will be easier to write and more likely to be accepted for publication than a broad-based manuscript on financial management. Your topic's focus will emerge as you review the literature and identify missing information.

When you know who the primary reader of a journal is (staff nurses, first-line managers, academic educators, or clinical nurse specialists), tailor your ideas to their needs for certain information. Find out who the primary reader of a journal is by reading the journal and its information for authors. If still in doubt, call or write the editor.

Finally, pick an idea that is personally interesting. The publishing process is lengthy, often 12 to 18 months from manuscript submission to publication. Your interest and motivation have to be sustained over a long period of time. Avoid writing about past experiences if they are not relevant to your personal or professional life. For example, if you were a practitioner involved in a complex clinical problem and are now in a new management position, removed from day-to-day clinical contact, it will become harder and harder for you to write the clinical paper. Your attention and commitment will be directed toward acquisition of new management skills.

Developing Your Idea

The best idea in the world can lack substance, interest, and clarity if it is poorly developed. Your comprehensive review of the literature occurs when you are committed to one topic. It is during this period that your ideas are refined. You should emerge from the literature review phase by being able to answer these questions:

- What purpose do you hope to achieve by writing on a particular topic with a particular slant? (e.g., you want to change the way administrators evaluate the performance of staff)

- What is the point you want to make? (e.g., this paper will show administrators how to establish a nonthreatening environment for evaluation of staff)
- How does your idea relate to trends that affect health care and nursing?
- How does your idea differ from present practice?
- What examples illustrate the idea and its usefulness?
- What aspects of your idea are original and unique?
- Who would be interested in reading about the idea? Administrators? Faculty? Staff educators? Staff nurses? Students?
- What information is not in the literature about your topic?

Answering these questions as you review the literature will give you an idea of the depth of your knowledge of the topic as well as gaps in your understanding. Answers to these questions also give you the information you need to query the editor, write a working abstract, and begin the paper.

SELECTING THE APPROPRIATE JOURNAL

Most people are aware of only the few journals that they read. By knowing all the journals that might be appropriate for your idea, you will increase your chances of getting your paper published. The most useful source of information about nursing journals is Swanson, McCloskey, and Bodensteiner's (1991) article. While this reference will not list journals established since 1991, it is a good beginning. In addition to listing 92 journals by specialty area (e.g., administration, gerontology, and maternal-child health, to name a few), the article provides demographics about each journal in 18 different categories, such as number of subscribers, issues per year, desired manuscript length, need for query letter, length of time for the review process, and length of time from acceptance until publication. McConnell (1995) provides similar information for 42 nursing publications outside the United States.

Use the Swanson et al. article (1991), as well as McConnell (1995), to identify potential journals that, by title, seem appropriate for your topic and target readers. For journals since 1991, access The National Library of Medicine's MEDLINE file (available through major Internet providers by typing MEDLINE at the "go to" or "keyword" prompt) or a nursing journal database such as SilverPlatter's RNdex Top 100 (Information Resources Group, Pasadena, CA, 818/405-9212). When potential journals have been identified, it is critical that you examine copies of the journals. Photocopy the information for authors' guidelines and note the editor's name and address from the most recent issue. Using the Swanson, McCloskey, and Bodensteiner article's (1991) demographic information as well as an actual copy of each potential journal, rank the best to the least likely fit of your topic with the journal. Consider the following items:

Readership

Know for whom you are writing and how your paper will meet the information needs of the journal's primary readership. Determine the audience's educational level, degree of expertise, and special interests by scanning journal article titles, abstracts, and contents. Note this information because later your query letter, your abstract, and your article will all have to be tailored to this particular group.

Circulation

How much of your target audience is reached by the journal? Only a small percentage of nurse executives subscribe to generic nursing journals such as the *American Journal of Nursing* (AJN) or *Nursing*. A manuscript with an administrative focus has a better chance of being accepted if it is submitted to a journal that is read only by administrators (e.g., JONA).

Publication Frequency

The more often a journal is published, the more manuscripts it can accept. All other factors being equal, choose a journal that is published monthly over one that is published quarterly or bimonthly.

Refereed Status

A refereed journal publishes manuscripts that have been reviewed by members of a journal's advisory board or manuscript review panel. These reviewers represent a broad range of expertise in the journal's subject matter. In academic settings, publication and promotion committees give more weight to articles published in refereed journals. If you now or ever intend to work in a school of nursing, this factor is an important journal selection criterion.

Format

Examine at least two issues of all your potential journals. Make a note of the style and the average length of an article, language complexity and style, length and format of the abstract, title, biographical statement, introduction, conclusion, structure of tables and figures, and use of photographs and illustrations. Will your topic, as you envision it being developed, fit into the journal's overall style and format? For example, if your article uses photographs to show how a procedure is done, does the journal publish photographs? If no, would the journal publish photographs if asked, or could you make your point through line drawings instead?

Type of Article

Is your article going to be conceptual, practical, how-to-do, or research oriented? Does it have a clinical, management, staff, or academic focus? Make sure your plan for developing an idea for a specific journal fits into the journal's approach to content.

Author Payment

Although some journals pay authors a certain amount of money per printed journal page, most simply provide reprints of the article or copies of the issue in which the article appears.

Time Frames

The length of time it takes to review and publish a manuscript is a critical journal selection criterion depending on the timeliness of your idea. For example, a manuscript on time management can tolerate a longer time frame than a paper dealing with a strategy to comply with a new federal regulation. If possible, write for journals with the shortest time frames.

Acceptance Rates

Specialty journals and new journals tend to have higher acceptance rates than generic journals (such as AJN or *Nursing*) and well-established journals (such as JONA and *Nurse Educator*). Two reasons contribute to this phenomenon: Compared with a generic journal, specialty journals have a smaller group of people with expertise in the subject matter; and mature, well-established journals are the first journals that come to authors' minds.

Interest in Your Idea

To assess a journal's interest in your idea, write the editor a query letter. In this letter, briefly explain the problem or issue that the readership faces and how the reader will be better off after reading your solution or approach. You can gauge interest in your idea by how quickly and in what manner the editor responds—from an impersonal form letter to a personalized, encouraging letter to a telephone call.

Decision Making

Assess these journal selection factors and their relative importance to you. Rank your potential journals from first to last choice. Write query letters to the editors of all your potential journals. As soon as your number 1–ranked journal responds positively to your manuscript query, finalize the draft of your paper with that journal's specific formatting requirements.

WRITING THE PAPER

There are several methods you can use to organize your content before actually writing. The most well known is the standard outline. The outline is useful, however, only if you outline with ideas rather than words. It is useless to have Roman numeral I of your outline be "Introduction." That doesn't assist you in writing the introduction or anyone else in knowing what you want to do. Instead, have each step of the outline highlight a major point. Now, Roman numeral I might be "Prospective payment plans could threaten the financial viability of home care agencies."

Another outline approach is the use of index cards. Each key idea of your content is written in a sentence at the top of the card. These key ideas are each paragraph's topic sequence. Below each sentence, jot down the key points you wish to make in the paragraph. Shuffle the cards to organize and reorganize the content, and start the writing process. This modular approach to organizing content allows you to write any part of the paper first. If one card's key concept eludes you, pick another card.

A good approach to organizing content for a visual person is the hurricane method. Using a brainstorming approach, quickly write all your ideas about your topic on a large piece of paper. Then, using different colored crayons or markers, circle similar concepts in the same color. To define each idea further, a second round might include taking each word in a color set, for example all the words marked in green, and repeating the exercise. You would quickly brainstorm all ideas related to the green words, and color code the subset. Do this until you feel you are ready to write using your color-coded pages.

For those who actually have to write the paper before they can do an outline, try the following methods for organizing content. Write your paper without much attention to fine details. Just get your ideas down on paper. Then copy the paper and cut it into pieces, grouping the paragraphs with similar ideas together and throwing away redundant information. As with the index card approach, rewrite the paper, and repeat the process.

For help with style, format, and grammar, refer to the style book recommended in your target journal's Information for Authors as well as Fondiller and Nerone's (1993) books, *Health Professionals' Style Book* and *The Writer's Workbook: Health Professional's Guide to Getting Published* (Fondiller, 1992). After writing the last draft of your paper, have it critiqued by the three types of reviewers previously discussed. When you are done writing, refer to the journal's information for authors and the most recent copy of the journal to prepare the manuscript for submission.

SUBMISSION CHECKLIST

If the information for authors' guidelines and an issue of the journal do not give you the following information, telephone the editorial assistant and ask for the journal's procedure.

Number of Copies

At a minimum, most journals require three copies of your paper; some require five or more.

Abstracts

There are three basic types of abstracts: descriptive, structured, and benefit oriented. The descriptive abstract is most often seen in a research journal. It outlines the major elements of the manuscript and can be up to 250 words in length. The structured abstract, again used most often by research journals, describes the content using these headings: objective, methods (sample, procedures, analysis), results, and conclu-

sions. The benefit-oriented abstract stresses the article's outcomes for the reader (how the reader will be better off after reading the content). It is usually 100 words or less and states the importance of a problem or issue to the reader and how the reader will be more effective after reading the author's solution to the problem. It does not give many details about the approach or solution.

Illustrations

Tables and figures should each be placed on separate pages that follow the reference list. Give a title as well as a page number to each illustration. Make sure every illustration has a reference in the text. Most journals require camera-ready illustrations, which are black type or ink on white paper or black-and-white glossy photographs. Diagrams, graphs, and line drawings should be professionally drawn or laser generated.

Reference Style

Make sure your references are formatted correctly. Although a number of journals use the style manual of the American Psychological Association, many journals use other styles.

Headings

Divide manuscript content by using headings and subheadings. This makes it easier for the reader to follow your main points. The subdivision of the content by headings is similar to a standard outline except that the Roman numerals, numbers, and letters are eliminated. All headings and subheadings should be grammatically similar.

Biographical Statement

Some journals use three- or four-sentence narrative biographical statements; others simply use name, credentials, title, and place, city, and state of employment. Some publish a photograph of the author. The ideal photograph is a black-and-white glossy photograph of the head and shoulders. For as little as $60, professional photographers will provide you with 10 wallet-size publicity photos.

Computer Disks

Most publishers will ask you to submit a computer disk containing your manuscript file. While each journal has specific formatting details for electronic copy, in general, you need to label the disk indicating which word processing software version you used and what you named your file. Unless the information for authors states otherwise, the computer disk is submitted only after review and acceptance of your manuscript.

Copyright Transfer

Just by producing a work, you hold its copyright. At some point, the editor will require transfer of your copyright to the journal's publisher. Some journals wish the transfer to be made when you submit the manuscript; others will require this only if the paper is accepted for publication. If transfer is to be made with your paper, the information for authors will provide the correct wording.

Use of Copyrighted Material

To use material already published by someone else, you must have permission from the copyright holder. It is your responsibility to write the copyright holder, requesting permission and indicating exactly how you will use the material. In addition to sending a copy of your manuscript highlighting the borrowed materials, send a copy of the original material indicating its source (because most copyright holders are publishers of many journals and books).

Copyright law does not specify how much material you can borrow without requesting permission. A general rule is that you need permission to borrow any element that is self-

standing (such as a poem, a cartoon, a photograph, a figure, or a table) or that represents a significant percentage of the whole (three words of a four-word poem). When you directly quote narrative, a general rule of thumb is to request permission when quoting more than 250 words.

Finally, if you are a published author, you still have to get permission to quote yourself. Even though your ideas are always yours, to be used at will, the exact words in published material belong to the copyright holder. Do not be guilty of self-plagiarism.

Cover Letter

When submitting your manuscript, include a cover letter. The cover letter should highlight the importance of the manuscript's content to the reader in two or three brief sentences. It should include the title of the article and with whom the editor should correspond if there is more than one author. If you previously queried the editor, refer to that correspondence.

Appearance

I often receive manuscripts with no cover letter, too few copies, incorrect formatting, hard to read photocopies, and no author address (except that the institution and city might be mentioned in the biographical statement or somewhere in the manuscript). Failure to adhere to guidelines and present yourself and your manuscript in a professional way at best reflects poorly on you and at worst is a cause of rejection. When two papers with equally good but similar content are being assessed, the editor will always choose the one that followed the information for authors' guidelines.

RESEARCH

Research reports, theses, and dissertations have a different style and format from those required by research or nonresearch journals. For example, most research reports have lengthy background narrative and literature reviews. These two items are dramatically reduced in papers written for publication.

Nursing journals vary in how they report research projects and in the emphasis each wants placed on major elements. Before writing a manuscript about your research, study articles in your target journals, and note how the article is formatted, how long various sections are, and what sections are stressed the most.

In JONA, which is not a research journal, we want the research reported in as brief a way as possible, with the author stressing the implications of the study, answering the "so what" question. We are not as concerned with a literature review section as we are with the literature being integrated into the narrative to support the author's ideas. Many other journals want a comprehensive but synthesized literature review section that highlights major literature in the topic area.

Student Research Projects

Publishing reports of research done as a student can be difficult. Because of limited resources, the student's sample is usually small, which hampers the ability to generalize the findings and limits the scope of the research problem. In this case, local publications (newsletters and journals published by area schools of nursing institutions, or professional associations) can be an appropriate outlet.

Also, the style and format for writing school papers, particularly theses and dissertations, differ from what is required by journals. The academic paper tends to be written in a passive, third-person voice ("It was believed that . . .) rather than the active first-person voice ("The investigator believes . . .) wanted by journals. The school paper's literature review is lengthy to show the professor that you have a full grasp of your topic. Editors of nursing journals assume that you know the published material and seek to have you add to the literature rather than repeat it.

School papers generally are lengthy and redundant because key ideas are said many times in different ways. Editors want concisely written papers; every extra word and redundant idea in a manuscript takes editorial space away from others waiting to be published. Use the smallest number of words to convey your message.

Last, many student authors are not members of the journal's readership group. This often leads to manuscript content that is not sufficiently sophisticated and relevant for the readers. This problem can be overcome through coauthorship with, or review of the manuscript by, a member of the journal's prime readership.

Although it can be difficult, it is possible to get work done as a student published in nursing journals. Those who wish to turn theses, dissertations, and research reports into publishable manuscripts will find Tornquist's work (1983, 1986) invaluable. Tornquist discusses each element of a research report and then highlights approaches to rewriting the material for nursing journals.

Agency Data

Every agency has research data (e.g., number of staff, number of visits, or type of client). Often, data are manipulated to see what will happen. Will the number of client visits increase if staff only come into the agency once a week? Will staff be any happier? Will patients be better off? Will office efficiency increase? Many times, the methods used to assess the intervention are informal. When this is the case, do not try to write a research article. The flawed methodology and inability to generalize the findings will lead to rejection.

The outcomes of your intervention probably are of interest to others, however. Many journals welcome manuscripts that discuss one agency's experience with an emerging problem or issue. It is acceptable to support discussion of the problem and the solution with agency data, even if data collection tools only had face validity. Readers can decide whether they want to test your ideas in their agency. Never feel hesitant about sharing what works for you with others, just do not try to disguise informal problem solving and data collection as a formal research project.

THE PUBLISHING PROCESS

When you submit your manuscript, it is critiqued by the editor and selected members of the manuscript review panel. If your manuscript is rejected, you will be told why. If you are not clear why your manuscript was unacceptable, write or call the editor.

Most accepted manuscripts require at least one revision based on the editor's and reviewers' feedback. If suggestions are extensive, you may actually have to rewrite the paper. All revision suggestions should be carefully considered while keeping two thoughts in mind: It is better to address a criticism or question before publication than after, and the point of review, feedback, and revision is to make your manuscript as good as it can be, thus making you and the journal look good.

Once your paper is acceptable to the editor, you will wait from six months to two years to see it published. The production process (copy editing, typesetting, proofing, and preparation of art work) takes approximately three to four months. The remaining time is accounted for by all the other manuscripts accepted before yours that are not yet published. If you did your preliminary work in selecting a journal, you should not be one of the people waiting two years.

Manuscripts are edited to improve clarity, conciseness, grammar, and expression of ideas. You will be asked to approve the copyedited manuscript before publication. The copyeditor will probably have questions for you, asking you to supply missing information or to clarify your intent. Because the published paper reflects your views, always feel free to contest copyediting that changes your meaning.

Up to four months before the scheduled publication date, information in the manuscript can be changed. Editors want manuscripts to be as up to date as possible. If there is a new development on your topic, ask whether you can add a paragraph to the paper. If new information has just been published on your topic, ask whether you can add the resource to your reference list. Finally, if you change jobs or addresses, notify the editorial office so that your biographical statement can be updated.

ETHICS

Authors make many decisions during the process of writing for publication. Some decision making is straightforward: Should a query letter be written? What graphs best illustrate the material? These decisions do not involve a moral right or wrong. Other decision-making points involve legal and ethical considerations. For example, all authors should know from reading the information for authors' guidelines and publishing agreements that editors assume that they are considering and publishing original material unless told otherwise (Blancett, Flanagin, & Young, 1995). Yet this is often not the case (see, for example, the April 1990 issues of RN and *Nursing* for similar articles on pain by the same author and the November and November/December 1991 issues of JONA and *Nursing Economics* for similar articles on bedside automation by the same authors). Because the authors in both examples did not cite the other article, there is the possibility of both illegal and unethical behavior.

First, it is illegal to use copyrighted material, even if it is your own, without permission. Second, the authors, even if pleading ignorance of the copyright violation, should have cited the other manuscript. Because both these journals serve the same readership, it is doubtful that the editors were informed.

To add another dimension to this issue, what should you do if you see almost identical articles in two journals by a colleague and note that neither article refers to the other? Notify the editor? Confront your colleague? Write an anonymous letter to your colleague or to your colleague's boss? Do nothing? Living with the possible implications of any choice is not easy.

Another problem area involves entitlement to authorship. There is a common assumption that people listed as authors have made a substantial contribution to the work. Yet many times this is not the case. A research director lists as an author a staff nurse, who did some peripheral work, to reward and motivate the nurse to continue scholarly pursuits. To thank an agency director for support, an author lists the director as an author.

Although it is noble and generous of the real authors to be so thoughtful, honorary authorship can also be viewed as diluting the work of the real author, giving credit where credit is not due, and deceiving the editor and readers. The ethical problem is whether to tell the editor that there are honorary authors.

Another area in which authors and editors make an ethical decision relates to informed consent. Should an author inform the editor, and the editor in turn inform readers, that the author of an article about a new and innovative staffing software package consults for the company that produced the software? If the content of the article is peer reviewed, accurate, and seemingly unbiased, does it matter that the author can gain financially?

Legal and ethical decision making is often difficult because there are always two or more interested parties, ethical principles can compete with each other in any given situation, and laws are open to interpretation. A key in making the right decision legally and the best decision ethically when writing and publishing is being informed and having a decision-making framework. I recommend that you read Silva (1990) for a clear decision-making framework and Blancett (1991), Ketefian and Lenz (1995), Skolnick (1991), Stevens (1986), and Susser and Yankauer (1993) for information about ethical issues in writing and publishing.

THE BENEFITS OF PUBLISHING

How often do you use ideas in your management practice that come from nursing books and journals? As you read and think about ideas in the literature, you probably adapt and further develop them so that they work better. However, did you take the final step in developing and refining nursing knowledge—that of disseminating knowledge? Our obligation to contribute to the ongoing development of the profession's body of knowledge implies that we should not only develop but also share our expertise. Writing for publication is the ideal medium through which nursing knowledge can directly advance professional practice and the health of the nation.

When we publish our ideas, we increase the effectiveness and efficiency with which professional, program, and agency development occurs. Publishing positively decreases the amount of time spent reinventing the wheel. As an additional benefit, published authors receive feedback from colleagues on their work and thus further develop their own ideas and approaches.

Writing for publication also brings recognition for your institution. As competition and concern with image increase, having details of an institutional program or event in the national press is a boost for public relations. Institutional visibility through the publications of staff implies a visionary, supportive environment and can be used as a recruiting tool for new staff.

Publications often lead to reader requests for more information. Authors are asked to speak and consult. Agencies are asked to share programs and tools.

Personal satisfaction with seeing one's name in print and claiming an idea as one's own is both a benefit of writing and a motivator to write. In addition, publication is a mark of professional skill and is often a performance evaluation criterion for nurse administrators and expert practitioners. A list of publications on a curriculum vita may assist in job security, promotion, and research funding.

CONCLUSION

Writing for publication can be an exciting process. Knowledge combined with experience and perseverance is a powerful tool for effecting change. Just as it works in your personal and professional life, it can work to make you a published author.

REFERENCES

Barnum, B.S. (1995). *Writing and getting published: a primer for nurses*. New York: Springer Publishing Co.

Blancett, S.S. (1988). The process and politics of writing for publication. *Clinical Nurse Specialist, 2*, 113–117.

Blancett, S.S. (1991). The ethics of writing and publishing. *The Journal of Nursing Administration, 21*(5), 31–36.

Blancett, S.S., Flanagin, A.F., & Young, R.K. (1995). Duplicate publication in the nursing literature. *Image, 27*(1), 51–56.

Camilleri, R. (1987). Six ways to write right. *Image, 19*, 212–219.

Flarey, D.L. (1991). Journal club: encouraging new authors. *Nurse Author & Editor, 1*(4), 6–8.

Fondiller, S.H. (1992). *The writer's workbook: health professionals guide to getting published*. New York: The National League for Nursing Press.

Fondiller, S.H., & Nerone, B.J. (1993). *Health Professionals' Style Book*. New York: National League for Nursing Press.

Ketefian, S., & Lenz, E.R. (1995). Promoting scientific integrity in nursing research, part II: strategies. *Journal of Professional Nursing, 11*(5), 263–269.

Knox, A. (1989). *Teaching writing to adults*. San Francisco: Jossey-Bass.

Mateo, M.A., & Meeker, M.H. (1992). Publication skill development in nurses: a vital role of nurse executives. *The Journal of Nursing Administration, 22*(4), 64–66.

McConnell, E.A. (1995). Journal and publishing characteristics for 42 nursing publications outside the United States. *Image, 27*(3), 225–229.

Rico, G.L. (1983). *Writing the natural way*. Los Angeles: Tarcher.

Rosenberg, H., & Lah, M. (1985). Tackling writer's block: suggestions for self-modification. *The Journal of Nursing Administration, 15*(3), 40–42.

Sheridan, D.R., & Dowdney, D.L. (1986). *How to write and publish articles in nursing*. New York: Springer.

Silva, M.C. (1990). *Ethical decision making in nursing administration*. Norwalk, CT: Appleton & Lange.

Skolnick, A.A. (1991). Maharishi Ayur-Veda: Guru's marketing scheme promises the world eternal "perfect health." *Journal of the American Medical Association, 266*, 1741–1750.

Stevens, K.R. (1986). Authorship: yours, mine, or ours? *Image, 18*, 151–154.

Susser, M., & Yankauer, A. (1993). Prior, duplicate, repetitive, fragmented, and redundant publication. *American Journal of Public Health, 83*(6),6–7.

Swanson, E.A., McCloskey, J.C., & Bodensteiner, A. (1991). Publishing opportunities for nurses: A comparison of 92 U.S. journals. *Image, 23*, 30–38.

Tornquist, E.M. (1983). Strategies for publishing research. *Nursing Outlook, 31*, 180–183.

Tornquist, E.M. (1986). *From proposal to publication*. Menlo Park, CA: Addison-Wesley.

CHAPTER 66

Student Placements in Home Health Care Agencies: Boost or Barrier to Quality Patient Care?

Ida M. Androwich and Pamela A. Andresen

The placement of students in a home health care agency has the potential to both help and hinder the work of the agency. In this chapter, these boosts and barriers to quality patient care are addressed by two nursing faculty members who have taught community health administration courses using home health care agencies as clinical sites (Androwich & Andresen, 1986). One faculty member was formerly the director of a Medicare-certified home health care agency involved with student placements and currently teaches graduate students in home health care administration. The other faculty member is the current director of Loyola University's faculty nurse-managed center and has extensive experience as a staff member in a large Visiting Nurse Association.

BOOSTS

A major benefit of student placements is the collaboration or marriage between education and service. Motivators for this union include the need for home care for the sick and the desire for faculty-student shared clinical practice. Opportunities for sharing of information and expertise between these disciplines are great. Nurse educators offer clinical expertise, research skills, the desire to test new models of nursing practice, and students who can make reimbursable home visits. Nursing service brings to the marriage an available clinical site with qualified nursing personnel and support services.

A second benefit to the agency is increased staff support. A typical group of 8 to 10 students is able to visit at least that number of patients during a clinical day. Not only can this produce revenue for the agency but it also allows staff to pursue other endeavors. For example, students making visits can permit staff to complete outstanding paperwork or attend continuing education programs without an accompanying drop in the agency's productivity.

Depending on the type or level of student (e.g., Associate Degree (AD), Bachelor's of Science in Nursing (BSN), or graduate student) and the length of the clinical experience, creative use of students can provide assistance to the agency in many other ways besides making visits. Home health agencies frequently receive requests to participate in community programs (e.g., health fairs, blood pressure screenings, and health education for community groups) that do not generate revenue for the agency but enhance good community relations. Students can be used to help meet these requests. This type of contact with community groups provides students with a well-rounded view of different roles in community health nursing.

Medicare provides coverage for medically ordered services; however, students may be used to fill the Medigap by providing additional visits for nonreimbursable services. For example, the health promotion needs of other family members may be addressed. Chronically ill adults could be visited by students after discharge by the primary nurse for reimbursable visits. The agency might also accept referrals for nonreimbursable visits that would otherwise be refused. These are just a few examples of how students can be used to expand the agency's services without placing further demands on the staff.

Harris (1984) describes two outcomes of student experiences that have the advantage of being mutually beneficial to both learner and service agency. Graduate students can provide assistance with several types of administrative projects, such as completing needs assessments and quality review audits, developing management information systems, and conducting program planning and evaluation of existing programs. Graduate students in clinical specialty programs can also assist with staff inservices and serve as consultants to the staff.

Staff usually benefit from student placements. They are given an opportunity to serve as role models for students and are typically rewarded with gratitude and admiration from those students. Students are impressed by the independent judgment and high degree of professionalism demonstrated by the community health nurse. Staff may feel renewed by exposure to student enthusiasm.

The nursing care plan for a patient cared for by a student is developed by the student in conjunction with the primary nurse and the instructor, a Master's-prepared or doctorally prepared expert in community health nursing. The patient then receives the benefit of staff, faculty, and student input with a fully comprehensive plan of care as a result.

Productivity, in terms of the number of patients whom students visit per day, is typically not a priority of nursing education. Therefore, a student who visits only one or two patients per day has much more time to spend preparing for the visit as well as more actual visit time than the staff nurse visiting five or more patients on the same day. This is another benefit to the client and can be particularly helpful with cases requiring lengthy teaching such as new diabetics.

After students have completed their clinical experiences, home health administrators may find that the best and most enthusiastic of the students return as employees after graduation. This can facilitate not only recruitment but also retention. The student and staff know each other. Expectations of the staff nurse role should be clear to the new graduates because they are familiar with the agency. Orientation time will probably be lessened.

Before graduation, students may be able to work temporarily as home health aides, offering flexible staffing in this area. The Loyola University Community Nursing Center has used students quite successfully for staffing periods of the year when clinical courses are not in session. Registered nurse (RN)-BSN completion students or graduate students looking for part-time or flexible hours may be hired on a fee-for-visit basis. Many of these students work in or have had experience in critical care settings and would be qualified to deliver high-technology care in the home. Again, because they are familiar with the agency, the quality of their work will probably be superior to that of a nurse hired on a contract basis who has never been oriented to the agency.

Beyond the contact with students and faculty during clinical experiences the home health administrator and agency staff can benefit from their relationship with a university and its school of nursing. Some degree of prestige is associated with having a university affiliation. Administrators are frequently offered clinical faculty appointments and are invited to participate in university programs and continuing education. Formal or informal consultations may be provided to the agency by faculty. An administrator can also develop working relations with faculty from other departments within the university (e.g. social work, psychology, medicine, and business). Unique experiences can be offered to students from these departments that fulfill their objectives as well as meet the needs of the agency. Graduate students from Loyola's School of Business provided the university's nurse-managed center with extensive consultation in the area of marketing. Students from the psychology department have visited caregivers of elderly family members in need of support. These are just two examples of the many possibilities available to an agency affiliated with a university.

BARRIERS

Despite the many benefits, there are drawbacks to student placements. Perhaps the greatest barrier is presented by the increasing complexity of technology delivered in the home. Staff nurses with or without critical care backgrounds often require extensive training in technical areas (e.g., intravenous (IV) therapy, Total Parenteral Nutrition (TPN)) in order to adapt these procedures to the home environment. Students and faculty without recent acute care experience may be unprepared to provide high-tech care in the home. Therefore, great consideration needs to be given to the individual nurse's skills when assigning a technically complex patient. RN students enrolled in BSN completion programs are not consistently prepared in these technical skills, and faculty may rely on one or two students to visit patients requiring, for example, venipuncture. Developing a caseload for a group of traditional undergraduate students can become an overwhelming task for both the instructor and nursing supervisor. Yet, the pairing of students with staff nurses for all home visits may be an unacceptable solution from the viewpoint of both the instructor and the home care supervisor. From the instructor's perspective, the student placed in the role of follower is unlikely to develop the case management skills necessary to meet the objectives of his or her community health nursing practicum. From the agency perspective, the decrease in productivity may be unacceptable since the

time demands this arrangement places on the staff nurse may be extraordinary.

While an adequate caseload must be available for student experiences, a second issue deals with orienting students to written documentation. If visits are not documented correctly, denials for Medicare reimbursement may follow. For example, a faculty member may request that students chart in-depth information on a family's psychosocial status. This could lead Medicare reviewers to believe that the patient is being followed primarily for nonreimbursable mental health needs rather than for an unstable physical condition. As previously mentioned, student visits do generate revenue for the agency. Although the instructor should review student documentation, the home health administrator must determine who within the agency, such as the primary nurse, will also review student charting.

In addition to communicating through written documentation, students need to have a mechanism for relating pertinent information to the primary nurse and physician. The danger of misinterpretation of patient data arises if information is relayed through a circuitous route. For example, communication may flow from the student (who actually made the visit and assessed the client) to his or her instructor to the nursing supervisor to the primary nurse to the physician, with each step increasing the opportunity for miscommunication. This is not an unlikely scenario, since a student's clinical hours often do not coincide with a primary nurse's time in the office. Further communication gaps may occur when students are not present in the agency on days when support staff, such as the rehabilitation team, are available.

Although the strengths and goals of nursing education and service complement one another, they may also create conflict. For example, a faculty member may wish to use the agency as a site for testing a new model for nursing practice. The time required to orient staff to assist with the research may conflict with the administrator's need for the nurses to maintain a certain level of productivity. Communications may be another pitfall. Community health nurses have long valued team conferences as a means for receiving input when managing caseloads. Students are continuously in a team environment that includes their instructor and other students. A student seeking advice from diverse sources may find it difficult to develop one comprehensive nursing care plan with clear long-term goals for the patient.

A quality of care concern is discontinuity. A student bringing much time and energy to a case may also create discontinuity because the patient wonders what has happened to his or her "regular" nurse whom he or she knows and trusts. Patient visits must also fit into the student's schedule since students are rarely in an agency five days per week. Students are also present in an agency for a limited number of weeks. A student may have just established a good working relationship with a client or family when it is time for the student to move on to his or her next clinical experience. Discontinuity may also occur when students are not present in the agency on days when support staff, such as the rehabilitation team, are available.

Environmental or space problems may be a minor but constant irritant. It is obviously not cost-effective for an agency to maintain more space than needed, so that, when a team of 10 or 11 students and their instructor is added to a space meant to house 11 people or fewer, crowding occurs.

GRADUATE STUDENTS

The above boosts and barriers apply to both undergraduate and graduate students from a variety of disciplines. There are certain differences to be considered when one is planning for a graduate student experience.

The graduate student experience is different from the undergraduate experience in two main ways. First, it is usually organized on a one-to-one basis with a specified preceptor. The preceptor, student, and faculty work jointly to outline the practicum parameters. The relationship

that develops between the preceptor and the student will have a major impact on the satisfactory outcome of the experience.

Preceptor Considerations

The preceptor serves as role model, facilitator, supervisor, educator, resource, and sounding board for the student. It is critical that the preceptor be committed to the experience and be aware at the outset that having a student will require additional time and reorganization of daily schedules. Different preceptors have successfully used a number of strategies to integrate the student's experience into the agency routine. Depending on the time parameters of the practicum, a preceptor might lay out his or her calendar for the student to select the most interesting and useful meetings to attend. One preceptor had the student begin each day as she did, by sorting the in basket and discussing plans to address each item on the calendar. There is wide variation in the techniques that can be used to promote the student's learning.

Lettow (1991), a graduate student in home health care, cited three aspects of the student-preceptor relationship: as a contract, with formal structure, guidelines, concrete objectives, mutually developed outcomes, and the preceptor as the senior member of the relationship; as a partnership, with mutual benefits and respect for the experiences and position of the other; and as a commitment, with respect for the other's time and efforts, self-direction on the student's part, and support on the preceptor's part.

The student-preceptor relationship develops as trust is established. A major ingredient in this trust building is the assurance of confidentiality. Strict confidentiality is stressed with the students as an essential component of the practicum and one that may not be violated. It is helpful to discuss this issue during the first joint meeting with the preceptor, student, and faculty present. On occasion, a potential conflict may develop when the student is employed at a competing agency. If this type of potential conflict is present, these competing interests should be addressed and managed with either an alternative placement for the student or clear guidelines as to what information is to be treated with confidentiality. In our experience, students at this level have uniformly responded with noteworthy sensitivity and discretion.

Another issue concerning preceptors is related to the evaluation of the experience. It is important for the preceptor to be clear as to the type and weight of any expected student evaluation. Thoughtful analysis of the student's strengths and areas and skills to enhance can be extremely useful to the student. A strategy that has proved successful is for the student and preceptor to discuss their perceptions of the experience before the final faculty conference. Most preceptors elicit student feedback about components of the practicum and the types of support that were most beneficial to the student. This allows for an open sharing without concern for the valuative nature of grading considerations to interfere.

Setting Objectives

The second major characteristic distinguishing graduate from undergraduate students involves the type of objectives and projects to be accomplished. Whereas the undergraduate students are concerned with visiting patients, the graduate student will be more apt to work on broader projects or programs. Preceptors and faculty must work together to assist the student in developing achievable goals.

The worst projects are those that are vague, amorphous, and linked to others' schedules and approvals with little opportunity for the student to exercise independent decision making. Frequently the student may arrive with the idea that he or she would like to do something in the area of quality improvement and monitoring (QI). If the agency has struggled for the last 10 years with developing continuous quality improvement (CQI) and has no more than a minimum QI program, help the student accept that such a program will not be achieved in the next three

months. It may be possible to accommodate the student's interests by carving out a discrete piece of QI, or it may be best to have alternative suggestions.

The best projects are small, self-contained, allow the student to work independently within broad parameters, and yield a tangible result. In addition to the projects mentioned earlier, some that have been successful for both the student and the agency are as follows:

- needs assessment for health care among retirement home dwellers
- developing an orientation/preceptor's book for new agency staff
- outlining a marketing plan for a new program
- reliability and validity assessment of a newly developed QA (Quality Assessment) audit tool
- cost-benefit analysis of a proposed hospice program
- assessment of mature nurses' employment needs
- specific policy development (e.g., do not resuscitate orders, home health aide program)
- pro forma business plan for opening a branch office

There are numerous others, and one that blends agency needs with student goals usually can be found.

It is important that the student be involved in a project that is perceived to be worthwhile, that is, not artificially created as busywork for the student. One way to avoid this is to discuss how the project output will be used by the agency. This will also ensure that the information the student produces is in a practical form.

RECOMMENDATIONS

From the above advantages and disadvantages, a set of recommendations has been developed. First, faculty need to be oriented to the agency before the student begins the experience. It is recommended that faculty not only be oriented to the organizational structure, policies, and documentation but also be given the opportunity to make joint home visits with a staff nurse. The administrator and educator should jointly develop a plan for orienting students in these areas, with each party's role in the orientation being clearly spelled out. Some agencies may use faculty in practice roles or to serve on various agency committees, such as the audit committee or the professional advisory committee. Faculty who are knowledgeable concerning the mechanics of operations and reimbursement benefit the agency by providing improved student guidance and decreasing the amount of time staff need to spend with students and faculty.

Orientation is only one area for which accountability must be determined. Accountability for documentation (other than progress notes), Medicare form completion, communication with support services and the physician, and case finding are just a few of the many points to be addressed. From the start, a plan should be developed for evaluation of the experience, including feedback from students, faculty, nursing staff, and administration.

Planning for the student experience must begin far in advance of its start. It is standard practice in universities to solidify contractual arrangements during the spring semester preceding a fall semester experience. During the summer months, faculty should meet with administrators to discuss the needs of each party in terms of case finding, space, the orientation process, and so forth.

Contractual Arrangements

It is to each party's advantage to have respective responsibilities clearly delineated in the form of a contract or letter of agreement. In many cases, this will be initiated (and required) by the school or university. Typically this contract is negotiated to outline each party's areas of accountability—the agency assuming primary responsibility for the quality of patient care and education assuming primary account-

ability for student supervision. In Bottorf v. Waltz, the Pennsylvania superior court ruled that teachers have three main areas of responsibility to their students (Van Biervliet & Sheldon-Wildgen, 1981):

- to provide adequate supervision
- to exercise good judgment
- to provide proper instruction, especially when potentially hazardous conditions exist

Implications of this ruling include the need for agency staff to assist faculty in meeting their responsibilities in this area. Often agency staff are in a better position to evaluate client needs and characteristics and can guide faculty in the selection of appropriate clients for the student's level of skill.

Other components of a contract or letter of agreement are the following:

- a statement as to the scope and duration of the agreement
- a nondiscriminatory statement
- liability and insurance documentation
- the agency's responsibilities (e.g., ultimate responsibility for patient care; provision of general orientation to aspects of the agency, policies, and procedures; emergency care, if needed; and space for faculty and students
- the educational institution's responsibilities (e.g., providing an educational program meeting accrediting body standards; providing appropriate, qualified registered nurse faculty as a specified faculty-student ratio and designated availability, such as on-call, etc.; informing the agency of the student and program educational objectives; and participating in joint evaluation)

Even with extensive planning, unanticipated problems are certain to occur. Not only must communication be open, but the channels of communication must be determined ahead of time. Considerations include whether students should communicate patient problems, issues, or questions directly to the staff nurse or to their instructor first. The second route may prevent the constant bombardment of staff with diverse student questions. A plan for reporting off at the end of the day should be developed for both students and faculty. Faculty should be advised of agency policy and preferences for reporting problems and communicating concerns.

Finally, assume that students will create a space problem to some degree. Even with unlimited space, students are often perceived as invading the staff's territory. During planning sessions, the administrator and educator should designate which space and telephones are available for student use.

COST-BENEFIT CONSIDERATIONS

It is extremely difficult to generalize a cost-benefit analysis from agency to agency because there are so many factors that are unique to each agency yet must be considered in an assessment of costs and benefits of student experiences. In a health care environment that is rapidly moving to managed care, individual agency incentives and ability to provide student placements will vary.

The first of these variables is the organizational structure and environment of the agency. At what stage of development is the agency? The stress of accommodating student placements in a new agency may prove to be overwhelming in an agency where systems have yet to become smooth. How adequate is staffing? Is there an individual with primary responsibility for coordinating student-faculty communications? An individual designated in this role can assist in the integration of students into the agency routine. Can provisions for alternative staff activities be made while students are in the agency? Unless the agency is seriously under-

staffed (not a desirable situation with students), staff will receive the same salary irrespective of student visits, and the total agency visits will not increase. If staff can be scheduled for continuing education/staff development, to use time as a "breather" and to catch up on documentation, or to assist with program/policy and procedure development or to audit records in the agency, the time can be maximized. The amount of documentation that is expected of students will also influence the time that staff spend with student cases. Does the agency desire or need the public relations exposure of a university affiliation? Is the potential for staff recruitment from student populations present?

A second major consideration is the type of faculty and students. Generic, RN-BSN completion, or graduate students may make a difference in the reimbursement. Medicare will reimburse for all nursing student visits, but other third-party payers may require registered nurse licensure for reimbursement; thus only RN or graduate students would be reimbursed for visits. The faculty supervisor's familiarity with the agency and its clients and his or her general proficiency and experience in home care will influence the time required by the agency in orientation and assistance with documentation and care planning. Faculty who can assume the bulk of the student's orientation and can oversee charting and client care services will reduce the amount of time spent by agency personnel in these activities.

Consequently, there is no single answer for every agency, or even for the same agency at different time periods. Overall, the consensus among the agencies with whom we have had the good fortune to be affiliated is that the boosts and benefits of having students in the environment far outweigh the barriers.

REFERENCES

Androwich, I.M., & Andresen, P.A. (1986, May). *Student placements in home health care agencies: Boost or barrier to quality patient care?* Poster presented at the Second National Symposium of Home Health Nursing, Ann Arbor, MI.

Harris, M. (1984). Student programs benefit nursing service agencies. *Home Health Care Nurse 2*, 34–35.

Lettow, J. (1991, February). *The preceptor role in home health care administration: The student perspective.* Paper presented at the University of Illinois College of Nursing, Chicago, IL.

Van Biervliet, A., & Sheldon-Wildgen, J. (1981). *Liability issues in community-based programs.* Baltimore: Brooks.

BIBLIOGRAPHY

Androwich, I.M. (1989). Creative utilization of staff. In L. Benefield (Ed.), *Home health care management* (pp. 180–199). Englewood Cliffs, NJ: Prentice-Hall.

Hackbarth, D., & Androwich, I.M. (1989). Graduate nursing education for leadership in home care. *Caring 2*, 6–11.

CHAPTER 67

A Student Program in
One Home Health Agency

Marilyn D. Harris

The Visiting Nurse Association (VNA) of Eastern Montgomery County/Department of Abington Memorial Hospital (AMH) has an active student program. Each year 8 to 10 educational facilities place students with the VNA for observational or practical experience. An average of 100 students affiliate with the agency for variable periods of time each year.

The VNA offers educational opportunities for diploma, baccalaureate, graduate, and doctoral student nurses; medical students and residents; and health care administration students. The

---

Exhibit 67–1 Student Program

PHILOSOPHY

We, the VNA/AMH, believe that our student program is a vital component of our home health and hospice program and is mutually beneficial to both the student and our agency. Furthermore, we believe that it is a valuable experience because it provides the student with a broader perspective of the health care system by incorporating a uniquely different health component. It also provides an opportunity for practical application of the theory gained through an academic program. Finally, we value highly the information exchange that occurs as a result of our experiences with the students.

PURPOSE

The primary purpose of the program is to provide the student with an opportunity to augment his or her perspective of the health needs of the aggregate population as well as of the client and family in the community setting. The program also allows the student an opportunity to gain a better understanding of the role of a community nursing organization in meeting these health needs.

OBJECTIVE

The individual student experiences are based upon and consistent with the course objectives of the various academic institutions that participate in our program.
Origin: 2/83
Revised: 6/93

Source: Reported with permission of Visiting Nurse Association of Eastern Montgomery County/Department of Abington Memorial Hospital, Willow Grove, Pennsylvania.

VNA has developed manuals that include a statement of the philosophy and objectives for the overall program (Exhibit 67–1). There are also goals and objectives for each level of the student programs. The educational facilities are also asked to submit program objectives and curriculum outlines to the agency. Contracts are approved and signed by both the VNA and the school. These are reviewed annually and renewed on a periodic basis. Sample contracts for baccalaureate (Exhibit 67–2) and graduate nursing students (Exhibit 67–3) are included in this chapter with the permission of the educational facilities. The contracts list the responsibilities of both organizations, the number of students to be assigned to the agency at any one

---

Exhibit 67–2 Agreement between the VNA/AMH and Gwynedd-Mercy College, Gwynedd Valley, Pennsylvania

---

AGREEMENT made and dated this 1st day of July, 1996 between Gwynedd-Mercy College, hereinafter referred to as the "College," and the VNA/AMH, hereinafter referred to as the "Agency." It is agreed:

1. That the College will provide instructors for teaching and supervision of students assigned to the Agency for clinical experience.
2. That the College will have the responsibility for planning the schedule of student assignments and participation in the selection of learning experiences in cooperation with the director and will notify the same 2 days before any change in schedule necessitated by an academic requirement.
3. That the College will assume responsibility for College faculty and students complying with all the rules and regulations of the Agency insofar as they pertain to the activities of both while in the Agency.
4. That the College will impress upon the faculty and students their obligation to respect the confidentiality of all records and information that may come to them with regard to the patient's and Agency's records.
5. That the Agency will provide orientation and instruction for college faculty relative to the administrative policies and equipment utilized by the center for treatment.
6. That the Agency will notify the Division of Nursing of the College of any illness or accident involving a student as soon as possible and that the College will promptly take appropriate action.
7. That the faculty and students will provide their own medical care, except in emergencies.
8. That the College will assume responsibility for nursing faculty and nursing students of the Gwynedd-Mercy College Nursing Program carrying professional liability insurance while participating in the teaching and learning experience provided at the Agency.
9. That the College will offer its cultural programs to the Agency's professional personnel.
10. This agreement shall be become effective September 16, 1996 to April 28, 1997.

This agreement may be modified upon request of either party but only upon the consent in writing of both parties.

IN WITNESS WHEREOF, the parties have duly executed this agreement and intend to be legally bound hereby.

President
Gwynedd-Mercy College

Director
VNA/AMH

Courtesy of Gwynedd-Mercy College School of Nursing, Gwynedd Valley, Pennsylvania.

Exhibit 67–3 Agreement

THIS IS AN AGREEMENT between LA SALLE UNIVERSITY, a Pennsylvania nonprofit corporation (hereinafter "University"), and VNA/AMH (hereinafter "Agency") from September 1, 1996 to June 30, 1997.

WHEREAS, University is an educational institution that prepares its students for careers in nursing; and

WHEREAS, University desires to have its students utilize Agency to provide its students with nursing experience; and

WHEREAS, Agency desires to associate with University and to make its facilities available to University and its students to provide nursing experience.

NOW THEREFORE, in consideration of the mutual promises contained herein, and intending to be legally bound hereby, University and Agency agree as follows:

1. Agency agrees to participate with University mutually in the implementation of a curriculum by University to provide nursing experience for students. The curriculum shall provide for a number of students, assignments, and schedules.

2. University will approve the students to be assigned to Agency and notify Agency of the identity of such students within a reasonable time in advance of the date but not less than 30 days when such students are required to report for experiences.

3. Agency will be responsible for ensuring that proper arrangements are made to permit students to report for experiences.

4. University will provide all supervision and instruction for the students, including the orientation of students to Agency. Graduate students will report to Agency preceptors during clinical experiences. Student will notify Agency of any absences.

5. Agency will report to University for disposition, any failure of students to offer proper nursing care, or failure to comply with Agency policies, regulations, and routines.

6. Agency will provide:

   a) Equipment and supplies needed for giving nursing care, including items necessary for student safety and health;
   b) Adequate conference room space, where feasible;
   c) Cafeteria facilities for use of the students and faculty of University, at their own expense;
   d) Orientation and instruction for University faculty regarding administrative policy and nursing procedures.

7. Agency will arrange for emergency health service to students and faculty of University while present at Agency for experiences, at their (faculty and students) own expense.

8. University will ensure that each student and faculty member who participates in the affiliation in all cases is a registered nurse who holds current state licensure and who will maintain nursing malpractice insurance coverage of at least $3,000,000 overall and $1,000,000 per occurrence. Such persons, and not Agency, will assume full liability for their own practice while in Agency. Agency may insist on proof of such coverage.

continues

Exhibit 67–3 continued

9. University will indemnify and defend Agency and its agents, employees, and staff from any claims, demands, actions, or expenses for damage, loss, or injury arising from or related to the negligence or misconduct of its students or faculty members; AND

   Agency will indemnify and defend University and its agents, employees, and staff from any claims, demands, actions, or expenses for damage, loss, or injury arising from or related to the negligence or misconduct of its employees or staff members.

10. Agency and University respectively agree that they will not discriminate against any student or faculty member on account of race, religion, national origin, age (40 years or older), sex, or non-job-related handicap, nor shall either require of the other any action that would violate this provision.

11. In the event of any difference of opinion concerning the care of a patient, the decision of the personnel of Agency shall prevail and control all parties involved.

12. The right and duties of this Agreement are not assignable by either party without the expressed written consent of the other party.

13. This Agreement shall be interpreted in accordance with the laws of the Commonwealth of Pennsylvania.

The term of this Agreement shall be from September 1, 1996 to June 30, 1997.

IN WITNESS WHEREOF, the parties hereto have executed this Agreement on the day and year first written above.

VNA/AMH   LA SALLE UNIVERSITY

_____   _____
Executive Director   Vice President for Business Affairs

Courtesy of La Salle University Department of Nursing, Philadelphia, Pennsylvania.

---

time, and other pertinent terms of the affiliation. The VNA has an interdepartmental arrangement with the AMH School of Nursing (Exhibit 67–4).

In some instances, guidelines for cooperative relationships between the clinical setting and the graduate program (Exhibit 67–5) are shared and agreed upon. These guidelines include information related to agency selection, qualifications of the preceptor, functions of the agency preceptor, expectations of the graduate students, responsibilities of the faculty preceptor, and the placement process.

The contractual relationships are the responsibility of the administrator at the VNA. The determination of the number of educational institutions and students that will affiliate at the VNA each year is the responsibility of the nursing supervisor in charge of education and quality assessment/performance improvement (QA/PI). This decision is made in consultation with the director of professional services, the clinical educator, and the clinical supervisors. The clinical educator is responsible for orientation of the faculty and students to the VNA each semester.

Evaluation of the student placements is an integral part of the total annual evaluation process at the VNA. As part of the evaluation process, students complete, and the schools forward to the VNA, evaluations of the experience.

Exhibit 67–4 Operational Agreement with the School of Nursing

Purpose: To provide a clinical facility for observation of the skills necessary for the nursing of clients in the home.

Services to be provided: Observational experience shall be limited to 2 days per student and subject to the procedures listed below.

Procedures:

1. The number of students sent to the VNA by the School of Nursing shall not exceed three or four on any one day.

2. The VNA will provide each student with orientation and observation under the direction of a registered nurse.

3. The School of Nursing will provide the VNA with a master schedule listing names of student nurses and dates of the planned experience before the beginning of observation. In the event of any change in schedules, either party may notify the other of the change verbally or in writing.

4. The School of Nursing agrees to have its students:
   a. abide by general policies of the VNA when visiting patients by direction of the registered nurse with whom the students are observing, and
   b. keep confidential all knowledge and records of patients

5. The VNA will make available to students and faculty all pertinent educational material during the period of observation.

6. In the event of accident, injury, or illness of a student on observation experience, the VNA will notify the School of Nursing, and plans for the student's return to the School of Nursing will be made on an individual basis dependent on the situation. The School of Nursing shall assume responsibility for care and emergency transportation of the student.

7. The faculty of the School of Nursing agree to present the terminal evaluation of the observation experience to the executive director of the VNA within 30 days of its completion.

8. School of Nursing students will provide individual malpractice insurance coverage.

Origin Date: 9/80
Revision Date: 6/96

Courtesy of the Visiting Nurse Association of Eastern Montgomery County/Dept. of Abington Memorial Hospital, Willow Grove, Pennsylvania.

These evaluations are shared with the staff. In general, the students, patients, and staff indicate that student affiliations are a valuable aspect of the total VNA service. The changing health care climate presents several areas of consideration for the home health agency administrator in relationship to student programs. Staff productivity is one of these areas. A majority of home care services are reimbursed on a per-visit basis.

Students do affect the productivity of staff. Even though a representative from the educational institution is on site, staff are involved in student orientation to both agency and patients. Having someone accompany the nurse on home visits on a regular basis slows down the nurse. This could result in fewer visits per day, which under the current per-visit reimbursement schedule would result in less income for the

Exhibit 67–5 Guidelines for Cooperative Relationships between Villanova University College of Nursing and Practicum Agencies

SELECTION OF AGENCY—The agency must be:
1. Willing to cooperate with the university in providing learning experiences for a graduate nursing student.
2. Willing to offer opportunities for a student to implement specified skills in an administrative, teaching, or clinical role.
3. Approved/accredited by the appropriate state/national agencies.
4. Willing to sign a contract or letter of agreement with Villanova University as per the criteria for selection of agencies.

QUALIFICATION OF THE AGENCY PRECEPTOR—The agency preceptor:
1. Must hold a minimum of a Master's degree in nursing.
2. Must have demonstrated expertise in the specific practicum area.
3. Must be willing to serve as a preceptor and be a role model for the student.
4. Is designated by the agency's nursing department head.

FUNCTIONS OF THE AGENCY PRECEPTOR—The agency preceptor is expected to:
1. Participate with the designated faculty member and student to plan the practicum experience.
2. Assist the student in achieving practicum objectives through facilitating his or her involvement in various relevant activities within the agency.
3. Assume a liaison role in clarifying the expectations of students as learners compared with expectations of employees.
4. Participate in the evaluation of the practicum process and the preceptorship program.

EXPECTATIONS OF THE GRADUATE STUDENT—The student is expected to:
1. Submit a resume and evidence of a current registered nurse license in the state where the practicum experience occurs, current malpractice insurance, a current health examination, and current certification in CPR (basic life support).
2. Write specific practicum plan, including personal learning objectives, process and outcome activities, a time frame, and how he or she will comply with the agency's expectations.
3. Serve as the liaison between the agency preceptor and the faculty member.

RESPONSIBILITIES OF THE FACULTY MEMBER—The Villanova University faculty member is responsible for:
1. Planning the practicum experience with the student and agency preceptor.
2. Monitoring the implementation of the practicum.
3. Evaluating the student's achievement of practicum objectives.
4. Conducting periodic supervision/teaching/consultation visits with the student at the agency and being available for interim consultation.
5. Assisting the student to reorder and reorganize current knowledge and to apply new knowledge throughout the practicum.
6. Evaluating the practicum experience.

PLACEMENT PROCESS—The following process is to be followed to arrange practicum placements:
1. The director of the graduate program will initiate contacts with the agency and determine the feasibility of placement of students in any given academic year.
2. The faculty member will initiate contacts with the agency preceptor for specific practicum planning.
3. The assistant to the dean will initiate interagency contracts or letters of agreement.

Courtesy of the Villanova University College of Nursing, Philadelphia, Pennsylvania.

agency. The Medicare regulations allow for student nurses to provide billable services under a general super-vision provision (U.S. Department of Health and Human Services, 1989). Physical therapy students must work under the direct supervision of the licensed therapist. Once again, this requires the time of the licensed therapist in the home and office.

Documentation is another area for consideration. Documentation must be reviewed to determine that it meets agency standards (e.g., use of the patient classification system and nursing diagnoses), professional standards, and reimbursement standards. Agencies cannot afford to have visits denied on a medical or technical basis. Therefore, additional supervisory time and expenses are incurred to review and verify that all student documentation meets established criteria.

Another consideration regarding documentation at the VNA is related to the implementation of a computerized clinical documentation system. Students do not have access to laptop computers; therefore, all manual documentation completed by the students has to be input into the computerized system by the VNA staff.

The financial impact of student programs must also be considered. To date, there is minimal or no financial compensation available to agencies that cooperate in student programs. Financial consideration for clinical experience should be discussed with each institution and included in the agreement whenever this can be negotiated. This compensation could be in the form of actual dollars or free attendance at continuing education programs for a specific number of staff from the cooperating agency. Another form of payment could be the free use of audiovisual equipment, services, or faculty participation in agency projects. This matter should be discussed each time the contract is renewed. Student programs in home health agencies are beneficial for staff, patients, students, and the educational facilities. Although administrators must be cognizant of the various challenges that exist, they should take the opportunity to participate in the education of future home care staff.

REFERENCE

U.S. Department of Health and Human Services. Health Care Financing Administration. (1989). *Medicare home health agency manual* (Transmittal 222, Section 205.1 (14)). Baltimore: Department of Health and Human Services.

CHAPTER 68

The Role of the Physician in Home Care

Kenneth W. Hepburn and Joseph M. Keenan

Beginning in the 1980s and continuing in the 1990s, home care led the health care industry in growth; home care administrators face important challenges if this trend is to continue into the next century. Perhaps the most important of these challenges will be finding ways to increase physician knowledge and understanding of modern home care and to strengthen physician participation in home care leadership and in the home care team.

Demographics, incentives, and available resources position home care to continue its growth and to reinforce its central position in the community-based long-term care continuum. The older population, which constitutes a significant user group in health care, will continue to expand. The number of frail individuals, those with deficits in activities or instrumental activities of daily living, will also increase. By recent estimates, the number of frail older persons will increase from 7.5 million in 1985 to 18.2 million in 2020 (U.S. Bipartisan Commission, 1990). The diagnosis-related group (DRG) prospective reimbursement system will continue to reduce the time patients spend in acute facilities and increase the need to provide restorative/rehabilitative care in alternative care environments. Vertically and horizontally integrated systems of care will expand the developing number of pathways that seek to optimize patient outcome while mini-

mizing the use of costly institution-based care. Available nursing home beds, an obvious alternative to acute beds in such pathways, will become ever more scarce. The present national supply of about 1.7 million nursing home beds is unlikely to increase to the 4.1 million projected as needed for the frail elderly (U.S. Bipartisan Commission, 1990), especially in the face of moratoria on construction of new beds in many states. Finally, a number of federal-, state-, and foundation-funded initiatives are encouraging innovative financial and organizational structures to meet the needs of persons who are frail and/or chronically ill.

Rapid and dramatic changes in the home care industry have fostered increased public and professional awareness of its capacities. Even more impressive than the attention-getting growth of the industry (a 50% increase in Medicare-certified agencies and a six-fold increase in Medicare billings (to $12.7 billion) from 1988 to 1994) has been the demonstration of innovation and ingenuity that has characterized home care in the last decade. This has been marked by the development and use of safe, technologically sophisticated, transportable diagnostic and therapeutic devices, the implementation of equally sophisticated clinical protocols, and the implementation of complex disease management strategies as product lines. Mobile medical offices and urgent care centers bring an extremely wide array of services to patients in their homes or in nursing home settings. These services foster cost-effective continuity of care (often delivered at a fraction of transport and hospital-based costs) and preclude the iatrogenic risks associated with institutional care. Home care has also thrived on meeting patient needs through the tailored use of multidisciplinary teams of professionals and other direct care providers. This practice has drawn into the field the interest of many forward-thinking professionals, especially in nursing.

Finally, home care provides community-based long-term care (Welch, Wennberg, & Welch, 1996), thus meeting the needs of patients (and their families) and their preferences as well. Patients want to remain in their homes for as long as possible, and they do not want to be placed in nursing homes if this can be avoided (American Association of Retired Persons, 1987). Family members, who play such an important role in the community-based care of the medically frail, similarly prefer home care. Furthermore, family caregivers display a capacity for working in concert with home care agencies. They are not scared off by the home care team; neither do they flee the scene when paid help arrives (Christianson, 1988). The relationship is a reinforcing one that works to the benefit of the patient and the care team, whose goal is to keep the patient at home.

PHYSICIAN INVOLVEMENT

Currently, physicians are not significantly involved in home care, a situation that has evolved for historical, educational, and economic reasons. This lack of involvement, should it continue, could pose a rate-limiting factor for home care growth. The patients for whom an expanding home care industry will provide care will represent increasingly complex cases. Although physicians are more frequently assuming upper management roles (e.g., as medical director), even greater physician involvement will be essential for managing these cases that entail multiple therapies and

procedures, require careful monitoring, pursue delicately balanced care goals, and extend over a long period. Such involvement must include case supervision, teaching, and appropriate home visiting. Ideally, physician involvement should also include serious participation in planning and leadership, in the continued reshaping of the vision of home care, and in the ongoing design of systems to respond to increasingly complex needs.

Historical trends help to explain why physicians are so little involved in home care. Physicians' perceptions about the standard of care have changed over time. In recent decades, physicians have come to perceive the home as a setting in which they cannot provide the best of care. As recently as World War II, the physician, armed only with a black bag, could feel confident that the care he or she could provide in the home was equivalent in scope and quality to what could be provided in the office. Rapid technological advances changed that situation; the therapeutic and diagnostic armamentarium of the hospital and the office became extensive. Physicians have been slow to recognize that much of this technology is portable and is increasingly available in the home setting.

During this same period, the economics of medicine changed along with the perceived standard of care, further removing home care from the physician's normal practice. Physicians have come to prefer the familiarity, professional comfort, and efficiency of a well-equipped and well-staffed medical office. An office practice incurs overhead costs that must be maintained through carefully managed office efficiency and productivity. In this context, a physician home visit is doubly disadvantageous: It is generally an inefficient and still poorly reimbursed use of physician time, and it does not utilize ancillary office staff and facilities productively.

Perhaps because the standard of care and the business of care have both been changing, a whole generation of physicians has been trained whose knowledge, skills, and attitudes about home care are out of sync with the reality of home care in the 1990s. Medical school and residency education seldom provide physicians in training with information about or exposure to modern home care practice. Similarly, these learners are exposed to few practicing physicians who can serve as role models to teach them about home care and to help them form positive attitudes about it. As a result, home care agencies report that physicians typically do not know what home care can do, do not know how to use home care to its full capacity, and are not skilled in participating in home care (either in terms of clinical skills or in the ability to document care in ways that help agencies gain reimbursement).

Some attitudinal barriers also keep physicians away from home care. These are complex and come from a number of sources but are primarily manifestations of the continuing struggle of physicians and nurses to learn how to work together. Many of the innovations in home care were stimulated by nurse-led agencies working independently of physicians. Home care offered nurses an opportunity to demonstrate their clinical skills and creativity as well as to exercise their leadership and entrepreneurial capacities. Physicians, having no part in this, felt no part of it: Home care was perceived as a nursing intervention. Similarly, nurse leaders in the field were reluctant to invite participation that might be based on physician expectation that nurses would resume a support role in this reinvigorated delivery system.

For physicians, home care still seems a situation in which the time and effort spent and the responsibilities assumed are not balanced by the returns. A 1990 American Medical Association national survey of physicians found that the principal barrier physicians expressed to home care use related to the disincentives built into the reimbursement structure. Physicians reported spending up to four hours a week providing service for which they were not reimbursed (Keenan et al., 1992). Despite recent improvements in the reimbursement system, Medicare continues to expect physicians to provide case management for home care, although there is no reimbursement for these services.

THE HOME CARE ADMINISTRATOR'S ROLE

To draw more physicians into home care and to foster the continued growth of the field, the modern home care administrator will need to adopt five major goals:

1. help build physicians' home care capabilities
2. expand concepts of teams and teamwork in home care
3. expand physicians' leadership and management roles in home care
4. support an enhanced physician role in home care
5. support an alliance for appropriate reimbursement for home care

The sections that follow detail each of these goals.

Build Physician Home Care Capabilities

Given physicians' lack of training about home care, the home care administrator can contribute significantly to the development of physician skills, knowledge, and attitudes related to home care. On a spectrum of home care skills and knowledge, physicians may fall anywhere from a rudimentary awareness to a high level of sophistication. It is important, therefore, that administrators be able to assess where a physician falls on this spectrum, have available a repertoire of instructional information and systems, and in some instances, bear the costs of special training to advance a physician's development. The following discussion outlines some of the elements making up this repertoire.

Home Care Information

Physicians beginning to work in home care need orientation as much as any other provider. Physicians need to be aware of what home care can do and that it includes a large array of professional and direct care services. They must understand that portable equipment (e.g., for radiography and infusion therapy) and durable medical equipment support a large and growing range of therapeutic capabilities. They need to be aware of the kinds of conditions that can be cared for at home, such as active rehabilitation, long-term maintenance of the frail elderly, and hospice care (including advanced pain management techniques).

Physicians deciding to make home visits may need guidance about the benefits of home visiting (Ramsdel, Swart, Jackson, & Renvall, 1989; Ward et al., 1990) and about the sophisticated evaluation they might take part in (Stuck et al., 1995). They may also need information about the kinds of supplemental assessments they can perform during the visit (e.g., of the environment), and they may well profit from tips of the trade from experienced home care nurses (e.g., how to get enough light for an examination). Physicians making their first visits may need concrete assistance in preparing for them; for example, agencies might assist with lists of what a physician should pack in the medical bag.

Agencies should be prepared to fill in the gaps in physicians' knowledge through a range of informational techniques. These can include standard written descriptive materials, but other strategies might prove more effective with physicians whose time is carefully linked to productivity. Scheduled briefings, before or after office hours, could provide a focused means of communication and help build rapport. Well-made audiotapes are convenient for listening during commute times and represent an effective use of that time. To enable key physicians to play pivotal roles in special programs, support for participation in continuing medical education programs may be beneficial.

Home Care Use Information

Physicians may need to be taught how to use home care: how to order it, how to interact with it, and how to document it appropriately. Agencies need to make it clear what they need and

expect from physicians and what physicians can expect in return. It is particularly important to negotiate the manner in which care plans are generated, altered, approved, monitored, and revised. In general, how are practice-preference conflicts resolved? Physicians need to be made aware of any established protocols that an agency might use and how their own practice style and preferences will interact with these protocols. Does, for example, the agency's pain management protocol typically involve patient self-regulation of morphine, and does it usually involve the use of certain equipment obtained from the home care agency's own pharmacy supply arm? What is the physician's role in this? Can the self-regulation order be changed? What about the use of another kind of device, perhaps from another supplier? Is the agency's rehabilitation protocol, for example, structured in a way that makes efficient use of agency personnel's time over the typical reimbursement period? If so, can a physician alter it, and under what circumstances? What if, for example, the physician should want to tailor the rehabilitation protocol to include greater than usual amounts initially? Can the agency accommodate this?

Systems That Facilitate Use

Mechanisms that improve efficiency and reduce physician's unreimbursed time will be appreciated. Among the systems that agencies can develop are the following:

- *Effective phone systems*: Phone calls between the agency and the physician must be timely and appropriate. Calls to physicians by agency personnel should be carefully triaged to ensure they are essential, calls about matters that really require a physician's attention. A system should be developed with the physician's office so that, when possible, essential calls can be scheduled and that, again when possible, office staff can handle matters through a message system. Use of fax and e-mail technology will also simplify office-to-office contact and reduce the time of contact.

- *Facilitation of home visits*: When the agency or the physician feels that a physician home visit is essential for care planning or management, the agency should provide as much assistance as possible to make the visit as efficient and effective as possible. This assistance might include providing brief summaries of the agency's most recent assessments of the patient situation, including the agency's agenda for the home visit, specifying why it is needed, what needs to be accomplished, and what the desired outcomes might be; scheduling appropriate family caregivers and home care agency personnel to be at the home with the physician; and making sure that any equipment or supplies the physician might need are on hand for the visit.

- *Management information systems*: Particularly because home care medical supervision involves management at a distance, timely and appropriate information and systems of information management are critical. The physician needs to know about significant changes in patient condition and in the care plan. Many changes in plan will be outside the medical realm and will not require physician approval (e.g., enhancing a patient's available nutrition through Meals-on-Wheels or having a spouse or caregiver attend a support group). Nevertheless, because such changes affect the overall situation in which the patient and family find themselves, the physician needs to be aware of them. The agency should have a system for providing the physician with brief summaries of such changes. Similarly, even when no care plan changes are instituted, brief progress reports on patient condition and response to care will keep the physician up to date on the patient. As with the system for phone contact, the management information system should emphasize brevity and pertinence and should be user-friendly: These systems should instill in participating physicians the confidence that time spent using them is time well spent. If an agency adopts an electronic medical record based in laptop PCs, provisions will be needed to link physicians to the system.

- *Quality assessment and outcome data systems*: Physicians, like other health care professionals, are motivated by the wish to provide beneficial care. They need to have information about the outcomes of care. In home care, because their role is often a distant one, physicians can be removed from direct knowledge of how things turned out with patients. Agencies should have systems that provide participating physicians with performance data. These data should indicate both how agency patients fare in general and how a physician's own patients have done.

Educational Involvements

Where it is possible to do so, home care agencies can provide opportunities for medical students or residents to rotate through the agency as part of their training. This provides physicians with important exposure to home care at a formative stage of their development.

Promoting Teams and Teamwork

One of the critical roles of the home care administrator is that of team builder. The virtues of working in teams to deal with the multiple biopsychosocial problems of frail or complex patients are well appreciated. It is also well appreciated, however, that developing, nurturing, and maintaining a well-functioning team require work and energy. This is especially true in home care, where the composition of the team varies from patient to patient. In particular, although a core nursing team might remain together across a large group of patients, it is likely that most of these patients will have their own physician. Hence the core team will be relating to many different physician team members.

A number of concepts define a health care team. Team members have specified roles and responsibilities that are all applied toward a shared goal or purpose that is pursued through interdependent work. Typically, teams develop their own ways of talking with one another, often employing a compressed form of communication that is both brief and precisely understood by those on the inside. There are usually shared standards—a common set of expectations about the intensity, quality, and outcomes of the work—as well as a shared way of doing things (common practices and procedures). Team members behave according to a code that combines trust, reliability, and respect: They can count on each other, there are no "dumb" questions, and everyone is important. The team often provides its members with a source of important intangibles, such as rewards, a sense of personal worth, and growth. Typically, teams know their own boundaries (e.g., who is a member and who is not, and whose knowledge and experience afford primary authority on which issues).

The home care administrator can play a key bridging role between the established regulars—the core nursing team—and the physician, whose task it is to provide medical care and supervision in the particular case. The administrator will accomplish part of this role by attending to the tasks outlined above (building physician home care capabilities). Quickly familiarizing the physician with what the agency can do and having established ways for the physician to participate will allow the physician to fit into the ways and mores of the team. In addition, home care staff orientation and training can provide regular team members with insight into and techniques for maintaining a team in which one key member is almost always an outsider. It is particularly important that orientation and ongoing staff development emphasize that a physician often has a long-standing relationship with a patient and family. This relationship can improve the receptivity of

the patient to the home care team and can add continuity to the overall plan of care.

A more subtle role for the administrator is that of listening post. Team functioning demands mutual respect, and the administrator is often in a position to hear when one player on the team is speaking or behaving in a manner that disregards or belittles another. Physician-bashing and nurse-baiting are equally destructive to effective team functioning and need to be addressed immediately to stave off specific negative consequences and the development of a more generalized negative environment.

A home care agency can foster team performance by physicians by building links to the local physician community. Such links help each side know the other: Local physicians get to know the agency and the core staff, and staff members have opportunities to meet and interact with community physicians.

Expand Leadership and Management Roles

As home care continues to take on increasingly complex medical management responsibilities and as it continues to integrate with more complex organizations, the need for physician involvement in home care leadership and management grows. A medical director or medical executive in a diversified modern home care agency is called upon to engage in a number of high-level program activities. These include participation in the agency's long-range visioning and planning; involvement in assessing the risks, feasibility, benefits, and personnel needs in developing new lines of service; leading in the design and development of new, medically complex products; instituting systematic staff and physician development programs; providing consultation on issues of complicated medical ethics; and participating in the agency's quality management program.

These roles go far beyond (yet do not obviate) the traditional roles of physician liaison (establishing and maintaining links with local physicians; providing direct intervention with a physician in instances where there is conflict in the team; and providing educational interventions to both staff and physicians that can help build, strengthen, or mend teams). They require skills and knowledge not taught in medical training and seldom learned in the normal course of practice. When an agency perceives the need for physician participation in top management, the agency must be willing to invest in the development that will be necessary for the physician to make the contributions that will be expected. As with enhancing physician skills for home care, enhancing physician skills for leadership will require added training—provided by the agency and/or through continuing medical education programs, such as those provided by the American Academy of Home Care Physicians.

Enhanced Physician Role

Of all the goals, this is the most intangible; it has to do with the home care agency's perception of the place of the physician in home care. Certainly, medical education has the major task ahead of altering curricula so that physicians emerge from training better able to work in home care. Under certain circumstances, the home care administrator may be able to cooperate with this educational process, but for the most part medical education is out of his or her control. What is under the control of the home care administrator, however, is the ambiance of the agency as it relates to physician participation.

For patients and families, physicians remain the principal point of contact with the medical system and are the professionals who are perceived as having the most knowledge and authority within the health care system. As such, their validation of the home care plan plays an important role in patient and family compliance and satisfaction. This can be a sticking point with other home care professionals, who may feel that it is their on-the-spot assessment and integration of information that make the plan work, not the blessing of a physician who may never have been in the patient's home.

Administrators well understand that home care professionals can feel slighted or demeaned by having physicians who appear only tenuously connected with their patients called home care team leaders. Similarly, administrators know that these professionals can bridle under mandated physician authority in situations in which they are essentially setting the care plan.

The administrator has to see to it that the physician is welcome in the agency. The system can breed or fuel resentment; the reimbursement system has vested accountability in the physician. Nor is this without reason: Although the home care staff's abilities in management may be greater than those of the physician, the physician has trained longer, and his or her fund of knowledge is greater in medical areas than the care staff's. The administrator must see to it that these system factors do not interfere with the home care agency staff's abilities to work collaboratively with physicians.

The modern home care administrator will see to it that the agency demonstrates an adequate physician presence in its management and decision making. As noted above, this presence can be established through the development and support of a meaningful medical director role within the agency. The use of medical advisors and consultants in specific roles (e.g., creating and maintaining a meaningful physician education or quality assurance function) will also support this presence. The message to the physician community should be that physicians are valued not only as members of the clinical team but as participants in the development of new programs and protocols. It is important to involve physicians in the agency's strategic and tactical planning. Physicians should be invited to participate in shaping the developing vision of home care. Equally, they should share in designing solutions for clinical problems that arise in pursuing these strategic directions.

Alliance for Appropriate Reimbursement

Home care agencies and physicians involved in home care have common cause in the matter of appropriate reimbursement. Despite the Health Care Financing Administration's recent increase in the reimbursement rates for physician home visits and its decision to reimburse care plan supervision (Department of Health and Human Services, 1994; National Association for Home Care, 1994), there is much in home care that remains poorly reimbursed or not reimbursed at all. In particular, physicians should be compensated for the time they spend in case management activities. Agencies have a particular need to reduce or eliminate the number of retrospective denials they receive.

While this alliance has been somewhat successful in bringing about appropriate reimburse-ment, the majority of physicians still feel reimbursement is inadequate. Home care agencies can provide leadership and technical know-how in the effort to improve the reimbursement picture. They can provide physicians with technical assistance in the area of care plan and progress note documentation. Agencies can work collaboratively with physicians who develop protocols of care that ensure optimal reimbursement and simplify documentation. Agencies can also encourage their organizations to link strategically with organized medicine in a common pursuit of health policy that supports appropriate home care development and reimbursement.

REFERENCES

American Association of Retired Persons, the Villers Foundation. (1987). *The American public views long-term care* (survey). Princeton, NJ: R.L. Associates.

Christianson, J.B. (1988). The effect of channeling on informal caregiving. *Health Services Research, 23*, 97–117.

Department of Health and Human Services. Health Care Financing Administration. (1994). *Federal Register, 59* (121). *Medicare Program: Refinements to geographic adjustment factor values and other policies under the physician fee schedule.* Friday, June 24, 1994. 32754–32794.

Keenan, J.M., Boling, P.A., Schwartzberg, J.G., Olson, L., Schneiderman, M., McCaffrey, D.J., & Ripsin, C.M. (1992). A national survey of the home visiting practice and attitudes of family physicians and internists. *Archives of Internal Medicine, 152*(10), 2025–2032.

National Association for Home Care. (1994, December). *Physician payment for care plan oversight services and home visits in the 1995 fee schedule.* Washington, DC: Author.

Ramsdel, J.W., Swart, J., Jackson, J.E., & Renvall, M. (1989). The yield of a home visit in the assessment of geriatric patients. *Journal of the American Geriatric Society, 37*, 17–24.

Stuck, A.E., Aronow, H.U., Steiner, A., Alessi, C.A., Bula, C.J., Gold, M.N., Yuhas, K.E., Nisenbaum, R., Rubenstein, L.Z., & Beck, J.C. (1995). A trial of annual in-home comprehensive geriatric assessments for elderly people living in the community. *The New England Journal of Medicine, 333*, 1184–1189.

U.S. Bipartisan Commission on Comprehensive Health Care (Pepper Commission). (1990). *Final report: A call for action.* Washington, DC: Government Printing Office.

Ward, H.W., Ramsdel, J.W., Jackson, J.E., Renvall, M., Swart, J.A., & Rockwell, E. (1990). Cognitive function testing in comprehensive geriatric assessment: A comparison of cognitive test performance in residential and clinic settings. *Journal of the American Geriatric Society, 38*, 1088–1092.

Welch, H.G., Wennberg, D.E., & Welch, W.P. (1996). The use of Medicare home health care services. *The New England Journal of Medicine, 335*, 324–329.

CHAPTER 69

The Physician Connection

Marilyn D. Harris

"Too much paperwork. Every order change must be accomplished multiple times (explain to family, home caretaker, nurse and sign). There must be an easier system."

Each year physicians who refer patients to the Visiting Nurse Association of Eastern Montgomery County (VNA) are given the opportunity to evaluate the agency, its services, and its personnel through a mailed questionnaire. On a questionnaire returned some months ago by one physician, the complaint quoted above was written. It correctly characterized the detailed requirements of the Medicare program's plan of care (POC) forms 485, 486, and 487 before the revised Health Insurance for the Aged (HIM 11) regulations took effect on July 1, 1989 (Department of Health and Human Services, 1989a).

One result of the revised HIM 11 has been to increase physician involvement in the patient's plan of care. It is important that HIM 11 revisions be shared with the physicians who refer patients for home care services. It is equally important for physicians to be informed about the many issues—clinical, administrative, and legislative or regulatory—that have an impact on their patients' care. Awareness of these issues leads physicians to appreciate the importance of a cooperative relationship with a home

health agency and its staff to use appropriately the Medicare benefit for patients.

LEGISLATIVE OR REGULATORY AND CLINICAL ISSUES

Under the Medicare conditions of participation (COP) (Department of Health and Human Services, 1989b; COP 484.30), the nurse is the coordinator of care. One aspect of the nurse's role is to keep physicians informed of the ever-changing health care climate as it relates to the Medicare program and the physicians' patients. This coordination process includes education related to the restrictions imposed by Medicare concerning homebound status, the need for laboratory studies for coverage for specific diagnoses such as pernicious anemia, the length of time Medicare or other third-party payers will pay for services, and what services and supplies are reimbursable, e.g., specific products for specific stages of wounds.

Home care nurses or the administrators of the agency must provide information that will help physicians understand the regulations under which the agency now provides services. When original POC forms were introduced in 1985, I shared copies of the instructions on completing

Source: Adapted with permission from M.D. Harris, The Physician Connection, *Home Healthcare Nurse*, Vol. 7, No. 6, pp. 39–41, © 1989, J.B. Lippincott Company.

the forms with selected physicians so that they would know why the order forms were changed and why they were being asked to comply with new requirements.

At that time we also developed a form letter that detailed why the physician was being asked to complete orders every three weeks on selected patients. Another letter, signed by the chairman of the professional advisory committee (PAC), advised physicians that it is important to the care of the patient that the physician write a meaningful progress note, sign it legibly, and return it to the agency in a timely manner. Still another type of letter that is sent to physicians addresses the regulation of the administration of vitamin B_{12} for the diagnosis of pernicious anemia and other specific diagnoses. It includes a reference to the section in the Medicare manual, the recommended dosage, and the administrative schedule for the selected diagnoses.

In July 1989, I wrote a letter to the chief of staff at the local hospital informing him of the recent changes in the Medicare program for home health services as a result of a national lawsuit. I included the following sections of HIM 11 (Department of Health and Human Services, 1989a):

- The plan of care must contain all pertinent diagnoses, including the beneficiary's mental status; the type of services, supplies, and equipment ordered; the frequency of visits to be made; prognosis; rehabilitation potential; functional limitations; activities permitted; nutritional requirements; medications and treatments; safety measures to protect against injury; discharge plans; and any additional items the home health agency or physician chooses to include (204.2).
- The qualified physician must sign the plan (a stamped signature is not acceptable) (204.2(c)).
- If the 62-day recertification form is not signed before the previous certification expires, there must be a verbal order

before service is provided in the subsequent period (204.2-E).
- Any increase in the frequency of services or additions of new services during a certification period must be authorized by a physician by way of a verbal order or written order before the provision of the increase or additional services (204.2-E(3)).

At that time, I also included a paragraph stating that, at present, Medicare did not provide for a method to reimburse physicians for their involvement in the plan of care for home care services. I did mention that the National Association for Home Care included support for this type of legislation in its annual Blueprint for Action.

The hospital's chief of staff called me and said he thought it was important to share these changes with all physicians. He invited me to prepare a one-page memo. He planned to include this with his next biweekly mailing to the entire medical, dental, and podiatry staff. Through this memo I was able to share important information with more than 600 physicians at one time and at no additional expense.

In 1994, another letter was shared with physicians to inform them of the availability of physician payment for care plan oversight that became effective January 1, 1995 (Health Care Financing Administration, 1994; National Association for Home Care, 1994).

ADMINISTRATIVE ISSUES

Administrative issues that affect the physician include the following:

- appreciation of the time frame for return of the signed order; this is most important for patient care as well as reimbursement for the home health agency
- the requirement by Medicare as well as other insurance companies that selected bills must be accompanied by a letter from the physician confirming homebound status; this letter is often associated with a

reopening or reconsideration of a Medicare denial of service

- the need to use specific wording on the POC for reimbursement purposes

I offer several suggestions that we have found useful to inform physicians about the administrative aspects of the Medicare program:

Invite additional physicians to serve on the agency's PAC. The PAC is a valuable asset to the agency as well as to the medical community. PAC members can share their expertise on home health issues with other physicians in the community.

Invite physicians to provide feedback to the agency on an ongoing or annual basis through the use of a formal questionnaire (Exhibit 69–1). At the VNA the questionnaires are mailed during one 62-day recertification period each year. Our response rate averages 50% each year. About 25% of the physicians take the time to include comments in addition to marking the checklist. We follow up on any suggestions for new services. Sometimes the suggested service is already in place, so that the follow-up contact serves to provide information about the service. We also follow up on suggested areas for improvement.

Home health nurses and administrators must also let physicians know the qualifications of the staff. Do your referring physicians know that you have certified pediatric and adult nurse practitioners and that your staff includes nurses certified in the administration of intravenous medications, feedings, and chemotherapy to care for their patients with special needs?

Formal educational programs with area medical schools for medical students and residents are another way to let new physicians know the importance of the home health care nurse in the care of the homebound patient. A day spent on home visits with the nurse is an excellent way for medical students and residents to become acquainted with the levels of care that can be provided in the community.

Information from national and state organizations can also be shared with physicians by means of an insert accompanying the POC when it is sent to the physician for a signature. This information may be helpful in explaining the current home health care environment and why the physician's cooperation is required and appreciated even though there may or may not be additional payment available to him or her (Department of Health and Human Services, 1994).

Through a cooperative effort between the hospital's chief of staff and the home care department, an annual letter is sent to all physicians who are on staff to update them on current Medicare regulations related to home health care and standards of the Joint Commission on Accreditation of Healthcare Organizations (Joint Commission, 1996). The Joint Commission Standard Care, Treatment and Services (TX 2.2.1) requires that the organization inform physicians managing patient medical care and services of its policies and procedures regarding the organization's and physicians' responsibilities in providing care and services. The home care administrative staff are also invited to the orientation program for new physicians who join the hospital staff. All new referring physicians who are not on the hospital's staff receive a letter from the director at the time that the POC is sent for signature.

CONCLUSION

The home health care nurse is a vital link between the patient and the physician when home care is needed. The sharing of information related to the clinical, administrative, and regulatory aspects of home care benefits the patient, the physician, the nurse, and the home health agency.

Exhibit 69–1 Physician Satisfaction Survey

Your patients have used one or more of the services available through the Visiting Nurse Association of Eastern Montgomery County/A Department of Abington Memorial Hospital. Would you please take the time to complete and return this questionnaire in the enclosed self-addressed envelope? Please comment and make suggestions for improvements you believe would be helpful in making this association more effective in the community. Thank you for your cooperation in this evaluation process.

Marilyn D. Harris, RN, MSN
Executive Director

Services are provided to more than 1,100 patients by more than 150 health care personnel each month, for a total of over 10,000 visits per month. These services could have included:

Skilled Nursing	Speech Therapy	Enterostomal Therapy	Home Health Aide
Medical Social Service	Psychiatric Nursing	Occupational Therapy	Maternal Child Health
Hospice	Physical Therapy	Continence Management	Hi-Tech Services

1. How satisfied are you with the quality of care given by this agency's personnel?

0	1	2	3	4
Not Applicable	Very Satisfied	Satisfied	Dissatisfied	Very Dissatisfied

Comments: _____

_____

_____

2. Communication is crucial to the coordination of patient care. Please indicate your level of satisfaction with access to patient specific/agency information.

0	1	2	3	4
Not Applicable	Very Satisfied	Satisfied	Dissatisfied	Very Dissatisfied

Comments: _____

_____

_____

3. In this era of shortened hospital stays, are there any other programs or services that you would want this department to provide for your patients?
Comments: _____

_____

_____

Signature: _____

Source: Reprinted with permission of the Visiting Nurse Association of Eastern Montgomery County/Dept. of Abington Memorial Hospital, Willow Grove, Pennsylvania.

REFERENCES

Department of Health and Human Services. Social Security Administration. Health Insurance for the Aged. (1989a). *Home health agency manual* (HIM 11, Transmittal 22). Baltimore: Author.

Department of Health and Human Services. Health Care Financing Administration. (1989b). Author. *Medicare program: Home health agencies: Conditions of participation and reduction in record keeping requirements.* Interim final rule (42 CFR Part 484). *Federal Register,* 54, 33371.

Department of Health and Human Services. Health Care Financing Administration. (1994). *Federal Register,* 59 (121). *Medicare Program; Refinements to geographic adjustment factor values and other policies under the physician fee schedule.* Friday June 24, 1994. 32754–32794.

Joint Commission on Accreditation of Healthcare Organizations. (1996). *1997–98 Comprehensive Accreditation Manual for Home Care.* Standard TX 2,2 1. Oakbrook Terrace, IL: Author.

National Association for Home Care. (1994, December). *Physician payment for care plan oversight services and home visits in the 1995 fee schedule.* Washington, DC: Author.

CHAPTER 70

The Role of the Medicare Fiscal Intermediary and the Regional Home Health Intermediary

Deborah A. Randall

PART I

The Medicare fiscal intermediaries (FIs) are private insurance companies that serve as the federal government's agents in the administration of the Medicare program, including the payment of claims. There are two primary functions for the FI: reimbursement review and medical coverage review. Hospital-based home health agencies are reviewed by the hospital's FI for reimbursement purposes. All home health agencies are assigned to a special FI, the Regional Home Health Intermediary (RHHI), for medical review issues. The same or a different FI may audit the hospital's cost report. Free-standing home health agencies deal with separate reimbursement and medical review divisions within a single RHHI's office. This chapter reviews the role of the Medicare FI and the RHHI and their relationship to home health agencies.

The FI's authority to impose requirements on home health agencies, to audit home health cost reports, and to determine coverage of Medicare claims submitted by the home health agency stems from the FI's contract with the Health Care Financing Administration (HCFA). HCFA annually reviews the six RHHIs as well as all other FIs for their compliance with their con-tracts and for their performance relative to one another, using measurements from the Contractor Performance Evaluation Program (CPEP).[1] FIs that score poorly on CPEP face possible cancellation of their contracts, or must bid against other insurance companies to regain the contract.

The six RHHIs and their assigned geographic areas are:

1. Associated Hospital Service of Maine: Connecticut, Maine, Massachusetts, New Hampshire, Rhode Island, and Vermont
2. United Government Services of Wisconsin: Michigan, Minnesota, New Jersey, New York, Wisconsin, and the Virgin Islands[2]
3. Palmetto (Blue Cross and Blue Shield of South Carolina): Kentucky, North Carolina, South Carolina, Tennessee, Arkansas, Louisiana, New Mexico, Oklahoma, Texas, Alabama, Florida, Georgia, and Mississippi
4. Health Care Service Corporation (Illinois): Illinois, Indiana, and Ohio
5. Blue Cross of Iowa: Colorado, Iowa, Kansas, Missouri, Montana, Nebraska, North

Source: Part I, Reprinted with permission from D. Randall, The Role of the Medicare Fiscal Intermediary Part I, *Journal of Nursing Administration,* Vol. 22, No. 6, pp. 47–53, © 1992, J.B. Lippincott Company.

Dakota, South Dakota, Utah, Wyoming, Pennsylvania, Delaware, District of Columbia, Maryland, Virginia, and West Virginia

6. Blue Cross of California: Alaska, Arizona, California, Hawaii, Idaho, Oregon, Nevada, and Washington.

Three of the RHHIs serve as alternate RHHIs, and can be assigned to a home health agency instead of the usual RHHI, if the agency proves to HCFA that it is in the best interests of the Medicare program.[3] Other than for chain operations or rare situations in which home health agencies demonstrate a persisting conflict with the assigned RHHI, HCFA has been generally resistant to granting requests for an alternate RHHI. The alternate intermediaries and the states to which they are assigned are:

- United Government Services of Wisconsin: Alabama, Connecticut, Delaware, District of Columbia, Florida, Georgia, Iowa, Kansas, Kentucky, Maine, Maryland, Massachusetts, Mississippi, Missouri, Nebraska, New Hampshire, North Carolina, Pennsylvania, Rhode Island, South Carolina, Tennessee, Vermont, Virginia, and West Virginia

- Blue Cross of Iowa: Alaska, Arizona, Arkansas, California, Hawaii, Idaho, Illinois, Indiana, Louisiana, Michigan, Minnesota, Nevada, New Jersey, New Mexico, New York, Ohio, Oklahoma, Oregon, Puerto Rico, Texas, Virgin Islands, Washington, and Wisconsin

- Blue Cross of California: Colorado, Montana, North Dakota, South Dakota, Utah, and Wyoming.

The central office of HCFA outside of Baltimore, Maryland, is responsible for policy development and contractor selections and monitoring. To accomplish this program management, HCFA works through its 10 Regional Offices that in turn, disseminate directions to the FIs and RHHIs. When home health agencies are experiencing difficulties with RHHIs/FIs

that cannot be solved at the upper levels of supervision within the FI's Medicare Part A program staff, home health agencies should first approach the Regional Office of HCFA, seeking out the Associate Regional Administrator for the Medicare Division. If there is not an acceptable resolution, or the resolution is too slow in coming, home health agencies should contact the central office of HCFA through their health care attorney. HCFA has reorganized its divisions along health industry specialty lines. Coverage policy and Medicare reimbursement or disallowance for home health or hospice costs are now handled in the Bureau of Policy Development. The same office handles coverage and reimbursement for nursing facilities.

FUNCTIONS OF THE FISCAL INTERMEDIARY

The principal tasks of the FI for home health providers are 1) information dissemination and education of providers; 2) coverage determinations and claims processing; 3) provider audit, including prepayment and postpayment claims audits and year-end cost report audits and settlement; 4) resolution of cost report disputes and appeals; and 5) program integrity reviews, including utilization analyses and responses to complaints or "tips" about fraudulent practices. (The degree to which this function will change in fiscal 1998 depends on whether the Office of the Inspector General takes over all integrity reviews.) The details of the FI functions are described in three Medicare health insurance manuals ("HIMs") published by HCFA. These are the Intermediary Manual (HIM-13), the Provider Reimbursement Manual (HIM-15), and the Home Health Agency Manual (HIM-11), all of which can be purchased from the federal government publishing offices.[4] A properly prepared home health agency staff should have ready access to all three of these manuals.

Information Dissemination and Education

Although state home care associations and various national associations in the home health field make strong efforts to keep their members abreast of Medicare requirements and developments, the FI is the formal, official source of information about rules, changes in rules, developments in regulations, and sometimes the text of Congressional laws.

The education and information dissemination function of the FI is accomplished by providing agencies with written materials, interpretations, and educative programming. The FIs distribute the Medicare bulletins that announce changes in the Medicare law and regulations, or advice of interpretations of policy. In the past, there have been numerous occasions in which the FI's interpretation of Medicare home health coverage as distributed in one area of the country has differed with the practice, or possibly the disseminated interpretations, of an FI in another area. The concentration of medical review function in six RHHIs and the quarterly meetings among those RHHIs have reduced these inconsistencies considerably since the late 1980s. (Many home health agencies feel the "consistency" is moving toward a narrower view of what is reimbursable.) A further, important change was HCFA's revision in April 1989 of the coverage sections of the Home Health Agency Manual and the subsequent revision of certain of the regulations in 1994. HIM-11 now provides better examples of covered care, forbids RHHIs from using their own self-developed "rules of thumb" to limit interpretations of Medicare coverage, and gives a greater presumption of correctness to the physicians who make the medical necessity decision when ordering home care for patients. By 1997, however, HCFA and the Office of the Inspector General, as well as the General Accounting Office, concluded that home health agencies in many states were providing too many services and that the coverage rules again needed tightening.

FIs have generally provided little written information and guidance concerning the reimbursement aspects of the home health agency's function, although they do pass on to agencies any HCFA directives on major issues. Because of increasing limitations in the FI contractor budget, written consultations for home health agencies have been much reduced. Frequently, home health agencies must push for an appointment and bear the administrative and travel costs to the FI's headquarters to seek guidance for a reimbursement matter. However, such efforts by the home health agency can be critical. For some issues, such as a home health agency's structuring its allocation of costs to assign costs more directly to certain cost report "cost centers" or companies, the Provider Reimbursement Manual requires the home health agency to obtain the FI's written consent to a unique approach or methodology to support cost allocations.[5] In-person on-site negotiation with the FI is strongly preferred for the home health agency if the reimbursement proposal is complex, and should be preceded by detailed written descriptions of the structuring approach. When FI prior approval has not been obtained, the home health agency may face significant cost disallowances during cost report settlement. Several distinct business operations costs may be "collapsed" into a single administrative cost pool and allocated among all the agency's functional areas. This could greatly reduce the Medicare reimbursement rate for the agency.

Should the FI show resistance to providing information or if it distributes apparently inaccurate interpretive materials, home health agencies should contact their state home care associations (for good networking) and the HCFA Regional Office.

Coverage Determination and Claims Processing

Review of Claims Submitted

Home health agencies bill on a monthly basis, using an electronic claims transmission format. As the initial plan of care, home health agencies create and submit to the referring physician the HCFA form and physician certification (Form 485). After the first month in which services were provided, the home health agency transmits its bill to the FI. The *signed* 485 must be in the agency's possession before billing. A verbal order also must be confirmed, in writing, signed, and returned before a bill is sent. The third month of service begins a recertification period, triggering another Form 485, and so on.

RHHIs are now graded on their capacity to coordinate their own organization's activities and their home health agency providers in electronic billing. The home health claims are screened by use of electronic computer "modules," initially developed by HCFA with United Government Services of Wisconsin and now used by all RHHIs. The module "kicks out" claims that profile as problems, which are then read by medical review staff. Questions about coverage usually result in the mailing to providers of Form 488, or a remittance inquiry which solicits further medical information.

A decade ago, home health providers could telephone intermediaries concerning denials of claims, and discuss through the inquiry process how the claim could be explained or better documented to permit payment. During the 1986–1988 period, FIs responded to perceived (but unwritten) changes in central HCFA's coverage policy, by generating enormous numbers of denials.[6] After court litigation was initiated by members of Congress, providers, patients, and the National Association for Home Care,[7] HCFA reached a settlement that involved rewriting the HIM-11 in consultation with providers. Subsequently, during the 1990–1996 period, denials of Medicare home health coverage by RHHIs have been low. However, HCFA also eliminated the informal "inquiry" practice which may force claims denials to a formal reconsideration process, discussed below.

Providers paid under the periodic interim payment (PIP) method, which relies on historical cost/visit volume data, do not experience an immediate change in monthly payment because of the RHHI's denials or slight changes in visit volume. PIP reimbursement is a fixed semi-monthly lump sum reimbursement. PIP status is maintained by quarterly statistical reports filed by providers with the FIs. Providers can request immediate adjustments in their PIP rates when volume rapidly increases and cash flow to pay for employee services becomes acute. Providers that do not inform FIs of decreases in volume face year-end cost report recoupment demands, that often are substantial. Cost settlement also requires the provider to account for denied Medicare visits as "other" visits, for which there is no Medicare reimbursement. The next year's PIP rate may be adjusted down by the FI by using a factor representing errors in the cost report, the claims denials, and 12 months' accounting by the provider. HCFA has announced its intention to eliminate the PIP payment system.

When the RHHI processes claims, it first verifies that the patient is eligible for the Medicare program and that the patient was homebound, in need of skilled nursing or home health aide services on an "intermittent" or part-time basis, or in need of physical or speech therapy, and had a plan of care properly established by the treating physician. Denials on any of these bases constitute "technical" denials. Assuming no technical error, the claim is then reviewed for medical necessity and appropriateness. Until the statute sunsetted December 31, 1995, "waiver of liability" permitted the RHHI to find that although services were not medically necessary, neither the patient nor the provider knew this was the case. The claim in question was paid if the provider's three-month (quarterly) error rate was less than 2.5% and all claims in that same quarter also were paid, as long as the provider was "faultless" and unknowing as to each claim.[8] In the rare instance when the RHHI found the beneficiary knew or had reason to know that the claim was not covered, the RHHI would deny payment to the provider but permit it to recoup from the patient. When the patient was unknowing, neither the RHHI nor the provider could bill the patient. As of January 1996, presumption of waiver was eliminated for medical necessity denials but remained in place for technical denials for allegedly non-homebound or nonintermittent cases.

For years, one of the chief complaints about the RHHI's claims processing and denials was the lack of specificity of the denial letters. Some improvements have been made but denials issued by FIs pursuant to certain investigations by the Office of the Inspector General have been very general, providing conclusions of noncoverage without real detail.

Since these cases also involve use of claims samples and projections of "error" rates onto an entire year's claims, they are particularly difficult and unfair to providers. Federal contractor budget cuts continue to force the RHHIs to limit their medical review staff's reviews of denials.

A second complaint was the delay in claims processing by RHHIs. Because of Congressional imposition of penalties on administrative contractor payment delays, if a claim is "clean" and can be reviewed by the RHHI without further development through request for missing documentation or supplemental documentation, it will be paid initially. In some cases, RHHIs did not record as "received" those claims a provider had sent, presumably so that the RHHI avoided starting the clock on the timely payment processing. Electronic billing has largely eliminated this problem, as has the dropping of requirements for the transmission of updates in patient status and orders. When long periods go by of payment without delay or questioning, some home health agencies have drifted into patterns of overutilization of services. They then may be the subject of "focused" review and devastating denials.

An FI's Role in the Appeal of Claims Denials

Considerable change has come to the Medicare Part A denial appeals area. Much tension exists between HCFA's desire to reduce appeal costs and the beneficiary/providers' push to protect appeal rights through independent administrative law judges and accountability of the RHHIs for their reversal rates on appeals.

Medicare beneficiaries have the right to appeal any denial of coverage of a Medicare claim. In the past, a provider could directly appeal only those claims that were not paid

under waiver.[9] By assisting a beneficiary or by serving as a beneficiary's representative in an appeal, a provider can vindicate the underlying issue in a "technical" denial paid under waiver. This protects the provider's ability to continue to interpret the regulations to allow serving both for future needs of that particular patient and for other patients who have "similar or comparable" circumstances.[10] To serve as a beneficiary's representative, the provider must agree not to go against the beneficiary for the amount in question should the appeal fail, not to take a fee from the beneficiary or his or her family/ friends for representing him or her, and not to put the administrative costs of serving as representative in a losing appeal on its Medicare cost report. The provider must also have the beneficiary sign an HCFA form for providers serving as patient representatives, and include the form when filing the appeal. HCFA has been considering a requirement for an original, new form for each appealed claim rather than allowing the current practice of using photocopies of the form.

When the FI sends a claim denial to the provider, it also sends one to the beneficiary. Within 60 days of receipt of this notice (presumed to be no more than 65 days from the date on the notice), the beneficiary or the provider must file with the FI a request for reconsideration of the denial,[11] and the representative appointment form, if applicable. This request should be sufficiently documented to offer the FI a factual basis for approving payment. A written statement from the treating physician, copies of nurses' notes, a statement from the patient (if appropriate), photographs (with patient consent), a recitation of and argument from the facts, and the regulations and the HIM-11 manual sections supporting the home health agency should all be part of this filing. These materials are reviewed by the FI/RHHI and an opinion reversing or maintaining the denial is sent to the parties filing the appeal. If the claim is still denied or partially denied and the amount at issue is at least $100, the provider and the beneficiary have another 60-day time limit from the date that the second denial is received (or 65 days from the date on the letter) to request an administrative law judge (ALJ) hearing.[12] A provider or beneficiary can "aggregate" or lump together various claims for the particular patient to meet the $100 limit.[13] Issues arose in the past when RHHIs reduced the denial during reconsideration to a single visit for a patient, in many cases bringing the amount in controversy below the hearing requirement of $100. Whether there is ALJ review for a single visit denial for a particular service could thus depend on whether the care was rendered in a major urban area where the cost limit is more than $100, or in a rural area where it is not.

The provider or beneficiary has the choice of a live hearing (rather than a review of the documents alone) before an ALJ, whose background generally is in Social Security proceedings. The provider or beneficiary must be able to explain to an ALJ how home care works and why the RHHI and its medical/nursing reviewers have misunderstood the Medicare regulations and the facts of the providers' care. The RHHI does not appear in person at the ALJ hearing. RHHI staff prepare an official file for the ALJ, including the RHHI's substantive responses to the reconsideration request. Although the RHHI has an obligation to be fair and accurate in representing the course of the claims review, the RHHI file may be incomplete or it may contain an internal consultant's review that has never been seen by the provider. The provider or beneficiary therefore should carefully review the contents of the file enough in advance of the hearing to prepare a response or bring the issue of missing documents to the ALJ's attention. If HCFA has issued a "ruling" governing certain aspects of the Medicare Program, the ALJ is required to follow it.

A party dissatisfied with the ALJ decision may request another review by the Appeals Council, a semi-autonomous body in Arlington, Virginia.[14] Technically, there is no right of appeal by the RHHI to the Appeals Council, but frequently the RHHIs have informed the Regional HCFA offices of "hot" cases lost to the provider at the ALJ level. The HCFA office then sends a memo to the Appeals Council suggesting the ALJ has made a mistake of fact or law, or that there is a serious impediment to acting on the ALJ's opinion. The Appeals Council takes these memos under advisement, as an administratively convenient substitute for its own authority to review any ALJ opinion. The Appeals Council may refuse to review any motion from a party, but usually accepts the case. It reviews written briefs submitted by the provider and the RHHI (or sometimes HCFA), and the underlying case record. This means that the *only* time to introduce evidence is at the ALJ level. The Appeals Council historically has supported ALJ opinions favoring providers and beneficiaries. One area where it has consistently ruled against them, however, is when a beneficiary has died and the appeal was originally brought in his or her name. The Appeals Council has held that if no money is owed anyone, there is no controversy that lives beyond the beneficiary. This is difficult for a provider seeking to gain support for its judgment about Medicare coverage interpretations.

Finally, the provider or beneficiary dissatisfied with the results of the Appeals Council or denied review by the Appeals Council may appeal to the United States District Court if the amount in controversy is $1,000 or more.[15] There is a 60-day time limit from receipt of the Appeals Council's decision. In federal court, attorneys from the Department of Health and Human Services (DHHS) will represent the RHHI. Two basic kinds of review can take place. If simply reviewing the medical facts of the denial, the court will decide whether there was substantial evidence to support the ALJ's decision. If the provider or beneficiary raises an underlying legal question of the actions of HCFA, the RHHI, or others and their legality as an administrative practice, the court will give this matter a full review. In all cases, the provider can expect that DHHS's attorneys will argue that DHHS is entitled to "deference" in the interpretation of its own regulations, including by its RHHI contractors. Appeal lies for both sides to the Federal Circuit Court of

Appeals and then to the Supreme Court, which may not agree to accept the appeal.

The informal review process is known as "reopening," but does not require an RHHI, an ALJ, or the Appeals Council to review a case on the written request of the provider or benefi-ciary.[16] HCFA has instructed its RHHIs to use the formal reconsideration process, not reopen-ing, for coverage reviews, largely for budget reasons. Timelines for reopening are within 12 months of a determination or decision for any reason; within four years for "good cause" stemming from new and material evidence or clerical error; or any time if fraud or similar fault is shown, or a clerical error on the face of the evidence is shown by the provider or benefi-ciary.

Although the majority of home health claims denials by RHHIs are Part A Medicare claims, there are occasional Part B claims for home health services, and home health agencies may submit Part B claims for durable medical equip-ment, prosthetic devices, and certain physical

therapy services. The Medicare Part B appeals system is a close parallel to the Part A system as a result of a 1986 Congressional action to pro-vide more protection to providers, including judicial review. The principal differences are a preliminary review by "fair hearing"[17] con-ducted by a hearing officer who is an employee of the Part B Carrier (the Part B side of the insurance company that parallels the FI role for Part A), and a $500 minimum for a provider or beneficiary to proceed to an ALJ review.

In all claims denials resolved by ALJ opin-ions, the case is considered restricted to a par-ticular patient and does not become a legal precedent for other ALJs or courts. However, many home health agencies can strengthen their written materials for an ALJ's review if they include copies of other ALJ opinions (with patient identifiers removed) as a suggested approach. State and national home care trade associations may be able to provide such opin-ions to providers and analyze helpful ALJ opin-ions.

REFERENCES

1. The CPEP requirements are reviewed and published annually in the Federal Register for public comment. CPEP scores are made available to Congress and to the Government Accounting Office, both of which have been generally critical of HCFA's ability to manage the FI's performance. Home health program criteria are only one portion of the CPEP measurements.

2. Originally there were 10 RHHIs, the maximum approved by Congress's act to centralize and make more consistent the FI activities in Medicare coverage. Prudential, Blue Cross of New Mexico, Aetna, and Independence Blue Cross had withdrawn by mid-1997. Litigation by hospi-tal-based home health agencies to resist transfer to the RHHIs for medical review was resoundingly defeated. New Britain General Hospital Home Health Agency, et al. v. Bowen, 702 F. Supp. 288 (DDC 1988).

3. In Volume 42 of the Code of Federal Regulations, Sec-tions 421.106 and 421.110 set out the process for requesting an alternate RHHI. Notice to HCFA with sup-porting proof of how the change will be "consistent with effective and efficient administration of the program" must be given at least 120 days before the end of the home health agency's cost reporting year.

4. NTIS, a government manual publishing service in Vir-ginia, sells HCFA manuals with updates as a subscription service. The NTIS subscription department's telephone number is 703-487-4630; the toll-free number for account customers is 1-800-336-4700.

5. Transmittal 336, revising the Provider Reimbursement Manual Sections 2307-2313 was issued in 1986 without any really useful examples of direct cost allocation in the free-standing home health area. However, the timeline requirements for FI approval are strict: new "unique" cost centers must be approved in writing before the com-mencement of the affected cost year, § 2313; direct assignment of general service costs must be requested for approval in writing at least 90 days before the new cost year, § 2307.

6. Randall DA. Home Health Services Under Medicare: The Need for Organized Responses to Growth and Change. *Pride Institute Journal of Long-Term Home Health Care.* Fall 1987.

7. Duggan, et al. v. Bowen, Civ. No. 87-0383, heard by Judge Stanley Sporkin of the U.S. District Court of the District of Columbia, resulted in only one published judicial opinion, which concerned the definition of

"intermittent" care. 691 F Supp 1487 (DDC 1988). There were no judicial findings on the major area of FI denial activity concerning medical necessity. However, HCFA's agreement to substantial changes in HIM-11 negotiated with the National Association for Home Care is widely regarded as having broadened the coverage interpretations. Subsequent large increases in home health Medicare expenditures have been blamed on this manual revision by critics.

8. Section 1879 of the Social Security Act sunsetted after many attempts by HCFA to eliminate home health waiver of liability for providers. Congress repeatedly acted to protect waiver of liability for home health agencies, including passage in the Omnibus Budget Reconciliation Act of 1990 of a waiver guarantee until December 31, 1995. The startling growth of home care visits in the early 1990s and concerns about provider exploitation undermined Congressional support. The waiver for "technical" denials remains, as of this writing, and provider associations are lobbying for the restoration of the full waiver section.

9. See, generally, the federal regulations on the Part A coverage appeal process, found at 42 CFR §§ 405.701– 405.750 (1990 codification).

10. 42 CFR § 411.406(b).

11. 42 CFR § 405.711.

12. 42 CFR § 405.722. The filing is made at the local Social Security office or with HCFA (preferably with both) and should include any further factual development and the request for a Part A hearing form, available from the Social Security office. The provider does not need to obtain a new provider representative designation; the previous form will remain in effect unless the beneficiary voids it.

13. 42 CFR § 405.740(e).

14. 42 CFR § 405.724 and 20 CFR § 404.967 (1995 codification).

15. 42 CFR § 405.730.

16. 42 CFR § 405.750. The request must go to the highest level of review that has issued an opinion.

17. 42 CFR §§ 405.801-872. The continued requirement of a fair hearing prior to an ALJ proceeding was not explicitly included by Congress, but litigation to remove it from the requirements on appeals was unsuccessful.

PART II

PROVIDER AUDIT

FI Cost Report Audits

A home health agency is required to submit an approved format for a year-end Medicare cost report within five months of the last day of the provider's fiscal year. Free-standing home health agencies file a stand-alone cost report. Hospital-based home health agencies' costs are accumulated as a cost center on the hospital's cost report, and the center is allocated overhead costs from various service and support areas of the total hospital. This process of allocating hospital center costs to its home care department has remained in place despite elimination in October 1993 of the add-on of 13% to the cost limit per service visit that the HCFA calculates for all home health agencies in rural state areas and metropolitan statistical areas.[1] How-

ever, FIs have begun to challenge whether home health agencies are in fact hospital-based when they are run very independently from the hospital corporation or are very great distances from the hospital with which they supposedly are "fully integrated." In August 1996, HCFA issued further definitions affecting hospital-based status and beginning January 1997, close review is made of all cases.

The Medicare cost report, which can be derived from computer software or manually created, sets out the total costs of the agency, the allocation of costs between reimbursable functions and nonreimbursable functions, the proportions of visits between Medicare-payable and all non-Medicare payers, and the total amount of Medicare reimbursement claimed by the provider for services to Medicare beneficiaries during the year. The home health agency's cost per visit in each of the dis-

Source: Part II, Reprinted with permission from D. Randall, The Role of the Medicare Fiscal Intermediary Part II, *Journal of Nursing Administration,* Vol. 22, No. 7–8, pp. 24–29, © 1992, J.B. Lippincott Company.

ciplines is derived from the cost report's aggregate data. The agency receives that rate or the area cost limit cap, whichever is less. Various schedules accompany the basic cost report document, which itself is signed and certified as accurate by the corporate officer assuming responsibility for the reimbursement claims of the provider. The Medicare cost report is a serious document that constitutes an aggregate claim to the Medicare program for reimbursement. If it contains information that is a misstatement, or a claim for reimbursement for costs not reimbursable under Medicare, the provider, responsible senior management, and the signer of the document might be at risk of a "false claims" charge. Intentional fraud in the submission of a cost report can lead to criminal prosecution. In many states the Medicare cost report is the basis for the Medicaid cost report, and thus the Medicaid rates and Medicaid investigations for home health services.

When the cost report is received, the FI first reviews the report in a "desk audit," checking the documentation provided by the agency to ensure that calculations are accurate and that, superficially, only appropriate claims for Medicare-reimbursable costs appear to have been made. The FI then decides which providers (from all provider types) should be scheduled for on-site audits using a variety of trends or measures, including whether the agency has recently entered the Medicare program, whether it has a large percentage of contract workers or large consulting fees, whether its overall Medicare service volume is large, and what percentage of its visits, supervision, and administrative costs are allocated to Medicare-intensive areas. The FIs also reaudit agencies where significant reimbursement recoupments have been sought in recent years, and when costs for chief executive officers (CEOs) or owner-administrators appear to be high compared with other agencies.

The question of comparative expense can raise two important Medicare reimbursement issues for the FI: Is the agency paying for unnecessary services because they are not truly related to patient care, and are the costs unreasonable because they either are "substantially out of line with similarly situated providers"[2] or are not what a prudent buyer would pay? One prime area for in-depth audit review in the 1990s has been comparative key executive compensation, including all aspects of fringe benefits. Because some home health agencies receive administrative services from a home office company that is related by ownership or common corporate control, the FI will receive and audit a home office cost report that includes management and administrative costs that are assigned to the home health agency provider. Under some circumstances, FIs will allow health systems with small volume and simple structures to dispense with a home office cost report; generally, the providers must follow HCFA's Manual HIM 15, the Provider Reimbursement Manual, which has a detailed requirement for a home office filing.[3]

During an on-site audit, the agency must make available to the FI auditors any requested documentation to support the costs claimed on the provider cost report. The provider should make all reasonable efforts to comply at the time of the audit to avoid potential problems that could result in cost disallowances. If the documentation is not readily available, the provider should arrange to have it forwarded to the FI's offices after the audit but before issuance of any formal reimbursement notice. Generally, the FI will give the provider written notice of the areas in which possible disallowances are likely by providing a set of on-site working audit adjustment papers. These may be (but are not always) produced during the exit conference, a time when the provider's administrator or CEO and finance personnel should make every effort to satisfy the auditors about cost reasonableness and necessity. It is appropriate to use the exit conference to vigorously press the provider's position on any matters in which the FI staff are taking unreasonable or unsupported positions. Providers should also educate inexperienced FI auditors about the way in which home health agencies function and how they differ from other provider types. Occasionally audit adjustments are received in reports mailed to providers but never mentioned during the exit conference. HCFA backs the FI's discretion to issue such "surprise" adjustments if review and consideration at the FI's office produces additional areas of concern.

The proposed disallowances on the audit adjustment reports may represent partial deductions for unreasonable amounts of cost, for example, extensive advertising in the Yellow Pages, or total disallowance for nonreimbursable kinds of cost, such as fund-raising expenses. The auditors may reduce the number of Medicare visits claimed by the agency in its patient statistical report, based on the FI's records of visits processed or based on records of Medicare denials during the period. Occasionally, there will be disagreement between the FI staff and the provider about lump sum or PIP payments during the fiscal year, making the provider's financial records and data retrieval capacities extremely important.

The exit conference may also be an opportunity for the provider to receive useful information concerning management issues relating to the operation of the agency. A provider should maximize the opportunity the exit conference presents to discuss FI perceptions, to clarify the bases for any proposed adjustments, and to solidify the FI's commitment to what further documentation would substantiate the challenged costs. If resolutions are achieved at this stage, the FI will not have to create a record of certain disallowed costs and seek reimbursement recapture when it issues the notice of program reimbursement (NPR). Once the FI issues an NPR, it creates a statistical document which is reflected in its contractor performance evaluation program record. Thereafter, the FI has to account to HCFA as to why these disallowances are later diminished or removed, if the provider negotiates to eliminate an adjustment.

Postpayment Compliance Audits

In addition to prepayment screening of claims, RHHIs may conduct postpayment audits of home health agencies' claims, including on-site reviews of case charts, sampled from a multimonth period. The RHHIs are measured by HCFA for accuracy in performance of audits; in various years HCFA budgets have not allowed many on-site compliance audits to be performed, so FIs generally target agencies with high-cost, high-utilization profiles.

Agencies may be selected for audit for one of several reasons, including the average Medicare cost per patient, the average number of visits per patient, the Medicare utilization rate of the agency (some agencies are close to a 100% Medicare patient census), or the rate or number of home health aide visits by the agency, all of which are compared with the other home health agencies in the RHHI's responsibility. Additionally, newly certified home health agencies or those with significant indications of coverage difficulties may be scheduled for the compliance review. Difficulties in the coverage area triggering the compliance audit could include poor performance on a prior on-site audit, or particular patterns of denials shown in the RHHI computer module screening guidelines. The FIs will not make these criteria public, lest agencies begin to game the system.

The on-site RHHI medical review auditors will examine the sampled cases and may include in-home visits to beneficiaries. The purposes of the audit are to verify the fundamental eligibility of patients served as being homebound and in need of intermittent skilled nursing services or a skilled therapy, that the plan of care and the nursing or therapy chart entries contained sufficient information to support the care billed to the Medicare program as medically necessary, and that the patients were receiving the services that had been billed to the program. After the review, there is an exit conference in which the medical review staff present their proposed findings and the agency can do its best to retrieve missing documentation or respond to criticisms. The RHHI staff should accept on-site further documentation but are not required to accept postaudit visit materials. An RHHI's refusal to accept other materials, however, may be counterproductive if the papers would be accepted by an administrative law judge as relevant to the coverage of the claim. A failed audit subjects the home health agency to 100% prepayment review of its claims, and the individual denials made are subject to the same denials appeal process as outlined above.

Sample Projection and Recoupment from All Medicare Claims

The HCFA has prevailed in its litigation to support the use of a random sample projection technique by FIs to recoup vast amounts of dollars from the "universe" of a provider's previous 12 months of Medicare billings. Random sample projection techniques have been supported by the courts in the Medicaid reimbursement and Medicare Part B physician reimbursement areas as an appropriate administrative tool because the burdens of processing a 100% claims review postpayment are too costly. In the home health field, the case of Chaves Co. Home Health Services, Inc., et al. v. Sullivan[4] posed the issue of whether the rights of beneficiaries to administrative and judicial review of their denied claims, and the provider's derivative rights, were obliterated by the use of the projection technique. In two levels of judicial review, the issue was resolved in favor of the HCFA, although with certain twists in judicial language suggesting that the courts did not fully appreciate the impact of their opinions on the ability of agencies to know Medicare coverage policy before rendering care.

In audits conducted by the Office of the Inspector General (OIG), the Department of Health and Human Services, as part of "Operation Restore Trust," 100 case samples were utilized during 1996 to project multi-million dollar recoupments of allegedly non-covered claims.

When combined with the suspension of ongoing Medicare payments (allegedly for abusive billing practices), sampling recoupments result in bankruptcy of providers before any reasonable access to an appeal process.

RESOLUTION OF COST REPORT DISPUTES AND REIMBURSEMENT APPEALS

Determinations Preceding an Appeal

Once the home health agency has received the NPR from the FI/RHHI that has reviewed its cost report, the cost report is considered settled, and its reopening (without appeal) is a discretionary act by the FI. Some home health agencies have experienced a rapid cutoff of postaudit discussion, a short timeline to submit further documents to the FI, and a rapid issuance of the NPR just before the federal September 30th fiscal year end, with a promise from the FI that things can change later. It seems apparent that this abrupt process is some FIs' response to HCFA's demand for rapid identification of overpayments and recoupment within a short time. Once again, a good performance in this area by the FI results in CPEP points. The HCFA has informed the FIs that no more than 30 days should be allowed for the provider to pay back the NPR recoupment demand; FIs may give a shorter time, and some give only 15 days from the date of the NPR. (In certain cases, providers can establish a payback schedule over several months or up to a year, with interest.)

Thus, an FI's assurance that negotiations of the disallowances can always proceed after the NPR issues ignores the negative effect for the provider of having to pay back first and talk second. Also, many audit adjustment reports that accompany the NPRs are not definitive descriptions of the bases for the disallowances. The FI is required to cite the section of the Provider Reimbursement Manual (HIM 15), HCFA's Medicare Home Health Manual (HIM 11), or the regulations on which it relies to claim recoupment. The provider must ask for the FI workpapers as well to have a clear picture of the auditor's interpretation of the provider documentation as it relates to the Medicare program requirements.

The second negative effect of receiving the NPR is that its issuance date begins the 180-day time period in which the provider must decide and act to file an appeal. The 180-day limit is statutory and not extendable. Reopening of a cost report does not provide more time to appeal issues from the first NPR that are not the subject of the revised NPR.[5]

Filing an Appeal of the FI's Disallowances

If the Medicare reimbursement effect of all the issues that the home health agency wishes to appeal is greater than $1,000 but less than $10,000, it must file its written request for an appeal with the FI's office that handles intermediary appeals.[6] If the amount at issue totals $10,000 or more, the written request for an appeal is filed at the Provider Reimbursement Review Board (PRRB), located in Baltimore, Maryland.[7] The request should include a simple statement of the issues and of the Medicare effect of the disallowance as to each issue and should attach the NPR and pertinent pages of the audit adjustment reports. Most providers have health counsel handle PRRB appeals; counsel files a letter from the provider to the PRRB appointing that counsel as its representative.

The PRRB's members are appointed by the Secretary of Health and Human Services and are semiautonomous in that they are subject to overrule by the administrator of the HCFA, who is permitted a right of review of their opinions. The PRRB's five members usually include accountants with FI background as well as individuals who have worked with providers. The PRRB members must apply the Social Security Act and formally promulgated HCFA rulings and regulations to decide the appeal, but they are not bound by the HCFA manuals. The FI's employees serve as hearing officers for the

intermediary hearing and must apply Medicare regulations, rules, manuals as written, and official interpretations of the department, making the independence of the latter appeal even more questionable. In both cases, the provider and intermediary file position papers, and call and cross-examine witnesses. There is a right of appeal to federal court for the provider dissatisfied with a PRRB decision, but there is no judicial review of the intermediary hearing decision.[8]

If an agency is one of a group of providers under common ownership or control, a PRRB appeal must be brought as a group appeal for any issue common to them all for which the Medicare reimbursement effect is, in the aggregate, $50,000 or more.[9] Several agencies in a small chain of home health agencies, however, might be affected by an FI's adjustment of a home office expense that is less than $10,000 to each of them and collectively is less than $50,000. Unless each agency also has other issues that will give the agency $10,000 or more at stake, all the agencies will be subject to the intermediary hearing rather than a PRRB hearing. A group appeal can also be organized by home health agencies that are not related but are being affected by the FI's interpretation of reimbursement policy in a manner consistent with each of them, therefore presenting the common question of fact and law necessary to the appeal. Group or individual provider appeals to the PRRB of reimbursement policy, which is stated in the HCFA regulations but is believed by providers to be illegal, are the first step and are absolutely necessary to bring a federal court lawsuit on a payment policy. Many providers have lost their cases by failing to go through the necessary administrative appeal process and trying to "leapfrog" into federal court. There is a regulatory provision for an expedited appeal to the PRRB for those issues where the legality of a regulation, an HCFA ruling, or a statute is at issue[10] and the PRRB acknowledges that it cannot act, moving the appeal more quickly to the courts.

If the PRRB's ruling is not satisfactory to the provider, the provider may request the HCFA Administrator's review and, if still unsatisfied, federal district court review. In each case, the provider has 60 days from the date of the decision by the PRRB or the Administrator[11] to file at the next level of appeal. The Administrator can and routinely does review PRRB decisions and is notoriously inclined to limit or reverse PRRB opinions favoring providers.

The federal district court determines whether the administrative decision of the Administrator or the PRRB was reasonable. Generally, courts will give great deference to a government agency's rulings under its own program, particularly in opinions dependent largely on factual details, such as whether costs are reasonable or documentation is adequate. Some providers, however, have successfully challenged PRRB or Administrator decisions by proving to the courts that the PRRB or Administrator improperly or arbitrarily interpreted the Medicare regulations or, on occasion, that the Medicare regulations were inconsistent with the Medicare statute. The Department of Health and Human Services is represented in court by federal attorneys, and the proceedings may take more than a year before the judge issues an opinion. Either the provider or the Department may appeal to federal circuit court and then to the U.S. Supreme Court,[12] which may decline to take the case, leaving the circuit court opinion as the final word. Each level of appeal is a complex and expensive undertaking by a provider.

Program Integrity Reviews

The FI is charged with a responsibility under its contract with HCFA to review all materials relating to the providers in its responsibility with an eye to possible program integrity concerns. Program integrity efforts for Medicare, and also for Medicaid, can include prevention of inappropriate utilization of Medicare program resources, submission of claims for services that are not covered by the program, submission of claims for services that have not been rendered as described in the claims (including miscodings), knowing submission of charges that are false or not customary for the particular provider, and kickbacks and other referral schemes prohibited under the Anti-Fraud and Abuse provisions of the Social Security Act. FIs are also supposed to identify circumstances that might lead to a program integrity problem. Finally, whenever the FI receives or deduces information that suggests a program integrity concern, the FI is charged with conducting a preliminary investigation of the facts and forwarding materials as appropriate to the HCFA Regional Office division in charge of program integrity that includes staff of the OIG.

Among recent FI program integrity focus areas has been the billing by home health agencies for services allegedly rendered by contractors to the agencies. These contract nurses, therapists, and home health aide paraprofessionals have in some situations fabricated their visit entries in patients' charts, shortened the visit time, or altered patient records. Although it can be extremely difficult for an ethical agency to become aware of particularly sophisticated scams by these contractors, some agencies have been doing nothing to spot-check the delivery of services to their clients. This quality assurance function, as well as careful review of chart entries, is imperative for good integrity management by providers. When FIs receive word through tips from disgruntled former employees of providers, from competitors of providers, or from patients and/or families, the FIs perform on-site agency reviews of charts, interview staff of providers, and make phone calls and visits to the homes of beneficiaries. If numerous charts are requested by the FI auditors, the provider may not know whose care is being investigated or why. FIs may also contact and interview subcontractors to the home health agency. Federal law requires that providers include in their contracts for services an access to records clause that obligates the subcontracting professional or company to provide the government access to its records concerning care that is ultimately billed directly or indirectly to the Medicare program.

Such preliminary FI investigations should be taken seriously by providers, which should review facts and legal issues with health counsel in conjunction with an internal self-audit and before permitting any staff interviews. The fast timing of FI program integrity audits may not allow a provider much opportunity to organize its responses, which is of course why auditors move rapidly. A home health agency is obligated under its provider agreement with HCFA to permit the inspection of its written records by any authorized agent of the government when requested, and a refusal can result in loss of certification of the agency. Records requested in writing by the OIG must be provided within 24 hours or else the agency may be terminated immediately from the Medicare program.

In some cases, it is the home health agency that discovers that improper billing has occurred, and a decision must be made after proper fact-gathering with legal counsel as to what communications are legally required. In many situations, even if an error such as changes to chart entries appears isolated, a rigorous review by the agency of a sample of its own cases and official reprimands of staff (recorded in personnel records) should occur immediately. Once the scope of a larger problem is revealed, counsel may recommend that the provider voluntarily approach the FI's integrity office to discuss what has been discovered, the actions that have been taken, and the provider's proposal for repayment to the Medicare program. The FI's integrity office will be required to make a report to the HCFA Regional Office/Office of OIG staff, who will decide whether the investigation and proposed settlement are sufficient or whether a further sampling of cases by the OIG or the FI is necessary. Sampling by the OIG to determine sanctions and penalties has been sustained in court challenges. As previously noted, litigation to overturn the general use of sampling methodologies to project overpayments in Medicare Part A

home health has not favored the home health industry.[13]

If a home health agency deliberately includes inaccurate information on the annual Medicare cost report or makes repeated claims of reimbursable costs for items or services that were unreasonable in price or not fully devoted to the Medicare business, these actions could serve as bases for an FI integrity audit and recommendation of adverse action and for a charge of submitting false claims. In that case, the agency would be penalized, and the Administrator or chief financial officer who knowingly included the information could be charged with fraudulent conduct. During 1995–96, several cost report investigations resulted in criminal proceedings against home health executives, large fines, and jail sentences.

FIs are required to review year-end adjustments and to send providers written warnings of audit adjustments, which, if repeated on future cost reports, might serve as bases for integrity actions. Naturally, if the providers believe their cost entries and allocations were justified, and especially if a reimbursement appeal is filed, there are defenses against an accusation that an agency has knowingly filed a demand for total-year reimbursement that is unsupportable.

Because of the increasing investigations and the Operation Restore Trust audits, it is wise for each home health agency to institute its own compliance audit and formal compliance program. The audit, conducted under the protections of attorney-client privilege by knowledge-able health attorneys, identifies areas of weakness. The compliance program establishes self-monitoring, standards of conduct and self-policing.

CONCLUSION

The relationship of a home health agency with its FI, whether as the reimbursement monitor or the RHHI for medical review, is pivotal in the agency's successful delivery of services to Medicare patients and its growth as a business entity. Good communications and identification of the proper contacts within the FI will help a large or small home health provider weather difficult Medicare program issues and get paid promptly. The FI that remembers its important function as a disseminator of accurate information and facilitator of service delivery serves as a model and a worthy agent for the federal government. FIs also must continue to be protectors of the Medicare program against fraud and waste. By careful self-monitoring, home health agencies will lessen the chances that FI surveillance might reveal provider failures.

REFERENCES

1. Beginning with cost report years for July 1, 1991, to June 30, 1992, the home health cost limits were derived from local and national home health cost data and shifted toward a national home health database and a hospital wage index multiplier over three years. There continues to be considerable controversy about the appropriateness of a home health–specific wage index multiplier, with the home care industry having lobbied first for statutory inclusion and then for repeal of such a process. Once a program for prospective payment is in place, the role of geographic wage modifiers (if any) will change.

2. The principal source for understanding of the reimbursement theories of the Medicare program is the Code of Federal Regulations, Volume 42, Part 413. The concepts of reasonableness, as including variation among providers' costs, and fairness to the providers are both included in 42 CFR § 413.9, the quoted section being 42 CFR § 413.9(c)(2).

3. Provider Reimbursement Manual HIM 15, Section 2150.

4. The Chaves case, 531 F.2d 914 (D.C. Cir. 1991), was filed on behalf of Chaves, the VNS of Albuquerque, and the VNA of Bayonne, NJ, in the federal district court of the District of Columbia after the three home health agencies filed appropriate administrative actions with administrative law judges in their geographic areas. Both the District and the Circuit Court held that there was no express statutory prohibition against use of a sample review and projection of a denial rate over Medicare Part A claims. The United States Supreme Court let the Circuit Court's opinion stand, 112 S. Ct. 1160 (1992).

5. Several courts have considered this important issue of the reopening of the cost report, and the majority of the opinions hold that the reopening does not allow a provider to raise any issue that was part of the first NPR's adjustments of costs but not an adjustment under the second NPR.

6. 42 CFR § 405.1809.

7. 42 CFR § 405.1835(a)(3).

8. 42 CFR § 405.1833.

9. 42 CFR § 405.1837.

10. 42 CFR § 405.1842.

11. 42 CFR § 405.1875.

12. 42 CFR § 405.1877.

13. See the discussion of Chaves County Home Health, et al. v. Sullivan.

CHAPTER 71

The Appeal Process: Reopening, Reconsiderations, Administrative Law Judge Hearings and Appeal Council

Louisa M. Jordan

INTRODUCTION

Home health agencies in the late 1980s experienced a drastic increase in the number of denied claims. This increase occurred at a time when home health visits should have been increasing due to the aging population and the impact of diagnosis-related groups (DRGs) on hospitals with quicker discharges of sicker patients.

Home health administrators attacked the problem on three fronts. Lawsuits were filed to clarify the definitions used for reimbursable home health care. Political action was taken that resulted in several acts further defining and clarifying actions of the Health Care Financing Administration (HCFA) and fiscal intermediaries (FI). The third step was the active pursual of the appeal process.

This chapter focuses on one aspect of the appeal process, the Administrative Law Judge (ALJ) hearing. During an ALJ hearing the expert nurse presenter should be able to testify in a concise manner on the agency's delivery of care based on standards of care, actual chart documentation, and Social Security regulations, not interpretations from the FI and HCFA. The expert nurse should verbally be able to persuade a judge, based on facts, that this patient's care was necessary, utilizing chart documentation, letters from the family, and attending physician letters.

BACKGROUND

The home health agency for which I am the administrator experienced a dramatic increase in the number of Medicare denials. From 1968 to February 15, 1987, the agency had only five visits denied on three cases or claims. From February 15 to the end of 1987, there were 82 claims denied for a total of 558 visits or 11.16% of our caseload. The agency had the exact same staff who completed the exact same forms. The same Conditions of Participation were followed. The agency was in financial trouble as a result of this loss of income. At the beginning of the denials the board determined that every denial should be appealed. Workshops were attended to learn the process. The appeal process was started. Today, as a result, most of these denials have been reversed in favor of the agency. The agency has recovered the funds that were withheld during that time. In speaking to many other home health agency administrators, this author was surprised to learn that many other administrators did not take this aggressive approach through all the stages of appeal, particularly at the ALJ level.

During the time frame from 1986 to 1988, Medicare certified home health agencies experienced a dramatic increase in the number of billed home health cases that were denied by the FI. This resulted in decreased funding to the agencies. In a tongue-in-cheek article, Marilyn

Harris (1987) addressed the dilemma felt by many home health agencies across the country. The patient needs the care; the doctor orders the care; the nurse delivers the care; the regulations say that the care is justified; the agency submits the bill; the FI may or may not pay for the care; the agency reviews the care and appeals and appeals and appeals. She noted the frustration and low morale of the nurses. The nurses needed to be superhuman, with every form filled out correctly. The nurses needed to know the unwritten rules of the FI. Even when a denial occurred, the nurse still did not know why. These were the same agencies with the same personnel in many cases and with the same Medicare regulations that prior to 1986 had received no or few denials. They were asking questions. The game was the same but the rules were different. They disagreed with the determinations of the FI. Since they disagreed with the FI, they needed to learn how to appeal the denials that were occurring at a phenomenal rate. Many individuals attended workshops to become more educated. Experience also taught them the process.

Home health administrators needed to make decisions. What information did they need? What was their financial situation? What could they do to prevent denials? How could they reverse this trend? Should they appeal? How did they appeal? Who could appeal? Nurses were in a pivotal position to change the Medicare home health benefit. It could be made stronger or dismantled depending on their actions.

CLIMATE FOR ACTION

Many changes were occurring in the home health care delivery system in the late 1980s. The over-65 population was growing from 16.5 million in 1960 to an estimated 31.7 million in 1990 (Moran, 1989). Cushman (1988) noted that in 1971 home health represented 1% of the Medicare budget. By 1985, it increased to 3%. The Omnibus Reconciliation Act of 1980 removed the three-day required hospitalization

and the 100-visit limit per year. In 1983, DRGs were implemented for hospitals (Cushman, 1988). From 1980 to 1986, home health became the fastest growing aspect of the Medicare budget with a peak number of home health agencies in 1986 of 6,000 (Cushman, 1988).

Cushman noted that government was working at cross purposes. Congress supported the expansion of home care services in the interest of cost containment and consumer preference. Meanwhile an administration ran amok with intent to curtail the same benefit because of that very growth. The Tax Equity and Fiscal Responsibility Act (TEFRA) mandated that the HCFA develop a fiscal target and evaluation criteria to measure the performance of the FI (Moran, 1989). HCFA developed a 5:1 cost saving standard for the medical review. This means that the FI needed to return $5 for every $1 spent on medical review.

The Gramm-Rudman Hollings Act attempted to balance the federal budget by reducing payments to most programs (Moran, 1989, p. 44). Home health was particularly hard hit since it is cost reimbursed with caps for maximum reimbursement. The reductions occurred on the costs, not the caps.

At this stage the National Association of Home Care (NAHC) reported the attempted dismantling of the Medicare home health benefit (NAHC, 1986, March 19). NAHC noted ". . . that some 30% of the patients receiving care under Medicare fell outside the home care box, that is they were either too sick, not sick enough, not homebound, or in the judgment of the Health and Human Service (HHS) officials, the care ordered by physicians and given by home health agencies was not reasonable and necessary." Home health agencies were self-limiting visits to avoid denials. Harris (1988) noted that there was a 27.5% increase in the intensity of home health services required between pre- and post-DRG implementation. This was due to increased documentation time, increased patient acuity levels, increased home visit time, and new on-call systems.

An unofficial redefinition of key terms such as skilled care, intermittent care, and homebound in Medicare regulations was occurring by the FI and HCFA across the country (Pini, 1989 #342). This resulted in such reasons for visits being denied as too many, too often, not necessary, not homebound because the patient could get out of bed, and even too many visits to the doctor.

Harris (1988, p. 20) referred to two studies that indicated the need for more home health visits, not less. The first study indicated that 1 in 10 patients felt their hospital stay was too short. About two thirds of the participants were readmitted for the same condition. In another study there was an increase of a 20% hospitalization rate and 10% mortality rate among the care receiving spouses within two to three months after discharge with the new definition of stable.

The stage was set for denials. (Moran, 1989, p. 30) noted that denials increased from 3.4% in 1985 to 7.9% in 1987. The increase in the rate of denied claims raised problems for beneficiaries and providers.

TYPES OF DENIALS

Claim denials occur when the FI concludes that Medicare cannot cover services performed, either because the beneficiary did not meet certain coverage compliance conditions or because the care was determined to be not medically necessary (Moran, 1989, p. 30). Most claims are submitted monthly for billing and contain several visits. A claim is considered denied if any portion is denied. If more than one visit is denied, it still counts as one claim. The denied visit may be in any of the six disciplines reimbursed by Medicare, which are skilled nursing, physical therapy, speech therapy, occupational therapy, medical social services, and home health aide services.

There are two types of denials—medical and technical. Medical denials are issued for excessive visits, care not recognized as reasonable or necessary, failure of documentation to support a

skilled need, custodial care, administration of a nonapproved drug, and noncovered diagnosis (Stone & Krebs, 1989). A technical denial is received if a determination is made that the patient is not homebound, the physician's orders do not cover services rendered, and if the required Physician Plan of Care (485) is completed incorrectly. Home health aide, medical social work, and occupational therapy will receive technical denials if a denial occurs on the qualifying service of skilled nursing, speech therapy, or physical therapy (Della Monica, 1994).

IMPACTS OF DENIALS

Waiver of Liability

Prior to January 1, 1996, agencies had Waiver of Liability (Medicare Provider Bulletin [MPB], 1996). There was a sunset of the favorable presumption provisions at that time. Currently there are actions in Washington to reinstate the Waiver of Liability retroactive to January 1, 1996. At present, it means that there is no favorable presumption to be used to make payment for a denied service until it is appealed. "The intermediary will apply waiver on a case by case basis. In most instances, it is assumed that the provider has knowledge of coverage issues, therefore no payment will be made for services denied by medical review. The appeal process continues to include a review of both the coverage decision and waiver determination." Even though this is currently repealed, the author feels that it will be resumed and therefore will describe it.

Denials affect an agency's Waiver of Liability. The Waiver of Liability principle was created by Section 213(a) of the Social Security Amendment of 1972 (Kohler, 1988). The purpose of the waiver is to hold harmless a beneficiary or provider who acted in good faith in accepting or providing services later determined to be noncovered because they were either not reasonable or necessary, or custodial in nature.

Specifically the program will make payment in those instances where the provider and beneficiary did not know, and could not reasonably have been expected to know, that payment would not be made for such items or services. The percentage for favorable waiver is less than 2.5% of the billed visits denied in a quarter. When the agency is under presumptive favorable waiver, payments are made for the denied visit. When the waiver status is unfavorable, payment is withheld immediately. A survey done by the Pennsylvania Association of Home Health Agencies (PAHHA) in July 1987 showed that 56.6% of the 106 responding agencies out of 285 were not on favorable waiver status. This caused a financial hardship for many agencies.

EXAMPLES OF DENIALS

References have been made regarding the denials, but what are some examples? Nursing procedures such as diabetic teaching and other follow-up procedures have been denied with the statement, "The patient should have been taught in the hospital" (Harris, 1988, p. 14). Fresca (1989) cited the following:

1. Patient does not need speech therapy because husband is deaf.
2. Terminally ill patient does not need to be monitored, because he is going to die anyway.
3. Home care social worker services are not necessary if the patient had any social work intervention provided in the hospital setting.
4. Patient does not need home health services as she has a good family support system.
5. Home health aide services are not needed as family can perform these duties.

Moran (1989) cited an example of a deep wound requiring daily visits for sterile packing over a period of 10 months. The wound did heal. The agency received a denial for care done 10 months earlier. She also noted a case where the daughter received a denial after the death of the parent for the home health aide services provided to a bedbound 91-year-old parent with an established intermittent skilled nursing need. Patients were fearful and apprehensive. A section of the denial notice read "therefore no further Medicare benefits can be paid." The reasons for denials seem to be no more appropriate today.

Time and Expenses Involved

These denials were both time-consuming and expensive. Fresca presented in her Senate testimony 27 cases. From the date service was provided, the initial denial occurred from two months to nine months after the care was provided. All reconsiderations were filed within the 60-day limit. The FI responded to the reconsideration appeal in from 1 month to 17 months with the exception of one case that was still outstanding after 8 months. In all of these cases, all or part of the denial was upheld by the FI. Again the appeal proceeded within the required 60 days for an ALJ hearing. From the date of the appeal until the hearing the time ranged from three to nine months. From the time of the hearing until notification to the agency of the decision the time frame was one week to nine months. Missing from this summary is when the agency received reimbursement for the services since the ALJ decision is sent to the regional HCFA office who then releases it to the FI for payment to the agency. The time frame from the care of the patient until a decision of the ALJ ranged from 11 months to 30 months with an average of 19 months. It was noted that the process was expedited at all levels as time passed. This means that in 1986, it required more time for decisions on all levels than in 1988 for the process to be completed. One case did proceed to the next level of the Appeals council and the denial was upheld. Of the 519 visits denied that could be counted in this summary representing at least three home health agencies, 496 were reversed in favor of the agencies for a reversal rate of 95.5%. The cost for this was $95/reconsideration to the FI. The cost for an ALJ hearing was $46 to the FI and $715 to the Social Security system in which the ALJ is located (Shikles, 1990). Based on these costs for 1987, this represents $23,112 in appeal costs to reduce the payment of just 23 visits. The agencies' expenses were unknown. We can only assume that the costs have increased today.

Moran (1989) noted that reversal rates increased over the years and varied throughout the country. Of the 186,138 denials in fiscal year (FY) 85, 21.1% were reversed at the reconsideration level. By the end of the first quarter of FY 88, there were 135,033 denials with 35.2% reversed. On the ALJ level in FY 85, 390 were presented at the ALJ level with a reversal rate of 5.6%. It should be noted that the family or beneficiary had to present most of these cases since the provider was unable to represent the beneficiary. By the end of the first quarter in FY 88 of the 135,033 denials, there were 1,022 ALJ hearings with a reversal rate of 76%.

Financial Impact

Home health administrators in 1986, 1987, and 1988 did not have reports such as the General Accounting Report. They knew that they were not being paid for care that had been paid in the past. They were losing their favorable waiver status. Problems were identified in the areas of unclear definitions of eligibility for the Medicare benefit, variation in the calculation of the waiver benefit status, agencies unable to represent a beneficiary who was afraid and did not understand how to appeal, and in many cases lack of knowledge for the agency to appeal. Administrators needed to make decisions. Some agencies closed, as noted previously by Cushman and Shikles, since there were 6,000 agencies in 1986 and 5,661 in 1988.

ACTIONS

The denial dilemma was approached on three fronts. These were legal via lawsuits for a long-term approach, political pressure for an interme-diary approach, and appealing for the short-term gain to the agency. National and state home health associations helped administrators and administrators helped these organizations.

Legal

In the August 1, 1988, decision of the District Court for the District of Columbia, the Duggan vs. Bowen decision set aside the continued use of part-time or intermittent care in section 206.6 of the Home Health Agency Manual HIM-11 (Medicare Home Health Provider Bulletin [MPHHB], 1989a). It did not change the Social Security Amendment 1814 (a) (2) (D) or 1835 (a) (2) (A). Part-time now meant any number of days per week. Intermittent care could be up to a total of 35 hours a week on a less than daily basis for the combination of nursing and home health aide visits. From 28 to 35 hours a week, care would be reviewed by the FI. The FI had to send form 488 requesting additional data before the denial could be made. There was also a retroactive review of some previously denied cases. Further examples were sent to the agencies in Medicare Home Health Provider Bulletins (MHHPB, 1989b). NAHC was instrumental in the case being brought to trial.

Political

Home health administrators were corresponding and meeting with local legislators during this turbulent time. These legislators were invited on home visits to patients that were being denied payment for care. Inquiries were being made to HCFA by the legislators on behalf of constituents and providers. Multiple bulletins were being issued to providers to clarify coverage with examples that were current. In other MHHPBs (1987d, 1987e, & 1987g) many other definitions were clarified and more specific examples were given such as homebound status based on communication disorders, therapy coverage for old onset diagnoses, homebound, intermittent, PRN visits, verbal orders, intravenous antibiotic therapy, and not-covered services for all therapies. OBRA expanded the right to appeal. Providers were now allowed to represent beneficiaries and appeal technical denials if they were liable (MHHPB, 1987a, 1987b, 1988c, 1989b). The denial letters received by the home health agency and beneficiary were more specific and in a language easily understood (MHHPB, 1988b). Clarifications were issued regarding payments following denials (MHHPB, 1988a). And finally, there were numerous updates for the calculation of the agency waiver status (MHHPB, 1987c, 1987f, 1987h). The last revision based on OBRA 89 does not allow a denial to be counted against an agency for at least 60 days. If there is a reconsideration in progress, it will not be counted until it is final. Also, additional information must be requested by the FI on a form 488 before a denial can be issued (MHHPB, 1990). The agency can also receive information via the computerized billing system that medical review is requested, and it has 35 days to submit the data until it is sent to the LIMO file. After 60 days the claim requesting data is purged from the LIMO file instead of a denial occurring (MPB, 1994a). If an error in billing is noted when data are submitted for review, the agency may note this and ask the claim to be adjusted. Then a denial will not be issued (MPB, 1994b).

National and state associations helped the home health administrator to inform politicians of the problems encountered.

Appeal Process

There was an immediate step that many administrators took in their agencies. This was the appeal process. It was necessary to recoup the funding that was lost during this turbulent period in the late 1980s. Denials are still occurring in agencies and agencies must continue to appeal them. There are at least four steps in the appeal process, which are reopening, reconsideration, ALJ hearing process, and Appeals Council review (Table 71–1). The exact regulatory language on any issue involving claims denials is located in the HIM-11, Home Health Agency Manual or the Code of Federal Regulation, Title 42-Public Health (1965).

STEPS IN THE APPEAL PROCESS

Reopening

The reopening is not in a legal sense appeals (MPB, 1993). They are actions that an agency can take after a claim is closed. The FI will evaluate the claim for appropriateness and

Table 71–1 Guidelines for Filing Appeals

Denial Actions	Reopening	Reconsideration	ALJ Hearing	Appeals Council Review
Time to file from denial date or date of last notification	1 year	60 days	60 days	60 days
Minimal amount of charges	$0	$0	$100	$1,000
Patient can appeal	Yes	Yes	Yes	Yes
Representative can appeal	Yes	Yes	Yes	Yes
Agency can appeal medical denial	Yes	Yes	Yes	Yes
Agency can appeal technical denial	No	No	No	No

Note: These guidelines summarize who can appeal a denial, the time involved for actions, and the dollar amount that is involved. The dollar amount is the agency charges, not the costs.

decide whether or not to honor the request. The reopening should only be used after the other appeal methods are exhausted. A reopening could be used to correct an error, in response to suspected fraud, or in response to the receipt of information not available or known to exist at the time the claim was initially processed.

Enhanced documentation skills have been a major factor in many home health agencies to prevent denials (Stone & Krebs, 1989). Staff have been given inservices on documentation. Utilization review nursing positions have been created. In September 1985, the Medicare program initiated the use of HCFA 485, 486, and 488 forms. Form 485 is the plan of treatment or care signed by the physician. It also contains other data such as supplies, visit frequency, laboratory work, medications, and dressing changes. The form 486 is used on admission and every 60 to 62 days to provide a summary of the patient care, projected number of visits, types of disciplines, significant changes, rehabilitation goals, homebound status, availability of a caretaker, etc. On both of these forms no area may be left blank or it will be denied. The summaries should tell a sequential story of the patient's response to treatment and care by the agency. The story should show evidence of services utilized that are included in the home health benefit. The FI is to request additional or missing data on the form 488 or electronic billing. This was not being done with regular frequency in 1986 and 1987. Reopenings are rarely being done today. In March of 1993, the submission of the 485 and 486 with billing was stopped, but they still must be completed in case a 488 inquiry occurs.

Reconsideration

Reconsideration is the next step in the appeal process and can be completed by resubmitting the patient information accompanied by HCFA form 2649 (Exhibit 71–1). The form does have an area where the provider or beneficiary may state the reasons why they disagree with the denial. Usually a copy of the chart at least for the time frame that was denied is submitted with this and references made in the summary to the chart. The information is processed by reviewers in a separate reconsideration department at the FI. These reconsideration nurses or other disciplines issue decisions without any consultation with the FI. The reconsideration reviewers make the decision to uphold the denial or reverse the denial (Stone & Krebs, 1989).

For reconsideration there is no minimum dollar amount in controversy necessary to file (Moran, 1989). The beneficiary or his or her assigned representative may appeal any denial. The form must be completed within 60 days from the date of the denial notice date. However, in a FI bulletin we were informed that the reconsideration must be received in 60 days (MHHPB, 1993). The date is the date on the notice, not the postmark date or the received date. There are a few exceptions to the 60-day filing period such as mental or physical impairment, death, over age 75 prior to date service began, incorrect information furnished by official sources, delay in obtaining supporting evidence, circumstances in which the individual would not have been aware to file timely, and damage to records (Levy, 1987). These exceptions also apply to the representative. Based on the Code of Federal Regulations 405.710(b)(40) F.R. 1025, Jan. 5, 1975, the provider may appeal when the individual on whose behalf the request for payment was made has indicated in writing on form SSA 1696-U4 (Exhibit 71–2) that he or she does not intend to request reconsideration of the FI's initial determination, or if the intermediary has made a finding that such individual did not know or could not reasonably have been expected to know that the expenses incurred for the items or services for which such request for payment was made were not reimbursable by reason that they are not reasonable and necessary or constitute custodial care. In addition, the provider must be liable. In other words, the provider may appeal if it is the representative on any denial, or if it is not on favorable waiver and the denial reason is not

Exhibit 71–1 Request for Reconsideration of Part A Health Insurance Benefits

INSTRUCTIONS: *Please type or print firmly.* Leave the block empty if you cannot answer it. Take or mail the WHOLE form to your Social Security office which will be glad to help you. Please read the statement on the reverse side of page 2.

1. BENEFICIARY'S NAME	2. HEALTH INSURANCE CLAIM NUMBER

3. REPRESENTATIVE'S NAME, IF APPLICABLE

(□ RELATIVE   □ ATTORNEY   □ OTHER PERSON)   □ PROVIDER FILING

4. PLEASE ATTACH A COPY OF THE NOTICE(S) YOU RECEIVED ABOUT YOUR CLAIM TO THIS FORM.

5. THIS CLAIM IS FOR

□ INPATIENT HOSPITAL   □ SKILLED NURSING FACILITY (SNF)   □ HEALTH MAINTENANCE ORGANIZATION (HMO)

□ EMERGENCY HOSPITAL   □ HOME HEALTH AGENCY (HHA)

6. NAME AND ADDRESS OF PROVIDER (*Hospital, SNF, HHA, HMO*)	CITY AND STATE	PROVIDER NUMBER
7. NAME OF INTERMEDIARY	CITY AND STATE	INTERMEDIARY NUMBER
8. DATE OF ADMISSION OR START OF SERVICES	9. DATE(S) OF THE NOTICE(S) YOU RECEIVED	

10. I DO NOT AGREE WITH THE DETERMINATION ON MY CLAIM. PLEASE RECONSIDER MY CLAIM BECAUSE

_____

_____

_____

_____

_____

11. YOU MUST OBTAIN ANY EVIDENCE (*For example, a letter from a doctor*) YOU WISH TO SUBMIT.	13. ONLY ONE SIGNATURE IS NEEDED. THIS FORM IS SIGNED BY: □ BENEFICIARY □ REPRESENTATIVE □ PROVIDER REP.
□ I HAVE ATTACHED THE FOLLOWING EVIDENCE:	SIGN HERE
□ I WILL SEND THIS EVIDENCE WITHIN 10 DAYS:	
□ I HAVE NO ADDITIONAL EVIDENCE OR OTHER INFORMATION TO SUBMIT WITH MY CLAIM.	14. STREET ADDRESS
12. IS THIS REQUEST FILED WITHIN 60 DAYS OF THE DATE OF YOUR NOTICE? □ YES □ NO	CITY, STATE, ZIP CODE
IF YOU CHECKED "NO" ATTACH AN EXPLANATION OF THE REASON FOR THE DELAY TO THIS FORM.	TELEPHONE DATE

15. If this request is signed by mark (X), TWO WITNESSES who know the person requesting reconsideration must sign in the space provided on the reverse side of this page of the form.

DO NOT FILL IN BELOW THIS LINE—FOR SOCIAL SECURITY USE—THANK YOU

16. ROUTING	□ INTERMEDIARY	18. SSA OR INTERMEDIARY DATE STAMP
	□ HCFA, RO-MEDICARE	
	□ BSS, ODR	
17. ADDITIONAL INFORMATION		

Exhibit 71–2 SSA Form 1696-U4, Department of Health and Human Services Social Security Administration

NAME (Claimant) (Print or Type)	SOCIAL SECURITY NUMBER

Section I   APPOINTMENT OF REPRESENTATIVE

I appoint this individual _____

(Name and address)

to act as my representative in connection with my claim or asserted right under:

☐ Title II (RSDI)   ☐ Title XVI (SSI)   ☐ Title IV FMSHA (Black Lung)   ☐ Title XVIII (Medicare Coverage)

I authorize this individual to make or give any request or notice; to present or elicit evidence; to obtain information; and to receive any notice in connection with my pending claim or asserted right wholly in my stead.

SIGNATURE (Claimant)	ADDRESS
TELEPHONE NUMBER (Area Code)	DATE

Section II   ACCEPTANCE OF APPOINTMENT

I, _____, hereby accept the above appointment. I certify that I have not been suspended or prohibited from practice before the Social Security Administration; that I am not, as a current or former officer or employee of the United States, disqualified from acting as the claimant's representative; and that I will not charge or receive any fee for the representation unless it has been authorized in accordance with the laws and regulations referred to on the reverse side hereof. In the event that I decide not to charge or collect a fee for the representation, I will notify the Social Security Administration (completion of Section III (optional) satisfies this requirement).

I am a / an_____

(Attorney, union representative, relative, law student, etc.)

SIGNATURE (Representative)	ADDRESS
TELEPHONE NUMBER (Area code)	DATE

Section III (Optional)   WAIVER OF FEE

I waive my right to charge and collect a fee under Section 206 of the Social Security Act, and I release my client (the claimant) from any obligations, contractual or otherwise, which may be owed to me for services I have performed in connection with my client's claim or asserted right.

SIGNATURE (Representative)	DATE

WAIVER OF DIRECT PAYMENT

I ONLY waive my right to direct certification of a fee from the withheld past-due benefits of my client (the claimant). I do NOT, however, waive my right to petition for and be authorized to charge and collect a fee directly from my client.

SIGNATURE (Representative)	DATE

medically necessary or custodial. Please refer to previous definitions of medical and technical denials and the rights of the home health agency to be the patient's representative. As previously mentioned, and demonstrated by the time delay, in the example of cases cited by Fresca (1989), there was no time frame for the FI to issue a determination of reconsiderations.

Administrative Law Judge Hearing

If the FI still denies the claim after reconsideration and the amount in controversy is $100 or more for Part A of Medicare, a request for a hearing may be filed (Levy, 1987). The $100 is the amount billed, not the costs, since home health agencies are cost reimbursed. A HA-5011-U6 Form (see Exhibit 71–3) must be mailed within 60 days along with the accompanying documentation to the local Social Security office. The provider, beneficiary, or representative may submit additional data at this time, such as a copy of the entire chart, pictures of wounds, a brief that summarizes care and/or progress of the patient (Exhibit 71–4), letters from the beneficiary or family members, reference to Social Security regulations that refer to the Medicare Home Health benefits, references to bulletins issued by FIs, copies of articles that show the provider was delivering care according to current standards, and letters from the attending physicians that support the chart documentation. At this stage the appeals process moves from the control of HCFA to Social Security. Additional data are requested from the FI Reconsideration Department by Social Security. This may include letters from the physician and physical therapist. The ALJ assigned to the case notifies the provider and beneficiary or his or her representative of a date and time for the hearing. The right to appear may be waived and the ALJ will determine the merits of the case based upon the written documentation on Social Security regulations.

Based on both experience and details by Levy (1987), the hearing is an informal process. A site is assigned near the provider or benefi-

ciary such as the Social Security building, a post office, or rented offices. There are tables and desks. All conversation is tape recorded. A lawyer does not need to be present. A registered nurse is considered an expert and is allowed to testify on behalf of the beneficiary and present the case. The judge has a file of information submitted by the provider, beneficiary, representative, and/or the FI. This chart may be reviewed prior to the hearing time, which is recommended. Data may be missing or there may be additional data in the file such as a letter from the FI physician or therapist that the presenter will need to address in the hearing.

Again, based on experience and Levy's seminar, the hearing usually proceeds in the following manner: The presenter is sworn to tell the truth. The ALJ will ask the qualifications of the presenter. This may include education, experience, current position, and relation to beneficiary, if appropriate. If additional persons are present, they will also be questioned. The ALJ will describe the format that is to be followed. The presenter is asked if the ALJ file is complete or if the presenter has additional information to submit. Additional data will be marked and dated as another exhibit. It will be added to the file or data previously submitted by the provider and FI. Usually the presenter will state the facts as to why the denial should be reversed. This material does not need to be memorized, but the presenter must be familiar with all of the material. The presenter may refer to any copies of information that are available. It is suggested that a copy be made of all material submitted. The presenter should paint a picture of the beneficiary and the circumstances at the time of care that may include the following:

- a description of the environment, such as the support system, that was viewed by home health personnel
- the location of the home from medical help
- specific documented care and the patient's response to that care that make the patient eligible for the home health benefit

Exhibit 71–3 Request for Hearing

HOSPITAL INSURANCE BENEFITS PAYABLE UNDER PART A OF TITLE XVIII
(Amount in Controversy, $100.00 or more - PRO $200.00 or more)
See Privacy Act Notice On Reverse Side Of Form.
Take or mail original and all copies to your local Social Security office.
*NOTICE - Anyone who misrepresents or falsifies essential information requested by this form may upon conviction be subject to fine and imprisonment under Federal law.

BENEFICIARY	CLAIM FOR
	☐ Inpatient Hospital Services
WAGE EARNER (Leave blank if same as above)	☐ Skilled Nursing Facility Services
	☐ Home Health Agency Services
HI CLAIM NUMBER	☐ Emergency Services
	☐ Other (Identify)

NAME AND ADDRESS OF INTERMEDIARY OR PROFESSIONAL STANDARDS REVIEW ORGANIZATION	PERIOD IN QUESTION FROM TO
	NAME AND ADDRESS OF PROVIDER (INSTITUTION)

I disagree with the determination made on the above claim and request a hearing. My reasons for disagreement are:

Check ONLY ONE of the statements below:	Check ONLY ONE of the statements below:
☐ I have additional evidence to submit (Attach such evidence to this form or forward to the Social Security office within 10 days.)	☐ I wish to appear in person.
☐ I have NO additional evidence to submit.	☐ I do NOT wish to appear at a hearing. I request that a decision be made on the basis of the evidence in my case.

Signed by: (Either the claimant or representative should sign—Enter addresses for both. If claimant has a representative, Form SSA-1696-U3 (Appointment of Representative) must be completed.)

SIGNATURE OR NAME OF CLAIMANT'S REPRESENTATIVE ☐ Attorney ☐ Non-Attorney	CLAIMANT'S SIGNATURE
ADDRESS	ADDRESS
CITY, STATE AND ZIP CODE	CITY, STATE, AND ZIP CODE
AREA CODE AND TELEPHONE NUMBER	DATE	AREA CODE AND TELEPHONE NUMBER

Claimant should not fill in below this line

TO BE COMPLETED BY SOCIAL SECURITY ADMINISTRATION

Is this request timely filed? ☐ YES ☐ NO If "No" is checked: (1) Attach claimant's explanation for delay. (2) Attach any pertinent letter, material, or information in the Social Security office.	Interpreter Needed_____ (Language, including sign language)

ACKNOWLEDGMENT OF REQUEST FOR HEARING

This request for hearing was filed on _____at _____
The Administrative Law Judge will notify you of the time and place of the hearing at least 10 days in advance of the hearing.

HEARING OFFICE COPY TO: ☐ Hearing Office_____ (Location)	For the Social Security Administration By _____ (Signature) (Title) (Street)
CLAIM FILE COPY TO: ☐ INTERMEDIARY ☐ HEALTH MAINTENANCE ORGANIZATION (HMO) ☐ PEER REVIEW ORGANIZATION (PRO)	(City, State, and Zip Code) Servicing Social Security Office Code _____
Form HA-5011-U6 (6-86)	ATTACH A COPY OF THE RECONSIDERATION DETERMINATION (IF AVAILABLE) TO THIS COPY
	CLAIM FILE

Exhibit 71–4 Guidelines for a Brief

Patient Name_____

HIC _____

Agency Provider Number _____

Period of Care in Question _____

Visits Denied and Reasons

Dates of Correspondence
Date of original 488 or computer request
Date on denial letter
Date of reconsideration
Date of letter from FI upholding the denial
Date of filing for hearing

Summary of Condition before Denial Period

Suggestion: Use summaries found on 486s if completed and on the chart. Paint a picture of the progress or lack of progress for the patient. Include patterns that the patient had before an acute episode. Include significant changes immediately before the denial period.

Care Denied

Be specific about what is documented and the subtle changes that occurred during this period. Emphasize the intermittent skilled aspect of the care. Usually do this visit by visit.

Care after the Denial Period

If the patient received care after the denial period, summarize this, including whether it was denied or not denied. If an acute episode occurred, provide details leading up to the acute phase, and compare them with those described for the denied time frame.

Reasons for Disagreement with the Denial

Use direct quotations from the HIM-11 for the regulation and example, FI bulletins, Social Security laws, articles from magazines for standards of care, and quotations from the attending physician letter if you have obtained one. Refer directly to the attached copy of the chart for specific examples of this patient's care that match these examples.

- matching this case to specific examples of covered care in the HIM-11 manual and FI bulletins and relating it to the covered home health benefits in the Social Security regulations

If additional data have been submitted by the FI, the presenter should clarify why there is dis-agreement with these additional data. The judge has reviewed the data previously submitted and may question the presenter on areas that were not covered in the opening statements and for which more detail is needed. The judge will also ask for definitions of medical terms that are unfamiliar to him or her. The judge will then ask for a brief closing summary. At this time it is good to reiterate the Social Security regulation and specifically why you disagree with the findings of the FI. During this presenter's experience, the time before an ALJ ranged from 5 minutes to 35 minutes on one case.

The denial can be affirmed or reversed. Written notification of this is sent to the provider, beneficiary, and representative. Receipt of the written notification will vary from a few months to over a year depending on the activities in your local region. Documentation of the decision is also submitted to the regional HCFA office, which forwards it to the FI. If the denial is reversed, the FI then pays the provider for previously rendered care and subtracts the number of visits involved in the decisions from the number of denied visits in the current quarter to be calculated the agency's waiver of liability (Moran, 1989).

Appeals Council

If the claim is denied by the ALJ and if the claimant and or provider is dissatisfied, they may request the Appeals Council to review the decision. HCFA does not have a similar right to appeal an ALJ determination. Claimants may submit new evidence to the Appeals Council that relates to the period reviewed by the ALJ or an earlier period. The Appeals Council review is otherwise limited to the ALJ record and no hearing is held. The Appeals Council evaluates the entire record, including new evidence, to determine whether the ALJ decision is contrary to the weight of evidence (Moran, 1989, p. 40). This action must be filed within 60 days after the mailing of the ALJ determination (Levy, 1987). Fresca (1989) cited only one case that reached this level.

Civil Action

If the Appeals Council does not reverse the denial there is still one more step in the appeal process, civil action. Levy noted one case, Gray Panthers v. Califano USDC (D of D) 466 Fi supp 117, March 6, 1979. At this level the dollar amount must be $1,000, the Appeals Council

must have made a ruling, and action must be filed within 60 days after the mailing of the Appeals Council's notice of denial unless good cause can be made. A nurse may not present the case at this level. It must be presented by a lawyer.

OPINIONS OF EXPERT NURSE PRESENTERS AT THE ALJ LEVEL

In order to solicit successful ideas from other administrators, a mailed survey was sent to eight known presenters at the ALJ level. Five nurses responded for a return rate of 62.5% (Jordan, 1990) and shared the following ideas on how to obtain a successful outcome with the ALJ process:

1. When your facts and rationale clearly demonstrate the need for skilled intervention and its necessity, your case should be strong
2. A good knowledge base coupled with the caregiver and family or patient testimony is the best defense
3. A letter from the physician is helpful, especially in cases where a "physician consultant" is utilized by the FI
4. Citing from the Code of Federal Regulations in your case presentation and summary is helpful since these are the regulations binding an ALJ
5. Include specific citations from the Social Security regulations and why you disagree with the FI

The ideal presenter should be able to testify verbally in a concise manner on the agency's delivery of care based on standards of care, actual chart documentation, and Social Security regulations, not interpretations from the FI and HCFA. The presenter should be able verbally to persuade a judge, based on facts, that this patient's care was necessary despite disclaimers from the FI representatives using other available documentation such as letters from the family and attending physician.

WHY SHOULD DENIALS BE APPEALED?

Nurses have been advocates for patients for a long time. This is another example of nurses still fulfilling this role. It is different from doing treatments, but vital. The appeal process at the ALJ level also has some vital elements that can be transferred to other areas and issues that are occurring. There are now, throughout the country, state review organizations that monitor patients being discharged from the hospital too early. The same argument as the brief may assist hospital and home health nurses who must summarize data when they are requested. Home health administrators will also use the same Social Security system of Administrative Law Judges should the state Department of Health issue a violation of a Condition of Participation to appeal the decision. In the recent Chaves case the courts ruled that the denials made during the compliance audit could be applied to all of the visits made during the fiscal year (NAHC #410, 1991). This has already had major financial impact on several agencies.

CONCLUSION

The appeal process is time consuming, expensive, and stressful for most nurses. Nurse administrators must make decisions on whether or not to appeal. They did make decisions to enhance documentation techniques, to educate nurses regarding the specifics of regulations, and to centralize functions in utilization review nurses. They needed to determine the beneficiaries' need for skilled care, their commitment to quality care, and financial solvency (Harris, 1988) to decide to proceed with the appeal process. Based on previous data, many appeals were made at the reconsideration level, but only a small percentage of the remaining denials proceeded to the ALJ level. Lack of education and fear seemed to be two hindrances to the next step.

Home health care denials have decreased, but they are still occurring and with the loss of Waiver of Liability may increase again. Based on the reversal rates cited in this study, this author would suggest that every agency should appeal to the highest level possible. Only one case was noted at the Appeals Council Level. An area that was not addressed is the agency's expenses such as the time involved in prehearing preparation, copies of the chart, time spent obtaining signed representative forms, mailing expenses, travel time to and from hearings, and approximate presentation times. If the objective of the denials by HCFA was cost containment, it was not effective based on the number of reversals that did occur. If the objective of the denial by HCFA was to clarify the home health care benefit, it was effective.

Effective decision making occurred by home health administrators. Pini (NAHC #342, 1989) noted 12 changes as a result of actions that occurred in the late 1980s. These are:

- there is advance written notice of policy changes from HCFA with a 60-day comment period
- home health agencies have increased involvement in policy and procedure development
- there is a set qualification criteria of reviewers of denials
- no denial can be issued without the request for additional data
- the release of the screening model is used by FIs for audit criteria
- the rewriting of the denial notice is less traumatic to the patients and more informative to the providers
- there is a continuance of the waiver of liability
- no denial can be included in the waiver calculations until after reconsideration or 60 days from denial
- there is an expedited appeal process for the FI
- there is maintenance of the ALJs in the Social Security system instead of HCFA
- there is a speedier appeal process for active beneficiaries

• there is approval of daily care when the patient's need is not finite and predictable.

These decisions will help protect the home health benefit and provide better financial sol-vency for home health agencies. As of January 1996 waiver was eliminated for medical necessity denials but remained in place for technical denials for allegedly nonhomebound or nonintermittent cases.

REFERENCES

Cushman, M. (1988). Political issues in home health care: a national perspective. In M.D. Harris (Ed.), *Home Health Administration* (pp. 604–611). Owings Mills, MD: National Health Publishing.

DellaMonica, E.D. (1994). Home health care documentation and record keeping. In M.D. Harris (Ed.), *Handbook of Home Healthcare Administration* (pp. 126–127). Gaithersburg, MD: Aspen Publishers, Inc.

Fresca, C. (1989, February 22). Testimony on Medicare claims denials. (Testimony presented before the HCFA Advisory Committee for the American Hospital Association, Baltimore, MD): IV-1-32, V-1.

Harris, M. (1987). Medicare and the nurse—the denial dilemma. *Home Health Care Nurse, 5*(5), 46–47.

Harris, M.D. (1988). The impact of DRGs on nursing care in community settings. (HRSA 87-339P) 5285 Port Royal Road, Springfield, VA 22161. (NTIS No. HRP-0907180): 15–18.

Jordan, L.M. (1990). *The opinions of expert nurse presenters in administrative law judge hearings for successful reversal of denied home health claims.* Unpublished master's thesis, Villanova University, Villanova, PA.

Kohler, C. (1988). Reimbursement. In M.D. Harris (Ed.), *Home health administration* (pp. 505–507). Owings Mills, MD: National Health Publishing.

Levy, M. (1987, April). *Handbook on Medicare appeals process.* (Conference conducted by Pennsylvania Association of Home Care, Harrisburg, PA): 17, 21–25, 31–32.

Medicare Home Health Provider Bulletin. (1987a, January 16). *Reconsiderations/reopenings.* (87–2). (Available from Blue Cross of Greater Philadelphia, 1901 Market Street, Philadelphia, PA 19107-1480.)

Medicare Home Health Provider Bulletin. (1987b, March 11). *Beneficiary representation by home health agency.* (87–10). (Available from Blue Cross of Greater Philadelphia, 1901 Market Street, Philadelphia, PA 19107-1480.)

Medicare Home Health Provider Bulletin. (1987c, March 16). *Home health agency denial adjustments.* (87–11). (Available from Blue Cross of Greater Philadelphia, 1901 Market Street, Philadelphia, PA 19107-1480.)

Medicare Home Health Provider Bulletin. (1987d, March 27). *Home health coverage issues.* (87–14). (Available from Blue Cross of Greater Philadelphia, 1901 Market Street, Philadelphia, PA 19107-1480.)

Medicare Home Health Provider Bulletin. (1987e, May 14). *Clarification of medicare coverage issues.* (87–18). (Available from Blue Cross of Greater Philadelphia, 1901 Market Street, Philadelphia, PA 19107-1480.)

Medicare Home Health Provider Bulletin. (1987f, May 22). *Denial rate determinations.* (87–19). (Available from Blue Cross of Greater Philadelphia, 1901 Market Street, Philadelphia, PA 19107-1480.)

Medicare Home Health Provider Bulletin. (1987g, July 22). *Clarification of medicare coverage issues.* (87–25). (Available from Blue Cross of Greater Philadelphia, 1901 Market Street, Philadelphia, PA 19107-1480.)

Medicare Home Health Provider Bulletin. (1987h, September 18). *Changes in waiver of liability provision.* (87–38). (Available from Blue Cross of Greater Philadelphia, 1901 Market Street, Philadelphia, PA 19107-1480.)

Medicare Home Health Provider Bulletin. (1988a, November 8). *Payment following reversal of denial.* (88–38). (Available from Blue Cross of Greater Philadelphia, 1901 Market Street, Philadelphia, PA 19107-1480.)

Medicare Home Health Provider Bulletin. (1988b, December 12). *Notice of medicare claim determination—denial letters.* (88–48). (Available from Blue Cross of Greater Philadelphia, 1901 Market Street, Philadelphia, PA 19107-1480.)

Medicare Home Health Provider Bulletin. (1988c, December 16). *Medicare part A appeal procedures.* (88–49). (Available from Blue Cross of Greater Philadelphia, 1901 Market Street, Philadelphia, PA 19107-1480.)

Medicare Home Health Provider Bulletin. (1989a, January 9). *Guidelines for Duggan vs. Bowen court decision (continued use of "part time or intermittent").* (89–1). (Available from Blue Cross of Greater Philadelphia, 1901 Market Street, Philadelphia, PA 19103-1480.)

Medicare Home Health Provider Bulletin. (1989b, April 26). *HHA's right to appeal initial determination under the limitation of liability provision.* (89–13). (Available from Blue Cross of Greater Philadelphia, 1901 Market Street, Philadelphia, PA 19103-1480.)

Medicare Home Health Provider Bulletin. (1990, April 30). *Calculation of denial rate to determine an HHA's qualification for a favorable presumption.* (90–13). (Available from Blue Cross of Greater Philadelphia, 1901 Market Street, Philadelphia, PA 19103-1480.)

Medicare Home Health Provider Bulletin. (1993, August 6). *Part A Appeals Process.* (93–25). (Available from Blue Cross of Greater Philadelphia, 1901 Market Street, Philadelphia, PA 19103-1480.)

Medicare Provider Bulletin. (1994a, December 9). *Change in procedure for records which are not received.* (94–48). (Available from Independence Blue Cross, 1901 Market Street, Philadelphia, PA 19103-1480.)

Medicare Provider Bulletin. (1994b, September 2). *Handling of provider billing errors on medical review claims.* (94–34). (Available from Independence Blue Cross, 1901 Market Street, Philadelphia, PA 19103-1480.)

Medicare Provider Bulletin. (1996, February 2). *HCFA ruling concerning expiration of waiver.* (96–6). (Available from Independence Blue Cross, 1901 Market Street, Philadelphia, PA 19103-1480.)

Moran, S. J. (1989). *Report to Congress and the administrator by the advisory committee on Medicare home health claims.* (U.S. Department of Health and Human Services, Health Care Finance Administration, July 1, vol. 1). Washington, DC: U.S. Government Printing Office: 40–41, 44, 94–95.

National Association for Home Care. (1986, March 19). *The attempted dismantling of the Medicare home health benefit.* Report to Congress.

National Association for Home Care. *NAHC Report #342*, December 15, 1989. Washington, DC: Author.

National Association for Home Care. *NAHC Report #410*, May 3, 1991. Washington, DC: Author.

Pennsylvania Association of Home Health Agencies. (1987). [Claims Denial survey, July 1987]. Unpublished raw data.

Pini, R. (1989, December 15). *Home health care claims committee reports to Congress on Medicare Denials.* Washington, DC: National Association for Home Care.

Shikles, J.L. (1990). *Increased denials of home health claims during 1986 and 1987.* (GAO/HRO-90-14BR). Washington, DC: General Accounting Office.

Stone, C.L., & Krebs, K. (1989). The use of utilization review nurse to decrease reimbursement denials. *Home Healthcare Nurse, 8*(3), 13–17.

BIBLIOGRAPHY

Bailey, J.T., & Hendricks, D.E. (1982). Decisions, decisions: guidelines for making them more easily. *Nursing Life. 2*(4), 45–47.

Denzier, J. (Ed.). (1991, May 3) *NAHC Report.* (Available from National Association of Home Care, 519 C Street, N. E., Stanton Park, Washington, DC 20002.)

Dozier, J. (Ed.). (1991, August 2) *NAHC Report.* (Available from National Association of Home Care, 519 C Street, N. E., Stanton Park, Washington, DC 20002.)

Fiesta, J. (1983). *The law and liability: guide for nurses.* (p. 3). New York: Wiley Medical Publication.

Medicare Home Health Provider Bulletin. (1987, July 17). *Recoupement of denials.* (87–24). (Available from Blue Cross of Greater Philadelphia, 1333 Chestnut Street, Philadelphia, PA 19107.)

Medicare Home Health Provider Bulletin. (1989, February 24). *Guidelines for Duggan vs. Bowen court decision (continued use of "part time or intermittent") delay in reporting requirements.* (89–6). (Available from Independence Blue Cross, 1901 Market Street, Philadelphia, PA 19103-1480.)

NAHC Report. (1988, Jan. 6, #244-A). *Special Report.* (Available from National Association of Home Care, 519 C Street, N.E., Stanton Park, Washington, DC 20002.)

O'Leary, J., Wendelgass, S.T., & Zimmerman, H.E. (1986). *Winning strategies for nursing managers.* (pp. 75–80). Philadelphia: J.B. Lippincott Company.

Pini, R. (Ed.). (1990, March 23). *NAHC Report.* (Available from National Association of Home Care, 519 C Street, N.E., Stanton Park, Washington, DC 20002.)

Pini, R. (Ed.). (1990, April 6). *NAHC Report.* (Available from National Association of Home Care, 519 C Street, N.E., Stanton Park, Washington, DC 20002.)

CHAPTER 72

Nursing Research in Home Health Agencies

Marilyn D. Harris

The American College Dictionary defines research as the "diligent and systematic inquiry or investigation into a subject in order to discover facts or principles." Research can be scholarly and abstract, or it can be down to earth and practical. In home care there are many practical subjects to investigate, such as the following: How many patients have decubitus? What treatment is used? What is the outcome? How many after-hours calls and requests for service does an agency receive, and at what hours? What is the cost of service by various classification systems?

I believe that research in such areas—clinical, administrative, and financial—is imperative. Whether it is the identification of a problem and the search for ways to alleviate it or a more formal analysis of one particular aspect of home care, a diligent and systematic inquiry, with findings carefully documented, can provide the data necessary to approve or reject ideas for new programs and services and to identify ways to contain costs without jeopardizing quality of care.

TYPES OF RESEARCH PROJECTS

A research project can be undertaken by the home health care agency either independently or in collaboration with others. To conduct independent research, it is essential that the agency's

principal investigator have a working knowledge of research principles and techniques. Whether it is independent or collaborative research, setting up a research project involves writing a proposal that addresses problem identification, study design, hypothesis, data analysis and evaluation techniques, and a plan to disseminate the findings. Such a proposal often becomes the basis for requesting funding to support the project (Exhibit 72–1).

Collaborative research offers several advantages to a home health agency as well as to the individual or group collaborator. Establishing an effective networking system with area educational institutions can be of benefit to the institutions, their students, the home care agency, and patients. For example:

- As collaborators, graduate nursing students can help the agency meet an identified need while at the same time meeting their own educational goals.
- Faculty members may have access to university grant monies for projects that can be conducted in home care agencies.
- Working with an educational institution may provide access to computer services that can be used for data analysis at no or low cost to the home health agency.
- Doctoral students can be permitted to collect data for their dissertations through the home care agency if the results will be of

Exhibit 72–1 Possible Funding Sources for Research in Home Health Agencies

---

American Nurses Foundation
600 Maryland Avenue SW, Suite 100
Washington, DC 20024-2571

Annual Register of Grant Support
Marquis Who's Who, Inc.
Reed Reference Publishing Company
121 Chanlon Road
New Providence, NJ 07974

The Foundation Center
79 Fifth Avenue
New York, NY 10003

The Foundation Reporter
B. Romaniuk, Editor—24th Edition 1993
The Taft Group
12300 Twinbrook Parkway, Suite 450
Rockville, MD 20852

National Institutes of Health Guide
Distribution Center
National Institutes of Health
Bethesda, MD 20892

Regional Foundations
Example:
Directory of Pennsylvania Foundations
Triadvocates Press
The Free Library of Philadelphia
Logan Square
Philadelphia, PA 19103

Sigma Theta Tau (national office)
1100 Waterway Blvd.
Indianapolis, Indiana 46202
(Or contact local chapter for information)

(Note: Refer to Chapter 62 on Resource Development for Home Health Care Providers for additional information.)

---

benefit to the agency's quality of care. Similarly, collaboration with an area medical school can be of mutual benefit; an example is a study conducted in the mid-1980s of medication use in the homebound—interactions, compliance, and cost—that was undertaken in a joint project by the Visiting Nurse Association of Eastern Montgomery County (VNA) and faculty and students from Temple University Medical Practice (Lavizzo-Mourey, Laskowsky, Harris, & Parente, 1987, 1989).

Other examples of projects in which this VNA has been involved are summarized in Exhibits 72–2 and 72–3.

Schools of education are not the only sources of collaborative efforts. Ideas that are directly or indirectly related to health care may originate within private businesses and require the expertise available in a home care agency staff to be brought to fruition.

PROJECT ESSENTIALS

Whether the agency engages in independent or collaborative research, certain basic requirements must be satisfied.

Agency Commitment

The agency's administrative staff must be committed to nursing research. Without that commitment, projects can too easily be set aside amid all their other responsibilities. Administrators should have an ongoing list of possible research projects on file, in order of priority, ready to present whenever staff members or students seek suggestions for such projects.

Project Validity

The problem to be addressed (or the objective of the research) must be clearly identified. Why is it a problem? What has been done about it in the past? What does the literature report? How will the results benefit patients and staff?

A Designated Overseer

Someone within the agency must be an appropriate appointee to oversee the research. It

Exhibit 72–2 Three Examples of Research Projects at the VNA

Independent Project Carried out with Foundation Funding

A Tape Recording and Transcribing System To Maintain Patients' Clinical Records. This project was funded with a $32,000 grant in 1980–1981. The goals of the project were to (1) reduce the amount of time that professional personnel spend on patients' recordkeeping by providing a portable dictating system to record clinical records, (2) increase the number of patients whom professional personnel will be able to visit in a day, and (3) increase the amount of time that professional personnel spend in direct patient care. The results of this project were published in *Nursing & Health Care*, 1984, Volume 5, Number 9, pp. 503–507. This research was related to a clinical issue but was beneficial to administration because the goal was to increase staff productivity while improving clinical documentation.

Doctoral Student Research

Communication Pattern between Health Care Providers and Clients and Recall of Health Information. In 1981, K. Kishi examined the verbal communication patterns that take place between health care providers and clients in well-infant clinics and then investigated how these patterns related to recall. Based on the outcome of her study, the VNA developed three in a series of brochures titled *Watching Your Baby Grow* to be used in the clinics. K. Kishi's dissertation is in the University of Pennsylvania's School of Nursing Library (1981). An article titled "Communication Patterns of Health Teaching and Information

Recall" appeared in *Nursing Research* 1983, Volume 5, Number 4, pp. 230–235.

M. Harris wrote an article on the development of the brochures, "Student Programs Benefit Nursing Service Agencies," which was published in *Home Healthcare Nurse* 1984, Volume 2, Number 5, pp. 34–35.

This clinical research was related to the health promotion aspects of the VNA's services.

Collaborative Research with Faculty and Student from a Major University, Funded by a University Grant

The Cost of Care by Nursing Diagnosis. This project was made possible through a grant from the Public Policy Initiative Fund at the University of Pennsylvania. One of the faculty, Judith B. Smith, PhD, RN, and a doctoral student, Donna Peters, RN, MA, CNAA, worked with the director and staff at the VNA to refine further a patient classification system to include the quantification of outcomes and the cost associated with providing care based on nursing diagnosis. The results of the 1-year study are included in *Home Health Administration*, a book edited by M. Harris, published by National Health Publishing, Owings Mills, MD, in 1988. Data collection continued after the initial study. These data, in addition to other outcome data such as the identification of the cost of care by goals within a patient classification system and the quantification of these outcomes, will be beneficial to the agency when reimbursement for home care changes from a per visit to another, yet undetermined method in the future. This research addressed both the clinical and the administrative aspects of home health care services.

can be the administrator, a supervisor, a nurse practitioner, or a staff person with research experience. (Such a designation can also be an excellent way to give additional responsibility to a staff nurse in need of completing course requirements for a degree.)

THE COST IN TIME

Regardless of how the research is accomplished, independently or collaboratively, the question must be asked: What will its impact be on agency productivity? It takes time to explain

Exhibit 72–3 Examples of Recent Research
Projects at the VNA

- Consumer Evaluation of Skin Protectants in the Management of Incontinent Patients
- Continence Program for Care-Dependent Community Elderly
- Patient Expectations and Satisfaction with Home Health Nutritional Care
- Animal-Assisted Therapy for the Home-bound Elderly (Harris & Gellin, 1990, 1992; Harris, Rinehart, & Gerstman, 1993)

a project to staff as well as to patient groups. Throughout the course of the project, considerable paperwork is involved. To illustrate this point, the following experience is summarized; it was involved in the aforementioned collaborative agency–medical school study of medication in the homebound.

Procedure for Collecting Data

The VNA's admission-to-service procedure includes completing forms, obtaining informed consent, and completing the nursing assessment, problem identification (nursing diagnosis), and billing information. The staff were asked to have each patient complete an informed consent specific to the medication study. There was to be a visual inspection of all medications, and patients or their families were asked to have all medications available for the nurse on the first visit.

Procedure for Record Abstracting

The clerical staff kept a list of all patients admitted to VNA services. The VNA had two offices, and during the study these lists were given to the medical record department of both VNA offices, where staff pulled the clinical records for these admissions and sent the records to a specific location in one office. Each Saturday morning during the study, one investigator and a student came to the VNA office to abstract the charts for patients admitted that

week. Charts were returned to the appropriate medical record department on Monday morning. The abstracting process took about three hours each week. Weekend time of the nursing supervisor was also spent in answering questions.

Summary

This example, which covers only a portion of the project, shows how important it is that every contemplated research undertaking be evaluated from several viewpoints, in terms of not only the time it will take but also the funds it will require, as suggested by the following list:

- staff time for development and education
- time for carrying out the project
- computer time (hours as well as possible costs)
- cost of equipment and supplies
- project staff time as well as benefits
- time spent in writing up results for publication

Hluchyi (1994) suggests that a home care agency is more likely to have a successful experience with research if it establishes a structure within which activities can be accomplished in a logical, professional, and consistent way. This structure includes a research policy that defines the principles the agency has adopted for participating in research, whether the research is conducted by agency staff or by persons outside the organization.

Home health care administrators need to be familiar with the guidelines and procedures included in their facility's Institutional Review Board's (IRB) review process. These guidelines will delineate certain categories of social, educational, and economic research that are exempt from the IRB's review under federal regulations.

CONCLUSION

It is appropriate and feasible for home care agencies to conduct research. They have a ready population and sample. Many aspects of home care need to be studied to improve the quality of care and the quality of life. The rewards of research can more than justify the perceived burdens. The practical benefits are the strengthening of staff knowledge and expertise through exposure to the process of investigation and to the clinical applications and implications of the findings. The bottom line will be improved patient care.

REFERENCES

Harris, M., & Gellin, M. (1990). Pet therapy for the homebound elderly. *Caring, 9,* 48–51.

Harris, M., & Gellin, M. (1992). The effects of weekly pet visits upon the circulatory system and the personal adjustment of homebound elderly persons. *The Pennsylvania Nurse, 47*(4), 12–13.

Harris, M., Rinehart, J., & Gerstman, J. (1993). Animal-assisted therapy for the homebound elderly. *Holistic Nursing Practice, 8*(1), 27–53.

Hluchyi, T. (1994). Structure of the research process. In: Balding, M., Hluchyi, T., Ira, P., Schins, I., Smith, A., (Eds.), *Home care. A research guide* (pp. 17–36). Ann Arbor, MI: Michigan Foundation for Home Care.

Lavizzo-Mourey, R., Laskowsky, R., Harris, M., & Parente, C. (1987). Improving drug regimens for the homebound. *American Journal of Nursing, 5,* 593–596.

Lavizzo-Mourey, R., Laskowsky, R., Harris, M., & Parente, C. (1989). Three drug management problems: Cost, confusion and adverse reactions. *Nursing '89, 19,* 62–63.

CHAPTER 73

Hospice Care

Rosemary Johnson Hurzeler, Evelyn A. Barnum,
Sandra J. Klimas, and Eugene G. Michael

INTRODUCTION

During the latter part of this century, the simultaneous development of high-tech advances in medical care that offer hope of cure, and the evolution of a hospice movement providing compassionate care for the terminally ill, have created a serious ethical dilemma for patients, families, and caregivers.

The difficult question confronting caregivers and patients in advanced stages of disease is: when is it appropriate to curtail aggressive treatment modalities and initiate palliative care under the auspices of a qualified hospice program?

The hospice movement has flourished in this country since its inception in 1974 when The Connecticut Hospice, Inc., initiated services to the first American hospice home care patient in New Haven, Connecticut.[1] There are now well over 2,000 hospices in the U.S. providing care to 250,000 patients and families each year.

Despite this phenomenal growth in less than 25 years, many hospice-eligible patients[2] are never referred to hospice programs and die in hospitals, often in pain and often in isolated intensive care units.[3]

The reluctance to refer patients to hospice care is partly explained by the fact that the term hospice has become associated with death, albeit a comfortable, compassionate, and loving end of life experience. For those patients and caregivers who are not yet ready to curtail hope of cure and wish to continue aggressive treatment, hospice care is seen as premature and therefore either avoided completely or withheld until the last possible moment.

Thus, the challenge to the hospice movement in the U.S. in this era of managed care and cost limitations is to find a way to redefine traditional hospice care, extending access to quality care at the end of life at an appropriate time while safeguarding the right of each patient to make appropriate, informed decisions on aggressive as well as palliative care measures. We must begin wherever people are; indeed, palliative care must begin in the hospital, even while active treatment continues. The challenge is to make hospice care an integral, seamless part of the health care delivery system.

In this chapter, we will define terms, present a historical perspective and explanation of hospice care, describe relevant regulatory and financing issues, and project trends and future challenges.

HOSPICE DEFINED

Hospice is a specialized program of health care for the terminally ill patient and his or her family. (See Commonly Used Terms.) For these patients, management of their end of life care requires clinical expertise and interdisciplinary resources to offer the patient/family the highest level of caring in a limited time period. The goals of hospice care are directed toward palliation of pain and control of other symptoms, rather than toward curative measures. Hospice care is appropriate for those patients with progressive disease who need the full complement of the hospice interdisciplinary approach, which extends beyond the traditional home care model to encompass medicine, pastoral, arts, volunteers, and bereavement in addition to skilled nursing, social work, and therapies.

The strength of the relationship between community physicians and the hospice team under the leadership of a hospice medical director is a critical aspect of the interdisciplinary team function. Close communication and interaction with community physicians and the caregiving community facilitates patient/family and staff education as well as the refinement of the patient care plan. See Ten Principles of Hospice Care.

The role of pastoral care in the interdisciplinary team is to offer support to meet the sensitive spiritual needs of the patient and family. The arts program also provides a venue that heightens the spiritual awareness of many hospice patients. The creative blend of music, literature, and the creative arts enhances the ability of patients and families to express themselves and the deep feelings they are experiencing.

Volunteers are an essential component of the hospice team. The commitment and the dedication of specially trained lay and professional volunteers augment the care staff.

An integral part of any hospice program is comprehensive bereavement follow-up to assist families with grief and loss. This is the dimension of hospice care that can be regarded as preventive care. An effective bereavement program enables individuals who have experienced loss to assimilate that loss and promotes wellness in the future.

Hospice care is primarily a home care program but necessarily includes an inpatient component to meet the more complex needs of some patient/families. The hospice program of care enables the patient to remain at home for as long as possible. Hospice caregivers encourage

Commonly Used Terms

Palliative care is comfort-oriented care directed to the alleviation of pain and control of other symptoms experienced by a patient in advanced stages of disease.

Terminal care refers to services provided at home or in a hospital for patients during the last days and weeks of life. It is often used by agencies and institutions who may not be certified to provide hospice care.

Hospice care incorporates both palliative and terminal care with a focus on family as well as patient and including an interdisciplinary approach in a comprehensive, structured program.

Ten Principles of Hospice Care

1. Patient and family are regarded as the unit of care.
2. Services are physician-directed and nurse-coordinated.
3. Emphasis is on control of symptoms (physical, sociological, spiritual, psychological).
4. Care is provided by an interdisciplinary team.
5. Trained volunteers are an integral part of the team.
6. Services are available on a 24-hours-a-day, 7-days-a-week, on-call basis with emphasis on availability of medical and nursing skills.
7. Family members receive bereavement follow-up.
8. Home care and inpatient care are coordinated.
9. Patients are accepted on the basis of health needs, not on ability to pay.
10. There are structured systems for staff support and communication.

Copyright © 1974.   The Connecticut Hospice, Inc.

and support the patient/family to participate in decisions about the patient's care and assist in caring for the patient.

Hospice home care can also be available to residents of skilled nursing and extended care facilities providing that the resident's room/board as well as care not related to their terminal illness are not reimbursed by Medicare. With the appropriate agreements in place to coordinate the work of the hospice home care team and with the work of facility personnel, full-scope hospice home care can be effectively rendered to residents of skilled nursing facilities.

REGULATION ISSUES

Federal Legislation

In 1983, Congress passed the Tax Equity and Fiscal Responsibility Act (TEFRA) in an effort to slow the rate of increase of federal expenditures for health care. At a time when virtually no other social or health care program legislation received congressional approval, TEFRA made "hospice care" a federally recognized and reimbursable form of health care with extraordinary bipartisan congressional support. With the enhancement of TEFRA, the word "hospice" entered the Medicare lexicon. The first case-managed reimbursement system, the Hospice Benefit, continues to be the model for reimbursement at the federal level.

Certification

To ensure that consumers are guaranteed to receive full scope and quality hospice services, Congress has mandated that organizations providing hospice care to Medicare beneficiaries must have certification demonstrating their compliance with federal standards. Certification is a minimum quality assurance device and controls payments to providers for hospice beneficiaries. The certification process for hospices, as a separate and distinct category of provider under Medicare regulation, began with the 1983

enactment of a special hospice reimbursement provision of TEFRA.

The Conditions of Participation, developed by the Department of Health and Human Services to implement the TEFRA Hospice Benefit, create regulatory requirements that are unique to the hospice legislation. These regulations are consistent with the hospice concept of care because they require centralized authority, medical direction, establishment of a patient-focused plan of care, provisions for staff development and performance improvement, use of the interdisciplinary approach, and emphasis on home care. Contrary to traditional Medicare requirements, a Hospice Benefit patient need not be "essentially homebound" in order to receive hospice care. This adjustment to the Medicare regulations supports the idea that the hospice concept and program of care encourages and supports the patient/family in living life as fully as possible for as long as life lasts. These provisions are intended to reinforce the concept of hospice as a program of home and inpatient palliative care for the patient and a program of bereavement follow-up for the family.

To encourage the development of hospice home care and maintain the emphasis on home care, all hospices certified under the Hospice Benefit are mandated to maintain a ratio of home care days to inpatient care days of 80:20. This ratio is reviewed in the aggregate annually.

State Licensure

State licensure plays an important role in monitoring quality of care and performance improvement and integrates with Medicare certification under the TEFRA legislation. In defining the term "hospice program," TEFRA requires that in any state that provides for the licensing of hospices, the hospice program seeking federal Medicare certification must be licensed pursuant to that state's hospice licensure law.

The licensure requirements for hospice were first adopted in Connecticut and serve as a model for home care and inpatient hospice care requirements. The requirements for each component of the interdisciplinary hospice care team are addressed in the State of Connecticut licensure.

While licensing and revocation of licenses are powerful weapons in ensuring quality, licensure regulations in any state are effective only to the extent that their implementation is ensured through regular inspections. Meticulous recordkeeping and rigorous monitoring of home care operations contributes to quality assurance and guarantees compliance with regulatory requirements.

Accreditation

The Joint Commission on Accreditation of Healthcare Organizations (Joint Commission) has reinstituted accreditation for hospice home care organizations by incorporating hospice as a dimension of care within the *1995 JCAHO Accreditation Manual for Home Care* (Joint Commission, 1994).

In keeping with the Joint Commission mandate for performance improvement, measurement of a hospice home care program through an ongoing evaluative process is critical to continuously improve service delivery to the hospice population. This should encompass documentation of hospice clinical and interdisciplinary processes as well as outcomes according to hospice standards of care. A hospice performance improvement plan must include ongoing assessment of patient/family satisfaction that delineates the patient/family's perception of the program and services provided as well as symptom management and process outcomes.

FINANCING

The Federal Hospice Benefit

To be eligible, an individual must be certified as terminally ill and be entitled to receive benefits under Medicare Part A. The patient must elect the "Hospice Benefit" and sign an election form. Each Medicare beneficiary is entitled to two 90-day election periods, one 30-day election period, and a fourth "lifetime" election period that extends for the duration of the patient's life. Under TEFRA, hospice-covered services include nursing care, medical social services, physician services, counseling services, short-term inpatient care, medical supplies (including drugs and biologicals for palliation), pastoral care, arts, services of home health aides, physical therapy, occupational therapy, and speech-language pathology. The Act requires that these services must be reasonable and necessary for palliation and management of the terminal illness and that volunteer hours account for 5 percent of all care hours. The hospice interdisciplinary team bears responsibility for designating the care necessary (see Exhibit 73–1).

The beneficiary elects the benefit and chooses to receive care from a hospice rather than from the standard Medicare program. The care provided by a certified hospice provider is comprehensive and includes full-scope interdisciplinary home care services, hospitalization related to the terminal illness, respite care and continuous care in the home on a short-term basis, durable medical equipment, and pharmaceuticals. The beneficiary does not pay for services related to the terminal illness, except a small copayment for outpatient medications.

The patient's attending physician and the hospice physician are required to certify that the patient is terminally ill. The certification must take place within 48 hours of the patient's admission to the hospice program. Admission does not occur until the patient has signed the election of the Hospice Benefit. This unique provision demands that a physician make a definitive statement with regard to the patient's prognosis. Physicians may be reluctant to certify such a speculative prediction, and accordingly, the resources of the hospice program may not be applied early enough to be effective in assisting the patient and family.

Exhibit 73–1 Medicare Hospice Benefit

The Tax Equity and Fiscal Responsibility Act of 1983 (TEFRA) enacted the Medicare Hospice Benefit, specifically designed to reimburse for care of terminally ill patients and their families through care provided by a core interdisciplinary team coordinated by a hospice provider as case manager.

Entitlement-Eligibility Requirements:

1. Physician Certification of six months or less prognosis
2. Patient Election of Medicare Hospice Benefit
3. Medicare Part A Coverage

Core Services Required of All Medicare-Certified Hospices:

1. Physician
2. Nursing
3. Social Services
4. Counseling (Bereavement and Pastoral)

Other Hospice Services Available Include:

1. Inpatient General Care
2. Respite Care
3. Physical, Speech, and Occupational Therapies
4. Homemaker/Home Health Aides
5. Medical Equipment
6. Medical Supplies
7. Drugs/Pharmaceuticals
8. Continuous 24-hour Coverage

Reimbursement:

1. Payment for hospice services is on the basis of all-inclusive inpatient or home care per diems, with physician services being reimbursed separately.
2. Deductibles do not apply.
3. Co-insurance is limited to 5% (up to $5.00) maximum on drugs related to the terminal illness.

Managed Care Financing

While the great majority of hospice patients (usually 80 percent) are Medicare eligibles covered by traditional Medicare, the remainder of privately insured patients under age 65 are increasingly covered by health maintenance organizations (HMOs) and other managed care networks. Historically, services to such patients were reimbursed on a fee for service basis. As managed care networks have increased, reimbursement has shifted to per diem, both for home care and inpatient care. More recently, capitation has entered the scene as a method of financing care. Capitation involves a spreading of the total cost of care (average total cost per patient times the expected number of patients in a year) across the total membership of the HMO or managed care network. Capitation involves financial risk and care must be carefully managed.

The significance of the national movement to managed care is that it not only affects private insurance patients, but, increasingly, also includes the Medicaid population in each state and Medicare-eligible patients.

The acute needs of patients and families in the last weeks of life are evidenced by the consumption of Medicare dollars in the days preceding death (Figure 73–1) and can be addressed by hospice programs in a manner that conserves Medicare dollars by emphasizing home care over less appropriate and more costly acute inpatient care.

Care of the Patient

Hospice care should be regarded and administered as a specialty within the context of home health care. It is, in a sense, the "intensive care" of home care. Given the acuity of needs, physical and emotional, experienced by patients and their families, a considerable level of services and intervention is required.[4]

The emphasis that the hospice concept places on home care facilitates cost contain-

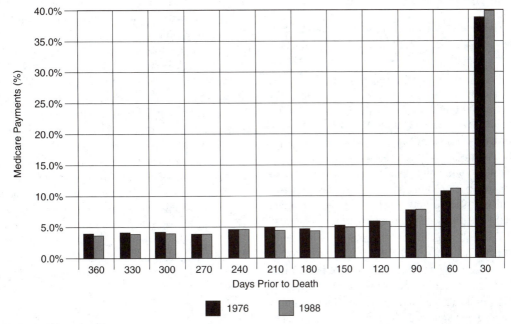

Figure 73–1 Distribution of Medicare Payments in the Last Year of Life. *Source*: "Trends in Medicare Payments in The Last Year of Life," James D. Lubitz, M.P.H., and Gerald F. Riley, M.P.H., *New England Journal of Medicine*, April 15, 1996.

ment without sacrificing quality of services. *Hospice care is offered regardless of ability to pay.* Accordingly, most hospice programs rely on contributions to supplement reimbursement. The high utilization of volunteers and the availability of integrated home care and inpatient services en-sure further continuity of care and cost control.

When one looks at the life continuum, birth is a critical event that changes a family. Likewise, terminal illness also dramatically impacts the family structure. Family members are encouraged and educated to be part of the caregiving team. The hospice care team formally acknowledges and incorporates patient and family teaching, counseling, and support.

Professional and lay volunteers augment the work of paid staff and greatly enhance the quality of services to hospice patients. Volunteers participate in all aspects of patient care and contribute at the interdisciplinary team meeting.

The services of hospice professional staff are supplemented in many programs by the use of contracted services for home health aides, physical therapy, speech therapy, and occupational therapy. The expanded staff available through contracted services enhances the core services of hospice that focus on skilled nursing care, counseling services provided by a social worker, care by a physician, pastoral care services, consulting dietary, and pharmacological services. Continuous care, i.e., around-the-clock skilled nursing care in the home, is available to patients and families for a limited time to address intensive needs of the patient/family. Home respite care, while not formally recognized under the Hospice Benefit, is an alternative to inpatient respite care and is designed to relieve the family and enable them to continue their caregiving role for the patient after a brief time away from their patient care responsibilities. Each family receives bereavement counseling and follow-up for a full year after the patient's death.

TRENDS IN HOSPICE CARE

Hospice care is continuously changing, consistent with changes in home care as well as the whole health care delivery system. The traditional concepts of care for the "terminally ill" have evolved to a proactive role for palliative and supportive care, especially to include those patients who wish to continue active treatment for their disease. A hospice model that includes the patient's physician, the acute care provider, and the community hospice team is essential to achieving care delivery that is full-scope and holistic. Accordingly, hospices have responded to the need to accept more "high-tech" patients.

Technological advances, such as video telecommunication via computer, permits professional caregivers to be "close to" the patient in a time of need and create a milieu for the patient and family to feel safe at home. Such systems connect decision making regarding patient care, symptom management, and ongoing evaluation. Hospice programs have enhanced their telecommunication capabilities. For the professional caregiver and also for the consumer, Internet communication offers the latest information on educational opportunities regarding hospice and hospice care.

Recently, a palliative care *International Classification of Diseases, Ninth Edition* (ICD-9) code has been established for selected hospitals to trial. This effort is seen as a possible precedent for a special palliative care DRG that would provide reimbursement for care that hospitals provide to their terminally ill patients. It remains to be seen whether the Health Care Financing Administration will establish such a DRG or whether the reimbursement will be in addition to or a replacement of other DRG reimbursement. Nevertheless, this development is another indication of the growing importance and recognition of essential care provided at the end of life.

Managed Care Organizations

Many hospices were initiated as community-based, specialized programs that broadened the array of services offered by home health agencies. Hospices are increasingly participating in the networks and coalitions that characterize the era of managed care. One of the key elements for financial survival of hospices during this extraordinary period of cost containment is the formation of strong relationships with managed care providers and provider networks who currently serve the non-Medicare populations. Understanding the uniqueness of the hospice population is difficult for many HMO case managers, not only for hospice-appropriate cancer populations, but also for those noncancer populations that may have a less predictable course of illness. There is an increasing need to define clinical pathways for these populations in order to assess the appropriateness for referral based on defined, objective clinical findings.

Challenges

As indicated in the introduction to this chapter, the central challenge to the hospice movement is to redefine hospice care, making it part of the mainstream of health care as opposed to a free-standing alternative.

A model approach to care of persons with irreversible illness and their families has been developed by The Connecticut Hospice, Inc. and is currently under trial in the state of Connecticut. The project, called "Advanced Care," employs nurse case managers who initiate contact with patients and families at an early, appropriate point in the course of disease progression, identified in the list of criteria at the end of this chapter. HMO case managers, physicians, and other caregivers use these criteria to determine the appropriate time to initiate contact and/or needed care from the hospice nurse case managers. It is important to note that the patient need not elect palliative care as a replacement for aggressive care, and active therapy may continue. While such care continues, the hospice nurse manager provides essential support and counseling and also arranges for any palliative care that may be required. Over time, as the disease and related care progress, informed decisions may be made, for example, to forgo an additional course of aggressive treatment in favor of palliative care that makes it possible to remain at home, close to family and friends.

The program is financed via capitation, that is, a managed care network payment per member per month to ensure complete coverage for an expected number of persons requiring end of life care. The care includes not only care at home or in a specialized hospice inpatient program, but also any needed community hospitalizations or emergency department use that is related to the terminal illness.

The "advanced care" is therefore not an alternative to active therapy, but rather, represents an integrated continuum of care with a blending of active treatment and palliative care. The capitation financing mechanism is used as an incentive to ensure that appropriate patients are referred as soon as they are identified by the managed caregivers.

Across the nation, many hospice programs are leading the effort to transform traditional hospice care, making it more relevant and responsive to today's advances in medicine and technology and seeking to more fully integrate the principles of quality hospice care into the mainstream of the health care delivery system.

Hospice care in the year 1999 will be 25 years young; the first quarter of the 21st century promises to be an exciting time in the maturation of this newest specialized health care delivery system.

NOTES

1. The first American hospice, The Connecticut Hospice, Inc., was incorporated in 1971, initiated hospice home care in 1974, and functions as a free-standing hospice program with full scope of hospice care provided at home, in a specially designed 52-bed inpatient setting and in a residential "cottage" program. The Connecticut Hospice is the nation's preeminent teaching hospice and serves as a clinical model for replication as well as a "laboratory" for hospice training and research.

2. Of 2.2 million deaths in the U.S. in 1994, an estimated 555,000 were hospice-eligible (U.S. Bureau of Census).

3. A recent study of over 4,000 dying patients in major teaching hospitals showed that 38 percent spent 10 days or more in an ICU and 50 percent reported moderate to severe pain more than half the time during their last three days of life (1995).

4. Severity of illness of hospice patients is reflected in the fact that hospice inpatients are in the 92nd percentile of patients serviced by all hospitals in the U.S. (Hurzeler, Barnum, & Abbott).

REFERENCES

Journal of the American Medical Association. 1995; 224(20).

Hurzeler, J.H., Barnum, E.A., & Abbott, J. (Date). Hospice: The beginning or the end?: The impact of TEFRA on hospice care in the U.S. *University of Bridgeport Law Review,* 5(1).

Joint Commission on Accreditation of Health Care Organizations. (1994). *1995 Accreditation manual for home care.* Oakbrook Terrace, IL: Joint Commission.

U.S. Bureau of Census. Statistical Abstract of U.S. National Health Statistics: Estimate based on percentages of contained disease.

Summary Guidelines for Initiation of Advanced Care

Advanced Care, Inc.
Developed by Catherine Sumpio, RN, MSN

Disease Category	Refer to Advanced Care Upon			
	Initial Diagnosis	**Recurrence**	**Progression**	**Critical Clinical Decision**
Cancer				
Brain/CNS Tumors	•			
Breast			• 2	
Colorectal			• 2	
Esophagus		• 1		
Gallbladder	•			
Head and Neck		• 1		
Leukemia			• 2	
Liver	•			
Lung		• 1		
Lung-inoperable	•			
Melanoma			• 2	
Ovarian-inoperable	•			
Ovarian/GYN			• 2	
Pancreatic	•			
Prostate/GU			• 2	
Renal		• 1		
Sarcoma			• 2	
Stomach		• 1		
End-Stage Diseases				
Neurological:				
Alzheimer's Disease			• 3	
ALS			• 4	
CVA				• 5
MS				• 4
Congenital, Infectious, or Traumatic Disability				• 6
Heart Failure			• 7	
Lung-COPD			• 8	
Liver Failure			• 9	
Kidney Failure				• 10
AIDS			• 11	

Important Note on These Guidelines
The footnotes on the following page are an integral part of these guidelines. They must be read in conjunction with the matrix above.

© Copyright, July 1996, The Connecticut Hospice, Inc.

Advanced Care, Inc.
FOOTNOTES TO SUMMARY GUIDELINES

(These footnotes are an integral part of the matrix presented on the previous page.)

Definitions

Initial Diagnosis	The first diagnosis of disease by a physician.
Recurrence	Subsequent diagnosis of same disease resulting from limited response to additional therapy expected and not durable.
Progression	Continuation of disease process.
Critical Clinical Decision	Consensus decision made by physician, patient, and family that want to forgo any continuing curative or rehabilitative treatment.

Footnotes

1. Limited response to additional therapy expected and not durable.
2. First-line salvage therapies have failed. Less than 20% response to second-line or other therapy expected and not durable.
3. Eementia beyond Stage 7 of the Functional Assessment Staging Scale for Alzheimer's Disease or Multi-Infarct Type. Optimal therapy reached (i.e. no further response to therapies expected), with major symptoms present and declining functional status (Karnofsky <50% and when there is partial or total dependence in ADLs).
4. Progressive nerve degeneration with resultant partial/total paresis or paralysis of extremities and muscles of respiration. Optimal therapy reached (i.e., no further response to therapies expected), with major symptoms present and declining functional status (Karnofsky <50% and when there is partial or total dependence in ADLs).
5. Massive CVA with no rehabilitation potential; patient unable to eat. Optimal therapy reached (i.e., no further response to therapies expected), with major symptoms present and declining functional status (Karnofsky <50% and when there is partial or total dependence in ADLs).
6. Congenital defects, complication of infections, or trauma based upon individual case review.
7. Long-standing history of congestive heart failure or multiple Ml. Class IV NY Heart Association symptoms and ejection fraction <20%. No further responses expected to medical therapy and no options for CABG, grafting, angioplasty, pacemaker, or transplant. Any one of the following: dyspnea, angina, othopnea, edema. Any two of the following: Karnofsky <50%, minimal activity tolerance, dependence on 2 or more ADLs.
8. Degradation of PFTs: FEV1 after bronchodilator <30% of predicted, decrease in FEV1 on yearly serial testing of >40 ml/year, Cor Pulmonale, Hypoxemia, significant CO_2 retention as measured by ABGs. Optimal therapy reached with multiple bronchodilators and steroid dependence with dyspnea (of any kind) and O_2 dependence. Declining functional status including Karnofsky <50%, chairbound, minimal activity tolerance, and dependence on two or more ADLs.
9. Worsening LFTs and documented evidence of disease (utilizing abdominal ultrasound, CT, HIDA Scan, Cholangiography, ERCP, or any appropriate diagnostic imaging demonstrating biliary obstruction), hepatic vein occlusion, hepatic artery thrombosis, hepatocellular dysfunction. No expectation of success from medical management and/or surgical intervention. Presence of any one major symptom and declining functional status (Karnofsky <50% and dependence on 2 or more ADLs).
10. Decision made to stop dialysis with one of the following conditions: chronic dialysis necessary to sustain life, disease progression despite interventions, intolerable associated medical complications of non-renal disease. In addition, at least one of the following: peripheral vascular disease degradation, hypotension, dementia, depression, resistance to dialysis Rx; and, declining functional status.
11. CD4 <50 with concurrent ongoing major infections, and the presence of at least one of the following: lymphoma, Kaposi's Sarcoma, PML, HIV encephalopathy, HIV wasting syndrome. Progression of disease on antiretroviral therapy and the presence of major symptoms with declining functional status.

PART **X**

The Future of Home Care

CHAPTER 74

Electronic Home Visits To Improve Care and Decrease Costs

Ilene Warner and Alexander S. Beller

THE HISTORY OF TELEMEDICINE

Some 30 years have passed since the first practical use of telemedicine in the U.S. was introduced in the health care field (Weissert & Silberman, 1996). During this event in 1962, the Nebraska Psychiatric Institute in Omaha was linked to the Norfolk Hospital in order to provide a psychiatric consultation between physicians. Telemedicine remained primarily a physician-to-physician service until the mid-1990s, when advances in technology provided other disciplines with the means of communicating with patients over these systems.

The term "telemedicine" has evolved over the past three decades. Perhaps the most inclusive definition is "the use of advanced telecommunications technologies to exchange health information and provide health care services across geographic, time and social/cultural borders" (Reid, 1996). Over the years, telemedicine grew as a result of federal funding for research and development. Although telemedicine programs encompass the specialty areas in medicine such as dermatology and psychiatry, teleradiology is the most common form of service provided by these systems. The primary benefit to date of telemedicine has been in improving access to health care providers by patients, particularly in rural areas. In these cases, specialists are frequently called upon to assist in the diagnosis and treatment of patients under the care of a primary physician.

"Telehealth" describes interactive telecommunications activities occurring directly between health care providers and their patients. Telehealth is defined as "systems to support the health care process by providing a means for more effective and more efficient information exchange" (Bennett, Rappaport, & Skinner, 1978). Telehealth moves away from the traditional diagnostic approach of telemedicine and, using the principle of increasing patient access, utilizes a system that allows for remote communication. Telehealth home care is a developing field that has been influenced by the availability of new technologies, market forces, plans in the shift in reimbursement by the federal government, the increased presence of health maintenance organizations (HMOs) as payers, the increasing aged population, and the supply of skilled nurses, physical therapists, occupational therapists, speech therapists, and medical social workers. These systems are designed to improve the delivery of care to patients by reducing travel time of nurses, therapists, and social workers as well as addressing issues of redundancy of documentation. They are intended to improve patient compliance with medications and treatments through a system that reminds and notifies patients of their scheduled activities. Finally, patient education and retention of information should be enhanced with a multimedia patient library resident in the patient's station. This library provides the patient with readily accessible information pertaining to a particular diagnosis.

The benefit of telehealth systems to home care agencies is to improve care quality and control costs. It will also improve the mechanisms by which health professionals can share health-related information with patients in such a way as to enhance their independence and knowledge in the management of their disease processes.

THE DESIGN OF TELEHEALTH SYSTEMS

Telehealth utilizes electronic visits to communicate from the patient to the nurse and from the nurse to the patient. The video and audio portions are delivered simultaneously, allowing the patient to actually see the nurse demonstrate a procedure or provide instruction. Some systems are designed to run over the cable television network into the home; others use wideband networks. Recent telehealth system announcements incorporate technological advances in data compression and computer modems enabling audio, video, and data to be simultaneously transmitted over a standard home telephone line or POTS (plain old telephone service). Since the majority of Americans have a basic telephone in their homes, telehealth systems can be plugged into their existing phone lines, allowing for remote access to nurses in a central location, such as the home health agency. High-resolution interactive video images allow the nurse to remotely assess the patient. Select images can be captured and stored to provide a record of a wound or condition of an infusion site. The patient's display should provide an adequate image size to deal with visual impairments.

Optimally, the patient's telehealth station should be ergonomically designed to require minimal operational and cognitive skills. The new patient stations should interact with the patient, informing, guiding, and instructing the patient through all procedures.

Many telehealth systems provide a means of creating a progress note and printing it for use in the clinical chart. Other systems directly integrate with proprietary software systems. The video visit is recorded in its entirety, allowing agencies to store and retrieve the visit. This can be critical when an agency is requested to provide documentation for third-party payers, legal inquiries, to provide intra-agency training, or to ensure compliance with the agency's standards of care.

SCOPE OF TELEHEALTH ACTIVITIES

Telehealth systems provide home health agencies with the ability to collect vital sign data from patients over a 24-hour or longer period. The patient is taught how to obtain blood pressure, pulse, and thermometer measurements. While on-line with the patient, the nurse can direct the placement of the stethoscope in order to auscultate heart, lung, and bowel sounds. Since the nurse can obtain a set of vital signs at any time, data can be collected to monitor a patient at preset intervals or when the patient feels weak, dizzy, or is experiencing other symptoms. In the case of a cardiac patient, the nurse can have the patient's station instruct the patient to take vital signs at specific intervals. The nurse can now determine the effectiveness of the medication regime, as well as detect orthostatic hypotension as a consequence of the medications.

A well-designed system provides an electronic reminder capability, through voice prompts, text messages, and graphics, to discipline medication compliance and inform of treatments, diet, exercise, and the scheduling of agency personnel in the home. Since noncompliance with drug therapy occurs in about 40% of the elderly population, attention to improving medication compliance can have a significant impact on long-term care placement and hospital readmission rates. The *Merck Manual of Geriatrics* (1995) further notes that up to 35%

of noncompliant older patients may experience some degree of health-related problems stemming from omissions or commissions in medication administration. In one study cited, 11% of all hospital admissions by the elderly were directly related to medication noncompliance issues. Providing patients with visual and audio reminders of what medication to take and when to take it can be a vital tool for the home health care agency.

A critical component of a telehealth system is the quality and number of educational modules in the patient station library to improve a patient's ability to self-learn health-related information as well as to improve the retention of this information. Modules should use a variety of text, illustration, and diagrams in audio, video, or a combination of these media to help the patient achieve mastery of the subject. For example, newly diagnosed insulin-dependent diabetics may need to view a video module on insulin preparation technique or insulin administration repeatedly until they feel confident enough to fill the syringe and inject independent of the nurse. Menus for a calculated diabetic diet can be reviewed, with sample menus made available on the system. Agency-specific policies for teaching can be incorporated into the system, allowing for improved compliance.

THE DELIVERY OF NURSING CARE

The primary focus of telehealth is to provide improved access and communication between the nurse and patient. Through a combination of physical visits and telehealth visits, a nurse can collect vital sign data, provide an electronic medication/treatment schedule, and provide general as well as specific teaching interventions for a particular patient. The number of physical visits that can be replaced with telehealth visits will largely be dependent on factors such as the patient's stability and ability to independ-ently interact with the system, and the primary diagnosis for which the patient is receiving home care services. For example, a patient with hypertension who is being seen because of a change in medications can receive the majority of his/her visits via the telehealth system. Visits will include gathering vital sign data multiple times during the day, providing an electronic medication schedule, as well as educating the patient concerning the disease process, specific medication use and side effect information, diet, exercise, and signs and symptoms to report to the nurse or physician. On the other hand, patients who require more "hands on" skilled visits for pressure ulcers, postoperative wound care, injections, or catheterizations are likely to require more physical visits and fewer telehealth visits. For these patients, electronic visits may be most beneficial in reinforcing patient or caregiver instructions or observing their return demonstration technique. If a catheter was to leak or become blocked, the nurse could demonstrate irrigation technique over the system, provide the patient station with a video clip of the process, or observe the patient's or caregiver's method of irrigation.

Home health aide supervision may be greatly enhanced by telehealth through the use of video visits when aides are providing care. Revisions in the home health aide plan of care can be made more frequently in the presence of the aide when changes in the needs of the patient become evident.

THE DELIVERY OF ANCILLARY SERVICES

Of all the therapies commonly provided by home health agencies, speech therapy has the greatest number of applications in the home care field. Interventions for dysarthria and dysphasia can be accomplished through the use of remote interventions between the therapist and the patient, replacing some of the physical visits with telehealth visits. To a lesser extent, physical and occupational therapies can be performed electronically, particularly after patients have had sufficient instruction in therapeutic exercise or specific techniques.

The impact of telehealth upon the practice of medical social work in the home will be significant in terms of enhancing the practitioner's ability to assess and meet the emotional and social needs related to the patient's health care issues. In particular, telehealth systems can increase the frequency of social work–patient counseling interactions in order to address specific issues such as depression, noncompliance, and isolation. The ability to identify client needs with reference to access issues such as transportation, rebates, and entitlement programs without making multiple visits to the home can enhance the quality of the services provided to the patient.

Additionally, telehealth can be used to link nursing, therapies, social services, home health aides, and administrative personnel in order to make grand rounds. The nurse, as the primary manager of the patient's care, can electronically meet with other members of the team in order to ensure that the goals of the patient are being met, the aide has sufficient instruction, and the care plan is kept up to date.

AGENCY CONFIGURATION

Home health agencies have two main options when launching telehealth as an adjunct to making physical visits. One alternative designates specific staff as "telehealth nurses." These staff members would make all of the telehealth calls for the patients served by the agency, with the primary nurses making the physical visits. Using this method, the agency could maximize the number of electronic calls made during the day; however, some degree of continuity might be sacrificed. The other option utilizes the primary nurse to make a blend of physical visits and telehealth calls. Using this scenario, the primary nurse maintains continuity with the patient; however, scheduling of both physical and telehealth visits becomes more complex. Agency administrators will need to take into account the number of patients receiving both physical and electronic visits, the distribution and availability of nursing staff in specific geographic areas, the number of patients who need to receive very early morning visits for insulin

preparation/administration, and the schedule of home health aide supervisory visits in order to determine the best use of nursing personnel and telehealth systems.

UTILIZATION BY DIAGNOSIS

Many of the diagnoses that are commonly seen in home health patients—hypertension, congestive heart failure, chronic obstructive pulmonary disease, diabetes, and coronary artery disease—require nurses to closely monitor vital signs and provide an assessment of the patient's status. Medication compliance and teaching are often key elements of skilled nursing interventions that can be accomplished by the use of electronic visits. Hospice patients and their families may benefit greatly from the use of telehealth systems in order to provide ongoing support, counseling, and teaching of medication changes, particularly as the condition of the patient declines. Agencies who experience high volumes of phone calls made after normal business hours may note a high proportion of these calls are from the families of hospice patients who are in need of reassurance or guidance from hospice professionals that can often be handled effectively using electronic means.

PATIENT SELECTION PROCESS

Patients who receive home care in the 1990s are certain to be less knowledgeable than subsequent generations of patients. The use of technology, for a majority of the population, is likely to be met with skepticism or apprehension. This can be diminished by examining who is the best candidate for the use of a telemedicine system. The patient must have sufficient hearing, vision, and physical dexterity as well as cognitive function in order to interact with the system.

For the newest systems the patient's standard telephone line is all that might be required. For cable and other network-dependent systems the patient must have accessibility to the required communication link. It has been noted that a patient who is capable of using a television remote controller should be able to effectively utilize the system.

In a study conducted in 1995, a group of 12 patients were provided with telehealth systems in addition to traditional home health care visits (Lenz & Mahmud, 1995). All 12 patients were able to successfully interact with the system, and there was a reduction in the number of physical visits required to meet the needs of 7 of the patients, resulting in a 58% decrease in the number of physical visits. While physical visits should be decreased through the use of telehealth, the actual number of interactions is likely to increase. Patients should be introduced to the use of electronic visits as a means of being able to capture vital sign data more frequently, being reminded when to take medications, and accessing educational modules using a number of media. Finally, it should be emphasized to patients that they will have increased autonomy through the use of telehealth, enabling them to gain the knowledge necessary for independence in their care.

QUALITY OF CARE ISSUES

One of the primary ways telehealth will enhance the quality of care for home health patients is to expand the "slice of life" usually obtained during a nursing visit. Instead of a physical visit providing data and interactions two or three times per week, the electronic visit can supply data on the vital signs throughout the day and can furnish nurses with the tools to assess the patient more frequently. The combination of physical and telehealth visits will assist nurses in meeting outcome objectives such as achieving stability of vital signs, having the patient be knowledgeable and compliant with medication regimes, and having the patient be able to verbalize information about disease processes and signs and symptoms to report prior to discharge.

In a study by Arthur D. Little, Inc., in 1992, telecommunications was seen as a method of enhancing care by reducing unnecessary emer-gency room visits, reducing unnecessary/unscheduled physician office visits, providing early intervention/prevention of repeat hospitalizations, and educating the patient in terms of early symptom management through a link to medical information. The role of telehealth in preventing rehospitalization, reducing readmissions to the agency, and preventing or delaying nursing home placement is yet to be fully researched; however, by the very nature of electronic visits, early symptoms and vital sign trends can be analyzed with interventions established.

The need for patient teaching and the amount of time nurses spend in providing instruction is substantial in the home care setting. The problem of literacy remains a issue, primarily for an elderly population of people whose education may have been cut short because of the war or family obligations. A recent study noted that 22.0–61.7% of participants had inadequate or marginal abilities to understand health information presented in a written format (Williams, Parker, Baker, et al., 1995). Since most patient teaching in the home has traditionally relied on the written word, telehealth systems will address these information and teaching issues using multimedia communications. The telehealth system informs the patient using a combination of selected video demonstrations, custom graphics, text messages, and audio.

LEGAL IMPLICATIONS

The legal dimensions of telehealth primarily center on the consequences for risk management generally and for professional malpractice specifically. The elements that compose the telehealth system and how these affect the scope of legal liability are of critical concern. The essential requirements for establishing malpractice are: 1) establishing a duty to care based on the patient–health professional relationship (evidenced by the agreement of the agency to accept the patient for services as well as the signed consent by the patient), 2) demonstration of a breach of that duty in terms of a violation of the standard of care, 3) showing of injury following the breach of the duty, and 4) evidence of a causal connection between the violation of the standard of care and the injury. All four requirements must be satisfied in order to effectively establish a legal basis for malpractice.

Legal liability for telehealth will be evaluated in relation to criteria similar to those used for any nurse–patient interaction, namely, how nurses perform their roles in accordance with agency policies, the state nurse practice act, and the standards of care of the industry. Although the telehealth system may augment the care provided by physical nursing visits, the added dimension of electronic visits introduces new types of information sharing and professional decision making. This enlarged scope will have a direct impact on agency policies.

Telehealth systems may potentially limit liability through their ability to ensure frequent communication between the nurse and the patient, a condition that enhances the nurse's capacity to monitor patient activity and provide interventions as warranted. The documentation of the patient's compliance with medications and treatments will likely be enhanced, and this can be used to demonstrate the degree to which the patient is able to participate in the detection of the signs and symptoms of the disease process as well as the intervention process to address these symptoms. Moreover, since telehealth visits provide the agency with an electronic record of the visit, administrators will be able to retrieve the visit record to justify the nurse's actions if legal questions arise.

Another aspect of the legal dimension of telehealth systems is that of privacy and confidentiality of the patient record—matters of concern to home health agencies, patients, and third-party payers. Electronic files may be secured through the use of passwords that authorize an agency to provide home care for the patient. These passwords can be changed regularly by administration in order to ensure the continued confidentiality of records. The same types of patient releases that are used to authorize an agency to provide home care for the patient can

be expanded to include the use of electronic visits, photographs, videotape, and other means to produce information regarding the patient's health status.

The legal rules governing the nurse–patient interaction remain the same for both physical and electronic visits. The requirements for malpractice and for safeguarding patient privacy remain constant across both physical and electronic visits. The critical difference is to be found not in the scope of the legal requirements but rather in the nature of the telehealth system, which introduces new levels of nurse–patient interactions and thereby influences professional decision making. It should be noted that improved recordkeeping, the documentation of all critical interventions, a record of patient compliance with medications and treatments, as well as the ability to note trends in collected data has the potential to positively affect the delivery of patient care, thus decreasing malpractice risk.

REIMBURSEMENT AND COST ISSUES

As we move closer to a prospective payment system (PPS), home health agencies will determine how best to position themselves in order to provide quality care, achieve outcomes, and control costs. Currently, telehealth systems are available at daily estimated costs ranging from $10 to $40. It is likely that basic telehealth systems may realize price reductions as the cost of cameras, modems, and software becomes more affordable. Proprietary telehealth companies may offer patient and nursing units equipment through rental/lease as well as purchase agreements.

Medicare currently does not reimburse for telehealth for home care visits, however HMOs that are under contract with home care agencies to provide care for patients using a specific dollar reimbursement may find the use of telehealth an attractive adjunct to physical visits. It is likely that managed care will take the lead in the health care arena as the impetus for the development of electronic patient systems. For example, if an agency authorizes a home care nurse to make seven visits to a diabetic patient, the nurse may find intermittent electronic visits with the patient between physical visits allow the nurse to gather more data over a longer period of time. This may allow the nurse to do more frequent interactions and improved teaching in order to ensure the stability of the patient and the attainment of education prior to discharge from home care. The management of a complex patient over a limited amount of visits becomes enhanced through the use of telehealth systems.

THE FUTURE OF TELEHEALTH FOR HOME CARE

The combination of advanced technology, the growth of the home health care market, and the need for cost-effective means of patient care will promulgate telehealth systems for home health care. Additional future remote capabilities of telehealth systems will likely include glucometers, pulse oxymetry, electrocardiographs (EKGs), and other sensors that will aid in the early detection of symptoms. Advances in home communication links should allow for full motion video and simultaneous high-resolution images. Patients will interact with nurses with image and voice quality similar to that of home television.

The acceptance of electronic visits will be dependent upon the quality of care promised versus the quality of care delivered, the ease of use by both patients and health care providers, the continued development of appropriate technologies designed to enhance the effectiveness and efficiency of providers, and the production of training for health care professions in the use of these systems. As nurses become more comfortable with the infusion of technology, patient acceptance is likely to follow. Telehealth systems hold promise as a means of improving the delivery of care to patients in their homes, whether for short periods of illness or for the ongoing management of disease processes.

REFERENCES

Bennett, A.M., Rappaport, W.H., & Skinner, E.L. (1978). *Telehealth handbook.* Bethesda, MD: U.S. Department of Health, Education and Welfare.

Lenz, J., & Mahmud, K. (1995). The personal telemedicine system: A new tool for the delivery of health care. *Journal of Telemedicine and Telecare,* 1(1), 15–20.

Merck manual of geriatrics. (1995). *2nd Ed.* Philadelphia.

Reid, J. (1996). *A telemedicine primer: Understanding the issues.* Billings, MT: Artcraft Printers.

Telecommunications: Can it help solve America's health care problems? Cambridge Reference 91810-98:A3-A9; Arthur D. Little, Inc., 1992.

Weissert, W.G., & Silberman, S. (1996). Health care on the information highway: The politics of telemedicine. *Telemedicine Journal,* 2(1), 1–15.

Williams, M.V., Parker, R.M., Baker, D.W., et al. (1995). Inadequate functional health literacy among patients at two public hospitals. *JAMA, 274,* 1677–1682.

CHAPTER 75

Using the Internet for Home Health and Hospice Care

Susan M. Sparks

Home health and hospice professionals are taking advantage of the unique communications opportunities afforded by the Internet, a web of computer networks that exchange and transmit data and information. The Internet is one major technology of several that are popularly referred to as the "information superhighway."

Until recently, the Internet has been used by health professionals primarily as a means of personal communication (e-mail) and to disseminate traditional text and graphics electronically. Some health professionals are beginning to take advantage of the Internet for the rapid transmission and distribution of information that includes sounds, and still and motion images in addition to text to their colleagues, patients, and the public.

The current functionality afforded by the Internet could be useful to home health and hospice professionals in the diagnosis, control, and management of conditions of patients and families in their care. The following are examples of Internet applications; some are already in use, and some are yet to be developed:

- To disseminate information about etiology and prevention interventions, especially for conditions such as urinary tract infections and urinary incontinence.
- To identify and diagnose diseases. Pictures of patient signs and symptoms, of radiological studies, or of pathological slides can be transmitted to or from anywhere in the Internet-accessible world. Activities such as telediagnosis can provide rare diagnostic expertise nearly instantaneously in even the most remote parts of the globe.
- To facilitate collaboration. Joint consultations, diagnostic and treatment plans, clinical trials data, and manuscripts for publication (either electronic or in print) are some of the activities that could be accomplished relatively easily using the Internet. Patients and families might also collaborate with home health nurses and other health care providers. They might also collaborate with others with a specific condition or disease, such as people having spinal cord injuries, perhaps in an electronic support group, over the Internet. Synchronous or asynchronous virtual conferences could be substituted for some traditional face-to-face conferences.
- To deliver care to patients in their homes or hospice. For example, patients and their families could be taught appropriate range of motion exercises, enterostomal care, or urinary catheterization using the Internet. A "virtual" home visit could be conducted. Using Internet technologies yet to be developed, studies using scopes and pressure measurements could be performed

Note: This chapter was developed in the public domain. No copyright applies.

and administered providing care to patients at a distance (i.e., telepractice).

- To provide rapid and large-scale dissemination of information. Health professional, patient, and public education about nearly any aspect of home health or hospice care, such as prevention of tuberculosis and other common secondary infections, can easily be done using Internet technologies.

JUST WHAT IS THE INTERNET?

Computers on the Internet are of various sizes and may be connected with each other by relatively expensive high-capacity fiber optics, telephone lines, and satellites. The Internet is global, although many third-world nations do not yet have access. However, should access become necessary in a situation, such as it was in the recent Ebola outbreak in Kikwit, Zaire, portable satellite phones and cellular technologies can be added to enable connectivity.

Internet connectivity is obtained via an Internet service provider (ISP), roughly analogous to a long-distance telephone service provider. Many educational and health care institutions give Internet access to faculty, staff, and students. In addition or instead there are other ISPs. Some are nationally accessible value-added ISPs such as CompuServe, America Online, and Prodigy. They primarily serve up a wide range of information, opinion, and products. They also provide some access to the Internet. Other ISPs may be national, regional, or local. Their primary purpose is to provide access to the Internet. Detailed information about thousands of ISPs and their direct access is available at http://www.thelist.com.

At least five types of Internet communication are supported. These are e-mail, file transfer protocol, telnet, Gopher, and the World Wide Web. All, except e-mail, require software specific to that kind of communication application. Some types of communication require that the address be in capital and lowercase letters. To avoid addressing inaccuracies, type or enter electronic addresses in exactly the form given.

E-mail

Everyone who has Internet access has electronic mail (e-mail). This means that to reach the largest number of people around the Internet world, e-mail is the Internet communication mode that should be used. E-mail can be used for memoranda or letter-type communications and short manuscripts. At this time e-mail supports text but no true graphics. E-mail can be exchanged one-to-one and one-to-several individuals.

There are more formalized applications of e-mail technologies, such as LISTSERVs and newsgroups. LISTSERVs are mailing lists of people who are interested in a specific topic. Some LISTSERVs have a handful of subscribers others have thousands. One e-mail message sent to a LISTSERV is distributed to the e-mail addresses of all subscribers. It is possible to identify subscribers to a LISTSERV. Newsgroups are e-mail postings, such as to a bulletin board, where interested people connect to share and exchange similar information. One newsgroup that carries messages related to home health care is sci.med.telemedicine. Individuals must connect with newsgroups purposely. And, unless a person leaves a message, it is impossible to know who is participating in the newsgroup. Newsgroups are public, meaning that anyone can participate. LISTSERVs may be public or private, allowing only certain people to subscribe, such as only the students in a home health nursing continuing education course.

There is a LISTSERV for the informational needs of home care and hospice nurses, HCARENURS. HCARENURS is designed to provide a place for discussion of issues pertinent to home care and hospice nursing including clinical issues, ethical concerns, and items related to home health nursing that differ from agency to agency.

To subscribe, follow the instructions below:

To subscribe, send an e-mail message
TO: MAJORDOMO@PO.CWRU.EDU
SUBJECT: (leave this line blank)

In the body of the message, type *only*:

subscribe hcarenurs (your e-mail address)

You might be interested in research-funding interests of several institutes of the National Institutes of Health (NIH). If so, it could be helpful to subscribe to the NIH (National Institutes of Health) Guide to Grants and Contracts via LISTSERV. Instructions for subscribing are given below:

The National Institutes of Health Guide to Grants & Contracts is a READ-ONLY LIST. To subscribe, send e-mail
TO: LISTSERV@LIST.NIH.GOV
SUBJECT: (leave this line blank)

In the body of the message, type only:
subscribe NIHGDE-L (Yourfirstname Yourlastname)

File Transfer Protocol

Another type of Internet communication, requiring special software, is file transfer protocol (FTP). Relatively large text documents may exceed e-mail capacity. To share these larger text documents and files that run computer programs, such as computer-assisted instruction software, FTP can be used. The file to be transferred is placed in a special computer directory. The intended file recipient(s) are notified of the file name, directory location, and any special passwords necessary to obtain the file. The intended recipient(s) access the host computer and the directory to electronically get the file themselves.

For example, you might be interested in obtaining any of the several Agency for Health Care Policy and Research Clinical Practice Guidelines. Most of the guidelines, such as Pressure Ulcers in Adults: Prediction and Prevention, Urinary Incontinence in Adults, and Post Stroke Rehabilitation are relevant to home health and hospice care. Many guidelines, which are posted in an electronic resource named HSTAT (Health Services/Technology Assessment Texts), come in four versions: the complete clinical guideline, a quick reference guide, and consumer guides in English and Spanish. Type in the FTP address:

nlmpubs.nlm.nih.gov

When asked for a password, simply enter the term "anonymous." Since this site is open to the public and no restrictions on use are applied, it is in network parlance referred to as an anonymous FTP site. Then choose the /hstat directory. From there you can select the index, which gives an explanatory title for each guideline; or you can select specific guidelines by their abbreviated titles.

Telnet

Telnet is another kind of Internet communication. Its popularity seems to be declining with the rapid development of more advanced, more functional Internet technologies. A telnet session is an interactive communication session with a host computer. The user connects with a computer and uses the files and programs provided there as though they were a terminal to the host computer. There is a constant electronic connection during a telnet session. America Online, CompuServe, etc., use telnet to provide their subscribers access to their proprietary forums and to the Internet.

Perhaps you want to do a free search of the National Library of Medicine's AVLINE database, which contains information about more than 25,000 audiovisual items, to identify a continuing education program related to home health nursing. Type in the telnet address locator.nlm.nih.gov and enter your login name as locator. Using search terms of your choice, you will retrieve bibliographic information about any audiovisuals included in the AVLINE database.

Gopher

Gopher, developed by the University of Minnesota (Golden Gophers!), is an Internet communication technology that supports hypertext.

Hypertext allows one to electronically leap from one text-based computer file to another. Hypertext does this, in networking parlance, relatively transparently (mouse point-and-click), without the user necessarily knowing any but the initial electronic address. Users have special software, a Gopher client, on their computer. The client software executes instantaneous connection with the chosen file on a chosen host computer, the Gopher server, then instantaneously transfers the text file to the client, and then disconnects from the server. The Gopher client also participates in formatting the text displayed.

You may wish to take advantage of the many resources available via PDQ, a database of the National Cancer Institute's CancerNet, which contains information in patient and health professional versions. To connect, enter the gopher address gopher.nih.gov:70/11/clin/cancernet/pdqinfo. From the menu, choose PDQ Treatment Statements for Patients. Here you will find information for the Breast Cancer Patient, the Pancreatic Cancer Patient, and for patients with many other oncological conditions. Take a look, too, at the health professional version of any of these statements. Home health and hospice professionals will find the Supportive Care Statements especially useful.

World Wide Web

The World Wide Web (WWW) is the technology with the most exciting developments. It has many similarities to Gopher. The major functional advantage currently is that WWW technology is hypermedia. Hypermedia allows the user to access a variety of computers easily. But, unlike text-based Gopher, the WWW accesses a variety of media, such as sound, still and motion pictures, graphics, and computer programs. The host computer has special server software; the user has special client software, generically referred to as a "browser." The browser participates in the formatting and display of digital information and data as text, sound, pictures, etc. WWW technology will also be capable of supporting the incorporation of computer files, such as interactive instruction and data modelling.

There are many brands of browsers all having similar functionality related to the WWW protocols, including Mosaic, Netscape, and others. But there are differences in the browsers' other functionalities. An important difference is whether the browser can also be configured to allow all the other Internet protocols such as Gopher, telnet, FTP, newsgroups, and e-mail.

It is the nature of telecommunications and networking technologies to be constantly changing, hopefully advancing and providing greater functionality. Readers should be aware that the information in this article will soon need to be updated.

For people involved with long-term conditions and diseases (experts and other health professionals, the public, and patients) the Internet can be tremendously valuable—like no tool we have had before. It should become an integral part of the scope of practice in the home health setting. There are probably thousands of sites pertinent to specific conditions encountered in home health and hospice care. The following are some of the sites of general interest:

Home Care Accreditation in Brief
http://www.jcaho.org/hhealth.html

Medicare Hospice Benefit
http://www.nho.org/medicare.htm

Homecare USA On-Line Homecare Directory
http://users.aol.com/health1636/hcusa.htm

SOME ISSUES

There are many issues involving the Internet and its applications that require astute professional attention. Some of these include:

- The quality of the Internet application or resource. Because the Internet culture allows anyone to put up nearly any material, professionals will need to decide how to safely identify the quality of resources to protect those least able to judge for themselves: their students, patients, and the public. There are some tips for assessing the technical and functional quality of resources available (Cybertourtorials, under Nursenet Resources at http://www.ualberta.ca/~jrnorris/nursenet/sparks.html). You are the expert in the urology content, its accuracy, its currency, its balance or bias, etc., and you are the expert in how the content and the functionality of the site interact. Much will depend on your applying your expertise in determining quality.

• Protecting confidentiality and privacy of personal or patient information. Before there can be useful clinical applications of the Internet, these security matters must be solved.

• Licensure of professional practice and reimbursement of services rendered. Is the professional practicing in the state or country where the patient is located or where the professional is located? Who will pay for what clinical services? How will this infrastructure be maintained?

As we exploit the technology in yet unexplored ways, unique issues will no doubt continuously arise.

SEARCH TOOLS FOR FINDING THE INFORMATION YOU WANT

Most Internet users have difficulty finding their way on the information superhighway until they discover tools to help them identify sites of interest and value. Before that, most are overwhelmed with the amount of information available and the chaos they perceive. Many get frustrated and give up on their pursuits of the information superhighway.

The remainder of this article will focus on the wonderful resources available on the WWW component of the Internet for urologic nursing or general health professional interests. Rather than "surf" around from someone's favorite

WWW site, the most useful starting point is one of the many search tools.

Most browsers have a search tool readily available to users right on the software interface. Some people prefer to use search tools prepared by other sources. Some tools only allow searching; others allow both searching and browsing. There are tools that focus on one database and others that encompass several databases. No one tool or combination of tools searches the entire WWW, much less the Internet.

As of April 4, 1997, according to the WebCrawler Top 100 most popular sites (of all kinds), Yahoo! was number 2, WebCrawler was number 3, and Lycos was number 8. Of the top 10 sites, 5 of them were search tools. AltaVista was number 10.

Each tool searches a different database of sites. Each offers different options. Each tool has a different interface. Before using any search tool, know the parameters of the database, how to use the options furnished, and how to interpret the results. This information is readily available on the interfaces of each search tool. Readers wanting more guidance in the use of search tools can access a Cybertourtorial on these four search tools at the following uniform resource locator (the URL is the WWW electronic address):

http://www.ualberta.ca/~jrnorris/nursenet/sparks.html

To connect and learn about each tool from the source, here are the URLs (case is important):

Yahoo!—http://www.yahoo.com
WebCrawler—http://www.webcrawler.com
    or
        http://webcrawler.com
Lycos—http://www.lycos.com/
AltaVista—http://www.altavista.digital.com/

Once a search is performed, the findings are presented as hyperlinks, or embedded electronic connections to other computers. So, to explore any findings, all that's needed is a mouse click or two to be connected. A general search term such as urology is likely to generate hundreds of resources (hits). For example, a search of Web-Crawler on September 6, 1996, retrieved 5,712 hits matching "cardiac rehabilitation." Some relatively rare search terms might not locate any resources.

As you use the search tools and look and learn, think about how these resources can enhance your work, your nursing or health care practice, and your education. Think about how they could be used in home health and hospice care to benefit patients, families, and significant others and to enhance professional practice. With these ideas and more experience using the Internet, experts, such as yourself, will be developing electronic resources and creating new applications for themselves.

If you are not already an Internet user or you want to change your ISP, contact http://www.thelist.com

OTHER INTERESTING SITES

Here are some sites of general interest to home health and hospice nurses and other health professionals:

- **Centers for Disease Control and Prevention**—http://www.cdc.gov
  (Access to reports, publications, guidelines, etc.)
- **National Library of Medicine**—http://www.nlm.nih.gov
  (Access to all MEDLARS databases, some of which require a fee, Online Images of

the History of Medicine, the Virtual Human, and other information resources)
- **World Health Organization**—http://www.who.ch/
  (Concerns of WHO countries, epidemiological information, bulletins)
- **University of Iowa Wound Care**—http://coninfo.nursing.UIOWA.EDU/www.nursing/virtnurs/chronwnd/!int.htm
  (Images of a variety of wounds and their care)
- **GOLDFISH**—http://www.gla.ac.uk/~ec19g/goldfish
  (A prototype testing a combined electronic patient record and patient education resource)
- **Interactive Patient**—http://medicus.marshall.edu/medicus.htm
  (A virtual patient that one can take a history of, do a physical exam and laboratory and radiological tests of, and submit a diagnosis for)
- **American Journal of Nursing Online**—http://www.ajn.org
  (Access to recent issues of the three premier journals published, forums for discussion, continuing education opportunities, etc.)
- **The Virtual Hospital**—http://www.vh.org/
  (A large database of teaching and testing materials on specific conditions and diseases, including interesting images and sounds)

CHAPTER 76

Developing a Home Page for the World Wide Web

Virginia K. Saba

Today, millions of health care professionals use the Internet to "travel" the information superhighway. They access the Internet resources to obtain information for research, educational, administrative, and clinical practice activities, as well as to support health care services in the community and other practice settings.

WORLD WIDE WEB

Many health care professionals who travel the Internet use the World Wide Web (WWW), the easiest, fastest, and most versatile Internet protocol. The WWW allows users to link to millions of on-line services or resources around the world. The WWW, the fastest-growing component of the Internet, supports a full range of multimedia that allow users to view text, graphics, and videos, or hear sounds. See Appendix 76–A for a glossary of Internet terms.

BROWSERS

Health care professionals access the WWW and navigate the Internet using a Web browser software package. Different browsers, also called "search engines," are used for different purposes. They are used to perform protocols such as process e-mail, upload and download files (file transfer protocol [FTP]), connect to remote computer system sites (telnet), or link to other search engines. A Web browser links to the first screen of a WWW site, called a home page.

THE HOME PAGE

A home page is designed to assist users in accessing information about a specific topic, professional organization, business (commercial), specialty organization, educational program, entertainment site, or individual. Each resource or service on the WWW opens with a home page that has its own address and, when accessed, resembles a book with a menu of items that link to additional Web pages that also contain information or additional links to other home pages. New home pages emerge daily as resources are added to the WWW and expand the Internet.

Health care professionals should take advantage of this relatively free source of information. This new technology offers new dimensions to their profession. It allows them to link and communicate their services and resources with other health care professionals around the world. Also, it offers health care professionals

Source: Reprinted with permission from V. K. Saba, Developing a Home Page for the World Wide Web, *American Journal of Infection Control*, Vol. 24, No. 6, 1996, Mosby-Year Book, Inc.

the opportunity to retrieve and share information about their specialty such as infectious disease.

For health professionals to create a home page, they must understand what computer hardware, software, and communication requirements are needed. They also must learn the skills needed to develop a home page, as well as how to create the overall design of one.

Home Page Requirements

A home page needs to be housed on a host computer (Web server) that is connected to the Internet. A Web server or host computer is generally available through a university, private organization, or commercial service. The host computer must have sufficient storage and processing capacity to process the home page information. Software is also required to transform and format text and multimedia information into digital data to link to the browsers as home and Web page screens.

Home Page Design

At least seven major rules should be considered when designing a home page for an Internet resource or service: purpose, scope, structure, enhancements, links, forms, and maintenance.

Purpose. Why do you want to share your information? Who is your audience? What does your audience want to know? Generally you create a home page to share and inform the world of your resources or services. Your home page should be designed to assist users in accessing information about what you have to offer. Remember, you should focus on the product being marketed.

Scope. What information do you want to share? Generally, it is the information that you disseminate and make available in a brochure, catalog, manual, or other printed documents. Such materials should serve as the primary focus of the home page menu, for example, a brochure that describes a course of study, an educational program, or your infection control manual. When sharing printed documents you need to consider copyright concerns.

Structure. How should the information to be presented appear? The best way to design a home page is to first review other home pages with similar information. Determine how you want to organize your information. Choose some overall guidelines for the format of your pages. For example: How should the home page menu items be organized—as boxes, listed alphabetically, color coded, or as graphical icons? Where should buttons for each screen be located? For example, should the "return to home page" button be placed at the bottom of the page or on the side of the page as a side tag? Sketching out your format on paper can speed up this process.

Enhancements. What graphics should be added that will enhance the information? How will the page look with and without the graphics? (Some users will view the home page using a text browser such as Lynx.) Test the graphics before including them on the home page. The transforming of graphics to a digital format requires a great deal of storage and takes a considerable time to appear on the home page and other Web pages.

Links. What internal and external links or connections should be made? Generally, the internal links listed on the home page menu relate to other Web pages for that specific resource, whereas the external links connect to outside resources. As a result, they pose different problems: Who should check and review their addresses to determine if they are correct? What policies should be established? What links should be included and why? How is quality addressed?

Forms. What types of forms might be included for users to request additional information? A form can be designed that can be downloaded by a user to mail or fax; however, it will require additional programs to run on the server. On the other hand, if a form is prepared as an e-mail request, then staff have to be assigned the task of processing the requests. Forms can serve as an excellent source of feedback on use by others.

Maintenance. What procedures should be established to maintain, update, and support the home page? Who will be responsible for keeping the information current, establishing procedures for its upgrade, and enhancing its features periodically? The information on the home page should always be dated so that a user will know how current it is.

Publish

What should be published to inform your users that you have a home page? Materials need to be prepared that disseminate what is available, what its universal resource locator (URL) is, and which browser(s) will access it most effectively. You should consider establishing a method for counting the number of users of your home page.

URL

A home page is the opening screen of a resource or service Web site. Each home page must have its own address, referred to as URL. Each URL has several basic components that are structured in a standardized manner. An example of a URL follows: **http://www.dml. georgetown.edu/schnurs**

- **http://** indicates hypertext transfer protocol server (the protocol used to connect the WWW to the Internet).
- **www** indicates World Wide Web links to the Internet.
- **dml.georgetown.edu** indicates location and type of WWW server site (Dahlgren Library at Georgetown University "edu" (educational) site). Other sites are "gov" for government and "com" for commercial.
- **/schnurs** indicates the path to the location of the particular document. (The document is located in the school of nursing directory on the computer.)

Hypertext markup language

Hypertext markup language (HTML) is the formatting language used to code WWW home pages and documents. It is a method used to organize and structure a document into sections. HTML allows the user to move from one site or resource to another by selecting (point-and-click) hypertext (text that is underlined or presented in another color). The marked hypertext then connects to another site or resource on the Internet.

HTML follows standardized rules to mark the basic blocks and sections of a document such as the title, body of the text, and lists of numbered items. The HTML consists of codes and tags that are inserted in the textual document to instruct how to format the text, paragraphs, and graphics, and how to link the document to other home pages. When designing an HTML document, you need to pay attention to how the document is organized logically, not visually. It may change depending on which browser is used to read the document.

Codes and tags

The HTML codes and tags control what the document will look like to the reader. They are used to mark the text or image. A HTML tag is composed of two codes—one that indicates the beginning of the tag and one that closes the tag. The text between the tags is formatted or translated according to which tag is used. Usually the opening tag appears in a box without a slash and closing tags with a slash, as follows:

<TAG> = opening tag

</TAG> = closing tag

Tags are used to mark (a) the entire document; (b) the header, title, and body of the text; (c) paragraphs; (d) unnumbered, ordered, and defined lists; (e) font size; (f) bold, italics, and center text functions; and (g) other features to enhance the visual appearance of the home and Web pages. See Exhibit 76–1 for examples of codes and tags.

Creating a home page is relatively simple. The HTML programming rules can be learned

Exhibit 76–1 Examples of Codes and Tags

<HTML>		Start document
<HEAD>		Start header
<TITLE>	GUNS Fall Courses </TITLE>	Title in header
<HEAD>		End of header
<BODY>	Courses include....	Body of text
<BODY>		End of body of text
<HTML>		End document

from continuing education courses, from textbooks, or individually from trade publications. Once you have created a home page for yourself or your organization you will be on the information superhighway and belong to the technological age.

RECOMMENDED READINGS

Levine, J.R., & Baroudi, C. (1994). *The Internet for dummies.* Foster City, CA: IDG Books Worldwide.

Mintel, J. (1995). *Easy World Wide Web with Netscape.* Indianapolis: Que Corp.

Shafran, A. (1995). *Creating your own Netscape Web pages.* Indianapolis: Que Corp.

Smith, B., & Bebak, A. (1996). *Creating Web pages for dummies.* Foster City, CA: IDG Books Worldwide.

Trauber, D., & Kierman, B. (1995). *Surfing the Internet with Netscape.* Alameda, CA: Sybex.

Glossary

Browser: A computer program used to search WWW resource documents. The most popular WWW browser is Netscape. Other browsers include Mosaic, Microsoft Internet Explorer, and those offered by on-line services such as America Online and CompuServe.

File transfer protocol (FTP): A protocol designed to transfer data files between computers connected to the Internet.

Graphical interface format (GIF): A format used to encode images to store and transfer over the Internet.

Hypertext markup language (HTML): The language used to mark text using codes and tags to format the text/image in a standardized manner.

Hypertext transfer protocol (http): A particular communication language or protocol used to connect the WWW to the Internet.

Home page: The opening page (first visual display screen) for an Internet site (resource or service) that a user accesses. It serves as the guide to its subsequent Web pages.

Uniform resource locator (URL): The address used to identify any file on the Internet. The URL consists of the name of the protocol, name of the server, and path name to the file.

Web page: A text/image document with HTML codes and tags used to specify how it is formatted.

Web server: A computer that connects to the World Wide Web and makes Web pages available on the Internet.

CHAPTER 77

Planning, Implementing, and Managing a Community-Based Nursing Center: Current Challenges and Future Opportunities

Katherine K. Kinsey and Patricia Gerrity

INTRODUCTION

The concept of a successful community-based nursing center is not new. In fact, the concept began with Lillian Wald and like-minded nurses in the 1890s. Ms. Wald founded the Henry Street Settlement House in response to the evident public health needs of New York City poor and émigré families. Through street outreach, culturally sensitive initiatives, and community activism, Ms. Wald and colleagues engaged community members in nursing and social services. Such services improved the well-being of individuals as well as the health of the community. The spread of infectious diseases and school absenteeism declined, obstetrical care became more of a norm, housing improved, and family life stabilized (Buhler Wilkerson, 1993).

Wald's vision of nursing practice moved beyond individualized care for the sick and infirm. Her prevention and advocacy perspective encompassed a reform agenda in the areas of health, education, industry, recreation, and housing. She actively campaigned for the social betterment of all (Reverby, 1993).

This nursing model of direct access to health care services in home and community settings when combined with social activism is as essential today as it was more than a century ago. In fact, given the changing health care delivery systems and funding sources, such a nursing service model may be the linchpin in planning and providing optimal health care to diverse populations in community settings (Barger, 1995).

Nurses and others who expand Wald's vision will create models of care that offer culturally appropriate preventive and primary health services. These proactive models will then engage the larger infrastructure of medical care and social institutions in the provision of cost-effective services.

Home health agencies are in ideal positions to develop such centers of care. In fact, many home health agencies have the needed resources to initiate such models. These resources include staff, internal agency structures, and recognized histories of successful clinical services in varied home and community settings.

Despite the current reimbursement limitations on holistic nursing practice in home and community settings, this is the opportune time for agencies to make prevention and social activism essential core activities. Agencies committed to change rather than the status quo may be better positioned to survive in this time of health care reform (Salmon, 1993).

The commitment to change and transformation is risky. It is also challenging. One challenge will be to create a nurse-managed public health and primary care service model in tandem with a sick care model. Another challenge will be to marshal the human resources and capital necessary for such risky transformation.

One of the most valuable capital investments that a home health agency has is in its staff. Wald contended that public health nurses were doers, educators, advocates, and creators. She saw their creative work as the start of broader community work. This broad work linked agencies and groups committed to the social betterment of all (Murphy, 1995). Home health agencies who view their staff as positive change agents will maneuver through and survive these uncertain times.

Maneuvering through any system is risky, particularly when there are few guidelines. In fact, there was substantial risk taking and no guidelines for faculty, students, and staff to fall back on when La Salle University Neighborhood Nursing Center (LSUNNC) was established in June 1991.

OVERVIEW

This chapter briefly describes the evolution of LSUNNC as a nurse-managed health center in a challenging urban setting. Strategies and issues influencing the ongoing development of this and other centers are highlighted. These include 1) conducting a practical assessment of community and agency assets, 2) prioritizing needs and interests of specific groups, 3) initiating a strategic plan, and 4) developing realistic service programs and evaluation criteria. The challenges to cost-effective administrative and fiscal management processes and sustainability are highlighted. Advocacy approaches and future opportunities are discussed.

EVOLUTION OF ONE URBAN ACADEMIC NURSING CENTER MODEL

La Salle University Neighborhood Nursing Center is unique in the city of Philadelphia. This public and primary health care model emerged from the School of Nursing and the university's commitment to the community and the community's interest in LSUNNC outreach, health promotion, disease/injury prevention initiatives, and primary health care services. The nursing center model extends Wald's model of culturally sensitive services and social activism in an at-risk community.

The evolution of LSUNNC built on the creative work of public health nursing faculty, students, and volunteers. There were limited opportunities to expose students to citywide public health nursing experiences; therefore faculty designed prevention and health promotion programs to actively involve students in community initiatives. Through these community initiatives, the health risks of individuals and families were further documented. It was evident that faculty and students should develop the resources to improve the health of community members over time.

A feasibility study to implement a nursing center was undertaken. This study was supported by a grant from the William Penn Foundation. This support enabled School of Nursing faculty to further examine community needs and resources, propose internal administrative restructuring, develop an initial mission statement and goals, initiate program planning for particular populations, establish a marketing plan, project financial support, and identify key community members to participate in the development of LSUNNC.

Based on this feasibility study, the Nursing Center was formally established in June 1991. It is one of the three divisions of the School of Nursing. The other divisions are the Undergraduate and Graduate Programs. Each program director reports to the Dean of the School of Nursing. School of Nursing faculty direct the LSUNNC programs. LSUNNC staff consists of full- and part-time faculty, public health nurses, nurse practitioners, substance abuse counselors, a business manager, an educational liaison, community health outreach workers, and affiliated graduate and undergraduate students in nursing, social work, business, and medicine. The diverse staff composition fosters collaborative work. Emphasis is placed on holistic services that focus on relevant and appropriate community health care initiatives. This model is adaptive and can be designed to meet the needs of other diverse urban populations as well as rural and suburban communities. It is not the traditional model of one-site primary care services or home health care administrative offices; therefore, it was critical to develop a mission statement that captured the essence of the model. The mission statement reflects the school and university's mission and represents the collective work of faculty, staff, students, and volunteers (see Exhibit 77–1).

Diverse populations and settings are targeted for services. Settings include the home; school; day care; Head Start programs; Women, Infants, and Children (WIC) nutrition sites; recreation centers; prenatal centers; etc. (Gerrity & Kinsey, 1996). Outreach, case finding, case management, quality public health nursing services, and collaborative community work are hallmarks of LSUNNC programs. The programs are framed by LSUNNC goals. The LSUNNC goals are dynamic in nature and are constructed on agency and community assets. Based on the dynamic processes of goal development, staff continually monitor community needs, interests, and the influences of external forces (i.e., natural disaster). These assessments reveal the

Exhibit 77–1 Mission Statement

> Through the development and implementation of exemplary systems of health care, the La Salle University Neighborhood Nursing Center supports and enhances the teaching, learning, and service mission of the School of Nursing and the University.
>
> Courtesy of La Salle University, Neighborhood Nursing Center, 1996, Philadelphia, Pennsylvania.

need for amendments or changes to goals. Exhibit 77–2 displays current LSUNNC goals.

Since the center's inception, emphasis has been placed on collaborative, multidisciplinary efforts to improve the health of underserved residents in this culturally diverse community. This work is demonstrated by the types of federal, state, regional, and city grants and contracts awarded to the center. These include Office of Minority Health: North Philadelphia Cancer Awareness Prevention Program, Pennsylvania Love 'em with a Checkup/Philadelphia Babies First, City of Philadelphia Maternal–Child Health: Perinatal Home Visiting Program, United Way: Greater Logan–Olney Support Services Center, Childhood Immunization Action Plan, Childhood Lead Poisoning Prevention Program, March of Dimes: Baby Talk at Health Center Nine, etc.

Exhibit 77–2 1996 Goals

- to improve the health of individuals, families, and their communities
- to provide direct access to nursing services to underserved residents in a multiculturally diverse community
- to emphasize disease prevention and health promotion as well as meet national health objectives established by Healthy People 2000

- to involve those who are highest risk and least likely to be served by existing health care services through outreach and case finding
- to evaluate program services
- to promote organizational, environmental, and public policy change
- to provide community consultation
- to provide optimal community-based educational experiences for students and clients

Courtesy of La Salle University Neighborhood Nursing Center, 1996, Philadelphia, Pennsylvania.

These collaboratives as well as the mission and goals have evolved from much inter- and intra-organizational work and time. Such work demands the input of others outside the university and the School of Nursing. The development of realistic goals relates to the contributions of community members. Community involvement continues to represent one of the most significant contributions to LSUNNC sustainability. No nursing center can sustain itself in a particular locale if community representatives are excluded from the processes of assessment and program development. In fact, it might be prudent to involve community representatives at every point of center work.

Yet such involvement can influence staff contributions and perspectives. These influences may be positive or negative. Skillful home health agency administrators must be sensitive to adverse or positive influences on staff productivity and relationships with community members. For example, staff who do not live in the immediate community (point of service) might be viewed by community members as less informed or insensitive to their concerns about daily life. In addition, staff and community members who do not share similar cultural or racial backgrounds, religious orientations, or work experiences may find it challenging to develop productive relationships. Common interests and bonds can be established. Yet, the labor to nurture productive relationships is time-consuming. Constructive outcomes may ultimately evolve only if all parties want things to happen. And often those at the table may not yet know what those "things" might be.

For example, one of the "things" that happened to create LSUNNC was the expressed community interest in ongoing public health nursing services. A neighborhood Bible institute committed space for renovation as a nursing center site. This site became the hub of faculty and student activity. Through such activity, it became evident that community members, in particular young women and their children, had unmet needs.

Interestingly, the opportunities for possible funding sources surfaced as the need for more services was documented. In part, these possibilities occurred in the form of request for proposals (RFP) calls from public and private organizations; however, much emerged through networking with community agencies and multidisciplinary collaboratives. The current LSUNNC programs have evolved from a variety of these possibilities. What the staff have realized is never to underestimate the value of relationship building and the potential to work together to create relevant health services for targeted populations.

Many LSUNNC services have taken much time and effort to build; others have seemingly evolved serendipitously. But in retrospect, even those services have emerged from much community and staff work. For example, the Rockland Street Immunization Initiative started from community and school work targeting minority children and their immunization needs. Funding to support outreach case finding and direct immunization services was provided by a 1995 American Nurses Foundation grant through the Pennsylvania Nurses Association. Although the funding has now ended, LSUNNC staff have incorporated the "Every Child by Two" campaign into other service programs targeting minority families with young children.

Although LSUNNC evolved from an academic model of teaching, learning, and service, the model could have just as well emerged from a home health agency. Different missions, goals, reimbursement structures, and program designs may appear obvious; yet the commitment across organizations to improving personal and family life is evident. What can influence the evolution of a similar model in a home health agency might be the agency's principal source of funds being linked solely to restorative and curative care. If sick care is the principal focus of an agency, a thorough community and agency assessment must be conducted before undertaking such a contrasting enterprise.

ASSESSMENT

Frequently, assessments are targeted outward toward the community of interest and do not include internal agency audits of resources, skills, interests, or needs. It is important to conduct concurrent internal agency review and external community assessments. Such information will be invaluable in constructing a realistic portrait of the feasibility of establishing a nursing model focusing on health, not disease and illness of a community (Henderson, McManus, & Morris, 1996).

At the community level, assessments focus on current health data, population demographics, specific needs by locale or neighborhood, resources, environmental characteristics, explicit and implicit needs, and interests of residents, workers, etc. In addition, barriers to services need to be identified. Such barriers may range from lack of public transportation to low literacy levels of adults to state changes in Medicaid coverage for low-income families.

The internal agency assessment will examine resources, staff skills, and limitations. This assessment should include 1) services currently in place, 2) services severely restricted by third-party payers, 3) services expanded to meet third-party requirements (i.e., more paperwork), and 4) services that have the potential to be more responsive and comprehensive to families.

Community assessments and resource analyses have always been strengths within nursing. Public health nurses in particular are prepared to take a holistic approach regarding health and ascertain the community's perspective on needs and problems. Holistic nursing assessments encompass more than health. Other factors that contribute to a community's health status include social, environmental, educational, employment, and demographic characteristics. Without such information, a community assessment is lacking, and powerless to support agency change.

The purposes of the community and agency assessment must be forthright. Community members involved in such assessments may be skeptical about the motive and, if suspicious, less inclined to contribute. Their skepticism may be due to past experiences with ineffectual community assessments. Open dialogue about agency interests and commitment can mobilize residents to work with staff throughout this phase.

The assessment phase should include careful consideration of locales for services. For example, should there be maternal–child health nurses who follow families until their youngest child has completed the primary immunization series? Should there be a source and site for free pregnancy tests and counseling, particularly for adolescents? Should there be open immunization hours for school-age children so they can be "caught up" and enrolled in school immediately? Should there be primary care providers closer to clients in need of such services?

This internal assessment may lead to some clarity about agency interest in establishing a site for one or multiple services. Or the audit may suggest that there should be an array of additional services but not necessarily more service sites. If there is an interest in establishing a site for services, the external assessment phase should not concentrate solely on "vulnerable" populations or socioeconomically depressed areas. All communities, be they urban, rural or suburban, have interests and needs for accessible primary health care services. Community members, if asked, often provide invaluable insights as to where such a service site could be established and perceived as "user friendly."

In addition, the assessment phase should not exclusively focus on what nurses offer to the community. The assessment forums must be open to community needs. It may be that in the eyes of the consumer, the concept of a "nursing center" is archaic. For example, LSUNNC has an array of staff. The staff includes nursing, medical, and allied health personnel and others. Such a multidisciplinary, collaborative model of preventive health care may be a difficult concept for the consumer to understand. And the name "nursing center" might limit consumers' ideas about what is available. Careful thought should be given to naming the center. What the service or site is called may influence consumer use and acceptance. It can also raise community awareness about what nurses and other health professionals can do in this era of change.

Further phases emerge if internal agency and external community data document need and interest. One phase can be viewed as a secondary process of assessment. It is now the time to gauge the amount of time, effort, and expertise necessary to develop a strategic plan. One essential step is to select a person or persons to spearhead this strategic plan. In addition, restructuring roles and responsibilities to lead this initiative must occur concurrently. Selected individuals must have sufficient time and resources to develop the strategic plan. If this work is simply added to a person's current responsibilities, there may be too little effort allocated to this initiative. This work must be viewed as essential and integral to moving the agency forward.

The secondary assessment phase allows for further examination of resources and possible influences on the development of this nursing service model. Is a site critical for the model? Are staff skills and interests sufficient in developing this model? Will other disciplines be critical to programmatic design? Are more staff needed? Can staff be retrained? How can the collaborative nature of this model be nurtured?

Professional barriers to model development might include lack of state prescriptive power for nurses, definition of "primary care provider" in managed care legislation, lack of or inadequate reimbursement for health promotion and health education, lack of physical space to provide on-site services, etc. Community barriers could be escalating violence in the immediate target areas, commuting distances to service sites, inadequate networking with other community and institutional services, the increasing acquisition of hospitals, and medical practices by for-profit companies.

The transition from secondary assessment into strategic planning may be effortless if the commitment to develop this model is clear, resources are available, and barriers seem surmountable. On the other hand, there will be agencies who will struggle with the question Should we or shouldn't we? The transition will then be more labor intensive. In fact, the process may be abruptly arrested.

STRATEGIC PLANNING

In the strategic planning phase, the agency's mission and vision need reexamination. The mission, vision, and values of the home health agency will strategically position the organization to develop a public health or a primary care model or blend features of each.

Current nursing centers, free-standing or housed within an academic center, are not alike. Some are based on the public health model in which services are designed for all those who need care, whether or not the consumers present themselves for such services, in a designated area. This public health model requires that outreach, case finding, and public health nursing case management be integrated components in any population- or health-focused service.

Primary health care services that involve on-site nurse practitioner service, be it pediatric, adult, or family, may develop accessible, affordable, user-friendly on-site programs. Such programs may not include outreach and community-based case finding. Other centers blend both. Population-focused outreach, case finding, case management, and primary health care services are essential elements in various sites.

The service sites also vary from center to center. Rural agencies may consider a mobile van an essential source of care. Thus, the van can be scheduled for services in strategic geographic points to reach the most people. An urban agency might consider multiple sites as point of contact. Some urban sites include schools, senior housing complexes, recreation centers, churches, and day care centers (Craig, 1996).

Throughout the strategic planning phases, the identification of agency collaborators will be critical. Home health agencies do not need to do this in isolation of other organizational resources. In fact, other organizations may have similar interests in extending relevant community services to those in need. Your agency may have to assume the risk in reaching out to other organizations and sharing ideas, but the yield might be great. For example, social service agencies and home health agencies have resources that complement each other. The nursing center model has the possibility of sharing resources. The sharing of such resources is economically sound and expands the nature of community-focused services.

The reimbursement struggle for newly proposed services now begins. The strategic plan and specific program development must constantly wrestle with this dilemma. Some state agencies provide direct reimbursement for primary care services to advanced practice nurses; thus, the idea of establishing a primary care site staffed by nurse practitioners may be immediately feasible. But health promotion, education, and disease prevention, hallmarks of public health and holistic nursing practice, are seldom directly reimbursable from state agencies. The possibility of contracting with local or regional agencies, public and private, for such public health services must be explored. These services could include immunization, outreach, and perinatal home visiting services (Elsberry & Nelson, 1993).

When direct reimbursement for proposed services is not evident, the agency must commit to moving forward with grant and contract proposals. Funding services through grants and time-limited service contracts allow for program implementation. But the lack of predictability of these funding streams is stressful. Agency staff must be continually vigilant about possible funding changes and other opportunities to seek alternative fiscal support.

PROGRAM DEVELOPMENT AND INFORMATION SYSTEMS

The transition to program development will be based on critical factors identified throughout the assessment and strategic planning phases. Agency resources and locus of services, be it one site, multisite, all community based, or in-home, will need to be built into each program developed. Therefore, staffing expertise, work patterns, familiarity with program development, strategic planning, the services the agency and its collaborators can provide, the community receptivity, and reliable reimbursement sources are all concerns.

Again, it may be prudent for the agency to determine what services could be shared with other providers. For example, social workers and public health nurses together can develop holistic care models that address individual and family issues. Rather than agencies working in isolation, communication and care patterns improve, and ultimately the client benefits from the dual nature of the work.

If there are one or more services in place, the agency must begin to measure client- or population-based outcomes. The methods of documenting the nature of services, client outcomes, and the costs of such services should be built into each program. Unfortunately, many outcomes have been based on medical models that do not capture the nature of public health work. Data will be needed not only to evaluate outcomes and improve quality but also to cost out services, to provide data for policy development, and to conduct research.

The struggle to simultaneously determine what data points to collect and at what intervals and what system to use will be ongoing. Centers that blend public health and primary care services, in addition to home health services, will be additionally challenged. Data from health promotion, disease prevention, education, outreach, and case finding activities should be maintained as well as the curative, restorative primary care data. What should be entered, how much should be entered, who enters the data, who analyzes the data, what are the data expectations of the funders, and what equipment is necessary to enter these data are major questions.

Some concerns may be dismissed early on but reemerge later as fundamental barriers to data analysis. For example, the assumption that the person who enters the data may be a low-level staff person may spell disaster. If there is lack of understanding of the nature of data and missing data, the retrievable information may be limited in scope. And many hours of professional labor may be invested later to retrieve data. In other words, cheap investments do not always pay off.

In addition, the scope of services may defy easy data computation. The complexity of nursing and allied roles continues to evolve. The escalating advances in the areas of telecommunication, including the Internet, raise serious questions about how to "capture" client encounters, the services provided, and client, family, and community outcomes. And despite the technological advances made, many staff and their clients may not be computer literate and may not have an interest in learning these skills despite agency advocacy. In addition, some communities do not have the resources to support or secure expensive technology.

However, home health administrators appreciate the programmatic demands placed on them by particular funders. Careful thought must be given to the modalities the agency can use for data collection and what would be wise investments. Two current possibilities are 1) to purchase a commercial computer product and customize data collection for particular programs with this product or 2) to have a consultant work with the staff to develop an agency-specific system.

Commercial products are now quite good in capturing primary care data, particularly as it relates to sick care and *International Classification of Diseases, Ninth Edition* (ICD–9) codes for billing purposes. Such products rarely include nursing and health promotion activities. On the other hand, the customized product may be quite costly. In addition, this product may require the ongoing services of that particular company or consultant. Does the agency want to have a continuing expense? Furthermore,

developing the customized computer program may be a tedious process requiring much staff work.

Another consideration will be the multiple sites that may be targeted for services. The more sites involved, the less manageable the data entry, collection, and analysis. Should data be entered into a portable system and moved from site to site? Should there be paper records and data entered later at a central site? What are the expenses involved in setting up computer support at each site? What happens if sites change? Multiple sites complicate an already complex issue. These issues and questions do not have easy answers.

It may be that resolution is directly related to agency resources and experiences with computerization and data collection. Another alternative is an agency directive to move forward. Then, there is no dispute about computerization. It is then a question of how much and when.

HUMAN RESOURCE AND FISCAL MANAGEMENT

Sound program development will be directly related to the agency's human resource and fiscal management services. This model is not inexpensive to initiate and sustain. For many home health agencies, such a model is beyond the scope of their services and mission. Other agencies may commit to this model because their resources are greater or the client/community need is so great.

For a nursing center model to be successful, the staff must envision themselves responsible and responsive to human need and interest without self-imposed boundaries. The attitude that "that is not my job" does not create the necessary esprit de corps. Flexibility, adaptability, the notion of transcending boundaries and bureaucracies, creativity, and commitment to the untried will be critical staff characteristics. Matching staff with new programs and the new ways of doing business at one or multiple sites is critical. The staff can make or break this new initiative. In fact, the agency and the staff must be risk takers together.

Part of the risk with introducing this model will be whether services are separated from or integrated into currently funded services. It may be a blend of each. On-site services for lead screening may be part of an overall lead toxicity prevention program. In-home services for mothers and their infants may also include education regarding lead and its effects on young children. This intervention may cross several programs. The nurse who understands that the intervention can be conducted several different ways, in several different places, and with multiple clients is the person for the job. The staff who want discrete roles and responsibilities, who become anxious with newness, and who are uncomfortable making independent decisions will undermine this initiative.

Agencies may be severely tested in recruiting staff for this model. Staff assignments without an interviewing and selection process may yield disappointing results. The staff must be the front-line marketers and representatives of this initiative and the agency. Putting the best foot forward is a necessary step in this process.

Also critical are sound fiscal management and solid grant writing skills. Home health agencies interested in developing this nursing model must reach out to nontraditional sources of funding. Grantsmanship will be critical as will staff investment of time, energy to write proposals, and the ability to accept the rejects with the accepts (Starbecker, 1996). In addition, agency administrators must know the costs and charges associated with such an endeavor. Nothing is for free, even if it appears so to the public.

Current knowledge about managed care contracts in your state, county, and city will be the responsibility of the fiscal manager and senior staff. In addition, how to project budgets based on certain health mandates or contract languages will increasingly be an expectation. Maximizing staff skills in these turbulent times will be challenging but is possible. Reallocation of resources, be they personnel, space, or equipment, is also the purview of the fiscal manager and senior staff.

Careful consideration of budgets, financial opportunities, and constraints must be ongoing. Conferences with the fiscal manager should be routinely scheduled. Senior staff should actively participate and be aware of productivity, client outcomes, program costs, personnel costs (including benefits), the status of accounts receivable, the prospects of future funding, etc. No one person should assume total responsibility for this model's fiscal viability. This should be a shared enterprise.

Nurses and other allied health professionals have seldom been involved in the planning and managing of budgets. This may be a first for some of the agency's staff. As such, staff may be reluctant to learn and may withdraw from the process. This would be detrimental to all. Through learning and sharing, expenses can be managed, programs can be provided, and positive outcomes can be documented.

Any plan for this nursing model must be realistic. Some voluntary programs may emerge from internal agency reserves but such reserves may not be sustainable. Long-term sustainability may emerge from productive provider and community relationships and their interests in working together to achieve common goals through shared resources.

THE FUTURE OF ADVOCACY AND NURSING CENTERS

Throughout the assessment, strategic planning, program development, information systems, human resource, and fiscal management phases, client advocacy prevails. If the agency loses sight of what the clients' needs and interests are, the viability and long-term sustainability of this nursing model is jeopardized.

Wald's advocacy prototype should be one of the agency's core activities (regardless of program, site of service, or targeted outcome). This activity should involve clients, staff, community members, and agency affiliates. Changes in staff roles and responsibilities can emerge through advocacy work. Even venues of services as well as the name for this nursing model may change over time. Being in tune with the community will help the agency move in concert with others interested in preserving and sustaining health.

It may be that the home health agency starting this nursing model is now better positioned to work with local health care institutions that plan major moves into the community. The institutions may be seeking practice opportunities, and the agency may need skilled staff. These are ideal opportunities to share rather than create more resources in isolation. Also, the hospitals might have an interest in funding some of the community-focused programs to meet their missions.

The evolution and future of nursing centers rest mainly on the targeted community, the agency, staff, and consumers. In the future, nursing centers may be hubs of health care with more work to accomplish than the large tertiary care institutions around the corner. Nursing centers will then be the stepping stones for other social and health enterprises.

The possibilities are limitless. Is your home health agency up for the challenge? Lillian Wald would say so.

REFERENCES

Barger, A. (1995). Establishing a nursing center: Learning from the literature and the experiences of others. *Journal of Professional Nursing, 11*(4), 203–212.

Buhler Wilkerson, K. (1993). Bring care to the people: Lillian Wald's legacy to public health nursing. *American Journal of Public Health, 83*(12), 1778–1786.

Craig, C. (1996). Making the most of a nurse managed center. *Nursing & Health Care: Perspectives on Community, 17*(3), 124–126.

Elsberry, N., & Nelson, F. (1993). How to plan financial support for nursing centers. *Nursing & Health Care, 14*(8), 408–413.

Gerrity, P., & Kinsey, K. (1996). Partnerships for health. *The Nursing Spectrum, 5*(7), 16–17.

Henderson, F., McManus, J., & Morris, A. (1996). *The making of a nursing center: Linking population based health care, community agencies and institutions.* Natchez, MS: Alcorn State University School of Nursing.

Murphy, B. (1995). *Nursing centers: The time is now.* New York: National League for Nursing Press.

Reverby, S. (1993). From Lillian Wald to Hillary Rodham Clinton: What will happen to public health nursing? *American Journal of Public Health, 83*(12), 1662–1663.

Salmon, M. (1993). Editorial: Public health nursing—The opportunity of a century. *American Journal of Public Health, 83*(12), 1674–1675.

Starbecker, M. (1996, April). *Grantwriting from the Division of Nursing.* Paper presented at the Nursing Center Regional Conference, Philadelphia.

CHAPTER 78

Adult Day Services—The Next Frontier

Joanne Handy, Judith A. Bellome, and Nancy Moldenhauer

Loosely defined, adult day services are understood to be services provided to the elderly or disabled, in a congregate setting, for fewer than 24 hours per day. A variety of services and levels of care allow programs to be tailored to meet specialty needs for diverse clients such as those with a diagnosis of Alzheimer's disease or the human immunodeficiency virus (HIV). Indeed, a center can be established to meet most identified community health needs.

The current surge of interest in adult day services can be attributed to the versatility and the cost-effectiveness of these programs. In fact, at an average charge of $40–$50/day, adult day care is the health care bargain of the decade. With health care costs soaring, the need for health care services growing, and the older population booming, adult day care is becoming the new "fair-haired child" of the health care industry. Adding to the popularity of the program is the fact that these programs, like home care, help to keep folks in their homes and communities—where they want to be.

HISTORY OF ADULT DAY SERVICES

In the United States, adult day care began in psychiatric day hospitals, such as the Yale Psy-

chiatric Clinic in the 1940s, primarily to assist patients following release from mental institutions. In the 1950s, Dr. Lionel Cosin's geriatric day hospital programs at sites in England inspired interest in creating adult day services in this country. He established his model of day programs in the Cherry State Hospital in North Carolina in the 1960s. During this decade, the day care concept shifted from its single psychiatric focus to other health maintenance issues. In turn the growth in the number of centers has been significant over the past two decades. In 1975, there were only 15 adult day centers. The number had grown to 1,200 in 1985; 2,100 in 1989; and 3,000 in 1994.

In the late 1960s, adult day service centers were a response to the need for supportive care outside of institutions. Then in the 1970s, it was held that institutions and nursing homes were being overused. The cost of this care was so high that adult day service centers began offering health and skilled services. Into the 1980s, Medicaid still remained the primary source of funding in addition to private pay clientele. Today, additional sources of revenue that should continue to foster growth include long-term care policies, Medicare Part B, insurance, and managed care reimbursement for skilled ser-

Reprinted by permission of the National Association for Home Care, from *CARING* Magazine, Volume XV, No. 12 (December 1996). Not for further reproduction.

vices including restorative and functional maintenance rehabilitation. The last frontier for adult day covered services is Medicare Part A.

THE ADULT DAY CARE SERVICE MARKET

Burton V. Reifler, MD, MPH, Director of Partners in Caregiving: The Dementia Services Program, supported by the Robert Wood Johnson Foundation, predicts a need for 10,000 adult day care centers by the year 2000. With only 3,000 adult day care centers existing in 1994, there is an abundance of business opportunity.

A profile of current providers reveals that two-thirds of the centers are affiliated with a larger parent organization including community-based service organizations, hospitals, and nursing homes. Fourty-four percent are located in urban regions, while 43 percent are in rural areas.

Centers provide a wide array of services, including substantial health care and rehabilitation (Figure 78–1). Services offered include:

- Recreational Therapy/Activities—93 percent
- Meals—92 percent
- Social Services—90 percent
- Transportation—81 percent
- Personal Care—80 percent
- Nursing Care—77 percent
- Rehabilitation Therapy—60 percent
- Medical Services—56 percent

The staffing mix reflects both the health focus and the range of services offered. Professional staff include Nurse—82 percent, Social Worker—64 percent, Occupational Therapist—24 percent, Speech Therapist—22 percent, Physical Therapist—20 percent, Art Therapist—4 percent, and Dietitian—2 percent (Figure 78–2) (Reifler, Henry, & Cox, 1995).

The average age of the adult day care client is 76. Not surprisingly, 62 percent of clients served are female of whom 81 percent are white, non-Hispanic. Forty-seven percent of the clients are widowed and 39 percent are married.

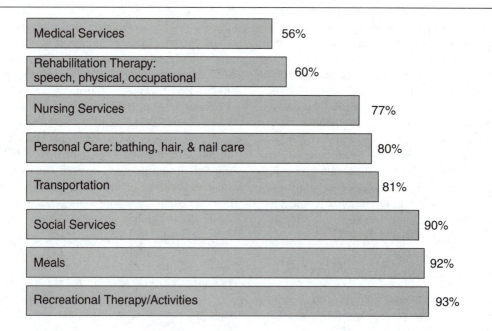

Figure 78–1 Variety of Services. *Source:* The Dementia Services Program, Department of Psychology and Behavioral Medicine, Bowman Gray School of Medicine, Winston-Salem, NC.

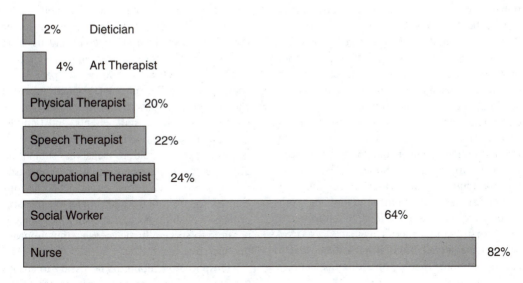

Figure 78–2 Professional Staff. *Source:* Reefler, B., Henry, R.S., and Cox, N. *Adult Day Services in America.* Robert Wood Johnson Partners in Caregiving. The Dementia Services Program, July 1995.

Levels of care have been recently integrated in the National Association of Adult Day Services (NADSA) revised *Standards and Guidelines for Adult Day Services* (1997) to respond to the increasing number of centers and clients as well as the increasing acuity levels and health care needs. Concurrently, over the last 10 years, there has been a noticeable decrease in functional level and independence among those served. There are three levels of need that describe more clearly the needs, care, and intervention required for individuals:

- The client at *Level of Need 1* is in need of socialization, some protective supervision, supportive service, and minimal assistance with ADLs. This client is medically stable and does not need nursing observation or intervention on a regular basis.
- The client at *Level of Need 2* is in need of moderate assistance and may need health assessment, nursing oversight, therapy services at a maintenance level, and moderate assistance with 1–3 ADLs. The participant

may have difficulty communicating and making appropriate judgments, and periodically demonstrates disruptive behavior that can be managed.
- The client at *Level of Need 3* is in need of maximum assistance. The participant's medical condition is not stable and requires regular monitoring or intervention by a nurse. Therapy services are needed at a rehabilitative or restorative level. There may be a need for total care in one or more ADLs. The individual may display frequent disruptive behavior requiring staff intervention and may be unable to communicate needs.

State regulation of adult day services varies, with only 25 states requiring licensure and 24 states with some type of certification regulations. Regulations regarding staff support ratios and square footage requirements are established by each state, but at a minimum, staff–participant ratio should be one to six (1:6). As the number and severity of participants with functional impairments increase, the staff–participant ratio should be adjusted accordingly. Average required space for participant usage ranges from 50 to 100 square feet per participant. In centers that serve a significant number of people with cognitive impairment or who use adaptive equipment for ambulation or medical equipment for support, the higher level of square footage is recommended. Other regulatory requirements may mandate minimum services and staff credentials. Some regulations may prevent adult day care centers from being part of an existing nursing home structure while others may require it. Standardization in the area of regulatory requirements is a goal of NADSA and is necessary if industry providers want to access additional funding opportunities.

FINANCING ADULT DAY CARE

Financing of adult day services is a challenge. The challenge includes an average start-up time of two to three years before full census is achieved, an operating cost of at least $200,000 to $250,000 per year, and poor third-party reimbursement. Traditionally, adult day care centers have been started and managed by not-for-profit organizations that served the low-income, Medicaid-eligible client. Since state Medicaid programs, the largest source of third-party payment, usually pay less than the cost of care, these providers covered their start-up, maintenance, service, and transportation costs with grants and fund-raising activities. As philanthropic dollars have "dried up," centers have looked to more and more private pay opportunities. Medicare does not cover the cost of adult day care, and affordable long-term care insurance policies that cover this kind of care are still fairly rare. Managed care and capitated rate opportunities will be addressed later in this article.

OPERATIONAL ISSUES IN ADULT DAY CARE

The physical facilities need to be in compliance with applicable state and local building regulations and zoning, and fire and health codes or ordinances. When possible, the center should be located on street level and have its own separate, identifiable entrance and space. The facility needs to have sufficient space to accommodate the full range of planned activities and services. Privacy and confidentiality needs must be ensured for staff, clients, and families with adequate attention to space.

Safety and sanitation measures should be implemented and assured on an ongoing basis. Economies of scale can be achieved by increased square footage and proper use of paraprofessional staff ratio. Such economies make it possible to serve a higher census, thus improving operating margins.

Transportation support is necessary to ensure the success of any center, but can be one of the greatest expenses and challenges to the program. The high cost to purchase multipassenger vans, especially those that are wheelchair-accessible, is only part of the expense when considering client transportation. High insurance rates, vehicle maintenance, driver availability/reliability, and scheduling can be time-consuming and a complicated task. Many centers recommend contracting for the transportation services with existing community businesses. Some centers assert that transportation is such an integral part of the program that they absorb the cost and assign regular staff as drivers. Facilities that are centrally located and close to major roads and highways make accessibility easy and convenient for the contracted transportation or family-arranged rides.

As in all successful business practices, marketing and sales must be adequately funded and implemented for success and growth of the center. Community awareness and name recognition of adult day services are low, so strong emphasis must be placed on media relationship-building. Human interest stories about clients and their families often attract immediate attention. Use of yellow page advertisement and wide distribution of attractive, professional low-cost brochures have seen the most success. Census development also depends upon strong community exposure through utilizing existing networks of social services and health care providers. Attendance at meetings and membership in service organizations helps to increase contacts that can lead to others. Targeting Family Practice Physicians, gerontologists, local Area Agency on Aging offices, and discharge planners in hospitals and long-term facilities is an important component of your marketing plan. Relationship-building with home health agencies, assisted living centers, and retirement communities may lead to an integrated system of referral and support. Establishing more formal alliances or networks can lead to managed care and insurance contracts.

As in all health service organizations, quality and adequacy of staffing is of primary importance. Recruitment and retention depends on proper attention to screening potential employee applicants with appropriately written job descriptions, offering appropriate salaries, and building a strong, professional team. Special attention to increased staffing for higher levels of care is important.

Financial management depends upon objectively setting your budget, knowing your expenses, and charging the cost of care (or more). Many adult day care organizations have historically charged less than the cost due to the mistaken belief that most clients and families are unable to afford the cost of care. In the past, fund raising and grant writing were used to subsidize the cost of care, but in today's market, many of those sources have disappeared, as well as the government entitlement programs of the 1960s.

The business of adult day care should follow the example of children's day care; that is, pay the service fee in advance and offer no refunds, even if the client does not attend as scheduled. Staffing requirements for scheduled clients remain the same. Also, hours of operation should reflect those of the local child care centers in order to accommodate working caregivers.

CONSUMER DEMAND

Consumer awareness is a primary determinant of consumer demand for adult day services. The Harvard/Harris Long Term Care Awareness Survey supported the notion that most Americans are uninformed about their long-term care options, other than nursing homes. Forty-one percent of adults over 50 have never heard or read about adult day care, compared with 28 percent who are unfamiliar with home care (Blendon et al., 1995). An earlier study found that 54 percent of households with a family member 60 years or older did not know about adult day centers.

The John Hancock Mutual Life Insurance Company/The National Council on the Aging Long-Term Care Study indicated that seven out of ten (70 percent) adults consider themselves familiar with long-term care services in general. While there is reported familiarity with the concept, there is far less familiarity with options available for providing or paying for long-term care options. Nearly all (84 percent) are very or somewhat familiar with nursing homes. However, only about half of the participants are at least somewhat familiar with options such as assisted living (51 percent), continuing care retirement communities (51 percent), and adult day care (49 percent). Two-thirds (67 percent) are very (28 percent) and somewhat (39 percent) familiar with Medicaid while 45 percent are familiar with long-term care insurance, and only 24 percent with reverse mortgages (Americans of All Ages, 1996).

Consumer demand appears to be stronger among caregivers seeking respite from the responsibilities associated with dementia care. The National Partners in Caring Project, supported by the Robert Wood Johnson Foundation, identified three target markets within the caregiver group: care seekers, who want full day, center-based services and are potential heavy users; respite seekers, who seek occasional breaks rather than daily care and are potential moderate users; and information seekers, interested in information but unsure if their loved one needs care. Despite consumer demand for day care services being somewhat higher among dementia caregivers, direct consumer referrals from family, friends, and coworkers accounted for only 19 percent of total referrals. Seventy-five percent of referrals typically come from formal sources: health care professionals, social service agencies, and the Alzheimer's Association (Reifler, Henry, & Cox, 1995).

In addition to the lack of consumer awareness, there are two other formidable barriers to use of adult day care. To many older people, the notion of regular attendance at a center, even when transportation is provided, is an unfamiliar one. Participation in most day care programs requires a commitment of a certain number of days per week; services are not provided on a drop-in basis. If a client has never visited a center, he or she may not be responsive initially to the service, expressing a preference to have services brought into the home. However, after attending the center for just a few days, a client quickly realizes the advantages of the group activities, social interchange, and the services available at the center. For this reason, most centers have prospective clients spend a few days on a trial basis so that both the client and the provider can determine the appropriateness of this type of service.

The out-of-pocket cost to the consumer is another formidable barrier. As noted above, Medicaid is the only significant third-party payer of adult day care at the present time, leaving most of the cost to be paid directly by clients and their families. Although a daily cost of $40–$50 per day covers several services and reflects an hourly rate of less than $10, families with fixed incomes or limited resources may find the total monthly cost to be substantial. Many not-for-profit centers have traditionally been reluctant to set their standard fee equal to or greater than cost for this reason, denying themselves the opportunity to have willing clients pay what the service actually costs.

THE HOME CARE–DAY SERVICE CONNECTION

Home care companies traditionally view day care as either a competitor or a service to which they can refer once skilled care is completed. The competitive view is reinforced by some fiscal intermediaries' interpretation of Medicare's homebound requirement in such a way as to render an adult day service client ineligible for home health agency services. The home care and day service industries are working together to remove this barrier. As home care assumes an increasingly important role within integrated delivery systems, incentives are created for home care companies to develop cooperative partnerships with day service providers. For example, a home care company operating under a capitated agreement would be interested in a home care–service care package if it effectively met clients' needs at a lower cost than home care alone. For a client receiving several skilled services per week, the cost of providing such treatment in a congregate group setting could provide significant savings. While a home care nurse might see 5 to 7 clients a day, a nurse in the adult day health center can provide skilled services to 15 a day. In this instance, the home care company would pay for the day services out of its capitation.

Most of the creative managed care opportunities for day service providers lie in the skilled services arena, stimulating interest on their part in developing the health services component of these programs. Home care companies can enter into contractual arrangements to provide nursing and therapy staff to day centers or provide additional training to existing center staff to strengthen their hands-on skills.

ADULT DAY CARE IN A NEW HEALTH CARE MARKET

Will the significant growth that the adult day services field has seen over the last few years be helped or hindered by health care reform and market changes? Can a traditionally public-funded and subsidized service attract both the private pay and insurance dollars required for expansion? These authors predict that adult day services will experience significant growth and development over the next five years as providers become part of integrated delivery systems and increasingly seek to manage chronic illness and disability through utilization of alternate levels of care.

Management of a stroke within an integrated delivery system provides an illustrative example. The traditional plan of care following the acute episode usually involves rehabilitation in a skilled nursing facility (SNF), followed by several weeks of home health care involving multiple disciplines. An alternative plan is to bypass or significantly shorten the skilled nursing facility stay, replacing it with a combined home care/day care plan that utilizes the time spent in the center for aggressive rehabilitation, skilled nursing, and personal care, supplemented by supportive home care services. Costs, based on charges, of the alternative options are presented in Table 78–1, assuming an eight week treatment period for each. The costs of a day service/home care package are significantly less than the costs of the SNF alone or home health care alone.

Although adult day service is not a covered Medicare or traditional insurance benefit, health maintenance organizations (HMOs), including Medicare HMOs, have the flexibility to "go outside of benefit." Some insurers will pay the cost of the rehabilitation component of adult day health under their policies' outpatient benefits. Likewise, provider delivery systems that operate under full capitation have incentives to pay for day service if it effectively substitutes for higher-cost services. To build the case, adult day service providers are busy trying to identify the types of clients and conditions that will benefit most from an alternative treatment plan. Outcome measurement is in its infancy in the adult day services field and the definitive data that HMOs want is generally not yet available.

Coverage under long-term care policies is much more common but less visible because of the small number of policy holders that currently use such benefits. California, for example, requires that adult day service be part of the benefit package under all its "certified" long-term care policies. The newer long-term care policies include adult day services and home care in addition to nursing home placement. The projected growth of long-term care insurance will undoubtedly expand the day service market.

Table 78–1 Cost Options

| | Option 1 | | | | Option 2: Combined Day Health/Home Care | |
	ADHC/CORF	HHA	SNF		ADHC/CORF	HHA
Weeks 1–4				Weeks 1–4		
	RN 5 x week	4 x wk	Daily		RN 3 x wk	1 x wk
	PT 5 x wk	3 x wk			PT 3 x wk	2 x wk
	OT 5 x wk	2 x wk			OT 3 x wk	
	SW	1 x wk		Weeks 5–8		
					RN 2 x wk	
Weeks 5–8					PT 2 x wk	
	RN 3 x wk	2 x wk	Daily		OT 3 x wk	1 x wk
	PT 3 x wk	2 x wk		Total Combined Cost	$7,160	
	OT 3 x wk	1 x wk			Compared with	
	SW	1 x wk			$8,000 ADHC/CORF only	
					$9,600 HHA only	
Total Cost	$8,000	$9,600	$13,020		$13,020 SNF only	

Source: Mount Zion Institute on Aging.

The national trend toward Medicaid managed care may well be the most significant factor fueling the growth of the day service field. Medicaid currently spends 74 percent of its budget on long-term care costs, primarily nursing homes. While the potential of adult day service to reduce acute care costs is yet untapped, its ability to prevent or postpone nursing home use for certain populations is well recognized. Since those states that have a Medicaid adult day service benefit usually require that the client be "nursing home certifiable" to be eligible, day service providers have substantial experience with this very frail population. When the states include long-term care under their Medicaid managed care initiatives, insurers and Medicaid nursing home providers will suddenly have huge incentives to utilize adult day services.

One of this country's leading examples of a fully capitated system of primary, acute, and long-term care for frail elders is the Program of All Inclusive Care for the Elderly (PACE). PACE is the national replication of the On Lok model, developed in San Francisco, and now conducted by select provider sites across the country. A PACE provider receives a monthly capitation for each client and is responsible for providing the full spectrum of medical, health, and social services, including acute and nursing home care if necessary, all aimed at making it possible for clients who would otherwise be in a nursing home to stay in the community. PACE services focus on clients' regular attendance at an adult day health center, combined with home care. All medical care and most skilled nursing care is provided on-site at the center.

Based on all these factors, several for-profit national providers have announced plans to enter the day health services market or significantly expand their existing presence. GranCare, one of the largest institutional long-term care providers, has plans to launch an adult day services initiative in certain of its cluster markets. Originally a nursing home company, GranCare has aggressively moved forward to develop its home health and pharmacy business. The addition of adult day services is part of its strategy to offer a full long-term care continuum. Caretenders HealthCorp, based in Louisville, Kentucky, provides both home care and day care. It currently operates 13 centers and plans to open 15 more within the next year. Deerfield, a Maryland-based company that exclusively focuses on the private pay adult day care market, plans to expand from its current 8 centers to 18 by 1997. Active Services Corporation, a newly formed Alabama-based company started with venture capital, has plans to open up 12 centers within the next two years in the Southeast (New Frontier, 1996).

CONCLUSION

Adult day services will continue to develop and expand as long-term care needs, managed care pressures, and integrated health care system trends exert their collective influence to shape new forms of care. For home care providers, adult day services represents a logical addition and a significant business opportunity. The combination of day services and home care services may well become the core of America's future long-term care system.

REFERENCES

Americans of All Ages Are Deeply Concerned about Long-Term Care. (1996). *Perspective on Aging, XXV*(3), 5–12.

Blendon, R., Hyams, T., Benson, J., Donelan, K., Leitnan, R., & Binns, K. (1995). *Harvard/Harris long term care awareness survey.* Harvard School of Public Health and Lewis-Harris Associates.

New Frontier for Home Care: Adult Day Care Comes of Age. (1996). *Home Health Business Report III, 5,* 12–14.

Reifler, B., Henry, R.S., & Cox, N. (1995). *Adult day services in America.* Robert Wood Johnson Partners in Caregiving: The Dementia Services Program.

CHAPTER 79

Basics for Beginning a Parish Nurse Program

Janice M. Striepe and Jean M. King

H.L. Mencken said, "For every complex problem or issue, there is a simple solution. However, it's usually wrong!" We would paraphrase, "For every question, there is a simple answer, but it is not always correct." What should you consider if you are asking the question "Should I be a parish nurse?" Admittedly the answer is not simple, but by hearing stories of other nurses' experiences, you will see the positive aspects of the complex and diverse methods involved in starting a parish nurse service. (See box: "General Topics for Parish Nurse Education.")

JAN'S STORY: CONGREGATIONAL-BASED MODEL

When I became interested in parish nursing in 1984, I talked with my pastor about being a parish nurse at Trinity Lutheran Church (350 members), and I spent many hours over four months laying the groundwork. There were no parish nurses in our rural area, and I wanted to ensure that our members, as well as the health and social work professionals, understood the role.

I wrote a proposal to our church council, outlining the role and my responsibilities for a five-hour-per-week parish nurse position. Since our church was unstable financially, I asked only for office space (I do not recommend this ap-

proach!). The council accepted the proposal, and I began communicating with community health nurses, social workers, physicians, and other key professionals in our area, informing them about the parish nurse role, asking if they had any questions, and listening to their comments. All reacted positively.

In our church I talked to various committees and groups, as well as asking members to complete an interest survey before a worship service. All expressed high interest in health education programs. I reviewed tools for recordkeeping and adapted them for my new parish nurse role. I wrote a parish nurse brochure, started a pamphlet library, wrote church newsletter articles, and read holistic health books and Bible studies about health and healing. My pastor and I planned together. I wanted to focus on two pri-

---

General Topics for Parish Nurse Education

1. Introduction to Parish Nursing
2. The Nurse as a Community Resource and Referral Person
3. Holistic Health and Wellness
4. Spirituality and Healing
5. Formal and Informal Support Systems
6. Listening and Adult Learning Principles
7. Holistic Aging: An Overview (or Topics Pertinent to the Demographics of the Community)

---

ority projects. We decided on a holistic health series for the adult Sunday school, followed by a series on grief.

We also felt that a special program, Individuals of Wholistic Awareness (IOWA), would be beneficial. Members who enrolled in IOWA would attend the health series, meet with me to write personal holistic health goals, and confer with me regularly for support and guidance. IOWA was a good kick-off activity for the new ministry. Other nurses choose to market their parish nursing with special events such as a health fair or an intergenerational program. One church with ample funds purchased copies of the book *Seeking Your Healthy Balance* by Donald and Nancy Loving Tubesing (Whole Person Associates, Duluth, Minnesota, 1991) and gave a copy to each family on the Sunday of the parish nurse's installation service.

During my first year as a parish nurse, the Social Ministry Committee agreed to expand its goals to include health, creating the Social and Health Ministry Committee. Later the congregation approved my request for Trinity to enroll in Iowa Lutheran Hospital's Minister of Health Program. I would attend their classes and be salaried for 20 hours per week (half being paid by the hospital) for one year. Although my education, teaching, and community health experience were a good basis for the parish nursing role, I wanted to learn more, especially about Clinical Pastoral Education. Every year since has brought new programs and opportunities for learning.

JEAN'S STORY: DIRECTOR OF RELIGIOUS EDUCATION MODEL

I first became involved with parish nursing in 1986 when Jan asked if I would be interested in assisting her in the development of educational programs for the Northwest Aging Association's (NAA's) Parish Nurse Project funded by the W. K. Kellogg Foundation. I have continued to be associated with parish nursing in the areas of education, evaluation, research, and resource development. Although I do not serve as a par-

ish nurse in my 2,400-member Catholic church, I have been involved in faith sharing and other activities.

Various nurses have been interested in serving as a parish nurse in this church since 1986, but for different reasons, the time was not right for them. Pastoral leadership has changed, and there is increasing emphasis on lay ministry and community building within the congregation. Parish staff has expanded to include pastoral ministers, a youth director, and a director of religious education (DRE).

Often church staffing includes a DRE. When a job description is developed for this position, it could be advantageous to select a registered nurse. The combined role of the DRE and parish nursing has evolved successfully in some churches in northwest Iowa. The nursing activities, which include caring, community building, nurturing, and healing and wholeness, would complement religious education and theology. A major advantage of this model is that it provides the opportunity to incorporate the entire congregation in the activities and interventions formerly reserved for children and youth.

SALLY'S STORY: CO–PARISH NURSE MODEL

When a member of my church and I read an article about parish nursing, we were convinced that this was needed in our 200-member church. During our planning phase, we decided that we would share the position of parish nurse. We wrote a proposal describing which activities each of us would be doing and a schedule of who would be there for the parish nurse office hours. We have developed a special friendship as we support each other in a shared parish nurse role.

EVELYN'S STORY: TEAM MODEL

I have a busy family and work schedule. But I've always been a teacher and a youth group leader, plus being involved in other church activities. When my pastor talked to me about parish nursing, I was excited, although also frightened and a bit overwhelmed. Over the weeks and months, a great team model evolved in our 600-member church. Because of the support and interest of other nurses and health professionals, I decided to be the parish health coordinator and to decrease my other church responsibilities. I work four to six hours each week planning, communicating, and coordinating, plus visiting my foster grandparent.

Since the parish nurse job is so broad, we decided to divide and conquer the role. Many nurses agreed to have a foster grandparent relationship with one to five frail elderly members. Other nurses agreed to do one of the following activities: 1) send get-well, sympathy, and thinking-of-you cards to persons on the 3-, 6-, 9-, and 12-month anniversaries of the death of a loved one, 2) conduct monthly blood pressure checks, and 3) make hospital and nursing home visits. An obstetrics/gynecology nurse volunteered to visit church families who had a newborn.

Some of the health professionals wanted to be involved only intermittently. I contact them for members who have short-term needs and for group presentations.

I utilize the youth group and women's circles for assisting members. For example, a family needed respite assistance because the pregnant mother was on bedrest and could not care adequately for their three-year-old. Since they had limited financial resources, they were thankful that I could arrange volunteers for three hours each morning to care for the child and do light housekeeping.

Team members record their activities on a form, and I compile them on a master report form, which is given to the council. For our church, this model has worked very well, and I'm thankful that we have been able to be of service to our congregation and community.

COMMUNITY MODELS

There are two types of community models in our network. In Marcus, Iowa, population 1,200, each of the five churches has a parish nurse. Obvious advantages are support, sharing expertise, referring clients to each other, offering programs together, and increased cooperation among the churches.

An important aspect of this model has been the development of community outreach programs. With all the churches cooperating on a project, they are able to help more people and identify community health priorities. When the need for a long-term care facility was recognized, the nurses and pastors were key people in the community's success in obtaining a certificate of need to build a nursing home.

The other community model involves two or more churches cooperating to hire one parish nurse. In one town, the two local denominational leaders simply met and agreed on the action. In another city, the ministerial association decided that each of its member churches would contribute money to hire a nurse.

NON–PARISH NURSE MODEL

Most nurses will never become official parish nurses. However, many nurses have told us what they do in their congregations. Even though they are not parish nurses, they are catalysts for holistic health and for enhancing caring in their churches.

Hearing about parish nurse activities and interventions has inspired nurses to be more intentional about using their nursing skills for fellow Christians in their local churches. For example, nurses have become Stephen Ministers, have led occasional health programs, or have facilitated an exercise class.

MARY'S STORY: BARRIERS

When I learned about parish nursing at a conference, I began exploring my options. I encountered several barriers during the planning stage. At the conference, the presenter stated that usually a parish nurse is an RN with at least two years of nursing experience, but there is no nationally recognized certification and no standards of practice nor educational requirements for parish nurses. Since I am an LPN with a degree in health education, I was unsure if I could call myself a parish nurse. Because of my work experience, I felt comfortable in the parish nurse role but did not want to be reported to the Board of Nursing for practicing outside the role of an LPN.

The problem was solved when an RN in our church agreed to supervise, guide, and support me. Other LPNs have told me that they do not call themselves parish nurses; they are care coordinators in their churches.

My pastor was supportive, but he was so busy that he wanted me to present the idea to the church leaders. My first presentation met with lukewarm response, and they had many questions. I suggested several actions: 1) I would give each of them articles about parish nursing to read, 2) at the next meeting, I would show the video *The Connecting Link,* and 3) at the following monthly meeting, I would have a parish nurse talk to them, using the speaker system on our phone so they could all hear her. It would have been better to have a parish nurse in person, but none were nearby.

After laying this groundwork, I had enthusiastic support that enabled me to continue with my planning. Two other barriers that needed to be addressed were accessible training and concern about liability. Using money from the Memorial Fund for tuition and expenses, my church sent me to the three-day conference in Chicago sponsored by the Parish Nurse Resource Center. My pastor and I alleviated members' fears about being sued by assuring them that I carried professional liability insurance and that the church could purchase a policy specifically designed for parish nurse service. Pastor also gently but firmly suggested, "Yes, we could get sued; however, that should not be a reason to deny this ministry." Since I focus on wellness activities and do not do physically invasive nursing procedures, the probability of being sued is low.

During the planning process, I learned how important it is to patiently listen and inform.

Because I did not push members to make a quick decision, they felt ownership of the new service, as well as being supportive.

ISSUES: FUNDING

In our experience, we have found funding to be a major issue. It would be ideal if all parish nurses could be salaried. But the reality is that not all churches can accommodate this type of expenditure. Once the congregation commits to establishing a parish nurse program, options can be explored.

The pastor or nurse could contact the chaplaincy department of the local hospital for financial support or for sponsoring educational classes. Other institutions that have supported parish nurse networks are denominational-based nursing homes and colleges. Fraternal insurance companies and individual denominational district, regional, or state offices have been funding sources. One example: the Health and Welfare Committee of the Iowa Conference of the United Methodist Church has budgeted money for parish nurses.

To spur interest in a collaborative, community-based network, the pastor or nurse may ask a hospital or college to sponsor a workshop on parish nursing. Community partnerships have often led to cooperative funding for a network.

Other options for funding include special church offerings and church fund-raisers, which have the advantage of involving members. Some networks have received grants from private foundations. Your local library will have a book that lists and describes all charitable foundations.

More than one nurse has written a proposal stating that he or she would be a volunteer parish nurse for one year, with the stipulation that the church provide funding after that, if the program is to be continued.

Sometimes none of these ideas are successful or feasible. Being a volunteer has its advantages. Many nurses who have been both a volunteer and salaried have said, "When I was a volunteer, any activity was greatly appreciated,

COURSES PROVIDING INTRODUCTORY AND SPECIALIZED CONTENT COLLEGE CREDIT

Gerontology Certificate Program
Iowa Lakes Community College
Spencer, Iowa
> Semester Hours Credit: 18
> Prerequisites: None
> Information: Marlene Donovan,
> 712/262-4171

Holistic Health
Grandview College
Des Moines, Iowa
> Semester Hours Credit: 2
> Prerequisites: None
> Information: 515/263-2800

Parish Health Nursing, Graduate Program
Georgetown Univ., Washington, D.C.
> Semester Hours Credit: 36
> Prerequisites include:
> > Baccalaureate degree in nursing from NLN-accredited school
> > Minimum undergraduate GPA 3.0 on 4.0 scale
> > One year clinical experience
> > Registered Nurse licenser
> Information: Norma Small, Director,
> 202/687-4637

Parish Nurse Program, Graduate Program
Azusa Pacific University
Azusa, California
> Semester Hours Credit: 58
> Prerequisites include:
> > Baccalaureate degree in nursing
> > Minimum undergraduate GPA 3.0
> > Registered Nurse licenser
> Information: Marsha Fowler, Director,
> 818/696-3434

OTHER PROGRAMS

A Parish Nurse Preparation Program
> Concordia University
> Mequon, Wisconsin
> Rosemarie Matheus, Program Director,
> 414/242-0162

Minister of Health Education Program
> Iowa Lutheran Hospital
> Des Moines, Iowa
> Kathleen Fleming, Nurse Coordinator,
> 515/278-2613

Northwest Aging Assoc. Parish Nurse Project
> Spencer, Iowa
> Jan Striepe, Coordinator, 712/262-1775

Parish Nurse Orientation
> The International Parish Nurse
> Resource Center®
> Park Ridge, Illinois
> Ann Solari-Twadell, Director, 708/698-4754

Northwest Parish Ministries
> Augustana Lutheran Church
> Portland, Oregon
> Barbara Connors, Regional Coordinator,
> 503/288-6174

The Parish Nurse Center
> Concordia College
> Moorehead, Minnesota
> Cindy Gustafson, Coordinator,
> 218/299-3976

Parish Nurse Program
> United Medical Center
> Moline, Illinois
> Harriet Olson, Coordinator, 309/757-2696

Valley Parish Nurse Program
> Ansonia, Connecticut, 203/732-4837

INDEPENDENT STUDY

Independent Study Program
> Northwest Aging Association
> Spencer, Iowa
> Jan Striepe, 712/262-1775

There is a wide variation in the length, structure, and cost of the educational programs. For specific information, contact the person listed with the individual programs.

but when I became paid staff, the expectations for activities and interventions were much higher." Church members often make unrealistic demands on their paid staff. Whether the nurse is salaried or not, a health ministry will need funds for resources and expense reimbursement. Any ministry requires some funding in order to be effective.

BE A PARISH NURSE PIONEER

In the book *The Parish Nurse* (Augsburg, Minneapolis, 1990) Granger Westberg gives steps to start a parish nurse program. He writes that you need to 1) learn all you can, 2) inform and talk with the pastor and key leaders, 3) form a health committee, 4) try to establish a link with a hospital, 5) select and orient the nurse, and 6) begin the program.

In addition, we think that it is very important to use the nursing process to determine the most appropriate model. Doing a reflective and detailed assessment of yourself, the pastor, leaders, the congregation, and community will help you decide your planning, implementation, and evaluation strategies, as well as deciding which model of parish nursing will work best in your church.

Throughout the process, remember the power of prayer. Request that prayer be offered during the worship service, as well as utilizing your personal prayer time and other previously existing avenues for prayer in the church.

There are no easy, simple steps to starting a parish nurse service. Parish nurses repeatedly say that the developmental process proved to be necessary and beneficial. They enjoy being pioneers. Parish nurses exemplify the saying "Don't go where the path leads; go where there is no path and leave a trail."

SUGGESTED READING

Lutheran General Health System. (1994). *Reaching out: parish nursing service. An institutional/congregational partnership*. 2nd ed. Park Ridge, IL: National Parish Nurse Resource Center.

Shelly, J.A. (1982). *The spiritual needs of children*. Downers Grove, IL: Inter-Varsity Press.

Shelly, J.A., & Fish, S. (1988). *Spiritual care: the nurse's role*. 3rd ed. Downers Grove, IL: Inter-Varsity Press.

Solari-Twadell, P., Djupe, A., & McDermott, M. (1990). *Parish nursing—the developing practice*. Park Ridge, IL: National Parish Nurse Resource Center.

Striepe, J., & King, J. (1992). *Parish nurse practice: An independent study*. Spencer, IA: Northwest Aging Association.

Westberg, G. (1990). *The parish nurse*. Minneapolis, MN: Augsburg Fortress.

RESOURCES

Journal of Christian Nursing
 Inter-Varsity Press
 Editorial Office
 5206 Main Street, PO Box 1650
 Downers Grove, IL 60515-4634

The International Parish Nurse Resource Center
 205 W. Touhy
 Suite 104
 Park Ridge, IL 60068
 1-800/556-5368 (phone)
 847/692-5109 (fax)

Stephen Ministries
 1325 Boland
 St. Louis, MO 63117

Surviving the Present Challenges and Thriving in the Future: A Personal Viewpoint

Marilyn D. Harris

There are many times when I feel that I know what a swimmer experiences when being pounded by unrelenting waves in a rough surf. Each year there has been one wave after another hitting home health administrators. There is hardly time to catch your breath before the next wave hits. Only the names of these waves change. In past years, the waves included DRG aftermath, Gramm-Rudman Hollings, technical and/or medical denials, and administrative law judge hearings. Today, the waves include new regulations related to the Clinical Laboratories Improvement Act (CLIA), the Occupational Safety and Health Administration (OSHA), health care issues, managed care/managed competition, redesign, and re-engineering. References to the current reimbursement climate and health care issues continue to appear in numerous places, including the editorial pages of local and national newspapers, television, lay and professional journals, and letters to the editors. As early as 1978, Partridge said: "In the face of mushrooming pressures, constituencies, and complexities, we have but three alternatives: we can muddle on with our unsatisfying, uneven national performance, we can succumb, or we can emerge into a tomorrow we helped fashion. This latter choice is within our grasp" (Partridge, 1978, p. 10). Home health care administrators and local, state, and national leaders have helped fashion the future of the home care industry, which has experienced major victories and is in the forefront of health care in the late

1990s. Our efforts, however, are not completed; they are ongoing.

TODAY'S HEALTH CARE CLIMATE

The changes in acute health care financing methods continue to have an impact on in-home services. One of the most obvious ones is that patients continue to be discharged more quickly and need more intensive levels of care. From the patient's and family's viewpoints, patients require skilled and support services, many of which they expect will be paid by Medicare or other third-party payers. This is not the case. For the administrator, more intensive levels of care may equal longer visits and decreased productivity for staff. Another consideration is fixed payment as determined by the third-party payer and increased costs that present the potential for exceeding the home health cost limits for Medicare-certified agencies. Although the homebound elderly represent a majority of home care patients, there are other age groups that benefit from home care services. Maternal and child health care services, specifically those related to the early discharge of a mother and newborn, vary as insurers promote or require early discharge programs for new mothers and infants, and legislatures and Congress enact laws that require specific lengths of stays for hospital admissions.

Although Medicare medical and technical denials may not be at the same overall high percentage experienced in the 1980s, these denials continue to present challenges to agency administrators. Focused medical review by the fiscal intermediary also occurs. More frequent admissions to and discharges from home care services continue. At the Visiting Nurse Association of Eastern Montgomery County/Department of Abington Memorial Hospital (VNA), readmissions represent approximately 35% of all admissions each year. This results in additional time and documentation for the visiting staff to complete the admission but shorter lengths of stay on service.

The administrator faces several challenges:

- to provide high-quality home health and hospice care in a continuously changing and uncertain economic and regulatory climate
- to continue to meet certification, accreditation, and licensure standards
- to keep the home health agency fiscally sound and solvent
- to attract and retain qualified professional and support staff
- to maintain the budgeted number of staff visits per day
- to keep the staff and supervisors content and happy
- to maintain a sense of humor and perspective
- to consider the ethical issues that affect patients, families, staff, and the home health agency. These issues include the increased responsibilities that are placed on families as a result of high-technology procedures in the home as well as administrative issues, such as who will receive care in light of shrinking financial resources and how this care will be distributed in order to meet the health care needs of patients.

The staff members face still other dilemmas:

- how to provide quality care to patients under increased pressures from internal and external sources

- how to keep up with all the regulations regarding the provision of care and the ever-changing coverage issues
- how to document care for reimbursement purposes, not only for clinical, legal, and professional purposes
- how to master computerized clinical documentation systems
- how to maintain productivity standards established by and communicated to them by their administrators and supervisors so that the agency remains solvent under the current per-visit payment method
- how to maintain their sense of humor and proper perspective amid all the internal and external demands placed on them

Patients and families face still other issues:

- increased responsibilities to care for acutely ill individuals in the home
- scattered nuclear family members, which makes it more difficult to coordinate care
- lack of financial resources to pay for needed services that are not covered by third-party payers
- lack of public or private funds to pay for long-term care

The future method of financing Medicare home health care services is currently under discussion. Bruce Vladick, director of the Health Care Financing Administration (HCFA), stated the HCFA is committed to a prospective payment system (PPS) for home health care, just not anytime soon. He predicted that it will take two to three years to develop the systems and gather the data necessary to implement the prospective scheme (Rak, 1996). Terms such as bundling and copayments continue to appear in Medicare payment proposals. The National Association for Home Care (NAHC) has expressed its strong opposition to both of these methods and supports a per-episode PPS for home care as a substitute for copayments and bundling and has presented the home care industry's unified PPS proposal to the Prospective Payment Assessment Commission (Pro-PAC) (NAHC, 1996).

In addition to the financial challenges and uncertainties that administrators face each day, there are the clinical issues. For those administrators who are nurses, the American Nurses Association's (ANA, 1995, p. 6) *Scope and Standards for Nurse Administrators* delineates five primary domains of activity—leading, collaborating, integrating, facilitating, and evaluating. As an administrator, the nurse executive promotes a practice environment that empowers nurses to provide effective, compassionate, and efficient nursing care.

STRATEGIES FOR SURVIVAL

In spite of the many uncertainties in the 1990s, I expect to continue to survive the present and thrive in the future. To accomplish these goals, both long- and short-term strategies must be in place and utilized. All the issues addressed in this book are important for administrators to use as survival strategies. In review, these include the following issues, which are not listed in priority order, except for number 1:

1. Provide cost-effective, high-quality care (which is an expectation), ever mindful that the main reason why a home health agency and/or hospice exists is that there are patients who need the services that the agency's staff can provide. This multidisciplinary care must be flexible to meet the needs of individual patients and their families.

2. Evaluate the care rendered in terms of patient-focused outcomes. Administrators must collect and analyze manual or computerized data that will assist with the documentation of these patient outcomes.

3. Be totally familiar with the certification and accreditation standards that affect home health and hospice services.

4. Establish or improve methods to maintain fiscal stability. This includes the use of a management information system to monitor the myriad activities, payer sources, and demographic data to provide vital information on which to base sound management decisions.

5. Attract and retain qualified staff and contractors.

6. Manage fluctuating caseloads that can be financially and psychologically devastating to administration and staff. This may include alternative staffing patterns as discussed in this book.

7. Consider undertaking diversification or corporate reorganizations as described in several chapters.

8. Use a patient classification system (PCS), standardized flow sheets (SFS), nursing diagnoses (ND), or a computerized system to document patient care and patient outcomes. The use of a PCS, ND, SFS, care maps, and/or clinical pathways makes it possible for staff to address all the parameters that contribute to quality patient care. Staff know what parameters have to be addressed to meet the agency's quality assessment/improvement program's patient outcome criteria, which are based on certification and accreditation standards.

9. Provide disease-specific management.

10. Be alert to legislative and regulatory issues that affect home care and hospice. It is most important to keep in contact with local, state, and national elected officials through letters and personal visits. It is also important to be a member of the state and national trade organizations that have established hotline communication networks to address pertinent issues on a timely basis.

11. Participate in research in the administrative and clinical aspects of home health and hospice care.

12. Develop and use patient education materials to maintain or increase the quality of care provided to patients because current and future payment methods dictate

that administrators need to become even more efficient in the delivery of services.

13. Select carefully the other providers with whom you do business. Home care staff need good equipment and services to meet patient and staff needs. The nurse or patient needs only one bad experience, such as not having the proper equipment in the home or all the supplies for a specific procedure, as reason not to use a specific company or contractor. Waiting for service or equipment affects patients, families, public relations, productivity, and everyone's satisfaction with the home care services.

14. Develop a sound business and marketing plan for your particular home care agency's services in this era of competition. This is especially important when the issue of cost or price is eliminated.

15. Network with other home care providers. This is accomplished through attendance at local, regional, state, and national conferences. This is also accomplished through sharing information about successes and failures, developing useful tools, sharing research findings, and making suggestions for improvements in the delivery of services through publication of these results in professional journals.

16. Understand the importance of the educational and professional preparation of the administrative and supervisory staff of the home health agency. Clinical staff must be skilled in their areas of expertise. Clerical staff are also of the utmost importance to the overall quality of the agency.

17. Know individual state professional licensing regulations and professional practice acts.

18. Establish positive working relationships with the regional fiscal intermediary and referral sources.

19. Embrace the new technologies that are available for patient care.

20. Benchmark with similar agencies.

As noted in the introduction to this book, there are primary and secondary cluster areas of knowledge and skills recommended for home care administrators. In addition to these cluster areas, textbooks indicate that a nurse administrator should be a leader of a clinical discipline, a problem solver, a facilitator, a teacher, a scholar, and a manager and should be able to do budgeting, staffing, and labor relations and meet regulatory demands. The basic attributes that are desirable in an administrator were listed 20 years ago in a 1977 National League for Nursing publication titled *Characteristics of the Home Health Agency Administrator.* Some of the personal characteristics listed are the following: exhibits a strong commitment to and abundant energy for the task (that "extra something" required to achieve goals), shows emotional stability, possesses the ability to operate under pressure, and shows initiative, enthusiasm, pragmatism, and creativity. These attributes are as important in the 1990s as they were in 1977. In reality, the administration of home health and hospice care services, plus the expanded areas of responsibilities, includes variable percentages of all the above. The stress level is often high for administrators, supervisors, staff, physicians, patients, and families. The important thing to remember is that the provision of high-quality health care services is a team effort. This is certainly evident when the concepts of total quality management, continuous quality improvement, and/or performance improvement are implemented in a home health agency. Staff must hear about those issues that could and probably will affect their work and stress level. Staff from all levels and departments within the agency must also be involved in the identification of the challenges that may adversely affect patient care and the solutions to meet these challenges. Working together as a team, successful administrators, staff, and governing bodies will be able to survive the current health care climate and progress into the 21st century.

In 1600 B.C., King Solomon said, "Have two goals, wisdom that is knowing and doing right and common sense. Do not let them slip away for they will fill you with living energy and bring you honor and respect" (Proverbs 3:21–26). These two goals—wisdom (including all the information that has been shared in this book) and common sense—are important to me as an administrator of home health and hospice care and health care in the community today and in the future.

Pulliam (1989) shared *Survival Skills for a Fast-Forward Society.* Three of her suggestions are essential in the 1990s:

1. Let go of what's no longer working. Make room for what will work.
2. Take risks. In an era of diminishing guarantees, it's necessary to do so in order to not only survive but to thrive.
3. Make friends with this changing world.

Carney (1997) noted that the home care marketplace is dynamic. It doesn't stand still. There are constant changes. New roads and relationships to build. New developments occur. Construction and maintenance along familiar routes might force some rerouting.

In her *Notes on Nursing,* Florence Nightingale (1859/1992) shared her thoughts on management:

> All the results of good nursing, as detailed in these notes, may be spoiled or utterly negatived by one defect, viz: in petty management, or, in other words, by not knowing how to manage that what you do when you are there, shall be done when you are not there. The most devoted friend and nurse cannot be always there. Nor is it desirable that she should. But, in both let whoever is in charge keep this simple question in her head, not, how can I always do this right thing myself, but, how can I provide for this right thing to be always done? (p. 20)

CONCLUSION

Administrators must manage the agency in an effective and efficient manner in spite of multiple internal and external changes, current economic conditions, regulations, and budget constraints. The information presented in this book should help students understand the many details involved with the administration of home health care and hospice services. The assimilation of the contents of this book into daily practice should enable administrators to be confident that the multifaceted responsibilities involved with home health care and hospice administration, as well as the expanded community-centered care, are carried out when they are present and when they have delegated these responsibilities to competent staff members in their absence.

REFERENCES

American Nurses Association. (1995). *Scope and standards for nurse administrators.* Washington, DC: Author.

Carney, K. (1997). Marketing: An overview. In M. Harris (Ed.), *Handbook of home health care administration.* 2nd ed. Gaithersburg, MD: Aspen Publishers, Inc.

National Association for Home Care. (1996). *Homecare News. ProPAC meets to consider Medicare payment proposals.* XI(6). Washington, DC: Author.

National League for Nursing. (1977). *Characteristics of the home health agency administrator* (Publication No. 21–1681). New York: Author.

Nightingale, F. (1859/1992). *Notes on nursing. What it is and what it isn't.* Philadelphia: Lippincott-Raven.

Partridge, K. (1978). *Community health administration in a cost-containment era.* (Publication No. 21–1743). New York: National League for Nursing.

Pulliam, L. (1989). *Survival skills for a fast-forward society.* Chapel Hill, NC: Pulliam Associates, Inc.

Rak, K. (Ed). (1996). *Home health line.* XXI(2), 2.

Abbreviations

AAA—Area Agencies on Aging

AAAHC—Accreditation Association for Ambulatory Health Care

AACPI—American Accreditation Program Inc.

ABC—Activity-Based Costing

ABM—Activity-Based Management

AD—Associate Degree

ADA—American Diabetes Association

ADA—Americans with Disabilities Act

ADLs—Activities of Daily Living

AHCPR—Agency for Health Care Policy and Research

AIDS—Acquired Immune Deficiency Syndrome

ALJ—Administrative Law Judge

AMA—American Medical Association

AMCRA—American Managed Care and Review Association

ANA—American Nurses Association

ANSI—American National Standards Institute

ASCII—American Standard Code for Information Interchange

AVPD—Average Visits per Day

AWP—Any Willing Provider

BP—Blood Pressure

BSN—Bachelor of Science in Nursing

CAPD—Continuous Abdominal Peritoneal Dialysis

CCO—Community Care Option

CDC—Centers for Disease Control

CEO—Chief Executive of Officer

CEU—Continuing Education Unit

CHAP—Community Health Accreditation Program

CHHA—Certified Home Health Aide

CHINs—Community Health Information Networks

CHIRS—Community Health Intensity Rating Scale

CL/WLA—Caseload/Workload Analysis

CLIA—Clinical Laboratories Improvement Act

CMV—Cytomegalovirus

CNA—Certified Nursing Administration

CNAA—Certified Nursing Administration–Advanced

COBRA—Consolidated Omnibus Budget Reconciliation Act

COPD—Chronic Obstructive Pulmonary Disease

COPs—Conditions of Participation

CPEC—Contractor Performance Evaluation Criteria

CPI—Consumer Price Index

CPI—Continuous Process Improvement

CPR—Cardiopulmonary Resuscitation

CPU—Central Processing Unit

CQI—Continuous Quality Improvement

CRT—Computer Readout Terminal

CVA—Cerebrovascular Accident

DHEW—Department of Health, Education, and Welfare

DHHS—Department of Health and Human Services
DME—Durable Medical Equipment
DRGs—Diagnosis Related Groups
EAP—Employment Assistance Program
EDI—Electronic Data Interchange
EEOC—Equal Employment Opportunity Commission
EKG/ECG—Electrocardiogram
EMR—Electronic Medical Record
EOB—Explanation of Benefits
EPA—Environmental Protection Agency
EPO—Exclusive Provider Organization
ERISA—Employee Retirement Income Security Act
FAI—Functional Assessment Instrument
FBI—Federal Bureau of Investigation
FI—Fiscal intermediary
FIM—Functional Independence Measure
FTE—Full-Time Equivalent
FY—Fiscal Year
GAO—General Accounting Office
GE—Graduate Equivalency Degree
GHAA—Group Health Association of America
GI—Gastrointestinal
GIGO—Garbage-In/Garbage-Out
GNP—Gross National Product
GQS—Generic Quality Screens
GUI—Graphical User Interface
H–HHA—Homemaker–Home Health Aide
HCA—Home Care Aide
HCCM—Home Care Case Manager
HCFA—Health Care Financing Administration
HEDIS—Health Plan Employer Data and Information Set
HHA—Home Health Agency
HHA—Home Health Aide
HHCC—Home Health Care Component
HIM—Health Insurance Manual
HIV—Human Immunodeficiency Virus
HMO—Health Maintenance Organization
HR—Heart Rate
I–9—Immigration and Naturalization Form
ICD–9—*International Classification of Diseases, Ninth Edition*
IDDM—Insulin-Dependent Diabetes Mellitus
IDS—Integrated Delivery System

IPO—Independent Physician Organization
IRS—Internal Revenue Service
IS—Information Services
JCAHO—Joint Commission—Joint Commission on Accreditation of Healthcare Organizations
LAN—Local Area Network
ICNP—International Classification in Nursing Project
LOS—Length of Stay
LPN—Licensed Practical Nurse
IV—Intravenous
MAE—Management and Evaluation
MBA—Master of Business Administration
MCH—Mathernal–Child Health
MCO—Managed Care Organization
MFCUs—Medicaid Fraud Control Units
MIS—Management Information System (Refer to Chapter 51)
MSN—Master of Science in Nursing
MSO—Management Service Organization
MSW—Medical Social Worker Title XVIII-Medicare
NADSA—National Association of Adult Day Services
NAHC—National Association for Home Care
NANDA—North American Nursing Diagnosis Association
NAPHN—National Association for Public Health Nursing
NAQA—National Association for Quality Assurance
NASA—National Aeronautical and Space Administration
ND—Nursing Diagnosis
NHCC—National Home Caring Council
NIC—National International Classification
NICU—Neonatal Intensive Care Unit
NLN—National League for Nursing
NPR—Notice of Program Reimbursement
OASIS—Outcome and Assessment Informaion Set
OBQI—Outcome-Based Quality Improvement
OBRA—Omnibus Budget Reconciliation Act
OIG—Office of Inspector General
OSHA—Occupational Safety and Health Administration

OT—Occupational Therapist
P.O.—Per Os (by mouth)
PAC—Professional Advisory Committee
PACE—Program for All-Inclusive Care for the Elderly
PCA—Philadelphia Corporation on Aging
PCA—Professional Care Aide
PCM—Payer Case Manager
PCO—Patient Classification Outcome
PCS—Patient Classification System
PHO—Physician Hospital Organization
PIP—Periodic Interim Payment
POC—Plan of Care
POR—Problem Oriented Record
POT—Plan of Treatment
PPD—Purified Protein Derivative
PPO—Preferred Provider Organization
PPS—Prospective Payment System
PRO—Peer Review Organization
ProPAC—Prospective Payment Assessment Commission
PRRB—Provider Reimbursement Review Board
PSDA—Patient Self-Determination Act
PT—Physical Therapist
QA—Quality Assurance
QA/PI—Quality Assessment/Performance Improvement
QI—Quality Improvement

QRR—Quarterly Record Review
QUIGs—Quality Indicator Groups
RAM—Random-Access Memory
REP—Request for Proposal
RHHI—Regional Home Health Intermediary
RN—Registered Nurse
ROM—Read-Only Memory
SHMO—Social Health Maintenance Organization
SN—Skilled Nursing
SOAP—Subjective, Objective, Assessment, and Planning
SOC—Start of Care
SP—Speech Pathology
SSI—Supplemental Security Income
SWOT—Strengths, Weakness, Opportunities, Threats
TEFRA—Tax Equity and Fiscal Responsibility Act of 1982
TPA—Third-party Administrator
TQM—Total Quality Management
UB–92—Uniform Bill–92
UPS—Uninterruptable Power Supply
UR—Utilization Review
URAC—Utilization Review Accreditation Commission
VNA—Visiting Nurse Association
WANs—Wide Area Networks

"Managed Competition 101" Syllabus

Mary M. Nearpass

Accountable Health Plan: Under the proposed management competition plans, these would be the insuring delivery systems and would offer a standardized, federally defined benefit plan set by the National Health Board.

All-Payer System: All payers of health care bills—the government, a private insurer, a big company, or an individual—pay the same rates, set by the government, for the same medical service. The uniform fees would bar providers from shifting costs onto those more able to pay. The Clinton administration is exploring the possibility of at least a temporary all-payer structure.

Alternative Delivery System: A method of providing health care benefits that departs from traditional indemnity methods. A health maintenance organization (HMO), for example, can be said to be an alternative delivery system.

Ancillary Services: Support services sometimes needed for diagnosis or treatment (e.g., X-ray, magnetic resonance imaging (MRI), computerized tomography (CT) scan, etc.). These services must be ordered by a physician prior to provision to patient.

Antitrust Enforcement Agencies: The Department of Justice's Antitrust Division, the Federal Trade Commission, and the various state attorneys general.

Budget Neutral Conversion Factor: A conversion factor that creates no net increase or decrease in aggregate private payer expenditures.

Capitation: The per capita payment for providing a specific menu of health services to a defined population over a set period of time. This payment is the same regardless of the amount of service rendered by the group.

Carrier: A private insurance organization that contracts with the federal government to handle claims from doctors and suppliers of services covered by Medicare medical insurance.

Catchment Area: The geographic area from which an HMO draws its patients.

"Clinic without Walls" ("group practice without walls"): A number of practices in separate geographic locations that have centralized ownership of assets and governance at various levels of independence to function as a single entity.

Closed Panel: Medical services are delivered in the HMO-owned health center or satellite clinic by physicians who belong to a specially formed but legally separate medical group that serves only the HMO. This term usually refers to group and staff HMO models.

Community Care Network (community health alliance): The coordination of providers within a regional area to provide integrated health care services paid by government or private insurers.

Community Rating: Setting health insurance premiums based on the average cost of providing medical services to all people in a geographic area without adjusting for each individual's medical history or likelihood of using such services. The White House is likely to call for some form of community rating in the insurance industry.

Composite Rate: A uniform premium applicable to all eligibles in a subscriber group regardless of the number of claimed dependents. This rate is common among labor unions and large employer groups and usually does not require any contribution by the union member or employee.

Coordinated Care Organization: In dealing with the new workers' compensation law recently passed by the state of Pennsylvania, a provider is limited to 113% of Medicare reimbursement levels if he or she is part of this type of group organization.

Deductible: A fixed dollar amount paid before a health plan will reimburse your doctor or hospital. Traditional health insurance usually requires you to pay a yearly deductible. Many HMOs require no deductible.

Employee Retirement Income Security Act: Sets federal requirements for private pension plans (see Third-Party Administrator).

Exclusive Provider Organization (EPO): Similar to a preferred provider organization (PPO) in that an EPO allows patients to go outside the network for care, but if they do so in an EPO they are required to pay the entire cost of care. An EPO differs from an HMO in that EPO physicians do not receive capitation but instead are reimbursed only for actual services provided.

Expenditure Limits: Targets established by the government for the total amount to be spent by a category of providers, a state, or a health plan.

Fee-for-Service: An arrangement under which patients pay physicians, hospitals, or other health care providers for each service and/or procedure rendered. The patient is billed at the time of service. Most then seek reimbursement from a private insurer or the government.

Formulary: The list of prescriptions/medications that may be used without authorization.

Foundation Model: A tax-exempt, corporate care provider (the foundation) is created that is governed by a combination of hospital, community, and physician board members. Physicians typically must be in the minority on this board. A separate physician group practice provides physician services to the foundation. The foundation purchases these services through an annual contract, often for a fixed percentage of gross collections. The group practice is self-governing. Examples are Friendly Hills Clinic and Kaiser Permanente Medical Group.

Gatekeeping: A name for the requirement in health care systems that your primary care physician (PCP: an internist, family practitioner, pediatrician, or obstetrician) authorizes all care from other doctors (specialists) except for emergencies.

Global Budget: The term commonly used by experts for placing a nationwide limit on overall spending for health care services. The cap would cover both public and private spending. President Clinton has said that he intends to propose a global budget set by an independent national health board.

Group Model HMO: There are two kinds of group model HMOs. The first type of group model is called the closed panel, in which medical services are delivered in the HMO-owned health center or satellite clinic by physicians who belong to a specially formed but legally separate medical group that only serves the HMO. The group is paid a negotiated monthly capitation fee by the HMO, and the physicians in turn are salaried and generally prohibited from carrying on any fee-for-service practice. In the second type of group model, the HMO contracts with an existing, independent group of physicians to deliver medical care. Usually, an existing multispecialty group practice adds a prepaid component to its fee-for-service mode and affiliates with or forms an HMO. Medical services are delivered at the group's clinic facilities (both to fee-for-service patients and to prepaid HMO members). The group may contract with more than one HMO.

Health Care Financing Administration (HCFA): Part of the U.S. Department of Health and Human Services. In addition to its many other functions, the HCFA is the contracting agency for HMOs that seek direct contractor/provider status for provision of the Medicare benefit package.

Health Insurance Purchasing Cooperatives (HIPCs): These are likely to be critical pieces of the restructured health care system that President Clinton will propose. They would be purchasing agents for large groups of employers in a region that would shop for the highest-quality health plan at the lower price. The hope is that the HIPCs would give small businesses the buying muscle they now lack.

Health Maintenance Organization (HMO): A prepaid health care plan under which people enroll by paying a set annual fee. They then receive all the medical services they need through a group of affiliated physicians and hospitals, often with no additional copayments or fees.

Indemnity Carrier: Usually an insurance company or benevolent association that offers selected coverages within a framework of fee schedules, limitations, and exclusions as negotiated with subscriber groups. Insureds are reimbursed after carriers review and process filed claims. Aetna, Connecticut General, and Prudential are examples of indemnity carriers.

Independent Practice Association: A type of HMO that contracts with individual physicians to provide services to the HMO's enrollees. Physicians maintain their own private practices and thus can contract with other HMOs or see regular fee-for-service patients as well.

Integrated Health Care System: A single organization or a group of affiliated organizations that provides ambulatory and tertiary care to its enrollees.

Inurement: Payments or other acts by a not-for-profit hospital that benefit a physician using prohibited, charitable funds.

Managed Care: A general term for organizing networks of health care providers, such as physicians and hospitals, to enhance the cost-effectiveness of their work. An HMO is a common form of managed care.

Managed Competition: A proposal for financing and delivering health care that is likely to be the cornerstone of President Clinton's plan. Developed by a group of academics and health industry experts who meet periodically in Jackson Hole, Wyoming, it attempts to meld the best features of government regulation and market competition. The basic idea is to blend employers into large purchasing networks to shop for the highest-quality health coverage at the lowest price. The government would require any insurance company, HMO, or other health plan bidding for government business to offer a standard package of benefits. The hope is that the networks' huge buying power would generate competition among health plans, lowering prices and improving quality. All employers would be required to contribute the cost of health coverage for their employees, and the government would subsidize the cost for the low-income unemployed.

Management Service Organization (MSO): In an MSO, network participants form a separate entity that provides administrative services to physician practices. It is frequently used to coordinate managed care contracts and to get diverse group practices together. Physicians, hospitals, HMOs, and entrepreneurs can be owners. This model is generally popular with physicians because they can help govern the entity. Some are free-standing and publicly traded. MSOs can also be a division of a hospital. An MSO's openness can be a liability because it is connected to physicians through a contract that can be revoked. MSO's also could face fraud and abuse scrutiny.

Medicaid: A jointly run program by the federal and state government to provide health coverage to low-income families and nursing home care for the low-income elderly.

Medicare: A jointly run program by the federal and state government to provide health coverage to those 65 years of age and older as well as for the disabled of all ages. Part A of Medicare represents hospital coverage and Part B of Medicare represents outpatient care.

Medigap: Private insurance carried by many Medicare enrollees. This insurance pays for out-of-pocket costs *not* covered by Medicare.

National Health Board: Under the proposed managed competition plans, this board would collect outcomes as well as pricing and quality information for general release and would also set risk adjustment factors. This board would design the federally defined standardized benefit package.

National Committee for Quality Assurance (NCQA): An accrediting body that surveys managed care organizations to determine whether these organizations meet agreed upon standards of quality.

Pay-or-Play: A proposal for restructuring the health care system so that all employers would be required either to provide health insurance for their workers or to pay a tax to finance a government plan to cover them and everyone else.

Physician-Hospital Organization: A corporation jointly owned and governed by the medical staff and hospital. It can joint venture to deliver medical services. It can be a new forum for shared governance of hospital and practice matters. Examples are the Mayo Clinic and Henry Ford.

Physician Payment Review Commission: Created by Congress to recommend changes in current reimbursement procedures and policies for physicians receiving payments from Medicare. The commission first met in 1986 and prepares an annual report to Congress.

Point-of-Service: This product may also be called an open-ended HMO and offers a transition product incorporating features of both HMOs and PPOs. Beneficiaries are enrolled in an HMO but have the option to go outside the network for an additional cost.

Portability: If you change jobs, you can continue your health care coverage or automatically qualify for coverage at your new employer.

Preferred Provider Organization (PPO): An insurance plan where the patient may go to the physician of his or her choice, even if that physician does not participate in the PPO, but the patient receives care at a lower benefit level.

Providers: Those institutions and individuals who are licensed to provide health care services (e.g., hospitals, skilled nursing facilities, physicians, pharmacists, etc.).

Quality Assurance Program: An internal peer review process that audits the quality of care delivered. The program should include an educational mechanism to identify and prevent discrepancies in care.

Safe Harbor: Standards developed by the U.S. Department of Health and Human Services to protect individuals and services from criminal and civil prosecution and/or exclusion from the Medicare and Medicaid programs.

Service Area: Or "catchment area" or "enrollment area." The geographic area that the HMO serves.

Single Payer: A system whereby one entity, usually the government, pays for all health care. Canada has the best known single-payer system. It is financed by taxes, and people go to the physician and hospital of their choice and bill the government.

Staff Model HMO: The staff model consists of a group of physicians who are either salaried employees of a specially formed professional group practice that is an integral part of the HMO plan or salaried employees of the HMO. Medical services in staff models are delivered at HMO-owned health centers, generally only to HMO members. The physicians in either form of staff model are usually limited in their fee-for-service activities.

Subscriber: An employer, union, or association that contracts with an HMO for its prepaid health care plan, which is offered to eligible enrollees.

Superbill: Form used by a doctor's office containing all the necessary procedure coding, diagnostic coding, and doctors' identification numbers, as well as signature blocks for billing the insurance company.

Third-Party Administrator: An administrative organization that collects premiums, pays claims, and/or provides administrative services for self-insured employers (see Employee Retirement Income Security Act).

Total Quality Management (also called continuous quality improvement): Uses the concepts originally developed by W. Edward Deming to study systems and processes at medical groups to identify and improve sources of error, waste, or redundancy. Uses input and feedback from all staff and patients to understand and improve problems in current procedures.

U.C.R.: "Usual," "customary," and "reasonable" charges. Code words to describe a practitioner's fee for a service. Insurers use this as a standard in determining the amount they will pay to reimburse for services.

Home Health Agency Reorganization Checklist

William J. Simione, Jr.

- Determine what services are to be included in the subsidiaries (agency).
- Determine tax status of subsidiaries (agency, legal, SCI).
- Determine size and composition of board and officers (agency, legal).
- Develop name; draft articles of organization and bylaws (legal, agency).
- Revise current articles of organization and bylaws (legal).
- Determine working capital needs and method of capitalization; identify assets to be transferred, if any (agency, SCI).
- Determine financial and tax accounting for assets transferred (SCI).
- Review documents, if any, relating to assets to be transferred (legal).
- Board and members to approve asset transfer, if any, and restated articles of organization of existing corporation, and board to approve bylaws amendments (agency).
- File restated articles of organization and new articles of organization with secretary of state (legal).
- File articles and bylaws with Division of Public Charities of the Attorney General's Office for parent and other nonprofit corporation, if required (legal).
- Finalize management structure and organization chart (agency, SCI).

- Prepare exemption application for new, nonprofit corporation and file with Internal Revenue Service (legal).
- Notify Internal Revenue Service of changes to existing corporation and request confirmation of public charity status (legal).
- Apply for federal and state tax identification numbers (legal).
- Determine sales and use tax status (legal).
- Obtain corporate seal (agency).
- Consult, as required, with Medicare, Medicaid, and Blue Shield with respect to provider number and treatment of new corporation (agency, legal, SCI).
- Perform conceptual review of new structure, as required, with Blue Shield and rate-setting commission, if applicable (agency, legal, SCI).
- Determine employment complement for each organizational entity (agency, SCI).
- Review Federal Insurance Contributions Act options and waive exemption as appropriate (agency, legal, SCI).
- Review pension plan and other benefit programs and amend or expand as required (agency, legal).
- Review and modify or expand personnel policies, general and clinical policies, and procedures and compensation programs, as necessary (agency, SCI).

- Apply for state unemployment tax forms (SCI).
- Apply for state workers' compensation forms (SCI).
- Arrange for federal and state income tax withholdings for new corporation (SCI).
- Identify any contracts, agreements, and leases to be transferred (agency).
- Review insurance coverages and changes as required (legal, agency).
- Send notices or obtain consents required by documents being transferred (agency, legal).
- Determine specific services or functions to be carried out by each entity (legal, agency, SCI).
- Determine relationships and lines of authority among entities (agency, SCI, legal).
- Determine accounting treatment, financial statements, systems of new structure, and asset transfers (SCI).
- Determine necessary changes and additions to banking relationships (agency).
- Develop new stationery, logos, and other related materials (agency).
- Determine space needs as necessary (agency).
- Prepare leases necessary to provide for space needs (legal).
- Establish new accounting systems, records, and methods of accounting as necessary (SCI).
- Establish new payroll systems for all new entities with employees (SCI).
- Identify financial reporting disclosure requirements as required (SCI).
- Develop interval educational presentation of restructuring (agency).
- Develop public relations materials for distribution to new media and designated agencies (agency).

- Conduct staff meetings to inform personnel of changes (agency).
- Prepare memorandum to employees informing them of new employer (agency, legal).
- Meet with employees to discuss new employer and job functions (agency).
- Notify all national, state, and local associations of restructuring and make appropriate changes in memberships (agency).
- Notify lessors and contractors whose documents are to be assigned to subsidiaries (legal).
- If agency owns any vehicles, are they to be transferred? If so, determine where (legal, SCI, agency).
- Establish new bank accounts as necessary (agency).
- Determine status of certification and certificate of need (agency, legal).
- Adopt pension plan by subsidiaries with the transfer of all vested rights (legal).
- Notify vendors concerning assumption of liabilities (legal).
- Transfer instrument of general conveyance of properties from existing corporation to subsidiaries (legal).
- Create new W-4 forms for employees of new corporation (agency).
- Obtain new postage permit number from U.S. Postal Service (agency).
- Prepare d/b/a certificates for subsidiaries to operate under different names if necessary (legal).
- Prepare intercompany agreements for utilization of personnel (legal, agency, SCI).
- Review endowment funds to determine existence of any reverters (legal).
- Notify health care facilities with which agency is affiliated, if any (legal).
- Review union contracts for possible conflicts.

Note: SCI stands for the agency of Simione Central, Inc.

Glossary of Insurance Terms

William W. Fonner

Additional insured employees coverage: The standard general liability policy only protects officers, directors, and stockholders of your company if they are personally named in a suit as the result of activities that further the company's interests. Additional insured employee coverage grants the protection of the policy to all your employees provided that they are acting on behalf of your business when such a claim occurs. This would remove the possibility of having a loyal employee lose his or her home and assets because the employee was personally named in a suit while involved in company duties.

Advertising injury liability coverage: Provides protection for nonphysical types of injuries arising out of an offense occurring in the course of an insured's advertising activities if such injuries arise out of libel, slander, defamation of character, violation of the right to privacy, piracy, unfair competition, or infringement of copyright, title, or slogan.

Agreed amount endorsement: An agreement obtained from the insurance company stating that the values being insured are in compliance with the coinsurance clause in your policy. In effect, the agreed amount endorsement waives the coinsurance clause in your policy, which relieves you of the burden of proving to the insurance company after a loss that you arc carrying insurance at least equal to the amount required by the coinsurance clause.

"All-risk" property insurance: Protects against all risks of direct loss or damage to contents unless specifically excluded by one of the exclusions in the policy. Most standard property policies provide only coverage for specific perils or hazards; if a loss is not caused by one of these hazards, then the policy will not cover the loss.

Blanket contractual coverage: The first exclusion in the standard general liability policy states that your insurance does not apply to liability assumed by the insured under any contract or agreement. Many jobs for which you contract will require that you assume the liability of others. These clauses in a contract that require you to assume someone else's responsibilities are referred to as hold harmless clauses. Blanket contractual liability coverage provides you with protection for any liability of others assumed under any written (or oral) agreement.

Buildings (real property): Buildings or structures including extensions; fixtures, machinery, and equipment constituting a permanent part of the building; building service equipment and supplies. Foundations, walls, retaining walls, and similar property may be included by endorsement.

Completed operations coverage: Provides coverage for bodily injury or property damage occurring after you have completed a job (or a portion of one at a job site) or abandoned it. Coverage while you are working on the job is covered by premises operations coverage.

Contents (personal property): Furniture, fixtures, office equipment, machinery, stock, product, etc.

Extended bodily injury coverage: The standard general liability policy does not provide coverage for bodily injury claims arising out of intentional acts on the part of the insured. Extended bodily injury coverage extends your policy to cover any intentional act by or at the direction of the insured that results in bodily injury if such injury arises solely from the use of reasonable force for the purpose of protecting persons or property.

Extra expense insurance: Pays for the necessary extra expense (over and above normal operating expenses) that the insured must incur to continue as nearly as possible the normal operation and conduct of business after damage or destruction to real or personal property by a covered peril.

Extra expenses: If your building was rendered untenantable by fire or by any other insured peril, it would probably be deemed necessary to secure other quarters to continue operations. The use of such buildings would undoubtedly involve many extra expenses, however, such as rent, installation of telephones, and the like. Additional expense coverage would provide the necessary money for such expenditures.

Host liquor liability coverage: Protects you for bodily injury or property damage claims arising from the serving or giving of alcoholic beverages to any person in violation of a liquor statute (e.g., a minor or an intoxicated person).

Independent contractor coverage: Provides protection in the event that you are sued because of a bodily injury or property damage claim caused by an independent contractor operating on your behalf. This coverage does not provide protection for the independent contractor, however.

Loss of income: The loss of income directly resulting from interruption of an insured's operations caused by loss or damage by perils insured against the building or the contents of the building.

Personal injury liability coverage: Provides you with protection against nonphysical types of injury, such as false arrest, libel, slander, defamation of character, and other similar allegations. If one of your employees apprehends a thief caught in the act of stealing and has this person arrested, your firm could be involved in a suit for false arrest, malicious prosecution, wrongful detention, or the like.

Premises medical payments coverage: Allows you to pay all the medical bills (incurred within one year of the date of the accident and not to exceed policy limits) incurred as a result of any injuries that a person may sustain because of a condition on your premises or because of any of your operations (except products and completed operations). There are a large number of exclusions in connection with this coverage, but basically it is intended to cover guests who are invited to come on your premises.

Premises operations coverage: Provides protection for bodily injury or property damage claims arising out of the premises (e.g., someone tripping or falling in your office or job site) and all operations of business both on and away from your premises except where specifically excluded by definitions, conditions, exclusions, or other clauses that are pointed out in the proposal.

Products liability coverage: Provides protection against any claim or suit brought against you for bodily injury or property damage arising out of any product manufactured, sold, handled, or distributed by you. Such claim must occur away from any place of business owned by or rented to you, and the product must physically be in the possession of someone other than an insured.

Replacement cost coverage: Eliminates the deduction normally taken for depreciation after any type of insured loss to property.

Index

A

Abington Memorial Hospital Home Care, documentation, 129, 134–143
Academic education, staff development, 514–515
Acceptance of patients, 40, 41
Accountability
  benchmarking, 419
  program evaluation, 326
Accountable health plan, defined, 935
Accounts receivable, management information system, 640, 642
Accreditation
  Community Health Accreditation Program, Inc., 67–75
    advantages, 73–74
    application, 74
    benefits, 68–69
    concepts, 71–73
    consumer focus for quality improvement, 71
    contract, 74
    determination of accreditation status, 75
    expert site visitors, 71
    process, 74–75
    purpose, 68
    self-study, 74
    site visit, 74–75

standards of excellence, 71–73
types of organizations eligible, 75
Foundation for Hospice and Home Care, National HomeCaring Council, 77–79
  process, 78–79
hospice, 875
Joint Commission on Accreditation of Healthcare Organizations, 57–66
Accrual basis statement, 607–608
Activity report, management information system, 643
Additional insured employees coverage, defined, 942
Administration, program evaluation, 329
Administrative law judge hearing, Medicare denial, 860–863
  brief guidelines, 862
  expert nurse opinion, 863
  forms, 861
Administrative priorities, 455–461
Administrator, credentialing, 90, 94–96
  American College of Healthcare Executives, 94–95
  nursing administration certification, 94
Admissions package, high-technology home health care, 268

Adult day services, 432–433, 913–920
  consumer demand, 917–918
  defined, 913
  financing, 916
  health care reform, 918–920
  history, 913–914
  home care-day service connection, 918
  levels of care, 915
  market, 914–916
  market changes, 918–920
  operational issues, 916–917
  staff, 914–915
  transportation, 914, 917
  variety of services, 914
Adult learner
  characteristics, 513
  principles, 513
Advance directive, 26, 28, 659–661
Advertising, 718
  staff recruitment, 497–498
Advertising injury liability coverage, defined, 942
Agency for Health Care Policy and Research, 321, 322
  quality improvement, 321
  urinary incontinence, 394–408
    guideline implementation, 394–408
Aging, 11, 678–679, 715
Agreed amount endorsement, defined, 942

All-payer system, defined, 935
All-risk property insurance, defined, 942
Alternative delivery system, defined, 935
Altruism, 673
American College of Healthcare Executives, 94–95
American Nurses Association discharge planning, 429, 447
  nursing diagnoses, 225–226
American Red Cross, 10
Americans with Disabilities Act, 662–667
  employment application process, 663
  hiring decisions, 663
  individuals with contagious diseases, 664
  office accessibility, 665
  promotion decisions, 663
  provisions, 663
  public accommodation, 665–666
  reasonable accommodations, 663
  standard, 663
  substance abuse, 664–665
  testing, 664–665
  termination decisions, 663
Ancillary services, defined, 935
Antibiotic therapy, 260–261
Antikickback laws, managed care, 539–540
Antitrust, 653–654
  referral, 454
Antitrust enforcement agency, defined, 935
Appeals Council, 863
Application program, defined, 628
Application software, defined, 628
Architecture, defined, 628
Area Agency on Aging, 556–557
  Philadelphia model, 557–559
Artificial intelligence, defined, 628
ASCII, defined, 628
Assembly of Outpatient and Home Care Institutions of the American Hospital Association, 3
Association, history, 99

Audiologist, credentialing, 93
Audit trail, defined, 628
Automobile/vehicle insurance, 568–569
Autonomy, 518
Average visits per day, 576, 577

B

Back-up, defined, 628
Balance sheet, 610–612
Batch processing, defined, 628
Battery, 655
Baud, defined, 628
Benchmarking, 322, 409–420
  accountability, 419
  action plan, 416–418
  application, 418
  benchmarking database, 414
  benchmarking databases, 414
  benefits, 419
  best practice benchmarking, 410, 414
  candidates selection, 413–415
  communication, 419
  Community Health Accreditation Program, Inc., 73
  concept, 409
  contact, 415–416
  defined, 409
  detailed interview guide, 414
  documentation, 419–420
  history, 410–411
  issues selection, 411–412
  keys to success, 419–420
  maintenance, 418–419
  performance improvement, 288
  performing internal analysis, 412–413
    analysis process, 413
    team members, 412–413
  potential sources, 414
  process, 411–419
  questionnaire, 414–415
  types, 409–410
Benefits, 493, 503

Best practice benchmarking, 410, 414
Billing and statement, defined, 628
Bit, defined, 628
Blanket contractual coverage, defined, 942
Board, defined, 628
Boot, defined, 628
Brainstorming, 283
Breach of contract, 654
Bridge, defined, 628
Broadband network, defined, 628
Browser, defined, 902
Budget neutral conversion factor, defined, 935
Budgeting, 572–583
  analytical budget controls, 583
  capital expenditure analysis budget, 583
  case mix analysis, 574, 575
  cash budget, 581
  cyclical vs. noncyclical operating year, 573–574
  departmental expenditure budget, 577–579
    administrative and general expenses, 578–579
    benefit analysis, 578
    combination, 579
    direct compensation analysis, 578
    direct contract services analysis, 578
    incremental, 579
    indirect cost, 579
    plant operation and maintenance expenses, 578
    zero base, 579
  expense classification, 576–577
  operational budget development, 573–583
  productivity, 575–576
    average visits per day, 576, 577
    full-time equivalent staff, 575
    home health aide staffing, 576
    nursing employment factor, 575–576, 577
  program evaluation, 572–573
  program planning, 572–573

revenue projection, 580–581
expense and revenue
summary analysis, 581,
582
nonoperating sources of
income, 580–581
patient care services revenue,
580
statistical budget development,
573–583
Buffer, defined, 628
Bug, defined, 628
Buildings (real property), defined,
942
Byte, defined, 628

C

Capital expenditure analysis
budget, 583
Capitation
defined, 935
geographic variations, 410
Care plan, 6, 40, 41
high-technology home health
care, 269
pediatric home care, 246
ventilator-dependent child,
275–277
Career counseling, labor-
management relations, 487
Carrier, defined, 935
Cartridge disk, defined, 628
Case finding, ethical issues, 675,
680
Case management, 525–529
components, 526–527
costs, 528
critical pathway, 365
defined, 525
quality assurance, 527
research on, 527–528
training, 528
types, 525–526
Case mix analysis, budgeting, 574,
575
Caseload
analysis, 204–214

Easley-Storfjell Instruments for
Caseload/Workload
Analysis, 204–214
administrative uses, 210–214
analysis graph, 209
analysis roster, 208
guidelines, 207
instrument instructions, 206–
210
process, 205–206
summary, 212
time allocation worksheet,
211
uses, 210–214
management, 204–214
Cash basis accounting, 607
Cash budget, 581
Cash entry, management
information system, 640, 642
Catchment area, defined, 935
Cause-and-effect diagram, 283,
284
Center for Health Care Law,
National Association for Home
Care, 105, 109–110
Central processing unit, defined,
628
Certificate of need
acquiring home health care
agency, 82–83
background, 81–82
feasibility study impact, 82–85
non-certificate of need state, 82
obtaining, 83–84
requirements, 81–85
review process, 84–85
Certification, hospice, 874
Certified nurse administrator, 94
advanced, 94
Change. *See also* Corporate
reorganization; Organizational
change
Charged-based reimbursement,
588
Chemotherapy, 262
Chip, defined, 629
Circuit board, defined, 629
Civil liability, 655–656
Classification, 192–201
classification theory, 192–193
Client flow sheet, 268

Clinic without walls, defined, 935
Clinical decision support, defined,
629
Clinical evaluation
analysis by ICD-9 code, 349–
350, 351
analysis by major disease
category, 352
analysis by nursing diagnosis,
349, 350
daily report form, 354–355
data analysis, 349
data collection, 354–364
forms, 353–364
quality assessment/performance
improvement staff, 348
standardized flow sheet,
development, 347–348
Clinical repository, defined, 629
Clinical simulation, orientation,
524
Clinical specialist, 94
Clinical-Link, 151–159, 635
field automation, 644–649
Closed panel, defined, 935
COBOL, defined, 629
Code of ethics, National
Association for Home Care, 104
Collective bargaining, 489–490
Communication, 740. *See also*
Writing for publication
benchmarking, 419
labor-management relations,
483–485, 488
marketing, 719
strategic planning, 704
Community, 6
defined, 4
Community care network, defined,
935
Community Care Option, long-
term care, 557–559
Community Health Accreditation
Program, Inc.
accreditation, 67–75
advantages, 73–74
application, 74
benefits, 68–69
concepts, 71–73
consumer focus for quality
improvement, 71

contract, 74
determination of accreditation status, 75
expert site visitors, 71
process, 74–75
purpose, 68
self-study, 74
site visit, 74–75
standards of excellence, 71–73
types of organizations eligible, 75
benchmarking, 73
documentation, 120
governance, 70
mission, 69–70
objectives, 70
philosophy, 69
program evaluation, 330
public disclosure, 71
staff development, 506
standards, 71–73
outcome measures, 73
vision, 69
Community health information network, defined, 629
Community Health Intensity Rating Scale, patient classification, 199–201
Community health nursing, nursing diagnoses, 225–239
concept, 225–228
effects, 234–239
process, 228–234
standardized flow sheet, 232, 233
Community outreach, staff recruitment, 498
Community rating, defined, 936
Community relations, 718–719
Community-based long-term care, 554–561
Community-based nursing center, 903–912
academic nursing center model, 904–907
assessment, 907–908
development, 903–912
feasibility study, 904
fiscal management, 910–911
funding, 906

future of advocacy and nursing centers, 911–912
goals, 905–906
history, 903
human resources, 910–911
information systems, 909–910
mission statement, 905
planning, 904–907
program development, 909–910
strategic planning, 908–909
targeted populations, 904
Compatibility, defined, 629
Competence, 27
Competency assessment, 160–181
application phase, 163–165
continuing education, 178
home health aide, 46–47
interview phase, 165–169
job description, 161–162
licensed practical nurse, 164
self-assessment form, 166–168, 171–174, 176–177
methods, 178–179
occurrence monitoring, 178
ongoing assessment, 175–178
organizational assessment, 160–161
orientation, 169–170
performance evaluation, 179–181
policies and procedures, 179
quality improvement, 178
self-assessment, 508, 512
sign-off, 175
supervisor, 162–163
Competition, 714
Competitive analysis, 711–712
Completed operations coverage, defined, 942
Complex services, 13
Composite rate, defined, 936
Computerized documentation, 128–129, 144–159
Clinical-Link, 151–159
commitment, 149
defined, 145
documentation process, 144–145
expectations, 147, 148
framework, 147–151
human factors, 149–151

impact of health care trends on documentation, 145–147
integrated care delivery, 147
outcome measurement, 146–147
regulations, 145–146
reimbursement, 147
site visit, 149, 150
standards, 145–146
successful computer implementation example, 151–159
technology, 147–149
vision, 147
workflow, 151
Conditions of participation, Medicare, 25–55
acceptance of patients, 40, 41
administrative review, 54
administrator, 31, 35
advance directives, 26, 28
agency program evaluation, 54–55
care plan, 40, 41
care plan periodic review, 40, 42
clinical record, 52–54
clinical record policy, 121, 131–133
clinical record protection, 53
clinical record retention, 53
clinical record review, 54
competence, 27
compliance with accepted professional standards and principles, 29, 31
compliance with Federal, State, and local laws and regulations, 29
confidentiality, 26, 28
conformance with physician's orders, 40–41, 42
coordination of patient services, 32, 36–37
disclosure of management information, 29, 30–31
disclosure of ownership, 29, 30–31
exercise of rights, 26
governing body, 31, 34–35
group of professional personnel, 39–40

home health aide, 45–52
home health care agency
  hotline, 27
institutional planning, 32–33, 38
laboratory services, 33, 38–39
licensed practical nurse duties,
  43
medical social service, 44–45
occupational therapy assistant,
  44
ongoing education, 506–507
organization, 31, 33–34
outpatient physical therapy, 52
outpatient speech pathology, 52
patient liability for payment, 26,
  28–29
patient rights, 25–29
personnel policies, 32, 35–36
personnel under hourly or per
  visit contracts, 32, 36
physical therapy assistant, 44
planning of care participation,
  26
policy and procedure manual,
  424
policy review, 54
registered nurse duties, 43
respect for property and person,
  26
right to be informed, 26
services furnished, 31, 34
services under arrangements,
  32, 38
skilled nursing services, 43
Subpart B: Administration, 25–
  42
Subpart C: Furnishing of
  Services, 43–55
summary report, 37–38
supervising physician, 32, 35
supervising registered nurse, 32,
  35
supervision, 44
therapy services, 44
written materials for patients, 27
Confidentiality, 26, 28
Configure, defined, 629
Console, defined, 629
Consolidation, 714
Consumer
  educated, 715

quality program, 320
Contents (personal property),
  defined, 943
Continuing education
  competency assessment, 178
  defined, 514
  quality assessment/performance
    improvement, 299, 300
  staff development, 514
Continuous form, defined, 629
Contract billing, defined, 628
Contract negotiation, 719
Control chart, 284, 286
Controller, defined, 629
Conversion, defined, 629
Coordinated care organization,
  defined, 936
Coprocessor, defined, 629
Core memory, defined, 629
Corporate liability of providers,
  654–655
Corporate reorganization, 723–727
  benefits, 724–726
  costs, 723–724
  decision to, 725–726
  market share, 725
  models, 726–727
  technology, 724–725
Cost center
  direct cost, 592–595
  indirect cost, 592–595
Cost-based reimbursement, 588
Cost-benefit analysis, student
  placement, 814
Council of Home Health Agencies
  and Community Health
  Services, National League for
  Nursing, 3
Credentialing, 90–97
  administrator, 90, 94–96
    American College of
      Healthcare Executives, 94–
      95
    nursing administration
      certification, 94
  audiologist, 93
  current guidelines for
    nonadministrator, 92–94
  home health aide, 92, 93
  licensed practical nurse, 92

National Association for Home
  Care, 95–96
  occupational therapist, 92
  occupational therapy assistant,
    92
  personal care attendant, 93
  physical therapist, 92
  physical therapy assistant, 92
  physician, 92
  program administrator, 91
  skilled nursing, 92
  social work assistant, 93
  social worker, 93
  speech-language pathologist, 93
  supervising physician, 90
  supervising registered nurse, 90
Crime insurance, 569–570
Criminal liability, 656
Criteria, quality program standard,
  320–321
Critical pathway, 128, 365–376
  benefits, 369–375
  case management, 365
  congestive heart failure, 369,
    370–373
  cost *vs.* quality, 375
  development, 365–367
  deviation, 366
  sample pathway, 369, 370–373
  utilization guidelines, 368–369
  variance analysis, 367–368,
    369, 374
Cultural shift, 554
Custom program, defined, 629
Customer analysis, 712–714
Cycle billing, defined, 628

D

Daily report form
  clinical evaluation, 354–355
  financial evaluation, 354–355
Data, defined, 629
Data collection
  clinical evaluation, 354–364
    forms, 353–364
  financial evaluation, 354–364
    forms, 353–364

nursing diagnosis, 346–347
  analysis by, 349, 350
nursing research, 870
program evaluation, 334
quality planning, 321
Data dictionary, defined, 629
Data element, defined, 629
Data item set, outcome-based
  quality improvement, 379–380
Data repository, defined, 629
Database, defined, 629
DBCDIC, defined, 630
DBMS, defined, 629
Debug, defined, 629
Decision making, 658–659
Deductible, defined, 936
Delta Health Systems, 634
Demographics, 11
  demographic shift, 554
Deontology, 673
Departmental expenditure budget,
  577–579
  administrative and general
    expenses, 578–579
  benefit analysis, 578
  combination, 579
  direct compensation analysis,
    578
  direct contract services
    analysis, 578
  incremental, 579
  indirect cost, 579
  plant operation and maintenance
    expenses, 578
  zero base, 579
Dependent care agency, 116
Developmental self-care, 116
Diagnosis-related group, nursing
  diagnoses, 238
Direct cost, cost center, 592–595
Director, liability insurance, 567
Director of volunteers, 768–770
  job description, 768–769
  requirements, 769
Discharge, 6
Discharge patient questionnaire,
  292
Discharge patient satisfaction
  questionnaire, 547, 549
Discharge planning, 427–444

Abington Memorial Hospital
  Case Management Review/
  Referral Form, 438, 439–440
    continuation form, 441–442
American Nurses Association,
  429, 447
assessment, 435–436
community expectations, 430
conceptual framework, 429
defined, 427
discharge plan components,
  430–431
documentation, 431
ethical issues, 443–444
evaluation, 437–438
goals and objectives, 429–430
high-technology home health
  care, 436–437
historical development, 427–
  429
home health agency interface,
  444
implementation, 437
institutional expectations, 430
integration, 434
Joint Commission on
  Accreditation of Healthcare
  Organizations, 428–429
length of stay, 428
maternal-child health program,
  243
models, 438, 439–442
multidisciplinary collaboration,
  431–432
patient expectations, 430
process, 435–436
quality assurance, 443
regulations, 433–434
research, 434–435
resources, 432–433
third party payer, 429
Discharge summary form, 188,
  189, 268
Disease, change in distribution, 11
Disk crash, defined, 629
Disk file, defined, 629
Diskette, defined, 629
Distributed client/server
  computing, defined, 629
Diversification, 728–735
  corporate structures, 730–731

  decision to, 728–730
  funding, 731–732
  model, 730–731
Documentation, 119–129, 519. See
  also Computerized
  documentation
  Abington Memorial Hospital
    Home Care, 129, 134–143
  benchmarking, 419–420
  client flow sheet, 268
  Community Health
    Accreditation Program, Inc.,
    120
  current trends, 127–128
  defined, 629
  discharge planning, 431
  discharge summary form, 268
  ethical issues, 676–677, 680
  high-technology home health
    care, 255–268
  individualized nursing care plan
    form, 264, 265–267
  initial patient assessment form,
    264
  Joint Commission on
    Accreditation of Healthcare
    Organizations, 120–121
  key to successful
    documentation, 124–125
  monitoring form, 264
  National League for Health
    Care, 120
  orientation, 508, 522, 524
  patient medication record, 268
  patient/family teaching record,
    268, 269
  physician's care plan, 264, 265–
    267
  problem list, 264
  progress report, 264
  reasons for, 121–124
  regulations, 120–121, 131–133
  skilled care, 125–127
  student placement, 809, 822
DOS, defined, 629
Down time, defined, 629
Downloading, defined, 629
Dumb terminal, defined, 630
Durable medical equipment,
  ventilator-dependent child,
  vendor selection, 273

E

Easley-Storfjell Instruments for
Caseload/Workload Analysis
caseload, 204–214
administrative uses, 210–214
analysis graph, 209
analysis roster, 208
guidelines, 207
instrument instructions, 206–
210
process, 205–206
summary, 212
time allocation worksheet,
211
uses, 210–214
workload, 204–214
administrative uses, 210–214
analysis graph, 209
analysis roster, 208
guidelines, 207
instrument instructions, 206–
210
process, 205–206
summary, 212
time allocation worksheet,
211
uses, 210–214
Eastern Montgomery County/
Department of Abington
Memorial Hospital Visiting
Nurse Association, student
program, 816–822
Edit, defined, 630
Education for All Handicapped
Children Act, 245–246
Education of the Handicapped Act
Amendment of 1986, 245–246
Effectiveness
defined, 472
productivity, 472
Efficiency
defined, 472
productivity, 472
Egoism, 673
Electronic data interchange,
defined, 630
Electronic data processing floater,
570
Electronic home visit, 885–891

Electronic medical record, defined,
630
E-mail, 893–894
defined, 630
Emergency funds support,
fundraising, 758
Employee handbook, 661
Employee relations, 494–495
Employee relations manager, 488–
489
Employee relations program, 488
Employee Retirement Income
Security Act, defined, 936
Employment agency, staff
recruitment, 498–499
Employment contract, 661
Enteral feeding, 260
Environmental Protection
Agency, 668
Equity
defined, 472–473
productivity, 472–473
Ethical issues, 671–682
ancient beginnings, 673
case finding, 675, 680
characteristics, 674–675
compatibility of public health
nursing and complex care,
677
discharge planning, 443–444
documentation, 676–677, 680
finality, 674
generality, 674
managed care, 537–538
nurse's role, 679–680, 681
ordering, 674
orientation, 523
publicity, 674
quality of life, 677–679, 680–
681
reimbursement, 676–677
universality, 674
volunteer program, 766
writing for publication, 805–
806
Ethical theories, 672–673
Ethics, defined, 671
Exclusive provider organization,
defined, 936
Executive Certification Program,
95–96, 109

Executive information system,
defined, 630
Expenditure limits, defined, 936
Expense and revenue summary
analysis, 581, 582
Extended bodily injury coverage,
defined, 943
Extra expense, defined, 943
Extra expense insurance, defined,
943

F

Family, 6
changes in social behavior, 12
defined, 4
Family teaching, orientation, 522
Fee-for-service, defined, 936
Field, defined, 630
Field agency agreement, quality
assessment/performance
improvement, 317–318
File, defined, 630
File transfer protocol, 894
defined, 902
Financial evaluation
analysis by ICD-9 code, 349–
350, 351
analysis by major disease
category, 352
analysis by nursing diagnosis,
349, 350
daily report form, 354–355
data analysis, 349
data collection, 354–364
forms, 353–364
program evaluation, 331
quality assessment/performance
improvement staff, 348
standardized flow sheet,
development, 347–348
Financial management report,
management information
system, 643
Financial statement, 607–615
accounts receivable aging
percentages, 608
accrual basis, 607–608

balance sheet, 610–612
cash basis, 607–608
cash flow, 614–615
income statement, 608–610
personnel, 608
schedule of statistics, 608
statement of functional
    expenses, 612–614
visits, 608
Fiscal intermediary, Medicare,
    836–850
claims denial appeal, 840–842
claims processing, 838–842
cost report disputes, 846–849
coverage determination, 838–
    842
defined, 836
determinations preceding an
    appeal, 846–847
education, 837–838
filing appeal, 847–848
fiscal intermediary cost report
    audits, 843–845
functions, 837–842
information dissemination,
    837–838
postpayment compliance audit,
    845–846
program integrity review, 848–
    849
provider audit, 843–846
recoupment from all Medicare
    claims, 846
reimbursement appeals, 846–
    849
review of claims submitted,
    838–840
sample projection, 846
Fixed disk, defined, 630
Flag, defined, 630
Flextime, 462–468
background, 462–463
eligibility criteria, 465
evaluation, 465
experience over time, 467–468
forms, 463
implementation, 465
pilot project, 464–465
pilot project results, 466
planning, 464–465
policy, 464

study limitations, 466–467
task force on, 463–464
Flow chart, 284, 285
defined, 630
For profit, designation, 16
Form 339, 595, 596
Formulary, defined, 936
Foundation for Hospice and Home
    Care
National Association for Home
    Care, merger, 76
National HomeCaring Council
    accreditation, 77–79
    process, 78–79
    history, 77
    standards, 77–78
    structure, 77
Foundation model, defined, 936
Fraud and abuse, 655
Medicaid, 656–658
Medicare, 656–658
Fundraising, 719, 740
capital support, 757
emergency funds support, 758
follow-up, 760
operating funds, 757
preparation, 755
programmatic support, 757
project types, 757
proposal development, 758–760
proposal elements, 758–760
proposal submission, 760
seed money support, 757
sources, 756
    improving probability of
        receiving funds, 756
    researching corporations,
        756–757
    researching foundations,
        756–757
    researching government
        sources, 757
stewardship, 760–761

G

Gatekeeping, defined, 936
Gateway tool, defined, 630

General liability, 567–568
GIGO, defined, 630
Gliding time, 463
Global benchmarking, 409–410,
    414
Global budget, defined, 936
Gopher, 894–895
Government home health care
    agency, 17, 20–21
Graduate student, 811–812
Graphical interface format,
    defined, 902
Graphical user interface, defined,
    630
Group model HMO, defined, 936

H

Hard copy, defined, 630
Hard disk, defined, 630
Hardware, defined, 630
Head crash, defined, 630
Health care
abbreviations, 932–934
acceleration, 715
changing health care
    environment, 119–120
costs, 530
history, 530
today's climate, 927–929
Health Care Financing
    Administration
defined, 937
form 485, 41, 119–120
form 486, 119–120
form 487, 119–120
long-term care, 555
management information
    system, 649–650
quality improvement, 321
Health deviation self-care, 116
Health insurance purchasing
    cooperative, defined, 937
Health maintenance organization,
    defined, 937
High-technology home health
    care, 250–270

acceptance criteria, 255, 260–262
admissions package, 268
care plan, 269
categories, 250
consent to therapy, 255, 263
coordination of pharmacy and/or equipment, 268
delivery process, 253
discharge planning, 436–437
documentation, 255–268
eligibility, 255, 256–259
financial plan, 253
intake procedure, 253–255
market or service analysis, 251
objectives, 251
patient information referral data, 254
planning, 251–253
service capabilities, 251–253
staffing, 252
timetable, 253
Hiring, 741
Histogram, 284, 287
Home Care Aide Association of America, 111
Home care case manager, 542, 543
role, 544–545
Home care nursing, defined, 516–517
Home care product management, 697–698
alternative definitions of product, 698–699
Home health aide, 45–52
assignment, 47, 51
competency, 48–50
competency evaluation, 46–47
credentialing, 92, 93
duties, 47, 51
evaluators, 50
inservice training, 46–47, 50–51
instructors, 50
performance review, 48–50
supervision, 47–48, 51–52
training, 45–46, 48–50
Home health care
abbreviations, 932–934
changes, v, xi, 823–834
chronology, 8–9
components, 215

customer audiences, 712–714
defined, 3–4
description, 4–5
early sources, 6–11
expanding services, 724–726
expenditures for federal government, 585
framework, 215
future trends, 927–931
goals, 3
history, 6–11
initiation, 5–6
insurance issues, 565–571
new decision-makers, 714–715
organizational form in 1950s, 10
payment mechanisms, 9–10
present challenges, 927–931
provider types, 22
reasons for growth of, 11–13
resources, 6
scope, 17
service periods, 6
survival strategies, 929–931
types of services, 585
Home health care administration
areas of knowledge and skills, xxxiii–xxxviii
overview, 3–13
Home health care agency, 5, 15–22
financial status, 16–17
growth, 585–586
growth in numbers, 16
historical overview, 15–16
licensure, 85–87
background, 85–86
legal considerations, 87
practical considerations, 87
typical licensure law, 86–87
organizational structure, 5
ownership, 585
range, 17–22
recent history, 15–16
reorganization checklist, 940–941
state trade association relationship, 99–102
types, 16–22
Home health care agency association
functions, 100–101
participation, 101–102

structure, 99–100
Home health care agency hotline, 27
Home page
defined, 898, 902
design, 899–900
hypertext markup language, 900–901
publish, 900
requirements, 899
URL, 900
Home visit, orientation, 521
Homemaker service, 432
Homemaker-home health aide agency, 19–22
Hospice, 19, 20–21, 432–433, 872–871
accreditation, 875
certification, 874
challenges, 878–879
characterized, 872–873
defined, 872–873
federal hospice benefit, 875, 876
federal legislation, 874
financing, 875–876
guidelines for initiation of advanced care, 880–881
managed care financing, 876
managed care organization, 878
Medicare, 589, 875, 876, 877
palliative care, 873
patient care, 876–877
principles of hospice care, 873
regulation, 874–875
state licensure, 874–875
terminal care, 873
trends, 878
Hospice Association of America, 111
Hospital affiliation, visiting nurse association, 736–747
accrediting organizations, 743–744
board impact, 744–745
budget/reports, 742
change in professional relationship with peers, 745–746
check requisition, 742
communication, 740
contracting agencies, 744

contract/policy approval, 742
decision process, 737–738
external contacts, 743
finance department billing
    activities, 742
financial intermediary, 743
fund raising, 740
hiring, 741
identification numbers, 744
medical record committee, 738–
    739
national associations, 744
negotiation process, 736–737
nursing administration, 738
orientation, 741–742
pastoral care, 739
payroll, 741
public relations, 740
quality assessment, 739
social service department, 738
staff, 740–741
staff adjustments, 745, 746
staff impact, 744–745
state associations, 744
state certifying agency, 743
state medical assistance office,
    743
therapy department, 738
transition process, 738–744
United Way, 744
utilization review, 739
volunteer, 739–740
Hospital Home Care Association
    of America, 111
Hospital information system,
    defined, 630
Hospital-based home care, 10, 15
Host liquor liability coverage,
    defined, 943
Human resources, 491–504
benefits, 503
community-based nursing
    center, 910–911
defined, 491–492
Hydration, 260
Hypertext markup language, 900–
    901
defined, 902
Hypertext transfer protocol,
    defined, 902

I

Income statement, 608–610
Indemnity carrier, defined, 937
Independent contractor coverage,
    defined, 943
Independent practice association,
    defined, 937
Index, defined, 630
Indirect cost, cost center, 592–595
Individual rights, 674
Individualized nursing care plan
    form, 264, 265–267
Indwelling catheter, 394, 395
bladder retraining, 398, 399
identification of catheter-
    related problems, 396–401
Infection control, 60
orientation, 521
Information resource management,
    616
Informed consent, 255, 263, 658–
    659
Infrastructure, defined, 630
Initial patient assessment form,
    264
Inland marine coverage insurance,
    570
Inservice education
defined, 508–509
home health aide, 46–47, 50–51
implementation, 513–514
planning, 513
quality assessment/performance
    improvement, 299, 300
staff development, 508–514
Institution-based agency, 18–19,
    20–21
Insurance
glossary, 942–943
types, 565–570
Insurance company, 10
Intake personnel, 450–451
Intake referral form, 448
Integrated delivery system, 715,
    748–752
assessment, 749
at-risk, 749–750
benefits, 748

computerized documentation,
    147
contracts, 749–750
defined, 748, 749
disease state management
    issues, 750
implications for home health
    care agencies, 751
survival recommendations,
    751–752
strategies, 750–751
Integrated health care system,
    defined, 937
Intentional infliction of emotional
    distress, 655
Intentional tort, 655
Interactive, defined, 630
Interagency referral form, 448
Interface, defined, 631
Interface engine, defined, 631
Internal analysis, market analysis,
    712
Internal benchmarking, 409
Internal memory, defined, 631
International Council of Nurses
    code of ethics, 671
Internet, 892–897
applications, 892–893
defined, 631, 893
issues, 895
medical uses, 892–897
search tools, 896–897
sites of interest, 895, 897
Interpersonal skills, labor-
    management relations, 483–485
Inurement, defined, 937
Investor relations, 719
IS, defined, 631
IT, defined, 631

J

Job description
competency assessment, 161–
    162
performance criteria, 161
registered nurse, 164
    physical requirements, 162

qualifications, 162
self-assessment form, 166–
168, 171–174, 176–177
working conditions, 162
supervisor, performance criteria,
163
Joint Commission on
Accreditation of Healthcare
Organizations
accreditation, 57–66
discharge planning, 428–429
documentation, 120–121
home care accreditation
program, 57–66
accreditation benefits, 65–66
accreditation decision grid,
63, 64
accreditation decision
process, 62–63
deemed status option for
Medicare certification, 65
early survey policy, 63–65
organization eligibility, 57–
58
random unannounced survey,
62
standards, 57, 58–60
unannounced survey, 62
unscheduled surveys, 62
program evaluation, 330
quality improvement, 321
staff development, 506
standards, 57, 58–60
assessment, 58
care, 58–59
continuum of care, 59
education, 59
environmental safety, 59–60
equipment management, 59–
60
ethics, 58
human resources
management, 60
improving organization
performance, 59
infection control, 60
information management, 60
leadership, 59
patient rights, 58
service, 58–59
treatment, 58–59

survey content, 61–62
survey process, 60–62
Justice, 673–674

K

Keystone Peer Review
Organization, 784
generic quality screens, 786–
794

L

Labor management committee,
489
Labor-management relations,
481–489
career counseling, 487
collective bargaining, 489–490
communication, 483–485, 488
conceptual framework, 481
cooperative environment, 488
economy, 482
employee relations manager,
488–489
employee relations program,
488
factors influencing, 481–483
formal grievance procedure, 489
grievance procedure, 489
informal staff meetings, 487
interpersonal skills, 483–485
labor management committee,
489
laws, 482
patient care committee, 487
personnel department, 495
positive reinforcements, 487
problem solving, 485–487
professional organizations, 482
public sentiment, 482
supervisor, 487–488
Leadership, 59
Legacy system, defined, 631
Legal issues, 653–669

advance directive, 659–661
antitrust, 653–654
attorney selection, 669–670
civil liability, 655–656
corporate liability of providers,
654–655
decision making, 658–659
environmental issues, 667–668
independent contractors *vs.*
employees, 662
informed consent, 658–659
labor and employment issues,
661–662
Medicaid denial, 855
orientation, 523
privacy, 658–659
referral, 453–454
agency policies, 453–454
referral information
collection, 453
referral information
maintenance, 453
tax matters, 667
telehealth, 889–890
tort, 655–656
volunteer liabilities, 764
Legislative process, 685–686
Length of stay
discharge planning, 428
patient outcome data, 392
Liability insurance, 567–568
director, 567
officer, 567
Liability issues, managed care, 539
Licensed practical nurse
competency assessment, 164
self-assessment form, 166–
168, 171–174, 176–177
credentialing, 92
performance evaluation, 180
Licensure
home health care agency, 85–87
background, 85–86
legal considerations, 87
practical considerations, 87
typical licensure law, 86–87
Medicare, 87
program evaluation, 330
Line surge, defined, 631
Linking, defined, 631
Load, defined, 631

Local area network, defined, 631
Local government, 684–685
Longitudinal patient record, defined, 631
Long-term care, 554–561
    becoming long-term care provider, 559–561
    Community Care Option, 557–559
    current policy, 555–556
    defined, 554–555
    Health Care Financing Administration, 555
    past performance, 560
    Philadelphia Corporation for Aging, 557–559
    physician, 560
    program trends, 555–556
    publicly financed, 556
    skilled care, differentiated, 560
Loss of income, defined, 943
LP, defined, 631

M

Main memory, defined, 631
Mainframe computing, defined, 631
Managed care, v, 530–541, 714
    advantages of contracting, 544
    antikickback laws, 539–540
    case management, compared, 542–543
    consolidation markets, 534
    contracting with, 536–537
    defined, 525, 937
    development, 531–532
    development stages, 534
    disadvantages of contracting, 544
    discharge patient satisfaction questionnaire, 547, 549
    ethical issues, 537–538
    evaluation of managed care organizations, 538–539
    future, 540–541
    geographic variations, 410
    growth, 531–532

history, 531
    in home care, 535
        strategic planning, 535
    hospice, 878
    legal issues, 539–540
    liability issues, 539
    loose-framework markets, 534
    managed competition, 534
    network, 535–536
    payment mechanisms, 534–535
    performance improvement, 547–552
    pricing strategies, 534–535
    problems, 537–540
    quality, 537
    quality assessment, 547–552
    referral, 539–540
    regulatory issues, 539–540
    research, 538
    safe harbor provision, 539
    Service Authorization Progress Note, 547, 548
    state regulation, 540
    structure, 532–534
    teaching, 538
    unstructured markets, 534
    working with managed care networks, success strategies, 545–547
Managed care information system, defined, 631
Managed competition, 534
    defined, 525, 937
    glossary, 935–939
Management information system, 550, 616–650
    accounts receivable, 640, 642
    activity report, 643
    ad hoc reporting, 640–643
    automation, selection, 618–622
    bundled systems, 621
    cash entry, 640, 642
    computerization, 616–617
        current computer technology, 617–618
        data analysis, 617
        rationale for, 622–623
        selection, 618–622
        timing of, 623–624
    daily report form, 638–640
    data collection, 635–636

data processing level comparison, 620
    example, 634–650
    existing software packages, 625, 626–627
        guarantees, 625
    expansiveness, 616
    features, 620–622
    financial management report, 643
    generalized system architectures, 634–635
    hardware needs, 622
    Health Care Financing Administration system, 649–650
    in-house software development, 624–625, 626–627
    master file maintenance, 636
    patient master update form, 636–638
    physician, 827
    program evaluation, 329
    quality assurance, 644
    scheduling system, 649–650
    selection committee, 619, 620
        issues, 621
    software, acceptance testing, 626
    statistical report, 643–644
    turnkey systems, 621
    types of systems, 620–622
    unbundled software, 621
    year-to-date visits, 640, 641
Management service organization, defined, 937
Market analysis, 711–714
    competitive analysis, 711–712
    customer analysis, 712–714
    elements, 713
    internal analysis, 712
Market share, corporate reorganization, 725
Market trends, 714–715
Marketing, 708–722, 717
    adaptation, 720–721
    benefits, 710–711
    communication, 719
    defined, 708–709
    focus, 720
    four Ps of marketing, 717–718

home health care role, 709–711
  implementation, 720
  local strategies, 720
  marketing structure, 720
  measurement, 720–721
  place, 717–718
  price, 718
  product, 717
  promotion, 718–719
  referral, 452–453
  sales, 719
Marketing plan, 715–716
  elements, 716
  living document, 720, 721
  planning, 715–716
  preparation, 715–716
Master patient index, defined, 631
Master person index, defined, 631
Maternal-child health program, 242–248
  discharge planning, 243
  funding, 243
  staffing, 243
Maxiflex, 463
Meals-on-Wheels, 432–433
Media relations, 718
Medicaid, 10–11
  defined, 938
  fraud and abuse, 656–658
  reimbursement, 12, 587
    changing reimbursement patterns, 12
Medical history, 256–259
Medical record, 52–54, 121, 131–133
  defined, 632
  program evaluation, 331–332
Medical record abstracting, nursing research, 870
Medical record committee, 738–739
Medical record department, 129
Medical record length, defined, 632
Medical social service, 44–45
Medical supplies, 589
Medicare, 5, 10–11
  conditions of participation, 25–55
    acceptance of patients, 40, 41
    administrative review, 54

administrator, 31, 35
advance directives, 26, 28
agency program evaluation, 54–55
care plan, 40, 41
care plan periodic review, 40, 42
clinical record, 52–54
clinical record policy, 121, 131–133
clinical record review, 54
competence, 27
compliance with accepted professional standards and principles, 29, 31
compliance with Federal, State, and local laws and regulations, 29
confidentiality, 26, 28
conformance with physician's orders, 40–41, 42
coordination of patient services, 32, 36–37
disclosure of management information, 29, 30–31
disclosure of ownership, 29, 30–31
exercise of rights, 26
governing body, 31, 34–35
group of professional personnel, 39–40
home health aide, 45–52
home health care agency hotline, 27
institutional planning, 32–33, 38
laboratory services, 33, 38–39
licensed practical nurse duties, 43
medical social service, 44–45
occupational therapy assistant, 44
ongoing education, 506–507
organization, 31, 33–34
outpatient physical therapy, 52
outpatient speech pathology, 52
patient liability for payment, 26, 28–29

patient rights, 25–29
personnel policies, 32, 35–36
personnel under hourly or per visit contracts, 32, 36
physical therapy assistant, 44
planning of care participation, 26
policy review, 54
record protection, 53
record retention, 53
registered nurse duties, 43
respect for property and person, 26
right to be informed, 26
services furnished, 31, 34
services under arrangements, 32, 38
skilled nursing services, 43
Subpart B: Administration, 25–42
Subpart C: Furnishing of Services, 43–55
summary report, 37–38
supervising physician, 32, 35
supervising registered nurse, 32, 35
supervision, 44
therapy services, 44
written materials for patients, 27
defined, 938
fiscal intermediary, 836–850
  claims denial appeal, 840–842
  claims processing, 838–842
  cost report disputes, 846–849
  coverage determination, 838–842
  defined, 836
  determinations preceding an appeal, 846–847
  education, 837–838
  filing appeal, 847–848
  fiscal intermediary cost report audits, 843–845
  functions, 837–842
  information dissemination, 837–838
  postpayment compliance audit, 845–846

program integrity review,
848–849
provider audit, 843–846
recoupment from all
Medicare claims, 846
reimbursement appeals, 846–
849
review of claims submitted,
838–840
sample projection, 846
fraud and abuse, 656–658
hospice, 589, 875, 876, 877
licensure, 87
orientation, Medicare home care
benefit, 522
program evaluation, 328, 329–
330
reimbursement, 12, 586–602,
604–605
administrative and general
expenses, 594
allocation, 592–595
changing reimbursement
patterns, 12
charged-based
reimbursement, 588
cost accounting, 589–590
cost finding, 589–590
cost limit, 595–598
cost report, 589–590
cost report appeal, 601–602
cost-based reimbursement,
588
customary charge, 598–599
depreciation, 594
discrete costing, 602–604
entitlement, 587
Form 339, 595, 596
home health aide, 587
increasing, 602–605
medical supplies, 589
methods of reimbursement,
588–602
nonallowable costs, 592–593
occupational therapy, 587–588
physical therapy, 587–588
PIP reimbursement, 598–600
prospective payment, 588
Provider Cost Report
Reimbursement
Questionnaire, 595, 596

Provider Reimbursement
Review Board, 602
reasonable cost, 588, 598–
599
restructured agency, 604–605
skilled nursing, 587
speech therapy, 587–588
Summary of Medicare
Uncollectibles, 595, 596
technical denial, 600–601
transportation cost, 594
waiver of liability, 601
staff development, 506
Medicare denial
administrative law judge
hearing, 860–863
brief guidelines, 862
expert nurse opinion, 863
forms, 861
appeal process, 840–842, 851–
865
Appeals Council, 863
background, 851–852
civil action, 863
climate change, 851–853
forms, 858, 859
guidelines for filing appeals,
856
reasons for appealing, 864
reconsideration, 857–860
reopening, 856–857
examples, 854–855
financial impact, 855
impact, 853–854
legal issues, 855
political process, 855–856
resulting actions, 855–856
types, 853
Medigap, defined, 938
Memory, defined, 631
Menu, defined, 631
Merge, defined, 631
Microcomputer, defined, 631
Microprocessor, defined, 631
Modem, defined, 631
Module, defined, 631
Monitor, defined, 631
Monitoring form, 264
Montefiore Hospital, 15
Monthly statement, defined, 628

Morality, traditional models, 671–
672
Motherboard, defined, 631
Motivation, 476
MS-DOS, defined, 631
Multicorporate organization, 726–
727
Multiplexon, defined, 631
Multitasking, defined, 631
Multiuser, defined, 631
Multivoting, 283

N

National Association for Home
Care, 95–111
affiliate organizations, 111
annual meeting, 109
Center for Health Care Law,
105, 109–110
certification, 109
code of ethics, 104
committees, 108–109
communications, 109
credentialing, 95–96
departments, 109–110
education, 109
Foundation for Hospice and
Home Care, merger, 76
functions, 95–96
goals, 105–107
governance, 107–108
Government Affairs
Department, 110
information dissemination, 109
legal symposium, 109
mission, 104
policy conferences, 109
regional conferences, 109
Regulatory Affairs Department,
110
reimbursement, 605
Research Department, 110–111
values, 104–105
National Association of Home
Health Agencies, 3
National Committee for Quality
Assurance, defined, 938

National Consensus Conference on the Educational Preparation of Home Care Administrators, xxxiii
National Health Board, defined, 938
National Home Caring Council, 3
National League for Health Care, documentation, 120
National League for Nursing, 10
  productivity calculation: home visits per day per employee, 577
National Medicare Quality Assurance and Improvement Demonstration, 387
National Organization for Public Health Nursing, 9, 10
Negligence, 655
Network
  defined, 631
  managed care, 535–536
Networking, 684–685
Nightingale, Florence, 7
Nonoperating sources of income, 580–581
North American Nursing Diagnosis Association, 226, 227
Not for profit, designation, 16
Nurse administrator, as author, 795–807
Nursing
  defined, 116
  historical aspects, 7
  partly compensatory system, 117–118
  supportive-educative system, 117
  wholly compensatory nursing system, 116–117
Nursing diagnosis, 216
  American Nurses Association, 225–226
  analysis, 219
  classification, 215–224, 220–221
    developmental strategy, 215–216
    implications, 219
    strategy, 216
    coding framework, 217

coding scheme, 220–221
community health nursing, 225–239
  concept, 225–228
  effects, 234–239
  process, 228–234
  standardized flow sheet, 232, 233
  data collection, 346–347
    analysis by, 349, 350
  diagnosis-related group, 238
  expected outcomes, 216
  North American Nursing Diagnosis Association, 226, 227
  nursing assessment form, 228–231
  Omaha Visiting Nurse Association, 226–227
  sample nursing diagnosis list, 235–238
Nursing interventions
  analysis, 219
  classification, 215–224, 222–224
    developmental strategy, 215–216
    implications, 219
    strategy, 217
  coding framework, 217
  coding scheme, 222–224
Nursing productivity, 204
Nursing research, 867–871
  agency commitment, 868
  collaborative research, 867–868
  cost in time, 869–870
  data collection, 870
  designated overseer, 868–869
  funding sources, 867, 868
  project elements, 868–869
  project validity, 868
  record abstracting, 870
  research project types, 867–868

O

Object code, defined, 632
Obligation, 674

Occupational Safety and Health Administration, 667–668
Occupational therapist, credentialing, 92
Occupational therapy assistant, 44
  credentialing, 92
Occurrence monitoring, competency assessment, 178
Officer, liability insurance, 567
Off-line, defined, 632
Older Americans Act, reimbursement, 587
Omaha Visiting Nurse Association, nursing diagnoses, 226–227
On-line, defined, 632
Open architecture, defined, 632
Operating income, 610
Operating loss, 610
Operating system, defined, 632
Operational planning, strategic planning
  linkages, 703
  participant selection, 703
  process, 704
Optical disk archiving, defined, 632
Organizational assessment, competency assessment, 160–161
Organizational change, 694–702
  environment manipulation, 694–696
  extraorganizational adjustment, 699–700
    from vertical to virtual integration, 699–700
  operational adjustment, 696–697
  product life cycle, 696–697
  strategic adjustment, 697–699
  strategic planning, 701–702
    assessment of external environment, 701
    clarifying goals and objectives, 701–702
    identifying phase strategy, 702
Organizational chart, 34
Orientation, 741–742
  clinical simulation, 524

competency assessment, 169–170

content areas, 520–523

documentation, 508, 522, 524

ethical issues, 523

family teaching, 522

home care nursing specialty, 520–521

home care nursing strategies for success, 523

home visit, 521

infection control, 521

legal issues, 523

Medicare home care benefit, 522

organization of home care system, 520

patient education, 522

role play, 524

self-directed learning, 524

specialized home care program, 523

strategies for effective clinical management, 522–523

teaching strategies, 524

update sessions, 487

Outcome, 6

types, 378–379, 387–388

Outcome and Assessment Information Set (OASIS), 127–128

outcome-based quality improvement, 379–380

Outcome measurement, 182–191

computerized documentation, 146–147

program evaluation, 331

Outcome-based quality improvement, 377–385

current demonstration programs, 383–384

data item set, 379–380

Outcome and Assessment Information Set (OASIS), 379–380

outcome report, 382–383

outcome types, 378–379

quality indicator group, 381–382

two-stage continuous quality improvement screen, 380–382

Outpatient physical therapy, 52

Outpatient speech pathology, 52

Output, defined, 632

Overhead, defined, 632

P

Pain management, 261–262

Palliative care, hospice, 873

Parallel, defined, 632

Parameter, defined, 632

Pareto chart, 284, 287

Parish nurse program, 921–926

barriers, 923–924

community models, 923

congregational-based model, 921–922

co-parish nurse model, 922

director of religious education model, 922

education, 924–925

funding, 924–925

non-parish nurse model, 923

parish nurse education, 921

team model, 922–923

Password, defined, 632

Pastoral care, 739

Patient assessment, 256–259

Patient care committee, labor-management relations, 487

Patient care services revenue, 580

Patient classification, 192–201

administrative management, 197–201

background, 345–346

classification theory, 192–193

clinical management, 194–197

Community Health Intensity Rating Scale, 199–201

critical indicators of care, 198

nursing diagnosis taxonomy, 193–194

patient classification systems, 193

program planning, 198

quality assessment/performance improvement, 295, 296

significance, 345–346

Patient classification outcome system, 182–191

advantages, 188–190

discharge summary form, 188, 189

objectives, 183–186

patient admission, 186–188

patient groups, 183–186

reliability, 190

Patient education, 519

orientation, 522

patient/family teaching record, 268, 269

Patient medication record, 268

Patient outcome data, 387–392

age, 389

AMH encounters, 390

diagnoses, 390–391

findings, 389–392

implication for home healthcare nurses, 392

insurers, 389–390

length of stay, 392

lifestyle, 390, 391

patients who expired following readmission, 391–392

procedure, 388–389

race, 390, 391

sex, 390, 391

Visiting Nurse Association visits, 390

Patient Self Determination Act, 659–660

Payer case manager, 542, 543

role, 544–545

Pay-or-play, defined, 938

Pediatric home care

adaptation monitoring, 246–247

care plan, 246

determining continuing needs, 245–246

goals, 244–247

patient stabilization, 245

transition from hospital to home and community, 244–245

Peer review, quality assessment/performance improvement, 299

Peer Review Improvement Act, 781

Peer review organization, 781–793
  agency-specific findings, 782–783
  generic quality screen, 781, 786–794
  national findings, 783
  process overview, 781–782

Performance criteria, job description, 161

Performance evaluation
  competency assessment, 179–181
  licensed practical nurse, 180

Performance improvement, 281–289, 290–302, 304–318
  acceleration, 288
  benchmarking, 288
  implementation, 282–287
  initiation, 282–287
  managed care organization, 547–552
  process improvement, 288–289
  process measurement, 288–289
  variation, 288

Peripheral, defined, 632

Personal care attendant
  credentialing, 93
  evaluation, 48

Personal injury liability coverage, defined, 943

Personnel administrator, 495–496

Personnel department
  goal, 492–495
  labor-management relations, 495
  personnel policies, 495, 496
  record retention, 495, 496
  role, 492–495
  services, 492–495
  size, 497
  staff, 495–497
  structure, 492–495

Philadelphia Corporation for Aging, long-term care, 557–559

Physical therapist, credentialing, 92

Physical therapy assistant, 44
  credentialing, 92

Physician, 719, 823–834

administrative issues, 832–833
clinical issues, 831–832
credentialing, 92
educational involvements, 827
enhanced role, 829
health insurance for the aged, 831
home care capabilities, 825–827
home care information, 825–826
home health care administrator, goals, 825–830
home visit facilitation, 827
lack of home health care physician involvement, 824–825
leadership and management roles, 828–829
legislative or regulatory issues, 831–832
long-term care, 560
management information system, 827
outcome data systems, 827
phone system, 826–827
physician satisfaction survey, 831, 834
quality assessment, 827
reimbursement, 829–830
teamwork, 827–828

Physician Payment Review Commission, defined, 938

Physician-hospital organization, defined, 938

Physician's care plan, 264, 265–267

PIP reimbursement, 598–600

Planning, program evaluation, relationship, 325–326

Platform, defined, 632

Point-of-service, defined, 938

Policy and procedure manual, 423–426
  approval process, 425
  conditions of participation, 424
  policy development, 423–424
  policy review procedure, 425
  professional advisory committee, 424–425

Political action committee, 687–688

Political process, 683–689
  legislative process, 685–686
  local government, 684–685
  political action, 687–688
  political action committee, 687–688
  regulatory process, 686–687
  relationship building, 683–684

Portability, defined, 938

Postpartum home care program, 247–248

Postpayment compliance audit, 845–846

Power surge, defined, 632

Preferred provider organization, defined, 938

Premises medical payments coverage, defined, 943

Premises operations coverage, defined, 943

Prenatal home care program, 247–248

Preventive health care, 118

Privacy, 658–659

Private home health care agency, 18, 20–21

Private long-term care insurance, 556

Problem list, 264

Problem solving, labor-management relations, 485–487

Process, program evaluation, 331

Product life cycle, 696–697

Productivity
  amount and quality of group work, 474
  budgeting, 575–576
    average visits per day, 576, 577
    full-time equivalent staff, 575
    home health aide staffing, 576
    nursing employment factor, 575–576, 577
  defined, 469–471
  effectiveness, 472
  efficiency, 472
  equity, 472–473
  evaluation, 469–479
    current productivity, 473–478
    process, 473–479

factors, 471–472
geographic area, 474
paperwork, 474
percentage of unnecessary
    activities, 475
program type, 474
resources, 470
service delivery analysis, 472–
    473
staff
    experience, 476
    length of service with agency,
        476
    motivation, 476
    scheduling, 474–475
standard, 473
    development, 473
valuation, environmental
factors, 473–475
Products liability coverage,
    defined, 943
Professional advisory committee,
    550
policy and procedure manual,
    424–425
Professional liability, 568
Professional relations, 719
Profit making, designation, 16
Program, defined, 632
Program administrator,
    credentialing, 91
Program development, cycle, 325,
    326
Program evaluation, 324–344
accountability, 326
administration, 329
areas to be evaluated, 331–332
benefits of, 336–337
budgeting, 572–573
characteristics, 324–325
clinical record, 331–332
Community Health
    Accreditation Program, Inc.,
    330
context, 327
data collection, 334
defined, 324–325
evaluation models, 332–333
external influences, 326–328
fiscal evaluation, 331
goal attainment model, 333

goals, 328–329
implementation considerations,
    337–338
industry influences, 326–328
internal influences, 328–329
interpreting results, 337
issues, 325–326
Joint Commission on
    Accreditation of Healthcare
    Organizations, 330
licensure, 330
management information
    system, 329
Medicare, 328, 329–330
operational considerations,
    336–338
outcome measure, 331
philosophy, 328–329
planned vs. actual performance
    model, 333
planning, relationship, 325–326
population served, 328
process, 331
program evaluation report, 335
program evaluation tool, 333–
    334
    formats, 338, 340–344
purpose, 327
quality assessment/performance
    improvement, 309–310
quality assurance, relationship,
    326
rules and regulations, 328
staff, 329
structure, 331
structure-process-outcome
    model, 332–333
system development, 329–332
systematic approach, 335–336
systems model, 332
Program for All-Inclusive Care for
    the Elderly, 555, 920
Program integrity review, 848–849
Program planning, budgeting,
    572–573
Progress report, 264
Property insurance, 566–567
Proprietary Home Care
    Association of America, 111
Prospective payment, 588
Protocol, defined, 632

Provider, defined, 938
Provider Cost Report
    Reimbursement Questionnaire,
    595, 596
Provider Reimbursement Review
    Board, 602
Public health nursing, historical
    aspects, 7
Public Health Title VI, 10
Public relations, 740
Purchasing insurance, 570–571
Purge, defined, 632

Q

Qualifying service, 34
Quality
    accrediting and certifying
        agencies' viewpoint, 294
    consumer's viewpoint, 291, 292
    home health agency viewpoint,
        294
    legislative and regulatory
        viewpoint, 293
    managed care, 537
    professional's viewpoint, 294
    telehealth, 889
    third party payer's viewpoint,
        291–293
Quality assessment, 739
    managed care organization,
        547–552
    physician, 827
    urinary incontinence, 397–400
        assessment tools, 403–408
        flow chart, 400–401
        intervention tools, 403–408
        patient education, 407–408
        planning, 397–399
        team implementation, 399–
            400
Quality assessment/performance
    improvement, 290–302, 304–
    318
    clinical evaluation, 348
    continuing education, 299, 300
    evaluating clinical data, 295–
        296

evaluation forms, 304–308
    policies, 304–308
evaluating financial data, 295–
    296
    evaluation forms, 304–308
    policies, 304–308
field agency agreement, 317–
    318
financial evaluation, 348
financial resources, 299–301
human resources, 297–299
    employment criteria, 297–
    298
    service/education
        collaboration, 297
inservice education, 299, 300
patient classification system,
    295, 296
peer review, 299
program evaluation, 309–310
quarterly record review, 311–
    316
resource analysis, 297–301
staffing, 298–299
Quality assurance, 281
    case management, 527
    defined, 290
    discharge planning, 443
    management information
        system, 644
    program evaluation,
        relationship, 326
    staff, 458–459
Quality assurance program, 319
    consumer, 320
    criteria, 320
        standard, 320–321
    defined, 938
Quality improvement, 319
    Agency for Health Care Policy
        and Research, 321
    competency assessment, 178
    Health Care Financing
        Administration, 321
    Joint Commission on
        Accreditation of Healthcare
        Organizations, 321
    urinary incontinence, 397–400
        assessment tools, 403–408
        flow chart, 400–401
        intervention tools, 403–408

patient education, 407–408
    planning, 397–399
    team implementation, 399–
        400
Quality indicator group
    description, 381
    examples, 381
    outcome-based quality
        improvement, 381–382
Quality of life, 13
    ethical issues, 677–679, 680–
        681
Quality planning, 319–323
    data collection, 321
    goals, 320
Quarterly record review, quality
    assessment/performance
    improvement, 311–316

R

RAM, defined, 632
Random, defined, 632
Reasonable cost, 598–599
Recordkeeping, 119–129. *See
    also* Documentation
Referral
    antitrust, 454
    criteria for service, 449, 450
    intake personnel, 450–451
    intake referral form, 448
    interagency referral form, 448
    legal issues, 453–454
        agency policies, 453–454
        referral information
            collection, 453
        referral information
            maintenance, 453
    liaison to referral sources, 451–
        452
    managed care, 539–540
    marketing, 452–453
    referral information, 448
    referral sources, 447–454
    rejection, 449–450
    seasonal trends, 452
    service acceptance policies, 450

Regional home health
    intermediary, 836–850
    geographic areas, 836–837
Registered nurse, job description,
    164
    physical requirements, 162
    qualifications, 162
    self-assessment form, 166–168,
        171–174, 176–177
    working conditions, 162
Regulations, computerized
    documentation, 145–146
Regulatory process, 686–687
Rehabilitation, changing patterns,
    12
Rehabilitation potential patient
    classification system, 346–348,
        350
    analysis by, 350–352
Reimbursement, 519–520, 585–
    606
    computerized documentation,
        147
    ethical issues, 676–677
    Medicaid, 12, 587
        changing reimbursement
            patterns, 12
    Medicare, 12, 586–602, 604–
        605
        administrative and general
            expenses, 594
        allocation, 592–595
        changing reimbursement
            patterns, 12
        charge-based reimbursement,
            588
        cost accounting, 589–590
        cost finding, 589–590
        cost limit, 595–598
        cost report, 589–590
        cost report appeal, 601–602
        cost-based reimbursement,
            588
        customary charge, 598–599
        depreciation, 594
        discrete costing, 602–604
        entitlement, 587
        Form 339, 595, 596
        home health aide, 587
        increasing, 602–605
        medical supplies, 589

methods of reimbursement, 588–602
nonallowable costs, 592–593
occupational therapy, 587–588
physical therapy, 587–588
PIP reimbursement, 598–600
prospective payment, 588
Provider Cost Report Reimbursement Questionnaire, 595, 596
Provider Reimbursement Review Board, 602
reasonable cost, 588, 598–599
restructured agency, 604–605
skilled nursing, 587
speech therapy, 587–588
Summary of Medicare Uncollectibles, 595, 596
technical denial, 600–601
transportation cost, 594
waiver of liability, 601
National Association of Home Care, 605
Older Americans Act, 587
physician, 829–830
telehealth, 890–891
Relational database, defined, 632
Relationship building, 683–684
Reliability, patient classification outcome system, 190
Reorganization. *See* Corporate reorganization
Replacement cost coverage, defined, 943
Report writer, defined, 632
Resource development, 755–761
preparation, 755
process, 756–760
sources, 756–757
Respite care, 432–433
Respondent superior, 654
Response time, defined, 632
Revenue projection, budgeting, 580–581
expense and revenue summary analysis, 581, 582
nonoperating sources of income, 580–581

patient care services revenue, 580
RFP, defined, 632
Risk management, 570
Role play, orientation, 524
Run chart, 284, 286
Rural Nursing Service, 10

S

Safe harbor
defined, 938
managed care, 539
Salary administration, 493
Save, defined, 632
Scheduling system, management information system, 649–650
Self-care
concept, 115
Orem's theory, 115–116
Self-care agency, 116
Self-care system, 115–118
Self-directed learning, orientation, 524
Senior transportation service, 432–433
Server, defined, 632
Service area, defined, 938
Service Authorization Progress Note, 547, 548
Sibling, ventilator-dependent child, 275–277
Single corporate organization, 726
Single payer, defined, 938
Skilled care
documentation, 125–127
long-term care, differentiated, 560
Skilled nursing services, 43
credentialing, 92
Smart card, defined, 632
Social service department, 738
Social work assistant, credentialing, 93
Social worker, credentialing, 93
Software, defined, 632
Sort, defined, 632
Source code, defined, 632

Special events, 719
Specialized home care program, orientation, 523
Speech-language pathologist, credentialing, 93
Spool, defined, 632
Staff, 719, 740–741
adult day services, 914–915
external forces, 455–456
high-technology home health care, 252
hiring in personnel shortage era, 457
hospital *vs.* home care nursing, 517–520
assessment skills, 517–518
autonomy, 518
determining frequency and duration of care, 518
direct care, 518–519
documentation, 519
home visiting, 519
patient education, 519
physician communication, 518
referral to community resources, 519
reimbursement, 519–520
safety, 520
work environment, 520
interviewing prospective, 457–458
job characteristics, 456–457
legal issues, 661–662
personnel characteristics, 456–457
personnel department, 495–497
productivity
experience, 476
length of service with agency, 476
motivation, 476
scheduling, 474–475
professional liability, 568
program evaluation, 329
qualifications, 550
quality assessment/performance improvement, 298–299
quality assurance, 458–459
recruitment, 456–459
retention, 455–459

collaboration, 460–461
issues within administrative control, 460
participation, 460–461
structural components, 459–460
transitioning hospital nurses to home care, 516–524
urinary incontinence, targeted staff education, 401
Staff development, 506–515
academic education, 514–515
ANA standards, 506–507
Community Health Accreditation Program, Inc., 506
competency self-assessment, 508, 512
continuing education, 514
educator responsibilities, 507
educator role, 507
inservice education, 508–514
Joint Commission on Accreditation of Healthcare Organizations, 506
Medicare, 506
necessity for, 506–507
orientation, 507–508, 509–511
defined, 507–508
Staff model HMO, defined, 938
Staff recruitment, 493, 497–499
advertising, 497–498
community outreach, 498
employee referral, 499
employment agency, 498–499
first impressions, 500
negligent hiring, 661–662
promotion from within, 499
Staff retention, employee relations, 503–504
Staff selection, 493
employment decision, 501–502
employment offer, 502–503
hidden agenda, 499–502
interview, 500–501
Staggered hours, 463
Standalone, defined, 633
Standard
Community Health Accreditation Program, Inc., 71–73

outcome measures, 73
computerized documentation, 145–146
defined, 633
Foundation for Hospice and Home Care, National HomeCaring Council, 77–78
Joint Commission on Accreditation of Healthcare Organizations, 57, 58–60
assessment, 58
care, 58–59
continuum of care, 59
education, 59
environmental safety, 59–60
equipment management, 59–60
ethics, 58
human resources management, 60
improving organization performance, 59
infection control, 60
information management, 60
leadership, 59
patient rights, 58
service, 58–59
treatment, 58–59
productivity, 473
development, 473
Standardized outcome and assessment information set, 388
Standards of Home Health Nursing Practice, 91
State licensure, hospice, 874–875
Statement, defined, 628
Statement of functional expenses, 612–614
Statistical report, management information system, 643–644
Strategic planning, 693–705
biased, 705
communication, 704
development, 702–705
incomplete, 704–705
operational planning linkages, 703
participant selection, 703
process, 704
organizational change, 701–702

assessment of external environment, 701
clarifying goals and objectives, 701–702
identifying phase strategy, 702
pitfalls, 704–705
resources, 702–703
unmonitored, 705
Streaming tape, defined, 633
Structure, program evaluation, 331
Student placement, 808–822
advantages, 808–810
barriers, 810–811
contractual arrangements, 813–814, 817, 818–819, 820
cost-benefit analysis, 814
disadvantages, 810–811
documentation, 809, 822
evaluation, 819–822
example, 816–822
graduate student, 811–812
guidelines for cooperative relationships, 821
objectives, 812
preceptor considerations, 811–812
recommendations, 812–814
student-preceptor relationship, 811–812
Student research project, 804
Subscriber, defined, 939
Substance abuse, Americans with Disabilities Act, 664–665
testing, 664–665
Summary of Medicare Uncollectibles, 595, 596
Summary report, 37–38
Superbill, defined, 939
Supervising nurse, 35
credentialing, 90
Supervising physician, credentialing, 90
Supervision, 44
home health aide, 47–48, 51–52
negligent supervision, 661, 662
Supervisor
competency assessment, 162–163
job description, performance criteria, 163

labor-management relations, 487–488
Surge protector, defined, 633
System development, program evaluation, 329–332
Systems analysis, defined, 633
Systems design, defined, 633
Systems integrator, defined, 633

T

Tax Equity and Fiscal Responsibility Act, 388
Technical denial, 600–601
Technology, 715
    corporate reorganization, 724–725
Telehealth, 885–891
    cost issues, 890–891
    defined, 885
    delivery of ancillary services, 887–888
    delivery of nursing care, 887
    future trends, 891
    home health care agency configuration, 888
    legal issues, 889–890
    patient selection process, 888–889
    quality of care, 889
    reimbursement, 890–891
    scope of activities, 886–887
    systems design, 886
    utilization by diagnosis, 888
Telemedicine, 885–891
    defined, 633, 885
    history, 885–886
Telnet, 894
Terminal, defined, 633
Terminal care, hospice, 873
Theory of individual rights, 674
Theory of justice, 673–674
Theory of obligation, 674
Third party administrator, defined, 939
Third party payer, discharge planning, 429
Third-party billing, defined, 628

Throughput, defined, 633
Time sharing, defined, 633
Tort, 655–656
Total parenteral nutrition, 261
Total quality management, defined, 939
Town and Country Nursing Service, 10
Training, 493–494
    case management, 528
    volunteer program, 773, 774
Transition process, 738–744
Transportable equipment insurance, 570
Transportation, adult day services, 914, 917
Turnkey system, defined, 633

U

U.C.R., defined, 939
Umbrella liability, 568
Unbundled, defined, 633
Uniform resource locator, defined, 902
United Way, 744
Upgrade, defined, 633
UPS, defined, 633
Urinary incontinence, 394–408
    Agency for Health Care Policy and Research, 394–408
        guideline implementation, 394–408
    behavioral interventions, 398
    bladder record, 406
    bladder retraining, 398, 399
    incontinence history, 404
    nursing research, 395–396
    quality assessment, 397–400
        flow chart, 400–401
        patient education, 407–408
        planning, 397–399
        team implementation, 399–400
    quality assessment
        assessment tools, 403–408
        intervention tools, 403–408
    quality improvement, 397–400

assessment tools, 403–408
    flow chart, 400–401
    intervention tools, 403–408
    patient education, 407–408
    planning, 397–399
    team implementation, 399–400
    staff, targeted staff education, 401
User-friendly, defined, 633
Utilitarianism, 673
Utilities, defined, 633
Utilization review, 739

V

Variable day, 463
Variance analysis, critical pathway, 367–368, 369, 374
Ventilator-dependent child, 271–277
    care plan, 275–277
    decision to discharge, 271–272
    developmental needs, 274
    durable medical equipment, vendor selection, 273
    emergency resources, 274–275
    funding, 272
    home assessment, 274
    nursing care, 273–274
    sibling, 275–277
    teaching plan, 272–273
Vicarious liability, 654
Virtual integrated delivery system, defined, 633
Visiting nurse agency, history, 7–10
Visiting Nurse Association, 15
    hospital affiliation, 736–747
        accrediting organizations, 743–744
        board impact, 744–745
        budget/reports, 742
        change in professional relationship with peers, 745–746
        check requisition, 742
        communication, 740

contracting agencies, 744
contract/policy approval, 742
decision process, 737–738
external contacts, 743
finance department billing
    activities, 742
financial intermediary, 743
fund raising, 740
hiring, 741
identification numbers, 744
medical record committee,
    738–739
national associations, 744
negotiation process, 736–737
nursing administration, 738
orientation, 741–742
pastoral care, 739
payroll, 741
public relations, 740
quality assessment, 739
social service department,
    738
staff, 740–741
staff adjustments, 745, 746
staff impact, 744–745
state associations, 744
state certifying agency, 743
state medical assistance
    office, 743
therapy department, 738
transition process, 738–744
United Way, 744
utilization review, 739
volunteer, 739–740
research projects, 869, 870
Visiting Nurse Association of
    Eastern Montgomery County/
    Department of Abington
    Memorial Hospital, 345–364
Voice recognition, defined, 633
Volatile storage, defined, 633
Voluntary home health care
    agency, 18, 20–21
Volunteer, 739–740, 762–780
    benefits, 764
    history of health care
        volunteerism, 763–764
    in home health care, 764–780

legal liabilities, 764
notion of volunteerism, 762–
    763
Volunteer program
    design, 768–770
    director of volunteers, 768–770
    ethical issues, 766
    evaluation, 772–773
    implementation, 774–779
    philosophical basis for, 765–770
    program goals, 765–766
    recruitment, 770–772
    relational premises, 766–768
    retention, 774–779
    structure, 770–779
    training, 773, 774

W

Waiver of liability, 601, 853–854
    denials, 853–854
Web page, defined, 902
Web server, defined, 902
Winchester disk, defined, 633
Windows, defined, 633
Worker's compensation, 569
Workload
    analysis, 204–214
    Easley-Storfjell Instruments for
        Caseload/Workload Analysis,
        204–214
        administrative uses, 210–214
        analysis graph, 209
        analysis roster, 208
        guidelines, 207
        instrument instructions, 206–
            210
        process, 205–206
        summary, 212
        time allocation worksheet,
            211
        uses, 210–214
    management, 204–214
World Homecare and Hospice
    Organization, 111

World Wide Web, 895
    browsers, 898, 902
    home page development, 898–
        902
Write, defined, 633
Write-protect, defined, 633
Writing for publication, 795–807
    abstracts, 802
    agency data use, 804–805
    appearance, 803
    benefits, 806
    biographical statement, 802–
        803
    blocks to writing, 795–797
    computer disks, 803
    copyright transfer, 803
    copyrighted material use, 803
    cover letter, 803
    ethical issues, 805–806
    getting started, 798–799
    headings, 802
    idea development, 799
    idea generation, 798
    idea selection, 798–799
    illustrations, 802
    inexperience, 795–796
    journal selection, 799–801
        factors, 799–801
    manuscript critique, 797–798
    manuscript rejection, 797
    process, 801–802
    procrastination, 796–797
    publishing process, 805
    reference style, 802
    research, 803–805
    student research project, 804
    submission checklist, 802–803
    workload, 796
Wrongful termination of
    employment, 661

X

Xenix, defined, 633